Fundamentals of
Family Practice

WILFRED SNODGRASS,

M.D., D.N.B., A.B.F.P.

Instructor, Family Practice Residency Program,
Santa Monica Hospital Medical Center, California

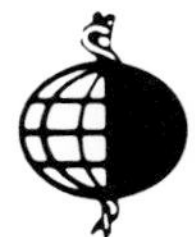

F.A. DAVIS COMPANY
PHILADELPHIA

Printed in the United States of America

Library of Congress Cataloging in Publication Data

Snodgrass, Wilfred.
Fundamentals of family practice.

Bibliography: p.
1. Family medicine. I. Title. [DNLM: 1. General practice. W89 S673f]
RC46.S65 616 74-11093
ISBN 0-8036-7960-2

Preface

Fundamentals of Family Practice is a new type of book for a new type of physician—the family physician. It is my hope that it will be used as an adjunct to the various textbooks from which the student has already learned the fundamentals of medicine.

It is intended for those who look for bearings in a new field and for all who feel in need of some orientation or updating in family practice. It is for the young and old, specialist and generalist alike.

As the text was being prepared I kept two objectives in mind: (1) to emphasize facts that a family physician should know regarding a discipline even though he may not intend to practice that discipline in depth and (2) to mark that which is important but sometimes difficult to understand in family practice, believing that if these major principles are understood other less important subjects will fall into place. While I fulfilled these objectives, I omitted discussions of the rarer and the most frequently occurring diseases included in more theoretic texts.

Clarification of my objectives can be recognized in the text's coverage of obstetrics. There may be family physicians who choose not to make deliveries. There is, however, a certain body of knowledge all family physicians should have regarding obstetrics. This information has been clearly presented in the chapter on obstetrics. As a further aid in achieving the objectives, the reader will find that no information regarding the actual technique of delivery is included. This information may be found in any standard textbook on obstetrics. Each medical and surgical discipline is covered in a similar fashion.

Choice of subjects has also been influenced by my experience as a teacher of family medicine at the Santa Monica Hospital Medical Center in California. I have included principles that have been difficult for residents to master or those they see so infrequently that they need reviewing. And last of all are subjects that may do duty as part of the American Board of Family Practice examination.

Because of the nature of the family physician's job and as the physician of first contact, and many times the patient's *only* contact with medical services, stress is laid on developing the reader's keenness in differential diagnosis, his awareness of the social implications of the initial complaints and his enthusiasm in preventive medicine. This is not to underrate his ability to handle catastrophic illness or accidents.

In his daily rounds, the family physician must be able to direct his thinking from one body system to another easily and frequently. His attention must range from the squalling newborn infant to the comatose geriatric patient, from a thrombosed hemorrhoid to an itchy ear. He is constantly faced with pains and symptoms that could originate in any body system.

Probably his greatest challenge and that which sets him apart from the other specialists is the fact that he has the responsibility of deciding from thousands of conditions the precise ailment affecting the patient in front of him. Consequently, the family physician's forte should be differential diagnosis. He must be intuitive. The other specialist who must develop the same approach is the radiologist. His thinking must also range from one specialty to another as he studies each radiogram.

This text, consequently, is organized to parallel the family physician's thinking. There is no attempt to cover definitions of diseases, their etiology, pathology, clinical signs and symptoms (the usual textbook format). Rather the text freewheels from subject to subject touching or enlarging on the problems family physicians face.

During the period of time it takes to write and produce a book, changes occur in the practice of medicine, some dramatic and others minor. Family practice cannot always be the first with the new nor can it afford to be the last to discard the old. The decisions as to what to retain of the old and what to add of the new were the most difficult for me to make. Such a book as this is bound to reflect in some measure the tastes and interests of the author. But I have chosen subjects which I hope point the way to the future while making use of the valid that survives from the past.

I have taken a rather dogmatic stand on several controversial subjects, believing that most readers will be persons of experience who will recognize my positive opinions as only one view of several solutions.

Finally, I am indebted to several coworkers for the production of this manuscript. I could never have produced and assembled the final copy without the tireless help and suggestions of my secretary, Linda Melber. Another friend and a fine artist, Linda Bright, prepared the illustrations and Reinette Heinley as a girl Friday ran errands and worked hours on the final assembly. Credit should go to my wife, Lula Berg Snodgrass, for all the photographs in the text. In addition, for more than two years, she calmly tolerated the many household and connubial annoyances that arise in a home when a book is being produced. The Department of Radiology of the Santa Monica Hospital Medical Center and its Director, Doctor S. K. Shearer, gave me permission to choose whatever roentgenograms I thought would enhance the text and I did so voraciously.

The F. A. Davis Company has my respect and sincere thanks for its guidance, cordiality and forbearance and my admiration for its skill in the difficult field of publishing medical texts. Of their staff and almost a co-author is Eleanor Mora, who corrected my syntax.

Wilfred Snodgrass, M.D.
Santa Monica, Ca.

Contents

THE FAMILY PHYSICIAN

He is the primary physician, the physician of first contact, the patient's entree into the health system

His forte is comprehensive—continuing care to the family and its members

He is able to diagnose and treat common ailments and he is a keen diagnostician of the uncommon

He constantly thinks in terms of prevention

CHAPTER 1

The Family Physician

PATIENT CONCERN

Unfortunately, medical education tends to distort youthful idealism and increasingly focuses on the exact sciences, losing sight of the behavioral and emotional aspects of the patient's life. However, the patient is a person—he has feelings, he needs care extending beyond mere physical treatment, and in time of illness he is very much afraid. Often the obstacle in a physician-patient relationship is the rejection of these needs because the physician thinks these needs are not important or he thinks he has no time for them.

Acquire early in your relationship, and always retain, a concern for the patient.

PATIENT COMMUNICATION

Many times young physicians do not realize they constantly communicate with their patients, even when they say nothing. Patients constantly catch the physician's communications by his appearance, a turn of his hand, a raised eyebrow or his silence. Patients search for signs of hope—good news or bad. Many patients decide their fate by methods of communication other than speech. Silence is communication, and to a fearful patient it spells hopelessness.

Don't be afraid to tell the patient you haven't made a diagnosis. Most patients want good medical care, not miracles. The failure to make a prompt diagnosis does not indicate incompetency. In fact, "No diagnosis," can be a sign of sincerity and honesty and may make the patient feel he is being treated with respect and dignity. At this point, however, you should explain what has been done and what needs to be done to arrive at a diagnosis. Unless the problem is insignificant, explain the problem to another family member by a three-way discussion.

Often patients ask, "What's wrong with me, Doc?" and do not expect a detailed case report. They mainly want to know whether their discomfort is serious or not. If you are not sure, but believe the problem a simple one and likely to be self-limited, merely reply, "Don't worry, you'll get better." Even though the question has been ignored, their relief at knowing the symptoms are not serious gives them the satisfaction they are seeking. This answer is not difficult to give since, in this age, modern medication often cures even when the physician's diagnosis is a little off target. Don't forget that your mission is to relieve distress, the emotional as well as the physical.

In order to be a sensitive family physician, do not hesitate to inquire into the impact his disability has on him, whether it be adolescent acne, alopecia, obesity or aging especially. Don't be afraid to ask, "How do you feel about your ______? Does it embarrass you around people?" Your knowledge of the patient's sensitivity is important in planning a comprehensive practical program of therapy for him. Some patients could care less and will not expend much energy carrying out your program; others shut themselves off from all social contact believing themselves repulsive and will overextend every suggestion you make.

THE PHYSICIAN-PATIENT RELATIONSHIP

Encourage the patient to express his ideas and feelings no matter how strange. Do not attempt to judge.

Give the patient support; recognize his dignity as a human no matter how troublesome or complaining he is. Do not, however, be afraid to set limits on what he can expect.

Maintain a professional attitude.

Recognize the dependent patient by the urgency of all his requests. He will monopolize your time and test you with his demands. He wants to be loved; he is fearful of being abandoned. All this generates anxiety. Assure the patient of your concern and your willingness to take care of him. Set limits on how much time he can demand from you but be willing to concede on minor points in order to get his full cooperation.

Recognize the controlled patient by his imposed discipline, his ritualism and his desire to know all details of his illness and its treatment. Anxiety in this circumstance is caused by the patient's loss of control of his environment and of his impulses. Sit down with this patient and explain what is known of his problem and the treatment plans. Allow him to participate in decisions and details of his treatment.

The captivating patient wants a warm relationship with the doctor. This may drive the woman patient to be sexually provocative. Be reassuring but not intimate. Be calm but firm regarding too tight an emotional bind.

The long-suffering patient may find satisfaction through suffering and subservience. For them, being sick evokes sympathy and attention. These are the patients who may be hospitalized over and over for ill-defined ailments. Recognition of this patient is of prime importance. Acknowledge the patient's suffering, but *do not* give the usual assurance that she will soon be better. Don't be pressured into unnecessary treatment, surgery or drugs.

You fall short of a patient's expectations when you fail to touch or examine a spot or place of which he is complaining. This is more than a symbolic gesture, "the laying on of hands." To the patient, you failed to examine him. Train yourself to reach over and palpate the spot no matter how obvious the problem. Besides you may be surprised at what you find. Take time to take off a shoe, a sock or a blouse and inspect and palpate. To the patient, you are a thorough physician, and, if the day comes when you do miss something, you'll be forgiven.

Attempt to be precise in recording the patient's medical history. Attempt to answer: What? Where? When? Kind? Range? Degree? Accentuated by?

There is nothing wrong with recording key words. For instance: Pain, precordium, clutching, severe, sustained, onset, abrupt, while walking, accentuated by exertion.

The key question in gaining an understanding of patients is *why?* You will find you are on safer ground if you understand *why* before you begin to give advice.

Why did the patient come?
Why did he come now?
Why did he say that?
Why does he think this?
Why does he feel this way?
Why does he ask?

Do not assume you understand what the patient means. Encourage the patient to be specific about the problem when he gives an evasive answer.

It is surprising how often some patient who puzzles you can be understood after he tells you what he thinks is the cause of his disorder. Ask him. He may at first deny he has any preconceived idea or he may be sarcastic and tell you that's why he came to see you. Keep your cool and ask again.

Find out what the disease means to the patient. Asking this question allows the patient to reveal his fantasies about his disorder.

You do not have to answer a patient's question. Occasionally it is wise to turn the question back to the patient by saying, "What do you think about this?" Or if the patient should suddenly ask, "Do you think I'm losing my mind?" ask the patient if he has been concerned about this or if there are any reasons why you should think so.

Do not try to explore or handle a patient's problems in an area that makes you feel uncomfortable. This requires that you understand your own inhibitions.

Questioning a patient in areas which he may dislike or resent takes courage. Do so with equanimity so as not to stir up excessive anxiety. Warm the patient up with preliminary questions, perhaps frankly ask the patient if you can ask a personal question. Indicate to the patient that all answers are confidential.

Be wary of the patient's spontaneous negative assertions. A depressed patient may admit to feelings of melancholy and then suddenly and spontaneously deny he would ever commit suicide. This type of negative assertion indicates the patient has been thinking of suicide. Don't accept these denials. They deserve careful evaluation.

Last of all, remember that a patient's behavior is often more significant than the words spoken by him.

PATIENT RECALL

No matter what other specialists do, the family physician should be a strong advocate of patient recall. In most busy physician's offices, patient recall is sadly neglected. Although most physicians feel a deep obligation to their patient's needs, in too many instances they neglect long-term follow-up care or, worse yet, do not recognize their obligation.

Many physicians excuse their neglect by flatly stating that recall isn't their responsibility. If recall isn't the responsibility of the physician who understands the patient's needs, whose responsibility is it? The patient can only know what he has been taught by his doctor who presumably is concerned about the long-term welfare of his patients.

Telling a patient to come back is not enough. Patients procrastinate. Admonishing a patient to recheck on a health matter in a month or year, particularly when the patient may be feeling relatively well at that time, falls short of proper care. Patients do not know the dangers of procrastination unless their family physician teaches them.

Is it unethical to recall patients for rechecks? As a matter of fact, I contend that, if the family physician claims to offer comprehensive, continuous health care and fails to recall his patients, that is an unethical practice. Patient recall for those patients who by their actions have contracted with a family physician for their health care is a doctor's obligation whether he recognizes it or not. If you have been led to believe that recall is unethical, resolve the matter by asking the patient whether he would prefer a notice of recall. Train your nurse or receptionist to do so if you are likely to forget.

To work properly, base your recall system on:

- –a sound patient education program of preventive care
- –conversion of the patient to an enthusiastic reception of the plan
- –tailoring of the program to the individual's needs, giving thought to whether his problems would better be checked in 6, 14 or 18 months
- –making the plan pay for both your attention and service to your patient

Determine the frequency of patient visits by:

- –safety of the drug which you are giving
- –course of the disease
- –anxiety quotient of the patient
- –patient's convenience
- –financial ability to pay

Determine the interval of visits by your knowledge of when complications are likely to occur. For instance, in pertussis, pneumonia is likely to begin during the third week; in measles, otitis media or pneumonia occur just as the rash begins to fade. Also keep in mind the natural course of the disease. An otitis media should definitely be better by the second day. If the disease is not following what might be reasonably expected, consider a change in treatment, further diagnostic workup or a consultation.

The art of medicine requires that you sense what the patient anticipates. Patient demands should not be your overriding guideline but patient cooperation is essential. If the matter can be serious, so state your case, but ordinarily a day or two one way or the other is a small price to pay for patient acceptance. If the patient is not well known to you, your attention to his case may need to be more intense.

The patient's return for a checkup may be inconvenient to the patient. Occasionally, more harm than good can result from a long and tiresome trip to your office. Talk this over with the patient and his relatives. Consider whether the patient can better be taken care of by home calls, hospitalization, referral or by a visiting nurse, your own nurse or paramedical personnel. Many times the interval between patient visits can be lengthened by the use of the telephone.

Never allow the financial factor to compromise your best judgment. You are in trouble when you begin developing two standards of care—one for the affluent and one for the poor. Take care of all alike. If your patient is unable to pay your fee and you do not wish to reduce it, refer the patient to a suitable clinic. Anything less than proper care can bring legal and ethical trouble. Occasionally adjustments can be made in your approach to the case without endangering the patient. For instance, the laboratory and x-ray studies may be started more sparsely with the idea that more may be required later. Hopefully, the first battery of tests may solve the problem and others can be dropped. This may take more time as an outpatient but, with the proper follow-up, it will save the patient some expense.

COMMUNITY HEALTH

The family physician has as much of an obligation to improve the overall community health as he has to treat the specific diseases of individual patients. Be actively concerned with the work of community health services and with the services provided by local hospitals and medical organizations.

You are the potential leader in any team effort. Take time to study the public health needs of your community, your county and your state. You can become an influential and effective public health influence.

Your participation in air and water cleanup, accident prevention, hospital planning and disaster programs can be the best assurance to your patients that you do not limit yourself to a narrow specialty but are truly a family physician interested in positive health for the whole man and the whole community.

ILLNESS AND THE FAMILY

Of all the specialities in medicine, the family physician stands alone in recognizing the patient as a member of a family unit. He recognizes and considers the close interpersonal interaction between members of the family. He knows that an illness or disability of one member of the unit will cause severe reactions in all other members and that interpersonal friction in a family can break the emotional health of its members. When one member is ill, the others may demonstrate fear and anxiety to such a degree to effect the outcome of the sick one's illness and their own equanimity.

Psychiatric illness may cause:

- Feelings of rejection in nonill members
- School absences to substitute for an ill mother
- Social stigma
- Feelings of isolation in teenagers and deprivation of their home as a status symbol
- Loss of self confidence in the mate of the alcoholic
- Anxiety over a suicidal partner
- Attempts to hide the mentally ill member
- Sacrifice of children when arguments arise between an alcoholic and nonalcoholic parent

The ordinary patient thinks of his heart as vital to life. Consequently, family physicians should recognize and assess the family's apprehension which arises when a member of the family has heart problems.

Parents of children with congenital heart disease build up anxiety about their newborn, the diagnosis and the child's symptoms. They may constantly worry about losing the child. Remember that situations which produce anxiety are: decisions concerning surgery, postoperative appearance of the child and postoperative wait to determine whether the surgery was successful.

Watch for anxiety in the families of adult cardiac patients. Apprehension can engulf the entire family and other close relatives. Survey the family and you may find anxiety and tension levels so high as to immobilize the entire unit and to prevent, even during a critical situation, the hearing of medical explanations. Your attempts to allay family anxiety may, indirectly, help the ill patient who caused the anxiety in the first place; less tension in the family may assist a cardiac patient during his rehabilitation period.

Tuberculosis and other pulmonary diseases probably disrupt the family unit more than other organic diseases. Family members may develop feelings of guilt or shame toward the sick person. This, plus the increased burden on the mate, are psychological stresses that can initiate anxiety reactions, phobias or behavioral disorders.

When a child develops diabetes, watch for reactions in his family, relatives, friends and even his teacher. Stress is engendered by: hereditary factors; harrassment by the daily routines of urine testing, medication and preparation of special diets at set intervals; overanxiety and hysteria of grandparents and sibling resentment of the special attention the diabetic child receives.

Again, attempt to allay the parents' fears and correct psychological attitudes, and you will hasten the patient's adjustment.

Every family with a chronically ill or handicapped child becomes somewhat emotionally disorganized, especially during the early period of adaptation. When the affliction is diagnosed, watch for fear, anger, guilt, confusion or bewilderment in the parents. Remember when parents find that their child is deaf or blind, the experience may be so overwhelming for the parents that they may need psychiatric help. Treatment of neurological problems such as epilepsy requires the family physician to give adequate emotional support to the parents in order to protect the afflicted child from developing secondary emotional problems.

Successful treatment of an emotionally disturbed child must include investigation and, often, treatment of the entire family.

If the defect is one that is not physically obvious, parents will attempt to deny its reality. The father and mother may pretend to each other that no handicap exists. This can lead to a failure in communication that spills over into other areas of their lives and even threatens their separation.

Even worse is the parent's discovery of a mentally retarded child. Parents may feel profound shock, suffer groundless personal guilt or blame their marital partner. Some mothers may blame an earlier sexual experience. The following problems must be discussed: whether institutionalization is best; emotional impact on normal siblings; handling of sibling's friends and visitors; and prevention of embarrassment when older sisters begin dating.

Take a searching family history in all patients with unresolved emotional problems. Start by asking the patient with whom he is living. This will shift the focus of the interview from the patient to his or her family. From this point it should only be a question or two more to sift out the family frictions that cause anxiety and tension. These areas of tension may stem from family members who are organically ill, from those who are psychosomatically disabled or from those with neurotic behavior patterns.

After obtaining insight into the family, choose targets for therapy. Frequently a separate or corporate family interview is wise. You will find that what one member exaggerates, another corrects, and what parents hide, children often blurt out. In any event, you can proceed with corrective measures, whether it be arranging therapy or quieting the fears of the patient at hand.

DIAGNOSIS

Think of the body as a whole, living in an environment. Knowledge of the environment is, therefore, as important as knowledge of the body, and knowledge of the whole body in its environment is more important than the most intimate familiarity with all its separate parts.

Attempt to diagnose a relievable condition. A diagnosis of an unrelievable disease, if wrong, may condemn the patient to invalidism or even death.

The initial stages of diseases sometimes need a period of observation. In some patients, you may need to await the appearance of subsequent symptoms before making a diagnosis. After a complete history and physical, wait and weigh.

Do not attempt to make up for an inadequate history and a sloppy examination by increasing laboratory tests.

When the diagnosis is uncertain but the patient is improving, do not interfere by ordering elaborate tests. Laboratory tests may be falsely positive and misdirect your attention from the problem at hand.

Your professional maturity may be measured by the amount of drugs you prescribe. You are in danger when you attempt overprescribing to make up for an inadequate diagnosis.

There is no better way to improve your medical ability than to put your knowledge to action. A young physician's ability increases in proportion to the number of patients he sees. Observation and reading is no substitute for doing.

Choose laboratory tests carefully but drain all information you can from the tests so chosen.

Learn from your own errors as well as from the errors of others.

Formulating a Diagnosis

Practice dividing your diagnosis into four parts: etiologic, anatomic, pathophysiologic and functional.

Etiology. State the predisposing factors whether they be infections, neoplastic, trauma, nutritional, drugs, congenital or socioeconomic.

Anatomic description. Summarize the nature, extent and location of the lesion.

Pathophysiological changes. Describe the disturbance in physiology.

Functional evaluation. Summarize the patient's overall physical functioning and emotional reaction to the disease.

Examples:

Case 1.

Etiology:
1. Carcinoma of right breast 4 years ago
2. Overeating

Anatomic:
1. Absence of right breast
2. Secondary osteoblastic lesion in left skull
3. Obesity

Pathophysiologic:
1. Severe headache

Functional:
1. Disabled physically and emotionally by disease and drug reactions
2. Husband supporting

Case 2.

Etiology:
1. Viral

Anatomic:
1. Atypical pneumonia right

Pathophysiologic:
1. Cough, fever

Functional:
1. Bed rest
2. Cheerful patient
3. Family helpful

Case 3.

Etiology:
1. Rheumatic fever

Anatomic:
1. Mitral insufficiency
2. Enlarged heart

Pathophysiologic:
1. CHF

Functional:
1. Class 111-C
2. Depressed, immobile
3. No family

CONSULTATIONS

A well trained family physician will need a consultation in approximately 10 percent of the patients who seek his help.

Consultations are often delayed because the family physician fears being discredited in the eyes of the patient, has an inherent anxiety of being criticized, or fears problems that might endanger his relationship with the patient.

Do not consider a consultation a personal defeat. The primary objective of a consultation is to seek the latest and best diagnostic and therapeutic aid for your patient.

Consider whether you are asking for a consultation to benefit the patient or to allay your own anxiety. Remember your consultant is more likely to criticize your method of referral than your treatment. This is under your control. Have all the basic work done and give the consultant a proper briefing. He should also know what you expect from him: diagnosis only, diagnosis and treatment, treatment suggestions, a specific test or a complete workup.

HANDLING CHRONIC PAIN

A recent study indicates that physicians give less analgesic medication to the patient who complains the most of pain. The same study revealed a tendency to give highly neurotic women more powerful analgesics than other patients. Attempt to overcome your prejudices and biases regarding analgesics. Base your decision regarding therapy on your patient's discomfort.

Do not rely on the presence or absence of organic pathology in evaluating the patient's need for pain relief.

In chronic pain do not rely on the physical evidence of pain, i.e. writhing, crying or sweating, as you do in acute pain. Patients adapt to pain and often show no physical evidence of how they suffer.

If a patient says he is in pain, accept the fact until you have positive proof he is a malingerer.

Consider the patient's reaction when considering the frequency of analgesic medication. Allow the patient to judge the interval unless he shows a tendency to overmedicate. Giving the patient a tranquilizer allows the narcotic to be given at longer intervals.

Do not be afraid to use narcotics when indicated. Supplement their use by potentiators to keep daily requirements as low as possible. If the patient begins to show a tolerance, switch to another narcotic.

Use and study three or four narcotics. There are three that may be alternated monthly, i.e. methadone, codeine and pentazocine.

Attempt to spot the potential addict by keeping account of the amount ingested. The addict-prone patient increases his dosage more rapidly than does the nonaddict.

Do not overlook the tricyclic antidepressants. They will frequently relieve physical as well as emotional distress.

Consider the following diagnosis when a patient complains of chronic pain of questionable origin—depression, hysteria, malingering, compensation neurosis and schizophrenia. Often patients with these conditions present with chronic pain as the chief complaint.

CALCULATED THERAPEUTIC RISKS

There is a risk in everything you do for and to a patient. Your acumen as a physician may well rest on your ability to calculate risks in therapy. Part of this ability depends on your innate common sense but this must be tempered with an accurate diagnosis, a knowledge of the natural course of the disease and an understanding of the action and side effects of the drug under consideration.

In addition, your knowledge must be continually updated. This takes time. It takes time, also, to think about a patient and his problem—to calculate the risk of what you are proposing to do to the patient. Either allow time for this contemplation when scheduling patients or put off therapy to a second visit when you can give the patient your best opinion.

PLACEBOES

Today we have specific and predictable drugs as well as definitive medical procedures. But the placebo can mimic the effect of active drugs, influence the course of organic disease or even reverse the action of potent, active drugs.

A placebo is any therapy that is deliberately used for its psychologic effect. A placebo may be inert or active; it is anything the physician does for or to the patient. It may be oral, parenteral or topical medication, inhalants, surgery or psychotherapeutics. However, all placebo effects are not favorable.

One of the most powerful placebo effects is the physician-patient relationship. In our society patients tend to relate unrealistically to doctors by the complicated psychological principle of transference. This transference of relationship between physician-patient and patient-physician influences the outcome of all treatment. A positive transference generates rapport, warmth, trust, faith, empathy, etc. The relationship is generated by the physician's interest in the patient and his personality, which may vary from positive warmth and friendliness to negative hostility and rejection. The relationship may also result indirectly as from a physician's interest in some theory or method of treatment rather than in a direct interest in the patient.

Some patients will respond better to a drug placebo, others to a psychotherapeutic placebo.

Drug placeboes are indicated in:

- Patients with degenerative or incurable diseases
- Patients with a confusing medical history in which active drugs may cause even more confusing problems
- Chronic or elderly patients who are on psychochemotherapeutic drugs and there is a need to differentiate between psychologic and nonpsychologic side effects
- Patients who are impatient with prolonged investigative procedures
- Patients who need weaning away from narcotics following surgery

Be cautious about the use of placeboes. There is considerable ethical and legal controversy regarding their use. Carefully examine all aspects of the case for the proper indications, particularly in hostile patients. Do not use placeboes when you can think of nothing else to do; there should be a positive indication for their use.

Everything you do for the patient has a placebo effect. For thousands of years physicians prescribed useless and dangerous drugs; this would have been impossible were it not for the various placebo effects, which did help patients.

HOSPITAL BED UTILIZATION

Considerable overutilization of hospital beds occurs because of inadequate planning of laboratory testing sequence. Rossman[1] presents a sequence of laboratory tests with which every family physician should be familiar.

Sequence of Laboratory Tests*

1. Any of the following tests which require a 24-hr collection of urine can be grouped together: Vanillylmandelic acid (VMA), aldosterone, serotonin, phosphorus, catecholamines, calcium, amino acid chromatography (acidify prior to collection with 15 ml of concentrated hydrochloric acid).
2. The following tests may be grouped for they do not require preservatives; however, the urine specimen should be refrigerated during the 24-hr collection time: creatine, creatinine, catecholamine, chloride, copper, sodium, potassium, alpha amino nitrogen (brown bottle required), diastase, estrogens, 17-ketosteroids, 17-ketogenic steroids, leucine amino peptidase.
3. The following tests requiring a fresh urine specimen may be grouped together: Bence Jones protein, cystine, cysteine, amylase, lactic acid dehydrogenase.
4. A protein-bound iodine (PBI) test should be ordered before the administration of iodides in any form to the patient. Some laboratories keep a specimen of the patient's

---

*Reprinted in part from Rossman, PL: Bed utilization improved by planned hospital procedures. JAMA 215:1483–1485, 1971, with permission.

serum, collected on admission, in case a PBI is later found to be necessary.

5. For greater accuracy in diagnostic problem situations the following tests should be ordered before the patient is given a blood transfusion: immunoprotein electrophoresis, iron-binding capacity (IBC), prothrombin consumption time, partial thromboplastin time, thromboplastin generation test, serum protein electrophoresis, blood smear evaluation, total lactic acid dehydrogenase, fractionation, and isoenzymes, reticulocyte count, coagulation time, prothrombin time, fragility tests, platelet count, blood indices, serum iron, bone marrow.

6. If vitamin B_{12} deficiency is suspected (pernicious anemia) a bone marrow study should be ordered and done before the Schilling test (see below).

7. Glucose tolerance test (GTT). (a) Avoid a GTT if meals have been withheld for roentgenographic studies or other tests. (b) Postoperative GTT's are unreliable because pain, narcotics, and salicylates affect the results. (c) For best results and to avoid a second test, a carbohydrate-loading diet should be ordered for at least three days prior to the test.

8. Cultures of sputum, blood, urine, etc. should be done prior to institution of antibiotic therapy.

Sequence of Tests in the Department of Radiology

Examinations Conflicting with Nuclear Medicine. If indicated, a thryoid ^{113}I uptake or a thyroid scan should be ordered before carrying out any of the following roentgenographic procedures: gastrointestinal (GI) tract series with diatrizoate meglumine (Renografin), intravenous pyelogram (IVP), intravenous or T-tube cholangiogram, gallbladder (GB) series, salpingogram, angiography, bronchogram, myelogram. All procedures involve the administration of iodine preparations. If in doubt regarding the contrast media used in any x-ray film examination, consult the Department of Radiology.

Examinations Conflicting with Clinical Laboratory Procedures. If needed, stool specimens, gastric analysis, gastric cytological or proctoscopic examinations should be accomplished before the following roentgenographic procedures: upper GI tract series, barium enema (BE), four views of chest with barium, small-bowel study, esophagogram. These procedures involve the administration of barium, which may interfere with these tests.

Barium Examination Conflicting with Visibility of Other Structures. Always order the following examinations before any barium study is requested: abdomen-scout x-ray film, lumbar spine, IVP, angiogram studies, retrograde pyelogram, myelogram. These studies require a barium-free abdomen. Radiopaque barium residue may be retained for as long as one week.

General Instructions for Ordering Routine Examinations. If the order involves an IVP, GB, upper GI, and BE series, the requests may be obtained in the following manner:

First day: IVP and BE
Second day: GB and upper GI series

A cathartic must be given prior to the IVP and BE. Therefore, the radiology department may do these two examinations the same morning. Gallbladder contrast medium cannot be given the same day as a cathartic because the contrast medium will be lost in the catharsis, and the test will have to be repeated. Therefore, do not request a BE and GB series for the same day.

Sequence of Nuclear Medicine Tests

1. The following nuclear medicine thyroid studies should be scheduled before doing any x-ray film procedures using iodine-containing media: Thyroid ^{131}I uptake, thyroid scintigram or scintiscan, thyroid stimulation test, thyroid suppression test. The accompanying notice, placed on the front of the patient's chart, has been helpful in preventing a conflict of tests.

PATIENT IS HAVING THYROID STUDIES IN NUCLEAR MEDICINE DEPT. DO NOT PERFORM GALL-BLADDER, IVP, BRONCHOGRAM, OR MYELOGRAM X-RAYS UNTIL THYROID STUDIES ARE COMPLETED. TEST WILL BE COMPLETED AT
________AM ON________19________.
________PM

2. Renogram: Intravenous urography should not be scheduled immediately prior to a renogram study.
3. Rose bengal liver function test: A sulfobromophthalein liver function test should not be scheduled immediately prior to this test.
4. Schilling test (for diagnosis of pernicious anemia): This test must be performed prior to all other nuclear medicine tests.
5. Red blood cell survival test and ferrokinetic study or iron study: These tests take two weeks. They may be started while the patient is in the hospital and completed on an outpatient basis to save hospital days.

Most other currently available nuclear medicine tests require no special timing. If the patient requires more than one nuclear medicine test, the doctor should consult with the Nuclear Medicine Department regarding a proper sequence as this can vary with each laboratory, depending on the type of equipment and isotopes available.

Electroencephalography

1. Male patients should have their hair free of hair tonic and female patients should be free of hair spray. Preferably the patient's hair should be washed the day before the test and no ratting or teasing allowed.
2. The patient should be warned not to take a sedative or diphenylhydantoin sodium (Dilantin) the night before the test. He should also be advised to have a good breakfast before the test to avoid any hypoglycemic effect.
3. Patients, especially psychiatric patients, should be assured by their personal physician that an electroencephalogram is harmless and is not shock therapy. This will allay their fears and save prolonged explanations and reassurances by the technicians.

Arteriography

1. Arteriography below the diaphragm, such as renal, femoral, or mesenteric arteriograms, requires the abdomen to be completely free of barium.
2. Anticoagulants should be discontinued at least five days prior to an arteriogram or cardiac catheterization to avoid risk of bleeding.
3. Blood should not be drawn from the antecubital veins of patients who are to have a right heart catheterization within a week. This avoids possible hematomas at the site of vein catheterization which, if extensive, could cause cancellation of the test.

Gastrointestinal Diagnostic Laboratory

1. Gastroscopy and gastric secretory studies: To avoid cancellations, be sure the patient has received nothing by mouth for at least 12 hours prior to the test. Anticholinergics should be discontinued 24 hours prior to gastric analysis.
2. Sigmoidoscopy: To insure a clean lower bowel, and to avoid having to reschedule the examination, be sure the patient has had enemas until the returns are clear at least two hours prior to the sigmoidoscopy. A barium enema may follow if the physician is careful not to introduce air during the sigmoidoscopy. This utilizes one preparation for both procedures.

THE FAMILY PHYSICIAN'S LIBRARY

A family physician who does not use books and journals or who thinks he does not need a library soon becomes medically outdated. Even if you have access to a large organized library, your private library will serve a constructive purpose in maintaining a reserve of medical information immediately at hand for emergency use and for hours of study and relaxation. No outside library can take the place of one's own books. Unless things are looked up at once, they are seldom looked up later.

I have found it wise to arrange my books by subjects rather than to number books serially on a shelf or assign them to a designated, fixed shelf. Develop some mark of ownership for your books and place it upon each book or journal in your library. Rubber stamps for journals and perforated stamps or bookplates for books are commonly used.

The acquisition of your library deserves careful planning and direction. A guide for the family physician who is planning a library or wants to upgrade his present library has been prepared by Doctor D. A. Lawrence of Riverside, California (see Appendix).

REFERENCES

1. Rossman PL: Bed utilization improved by planned hospital procedures. *JAMA* 215:1483–1485, 1971.

CHAPTER 2

The Obstetric Patient

The family physician will find obstetrics a healthy addition to his practice and its growth if he masters a few concepts and techniques. He may or may not, according to his talents and abilities, want to master the more sophisticated techniques such as cesarean section or forceps rotation, but in any event obstetrics offers him a delightful and challenging area of practice.

A family physician, who is not an obstetrician, may need consultation five or six times out of a hundred deliveries. There will be need for fewer consultations in obstetrics than in an equal number of medical or surgical cases.

Family physicians are in a position to change the infant mortality statistics in the United States. Improvement in infant mortality in the past has been attempted by focusing on more skillful delivery techniques and the knowledgeable handling of the parturient woman during labor. However, the family physician has an exceptional opportunity to seek out and correct significant prenatal events wherein lay the key to further reduction in infant mortality.

HIGH RISK PREGNANCIES

Wallace[1] recommends focusing on women of high risk. She gives characteristics of high risk women as follows:*

–lower socioeconomic status
–little education
–disadvantaged groups
–under 20 and over 30 years of age
–pregnant out of wedlock
–history of unfavorable outcome in a previous pregnancy
–pattern of late or no prenatal care
–marital or social problems
–malnutrition or undernutrition
–history of obstetric or medical complications in a previous pregnancy or in present pregnancy
–history of a previous operative delivery or a prolonged labor (24 hr or more)
–history of isoimmunization
–do not have easily available or accessible maternal health care
–previous induced abortion

RESPONSIBILITY TO THE TEENAGER

Whether a family physician does his own deliveries or not he owes the young female patients in his practice certain services that will prepare them psychologically and physiologically for pregnancy. These obligations begin in the early teens.

Sex and Family Education[2]

Most family physicians believe that sex and family life education is the combined duty of parents, schools, churches and themselves. Unfortunately, not all do their share. In preparing teenagers for family life

*Reprinted in part from Wallace H: Factors associated with perinatal mortality and morbidity. Clin Obstet Gynecol 13:13, 1970.

and a happy pregnancy, family physicians may have to fulfill the duty of parents or others.

In this regard, the following are the minimum obligations the family physician has to his young female patients in preparation for future pregnancies:

- –Establish a warm physician-patient relationship in which she is encouraged to discuss her problems; suggest she telephone for answers to her questions
- –Listen to her even if she does not listen to you
- –Schedule physicals for teenagers with idea of getting them to talk
- –Use as much common sense as possible; keep moralizing at a minimum
- –Inform the patient what you intend to say to her parents
- –If it is difficult to offer sex education to a young female give her an appropriate booklet to read; ask her to come back and discuss any questions
- –If she has not been taught at school, discuss with her the physical changes which occur during maturation
- –As she approaches marriage discuss the things that strengthen and build family life
- –Give her support during a crisis such as when she contracts venereal disease or becomes pregnant while unwed
- –Whether you give an unwed young woman contraceptive advice or not, she deserves careful consideration as to her request

(See the appendix for reading list in sex education for teenagers.)

Good Nutrition

Good nutrition of young females (Table 2-1) produces healthier, heavier and more mature infants when the teenager becomes pregnant. There is historic as well as experimental evidence to substantiate this observation. The siege of Leningrad in World War II produced infants weighing 49 percent less than 2500 g at birth and measuring 41 percent less than 47 cm in length.

Table 2-1. Recommended Dietary Allowances for Women Before Pregnancy

Calories	2300
Protein, g	55
Calcium, g	0.8–1.3*
Iron, mg	18
Vitamin A, I.U.	5000
Thiamine, mg	1.0–1.2*
Riboflavin, mg	1.5
Niacin, mg	13–15*
Ascorbic acid, mg	50–55
Vitamin D, I.U.	400

*For 16- to 18-year olds

A considerable amount of psychological and physiological evidence indicates that low birth weight infants are significantly over-represented later in life among the mentally subnormal.[3]

American female teenagers generally have poor habits of nutrition, i.e. inadequate breakfasts, poor calcium, iron and protein intake and bizarre methods of achieving weight control. Considering these are habits developed during the age when good nutrition is important for their own growth and maturation, it is of little wonder that the extra nutritional strain of pregnancy results in toxemias, hypertension, anemia and prematurity. Two of every five babies are born to these women under 20 years of age, which compounds the problem.

Basically, the young teenager should add 5 to 5½ cups of milk or an ounce of American or Swiss cheese daily to the four basic food groups to meet her calcium allowance. Skim milk may be substituted for whole milk if obesity is a problem.

Basic Menu Plan

Breakfast
- Citrus fruit
- Cereal
- Egg
- Bread
- Milk

Luncheon
- Meat, fish or poultry
- Bread
- Fruit
- Milk

Dinner
- Meat, fish or poultry
- Potato
- Vegetable (green or yellow)
- Bread

Iron

Do not allow one of your family practice patients in the childbearing age for whom you have been caring to become pregnant while anemic. Nonpregnant women have a 12 percent incidence of iron deficiency anemia. Pregnant women have a 15 to 58 percent incidence of the same type of anemia. In fact, 84 percent of pregnant women have absent iron stores and therefore are iron deficient. There are good reasons to believe that every woman who is likely to become pregnant should have an iron supplement for 9 to 12 months before each pregnancy.

The average American diet contains about 15 mg of iron per day (6 mg/1000 calories). Both males and females absorb about 1 mg per day but, while the male loses only 1 mg per day, the female will average about 1.5 to 2 mg per day loss, including the loss of blood from menstruation. The normal iron stores of 1.0 g must be lost before anemia can occur. This would take over three years if no iron were taken in the diet.

Diagnosis of iron deficiency anemia is not difficult. Although the first evidence may be the loss of stainable iron in the marrow, this check is not frequently needed. In pregnancy, a diagnosis of iron deficiency anemia can be made when the hemoglobin drops below 11 g/100 ml of blood and erythrocytes below 3,500,000 to 4,000,000 per cu mm. Microcytic hypochromic red cells on blood smears may appear much later than the loss of stainable iron in the marrow. The serum iron decreases and iron binding capacity increases.

If the diagnosis is in doubt, a patient may be subjected to a therapeutic trial of ferrous sulfate. With proper iron therapy, the hemoglobin should increase two g in three weeks. If this response is not obtained, the diagnosis must be reworked using more sophisticated tests and ruling out the macrocytic anemias that usually respond to folic acid but on occasion respond to both folic acid and vitamin B_{12}. Macrocytic anemias usually clear quickly and spontaneously in the postpartum period but tend to recur in subsequent pregnancies.

Transfusions are almost never indicated in a patient with iron deficiency anemia, pernicious anemia or folic acid deficiency. The hazards of transfusion are greater than the hazards of waiting for hemoglobin response to specific therapy.

Administer at least 200 mg of elemental iron per day. This is accomplished by giving ferrous sulfate (plain) 325 mg t.i.d. As indicated, this should be plain ferrous sulfate because the enteric-coated tablets interfere with absorption. For the 15 percent who do not tolerate ferrous sulfate, reduce the dose to one tablet per day and increase as tolerated. Other patients may need a change: ferrous gluconate may be tolerated better by some but mg/mg of iron it is little different than ferrous sulfate.

Radiation Protection

Family physicians are in a position to protect the young from excessive radiation in preparation for a healthy pregnancy. One such way: insist that the patient's gonads be protected from radiation even when taking x-ray pictures of the chest. All that needs be done is to place a heavy rubber shield over the gonadal area.

Rubella Immunization

Every family physician will save himself and others considerable frustration if he makes it his business to immunize all children, especially females, against rubella before the age of 12 years. (See Child Growth and Development.) One convenient way to make sure all young patients are immunized is to have your office nurse check for a history of laboratory confirmed rubella or previous immunization when children show up for routine examinations. A history of rubella without laboratory confirmation is not reliable.

If it becomes necessary to immunize a postpubertal female, follow these steps and record each step on the patient's chart:[5]

Have an HI test done to see if the patient has natural immunity. In case the patient has immunity nothing more need be done except to reassure the patient. Laboratory reports are available in 24 to 48 hr.

Rule out pregnancy. (The U.S. Public Health Service does not recommend mass immunization of adult females because of the chance of inadvertently immunizing a pregnant woman.) No pregnant woman should receive the live rubella vaccine. Since pregnancy tests are not accurate until 40 days after the last menstrual period, wait that long before ruling pregnancy out and giving the vaccine. Malformations occur in 3 percent of births. It would be easy to mistakenly attribute any malformation to vaccine-induced rubella.

Before immunization warn the patient that she must not become pregnant for the following 2 months; give contraceptive advice.

If immunization is given warn the patient of aching joints with or without effusion beginning 2 to 4 wk after immunization. Symptoms subside quickly on symptomatic treatment.

Rho Gam Administration in Early Miscarriages and Abortions

Unwed teenagers frequently turn to abortions as a way out of their dilemma. In recent years, many of these abortions are being done by skilled operators in good hospitals where Rh-negative problems are not overlooked. But because of social pressures, some abortions are still being done by the unskilled who makes no effort to determine the Rh status of the patient. Many times the family physician is the only one who knows an abortion has been done. In these cases, and in cases of miscarriage that he treats, the family physician is responsible for an Rh determination and Rho Gam administration if the patient is Rh-negative.

THE FIRST TRIMESTER

First Visit

Diagnosis of Pregnancy

An experienced family physician should be able to make a diagnosis of pregnancy as early as 6 to 8 weeks after the first day of the last menstrual period. Clinical diagnosis depends on careful bimanual examination of the uterus, a positive Hegar's sign and physiological changes in the vagina, cervix and breasts.

Positive signs are: fetal movement at 18 to 20 weeks, detection of fetal heart tones at 17 to 18 weeks using fetoscope, ultrasound using Doppler's principle at 10 to 13 weeks and fetal electrocardiograms at 12 weeks.

If there is need for an earlier diagnosis the urinary chorionic gonadotropin (hemagglutination inhibition) test will suffice and is probably the most accurate. (The latex particle agglutination inhibition test takes only two minutes but is not available everywhere.) The result can be obtained in less than 2 hours. This test is not dependable until 10 days past the previous missed period. False positives have not been reported; false negatives are less than 3 percent. The use of serum instead of urine is not recommended.

The hemagglutination inhibition test is positive in chorionepithelioma and hydatiform mole. In normal pregnancy the human chorionic gonadotropin (HCG) begins a rise 9 days after insemination and continues a rapid rise reaching a peak of 100,000 IU/L of HCG between the eighth and tenth weeks. It declines sharply between the twelfth and fifteenth weeks remaining at a constant 20,000 IU/L throughout the second and third trimesters.

In choriocarcinoma and hydatid mole the HCG rises to high levels reported to be 300,000 IU/L or higher of urine. Titers of 200,000 IU should lead one to suspect hydatid mole or choriocarcinoma. It is also significant if the high levels of a normal pregnancy (300,000 IU) persist beyond the fifteenth week. When a mole is removed the HCG should drop to 0 within 2 to 3 months.[6]

Setting Date of Confinement

Establish the first day of the last menstrual period early and firmly. The estimation of gestational term based on the menstrual history as obtained from the mother is more reliable than most obstetricians have been inclined to believe. The use of this date in computing expectant date of confinement is apparently as valid as other more exhaustive investigations.

Use Nagele's Rule to calculate length of pregnancy. Add 7 days to the first day of the last menstrual period and then check back 3 calendar months. For example, if the first day of the last menstrual period was July 10, 1974, add 7 days arriving at July 17th. Now check back on the calendar 3 months, which would give the patient an expected date of confinement on April 17, 1975.

The average duration of pregnancy is about 40 weeks. Now you may determine the immediate duration of pregnancy in weeks by counting the weeks from July 17, 1974 to the date in question, say November 1, 1974, in which case it would be about 15 weeks.

The average duration of pregnancy, calculated from the first day of the last menstrual period, is 40 weeks. The mean duration of actual pregnancy, calculated from the day of ovulation, is 267 days. Using basal temperature, it has been estimated that the average pregnancy from ovulation to term is from 266 to 270 days.

It is well to recall that only 4 percent of all patients deliver on the calculated date of confinement.

History and Physical Examination

Request pregnant women without complication to come for office visits monthly until the twenty-eighth week, every 2 weeks from the twenty-eighth to the thirty-sixth week, and weekly thereafter. At the first prenatal visit take a full history and do a physical examination including a PAP smear. Include in the history the details of the patient's menstrual and natal history. If a positive PAP smear is reported, Class III or better, repeat the smear. A definitive diagnosis of carcinoma should be made by cervical biopsy or coning after the 12th week.

Predicting Sex

Family physicians are often urged to predict the sex of the unborn child. The theory has been advanced that a consistent fetal heart rate of over 140 indicates a girl and a rate below 140 a boy. In practice this is not an accurate method of prognostication.

The most accurate method comes from a chromosome analysis of the mother's peripheral lymphocytes, which may be made as early as the fourteenth week of pregnancy.

Important Pelvic Measurements

Do a careful pelvic examination with an estimation of all pelvic measurements. However, external measurements mean little in prognosis. Most obstetricians agree that, as a minimum, the following are most significant determinations: the size of the pelvic inlet, the size of the midpelvis and the pelvic conformation. At the time of delivery other factors become important: the size and presentation of the fetal head and the quality of the uterine contractions.

Inlet contraction is present when the anteroposterior diameter (obstetric conjugate) is less than 10.0 cm or the transverse diameter less than 12.0 cm.

Midpelvic contraction is a reduction in the plane of least dimension and is present when the distance between the ischial spines is less than 9.0 cm. Obtain an accurate measurement of these diameters by x-ray pelvimetry. A family physician may be suspicious when on bimanual examination he finds a small pelvis with large ischial spines jutting into the birth canal.

Outlet contraction is present when the distance between the ischial tuberosities is less than 8.0 cm.

The pelvic conformation is more important than its size in prognosis. Classify the female pelvis as:

–Gynecoid (normal configuration)
–Android (male configuration)
–Anthropoid (reduced transverse diameter)
–Platypelloid (interference with entry into the inlet. Within this classification occurs the highest incidence of cesarean sections.)
–Mixed

Using Fundal Height to Determine Fetal Age

The traditional method of estimating fetal age from the height of the fundus is not very reliable. An error of up to 8 weeks is possible using this technique. It has been said that the fundus reaches the umbilicus at 24 weeks. In one study this landmark was reached any time after 18 weeks. The most accurate assessment of fetal maturity is made by pelvic examination during the first trimester.

Advising the Unwed Mother[7]

Family physicians are being confronted more frequently by the problems of the unwed mother and the proper disposition of her problems. The teenage girl who is pregnant faces serious problems and needs the sympathetic assistance of a physician.

The alternatives to getting married and proceeding naturally are the following:

Abortion: Legal and ethic bars to abortion appear to be relaxing and probably abortions will be used more frequently in the future to solve the unwed teenager's problem. Before advising an abortion, the family physician should familiarize himself with the state and local laws and the patient's attitude regarding abortion.

Keeping the infant though unwed. More and more young mothers are opting for this alternative. When parents and friends are accepting, this option has often worked satisfactorily. A few unwed mothers have a strong commitment to their pregnancy. They refuse any consideration of an abortion even when it is urged by the infant's father, her parents and other counselors. They may feel they have done wrong, but they are not about to compound their first mistake by a second.

Adoption of the infant. Most doctors and social workers would recommend this course of action.

Marriage. Occasionally when all facts are brought out and there seems to be a genuine relationship between the unwed girl and the infant's father, a hasty wedding solves the problem.

Steps in Solving the Problem

Determine why the girl is pregnant. Is she rebelling? Is she trying to run away from the family? Does she need someone to identify with? Is she trying to get attention? Is she having trouble at school? Psychiatrists, rightly or wrongly, claim the following motivations in single women for becoming pregnant: (1) the desire to become pregnant may be an unconscious need to which a girl may be driven. (2) an unsatisfactory relationship with her mother may cause a girl to seek pregnancy to prove that she is the equal of her mother and to punish her mother; and (3) with guilt feelings about having had intercourse outside marriage, she punishes herself by becoming pregnant.

Listen to the girl without censuring or excusing her behavior. Urge her to tell her parents. She must learn to be responsible for her actions.

Fight the inclination to rely on the girl's parents for a solution. Remember the girl is now the patient and the final decision should be made by her.

Do not neglect the teenage father. Some are irresponsible; others have a deep commitment. He should be interviewed and his motives explored. Occasionally a teenage father attempts suicide.

Twenty to fifty percent of teenage marriages end in divorce within four years; consequently, forcing a young couple into marriage may only compound their problem by increasing the number of children before the final separation.

Urge the girl to stay in regular school for at least 4 to 5 months, her health and the school authorities permitting. In school districts where continuation high schools are established, a transfer to one of these schools may be in order. Other alternatives are home study and special classes.

Contrary to past advice to unwed mothers, most authorities now feel that the young mother should see and hold the baby before giving it up for adoption. After all, there is no advantage to a hurried decision which may be later resented. Under these circumstances a girl makes a more reasoned judgment.

Sometimes a referral to an agency and its case workers is wise. The Florence Crittenton Association is a national organization devoted to helping pregnant unwed mothers. They may arrange for the mother to enter one of their institutions or be cared for on an out-patient basis. They can arrange for her to continue her education. There are case workers to help the girl decide whether she wants to keep her child or give it up for adoption. The fees in all Crittenton Agencies are scaled to the ability of the girl and her family to pay. Florence Crittenton organizations may be found in local phone books but the home office address is: 608 S. Dearborn St., Chicago, IL 60605. It will provide the names of facilities in the girl's area.

Obtain the parents' consent before accepting an unwed pregnant teenage girl for obstetrical care.

Genetic Problems

The family physician is usually the first professional counselor consulted by the family of an abnormal child. After the shock of having an abnormal child, the next question the parents want answered is "Will it happen again?" In some instances the answers are best made after study by a genetic expert. But there are many times the family physician may answer the questions authoritatively without expensive and time consuming genetic studies.

The causes of congenital malformations, in so far as they are known, fall into two main categories (Table 2-2).

The syndromes mentioned in Table 2-2 are best diagnosed by cytogenetic studies of the child and, if necessary, the parents. For this reason these cases are best referred to a specialist in human cytogenetics.

There are approximately 1500 conditions now thought to be governed by the first four simple genetic mechanisms in the table. If the family physician can diagnose the genetic problem he may well counsel patients as to the inheritability of the disease.

Most of these genetic disorders are inherited in one of three ways: as autosomal dominant; the sex-linked recessive; and the autosomal recessive. Most of the inheritable disorders have been classified, and you only need refer to a chart to find which of the three genetic routes the disorder will follow.

For each mode of inheritance, the risk to a subsequent child is known. In clear cut cases of sex-linked disorders, 50 percent of the sons will have the disorder and 50 percent of the daughters will be carriers. In autosomal dominant disorders the chance of a parent transmitting the abnormality to an offspring is 50 percent. In autosomal recessive conditions, the probability of a second child having the disorder is 25 percent, but all offspring will be carriers. Fraser elaborates on these phases of genetic counseling and the family physician.[8]

Autosomal Recessive Inheritance

The most common of these congenital traits is the autosomal recessive wherein the following diseases* and others are passed from one generation to the next:

Phenylketonuria—4/100,000; 15% parental consanguinity
Sickle cell anemia—2/1,000 American Negroes
Cystic fibrosis—1/10,000
Albinism—1/15,000
Adrenogenital syndrome—female pseudohermaphroditism; precocious puberty in male
Ataxia—telangiectasia

*Reprinted from Fraser FC: Genetic counseling. Hosp Practice 6:49–56, 1971, with permission.

Table 2-2. Causes of Congenital Malformations

Environmental Factors (Intrauterine)	*Genetic Factors*
Radiation Maternal infections (rubella, cytomegalovirus, herpesvirus hominis, toxoplasmosis, tuberculosis, syphilis, gonorrhea, listerosis and malaria) Maternal dietary deficiencies Drugs and poisons	Dominant genes Recessive genes Intermediate genes Sex-linked genes Mutations and abnormalities of chromosome behavior (Down's, Patau's, Edward's, Turner's and Klinefelter's syndromes)

Niemann—Pick Disease—chiefly in Jews
Cretinism—familial goitrous
Homocystinuria—usually urinary stone formers
Tay-Sachs (infantile amaurotic idiocy)—1/250,000; onset 1 to 6 mos; death within 2 yr; 25% have first cousin parents; mostly Jews
Progressive spinal muscular atrophy (Werdnig-Hoffmann's disease)—13% parental consanguinity
Familial dysautonomia (Riley-Day syndrome)
Laurence-Moon-Biedl syndrome
Alkaptonuria (pentosuria)
Wilson's disease (hepatolenticular degeneration)

In these autosomal recessive conditions the presumption following the birth of an affected child is that both parents are carriers. Advise the parents that the risk of a second child being affected would be 1:4 (25 percent). Because of the recessive nature of the condition, an affected individual cannot produce an affected child unless the other parent is a carrier but all his offspring will be carriers. If two affected persons marry, all their children will be affected. There is frequent consanguineous marriages among the parents of affected persons, usually between first cousins. Most of us carry three to five recessive genes of potentially serious defects, but most of us are also lucky enough to marry someone with three to five *different* serious recessive genes.

Eugenic advice for severe disease such as Tay-Sachs, cystic fibrosis or Werdnig-Hoffmann may be different from that for benign conditions like pentosuria or for diseases amenable to treatment such as phenylketonuria, galactosemia or Wilson's. Reproduction may be undesirable for parents who both carry the mutant gene of one of the severe diseases. Birth control by contraception or ovulatory suppression may be indicated. Sterilization is not justified for heterozygous carriers of any autosomal recessive gene, particularly not in a society with a high rate of divorce because mating partners may change. Termination of an existing pregnancy may be advisable.

Sex-Linked Recessive Inheritance

Less common are the sex-linked recessive conditions typified by the following diseases:*

Hemophilia A and B—4/100,000
Color blindness
Hurler's syndrome (gargoylism)
Duchenne's and Becker's muscular dystrophy
Ocular albinism
X-linked ichthyosis
Agammaglobulinemia (Bruton's disease)
Nephrogenic diabetes insipidus
Lesch-Nyhan syndrome
G-6-phosphate deficiency—sensitivity to java beans, primaquine or mothballs
Ectodermal dysplasia anhidrotic

An x-linked (sex-linked) genetic disorder is found almost exclusively in males and the gene must have been transmitted by the

*Reprinted from Fraser, FC: Genetic counseling. Hosp Practice 6:49–56, 1971, with permission.

mother except when a fresh mutation occurs. Male-to-male transmission of an x-linked gene does not occur. An affected male will transmit the x-linked gene to all his daughters and to none of his sons.

According to Fraser[8], counseling in x-linked disorders usually depends on whether the mother is a carrier. If she has two or more affected sons or one affected son and an affected male relative (brother, father, maternal uncle), consider her a carrier. If the mother as a carrier is known and the diagnosis is clear, counseling can usually be done by the family physician.

Thus when a family has produced a son manifesting a sex-linked disease, for example hemophilia, the mother may be a heterozygous carrier for the mutant gene. If the disorder has also turned up in one or more of the mother's male relatives the probability becomes a near certainty. Any future sons she produces will then have a 50 percent chance of hemophilia. Her daughters will be quite safe but will have the same 50 percent chance of being carriers.

If the first hemophiliac child is apparently unique in the family tree, the genetic situation is a good deal less certain. In this case the risk would be somewhere between 0 and 50 percent. The best one can say is that the greater the number of unaffected male relatives in a hitherto hemophilia-free family, the lower the probability that the mother is a carrier.

If you need to be more accurate, refer the patient to a genetic counseling center where it is now possible to determine whether a suspect female is or is not a carrier. This applies to both the sex-linked and autosomal recessive problems.

Prescribe birth control for women who are conductors of severe x-linked diseases such as Duchenne muscular dystrophy and gargoylism. Consider sterilization of women who are proven gene carriers. Do not advise sterilization of men affected with these diseases because they will not have affected sons. All his daughters, however, will need eugenic advice.

Consider termination of an existing pregnancy. Pregnancy may be an unbearable psychological experience for a mother who has already had a child with severe disease. In this situation, and before a decision is made, determine the sex of the fetus by amniocentesis. If the mother could be assured that she is expecting a girl, she would have no worry.

Autosomal Dominant Inheritance

The most easily identifiable of the inherited disorders are those which follow the autosomal dominant inheritance pattern.*

Huntington's chorea—onset at about 35 years of age
Lobster claw deformity of the hands
Achondroplasia—1/10,000; many sporadic cases probably mutations
Acute intermittent prophyria (Jegher's syndrome)—one third of cases sporadic; always becomes malignant so check relatives
Friedreich's ataxia
Neurofibromatosis (Recklinghausen's disease)—presence of 6 or more cafe-au-lait spots 1.5 cm or more in diameter is diagnostic
Hereditary hemorrhagic telangiectasia (Osler's disease)
Aniridia—1/100,000
Marfan's syndrome
Ehler's-Danlous syndrome (hyperelastica cutis)—rubberman contortionists
Gaucher's disease, adult type
Polydactyly, syndactyly, ear tags
Retinoblastoma—3/100,000; sporadic cases will transmit the disease to their children 50:50 risk. Very unlikely to occur in siblings of affected child with normal parents
Osteogenesis imperfecta
Any condition showing a mandelian dominant pattern in a concerned family

Within this group only a simple mutant gene is required to produce frank disease, so that the identification of carriers is

*Reprinted from Fraser FC: Genetic counseling. Hosp Practice 6:49–56, 1971, with permission.

normally not a problem. An affected individual with one normal parent is presumably heterozygous for the mutant gene, and the chance of it being transmitted to his offspring is one in two. What is comforting is that those who appear normal are probably genetically normal. It is possible, however, for the disability to skip generations due to poor *penetrance* of an apparently normal carrier.

Every affected patient has an affected parent unless the mutant occurred in the patient himself. Affected persons married to normal persons have, on the average, equal numbers of affected and normal children. Normal children of affected persons have only normal children.

Parents cannot be allowed to expect that because their first child was affected that their next will be normal to complete the usual ratio. Each child has a 50 percent chance of being affected if one parent is affected.

Many autosomal dominant traits are quite compatible with a normal life. Preventive eugenics may be indicated for serious conditions such as severe osteogenesis imperfecta, for some of the neurological conditions, for familial polyposis and for retinoblastoma.

You would be wise to suggest an abortion for severe disease. Prevention of pregnancy, in some instances even sterilization, may be considered. Needless to say, sterilization is justified only for the gene carrier, never for the healthy and genetically normal mate. If the husband is the carrier of the trait and the family wants children, consider artificial insemination of sperm from a healthy man. Suggest adoption if the woman is the carrier.

Multifactorial Diseases

Prognostication of the multifactorial diseases that are produced by a combination of genetic and environmental factors are best left to the specialist. The probability of their occurrence should be estimated from empirical data for any particular case.

The following are multifactorial diseases seen by the family physician:* cleft lip and palate, diabetes mellitus, schizophrenia, Hirschsprung's disease, congenital heart disease, spina bifida cystica, infantile autism, congenital dislocation of hip, pyloric stenosis, celiac disease, Crohn's disease, congenital deafness, anencephaly, multiple sclerosis, mental retardation and hypospadias.

Study this class of congenital problem by a review of mental retardation, which accounts for 3 percent of the total population. Mental retardation is found in a number of single-gene inherited conditions such as PKU, neurofibromatosis and muscular dystrophy. These account for only a small percentage of the mentally retarded. Other causes are either chromosomal aberrations or environmental factors as in cerebral injuries, anoxia and hypoglycemia.

The largest fraction of the retarded population are the so-called familial mental retarded of multifactorial origins. The retardation of this group is due to cultural deprivation or to multifactorial inheritance or a combination of both. The exact pattern of its hereditary transmission is not known. Remember, it is not always possible to distinguish between genetically-determined and environmentally-caused mental subnormality.

Counseling

Counseling is difficult. These statements are probably justified: (1) A mentally subnormal parent has an increased risk of having a mentally subnormal offspring (Table 2-3). If both parents are subnormal, the chance of subnormality in their children is high, perhaps around 50 percent. (2) Polygenic traits tend to regress toward the mean; in other words, children of moderately retarded parents have a chance of being, on the average, somewhat more intelligent than their parents.

Fraser offers sound advice when he summarizes the family physician's responsibil-

*Reprinted from Fraser FC: Genetic counseling. Hosp Practice 6:49–56, 1971, with permission.

Table 2-3. Common Risk Factors

Cleft palate (1/2500)
Risk for a child whose sibling is affected—3%
Risk for a child who has 1 affected parent—7%
Risk for a child who has 1 affected parent plus 1 affected sibling—17%

Cleft lip with cleft palate (1/1000)
Risk for a child whose sibling is affected—5%
Risk for a child who has 1 affected parent and 1 affected sibling—15%

Diabetes mellitus (5/1000)
Risk for a child who has 1 affected parent—5% or more
Risk for a child who has 1 affected sibling—5% or more
If both parents affected—about 25% of offspring (warrants eugenic counseling)

Meningomyelocele or Anencephaly
Risk to child with 1 sibling—1 to 2%
Risk to child with 2 siblings—10%

Pyloric stenosis (60% in males, 90% in females)
Of affected male patients—5 to 7% of sons, 1 to 3% of daughters
Of affected female patients—20% of sons, 6 to 11% of daughters

Inguinal hernia
Of affected male patients—10% of sons, 1% of daughters
Of affected female patients—15% of sons, 10% of daughters

Congenital deafness
If both parents are deaf—Risk of first child, 50%; after 1 unaffected child, 10%

Multiple sclerosis
Risk to all children—1%

Major psychosis (schizophrenia)
Risk to all children—10 to 15%

Congenital dislocation of hip
Of affected male patients—5% all children
Of affected female patients—1% of sons, 7% of daughters

Pernicious anemia
Presence of parietal cell antibodies—13 to 25% sons, 33 to 41% daughters

Allergy
All children—25 to 50%

Asthma
All children—5 to 10%

ities in genetic disorders.[8] First, take leadership in making an accurate diagnosis of the disorder under consideration. This is undoubtedly a rigorous requisite and may require specialized techniques and consultations. He wisely states that what on first glance appears to be a genetic disorder often becomes an acquired or environmental disability on closer scrutiny and thus not susceptible to genetic laws at all. He also warns against falling into the "genetic heterogeneity" trap wherein clinically similar diseases may show different patterns of inheritance.

Fraser's second precaution to the family physician is that he make clear to the patient just what the risk means. He warns that the patient's reaction might be different from the physician's, either over- or underreacting to the disorder and its probability of recurrence. As a rule of thumb, however, parents are willing to take a relatively high risk if the disability is mild but may be unwilling to take a small risk with severe disabilities.

In this regard, Fraser suggests that, with a little experience and forethought, family physicians should not hesitate in giving rather forceful advice. He demurs at, "thou shalt nots" but suggests that the family physician be prepared to tell what he, the counselor, would do under the circumstances.

Giving numerical risks alone is not really sufficient counseling. In most cases, account must be taken of emotional, religious, social, intellectual and age factors. In any event, the decision of how far to go in counseling differs from counselor to counselor and from case to case.

In the event a family physician chooses to refer the patient to a professional genetic counselor, whether he be an M.D. or not, the referring physician is obligated to make a proper referral. This should include a summary of his tests and findings, emphasizing particularly the basis of his diagnosis. It may save the family physician's time as well as preventing marital discord or divorce if some family background is included, especially information regarding sensitive members of the family, including grandparents.

Last of all, the family physician, after he understands the problem, owes a follow-up call to the patients to check on the family's comprehension of the counselor's findings.

In the future, genetic counseling may become more complicated because of two medical developments now taking place—liberalization of the abortion laws and genetic study of the fetus-en-utero. Consequently, in the future the family physician may be confronted with the rather abrupt question, "Should I have *this* baby?" rather than the speculative question of the probability of having another abnormal child. In an increasing number of cases, amniocentesis can help provide the answer.

Amniocentesis

DIAGNOSABLE GENETIC DISORDERS. As of this writing, more than 27 neurological diseases accompanying severe mental retardation may be diagnosed during the fourth and fifth months of pregnancy.[9] The diagnosis can be made early enough for safe termination of the pregnancy if the parents desire. The diseases are:*

Arginosuccinic aciduria
Citrullinemia
Cystathioninuria
Cystinosis
Fucosidosis
Galactosemia
Gaucher's Disease
  Infantile
  Adult
Juvenile GM_1 gangliosidosis
Glycogen storage disease, type 2
Homocystinuria
Hypervalinemia
I-cell disease
Isovalericacidemia
Lesch-Nyhan syndrome
Fabry's disease
Maple syrup urine disease
Hurler's disease
Hunter's disease
Sanfilippo's disease
Metachromatic leukodystrophy
  Late infantile
  Juvenile and adult
Methylmalonic acidemia
Nieman-Pick disease
Orotic aciduria
Refsum's disease
Tay-Sachs disease
Sandhoff's disease
Wolman's disease
Adrenogenital syndrome

*Reprinted in part from O'Brien JS: How we detect mental retardation before birth. Med Times 99:103–106, 1971, with permission.

The procedure involves taking a sample (10 ml) of amniotic fluid from the uterus between the twelfth and sixteenth weeks of pregnancy. The procedure is an outpatient one; does not require a general anesthesia; is relatively painless; and in skillful hands, can be carried out successfully with a very low risk to the fetus. Cells floating on the fluid come from the fetus and can be used for enzyme assay.

DIAGNOSTIC USES. There is increasing evidence that amniocentesis should be offered to every pregnant woman over 40 years of age in order to make the diagnosis of mongolism as early as possible. Other uses are:

- –Measurement of bilirubin, creatinine levels and examination of cells to determine fetal maturity
- –Visualization of amniotic fluid by amnioscopy for meconium
- –Determination of fetal sex for ruling out the presence of familial diseases
- –Cultivation of amniotic fluid cells to detect Down's syndrome and other metabolic problems
- –Analysis of hemoglobin products to determine need for fetal transfusions
- –Visualization of fetal skeleton, placenta and fetal gastrointestinal tract for intrauterine transfusions

Resources

The National Foundation conducts an active program of disseminating knowledge in the area of birth defects. It makes reprints available and, most importantly for the family physician, publishes the "International Directory of Genetic Services." In this book are listed genetic units throughout the United States and the world, along with the names of their directors, their addresses and specialized services provided. Copies available without charge upon request to the National Foundation, 800 Second Avenue, New York, NY 10017. Telephone number (212) 265-3166.

Counseling Regarding Abortions

Not only does the family physician have the problem of the unwed mother but also he sees an increasing number of married women who choose to terminate their pregnancies. Probably any healthy married woman who has made this decision should be seen two or three times for short office visits to explore her motivations, to discuss alternatives and to explain procedures. A few women may only be temporarily exasperated or overwhelmed by seemingly unsolvable family problems.

In any event the woman should have an opportunity to discuss the reasons leading to her request for an abortion and, if she has sought her family physician's counsel, she is entitled to his seasoned judgment. The physician should keep himself emotionally unengaged; the patient's decision should not be dictated by the attitudes of her physician. The woman, after an exchange with her doctor, should feel the decision is hers and that it is the best one for her family and her. The family physician has failed if he leaves the woman feeling guilty or culpable in whatever decision she makes.

One rule will stand the family physician in good stead. If, during these discussions, you uncover any clues that indicate that continuing the pregnancy would be valuable to her, wisely warn against termination of pregnancy.

If there is controversy in the family regarding a proposed abortion, the best course is to invite the husband and wife to the office for a mutual discussion.

Techniques of Abortion

If the patient is less than 13 weeks pregnant, calculated from the date of the last menstrual period, vacuum aspiration is the technique of choice because:

- –the procedure is completed in 3 to 5 minutes
- –paracervical block is sufficient anesthesia
- –minimal cervical dilatation is required
- –blood loss rarely exceeds 60 ml, if termination is before 10 weeks, but 200 ml at 11 to 13 weeks
- –uterine perforation is less likely to occur
- –risk of retained secundines is minimal
- –patient feels well in about an hour

Dilatation and curettage as a technique for abortion carries more risk because:

- –more cervical dilatation is needed
- –amount of blood lost is tripled
- –perforation of uterine wall is more common
- –general anesthesia is needed more frequently
- –more secundines retained

In the vacuum technique one end of a cannula is attached to a suction pump and the other end is introduced into the partially dilated cervix. Suction should be off before introducing the cannula into the uterus and before it is removed from the cavity. The maximum suction usually required is 25 to 30 inches of mercury.

Patients whose pregnancies are between 14 and 18 weeks are best aborted by the salting or saline injection method, which requires hospitalization. The hypertonic solution induces labor that may need medical support. The technique requires transabdominal removal of 75 to 100 ml of amniotic fluid from the amniotic sac and injection of 200 ml of 20 percent saline solution. About 150 ml is usually adequate to induce labor. The technique requires special training in amniocentesis.

As an abortion technique, hysterotomy is least often used. It is similar to a cesarean section as to risks. Hysterotomies are usually coupled with sterilization.

The most common complications of aspiration or D. and C. induced abortions are retained products of conception and infection. Any bleeding of more than an average menstrual period may signal an incomplete abortion. In this case, give ergonovine (Ergotrate) 0.2 mg orally. In many cases this causes the uterus to expel the tissue. When the patient is febrile (100 to 102°) for 2 to 3 days and has a large soft uterus, a D. and C. or repeat aspiration is probably indicated but not before cultures, antibiotics and possibly ergonovine is given. (See Prevention and Treatment of Septic Shock.)

Watch for a twin or ectopic pregnancy if uterus remains firm and enlarged or the patient complains of pain in her side. These possibilities can be supported by a pregnancy test at least 7 days after the abortion. Rho Gam should be administered to every Rh-negative woman within 72 hours after the abortion.

Aftercare involves helping the woman avoid another unwanted pregnancy. This can be started 2 weeks after an abortion.

Most patients are given Methergine and ampicillin for at least 24 hours following the abortion. They are cautioned to use sanitary pads only (no tampons) for 2 weeks; no intercourse for 2 weeks; no baths or douches for 2 weeks; to take their temperature AM and PM for 1 week; and to contact the physician if bleeding in one day exceeds a normal period, if bleeding continues longer than 2 weeks, if temperature is over 100.4° F, if discharge becomes foul smelling or if unusual pain develops.

The adverse psychological effects of an induced abortion seem to have been overemphasized. The emotional disturbance resulting from forcing a woman to carry an unwanted baby appears to be greater and persists longer than the disturbances resulting from a wanted abortion. Brody and coworkers[10] suggest women who were subjected to induced abortions showed a great decline in psychopathology within 6 weeks and were close to normal after 1 year.

When one considers that three-quarters of the abortions are done for psychiatric reasons, it follows that some type of psychiatric follow-up would seem desirable. Strangely enough, neither psychiatrist nor patient desires follow-up. Everyone seems to feel an abortion solves the problem.

Prevention and Treatment of Septic Shock[11,12]

The majority of cases of septic shock are due to infected abortions. The common agent is an endotoxin from the coliform group of organisms. Successful treatment is based on early recognition or suspicion. Septic infection precedes shock and is manifested by a temperature of 100.4° F or more for 16 consecutive hours and systemic manifestation of infection. For shock, the blood pressure must be below 90 mm of mercury and the pulse above 110. Be on alert in cases of:

- –late infected abortions (more than 10 wk gestation)
- –minimal blood loss by history and examination
- –hyperpyrexia (more than 103° F)
- –chemical douche (soap, turpentine, etc.)
- –minimal abdominopelvic tenderness
- –gram-negative organisms on cervical smear
- –diminishing urinary output

In speculum examination the cervix may be patulous with a foul-smelling tomato soup discharge. Other findings are not diagnostic.

Clinical staging:

Stage I Endometritis
Stage II Parametritis and adnexal involvement
Stage III Generalized peritonitis

TREATMENT. Massive doses of antibiotics: In 24 hr, give 40,000,000 units of penicillin, 3 to 5 g of chloramphenicol, and 1 to 2 g of streptomycin. Then reduce to a maintenance dose. Change as later indicated by cultures. Do culture and sensitivity tests on the cervix, endometrial cavity, urine, blood and throat.

CVP monitoring: At values 6 to 12 cm, fluids can be given cautiously. If CVP is above 12 cm, discontinue fluid administration. Monitor vital signs hourly, including urinary output.

Curettage is done after 6 to 8 hr of antibiotic therapy, sooner if septic shock threatens. Delay in performing a D. and C. may lead to irreversible deterioration.

X-ray study of abdomen may show signs of perforation, foreign body, or gas bubbles suggesting Clostridia. Order an x-ray film of the chest to rule out pulmonary complications such as pneumonia and infarction.

Antishock therapy: Look for septic shock by a decrease in urinary output. With the aid of a Foley catheter a urinary output of about 30 ml an hour is the minimum desirable. Intake and output should be strictly recorded. If the patient is in shock, indicated by a systolic blood pressure of less than 90, administer 0.5 to 1 g of hydrocortisone by direct intravenous injection and 100 mg every hour thereafter. A concentration of isoproterenol 0.4 mg per 100 cc is given by continuous infusion titrated against blood pressure and urinary output.

If the patient is found to be Rh-negative (unless the biologic father is known to be Rh-negative also) the fetal blood type must be considered Rh-positive. Administer Rho Gam after curettage to prevent maternal sensitization.

Indications for hysterectomy in treatment of septic abortion are: (1) the presence of c. welchii, (2) evidence that soap or lysol infusion was used to produce abortion, or (3) uterine perforation during the abortive attempt.

The Rh-Negative Mother

All pregnant women, whether the pregnancy is to terminate in successful childbirth or a spontaneous or induced abortion, should have their Rh status determined. An Rh-negative woman whose husband is Rh-positive may develop an Rh-positive fetus. In some of these women, the Rh factor of the fetus stimulates the formation of Rh antibodies in the Rh-negative mother.

Earlier transfusions of Rh-positive blood to an Rh-negative woman may also cause the formation and storage of Rh-antibodies. Should this mother receive a second transfusion of Rh-positive blood, a dangerous hemolytic reaction may occur. Erythroblastosis fetalis occurs when the Rh antibodies produced by the mother penetrate the placenta and attack the Rh-positive fetus. As prevention, no Rh-negative female should receive Rh-positive blood. If she does become sensitized to the Rh factor, erythroblastosis could be produced in the firstborn Rh-positive child, which is not ordinarily the case.

On the first visit of any obstetric patient take a careful history, noting previous pregnancies, abortions or transfusions. The history of these events may have initiated sensitization. Evaluation of the events surrounding a previous stillbirth should be thorough because the possibility of erythroblastosis fetalis in the infant is a good possibility. The expectant date of confinement should be set with accuracy. Interpretation of amniotic fluid analysis depends on this date. Continue to validate the date during the pregnancy.

Determine ABO blood type and Rh type. If screened as Rh-negative, check for D'' factor. If D''-negative, consider the patient Rh-negative. If Rh-negative primipara: Determine ABO and Rh type of husband. If husband is Rh-positive, check the patient's serum for antibodies. Recheck for antibodies or rising titer once in first trimester, twice in second trimester and every two weeks in third trimester. A family physician should not be lulled into a false sense of security by a fixed antibody titer. In two-thirds of all cases of stillbirth there is no rise in antibody titer.

Once a gravida presents with a positive anti-Rh titer, the present pregnancy and all future pregnancies are at risk for fetal survival. The first affected pregnancy may be the last good chance for the patient to have a live baby.

If the pregnant woman does not demonstrate circulating anti-Rh antibodies, routine prenatal care is given. Order a direct Coombs test on the infant's cord blood at delivery in addition to ABO and Rh typing. In the event the direct Coombs is negative and the infant Rh-positive, administer Rho Gam within 72 hours. (See Rho Gam administration.) If Rh-negative multipara: Check all tests mentioned above and, in addition, determine Rh type of all surviving children. Do an indirect Coombs two or three times during the second trimester and biweekly in the third trimester. A critical titer level indicating sensitization should be established by the laboratory. This may vary from 1:2 to 1:64 depending on the laboratory.

If the Rh-antibody studies reveal that the mother is sensitized, the first amniocentesis is done between the twenty-eighth and thirty-second week of gestation. If there has been severe involvement in previous pregnancy, amniocentesis is done between the twenty-sixth and twenty-eighth week. Tests are repeated weekly or biweekly, depending on initial analysis. The value of amniocentesis lies in determining the optimal time for delivery of infants with proven erythroblastosis.

Using spectrophotometric analysis of the amniotic fluid, investigators describe three zones or deviations of optical density. *Low Zone:* One can expect an Rh-negative infant or mildly affected Rh-positive infant. There is no fetal jeopardy and the pregnancy can be allowed to go to term. *Mid Zone:* Amniocentesis should be repeated weekly until a trend is established. If titer falls, amniocentesis can be done every two weeks. If the titer falls into low zone, delivery can be done near term. The infant may need one or more exchange transfusions, however. If mid zone readings persist, the infant should be delivered within the thirty-fifth week. A moderately ill infant should be expected and pediatric consultation arranged before delivery. When the pregnancy is less advanced than the thirty-fourth week, an intrauterine transfusion is recommended. *High Zone:* A high zone reading, especially when there is a history of previous stillbirth, indicates the need for intrauterine transfusion or immediate delivery, depending on the stage of gestation. The transfusions are repeated with an attempt to maintain pregnancy to at least the twenty-fourth week when delivery should be accomplished in the least traumatic manner.

Researchers have found that by amniocentesis perinatal mortality has been reduced from 22 to 30 percent to 9 to 10 percent. With the knowledge that the fetus is moderately or severely affected at 35 weeks, the physician can induce delivery. This has resulted in a 50 percent decrease in stillbirths in patients with a previous history of stillbirths or affected infants. In addition, amniocentesis has eliminated the induction of labor of premature infants who are Rh-negative or who are unaffected Rh-positive.

If the mother is Rh-positive and has received previous transfusions or intramuscular blood or had infants suggesting erythroblastosis, treat in the same way as an Rh-negative female. A miscarriage can cause primary immunization by entry of even a small amount of Rh-positive fetal cells into the Rh-negative woman's blood. Therefore, if an abortion occurs in an Rh-negative woman whose husband is Rh-positive, she should consider protective therapy with Rho (D) immune globulin within 72 hours of the abortion.[13,14]

Use of Drugs During Pregnancy

Every medication is a potential poison and should be given only when indicated. At no time is this axiom more appropriate than during pregnancy. However, there isn't a therapeutic drug you should withhold from a pregnant woman if the risk to the mother without the drug is greater than the risk to the infant. The basic problem lies not in avoiding drugs but in giving drugs without justification or without knowledge of contraindications, dosages and adverse reactions.

Recent attention has been called to the fetal danger of commonly used drugs such as aspirin, barbiturates, appetite depressants, sulfonamides and antacids. Nelson and Forfar[15] advise not administering any drug that carries a suspicion of teratogenicity unless that drug is specifically indicated and avoiding self-medication with common household remedies such as aspirin and antacids. As for antibiotics, penicillin has stood the test of twenty years use and appears to have the lowest incidence of toxic manifestations. It is hoped the cephalosporin will prove as good.

Some common problems and their treatment:

Hypertension: Administer a thiazide diuretic. If further help is needed, add hydralazine (Apresoline), 25 to 75 mg q.i.d. An alternate antihypertensive could be methyldopa (Aldomet) 250 mg 2 to 4 times daily. Reserpine may cause respiratory obstruction in the fetus.

URI in pregnancies: Treat symptomatically with aspirin, rest and fluids. Avoid antihistamines. If bacterial invasion is suspected, culture and treat with appropriate antibiotics. A gram-positive coccal or pneumococcal infection responds to ampicillan 250 mg q.i.d. for 3 to 5 days or until culture is negative.

Urinary tract infection: E. Coli, the most common GU infection, probably should be treated with ampicillan 250 to 500 mg q.i.d. providing the patient is not hypersensitive to penicillin. Furadantin may produce a hemolysis in the fetus. Tetracyclines should be avoided as they may inhibit fetal bone growth or produce discoloration of the teeth. Sulfonamides should be avoided at or near term when neonatal jaundice may be produced.

Many drugs readily cross the placenta; therefore, there is no placental barrier in medication. Whether a drug adversely affects the fetus is dependent on several variables, including the type of drug, the dose and the time given. Table 2-4 lists drugs reported to have adverse effects on the fetus. This does not mean these drugs are contraindicated, but they are listed to alert the family physician to their potential harm. This list is from the Division of Congenital Malformations. The National Foundation–March of Dimes.

Drugs in Infectious Disease

Mumps: Give hyperimmune human mumps gamma globulin, 1.5 ml up to 90 lb, 3.0 ml for patients between 90 and 140 pounds, and 4.5 ml for those over 140 pounds within 1 week of exposure. Repeat at 2-week intervals if exposure continues.

Influenza: Vaccination of pregnant women is advisable in epidemic years; tailor the vaccine to the epidemic strains. Immunize at any stage of the patient's pregnancy as the virus is inactivated. Immunize the pregnant woman in nonepidemic years if she needs the protection.

Hepatitis: Administer immune globulin in does of 0.02 to 0.06 ml per pound of body weight as soon as possible after exposure, preferably within 1 week. For single exposure the minimum dose is suggested; for continued exposure the larger dose. For delivery, omit drugs metabolized by the liver; nitrous oxide is safe. If the mother has had the disease, the virus may cross the placental barrier; consequently, you should observe the infant for 4 to 6 months for signs of the disease.

Chicken pox: On exposure administer gamma globulin, 0.1 to 0.2 ml per pound of body weight within 3 days. Zoster immune globulin holds greater promise of effectiveness if given in 10 ml doses.

Measles: If within 6 days of exposure, give gamma globulin, 0.2 to 0.1 ml per pound of body weight. If after 6 days of exposure, increase the dose to 0.2 ml per pound of weight. Live attenuated measles vaccine is contraindicated.

Recognizing the Dangers of Undiagnosed Infections

Alford, Jr.[16] screened umbilical cord blood of 7000 newborns for total and specific immunoglobulins. He found evidence of cytomegalovirus infections in 17, toxoplasmosis in 11, rubella in 8 and syphilis in 6 of these babies; only two cases could be diagnosed clinically.

The high frequency of maternal infections which can damage the fetus is just beginning to be recognized. Sever, Head of Research on perinatal infectious diseases at the Neurological Diseases and Stroke Institute, stated that not only rubella but also cytomegalovirus, Herpesvirus Hominis, toxoplasmosis, tuberculosis, syphilis, gonorrhea, listerosis and malaria are responsible for fetal damage. Others suspected of causing damage are influenza A, mumps, Mycoplasma hominis, Coxsackie B, and hepatitis viruses as well as generalized maternal infections.

Treatment Following Exposure to Rubella

Investigate the mother's degree of exposure, whether brief out-of-home exposure or an intense exposure to one of her own children with rubella. Do not accept the diagnosis of rubella without laboratory confirmation. Do not accept your own previous diagnosis of rubella as proof of immunity when pregnancy is involved.

Table 2-4. Drugs Having Adverse Effects on the Fetus

Maternal Medication		*Fetal or neofetal effect*
Analgesics	Heroin	Neonatal death
	Morphine	
Androgens, estrogens and oral progestogens		Masculinization and advanced bone age
Antianxiety agents	Meprobamate (Equanil, Meprospan, Miltown)	Retarded development
Anticoagulants	Bishydroxycoumarin (Dicumarol) Ethyl biscoumacetate (Tromexan ethyl acetate)	Fetal death; hemorrhage
	Sodium warfarin (coumadin sodium, Panwarfin, Prothromadin)	
Anticonvulsants/sedative-hypnotics	Phenobarbital (Luminal) in excess	Neonatal bleeding; death
Antihistamines		Anomalies; infertility
Antihypertensives	Reserpine	Stuffy nose; respiratory obstruction
Antimalarials	Chloroquine (Aralen) Quinine	Retinal damage; death; thrombocytopenia
Antimicrobials	Chloramphenicol (Chloromycetin)	Grey syndrome; death
	Erythromycin (Erythrocin, Ilosone	Liver damage
	Nitrofurantoin (Furadantin)	Hemolysis
	Novobiocin (Albamycin, Cathomycin)	Hyperbilirubinemia
	Streptomycin	Possible eighth nerve deafness
	Sulfonamides	Kernicterus
	Tetracyclines	Inhibition of bone growth; discoloration of teeth
Antineoplastics	Chlorambucil (Leukeran Methotrexate (Amethopterin) Aminopterin	Anomalies and abortion
Antipsychotics	Phenothiazines	Hyperbilirubinemia
Antithyroid agents	Methimazole (Tapazole) Propylthiouracil Radioactive iodine Thiouracil	Goiter; mental retardation; hypothyroidism
Corticosteroids	Cortisone (Cortogen, Cortone)	Cleft palate
Diuretics	Thiazide diuretics	Thrombocytopenia
Expectorants	Ammonium chloride	Acidosis
	Potassium iodide	Goiter; mental retardation; cyanosis; respiratory distress
Ganglionic blocking agents		Neonatal ileus
Hypoglycemics	Phenformin (DBI)	Lactic acidosis
	Sulfonylurea derivatives	Anomalies
Salicylates		Neonatal bleeding
Thalidomide		Phocomelia; death; hearing loss
Vaccinations	Influenza	Increased anti-A and anti-B titers in mothers
	Smallpox	Fetal vaccinia
Vitamins	Vitamin K analogues in excess	Hyperbilirubinemia

In previous years, obstetricians believed that an unborn child was only harmed if the mother had rubella during the first 3 months of pregnancy. A Johns Hopkins study has noted that there is a considerable number of smaller than average infants born during a year when rubella is epidemic. Post-delivery blood studies of these mothers show that they had rubella in the second 3 months of their pregnancy. The Hopkins study shows that these infants had a reduced number and smaller cells in their muscles. The same study shows other insidious disabilities, i.e. there is a larger number of minimal brain dysfunctional children as well as a generally lower degree of intelligence.

Order HI (hemagglutination-inhibition test for rubella antibodies) to determine presence of antibodies. For proper interpretation the exact dates of exposure and of obtaining blood specimens must be recorded.

If the first HI is positive and has a good titer (significant titers will vary with laboratory technique) and the specimen was obtained within 2 to 3 days after exposure, the patient is probably immune because of a prior active infection.

If the first HI titer is low, the mother is susceptible and may contract the disease, even subclinically, and is at risk. In this event, order a second HI 3 weeks later. If the mother contracted the disease, the titer will have increased.

If this does not clear the diagnosis, order a complement fixation test. Reliance on HI tests alone in diagnosing rubella in pregnant women is inadequate. Goldfield[17] calls attention to the appearance of antibodies extremely early following infection; consequently, if the HI titer is obtained 7 or more days after the onset of the rubellalike eruption, the titer will be of no value. He emphasizes only if the sample is taken in the first 2 days after the rash could 100 percent of cases be diagnosed. As early as the third or fourth day, 18 percent will exhibit maximum antibody titers. By the fifth or sixth day, 58 percent show maximum antibodies. Goldfield suggests that, under these circumstances, complement fixation tests can be used as late as the third week after onset of eruption. Better yet, a combination of the two procedures would permit a fairly reliable diagnosis with one sample drawn early and one late.

The risk of the infant being affected is 20 to 25 percent if rubella has occurred during the first trimester and was confirmed by laboratory tests. Infection during the fourth to eighth week produces the most serious results. Infection after the first trimester can also produce abnormalities but at a lower rate and predictions are more fallible. Consequently, consider the termination of pregnancy if rubella in the mother is subclinical but confirmed by laboratory tests. Advise the type of abortion consistent with the number of weeks pregnant. Every effort should be made to have the abortion done under 10 weeks (See Counseling Regarding Abortions in this Chapter).

Discuss in detail with the patient and record discussion and decision for medicolegal purposes. Explain the odds of a child being born normal are 4:1 or 5:1 and that the odds of continued infant health during the first year are 3:1 or 4:1. Explain the most likely defects. (See rubella syndrome.) Take into account religious and legal problems as well as parents' ages and number of living children. If all cannot agree, it is prudent to follow the mother's wishes.

If the mother refuses abortion, administer 20 ml gamma globulin. This is controversial. It may modify the disease in the mother, but the fetus has about the same chance of malformation after the gamma globulin as before.

If the decision is to allow pregnancy to continue and the baby is born with obvious or suspected rubella syndrome, or even if the infant appears normal, a pediatric consultation is mandatory. Some infants appear normal at birth. Examine the infant periodically and, when 6 to 8 months older, order a HI test. Assume the child has escaped infection if there are no antibodies at that age.

If the fetus has been infected, some infants will shed the virus for as long as 2 years. Warn the parents of this possibility and have them take precautions to avoid contact with any pregnant woman.

When a Pregnant Woman's Child Is Exposed to Rubella

Draw blood specimens immediately from both. If the tests show that the woman or child is immune by virtue of preexisting antibodies, she has nothing to worry about. If neither has antibodies, the woman should be followed carefully.

Since the child was exposed first, his rubella infection can be confirmed earlier with a second specimen drawn at least a week later. Absence of infection in the child should dispel all fears. Finally, if rubella infection is detected in the mother early in pregnancy, the family must be informed of the possible consequence and the alternatives available.

Wearing Seat Belts During Pregnancy

Urge pregnant women to wear seat belts. There is no evidence that seat belts are a hazard to the fetus. Instruct the patient to wear the belt low across the pelvic bones and upper thighs. Have her adjust the buckle to one side. Warn the patient not to stretch the belt over the uterus. Urge her to wear a shoulder belt too.

The Cigarette Smoker

It has been established that cigarette smoking is directly related to low birth-weight babies. Urge young mothers in whom the habit has not been fully developed to stop smoking. If this is not possible, suggest moderation in smoking.

Redouble your efforts to discourage smoking in mothers-to-be who have a history of reproductive failure; are hypertensive or prone to toxemia; or have a history of previous perinatal death, especially if low birth-weight and/or prematurity were involved.

Buncher[18] has reported there is significant evidence that cigarette smoking shortens the gestation time. He reports the difference in gestation of a nonsmoking woman and one smoking one package per day as 1 to 2 days. Further, he claims that 10 percent of reduced birth-weight babies were caused by shortened gestation.

X-Rays During Pregnancy

According to Stewart and Kneale[19] of the University of Oxford, even one x-ray picture taken during pregnancy can significantly increase the risk of a child's developing cancer in the first 10 years of life.

Their figures would indicate a direct relationship between cancer and the number of films exposed. If only one x-ray picture had been taken, the increased cancer risk to the child was 1.26 to 1. If five films had been taken, the increased risk was more than doubled, 2.24 to 1.

The radiation risk is highest during the first trimester of pregnancy. X rays during the first trimester led to more than eightfold increase in childhood cancer. No significant differences were found from radiation during the second and third trimester.

The American Dental Association recommends that women in the reproductive age and children be protected by a lead apron during dental radiography. This precaution is doubly true during pregnancy because the mother may be exposed to scattered radiation.

With these facts in mind, if x-ray films *need to be taken,* shield the patient with a lead apron. Delay elective x-rays, but if something has to be done do it.

Diet and Weight

Controlling the obstetrical patient's weight is an important function of the family physician. With a patient of normal weight and whose control is satisfactory expect the following gain:

First Trimester — no weight gain
Second Trimester — 9 to 10 pounds gain
Third Trimester — 9 to 10 pounds gain

This gain would amount to approximately 3 pounds per month during the second and third trimesters. Weight gained over this is fat or fluid. Physiological weight gain may be accounted for as follows:

Reproductive Weight Gain:	
Fetus	7.5 pounds
Uterus	2.0
Placenta	1.5
Amniotic Fluid	2.0
30% increase in blood volume (1.5 liters)	4.0
Extracellular fluid	2.0
Breasts and other organs including heart	1.0
Normal physiological weight gain	20 pounds

In an ongoing study by the National Institute of Neurological Diseases and Stroke, 56,000 mothers and 40,000 of their children have been observed since 1959. The mother's weight gain during pregnancy emerged as the most important factor in the weight of the infant at birth. Her weight before becoming pregnant was second.

The study appears to demonstrate that 25 to 30 pounds is the optimal weight gain both in terms of perinatal mortality and birth weight.

Flowers, Jr.,[20] asks patients who are gaining excessive weight and have fluid retention to calculate their diet and restrict it to approximately 2 g of sodium per day. He combines this with modified bed rest, including bed rest in the mornings and afternoons. Other obstetricians believe that only patients who have an excessive salt intake should have their salt curtailed.

For the anxious woman who eats excessively and consumes excessive calories, Dr. Flowers suggests a simple caloric calculator. He suggests a weight gain of no more than 22 pounds. Others recommend 18 to 20 pounds. He gives the woman a sheet listing salt and calorie content of the usual foods (see table in Appendix) and suggests she keep the tables where they can be seen easily and frequently. He advises the planning of menus in advance, giving concern to the total calories and sodium content, and urging that food choices be low in both. (In his chart one salt unit equals 50 mg of sodium; therefore sodium units should be kept between 40 and 80 units.)

Dr. Flowers believes the patient gives more concern to her diet if the doctor is careful to explain all features of the diet; consequently, he reads over with her a typical day's diet (see Appendix) and attempts to individualize the diet, taking into account the patient's cultural and family nutrition patterns.

General dietary suggestions should include the following:

Diet high in protein, low in sugars and starches.

Drink no more than one pint of milk per day because of the high phosphate content of milk. It is better to supplement with calcium in gluconate form or a Vitamin D and calcium preparation (Spar-Cal by Mead Johnson Laboratories). Each tablet of Spar-Cal contains 500 mg of elemental calcium and 200 USP units of vitamin D which will dissolve in six ounces of water. One half of the fetal calcium (25 g) is deposited in the last month of pregnancy. If the mother ingests 1.5 g daily during pregnancy, she will store more calcium than needed except during the last month. During the last month, the fetus absorbs more than two times as much as the mother can absorb. The Food and Nutrition Board of National Research Council recommends 2 g of calcium per day in the mother's diet. Most obstetricians recommend 1.5 g per day.

A full vitamin preparation daily and iron supplementation as suggested earlier.

Liver once a week and extra fruits and vegetables.

On occasion Flowers asks the patient to write down all foods eaten for 5 days and to calculate the calorie and sodium content. Many times this review is all that is necessary to stop a runaway gain.

The National Society for Medical Research warns that evidence is accumulating that pre- and post-natal malnutrition may inhibit division of cells in the growing brain, a conditions directly related to mental retardation.

Recognizing and Treating Bacteriuria[21]

Researchers have established the occurrence of fairly constant anatomical changes in the urinary system of the pregnant woman. These are: (1) dilation of the pelvis and calyces of one or both kidneys; (2) a dilatation, tortuosity and kinking of one or both ureters; and (3) a lateral displacement of these structures. Every pregnant woman shows some of these changes—marked hydronephrosis as a maximum and hydroureter as a minimum. Following delivery there is a return of the urinary system to normal in about a month.

Chronic pyelonephritis in pregnancy is a common cause of hypertension and a significant cause of perinatal mortality and morbidity often associated with prematurity and toxemia of pregnancy. Because asymptomatic bacteriuria in pregnancy leads to pyelonephritis, the best prevention of the disability would be to find and treat asymptomatic patients.

The incidence of asymptomatic bacteriuria in pregnancy varies from 3 to 10 percent. To diagnose, examine all clean-voided urine specimens microscopically for (1) bacteria in a gram-stained sediment of uncentrifuged urine and (2) white blood cells in a drop of unspun urine under the high-power objective. Most clinicians find a high correlation between the more expensive quantitative colony count exceeding 100,000 per ml and the finding of bacteriuria in the gram-stained urinary sediment or one or two white blood cells per high power field of unspun urine, or both.

If there is doubt, order a cultured quantitative colony count. A colony count greater than 100,000 per ml either in a single specimen of urine obtained by catheterization or in each of two consecutive clean-voided specimen makes the diagnosis of urinary tract infection 95 percent certain.

Asymptomatic and symptomatic bacteriuria should be treated by a 10-to 14-day course of ampicillin or possibly with a short-acting sulfonomide derivative. In both cases, do a careful follow-up. On recurrence, give another 2-week course before resorting to continuous suppressive therapy. In all symptomatic cases, order urine protein, white blood cells casts and urea nitrogen or serum creatinine.

In patients with chronic pyelonephritis administer continuous suppressive therapy with ampicillin or with a short-acting sulfonomide in low dosage.

Obviously, many times it becomes necessary to prescribe other antibiotics, even the nephrotoxic ones such as kanamycin, polymyxin B and gentamicin. Remember nephrotoxicity is usually dose related. Antibiotics may be used in lower dosages if the urine is alkalinized. With the advent of potent antibiotics, alkalinization of the urine has been neglected.

Where possible, avoid intravenous pyelography during pregnancy. Diagnose chronic pyelonephritis by the following: (1) increased proteinuria to between 200 and 1500 mg largely globulin; (2) serum electrolytes may show a hyperchloremic acidosis in mildly azotemic patients; (3) persistent failure to concentrate the urine after 12 hours without fluids.

Because the urinary system is susceptible to infection in the parturient woman, refrain from routine catheterization in the post-delivery phase.

The handicap in all this is the expense, particularly when cultures are involved. Several commercially prepared office tests are available for mass screening of asymptomatic patients. These tests are not advocated in symptomatic patients or in those suspected of having a urinary infection.

Filter paper test: This test may be somewhat more desirable than the dye tests. Simply dip standard filter paper in urine and place on a small plastic disk containing a nutrient agar. Two or less colonies is read as negative; three or more colonies as positive.

Glucose oxidase method: The multiplication of organisms in the urine uses up the small amount of glucose in urine which is not easily detected by usual methods. By using the glucose oxidase method any glycosuria which indicates the absence of bacilluria is detected.

Griess nitrite test: Bacteria reduce nitrates to nitrites indicated by a pink to red color.

Minicultures are available commercially and are less expensive than the regular culture and colony counts.

Plastic dip-slide method: (Dip-slide method of Guttmann and Taylor varies in technique.) Two slides are used. One slide is covered with a nutrient agar that supports common organisms. The other slide is covered with a nutrient that only supports gram-negative organisms. Slides are dipped into the urine, incubated 12 to 24 hours and read. These tests are precise and simple and perhaps the most useful.

TTC (Triphenyltetrazolium chloride): In presence of gram-negative organisms, TTC is reduced to triphenylformazan. The dye of TTC salt is used to indicate the presence of bacterial dehydrogenase activity. This test is not 100 percent accurate and cannot be used effectively if the patient has been treated with an antibiotic. Test is best in detecting E. Coli; with other organisms it may not be any more than 60 percent accurate.

None of these tests is very accurate, but one may be used as a screening test on asymptomatic pregnant women.

Complications

Spontaneous Abortion

The cause of spontaneous abortion varies with the stages of pregnancy:

- –first eight weeks: defective germ plasma
- –at twelfth week: impacted retroverted gravid uterus or progesterone deficiency
- –from fourteenth to twentieth week: incompetent internal os or occasionally a bicornuate uterus. Promp treatment (Shirodkar procedure) may save the pregnancy

Abortion usually refers to the loss of a fetus during the first 20 weeks of pregnancy or when the weight of the lost fetus is less than 500 g. Abortion usually begins with bleeding from the uterus and low abdominal pain. Another sign of impending danger is excessive Braxton-Hicks pains after 15 weeks as a result of an incompetent cervical os.

A rapid course usually follows an abrupt placental separation and the fetus dies from asphyxia or trauma. In this case, a D. and C. is not always necessary. A much slower course occurs when metabolic, genetic, enzymatic or hormonal factors are involved; in this situation, a D. and C. usually is necessary. Cervical incompetence may lead to increasing vaginal pressure without bleeding until the amniotic sac ruptures and the conceptus is lost.

Pregnancy tests remain positive 5 to 7 days after abortion. Watch for sepsis (See Septic Shock)

Vaginal cytology has a greater overall value in the prognosis of threatened abortion than does HCG immunoassay. Take vaginal smears before and after intramuscular injections of 5 mg of estradiol dipropionate (Ovocylin) for 3 consecutive days. If the pre-estrogen and postestrogen smears are good a successful outlook may be predicted. If the postestrogen smear is bad, even if the pre-estrogen smear is good, abortion is likely.

The HCG test is of definite prognostic value only when it is initially negative or becomes negative when repeated. In this instance spontaneous abortion occurs regularly. But if you are only requesting one test, do vaginal cytology.

Habitual Abortion

Habitual abortion is defined as the occurrence of at least three consecutive spontaneous abortions with no interposed viable pregnancy. The causes are divided into nine main groups: anomalies and tumors of the uterus; cervical incompetence; pathologic conceptus; vascular disorders; improper placentation; relative thyroid deficiency; abnormal gonadotropin, estrogen and progesterone metabolism; psychogenic factors; and miscellaneous (nutritional deficiencies, lues, chronic diseases).

Obstetricians have not standardized the treatment of habitual abortion. Treatment varies from simple bed rest to a variety of hormonal and vitamin medications. Attempt to diagnose the cause and then focus treatment on preventing the abortion.

Besides the usual clinical investigation, order such special tests and procedures as the petechial test for capillary fragility, a

PBI, cholesterol determination, hysterosalpingography, endometrial biopsy and examination of the husband's semen.

Ectopic Pregnancy

The symptoms of an ectopic pregnancy usually occur before the diagnosis of pregnancy has been verified. Consequently, be alert to the possibility of an ectopic pregnancy in a woman of childbearing age who develops lower quadrant pain or whenever there is a change in menstrual habits. Ectopic pregnancy does not depend upon a period of amenorrhea for diagnosis. Biologic and immunologic tests for pregnancy are positive in 50 to 60 percent of cases.

Common differential diagnosis: appendicitis, pelvic inflammatory disease, twisted ovarian cyst, pyelonephritis of pregnancy, and threatened or incomplete abortion.

One of the most difficult differential diagnosis is that of ectopic pregnancy versus pelvic inflammatory disease (PID). An important point in the differential is the fact that pain is unilateral (the tenderness and possibly the tubal mass of an ectopic pregnancy). The pain of an ectopic pregnancy (stabbing or cramplike) is seldom related to the menstrual cycle, while in PID the pain is coincident with the period. A fullness and tenderness in the cul-de-sac is significant. Blood pressure, pulse and hemoglobin are more likely to indicate shock in ectopic pregnancy. The leukocytosis of PID may be 15,000 or more.

Culdocentesis is a simple and valuable diagnostic procedure and should be done on nearly every patient suspected of having an ectopic pregnancy. Demerol is given to induce analgesia. Use a No. 17 needle attached to a 10 cc syringe to perform the culdocentesis. The withdrawal of nonclotting blood is characteristic of intraperitoneal bleeding; clotting indicates a traumatic tap. Posterior colpotomy and culdoscopy require more training than the usual family physician has received. Culdocentesis does not always solve the differential diagnosis.

The simple, most important aid in diagnosis of ectopic pregnancy is to keep its possibility in mind. If diagnosis is not clear, hospitalize the patient and, if necessary, request a colpotomy or culdoscopy. There should be no period of expectant observation; diagnose promptly.

Schedule for surgery once the diagnosis is made. Salpingectomy is the procedure of choice. There has been some argument as to whether the ovary on the ipsilateral side should be removed along with the tube to prevent future cystic degeneration of the ovary. But most authorities believe in a conservative approach, thinking that in ruptured or unruptured ectopic gestation the tube can be removed without compromising the circulation to the ovary.

If the ectopic pregnancy is located near the fimbriated end of the tube, attempt to express the products of conception manually from the tube, gently curet the area of implantation and preserve the entire tube.

If the pregnancy is implanted in the middle or inner one third of the tube, it is sometimes possible to incise the tube in a linear fashion directly over the implantation, excise the ectopic pregnancy and close the incision with fine suture material. Usually, however, it is not possible to save the tube.

Remember that following an ectopic pregnancy, the patient has a 50 percent chance of a subsequent pregnancy, a 30 percent chance of a successful term pregnancy and an 11 percent chance of a second ectopic pregnancy.

Heart Disease

During the second month of pregnancy there is an increase in cardiac output and some retention of sodium and water. These changes may result in a tachycardia with warm and flushed extremities. There may be some ankle edema which must also be differentiated from toxemia.

The cardiac apex beat may become more forcible and displaced to the left. The jugular venous pressure is slightly raised. The increased cardiac flow produces pulmonary and aortic systolic murmurs. A physiologic third sound is not uncommon because of rapid ventricular filling. Keep all these physiologic changes in mind before diagnosing heart disease during pregnancy.

With proven heart disease the following rules may prove helpful in recommending a continuation of pregnancy: Patients with no symptoms nor evidence of cardiac enlargement will usually go through pregnancy without trouble. Patients who have had heart failure or who have severe effort intolerance should be advised against pregnancy; if they have already conceived, the pregnancy should be terminated in the first three months. The group between these extremes presents difficulty in prognosis; cases in this group must be judged on their own merits.

Management during pregnancy: Observe closely. If dyspneic, full nights rest with afternoon naps. If failure develops, treat in the usual way. First evidence of failure is pulmonary congestion with rales. Confirm with x-ray studies. Filling of neck veins and edema may or may not be physiological.

Management during labor: Try normal delivery with forceps assist at earliest time. Do cesarean section to prevent rupture in coarctation of aorta.

Diabetes Mellitus

Diabetic women are less fertile, more likely to miscarriage, and more subject to toxemia of pregnancy and hydramnios than their healthy sisters.

Diabetes may be unmasked for the first time or become more severe during pregnancy. Insulin requirements increase during first trimester, level off during the second, and may increase or decrease during the third trimester. After delivery, watch the patient carefully for insulin-induced hypoglycemia. Breast feeding nearly always fails.

Sutherland and coworkers[22] offer a tip on which women should have a glucose tolerance test (GTT). The frequency with which women have glycosuria during pregnancy nearly precludes checking them all with a GTT. They suggest that GTT is more fruitful if it is done on all women who have glycosuria on a second fasting morning specimen. The suggested technique: check a fasting morning urine specimen for sugar; if it is positive, discard the entire overnight specimen and check the second fasting urine specimen. One sixth of the women with a positive second fasting urine had chemical or subclinical diabetes. None of those with only positive random glycosuria had an abnormal GTT.

In presence of diabetes or a positive family history of diabetes, 4 to 7 percent of the women had chemical diabetes whether glycosuria was noted on a random urine specimen or not. If glycosuria was present on a second fasting sample and there was obesity or a positive family history 17 percent had chemical diabetes.

Maternal mortality in diabetes mellitus has declined in the last 25 years, but fetal mortality remains at about 20 percent. Babies of diabetic mothers are prone to dying in utero, overweight, congenital malformations and death shortly before or after birth.

Maillard and associates[23] studied 79 newborn infants of diabetic mothers with the following findings: 19 had no problems; 14 had clinical signs of respiratory distress; 12 had convulsions; and 6 heart failure. The main laboratory findings were acidosis, serum bilirubin higher than 120 mg/L, and serum potassium higher than 6 mg/L. Eleven babies died of hyaline membrane disease or congenital abnormalities.

Because of the dangers of intrauterine death, consider the termination of the pregnancy either by induction or cesarean section at 36 weeks. This is a problem for a specialist.

Acute Appendicitis

The tenderness of appendicitis is usually a little higher in the abdomen of a pregnant woman and the course of the disease is more rapid. An appendectomy should be performed as early as the diagnosis is probable. The peritonitis of a ruptured appendix in pregnancy is more virulent and more difficult to handle than in the nonpregnant patient. Pregnant patients tolerate an appendectomy well unless the appendix has ruptured.

THE THIRD TRIMESTER

Lamaze Training

Lamaze training is 6 weeks of training sessions for the patient and her husband taken during the last 2 months of pregnancy. When the husband is certificated by Lamaze inst. uctors, many hospitals will allow him to be present at the delivery providing the doctor in attendance agrees.

Part of the Lamaze method is conditioning the mother, helping her develop breathing and relaxation responses that will function automatically during each stage of labor. The father has an active part to play in the delivery of his child by checking his wife's neuromuscular control and guiding her breathing.

Fetal Maturity

As indicated early in this chapter, a combination of an accurate determination of the first day of the last menstrual period combined with the dates of beginning fetal heart sound with the fetascope and fetal movement can give excellent prognostic data regarding fetal maturity.

As often happens, one or two of the above dates may be missing or inaccurate. In cases in which fetal maturity should be determined with accuracy there are two other measures available: (1) Ultrasound measurement of the biparietal diameter of the fetal head (91 percent of infants will weight 2500 g or more if this measures 8.5 cm or more) and (2) Creatinine level determination of the amniotic fluid (100 percent of cases will be 37 or more gestational weeks if this level is 1.8 mg percent or more). Rarely is it necessary to induce labor for postmaturity or postdatism.

Vaginal Bleeding

Placenta Previa

The placenta may be implanted completely or partially across the cervix. Bleeding usually is painless and comes in bright red gushes.

The prognosis for both mother and fetus has been improved by accurate localization of the placenta when time, fetal viability and circumstances permit. The most frequently used diagnostic techniques are soft-tissue radiography and radioisotopes. Other techniques sometimes tried are:

- –Arteriography: Equipment is expensive and available only at large medical centers.
- –Doppler's Technique: Uses the sonar principle and has a rather large margin of error (30 to 40 percent). Because of its availability, however, the technique may be used when there is active bleeding and the patient is in labor.
- –Ultrasound.
- –Amniography: Transabdominal injection of a radiopaque medium into amniotic sac. When the dye does not appear below the presenting vertex the test indicates a placenta previa. The test tends to cause uterine irritability and may start labor, an undesirable side effect.
- –Thermography.

Soft-tissue radiography will locate the placental implantation as anterior or posterior and in the lower or upper poles of the uterus. If there is still doubt, combine radiography with a cystogram. With a cystogram, if the presenting part and bladder are more than 1 cm apart, the radiogram is interpreted as indicating placenta previa. With these combined techniques placental localization is 98 percent accurate.

Radioisotope technique using I^{131}-labeled serum albumin (RISA) in 3 to 5 mc doses is preferred by many. The accuracy is similar to radiography but the mother and fetus receive only about 1/100 the number of rads. I^{132} causes even less exposure to the fetus than I.^{131} Tc^{99m} offers speed. Diagnosis can be made within 15 minutes, but material must be produced daily because of short half-life.

The most important point in making the diagnoses by these localization techniques is verifying the cause of the bleeding, but these techniques also aid in selecting the appropriate method of delivery. With this type of information, about a third of the patients with placenta previa respond to conservative management and the physician is able to prolong the gestation period.

At the onset of labor or at 37 weeks of gestation (whichever occurs first), each patient should be prepared for abdominal surgery and given a vaginal examination using the double setup technique. The patient's blood should be crossmatched and units reserved. The patient who has had excessive bleeding (more than 500 ml in a single episode) and is judged to be in labor is delivered by cesarean section. Whenever the placental mass appears to be in a position to cause dystocia and creates doubt as to feasible vaginal delivery (even in partial placenta previa) a cesarean delivery should be carried out. It must be remembered that the incidence of abnormal presentation is increased significantly in placenta previa. Approximately half the cases of placenta previa will benefit from this expectant management.

Abruptio Placentae

Abruptio placentae is a premature separation of the placenta. The cause is unknown but separation is more frequent in the anemic, hypertensive or eclamptic patients.

The condition usually starts with severe abdominal pain with or without low backache. This is followed shortly by vaginal bleeding. The uterus may be tender or it may be irritable, boardlike and enlarging. Palpating the fetus is nearly impossible. Fetal heart tones may indicate distress. Symptoms and findings vary in intensity depending on how extensive the separation has been.

If the fetus is premature and the bleeding is painless a study should be made to rule out placenta previa.

In suspected cases do the following:

Type blood, crossmatch and reserve at least 3 units of blood. Do a complete blood count, a plasma fibrinogen determination and observe clot formation and lysis.

Start two intravenous infusions: one arm to be used for CVP monitoring and infusion of Ringer's lactate. In other arm, place a 16 gauge plastic intravenous cannula for more Ringer's and blood when needed. Blood loss may be massive and can be monitored by CVP.

Order vital signs including pulse, blood pressure, central venous pressure and fetal heart rate every 5 minutes.

Place a Foley catheter and check the hourly urine output. Observe the patient for uterine tetany, fetal bradycardia, vaginal bleeding and the progress of cervical dilatation.

For a definitive diagnosis and treatment, prepare the patient for surgery using double setup technique. Examine the patient vaginally. Have anesthesia ready, operative pack opened and blood available.

If the cervix is open, do an amniotomy after exclusion of placenta previa. Supplement amniotomy with administration of an oxytocin. These two measures will decrease intra-amniotic tension and reduce extravasation of blood into myometrium.

Many times this conservative approach will cause a prompt vaginal delivery of the infant. If the delivery is not prompt or the cervix remains undilated, do a cesarean section promptly.

How to Delay a Premature Labor

A four-year experimental program at Cornell Medical College[24] pioneered in the use of alcohol infusion to delay premature labor. The technique is not generally accepted, but it may prove useful in certain cases.

The technique is not recommended for patients with ruptured membranes or a cervical dilatation of more than 5 cm or who are alcoholics or have damaged livers. The attendent must first determine whether the mother is in labor or whether she is having false labor pains. Determine this by putting the mother to bed for an hour or two and observing her labor.

The infusion fluid is 100 ml of sterile 95 percent (v/v) ethanol mixed with 900 ml of 5 percent dextrose and water to get 1000 ml of a 9.5 percent alcohol solution. This will contain 75.4 g of alcohol per liter. The Cornell group then proceeds as follows: a loading dose of 7.5 ml/kg of body weight per hour for 2 hours is given, and then reduced to a maintenance dose of 1.5 ml/kg per hour for 10 hours or more. This produces a blood alcohol concentration of 0.12 and 0.16 percent. Larger doses cause nausea and vomiting.

If contractions continue and become stronger after 2 hours of the infusion, the alcohol regime should be discontinued. Patients do not get drunk on intravenous alcohol; it seems to cause sedation and even depression.

Inducing Labor

The safest procedure for induction of labor at term is an intravenous drip consisting of 10 units of a oxytocin in 1000 ml of 5 percent dextrose. Adjust the rate of administration to 8 or 10 drops per minute until uterine response is observed. Initiation of rhythmic contractions with intervals of relaxation should follow in a short time. The frequency of contractions, their duration and the absence of fetal distress will determine the speed with which the drip is increased. Always use the pure oxytocic principle of natural or synthetic posterior pituitary.

Ideally a physician should be in attendance; at least he should be readily available while a competent person is observing the patient.

Do not use intramuscular sparteine sulfate or oxytocics because control of absorption is poor and continued absorption cannot be prevented if withdrawal is indicated.

Some physicians prefer Buccal Syntocinon. After the first dose of Buccal Syntocinon observe the patient every half hour for sensitivity to the drug. Increased doses are administered at half-hour intervals, and a full course is spread over 5 hours. If needed, give a second course after not less than 4 hours. Once uterine action is established, maintain the dose at the level of the previous administration. If contractions become too intensive, stop the medication and wash out the tablet fragments in the mouth with water.

Either procedure is more effective if preceded by artificial rupture of the membranes.

The use of sparteine sulfate for induction and stimulation has been praised and condemned. Studies show, however, there is no way to predict an individual patient's response to the drug. Sensitivity to sparteine sulfate varies from patient to patient. Any patient receiving sparteine sulfate for induction of labor must be under constant supervision. Smaller test doses are recommended, 75 to 100 mg rather than 150 mg intramuscularly.

The most recently proposed labor inducing drug is prostaglandin E_2. It does not appear to induce labor near term with any greater efficiency than does oxytocin (Syntocinon). About 75 percent of patients who receive these drugs will have delivered or reached 6 cm of dilatation within 12 hours of the start of the infusion.

Premature Rupture of Bag of Water

There have been few strict rules regarding the treatment of premature rupture of the bag of waters. Most obstetricians and family physicians have followed a laissez faire approach to the problem. Perhaps obstetricians can take a lighter approach, but Salzmann[25] of the New Jersey College of Medicine recommends the following, which would seem a wise course for family physicians to observe.

Admit the patient to the hospital for bed rest as soon as possible following the rupture. Determine the fetal position by clinical examinations and radiography.

Make only one vaginal examination and do it under sterile conditions. In addition to determining the cervical effacement and dilatation take a cervical bacteria culture.

What is done at this point depends on the findings of the vaginal examination. If the cervix is effaced and dilated one fingertip or more, start intravenous oxytocin (Pitocin) using 2 to 5 units in each 1000 ml of IV fluid. Do a cesarean section if labor is not established within 24 hours with oxytocin induction. If infection starts during the 24-hour oxytocin test, wait no more than 4 hours before doing the cesarean section.

If on the other hand the vaginal examination does not reveal any cervical effacement and dilatation, continue the patient on bed rest. As the risk of infection is proportional to the number of vaginal and rectal examinations, prohibit these checks until active labor starts.

The Salzmann regime demands that oral temperature be taken every 4 hours. If the temperature rises above 100° F, start oxytocin. After the temperature begins and induction fails, wait no longer than 4 hours before doing the cesarean section. If the patient comes to the hospital with fever, attempt induction for no longer than 4 hours before doing the cesarean section.

General Principles of Eclampsia Control

Early detection and treatment of mounting diastolic blood pressure, increasing proteinuria, edema or weight gain may prevent the development of eclampsia. Treatment of these early symptoms revolves around diet, sodium restriction and bed rest. A family physician may attempt to treat a *mild* eclampsia medically for no longer than 5 days. If signs and symptoms do not improve a consultation is in order.

The general principles in treatment of eclampsia have not changed in several years. They are:

Control of the initial convulsive episode by intravenous short-acting barbiturates and of central nervous system irritability by magnesium sulfate. This can be done by giving two of the following, preferably the first two:

Amobarbital (Sodium Amytal): 0.25 to 0.5 g (4 to 7½ gr) subcutaneously every 4 to 8 hr.

Magnesium sulfate 50 percent solution: 12.0 ml intramuscularly; then 6.0 ml after each convulsion. Maximum dose: 40 ml in 24 hr.

Chloral hydrate: 3.0 g (45 gr) in 100 ml of starch water administered rectally every 12 hr.

Morphine sulfate (least desirable): ¼ gr (16 mg) intravenously repeated until convulsions cease or respiration drops to 12 per minute.

Administration of an antihypertensive agent if the diastolic blood pressure exceeds 100 mm of Hg. Administer an intravenous drip with 20.0 mg hydralazine hydrochloride (Apresoline) and 5.0 mg of cryptenamine acetate (Unitensen Tannate) in 500 ml of 20 percent glucose. Start the drip with 15 drops per minute and adjust flow as needed to control the blood pressure. This may be continued 24 hr or until the hypertensive crisis is over.

Establish diuresis and control electrolytes. Diuresis may be established by using a chlorothiazide or hypertonic glucose. Many prefer the use of glucose. Administer one L of a 20 percent hypertonic glucose intravenously in 40 minutes. If necessary repeat in 8 hr and as long as there is a net loss of water and the concentration of electrolytes are not below normal range. *Do not overhydrate.* If you choose to use chlorothiazide for diuresis, order serial serum electrolytes and administer potassium. Give the chlorothiazide intramuscularly or intravenously. It is more effective if plasma volume is kept up by the use of hypertonic glucose or hypertonic mannitol. Use plasma albumin but remember it is expensive. Attempt to keep urinary output above 700 ml per 24 hr.

General supportive measures: Constant observation of the patient in room with dampened extraneous stimuli; retention catheter with urinary output checked every 2 hr; oxygen for cyanosis; mouth gag and suction; intubation or tracheostomy as needed. If acute asphyxia develops from a prolonged seizure, give intravenous thiopental sodium (Pentothal Sodium) until controlled. Order artificial respiration 1 to 2 hr.

Delivery of the patient within 24 hr after control of convulsions. If in labor stimulate contractions by rupturing the bag of waters. If not in labor within 8 to 10 hr after convulsions are controlled and diuresis established, or if it appears that vaginal delivery can not be accomplished within 18 to 24 hr, perform a cesarean section. Section is indicated if cervix is not dilated, induction fails, there is uterine inertia in spite of stimulation or there is obstetrical indication for abdominal delivery.

Severe eclampsia is indicated by:

- –a deepening or persistent coma
- –temperature of 102.2° F or more
- –a pulse rate over 120
- –a respiratory rate of 40 or more
- –more than ten convulsions
- –cardiovascular impairment indicated by pulmonary edema, cyanosis or falling pressure

Prolapsed Umbilical Cord

In about 0.6 percent of obstetrical patients, particularly in those with an abnormal presentation, the umbilical cord will prolapse. Do frequent examinations in breech or transverse presentations, especially after the membranes rupture. If a prolapsed cord is found and it is pulsating, place the mother in a deep Trendelenburg or knee-chest position and hold the baby's presenting part back. If the gestational age of the baby is adequate for survival, do an immediate cesarean section unless the cervix is dilated enough for an immediate vaginal delivery.

Fetal Heart Monitoring

Fetal heart monitoring is still in the experimental stage. Monitoring is a valuable aid for teaching the physiology of labor and its effect on the fetal heart rate, but as a technique to be used in routine labor room practice it is not recommended. If monitoring is available use it in high risk cases and as an aid in delivering premature infants.

Principles of Analgesia and Anesthesia

The ideal method of inducing obstetric anesthesia remains to be discovered.

The most popular drugs for analgesia during labor are secobarbital (Seconal), administered by injection or taken by mouth, combined with meperidine (Demerol) and an amnesic agent, usually scopolamine. Demerol and scopolamine seem to be less depressing to the infant than other agents.

These agents can be given simultaneously or the physician may start with half doses or by administering one at a time and observing the effects. Take care not to give the medication too close to the actual delivery. Remember these drugs pass through the placenta into the blood and tissue of the fetus.

Other less popular methods of analgesia are the intermittent self administration of certain anesthetics in low concentration under supervision of a trained observer. The common ones in use are nitrous oxide, trichloroethylene (Triline) and methoxyflurane (Penthrane).

During a contraction the patient breathes the analgesia from an inhaler. Use the Duke inhaler for Triline as well as Penthrane. The Analgizer is recommended for Penthrane alone.

Remember the concentration of gas varies with the temperature of the room, the patient's tidal exchange, the interval between inhalations, and even the warmth of the patient's hand on the inhaler.

Probably the best inhalation agent for anesthesia during delivery is cyclopropane. Its one drawback is its flammability. Otherwise it is rapid-acting, labile, and potent enough to produce the depth of anesthesia required for suturing an episiotomy. Cyclopropane is ideal following the Seconal-Demerol-Scopalamine analgesia.

Many of the new agents that are being used in surgery such as methoxyflurane, fluroxene and halothane have not replaced older agents in obstetrical anesthesia such as nitrous oxide and cyclopropane.

The newborn is narcotized by drugs in the same manner as an adult. The degree of depression is dose-dependent and varies with the potency and solubility of the drugs.

Regional Techniques

Both the older and newer drugs penetrate the placental barrier. The amount of anesthesia in the fetal blood is about 30 percent less than that in the maternal blood. The older drugs are procaine, tetracaine, chloroprocaine and piperocaine and the newer ones are lidocaine (Xylocaine), mepivacaine (Carbocaine) and prilocaine (Citanest). The newborn infant appears to metabolize lidocaine at approximately the same rate as the mother does with peak levels reached within 30 to 40 minutes following injection.

Procaine appears to be less toxic than lidocaine to the mother as well as to the fetus.

Spinal anesthesia or the saddle block (low spinal) is a satisfactory terminal anesthesia for vaginal delivery or for a cesarean section. Procaine may be used. Some anesthesiologists are using 50 mg of lidocaine in dextrose.

Caudal block by a single injection or the continuous technique is satisfactory if performed by one familiar with the method. Systemic reactions may occur in both mother and infant because the amount of drug used is many times that given for spinal or saddle block. Hypertension is as liable to occur as with saddle block.

Pudendal and paracervical block has few advantages because of the excessive amounts of drug needed and nonexpert placement of the drug.

Actually in some centers paracervical nerve block is being used less and less because of the toxic effects of the long-acting nonamide anesthetic agents. There is a definite risk to the infant whenever prilocaine (Citanest), lidocaine (Xylocaine), mepivacaine (Carbocaine) and others are used. The precautions in their use are:

–use no more than 10 ml of 1 to 1.5 percent in each side.
–do not give if delivery is expected within an hour; wait for metabolization.
–inject one side and wait 10 minutes before injecting the other side. In the meantime, observe the fetal heart rate for bradycardia.
–use only on normal obstetrical cases.

It is surprising how many mothers are quite satisfied with the local infiltration of 10 ml procaine in and around the site of the proposed episiotomy. Multiparas and others who want little or no anesthetic are particularly good candidates.

For breech deliveries: Cyclopropane. If more relaxation is needed, give halothane or ether.

For prolapse of cord: Cyclopropane has no equal.

For cesarean section: Cyclopropane or spinal. If cyclopropane cannot be given, administer nitrous oxide with ether or halothane. Occasionally in poor risk mothers use only a local anesthesia.

For prematurity: Use as little anesthesia or analgesia as possible.

Normal Descent of Presenting Part

Protracted descent of the presenting part may be defined as a rate of descent of less than 1.0 cm/hr in primiparas and 2.0 cm/hr in multiparas. Common cause for protracted descent are cephalopelvic disproportion, minor or major malpositions, excessive sedation and cervical dystocia.

Conservative expectancy and support results in better perinatal outcome than does uterine stimulation. Infants delivered by midforceps fare poorest, and results of midforceps used in cephalopelvic disproportion are even worse.

Trial of Forceps

Trial of forceps usually means that the physician attempts vaginal delivery with the realization that a certain degree of midplane or outlet disproportion may make this incompatible with a safe outcome for the infant. If modest efforts at vaginal delivery fail and midpelvic disproportion becomes more apparent, consider a cesarean section.

If patients are properly evaluated before delivery, a trial of forceps should seldom be necessary. Appraise contraction pattern, fetal size, fetal position and the internal pelvis and its relationship to the presenting part. If still undecided as to whether disproportion exists, order a lateral pelvic x-ray. Fetal mortality has been set at 25 percent where delivery was undertaken when the presenting part was at the level of the ischial spine.[27] Unless a family physician has had considerable training, midforceps extraction is best left to the specialist. Statistics show a cesarean section to be far safer for mother and baby. Trial of forceps is not to be confused with outlet or prophylactic forceps.

Reason for failure of forceps: (1) the physician is misled by marked molding and caput formation leading him to believe there has been cephalic descent; (2) premature attempts at vaginal delivery by an impatient physician or before the head is engaged or cervix dilated properly; (3) midpelvic arrest involving persistent occiput transverse or posterior positions wherein delivery could be easily accomplished after rotation of head to a proper anterior position; or (4) midpelvic disproportion.

Trial of forceps, however, is good obstetrics if properly done in selected cases when labor is weak and with the presenting part below the level of the ischial spine.

Episiotomy

Median episiotomy has the following advantages over a mediolateral incision:

- –median raphe is more easily repaired
- –elective perineorrhaphies may be done when indicated
- –less ragged lacerations if extension of incision does occur
- –less postpartum pain
- –less trauma to incision as patient moves about

The main criticism of median episiotomy is that a laceration might occur into and through the sphincter ani and rectum. For an inexperienced accoucheur, however, a mediolateral episiotomy has the advantage of extending the episiotomy to suit the need without the fear of an extension into rectum. The repair of the sphincter and anus takes more skill to repair if an extensive laceration occurs.

Prophylactic Forceps

Mines[28] believes that the proper use of prophylactic or outlet forceps on a virtually routine basis could sharply reduce all head injuries during the birth process. He thinks of forceps as a sort of a helmet that can protect the baby's fragile head as it descends through the birth canal.

Mines points out that damage is produced both by improper use and by nonuse of forceps. As to proper use, he says excessive compression is the chief hazard of using forceps but, since pressure is directly proportional to the amount of traction, the doctor can minimize this danger by pulling gently. He suggests that no more force than that necessary to flex the forearm be used, never bracing the feet or moving the mother.

His other suggestion is that the doctor lift the blades of the forceps after application so that the locking point of the forceps is directly over the midpoint of the posterior fontanel. Locked in this position, the blades will press directly on the bony base of the skull and cause little stress on the compressible cranium.

The purpose of outlet forceps is to aid the natural forces of labor, in which the back of the head slides under the pubic arch by internal rotation and is then pushed out by muscle action. The physician with the aid of the forceps must mimic this mechanism.

Shoulder Dystocia

It is frustrating to the inexperienced accoucheur to discover that after delivering an infant's head he is unable to complete the delivery because of shoulder dystocia.

Shoulder dystocia occurs when the anterior shoulder overrides the pubic symphysis and the posterior shoulder becomes wedged at the level of the sacral promontory. This is likely to occur if normal labor has been interfered with too early by an impatient doctor. Usually the infant is large, which complicates the situation. Obviously the physician must act promptly.

The following suggestions, given by Hibbard,[29] seem less hazardous than other methods for a family physician. Perform an exceptionally large episiotomy or extend a small episiotomy. After the head is delivered and is lying transverse, use it for manipulating the forces of labor. Place the flat of the hand on the anterior side of the presenting head with the index and middle finger straddling the infant's neck. While holding the infant's head in this position, push the jaw and neck downward towards the mother's anus. At the same time have an assistant make fundal pressure, increasing the pressure as the shoulder seems to give. Continue strong fundal pressure and and jaw and neck pressure. Fundal pressure finally results in an upward-inward rotation of the shoulder on the clavicular pivot, allowing more room and establishing the anterior shoulder under the pubis. At this point downward pressure on the infant's jaw and neck should be released. Delivery is now completed by lifting the infant's head (actually lateral flexion of head because head is transverse) and with fundal pressure the posterior shoulder descends into the hollow of the sacrum.

Principles of Breech Delivery

Determine three important points promptly: the size of the pelvis, the size of the baby and the type of breech presentation. To determine the size of the pelvis, order x-ray pelvimetry. Pelvic adequacy could be expected if the anteroposterior diameter of the inlet is more than 10.0 cm or the transverse diameter of the midpelvis is more than 9.5 cm. Clinical and x-ray examinations will help to determine fetal size and confirm the type of breech presentation.

If there is reasonable doubt of the adequacy of the pelvis, do a cesarean section since there is no time for a trial of labor. If, however, the pelvis is clearly large enough, attempt a vaginal delivery. Constant attendance during labor is essential. Analgesia should not be excessive. At delivery the most important principle is to permit a delivery as far as possible before giving assistance. Assist delivery of the head with the use of head forceps if there is delay. Adequate facilities for infant resuscitation are essential.

Indications for Cesarean Section[30]

Advances in surgical techniques, blood transfusions and principles of anesthesia have made cesarean section a safe and useful method for manipulation of certain obstetrical problems (Table 2-5). However, cesarean section is not the panacea of all complications in obstetrics.

POSTPARTUM CARE

What the Placenta Tells the Physician

If the umbilical cord has a single artery or the cord is abnormally long or is velamentous or if the placenta is circumvallate or has infarctions, examine the infant closely for congenital abnormalities.

If there has been an intrauterine infection because of premature rupture of the bag of waters look for infections, jaundice, lethargy, pneumonia or convulsions in the infant.

Diabetes with an immature placenta or toxemia with degenerative infarctions in the placenta may cause neonatal distress. Postmaturity may also cause degenerative infarctions in the placenta with resultant malnutrition in the infant.

Amnion nodosum is also a good reason to search for infant abnormalities. Tumors of the placenta, i.e. chorionepithelioma, chorioangioma or metastases from maternal malignancies, may not only cause metastases in the newborn but malformations, hemangiomas or fetal hypoxia.

Fetal hypoxia and distress may be caused by a variety of difficulties which interfere with the fetal circulation. Consider infant hypoxia whenever there has been a placenta previa, abruptio placentae, prolapse of cord, a long cord around infant's neck, torsion, knot or stricture of cord, short cord, entwined cords of single ovum twin, or tumors of cord.

Anemia, shock or infant death may follow maternal hemorrhage with fetal blood loss as in placenta previa; cesarean section with anterior placenta; rupture of vessels of cord; ruptured placenta, vessel or varix; abruptio placentae; or vascular anastomosis with twins.

Apgar Scoring

Apgar scoring (Table 2-6) is a method of grading the physical condition of the new-

Table 2-5. Indications for Cesarean Section

Fetal	*Maternal*
Fetal distress before feasible vaginal delivery	Fetopelvic disproportion (generally after a trial of labor)*
Diabetes mellitus	Previous uterine scar
Isoimmunization	Third trimester bleeding accompanying placenta previa or abruptio placentae
Cord prolapse early in labor	Uterine inertia with failure of stimulation
Valuable baby†	Failed forceps
	Abdominal presentations
	Toxemia (after control)
	Maternal distress (cervical carcinoma, fistulas or pelvic tumors)

* Most common indication

† Section done when an older woman has had several stillbirths

born. Five signs are scored 0, 1 or 2 points depending on their presence or absence. The grading is done 1 minute after birth and if indicated repeated in 5 minutes.

A score of 10 indicates an excellent condition of the newborn without any asphyxia. A score of 5 to 9 indicates a mild asphyxia calling for modest support measures. A score of 4 or less indicates a severe asphyxia. Act promptly.

Immediate Care of the Newborn

The first moments after birth are the most important and most dangerous of the child's life. Clearing the airway is the accoucheur's first duty to the infant.

If the baby does not cry spontaneously, stimulate his respiration by slapping his feet or brusquely rubbing his back with your knuckles. Try lightly blowing oxygen into the baby's face.

If the baby is not crying in *one minute*, use more effective resuscitative methods, i.e. positive pressure breathing with a closed mask (30 to 40 cm water) or start positive pressure breathing by intubating the infant.

Presently sodium bicarbonate therapy for acidosis is controversial in newborns. If it is used, introduce the bicarbonate solution through an umbilical artery (31.5 mEg/kg weight).

Postpartum Hemorrhage

Postpartum hemorrhage is defined as a blood loss of more than 500 ml in the postpartum period. Death from postpartum hemorrhage is almost always preventable, but it remains the leading cause of maternal deaths in the United States. The average time from delivery to death is 5 hours and 20 minutes.

Table 2-6. Apgar Score

Sign	*Points* 0	1	2
Heart rate	absent	under 100	over 100
Respiratory effort	absent	slow, irregular	good, crying
Muscle tone	limp	flexion of extremities	active motion
Reflex irritability: response to catheter in nostril	no response	grimace	cough or sneeze
Color	blue-white	body pink; extremities blue	completely pink

Uterine atony accounts for 80 to 90 percent of early cases. Other causes are lacerations, retained placental fragments, inadequate involution of the placental site (usually occurs 1 to 2 weeks postpartum), postpartum hematomas, placenta accreta or percreta with inability to separate from uterine wall and hypofibrinogenemia.

After delivery of the infant the uterus should be routinely expored and the placenta manually removed if needed. If fragments remain, an opened gauze bandage over the gloved hand may help remove them. Inspect cervix and the vaginal vault using ring forceps. Intrauterine packing usually is not helpful but may be tried. If blood seeps through the packing a hysterectomy is mandatory. The uterus should not be packed twice.

Usually there is not enough time for determination of the fibrinogen level. Substitute: put 2 drops of thrombin in a suitable tube and add 1.5 ml of blood. Examine in 10 minutes. If the clot formed contains most of the red cells and constitutes half the original volume, the fibrinogen level is over 150 mg per 100 ml.

Precautions in Delivering the Rh-Negative Mother

The family physician can do several things during the third stage of labor to prevent fetal/maternal hemorrhage and the resulting maternal sensitization to the Rh factor. First, any type of interference with the third stage of labor or any mechanical means for termination of pregnancy increases the possibility of sensitization. This is true for induced abortions (curettage, vacuum aspiration and hysterotomy) in which 20 to 25 percent of mothers become sensitized. Peculiarly enough, spontaneous abortions rarely produce sensitization.

Second, the usual practice of double clamping the cord and cutting between the clamps promotes fetal/maternal hemorrhage. In addition, early clamping deprives the newborn of 40 to 50 ml of blood which is rightly his. Clamping the cord with a single clamp on the fetal side and allowing some blood from the placental side to run would seem desirable practice in Rh-negative mothers.

When to Administer Rho Gam[31]

Use Rho Gam to prevent the formation of active antibodies in the Rho (D) negative of D^u negative mother who has delivered a Rho (D) positive or D^u positive infant. With an injection to the postpartum mother of passive Rho (D) antibody (Rho Gam), the mother's antibody response to the foreign Rho (D) positive fetal cells is suppressed. Thus the Rh hemolytic disease in subsequent pregnancies is prevented.

Administer Rho Gam within 72 hours of the birth of the baby. The postpartum mother should meet the criteria in Table 2-7 in order to be considered a candidate for Rho Gam. Pre-administration directions should be followed carefully as described by the manufacturers.

A miscarriage or abortion can serve as a primary immunization by virtue of the entry of a small amount of Rho (D) positive fetal cells into the Rho (D) negative mother's blood stream. Therefore, if a Rho (D) negative mother has a miscarriage or abortion, consider her a candidate for protective treatment with Rho Gam. Since the baby's blood type might not be known, assume that it was Rho (D) positive and administer Rho Gam within 72 hours after the miscarriage or abortion.

Contraindications are listed in Table 2-7.

Recognition and Preliminary Treatment of Thrombophlebitis and Pulmonary Embolism

Thromboembolic disease occurs rarely during or immediately after pregnancy. Although a relatively benign process it accounts for a large proportion of maternal deaths. Consequently, when phlebitis or pulmonary embolism is suspected, treat it vigorously.

Thrombophlebitis

The diagnosis of thrombophlebitis is usually not difficult and may be obvious if the physician keeps the possibility in mind.

Table 2-7. Rho Gam Administration

Criteria for mother to receive Rho Gam	*Do not administer to*
Rho (D) negative or D^u negative mother	An infant
Mother already immunized to Rho (D) factor*	A Rho (D) positive of D^u positive individual
Baby must be Rho (D) positive of D^u positive	A Rho negative patient who has received a Rho (D) positive blood transfusion
Baby should have a negative direct Coombs test	A patient previously immunized to the Rho (D) blood factor

*This can be determined by a laboratory test using a product such as Selectogen Reagent Red Blood Cells (Human).

Findings are usually a tenderness along the involved vein with or without edema of the extremity. Pain in the calf on dorsiflexing the foot (Homan's sign) is an excellent indication of the disease.

With involvement of the lower extremity, the foot of the bed should be elevated 2 or 3 notches on the gatch frame with no flexion at the knees. The head of the bed is kept flat except when the patient is eating. Continually apply warm, moist compresses from the ball of the foot to the groin during waking hours. Institute ambulation only after the edema is subsiding and clinical improvement is evident. Do not allow the foot to hit the floor without elastic compression on the leg from the ball of the foot to the knee or midthigh as indicated.

The treatment may range from heat and bed rest to anticoagulants. In most cases it is wise to treat with intermittent intravenous heparin for 10 days. This can be given intermittently via an in-lying Hepacath. 7,500 to 10,000 units (75 mg to 110 mg) every 6 hr. Most patients will have prolongation of the Lee-White coagulation time to the desired 2 to 3 times normal range (20 to 30 min) with a 24 hr total dose of 20,000 to 40,000 units (200 to 400 mg). Check a Lee-White coagulation time just prior to a subsequent dose of heparin. If symptoms persist, change to oral bishydroxycoumarin (Dicumarol). In some cases, as a protection against pulmonary embolism, consider femoral ligation or even vena cava ligation.

Pulmonary Embolism

This pulmonary complication may be difficult to diagnose depending on whether there has been a pulmonary infarction. In cases of infarction the symptoms are distinguishable: pleuritic pains in the chest, hemoptysis, cough, fever and tachycardia. A radiogram of the chest may show a pulmonary consolidation resembling pneumonial pleural effusion or atelectasis. Pulmonary radiophotoscanning or, better still, pulmonary angiography will settle the diagnosis. False positive scans can be caused by pneumothorax, atelectasis, pneumonia or any parenchymal lung disease.

I must emphasize that the symptoms and findings in cases of acute pulmonary embolism follow no consistent pattern. In one study only 62 percent of the patients had pleuritic pains, 27 percent had hemoptysis and 17 percent had a pleural rub. Fifteen percent had a normal x-ray film. Only 42 percent presented with a phlebitis. Dyspnea was the most common symptom (80 percent). Tachypnea and tachycardia were the most commonly observed signs and occurred respectively in 88 percent and 63 percent of the patients.[32]

A significant number have no symptoms; and a greater number may present with only one finding. This lack of classical findings accounts for the poor identification of patients with a recent pulmonary embolism.

Pulmonary embolism without infarction is more difficult to diagnose. Symptoms are less spectacular but the patient nearly always complains of substernal distress. Findings are dyspnea, tachycardia, hypotension, apprehension and sweating. Later, depending on severity of the case, the blood pressure continues to fall. As the disease progresses, the right heart dilates as indicated by progressive electrocardiographic findings and a rising CVP. Treatment may become complicated, but it is wise to start the patient on intravenous heparin.

Don't hesitate to anticoagulate even if borderline contraindications to anticoagulation exist. Anticoagulation therapy will increase the survival rate after an initial pulmonary embolus and lower the incidence of and the mortality from recurrent pulmonary emboli.

If absolute contraindications to anticoagulation exist, surgically interrupt the inferior vena cava. Remember that interruption below the inferior vena cava is accompanied by a higher incidence of recurrent pulmonary emboli.[33]

Recently a Frenchman advocated treating major pulmonary emboli with urokinase in addition to intravenous heparin. He advocates urokinase perfusion for 24 hr at an average dose of 2,700,000 CTA units. With this combination therapy only 1 patient out of 6 died who had severe bilateral disease. In severe disease this addition to the usual heparinization might be tried before resorting to surgery.[34]

The Rubella-Susceptible Woman

While this is being written the practice of checking women routinely for rubella hemagglutination inhibition (HI) antibodies has started. But little or nothing is being done about the women who are identified as susceptible to rubella.

Family physicians should take the lead in immunizing the rubella-susceptible woman in the immediate postpartum period while the woman is still in the hospital.

Check all pregnant women for HI titer when doing the other routine laboratory tests. As a reminder, mark all your charts of women who prove to be rubella sensitive. Immunize all women immediately postpartum. Warn the patient that postpartum women can become pregnant; suggest contraception. Request postvaccination HI check to determine if vaccination has been successful.

Rehabilitative Exercises[35]

Rehabilitative exercises are not as important with immediate ambulation as in the past when women spent several days in bed postnatally. A certain number of women, however, still prefer exercises with the hope of firming muscles and helping posture. The following three exercises are adequate in most cases.

Pelvic floor muscles: In a crosslegged supine position, contract and relax the glutei, press thighs firmly together and draw in the anus strongly as though preventing a bowel movement. Continue this muscular effort with the vagina and urethra.

Abdominal muscles: Rectus—Lying supine, raise legs alternately and progress to raising both legs simultaneously. Oblique—While lying supine with the knees flexed, rotate the pelvis by retracting the abdomen and rolling the knees from side to side, trying to touch them to the floor.

Spinal extensor muscles: While lying prone, alternately hyperextend the lower extremities while raising the head and shoulders with the arms stretched backward.

Postpartum Follow-up

The traditional interval between delivery and first postnatal examination has been 6 weeks. Because of developments in contraception many physicians are now seeing patients in 4 weeks, particularly those who do not wish to become pregnant again.

Ovulation will almost certainly have occurred prior to any 6-week examination; consequently, many women may not be receiving family planning instruction at the time they need it. It is wise to tell the mother not to douche or have intercourse until after a 4-week check.

CHOOSING A CONTRACEPTIVE PILL

Contraceptive pills are individually selected. The family physician must first know the relative estrogen-progestogen dominance of each pill. He then selects the type of pill to fit the characteristics or conditions of his patient (Table 2-8). Sequential pills are estrogen-dominant during the first 15 days and progestogen-dominant the last 5 days of the pill cycle.

Choose estrogen-dominant pills for women who have less feminine characteristics: flat chest, scanty periods, hirsute-acne, early cycle spotting and premenstrual syndrome. Also those women who are depressed and those who tend toward alopecia and moniliasis. Estrogen-dominant pills produce more nausea than the progestogens as well as fluid retention and irritability, clusters of nevi, headache, visual abnormalities, heavier periods, increased blood pressure, triggering of diabetes, thrombophlebitis, breast tenderness, chloasma and vaginal secretions.

Choose progestogen-dominant pills for those women who tend toward excessive moisture, fibroids, cervical erosions, bloating, nausea, fibrocystic breast disease, dysmenorrhea, hypermenorrhea or venous engorgement. The progestogen-dominant pills tend to be safer. Choose contraceptives from the midspectrum for most normal women.

Table 2-8. Contraceptive Pills

Agent	*Combined*	*Sequential*
Estrogen dominant	Enovid-E Enovid-S (lesser degree than Enovid-E)	Oracon
Estrogen-progestogen balanced		Norquens C-Quens Ortho-Novum SQ
Progestogen dominant: Strongly progestogen	Norlestrin 2.5 Ovral	
Medium progestogen	Provest Demalon Ortho-Novum 1, 2 Norinyl 1/50	
Slightly progestogen	Ovulen Norinyl 1/80 Ortho-Novum 1/80 Norlestrin 1	

REFERENCES

1. Wallace H: Factors associated with perinatal mortality and morbidity. *Clin Obset Gynecol* 13:13, 1970.
2. Round-table discussion: Dealing with teenage sexual problems, the pill, pregnancy, marriage and sex education. *Patient Care* 2:14, 1968.
3. Birch HG: Functional effects of fetal malnutrition. *Hosp Pract* 6:134, 1971.
4. Robinson CH: Basic Nutrition and Diet Therapy, ed. 2. New York: Macmillan, 1970, p 127.
5. Symposium: The Rubella vaccine: new hope, but lingering problems. *Patient Care* 3:99–102, 1969.
6. Ellegood JO, et al: Chorionic gonadotropin tests for diagnosis of pregnancy and chorionic tumors. *Postgrad Med* 46:105–109, 1969.
7. Fitzgerald JA: Single but pregnant: your patient's personal committment offers the alternative. *Med Insight* 3:65, 1971.
8. Fraser FC: Genetic counseling. *Hosp Pract* 6:49–56, 1971.
9. O'Brien JS: How we detect mental retardation before birth. *Med Times* 99:103–106, 1971.

10. Brody H, et al: Therapeutic abortion: a prospective study. *Am J Obstet Gynecol* 109:347–353, 1971.
11. Keith LG, Poma-Herrera P: Aggressive treatment of septic abortion. *AFP* 3:99–103, 1971.
12. Gordon M, Horowitz A: Septic shock in obstetrics and gynecology. *Postgrad Med* 46:144–148, 1969.
13. White CA, et al: Rho (D) immune globulin to prevent Rh hemolytic disease. *AFP* 3:85–89, 1971.
14. Charles AG, et al: Management of the Rh-negative gravida. *AFP* 3:104–119, 1971.
15. Nelson MM, Forfar JO: *Brit Med J* 1:523, 1971.
16. Alford, Jr, CA: Symposium: *MD* 101, 1971.
17. Goldfield M: Problems in rubella diagnosis. *Infect Dis* 1:19, 1971.
18. Buncher CR: Cigarette smoking and duration of pregnancy. *Postgrad Med* 46:178, 1969.
19. Stewart A, Kneale GW: Radiation risk. *Lancet* 1:1185, 1970.
20. Flowers, Jr, CE: How to persuade pregnant women to diet. *Consultant* 7:20–22, 1967.
21. Lein JN, Bulgar RJ: Why bacteriuria in pregnancy should be treated. *Postgrad Med* 45:201–205, 1969.
22. Sutherland HW, et al: Glycosuria problem. A review in *MD* 14:77, 1970.
23. Maillard E, et al: The newborn of diabetic mothers. *Ann Pediatr* 181:450, 1971.
24. Fuchs F: One for the slow road. *Emerg Med* 3:68, 1971.
25. Salzmann B: The day the waters broke. *J Med Soc NJ*.
26. Adriani J: Obstetric analgesia and anesthesia. *AFP/GP* 1:60–74, 1970.
27. Kalstone CE, Morley GW: Forceps: trial and fail. *Postgrad Med* 46:222–226, 1969.
28. Mines JL: Application of the obstetrics forceps. *Obstet Gynecol* 36:680, 1970.
29. Hibbard LT: Shoulder dystocia. *Obstet Gynecol* 34:424, 1969.
30. Lang WR: What are indications of cesarean section? *Consultant* 11:10, 1971.
31. Information from Ortho-Diagnostics Company literature.
32. Wenger NK, et al: Massive acute pulmonary embolism—the deceivingly nonspecific manifestations. *JAMA* 220:843, 1972.
33. Pollak EW, et al: Pulmonary embolism: appraisal of therapy in 516 cases. *Arch Surg* 107:66–68, 1973.
34. Brochier M, et al: Urokinase thrombolytic treatment of severe pulmonary embolism. *Sem Hop Paris* 49:1825–1836, 1973, as reviewed in *JAMA* 225:332, 1973.
35. Knapp ME: Physical medicine and rehabilitation in obstetrics. *Postgrad Med* 47:19–24, 1969.

CHAPTER 3

Child Growth and Development

Pediatrics offers the family physician a challenging opportunity for prevention of physical and emotional diseases. But preventive know-how has been spotty. More has been accomplished in the prevention of communicable diseases and the correction of congenital anomalies than in the prevention and treatment of disorders of reading, learning, speaking, spelling, writing and the social and emotional conflicts resulting from these disabilities. Even many pediatricians are unfamiliar with the prevention and treatment of delinquency, promiscuity, suicide, dropping-out and drug abuse. When these problems first come to the attention of the family physician he should be knowledgeable in their solution.

Consequently, the family physician should be skilled not only in diagnosing and treating physical ailments but also, because of his position as family physician, in recognizing aberrant behavior in families and the children they produce.

THE NEWBORN

Examining the Newborn

Whereas many residents in family practice are skilled in the examination of the adult, few have seen or examined a newborn. To recognize the abnormal in the newborn you must obtain experience in observing and handling the normal infant. Experience helps overcome the lack of communication. The infant speaks through body language; this language the family physician must learn to interpret.

A thorough examination of the newborn cannot be overemphasized. The first examination in a person's life could well be his most important. The overlooking of an abnormality in the newborn may allow a handicap to persist, which cannot be overcome in later life.

History is the key to diagnosis when examining adults. The family physician has no such aid when examining the newborn. You must rely on your ability to do a meticulous and thorough physical examination. You will have little on which to rely outside of the mother's obstetric history and the baby's Apgar score. Too often the Apgar score (Chapter 2) is ignored or unavailable.

First correlate the birth weight with the gestational age and identify the low birth weight infant (see Low Birth Weight Infants later in this chapter).

Inspect the Total Infant

Observe the baby while he is completely naked. Are the infant's arms and legs in partial flexion or does he have the pithed frog posture of the premature? Study the body's proportions; a large head and big abdomen with short extremities are normal for the newborn. Facial features are important. Is there asymmetry of the face? The upsloping eyes and the darting tongue of Down's syndrome? The wrinkled forehead? The flattened nasal bridge or the large protruding tongue of the cretin?

Is the infant's color satisfactory? A pink baby is a sign of health but the examiner must allow for vasomotor changes from time to time. Examine the baby in natural light for slight degrees of jaundice, pallor or cyanosis. What is the respiratory pattern? A normal respiratory excursion involves both the diaphragm and abdominal muscles. There should be no retraction of the ribs or xiphoid on inspiration.

Check the infant's temperature. The normal temperature for a baby lying covered in a bassinet is 98° to 99° F. The premature's temperature is lower, 96° to 98.6° F.

Before beginning the examination of special organs inspect the skin of the entire body for nevus flammeus, milia, mongolian spots, cutis marmorata, nevi, hemangiomas, sinus openings, skin turgor and general or local edema that occurs on the dorsum of the hands and feet in Turner's syndrome.

Head and Neck

Check the size, shape and symmetry of the head and face. How much molding has occurred? Are the fontanelles sunken or bulging? Distinguish between a cephalhematoma with bleeding over one cranial bone and caput succedaneum with edema crossing suture lines.

Do not attempt to force the eyelids open. Most infants will open their eyes if they are rocked from a horizontal to an upright position. Look for subconjuctional hermorrhage, nystagmus, ocular palsies and pupil inequality.

While inspecting the ears, notice their placement. Low placement or other malformations should cause the examiner to suspect renal or chromosome abnormalities. Look for small sinuses in or about the ear, the vestiges of branchial cysts. They are difficult to treat.

Checking the infants hearing by clapping the hands near his ears and noticing his response is insufficient. Vicon has manufactured a soundproducing instrument, Apriton, which produces flat noises between 100 and 6000 hertz. Touching or uncovering the baby is not necessary for testing. Nursery personnel can do the test by holding the soundproducing system 4 in from the infant's ear.

Examine the mouth for palate defects. If necessary use a gloved finger to investigate areas not clearly visible. Newborn infants are nose breathers; they must learn to mouth breath. Holding a baby's nose shut will cause degrees of suffocation.

Chest

The respiratory rate of a newborn at rest or when mildly active is anywhere from 20 to 60 respirations per min. With vigorous crying the rate will increase to 60 to 100/min. Apnea longer than 20 sec is always abnormal. Note the following physical findings:

- –synchrony of chest and abdominal motion
- –intercostal retraction
- –xiphoid retraction
- –flaring of alae nasi
- –expiratory grunting

Grade each of these findings according to severity and score as 0, 1 or 2. Obviously, a total score of 0 indicates no respiratory distress whereas a score of 10 signifies extreme respiratory distress.

The normal breath sounds are bronchovesicular. Always use a stethoscope to which the diaphragm for infants is attached. Carefully examine the exterior chest wall for the widely spaced nipples (shield chest) of Turner's syndrome. The breasts are nearly always engorged, but not truly hypertrophied. Check the clavicles for a fracture.

Heart

The heart rate 1 min previous to delivery varies from 80 to 130 beats per minute. After the delivery the rate ranges from 90 to 160 and the sleeping heart rate is 100 to 140. Blood pressure determination is a difficult procedure in an infant if the examiner attempts to use the conventional method.

Use the flush method. Equipment needed is a sphygmomanometer with a 2.5 or 5.0 cm cuff and a strip of elastic wrapping material 2 to 4 cm wide and 40 to 50 cm long. The infant may be prone or supine and should be relaxed (not crying) and warm. Good lighting is essential and two observers are desirable. Apply the cuff to the distal leg or forearm. Keep the manometer at heart level. Snugly wrap the distal extremities (hand or foot) with an elastic or rubber bandage. Inflate the cuff to 150 to 200 mm/Hg. Remove the elastic bandage. The hand or foot should be blanched. Lower the pressure 5 mm/Hg and observe for 3 to 4 sec. Continue the lowering procedure until flushing is first observed. Read the blood pressure in the usual way.

While examining the heart, keep the first signs of heart disease in mind, i.e. cyanosis, pallor and respiratory distress. Signs of cardiac failure are the above signs plus tachycardia, cardiomegaly, hepatomegaly, rales, rhonchi, gallop rhythm and occasionally edema. A murmur at birth may signify a late closing ductus arteriosus. An infant may have severe heart disease without an audible murmur. With respiration a normal sinus arrhythmia may occur; a splitting of the second sound in the pulmonary area on expiration is also normal.

Do not forget to examine for dextrocardia. The normal apex beat (PMI) should be on the left in the fourth costal interspace. Check the peripheral pulse for the bounding thrust of a ductus or aortic valve insufficiency. (See Congenital Heart Disease later in this chapter).

Abdomen

Careful examination of the abdomen is necessary in the search for various anomalies (Fig. 3-1). A skillful examiner will learn to examine the infant's abdomen with one or two fingers rather than with his hand. When palpating the liver 1 to 2 cm below the costal margin, the lower poles of the kidneys and occasionally the spleen are normal findings.

Evaluate the umbilical stump before the cord dries up. *A tip:* Normally an examiner detects a central vein with two peripheral arteries. If one artery is missing, search for a total or partial obstruction of the esophagus or anus.

You will find a single umbilical artery in about 1 percent of newborns providing you look for the abnormality. Of these infants, about 30 percent will have congenital abnormalities of one type or another, i.e. low birth weight, trisomies, tracheobronchial fistulas, cardiac anomalies and urinary tract abnormalities. A common urinary tract problem is the absence of one kidney. Learning to palpate both kidneys in infants might save unnecessary intravenous pyelograms. Give thought to ordering an intravenous pyelogram on these infants with a single umbilical artery.

If a careful examination is given the infant when he is born you usually will find the abnormality. Always inform the parents of the anomalous cord and discuss the problem with them.

An inguinal hernia may slip in and out unobserved and be almost impossible to demonstrate on examination. Examine the abdomen this way: ask the nurse or parent to hold the infant upright; then with the full surface of the examining hand, pump the abdomen in and out with gentle but frequent strokes. This procedure will cause the herneal sac to fill and become visible in practically all cases.

Rectal examinations need a special word because of the reluctance of examiners to cause the baby distress. The incidence of congenital anorectal anomalies is 1 in 1,675. The most common defect is the blind rectum which accounts for 67.5 percent. Next most common is an unabsorbed anal membrane, 20 percent. A variety of other anomalies make up the remainder (Fig. 3-2).

The newborn is examined digitally by slowly inserting the lubricated little finger. Finding green sticky meconium on the finger assures one that the intestinal tract is almost certain to be patent. If only a small plug of gray material is found, further examination is necessary. For visual examination procure special anoscopes or proctoscopes.

Genitalia and Perineum

The examiner's first concern in examining the genitalia should be the identification of the child's gender. Does the infant need the

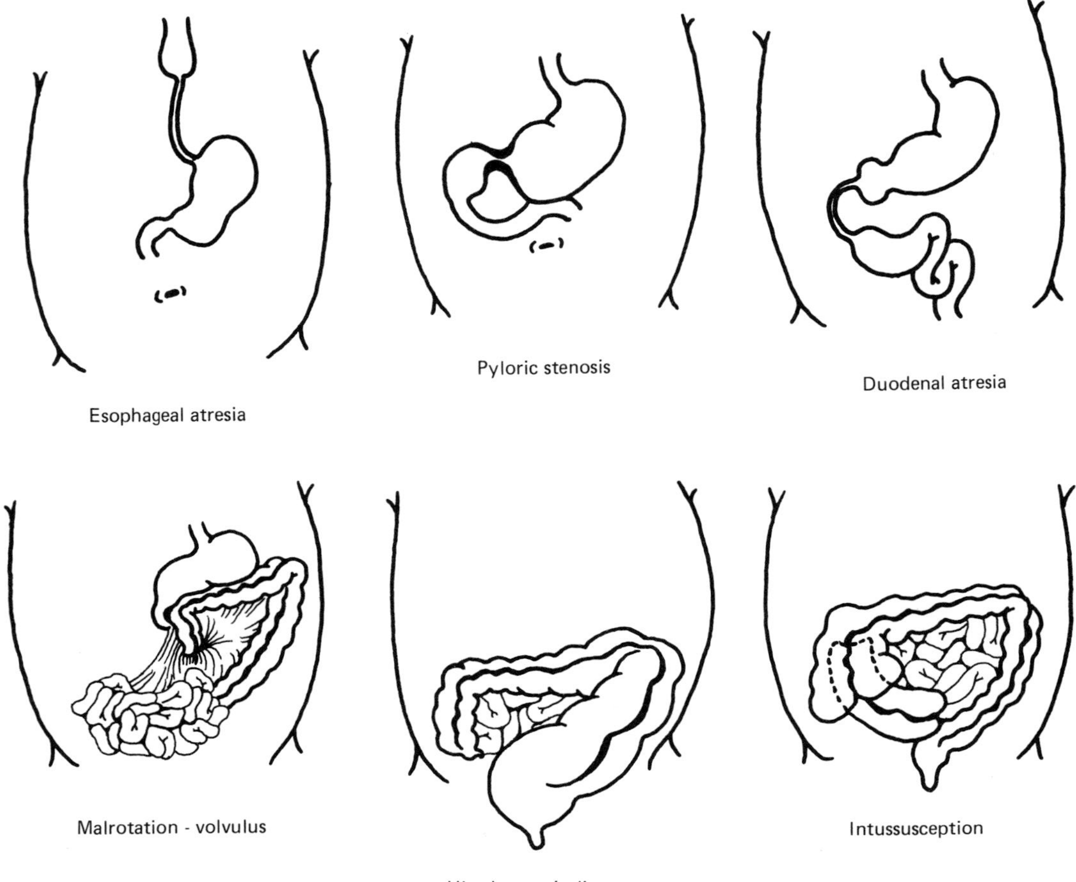

Figure 3-1. Abdominal anomalies.

Barr-Bertram check of cell chromatin to establish sex? Examine the penis for hypospadia, hypertrophy or atrophy. Palpate the scrotum for the testicles. Inspect the scrotum for edema. Does the infant have a hydrocele? Transillumination will help differentiate between hydrocele and hernia. Female infants will occasionally spot menstrual blood because of prenatal maternal hormonal influence.

Musculoskeletal System

Inspect and palpate the infant's spine for scoliosis, spina bifida (Fig. 3-3) or a pilonidal sinus. Spontaneous movement of all extremities is normal as well as the withdrawal of a limb from pain or discomfort. A healthy baby has good muscle tone.

Two abnormalities require special mention, i.e. metatarsus varus and congenital dislocation of the hip. Consciously search for both (see Infant Foot and Leg Problems later in this chapter). Determine the range of motion of all joints. Remember a fat pad fills the infant's arch and consequently the arch is flat or even bulging.

Central Nervous System

Evaluating the nervous system takes more skill and experience than other body systems. Even the most experienced examiner cannot differentiate intracranial hemorrhage, anoxia or cerebral edema. A detailed obstetrical history helps to diagnose CNS abnormalities.

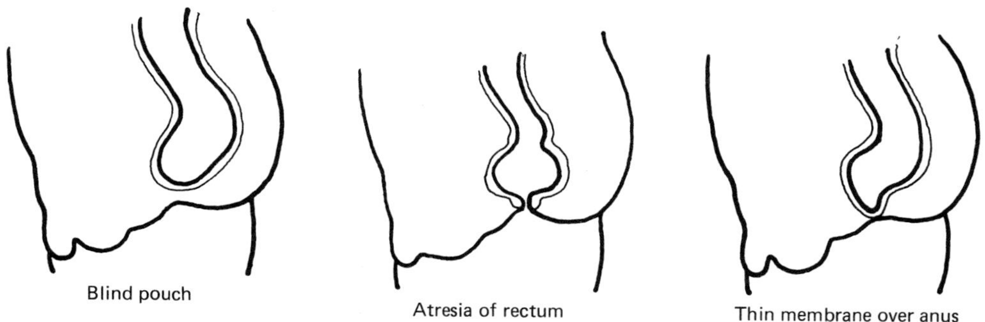

Figure 3-2. Congenital anomalies.

Start the examination by evaluating the infant's alertness, his activity, and his spontaneous use of all four extremities. Is excessive flaccidity or paralysis present? Is the child unusually sleepy or lethargic? Listen to the strength and character of the cry. A high-pitched, shrill cry is an unfavorable sign. Does the infant nurse vigorously? Observe again his reaction to stimuli. Does he withdraw his extremities from pain? Does he respond to stimuli with mass movement of all extremities? This is an unfavorable sign. Is there a tremor? The coarser the temor the more guarded the outlook.

The following reflexes are important in the newborn and should be provoked (Table 3-1).

Moro reflex. This is the most significant of the special responses. The reflex can be elicited in all infants except some prematures. Support the infant's head and shoulders on the hands and forearm then suddenly allow the head to drop back 20° to 30° from the trunk. A positive normal reaction is a sudden extension of the upper extremities followed by a slower drawing together of the extremities as in an embrace. Evoke the Moro also by suddenly striking the examining table or jerking the infant's feet. The reflex disappears in 1 to 3 months. Retention of the reflex may indicate CNS disability.

Rooting reflex and *sucking reflex*. These are automatisms present in the normal infant. Obviously, the sucking reflex is evoked by putting a finger or the tip of a tongue blade in the baby's mouth. The absence of these reflexes suggest CNS depression due to anoxia, anesthesia or congenital defects.

Palmar and plantar groups. Elicit these automatic reactions of fullterm newborns by firmly placing a finger in the infant's palm or at the base of his toes. The hand grasp reflex may be strong enough to allow the examiner to lift the baby from the examining table —the grasp and traction reflex.

Trunk incurvature (Gallant's response). Place the baby in a prone, horizontal position. Stroke the paravertebral muscles with a finger or pin. In a favorable response the infant swings his pelvis toward the stimulated side. Its absence indicates a spinal lesion or general depression of the nervous system.

Stepping. Support the baby in an upright position and as he is moved forward he will make stepping movements. While in the upright position place the dorsum of the infant's foot under the edge of the examining table. Expect him to lift his foot and place it on the table.

Eliciting these reflexes does not comprise a complete neurological examination but only a sketchy neurological screening, assessing mainly the motor function of the infant. To completely evaluate the motor and sensory systems plus the c.anial nerves is, indeed, a difficult task requiring patience and skill. In addition, physiological normals have not been set and available tests are not sensitive enough to detect the minor alterations of the child with minimal brain dysfunction.

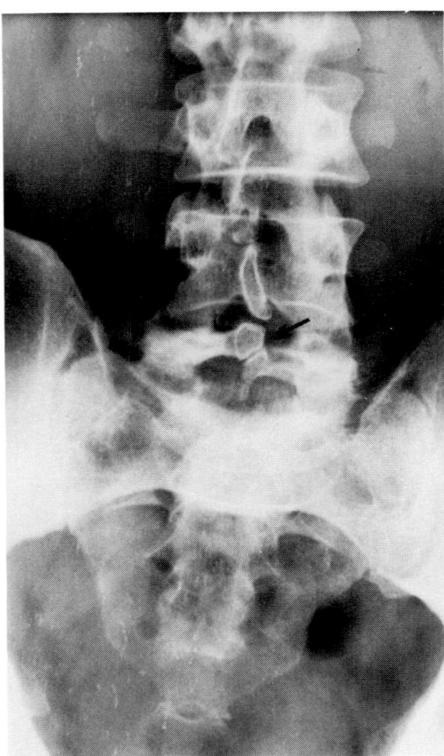

Figure 3-3. Spina bifida occulta. Failure of fusion of the neural arch of a vertebra is spina bifida. In occulta there is no protrusion of the meninges. The only external manifestation may be a dimple in the skin, a patch of hair or a lipomatous nevus.

Respiratory Distress

Causes of respiratory distress in the newborn are:

Obstructive lesions of larynx and trachea (Figure 3-4)
Obstructive lesions of neck
Airway obstruction by aspiration
Diseases of the nervous and muscular systems
–cerebral hemorrhage
–phrenic nerve paralysis
–cervial cord injuries
–immaturity
–drugs
Decreased pulmonary function
–respiratory distress syndrome (RDS) (hyaline membrane disease)
–massive aspiration of meconium
–transient respiratory distress
–atelectasis
–pulmonary dysmaturity (Wilson-Mikity syndrome)
–immature lung of the premature
–pneumonia
–pulmonary hemorrhage
–pneumothorax
–pulmonary tumor or cysts
–pleural effusion
–paralysis of diaphragm
–diaphragmatic hernia
–abdominal distension from pneumoperitoneum ascite tumors
Miscellaneous causes
–congenital heart disease
–cardiac and circulatory failure
–myocarditis
–hypoglycemia
–anemias

The three pulmonary abnormalities that account for most cases of respiratory distress are respiratory distress syndrome (hyaline membrane syndrome), meconium aspiration and transient respiratory distress.

The family physician should understand the pathophysiology of these three diseases. To clinically differentiate the three is difficult. The diagnosis is simpler with the aid of an x-ray picture of the lungs. Each disease has a typical roentgenographic finding. Therefore order an x-ray immediately whenever inspiratory retraction is observed.

Fortunately transient respiratory distress is a selflimiting disease usually resolving in 2 to 3 days. Supportive treatment with oxygen and controlled Isolette environment is sufficient treatment. The abnormality is more frequent in premature newborns or those delivered by cesarean section or by breech extraction. Transient respiratory distress starts within 6 to 8 hours after birth.[1]

Meconium aspiration does not often require treatment. The danger is pneumonia. If the disease develops treat with the appropriate antibiotics and with respiratory support.

Treat a cyanotic infant with a diffuse spotty atelectasis with oxygen and with

Table 3-1. Normal Ages of Neurologic Signs Peculiar to Infancy

Response	*Age normally appears*	*Age normally disappears*
Spontaneous stepping	Birth	2 to 6 wk
Positive supporting (neonatal type)	Birth	3 to 6 wk
Crossed extension (allongement croises)	Birth	1 to 2 mo
Trunk incurvature	Birth	1 to 2 mo
Moro	Birth	1 to 3 mo
Redressement du tronc	Birth	Variable
Leg flexion in vertical suspension	Birth	4 mo
Rooting	Birth	3 to 4 mo awake, 7 mo asleep
Palmar grasp	Birth	6 mo
Adductor spread of knee jerk	Birth	7 mo
Plantar grasp	Birth	9 to 10 mo
Tonic neck reflex	2 mo	5 mo
Landau	3 mo	12 to 24 mo
Neck righting reflex	4 to 6 mo	12 to 24 mo
Positive supporting (weight bearing)	6 mo	Persists
Parachute reaction	8 to 9 mo	Variable

Adapted from Paine RS: Neurological examination of infants and children. Pediatr Clin N Am 7:471, 1960, Philadelphia: W. B. Saunders Co., with permission.

other measures directed toward correcting the underlying cause. Give oxygen as needed to control cyanosis in an infant with a segmental atelectasis. Aspirate mucus from the airway and position the infant with the diseased lung side up.

Hyaline Membrane Disease

In contrast to transient respiratory distress, hyaline membrane disease starts at or shortly after birth. It is the most common cause of death in the newborn (Figure 3–5). The infant with the disease usually is premature, and the disease accounts for 20 to 40 percent of deaths in prematurity. The first sign is usually retraction of the chest wall with each inspiration, because the lung has abnormal resistance to expansion. As respirations become more labored, expiratory grunting develops accompanied by flaring of the nostrils.

Respiratory rate increases to 60 a min within 4 hr. If the disease continues to develop, cyanosis appears and deepens even with oxygen administration until finally the peripheral circulation collapses. Further complicating the disease is the development of a mixed respiratory and metabolic acidemia.[2]

Place the infant in an incubator and keep the temperature at 88° to 92° F and the humidity above 80 percent. Administer oxygen, 30 to 40 percent, to control cyanosis (see below). Give an antibiotic if infection is present. Penicillin is as good as any pending bacteriological studies—20,000 units/kg body weight per day.

At this point specialty care may be necessary unless the family physician is trained in intravenous administration. If so, start intravenous glucose, 40 to 50 mg of a 10 percent aqueous solution/kg of body weight.

Give sodium bicarbonate to keep the blood pH between 7.35 and 7.40. Start with 2 mEq/kg intravenously and then adjust according to the needs established by monitoring the pH, pCO_2, bicarbonate, glucose and electrolytes. Consider giving THAM-E or TRIS if constant monitoring is available. This is usually a job for the specialist.[3]

Oxygen Administration

Keeping the oxygen concentration in the incubator at 40 percent or below is no longer acceptable treatment. When this method was used, many infants were not getting therapeutic amounts of oxygen into

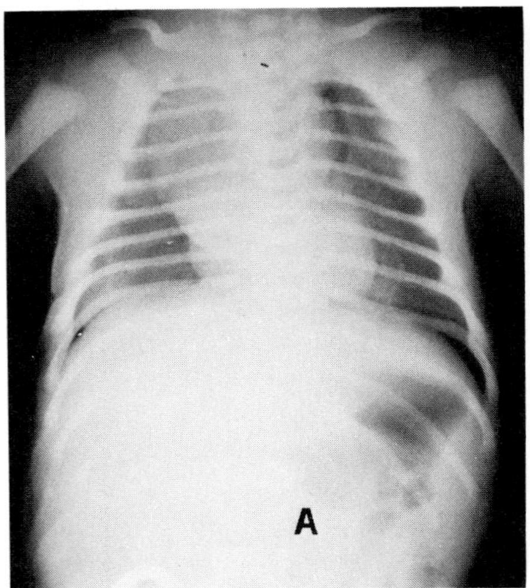

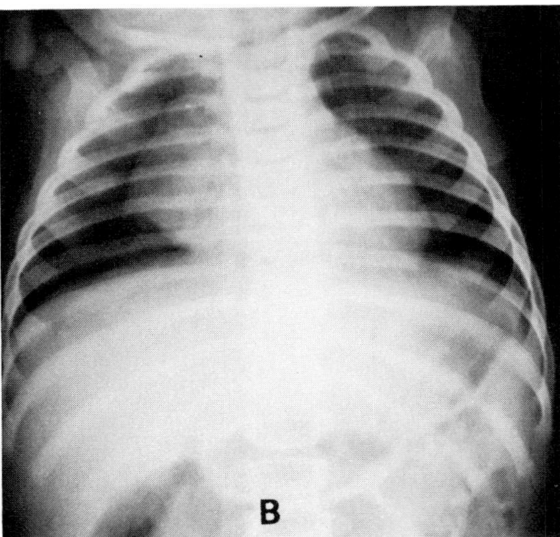

Figure 3-4. *A*, A prominent thymus is normal; *B*, PA view of the chest of an infant showing asymmetric enlargement of the thymus to the right, the so-called "sail sign."

the blood stream while others were absorbing enough to cause retrolental fibroplasia. The American Academy of Pediatrics' guidelines now emphasizes that the oxygen tension of arterial blood is the important factor. Manipulating the oxygen concentration of the inspired air is insufficient.

Many doctors and hospitals will find the new guidelines difficult to follow but they will not be able to do otherwise. In every hospital where oxygen is to be given to prematures, blood-gas microanalysis and appropriate personnel must be provided for monitoring. Otherwise the premature should be transferred to a hospital where monitoring can be done. Their guidelines provide one exception: mature infants who are cyanotic but not apneic may be given just enough oxygen to relieve the cyanosis.

Administer oxygen by whichever method is most suitable under the circumstances, i.e. funnels, hoods, incubators, masks or endotracheal tubes. The oxygen should be kept at 88° to 92° F and the humidity above 80 percent. Check the equipment for mixing the oxygen and air every 2 hr with the oxygen analyzer. Calibrate the same equipment daily with room air and 100 percent oxygen.

Administer enough oxygen to keep the arterial oxygen tension between 60 to 80 mm/Hg and never over 100 mm/Hg. The Academy suggests the temporal or radial arteries as the best sites for sampling arterial blood. As second choice, and always more available, is an arterial catheter placed in an umbilical artery.

If an infant improves rapidly, promptly discontinue the oxygen. If the infant is improving gradually, reduce the oxygen 10 percent and determine further oxygen concentrations by blood-gas determinations.[4]

Vitamin K_1

The American Academy of Pediatrics now recommends the routine use of vitamin K_1 for premature infants. The Academy does not consider maturity a counterindication and many are using vitamin K_1 for newborns. Their recommendation is based on the generally low prothrombin levels during the first 3 or 4 days of life. An infant gradually develops normal levels by the eighth or tenth day.

Give vitamin K_1 orally or intramuscularly (0.5 to 2.0 mg vitamin K_1, Konakion intramuscularly); both give equally good results. Most doctors prefer the oral route.

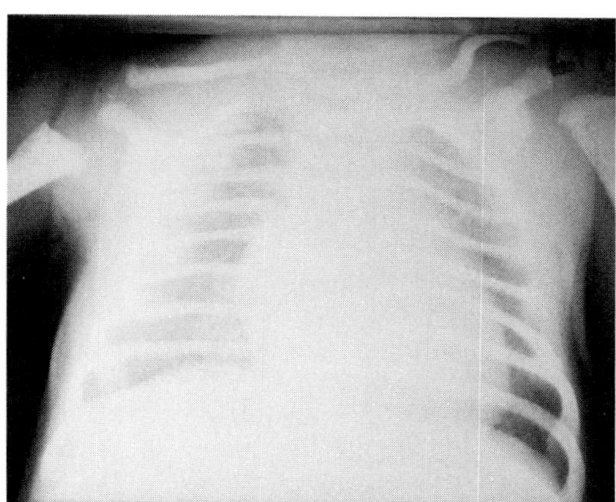

Figure 3-5. Early hyaline membrane disease.

Consultation in Rh Problems

The rules for treating a baby born of an Rh-negative mother are simple. (Care of Rh-negative mothers was discussed in Chapter 2.)

The obstetrical history is important. Obtain all the pertinent prenatal information including antibody and titer checks. In the event all the recommendations for the mother's care have been followed, the infant's care will be fairly well programmed.

Order a direct Coomb's test, ABO and Rh typing on the infant's cord blood. If the direct Coomb's test is negative and the infant Rh-positive, a hazard exists.

A consultation by a pediatrician familiar with the treatment of Rh problems is needed for the following:

–if serum bilirubin is 10 at 24 hr
–if serum bilirubin is 12 at 48 hr
–if serum bilirubin is 15 anytime
–if the hemoglobin falls below 14

A positive Coomb's test does not require a consultation unless the above criteria are met.

Low Birth Weight Infants

In recent years, the concept of the low birth weight infant has given new insights into perinatal problems. Low birth weight infants are divided into two groups: The true premature and the mature but low birth weight infant who has had intrauterine growth retardation. Be alert to this differentiation: treatment and prognosis depends, in large measure, on this classification.

The following characteristics help to identify the mature infant: silky hair; firm, well-formed pinnae; creases on the soles of the feet and extending over the heels; breast tissue of 7 mm or more; complete Moro reflex; complete crossed extension reflex; complete recoil on extension of extremities; strong grasp reflex; reflex standing when placed upright on a table; and testes in scrotum or well developed labia that cover the clitoris.

Weight and gestation age are two factors involved in determining infant mortality. Of the two, birth weight is the more important factor. The lower the birth weight, the higher the infant mortality subject to the secondary influence of gestational age. Yerushalmey's five categories[5] give a useful and practical method of gauging prognosis for survival (Table 3-2).

Phototherapy for the Premature Infant

Studies indicate that phototherapy helps control hyperbilirubinemia in the premature infant. The technique of treatment has not been standardized. In Southern California, the popular method is to place a light cradle over an Isolette which contains 10 20-watt cool white fluorescent bulbs with

Table 3-2.

Group	*Birth weight (grams)*	*Gestation (weeks)*	*Mortality (per 1000 live births)*
I	1500 or less	all	707.03
II	1501 to 2500	less than 37	104.7
III	1501 to 2500	37 or more	32.0
IV	2501 or more	less than 37	13.7
V	2501 or more	37 or more	4.7

Reprinted from Diamond EF: New insights from fetology. *Med Times* 98:115–118, 1970, with permission.

energy peaks in the 420 to 480 Mu wavelengths.

This produces 450 foot-candles at the baby's level. Do not confuse this light source with ultraviolet radiation which would be catastrophic. The treatment is continued for 6 days. For treatment, babies are nude except for eye coverings.

Use phototherapy for the slow development of hyperbilirubinemia associated with prematurity rather than with the precipitous accumulation of serum bilirubin of erythroblastosis. Evidence suggests that infant brain damage may occur when bilirubin levels reach 12 to 15 mg percent. In controlled studies, few infants develop higher concentrations than 15 mg percent when treated by phototherapy. Remember that two thirds of all fullterm infants have some jaundice during the first week of life. The serum bilirubin level may reach 7 to 10 mg/100 ml by the fourth day of life and then gradually subside.[6]

Hypoglycemia

Pediatricians have recently been studying blood sugar levels in the newborn as an explanation for symptoms in the premature infant. The incidence of neonatal hypoglycemia is 6 percent during the first 5 days of a premature's life. The rate rises to 15 percent in symptomatic infants whose birth weights are less than the fiftieth gestation percentile.

The onset of signs and symptoms varies from 2½ hr to 7 days of age and includes the following: tremors (most common symptom), episodes of cyanosis and convulsion, respiratory distress and eye rolling.

The normal mean level of glucose during the first week of life is 39 to 49 mg/100 ml. Measurements can be made on blood obtained by heel puncture in early morning 3 to 4½ hr after the last feeding.

Treatment is 10 percent glucose (orally) either as a supplement to their regular feedings or as intravenous therapy. If symptoms persist and blood sugar remains low, ACTH or cortisone will boost the blood sugar.

Circumcision[7]

Circumcision (Table 3-3) is a controversial procedure. The anticircumcision physicians claim the operation is unnecessary. The following statistics would appear to back their claims: At birth only 4 percent of boys have a fully retractable foreskin; at 6 months of age 15 percent; at one year 50 percent; and by 3, 90 have a completely retractable prepuce.

To diagnose phimosis a doctor must find a nonretractable foreskin and a small perputial opening. Ballooning of the prepuce may occur on micturition.

Do not perform a circumcision to prevent carcinoma of the cervix, penis or prostate. Substantial evidence to prove these benefits is lacking.

Not withstanding disagreement by many physicians, the majority of physicians and parents prefer to have their children circumcised. And all agree that circumcision should be done when medically indicated. Circumcised men prefer the cleanliness provided.

PKU Screening

Phenylketonuria (PKU) is an inherited disease transmitted by a single autosomal recessive gene. The disease occurs as a result of a deficiency of a liver enzyme whose function is to convert phenylalanine to tyrosine. Consequently, phenylalanine increases in the blood and spinal fluid. By some yet undetermined way the excess leads to mental retardation.

The pathophysiology and laboratory tests for PKU are constantly being revised. The information here presented is the method presently in use. The literature should be consulted from time to time in order for the doctor to stay up to date.

All states have passed legislation requiring PKU screening. The Guthrie test is popularly in vogue. In this test, puncture the infant's heel and blot the drops of blood obtained with filter paper and dry. The technician punches out a disc of dried blood and places it on agar medium containing Bacillus subtilis and B-2-thienylalanine. If

TABLE 3-3. Circumcision

Indications	*Techniques*	*Contraindications*	*Complications*
Congenital phimosis	Clamp method	Active infections	Hemorrhage*
Adherent prepuce	Dorsal slit and circumcision	Anomalies of the penis or meatus (hypospadias, etc.)	Infection
Redundant prepuce (inferfering with urination and collecting smegma and other secretions)	Gonco clamp technique		Surgical trauma and mutilation
Recurrent attacks of balanoposthitis	New disposable device available from Cluth-Circ, 1541 Wiltonway, La Habra, Calif. 50631		

* Check infant for blood coagulopathies before circumcising. Instruct nurses and parents to inspect the area for bleeding at four 15 minute intervals following surgery.

bacterial growth appears on the spot after 18 hours incubation, the physician may presume the infant has PKU. (B-2-thienylalanine inhibits bacterial growth unless phenylalanine, phenylpyruvic acid or phenylacetic acid is present.)

If the Guthrie test is positive, a quantitative determination of blood phenylalanine is necessary not only to confirm the bacteriologic diagnosis but also to establish the proper phenylalanine diet content.

The National Collaborative Study has established the following criteria for the diagnosis of PKU:

–blood phenylalanine levels greater than 20 mg percent on more than one occasion during the first 121 days of life
–persistence of these levels when challenged with evaporated milk at 3 mo of age
–urine showing the presence of phenylketones during the newborn and challenge periods
–normal blood tyrosine levels

The diagnosis of PKU cannot be absolutely established by considering blood levels alone.

An elevated blood phenylalanine may represent other entities: transient PKU, phenylalanine transaminase deficiency, transient or permanent hyperphenylalaninemic variant, hypertyrosinemia and laboratory errors. Consider the following guide lines:

–values over 25 mg percent have classic PKU
–values under 15 mg percent probably have a variant form
–values between 15 and 25 mg percent, diagnosis depends on family history, the course and the response to phenylalanine challenge.

A family physician should consult with someone of experience before launching long term treatment of PKU. Testing techniques and treatment regimes are yet unsatisfactory.

Place the child on Lofenalac (1:2) and adjust his diet to 25 mg/kg for 2 days, then change to 60 to 80 mg/kg for the next few days. At 3 mo challenge all children with evaporated milk and retest. If the phenylalanine level rises above 20 mg percent, resume the Lofenalac diet. Phenylalanine content of foods can be found by consulting proper tables. Warn parents to expect a diarrhea when starting Lofenalac. As the child grows he may lose his taste for Lofenalac. Suggest to the mother that she make cookies and pudding with it.

Keep children with PKU on a special low phenylalanine diet until they are 5 years old. Then gradually decreased, the diet for myelinization is about complete at this age.[8]

The Rubella Syndrome

The mortality from rubella during the first year of life is 10 to 20 percent. The following are defects associated with the rubella syndrome and are listed in order of their incidence. An infant may have one to five of these problems.

Eye defects: Blindness, glaucoma, cataracts. Rubella is the most common cause of congenital cataracts.

Hearing defects: In one study[9] 58.5 percent of children with history of prenatal rubella had significant hearing losses, 38 percent to a profound degree.

Mental retardation: Slight to severe. Gestational age at onset of maternal rubella is a significant factor in etiology. Maximum impairment falling between 14 and 60 days.

Congenital heart defects: Chiefly patent ductus arteriosus but ventricular septal defects and pulmonary stenosis as well.

Miscellaneous defects: Growth retardation, thrombocytopenic purpura, enlarged liver and spleen, microcephaly, bone marrow disease, transient long bone abnormalities.

For proper follow-up of a suspected rubella infant, see Chapter 2.

Planning The Infant's Diet

Breast Feeding

During the first 8 hr, give nothing by mouth. Start breast feeding on the second day with 5 min feedings QID, alternating breasts. After feedings, offer 5 percent glucose water. On the third, fourth and fifth day increase feeding time to 10 min six times a day. After the fifth day increase feeding time to 20 min. Do not exceed 30 min. Continue six feedings per day until the fourth week then discontinue the 2 AM feeding. Premature infants have more cellular fluid and poorer kidney function than mature infants, therefore delay oral feedings until the thirty-sixth to seventy-second hour. The main advantages of breast feeding are lower mortality; improved resistence to infection; better acceptance and tolerance; lower solute load and greater margin of expendable water and breast cancer protection for the mother.

Formulas

During the first 8 hr, give nothing by mouth. Between 8 and 24 hr, offer two feedings of 30 ml (1 oz) of 5 percent glucose water and follow with the third feeding of 30 to 60 ml (1 to 2 oz) of half strength formula six times a day for 10 min. Have the mother or the nurse hold the infant for each feeding. On the third, fourth and fifth days increase the formula to full strength and the quantity to 60 to 90 ml (2 to 3 oz) six times a day for 15 min. After the fifth day, adjust the amount of formula to the infant's demand. Continue six times a day for 4 weeks, then discontinue the 2 AM feeding.

EVAPORATED MILK. This offers flexibility that prepared formulas do not provide. If necessary the physician can vary the type and quantity of carbohydrates; if stools are loose, reduce carbohydrates; if stools are hard, increase carbohydrates. The most frequently used carbohydrates are Dexin, Dextra Maltose (Mead Johnson), granulated sugar, honey, Karo syrup and lactose. Keep in mind that Dextra Maltose is 4 T/oz; sugar and Karo are 2 T/oz.

The following is a simple method for preparing formula. For an 11 pound baby proceed as follows:

calculate total fluid needs:
  2½ oz/lb body weight (about 28 oz)
calculate amount of milk:
  –evaporated milk
    body weight x 1 oz = 11 oz
  –for whole milk
    body weight x 2 oz = 22 oz
calculate amount of water to add:
  –evaporated milk
    total fluid—evaporated milk or 17 oz
  –whole milk
    total fluid—whole milk or 6 oz
calculate needed carbohydrates:
  always add 1 oz

Evaporated Milk	11 oz
Water	17 oz
Dextra Maltose	1 oz (4T)
Whole Milk	22 oz
Water	6 oz
Dextra Maltose	1 oz

Some physicians prefer larger amounts of sugar and will give 1 oz up to 10 lb, 1¼ oz to 12 lb, and 1½ oz after 12 lb. Then later when the infant is taking other carbohydrates in solid foods, the carbohydrate is reduced to 1 oz.

PREPARED MILK FORMULAS. Prepared formulas on the market are Baker's (Roerig), Bremil (Borden), Enfamil (Mead Johnson), S-M-A s/26 (Wyeth) and Similac (Ross).

Mix all standard prepared milk formulas similarly: One T or one measure of the powder to 2 oz water or equal parts of liquid formula and water. These will all provide approximately 20 cal per oz. Start with 2½ oz per pound of body weight per day, and adjust quantity to infant's demands.

STERILIZATION. Sterilization of formula and bottles is important especially when the purity of the water supply is in question or the family's hygiene is poor. Terminal sterilization is convenient and probably most effective. Many physicians discontinue sterilization when prepared milk formulas are used and if the feeding is prepared in clean bottles at time of feeding.

A recent Philadelphia study[10] of mothers who prepared their infant's formula by an aseptic technique demonstrated contamination with enteric organisms in approximately 50 percent of formulas in bottles and in more than 50 percent of formulas stored in bulk containers.

STOOL EXAMINATION. The color, consistency and frequency of the infant's stools vary from infant to infant and change with increasing age. A doctor should know the difference between the stools of a breast fed and an artificially fed infant.

The breast fed infant's stools are soft, tend to be yellow-green in color and are of relatively low pH (4 to 6). Defecation occurs three or four times a day although stools may vary from eight per day to one every other day. Appearance is of greater significance than frequency. The stool flora contains Lactobacillus bifidus, a fermentative organism.

The artificially fed infant's stools are firmer than the breast fed infant's and yellow-brown in color. The Ph is alkaline (6.5 to 8.7). The stools have a fecal odor because of the mixed flora including putrefactive, fermentative and coliform organisms engendered by cow's milk.

The main difference in the two types of milk lies in the higher lactose content of mother's milk. Lactose supports the growth of the Lactobacillus with production of acid stools. The inoffensive odor comes from the fermentation of carbohydrates rather than the putrefaction of protein. The breast fed has more stools and they are softer because of the ease with which the softer stools are moved through the colon.

Examination of stools are a good indicator of how well the formula is agreeing with the infant.

SPITTING UP. A cause of spitting is inadequate burping. Teach mothers to burp their babies halfway through the feedings and again at the end.

Reduce air swallowing by using disposable plastic bottle inserts that collapse during feeding, valves that allow feeding by biting the nipples as well as by sucking and wing-type nipples that keep air from entering the sides of the baby's mouth.

COLIC. New mothers frequently complain of colicky infants and a family doctor should develop a routine of diagnosis and treatment. First do a thorough history and physical examination to rule out organic causes of paroxysmal pain. Determine whether the child is hungry by closely checking the infant's weight gain. Other signs of underfeeding are constipation, irritability and the sucking of his fingers or hands.

Investigate the mother's feeding technique, the mechanics of nursing. Is the nipple hole too large or too small? Does the infant empty the bottle and swallow air?

Is the positioning of the baby correct? Is the infant burped properly? Is the nipple placed deeply enough in the infant's mouth? What of the mother's emotional state?

Change formulas if necessary. Eliminate added carbohydrates and butterfat; substitute a demineralized (electrodialyzed) whey protein formula (Similac PM 60/40) SMA/S-26; or remove cow's milk protein by using milk substitutes (Similac Isomil; Soyalac).

Whole Milk

Give whole milk when the baby's weight reaches 15 or 16 lb, even if this occurs before the fourth month. Most physicians change to whole milk when the baby is 4 to 6 mo old.

Vitamins

Artificially fed infants may require supplements of vitamins C and D since cow's milk contains low levels of both. Breast fed infants often require supplements of vitamin D, especially if they are not adequately exposed to sunlight.

ORANGE JUICE OR VITAMIN C. Introduce orange juice anytime after the second week. A convenient time is following the baby's first office call when 3 to 4 weeks old.

If the baby reacts to orange juice (regurgitates or develops a rash) give a vitamin C supplement. (Ce-vi-Sol, Mead Johnson, 0.3 ml or 25 mg, later increasing to 0.6 ml or 50 mg.)

VITAMINS A AND D. Start vitamin A and D on the first office visit at 3 to 4 weeks. A commonly used preparation is Mead Johnson's Poly-vi-Sol. 0.6 ml supplies vitamin A, 3000 units and vitamin D, 400 units. This preparation also has significant quantities of thiamine, riboflavin and niacinamide. Begin with one drop on the baby's tongue and increase by one drop daily until infant receives 0.6 ml daily.

TOXIC VITAMINS. Three vitamins are toxic if supplied in large doses: A, D and menadione, an artifically synthesized type of K. Vitamin A should not exceed 4,000 units daily, to avoid toxic manifestations such as skin lesions, enlargement of the liver, hyperirritability, retarded or arrested bone growth and bone spurs. With normal infants, limit vitamin D intake to 400 units daily. Excessive vitamin D may induce hypercalcemia with calcifaction of tissues and renal damage.

In geographical areas where the fluoride content of drinking water is below 0.7 ppm, Poly-vi-Flor may be substituted for Poly-vi-Sol. Poly-vi-Flor is similar to Poly-vi-Sol plus 0.5 mg of fluoride per 0.6 ml. Calculate dosage for specific areas after determining the fluoride content of the area's drinking water. Do not give more than one ppm including drinking water and supplement. Do not use in children with dental fluorosis. Keep the bottle out of the reach of children.

In one study of 350 children given fluoride and 350 given only the regular vitamins A and D,[11] there were 57 percent less cavities in the fluoride group by age 3. By 7 and 8 the incidence of decay was reduced 70 to 80 percent in those receiving fluoride.

Solid Foods

Start solid foods when 30 oz of formula in 24 hr does not satisfy the infant. This usually occurs when the baby is about 12 lb and is between 2½ and 3½ months of age. Some researchers believe that semisolid foods do not become a useful source of nutrition until the infant is 4 to 6 mo old, but it may be given earlier to accustom the infants to foods other than milk.

Begin solid foods with cereals, preferably rice, barley or oatmeal. Rice probably is the least allergenic. Mix one tsp to 30 ml (1 oz) of formula and increase by ½ tsp daily until the baby receives 4 tsp to 30 ml (1 oz). Give cereal feedings twice daily, before the morning and evening formula feedings. Forcing semisolids before the ninth to twelfth week tends to increase the incidence of feeding problems and food dislikes in the infant.

Appropriate first fruits are bananas, pears and apples given after the cereal, morning and evening feedings. If stools are hard, prunes, apricots and plums may help. Begin only one new food each week. Start fruits at 4 mo.

Appropriate first vegetables are potatoes (first choice), squash, carrots, beets, spinach and broccoli started at the midday meal. Start vegetables at 5 mo.

Start strained meats and egg yolk last (6 mo) at midday along with vegetables. Lamb is less likely and pork or liver the most likely to cause a reaction. The following is a list of meats in order of their frequency of reaction: lamb, veal, liver, chicken, beef, bacon and pork.

For desserts use jello and nonchocolate junket with the main meal until near the end of the first year. Introduce eggs near the end of the year with custards, puddings and ice cream.

Potentially allergic foods: fish oils, orange juice, wheat, corn, eggs, tomatoes, leguminous vegetables and chocolate.

	Weight Gain
Birth to 3 mo	approximately 2 lb/mo (1 oz/day)
4 to 6 mo	approximately 1 lb/mo (½ oz/day)
4 to 6 mo	Double birth weight
1 yr	Triple birth weight

Supplementary Iron

The American Academy of Pediatrics has issued the following guidelines for the prescribing of iron: by the time an infant is 2 mo old, he should have a daily intake of 1 mg of iron/kg of body weight to a maximum of 15 mg/day. Meet this requirement by including in the diet iron-enriched infant cereals and milk formulas. (Similac w/iron, Ross; Enfamil w/iron, Mead Johnson).

In cases of low birth weight or those infants with low hemoglobin levels, give 2 mg of iron/kg of body weight by the third month. Ordinary infant diets will not meet this quota; therefore medicinal iron should be prescribed and continued for a month after a normal hemoglobin has been attained. (Chel-Iron Pediatric Drops, 25 mg elemental iron per ml, Kinney).

Salt

Mothers often ask whether to salt baby's food. Fomon and his associates[12] have studied the effect of salted and unsalted diets and have come to the following conclusion: cow's milk supplies three times as much sodium as human milk and unsalted strained foods have more sodium than does human milk. Consequently, there is no justification for adding salt to the baby's strained foods.

Congenital Heart Disease

The family physician should remember a few aphorisms regarding congenital heart disease. Nine tenths of the murmurs heard among newborns will disappear. Many newborns' murmurs are functional or represent an open foramen ovale or a patent ductus arteriosus and will fade as the pulmonary circuit pressure falls.

There will be times when the family physician will not know he is dealing with a serious cardiac defect until cyanosis or congestive failure develops. The diagnosis seldom is made before these overt signs appear.

Congenital heart disease more commonly affects the right side of the heart than the left. The heart chambers are often paired, the right side with low pressure and low oxygen content. Consequently shunting of blood from left to right does not cause cyanosis, while shunting from right to left does. A few congenital lesions do not produce shunting but cause other cardiac disabilities such as coarctation of the aorta, aortic and subaortic stenosis, primary endocardial fibroelastosis and vascular rings (double aortic arch).

Systolic murmurs by themselves rarely indicate the presence of valvular heart disease. In significant systolic murmurs, search for a thrill, a coexistent diastolic murmur, a history of a rheumatic infection, enlargement of the heart, signs of an overactive heart and changes in the heart sounds. Because the right heart is more commonly affected, increases or decreases in pulmonary artery flow are important.

This is best evaluated by listening to the pulmonary second sound and recording reduplication or splitting of the second sound.

Although murmurs are not always helpful, loud abnormal heart sounds are. Together with a rapid rate, unusual heart sounds may constitute the first sign of a serious congenital defect. Consider any abnormal heart sound which persists beyond 12 hours from birth as a warning.

Symptoms are important. Cyanosis in the newborn is more commonly due to pulmonary problems or cerebral damage than heart disease. Deep cyanosis that does not improve with oxygen and worsens on crying should cause suspicion of a right-to-left shunt. Order x-rays and electrocardiograms. Although the tetralogy of Fallot may not cause cyanosis until the third to sixth month, the patient may suffer apneic and blue episodes but not cardiac failure. Pulmonary stenosis, however, may cause cardiac failure after an insidious cyanosis.

Apnea may be from pulmonary or cardiac causes but, if associated with a tachycardia and/or hepatomegaly, cardiac failure is likely. Aortic stenosis is the most common cause of failure in the first week of life.

Edema is not common but when it is present check for coarctation of the aorta by arm and leg blood pressure measurements.

Functional Murmur

In infants and children, listen for functional murmurs over the great vessels left of the sternal border in the second and third interspaces and above the right clavicle. Auscultate in the neck and find the murmur's point of maximum intensity (PMI). When listening to a functional murmur, pressure over the artery at the murmurs PMI will cause the murmur to decrease or disappear altogether. The same diminution of sound will occur on moving the baby's head from one side to another.

In other instances, a common systolic functional murmur along the left sternal border will decrease if firm pressure is made over the area with the hand. Elicit the same effect in an older child by having him hold his head up while lying in a supine position. This position will fix the thorax and minimize any vibratory reverberations in the chest.

Types of Congenital Heart Disease (Table 3-4)

It is difficult to describe the five most common congenital heart lesions. The family physician must recognize that the severity of the lesions may vary from a maximum to a minimum degree and with each degree of change the infant's signs and symptoms will vary in gravity. Consequently, the examiner will find few typical clinical pictures. In addition, many entities do not occur in pure form but in combinations, again altering the typical findings. Therefore descriptions of the cardiac anomalies vary from author to author depending on these variables.

If a family physician has made a reasonably secure diagnosis as subsequently outlined, the decision to refer for cardiac catheterization depends on the clinical impact of the disease. Seldom does asymptomatic heart disease require cardiac catheterization.

VENTRICULAR SEPTAL DEFECTS. Common concurrence cites ventricular septal defects as the most common congenital heart disease. The infant is often asymptomatic and the examiner may miss the diagnosis because he may not hear the murmur until the third or fourth month. When audible, a systolic murmur can be heard left of the sternal border in the fourth and fifth interspace, which radiates into the upper chest and into the back. The murmur rapidly becomes loud, harsh, high pitched and holosystolic in time. A thrill usually accompanies the murmur.

Listen to the heart sounds for an important differential point: in an uncomplicated ventricular septal defect, a wide splitting of the second sound, which varies physiologically with respiration, is distinguishable. Inspiration delays P_2 and widens the degree of splitting while expiration narrows the A_2 to P_2 interval and quickens the splitting. Electrocardiographic, roentgeno-

Table 3-4. Types of Congenital Heart Disease Listed in Order of Frequency

Noncyanotic types	*Cyanotic types*
Ventricular septal defect[1]	Tetralogy of Fallot[2]
Persistent ductus arteriosus[1]	Complete transposition of great vessels[2]
Auricular septal defect[1]	Pulmonary stenosis with auricular septal defect[2]
Coarctation of aorta[3]	Pulmonary stenosis with ventricular septal defect[2]
Pulmonary stenosis	Eisenmenger's complex[2]
Aortic and subaortic stenosis[3]	Tricuspid atresia[2]
Primary endocardial fibroelastosis[3]	Persistent truncus arteriosis[2]
Idiopathic dilatation of pulmonary artery	Levocardia
Vascular rings (double aortic arch)[3]	
Aortic pulmonary window[1]	

[1]Left to right shunt; pulmonary markings increased
[2]Right to left shunt
[3]No shunting

graphic and fluoroscopic findings are important aids to diagnosis.

In managing ventricular septal defects, the family physician should have two concerns—possible heart failure and development of pulmonary hypertension and pulmonary vessel pathology.

At this point x-ray pictures may be helpful because the chief characteristic of the cardiac shadow will be an increase in the size of the pulmonary artery and its central and peripheral branches. A hypoplastic aortic knob will be associated. Fluoroscopically there will be vigorous pulsation of the pulmonary arteries. A diastolic murmur ushers in pulmonary artery involvement.

Fortunately many infants with ventricular septal defects improve and pulmonary complications do not develop. Solicit specialty help and possibly a cardiac catheterization (1) if the right ventricle enlarges, (2) if the EKG indicates an abnormal right ventricle hypertrophy and, (3) if the second sound in the second left interspace becomes brisker and accentuated. Symptoms which suggest need for consultation: severe hypoxemia, failure to thrive, paroxysmal dyspnea, decreasing murmur and rising hematocrit.

If cardiac signs and symptoms persist, surgical closure of defect is indicated between 5 and 6 years of age.

ISOLATED PULMONARY STENOSIS. This is about the fourth most common cause of congenital heart disease. We will discuss it in juxtaposition with ventricular septal defects because of the difficulty of distinguishing between the two in the newborn. Both anomalies present with loud, harsh systolic murmurs to the left of the sternal border. The murmur of pulmonary stenosis, however, is higher along the border, and in older children becomes localized in the second interspace. A thrill does not accompany the murmur of pulmonary stenosis as often as in ventricular septal defects. There are no diastolic murmurs.

The first heart sound is usually normal. Listen for an ejection click in the pulmonary area in early systole. This click may decrease as the disease progresses. While the disease is mild, the second heart sound may split in both phases of respiration but widen with inspiration as the stenosis tightens. In the severe forms of stenosis the second sound may become almost audible.

As the infant grows, x-ray findings become more helpful. Poststenotic dilatation of the pulmonary artery and its left main branches are classic x-ray findings in this condition. Fluoroscopically, the dilated pulmonary artery always has increased pulsations. In infants, the x-ray reveals decreased pulmonary vascular markings. Right ventricular and atrial enlargements are fairly consistent findings in functionally significant pulmonary stenosis.

Clinically, pulmonary stenosis may lead to cardiac failure following an insidious cyanosis. Other symptoms suggesting need for consultation are: persistent, intractable congestive heart failure and severe, recurrent lower respiratory tract infections.

The outlook varies from a normal lifespan for patients with minimal lesions to acute right heart failure in those with maximal lesions. Surgery offers complete relief from the obstructive symptoms and can be performed at any age.

ATRIAL SEPTAL DEFECT. The second most common cause of congenital heart disease is atrial septal defect. Rarely does the malformation cause a murmur loud enough to deserve investigation for three or four years.

One fact will help the family physician understand the pathophysiology of the findings in atrial septal defects: the flow of blood through the septal defect is silent and does not account for any of the auscultatory findings. The increased blood flow through the right cardiac chamber and pulmonary arterial tree produce all the sounds. Consequently, listen for a systolic ejection murmur loudest over the second and third interspaces adjacent to the left sternal border. In all likelihood the murmur comes from an increased blood flow across a normal pulmonary valve. As the disease progresses listen for two diastolic murmurs along the sternal border from dilatation of the pulmonary artery and pulmonary valve ring.

Patients with an atrial septal defect usually have a loud first heart sound over the apical area. But more important and virtually pathognomonic is the detection of a fixed splitting of the second heart sound not affected by respiration.

Again the electrocardiogram, x-ray and fluoroscopic examinations may help confirm the diagnosis of left-to-right shunt. As with the ventricular septal defect and a patent ductus the x-ray examination discloses an increase in the size of the main pulmonary artery and its central and peripheral branches. Again, the examiner will find the anomaly associated with a hypoplastic aortic knob and pulsations of the pulmonary arteries as determined fluoroscopically. Again, signaling the need for consultation are cyanosis, failure to thrive, paroxysmal dyspnea, decreasing murmur and a rising hematocrit.

The defect in the midposition of the atrial septum (foramen secundum defect) requires open-heart surgery only if cardiac enlargement is progressive. Have the defect in the lower portion of the septum (ostium primum defect), surgically corrected preferably at 5 to 8 years of age as it carries a poorer prognosis.

TETRALOGY OF FALLOT. This is the third most common cause of congenital heart disease. Frequently the cyanosis of this malformation does not appear until the third to sixth month of life. This anomaly commonly causes apneic and cyanotic episodes rather than cardiac failure because of the shunting of unsaturated blood from the right ventricle directly into the aorta. The cyanosis deepens and dyspnea occurs with increased activity. Fainting due to cerebral hypoxia is not uncommon. After exertion, these children assume a squatting position. Watch for clubbing of the fingers and toes as well as a polycythemia.

The tetralogy of Fallot comprises four defects:

- pulmonary stenosis, involving either the infundibular outflow tract of the right ventricle or the pulmonary valve or both
- right ventricular hypertrophy, secondary to pulmonary stenosis
- a defect high in the membranous portion of the interventricular septum
- overriding of the aortic arch

The systolic ejection-type murmur heard along the left sternal border at or near the third interspace has its origin in the stenotic area of the right ventricular infundibulum or pulmonary valve. The tetralogy has no diastolic murmurs. The heart sounds do not have any audible characteristics except a diminution of the second sound in the pulmonic area.

Unfortunately, from the diagnostic standpoint, the x-ray manifestations of tetralogy of Fallot are variable. The degree of pulmonary stenosis varies. Only about 20 percent of tetralogies present a so-called typical picture. They are:

- –coeur-en-sabot configuration with elevation of the cardiac apex
- –clear lung fields with flat or concave pulmonary artery segment
- –right-sided aortic arch

Early in infancy, nearly all cases will show electrocardiographically either a right ventricular hypertrophy or right bundle branch block or both.

There are two complications which occur with the tetralogy not commonly seen in other types of congenital heart disease: cerebral thrombosis and brain abscess. Consequently treat infections promptly and check hemoglobin levels occasionally.

If syncope occurs before the age of 4, consider Blalock's procedure as palliative treatment. Suggest open heart repair of the defects after 4 years of age.

PATENT DUCTUS ARTERIOSUS. This is the fifth most common congenital heart lesion. The ductus of Botalli may not close until the second year of life. The degree of disability varies with the diameter of the ductus. A bounding pulse should make the examiner suspicious of a patent ductus. Listen for a systolic murmur soon after birth. The diastolic component may not become audible until the sixth to twelfth month of life. The murmur is a characteristic, continuous, harsh machinerylike murmur louder during systole and radiating upward into the chest. Watch for the murmur along the left of the sternum in the second and third interspaces. A palpable thrill accompanies the murmur. Again, the x-ray discloses increased pulmonary arterial vascularity with an enlargement of the pulmonary artery segment, an increase in vascular pulsation, and cardiac enlargement all in various combinations. A radiologist should interpret the x-ray to help differentiate the anomaly from other malformations that cause increased pulmonary arterial vascularity. Have every patent ductus closed, even if asymptomatic after the child is 2 years of age. If, however, cardiac failure occurs at any age have the appropriate diagnostic studies done. After verification, advise surgical closure.

The Family Physician's Responsibility

The family physician has a weighty responsibility to the patient and his family besides making the diagnosis and managing the cardiac abnormality. His responsibilities include the treatment of infections; preventive inoculations; and guidance in diet, activity, discipline and schooling. Offer this medical guidance without creating undue alarm, especially when anxiety is unnecessary.

A child with congenital heart disease will voluntarily limit his activities. Allow the patient with pulmonary stenosis, atrial septal defect, coarctation, patent ductus arteriosus or mild ventricular defects to choose his own activity level as long as his choices are within the bounds of good hygiene. One exception: vigorous exercise in aortic stenosis may cause sudden death, especially in adolescence.

In infancy, in order to combat fatigue, suggest easily digested formulas every 3 hr instead of the usual 4. Give vitamins and supplementary iron, keeping the hematocrit around 50 to 60 percent if possible.

Encourage the parents to teach these children proper discipline. Brief periods of crying do not harm the child with congenital heart disease. Naturally, parents tend to spoil a child who has dyspnea or cyanosis. From a disciplinary standpoint most parents find assurance in learning that the child can be treated like normal siblings.

Give immunizations on schedule. Treat respiratory infections promptly. Do not hesitate to use prophylactic penicillin, 200,000 units twice daily. Treat other congenital or acquired defects as indicated using sound principles and preventive antibiotic preparation. Do tonsillectomies when indicated.

Most parents of children with congenital heart disease appreciate genetic counseling. They find reassurance in knowing that subsequent children may not inherit the disease. On the other hand, if a genetic hazard does exist, parent's value the opportunity to make their own choice.

General Indications for Complete Cardiac Study in Infancy[13]

- –significant cardiac enlargement
- –cardiac failure
- –cyanosis
- –apneic spells
- –growth failure (not based on a nutritional or other congenital defect)
- –marked right or left ventricular strain on EKG or a changing EKG pattern
- –severe repeated respiratory infections with evidence of heart disease or wheezing in infancy

Prevention of Congenital Heart Disease

The incidence of CHD is 6 to 8 per 1000 live births, and the prevalence is 2 to 6 per 1000 school age children. In 95 percent of the cases, the cause is not known. The causes of the other 5 percent are known and prevention is definitely in order. The family physician's responsibility lies in preventing exposure to environmental teratogens such as licit and illicit drugs, rubella, virus infections and irradiation.

The family physician should advise parents who have had a child with a congenital heart lesion to seek genetic counseling. A threefold risk exists for subsequent children born to the parents.

Continuing personal and community education by the family physician should point out the hazards of general environmental irradiation, poor radiologic technique which does not protect the gonads nor the embryo's heart, languishing rubella immunization program, needless medications during pregnancy and drug abuse.

Transporting Infants and Children by Automobile

Burg and others[14] reported as many children between the ages of 1 and 15 died of the effects of automobile accidents as of cancer in 1969. To combat this loss of life they recommend the following restraining devices for transporting children in automobiles.

For children up to 12 lb they suggest two plans. If an infant carrier is available put the child in the front seat. Place the carrier with the child's back toward the front of the car. The safety belt should hold the carrier in place.

If a carrier is not available place the infant in a car bed. Place the bed parallel to the car's axis and position the baby with his feet pointing toward the front of the car. Place a strong netting over the bed. Fasten the middle seat belts of the front and back seats. When once adjusted, leave the bed in place because of the difficulties in placing and removing.

For the child between 12 and 24 lb, two choices are also available. The toddler's seat, when fastened securely by the seat belt, does not give the child much freedom. Consequently most parents prefer an adequately designed safety harness which restrains the child across the high chest and pelvis. The harness design allows the child to stand or sit. The harness has a strong webbing which encloses the abdominal area and connects the chest and pelvic straps. Do not use the abdominal strap harness.

For children from 25 to 50 lb recommend a good safety childseat. A shield-type seat probably affords the best protection but limits what the child can see.

For children over 50 lb and less than 55 in tall, an adult type belt can be used.

Determining Children's Doses from Adult Doses

Family physicians too often prescribe medicine for children and infants without careful regard to dosage. Obviously children's dosages should be a fraction of an adult dose but merely dividing the adult dose by 2 or 4 is not accurate enough.

Ordering mg of drug/kg of body weight is a common rule and certainly far better than no rule at all. Better still is to determine dosage by body surface. In order to avoid the cumbersome arithmetic involved in arriving at dosage/sq meter, Table 3-5 may be consulted.

Table 3-5. Determination of Children's Doses from Adult Doses on the Basis of Body Surface Area

Age	*Weight**		*Surface area**	*Fraction of*
	(kg)	*(lb)*	*(sq M)*	*adult dose†*
	2.0	4.4	0.15	0.09
Birth	3.4	7.4	0.21	0.12
3 weeks	4.0	8.8	0.25	0.14
3 months	5.7	12.5	0.29	0.17
6 months	7.4	16	0.36	0.21
9 months	9.1	20	0.44	0.25
1 year	10	22	0.46	0.27
1½ years	11	25	0.50	0.29
2 years	12	27	0.54	0.31
3 years	14	31	0.60	0.35
4 years	16	36	0.68	0.39
5 years	19	41	0.73	0.42
6 years	21	47	0.82	0.47
7 years	24	53	0.90	0.52
8 years	27	59	0.97	0.56
9 years	29	65	1.05	0.61
10 years	32	71	1.12	0.65
11 years	36	78	1.20	0.70
12 years	39	86	1.28	0.74

*Approximate average for age
†Based on adult surface area of 1.73 sq M
Reprinted from Done AK: Drugs for Children in Modell W (ed): Drugs of Choice 1972–1973. St. Louis: C. V. Mosby Co, 1972, p. 55, with permission.

However, the AMA Drug Evaluations, 1971, warned there is no absolute rule for determining dosage. Even milligrams/square meter must be verified by clinical practice. The smaller the child the more care should be used in setting dosages.

Infant Foot and Leg Problems

A complete range of motion is present in a normal foot. If a foot appears to be deformed, attempt to place the foot in its normal position. A structural deformity is present if the examiner cannot correct the deformity with his hands.[15]

The Pigeon-toed Infant

CLUBFOOT (TALIPES EQUINOVARUS). Clubfoot occurs in about 1:1000 births. It is bilateral in about 50 percent of cases and twice as common in males. This abnormality will need correction. The family physician should refer the infant for immediate orthopedic correction which includes frequent casting, splinting and possibly surgery.

A number of clubfoot variations occur which should not present a troublesome differential diagnosis to the informed physician. In order not to overlook other pathology, first examine the infant's hip for the uncommon infantile anteversion of the femoral neck. With the child supine, rotate the hips inwardly and outwardly. With femoral anteversion the inward rotation may go as far as 90° but external rotation is limited. Treat with outflare shoes attached to an abduction bar during sleep. Rotation straps are useful and allow more motion. Rarely is casting needed.

Next check for internal tibial torsion which sometimes accompanies clubfoot or metatarsus adductus. Correcting poor sitting and sleeping positions may help correct tibial torsion. Draw a line from the iliac spine through the center of the patella; if there is no torsion the line will intersect the second toe. If tibial torsion is present the line will intersect the fourth or fifth toe.

As the child grows he attempts to compensate for pigeon-toeing by externally rotating his hips giving the appearance of bowleggedness. Another test: since the cause of this pigeon-toe-bowleg complex is below the knee, examine the child while sitting with his knees flexed and legs hanging over the edge of a table. With the patellae placed forward, the feet will turn toward each other 30 or 40°. Passively dorsiflexing the feet does not correct the deformity.[16]

For correction try a Denis-Browne splint with the feet in external rotation or a metal bar to which the infant's shoes are attached and externally rotated about 35°. For older children, nail a pair of old shoes to a ¼ in plywood board (10 in x 1 in) and have the brace worn while the child sleeps. For 24 hr use, suggest a Brackman skate. A child can wear this even while walking. Continue splinting for a month after correction.

If no evidence of the above described conditions (tibial torsion and infantile anteversion of the femoral head) exist, concentrate on metatarsus adductus or varus with or without tibial torsion. Occasionally metatarsus varus involves only the big toe and in this instance is called metatarsus varus primus.

METATARSUS VARUS. Diagnostic signs of metatarsus varus are: concave inner border of the foot, straight or convex outer border, and with knee caps forward the foot hangs in a varus position. A heel in a valgus position helps to establish diagnosis.

In the *flexible* metatarsus, if the inner concavity can be aligned with the ball of the foot or the foot overcorrected, put the right shoe on the left foot (outflared shoes) and vice versa for correction. More correction can be made with an internal tibial torsion bar. Overstretching by parental manipulation keeps the foot flexible.

For the *inflexible* metatarsus varus, the family physician may need speciality help. Apply a series of pressure casts changing them every two weeks and stretching the foot further and further into a normal position.

The following method is used in applying casts. Cast from toe to knee and apply adhesive liquid to keep cast from slipping. Wrap leg in 2 in webbing roll for protection and quickly wrap the leg with a 2 in plastic roll. As the cast dries, mold it correcting the deformity as much as possible. Hold the heel in the right hand and press into a neutral position, while the left hand pushes the forefoot out, overcorrecting if possible. When the plaster is hard enough to hold, wrap the leg in the second roll for reenforcement. Leave the toes visible for circulatory inspection. Change the cast every 2 weeks, overcorrecting each time for 3 to 4 months. Subsequently follow the treatment suggested for the flexible metatarsus varus.

Flatfeet

The most common pediatric foot problem is pes valgus (flatfeet); at least it is the most misdiagnosed. The question of pes valgus comes up when the child begins to walk. The condition is often over- or undertreated. The misconception stems from the foot's normal delay in forming a longitudinal arch until the child is about 2 years old. The diagnosis depends on observing eversion of the foot, prominent internal malleoli, and bowing or tightness of the Achilles tendon.

Generally no treatment is necessary but, if symptoms occur, simple exercises help. Teach older children to walk on the outer borders of their feet and on their toes and to spread their toes 5 minutes twice daily. Consider arch support only for the relief of symptoms. If considerable pronation is also present try an orthopedic shoe with a Thomas heel plus an additional ⅛ in wedge on the inner border of the heels until the child is 3. Check shoe wear from time to time. If wedging is satisfactory, the posterior lateral quadrant of the heel will wear down. More wedging is necessary if the wearing down is posterior or lateral.[17]

Congenital Dislocation of the Hip

Early treatment of congenital dislocation of the hip offers the only possibility of obtaining good results almost regularly (Fig. 3-6). The delay in ossification of the hip in this disease seems to be due to insufficient pressure of the femoral head into the acetabulum during fetal life. The condition occurs in females 8:1 and often is bilateral. Diagnostic signs are:

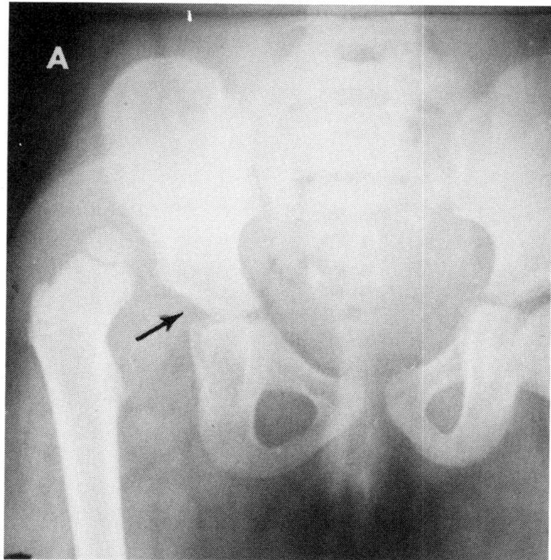

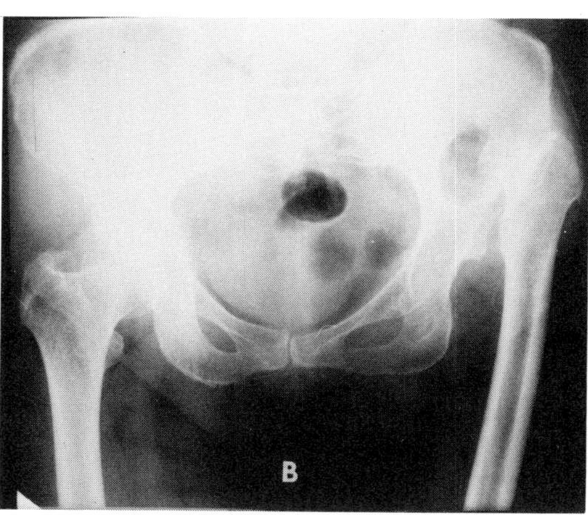

Figure 3-6. *A*,.Congenital dislocation of the hip; *B*, Dislocation of the hip in an adult. Diagnosis should be made as early as possible for optimum therapy.

- –asymmetric skin folds on the posterior thighs, particularly in female infants
- –limited abduction of the flexed thigh
- –inequality of knee height
- –Ortolani's snapping or clicking sign

The latter unequivocally denotes early dislocation. Eliciting the sign requires no special skill. Simply grasp the infant's thigh with thumb on inner side of the upper thighs and middle finger over the great trochanter and lift the great trochanter. This maneuver will reduce a dislocated hip with a visible movement and a palpable click.

Take x-rays to prove the diagnosis. Have the x-ray films interpreted by a specialist.

Diagnosis should be made in the first few weeks of life. If so, the wearing of an abduction brace with the legs in 90° flexion and 70° abduction for 2 to 4 months will cure most cases. Seek consultation. Consider traction before splinting. A diagnosis made after the child begins to walk requires the attention of an orthopedic specialist familiar with the problem.

How to Tell Whether a Child's Shoe Fits

Mothers usually consult the family physician prior to buying the child's first shoes. Be prepared to tell the parents how to select proper fitting shoes.

The length of a child's shoe should permit free movement of the toes. Allowing ½ to ¾ in from the tip of the longest toe to the tip of the shoe during weight bearing gives enough room for the toes as well as space for growth. The shoe with a rounded toe gives more toe space.

Have the width determined while the child is standing. The widest width of shoe which does not allow wrinkling across the top of the metatarsophalangel area should be chosen. The shoe will be about ¼ in wider than the foot.

The ball of the shoe should fit the ball of the foot, the first metatarsal head resting at the point of rounding of the medial aspect of the sole.

A properly fitted shoe should fit the foot trimly. There should be no large wrinkles running from one point to another. Palpate the heads of the first metatarsal bones to see if there is too much tension on the leather at these points and to determine if the first metatarsal head is at the point of rounding at the medial aspect of the sole. Lines running straight across the shoe should indicate the break of the shoe when the foot is bent. Ascertain the position of the distal ends of the first and second toes by palpation or by asking the child to force his toes against the shoe top. Examine the shoe at the heel to see if it clings properly.

If one foot is larger than the other, either broader or longer or both, fit the shoes to the larger foot. Have the mother check the fit of the shoe often. As soon as the toes come within ¼ in of the end of the shoe buy larger shoes.

Immunization

Don't give vaccines to a child with an acute infection. To prevent convulsions, wait until a cerebrally damaged child is past 1 year of age. Don't give measles or smallpox vaccine to anyone receiving antimetabolite or steroid therapy. Don't vaccinate a child for smallpox if he has a skin eruption.

DPT

Give diphtheria, pertussis and tetanus combination vaccine at 2 mo of age. Repeat twice before the infant is 6 mo old and at intervals of 4 to 8 wk. Give boosters at 18 mo and again before the child goes to school. Administer 0.5 ml doses intramuscularly in the anterolateral thigh. DPT given subcutaneously increases the frequency of reactions. This basic DPT course will produce 100 percent immunity to diphtheria and tetanus and 85 percent immunity to pertussis. Introduction of the basic course of immunization may be continued where interrupted anytime within 9 mo.

Immunize children with cerebral damage after 1 year of age and then give immunizations individually, administering pertussis last.

Do not give the adult type DT under 6 yr of age, and only the adult type DT after 8 yr of age.

The recommended intervals between boosters is 10 yr. If injury occurs give a tetanus booster after 4 yr. In the event of injury and if prior active immunization cannot be verified, give human tetanus antitoxin and penicillin as the primary means of preventing tetanus.

Oral Polio

Use a live trivalent oral polio vaccine (OPV) following the DPT schedule. Start the initial OPV series at 2 mo, giving the second and third dose before the infant is 6 mo old and at 6- to 8-wk intervals. Give the fourth dose at 18 mo and a fifth when the child enters school. After this last dose at age 5, do not give more routine boosters.

Give boosters to those at increased risk because of their contact with a known case, those planning to visit areas where polio is epidemic or those employed in a hospital, medical laboratory or sanitation facility when poliomyelitis is present in the area.

Measles and Rubella (MR) or Measles, Mumps and Rubella (MMR)

At present controversy exists over which combination is the wisest to give. A simple dose or rubella vaccine should provide long-term immunity for about 98 percent of inoculated children. The major objective now is to routinely immunize girls and boys in the 1-to-12 age group, and susceptible women of childbearing age on an individual and selective basis. A history of rubella infection does not negate the need for vaccination.

CRITERIA FOR RUBELLA VACCINATION OF WOMEN IN THE CHILDBEARING AGE. First test for susceptibility by performing a rubella hemagglutination-inhibition test. If the patient is immune do not vaccinate; if susceptible, vaccinate only those women who can avoid pregnancy during the subsequent 2 mo.

Failure of the rubella vaccination may result from immunizing children before 12 mo of age when maternal antibodies are still present. Failure also results from using vaccine virus inactivated by inadequate refrigeration or excessive exposure to light or by using a diluent containing a virucidal preservative.

Adverse reactions occur in up to 15 percent of vaccinated children. The incidence of joint reactions with Rubella Virus Vaccine, Live, and Rubelogen (HPV-77 dog kidney cell vaccine) is as high as 7 to 15 percent compared to the 5 percent reported by Meruvax (HPV-77 strain cultured in duck embryo cells) or Cedevax (Cendehill strain attenuated in rabbit kidney cells). When reactions occur, joint symptoms, or nonjoint pain and paresthesia in arms, hands or in the popliteal fossae, begin 2 to 10 days after immunization. With the less reactive vaccines, the symptoms persist for 1 to 3 days.

The live attenuated virus vaccine is 95 percent effective in producing rubella antibodies.

Mumps

Mumps vaccine is now being added to the immunization routine. The vaccine is safe and nontransmissable and gives virtually 100 percent protection for at least three years. Some physicians are giving the vaccine only to prepubertal males with no history of the disease. They argue that if the vaccine does not confer life-long immunity, the child may be left vulnerable to mumps later in life when complications are much more serious.

With the above in mind, the family physician must choose whether he prefers to give the rather noncontroversial MR or the more controversial MMR (see above). Perhaps more definite guidelines will be forthcoming shortly. In any event give one dose of MR or MMR after the infant is 1-yr old. Although polio may be given with DPT, it should not be given closer than a month to MR or MMR.

The mumps virus is grown on chicken virus, consequently the vaccine is contraindicated in persons sensitive to eggs or to neomycin. Immunization with live vaccine on the day of exposure will probably not protect against mumps but no harm results from the administration.

Measles

The vaccine is a live further attenuated (Schwarz) strain. Give without gamma globulin. This vaccine is 95 percent effective and antibodies continue undiminished through 6½ years. Five percent of those immunized will develop a rash and 15 percent may have a fever of 103° F or more. The Edmonston strains cause even a higher percentage of reactions. Inactivated measles vaccines should not be used.

An occasional child may have an undiagnosed tuberculosis which may be aggravated by measles immunization. A wise routine then is to tuberculin skin test a child before immunizing him to measles. Measles immunization given the patient within the first 24 hours after exposure may prevent the disease. After 24 hours give gamma globulin (0.25 ml/kg) to prevent measles. Actively immunize the child 6 weeks later.

Table 3-6 lists other vaccines that may be given in occasional overseas travel, epidemics, and emergencies.

THE CHILD

Developmental Landmarks of the Normal Child[19]

Study the developmental landmarks in Table 3-7. Variations from these norms may be the first clues to the diagnosis of such conditions as cerebral palsy, hemiplegia, mental retardation and defective vision. From birth to age 1, the mildly retarded are often difficult or impossible to assess because of variations in developmental patterns. Children who will develop familial retardation usually remain within normal ranges in their first year.

The Visually Handicapped Child

The Snellen Test

The vision screening test most widely used is the Snellen test. Use the test to check the distant and central visual acuity. The examiner can detect almost all cases of

Table 3-6. Vaccines Occasionally Employed for Active Immunization

Disease	*Produce*	*Live*	*Killed/ Toxoid*	*Dosage and Route*	*Hazards*
Cholera	Bacterial suspensions, fluid		X	Three doses 7 to 10 days apart SC 6 mo to 3 yr: 0.06, 0.12, 0.12ml 3 to 6 yr: 0.12, 0.25, 0.25ml over 6 yr: 0.25, 0.5, 0.5ml	None
Influenza	Multivalent chick grown viruses		X	0.1ml ID two times, 14 days apart, or 0.5 ml SC	Do not use in children with egg allergy
Plague	Bacterial suspensions, fluid		X	6 mo to 3 yr: 0.06, 0.12, 0.12ml SC	None
Rabies	Rabbit brain or duck embryo fixed rabies virus		X	0.5 to 1.0ml SC each day for 14 to 21 days	1. Allergic reactions 2. Encephalopathies, not found with duck vaccine
Tuberculosis	BCG organisms	X		0.1ml ID	1. Do not use in premature or malnourished children under 3 years old. 2. Any tuberculin-positive child
Typhoid-Paratyphoid	Bacterial suspension, fluid		X	0.1ml ID, three times 1 to 3 weeks apart; annual booster	None
Typhus	Chick embryo grown R. prowazekii		X	6 mo. to 3 yr: 0.12 ml SC 3 to 6 yr: 0.25ml SC over 6 yr: 0.5ml SC	None
Yellow Fever	Chick embryo grown virus	X		0.5ml SC	Mild febrile reactions usually about seventh day

Adapted from Kempe CH: Current Status of immunization. Drug Therapy 1:49, 1971.

myopia (nearsightedness), some cases of astigmatism, and occasional cases of hyperopia (farsightedness).

The room or hallway should be large enough to hold the Snellen chart 20 feet from the patient to be tested. With the aid of a mirror the distance can be reduced to 10 feet. The recommended standard of illumination on the Snellen chart is 10 foot candles of evenly diffused light. Avoid glare and shadows on the chart. Be careful to position the chart so that the patient being tested will not be looking into a light such as that from a window or a lamp. Be able to raise or lower the chart to bring the "20" line on a level with the eyes of the pupil being tested.

In testing, adopt a standard routine by testing the right eye first. If the child wears glasses, first test with his glasses on and then test with the glasses removed. Test the vision in one eye at a time. Hold a small cover card 3 x 5 in, obliquely along the nose of the pupil covering the eye not being tested. Both eyes, the one being tested and the one covered by the card, are to remain open during the test. Start with the line having the larger symbols to help the child develop confidence in himself. Proceed to the lowest line the child can read. If no visual difficulty is suspected, start with the "50" line to expedite the testing. If the child responds readily and correctly to this line, then check his performance on the "20" line.

Record responses for the right and left eye separately. The response is recorded in the form of a fraction. The numerator is the distance the child stands from the chart; the denominator is the lowest line read satisfactorily by the child. Allow one mistake per line. If the child reads the "20" line at 20 feet, the fraction set down is 20/20 for the eye tested. If the "40" line is the lowest one the child reads, record the fraction 20/40. "R" indicates the right eye and "L" the left eye.

If the child wears glasses, record results for the test with his glasses on and with his glasses removed.

The Plus Sphere Test for Hyperopia

Test all children who do not wear glasses and who are able to read the "30" line or better on the Snellen test. Place the plus sphere glasses on the pupil (+1.50 lenses for primary children, +1.00 lenses for junior high school) and allow him to wear glasses for a few seconds before starting the test. This permits the relaxation of the muscles of accommodation. Ask the child to read only the "20" line on the chart at 20 feet from the Snellen chart. First test the right eye and then the left. Children wearing the plus sphere glasses should not be able to read the "20" line on the Snellen chart. A child who is able to read the "20" line through the plus sphere glasses may be significantly farsighted. Record FT (Falls test) if he is able to do so.

Referral to an Ophthalmologist

In the *Snellen test failure,* refer children 12 years of age or under with 20/40 vision or less in one or both eyes for a diagnostic examination, children under 12 years of age who miss more than one symbol on the "30" line with one or both eyes and children with unequal vision.

In *plus sphere test failures,* refer all children who are able to read the "20" line on the Snellen chart with either eye while wearing plus sphere lenses.

Classification of Blindness[20]

The blind: A minor who comes within either of the following descriptions: if his visual acuity in the better eye after the best correction is 20/200 or less or if his visual loss is so severe that for educational purposes, vision cannot be used as a major channel of learning.

The partially seeing: A minor who comes within either of the following descriptions: if his visual acuity is 20/70 or less in the better eye after the best correction and he can use vision as a major channel of learning or if his vision deviates from the normal to such an extent that, in the combined opinion of a qualified educator and either physician and surgeon or an optometrist, he can benefit from the special educational facilities provided partially seeing children.

The Child with Impaired Hearing

One of the first pieces of diagnostic equipment the family physician should buy is a pure-tone screening audiometer which has a minimum frequency range of 500, 1,000, 2,000, and 4,000 cycles per second. If the family physician wants to do more accurate diagnostic testing, he should purchase a pure-tone audiometer for general diagnostic purposes (for threshold testing, which can provide the basis for medical referral), a frequency range of 126 through 8,000 cps, and a masking circuit.

Every complete examination on a child should include audiometry testing. This simple examination, which the office nurse can give, will identify children with early hearing losses. Many hearing losses in school age children can be improved by the removal of hypertrophic tonsils and adenoids.

Most family physicians bungle the diagnosis of deafness or decreased hearing in infants. Even without special equipment, a diagnosis may be suspected when a child sleeps through unusual noise or there is delay in speech or normal voice sounds. A physician would do well to heed a mother's concern regarding the possibility. There are simple clinical tests: for the infant less than a few months old, the eye-blink or startle reflex to sudden loud sounds. After 7 months, some suspicion may develop by watching the child's searching for rattling paper out of his field of vision; and over one year, the visible response to the calling of his name.

Suspect deafness in a young child when there is a history indicating a high risk of hearing loss. The failure to turn or coo in response to ordinary sounds by six months of age or to respond to loud noises about the home should cause a suspicion of impaired hearing. As soon as a hearing loss is sus-

Table 3-7. Developmental Landmarks of the Normal Child

Age (months)	Equipment	Progress*
1		Briefly follows moving stimulus Regards examiner's face momentarily Holds head erect briefly when supported in upright position Avoids mildly annoying stimuli, i.e. cloth lightly placed over face *Lifts head slightly when prone* *Quieted when picked up*
2		Holds head erect with bobbing when supported in sitting position Eyes follow moving person *Vocalizes other than crying* *Smiles at times*
3		Follows moving objects with eyes in all planes Searches for sound with eyes Lifts head and chest when prone *Vigorous body movements* *Anticipates actively feeding upon sight of bottle* *Coos and chuckles*
4	pencil	Grasps pencil with both hands and holds briefly Follows moving object when held in sitting position Enjoys play activity *Rolls from side to side but not completely over* *Initiates smiling and laughs aloud*
6	cup, toys (spoon, tongue blade), mirror	Sits with minimal support with stable back and head Lifts cup Attempts to attain toy held beyond reach Responds to image in mirror Exploits possibilities of play material (hand-to-hand transfer, banging, transfer to mouth) *Rolls over, supine to prone position* *Babbles in more than two distinct sounds* *Differentiates strangers from family*
9	test-tube corks, toys	Uses thumb when grasping tiny objects Holds and manipulates two objects at a time Sits alone and can change position without falling *Says "mama" or "dada"* *Plays interpersonal games like peek-a-boo and pat-a-cake*
12	toys, cup, corks, metal or paper pillboxes or blocks	Hands toy to examiner when requested to do so Puts small objects in, and removes them from, cup Will retrieve hidden toy (under box, cup, or cloth) Stands with support and takes steps when supported *Uses 2 or 3 words in addition to "mama" and "dada"* *Gives affection* *Holds cup with assistance for taking fluids*

*Italicized items may be observed or reported by parent.
Adapted from Caldwell BM, Drachman RH: Comparability of three methods of assessing the developmental level of young infants. JAMA 191:153, 1965.

Table 3-7—*continued*

Age (months)	*Equipment*	*Progress**
15	blocks, narrow-neck bottle, small objects (pencil, eraser), paper and pencil, book with large single object on a page	Stack two pillboxes or blocks one on top of the other Can imitate placing small object into small bottle (aspirin-size object into bottle) and if demonstrated can "pour" object out of bottle Scribble by imitation Walks without support *Climbs onto stairs or low chair* *Uses about 5 words* *Shows interest in picture books*
18	chair, pulltoy	Walks well and runs a bit Can seat self and climb into chair *Walks with pulltoy* *Goes up and down stairs* *Likes to be read to and interested in picture books* *Bowel training reasonably established* *Uses about 10 words* *Handles spoon reasonably well and partially feeds self*
24	picture book, ball	Can deal with a few mechanical contrivances (door knob, faucet) Identifies a few simple pictures by name Asks for things (food, drink, toilet) by combination of words and gestures *Throws or kicks a ball* *Walks up and down stairs alone* *Sits and "reads" little picture books, turns pages by self* *Makes 2-to-3-word sentences* *Imitates household tasks* *Identifies familiar objects seen on TV* *Engages in play activities similar to those of playmate, i.e. parallel play* *Daytime bowel and bladder control established*
30	paper and pencil	Imitates vertical and horizontal strokes on paper Folds letter-size paper in half to make a little book (demonstrated) Repeats two digits (4-7, 6-3, 5-8) and at rate of one per second Walks on tiptoe (demonstrated) and stands briefly on one foot Relates experience in simple language Can tell name and age (if taught) *Uses pronouns* *Helps to dress and undress self* *Perceives certain dangerous situation (not likely to walk into moving swing, aware of street as danger zone)*
36	paper and pencil	Copies a circle reasonably well Repeats three unrelated digits (one correct out of three trials) Relates what produces certain actions (barks, flies in the sky, gets hot, etc.)—any appropriate answer acceptable Knows last name when asked by examiner Handles most of dressing including shoes and accessible buttons *Goes up and down stairs one foot on each stair* *Can be trusted in room alone for short periods* *Rides tricycle using pedals* *Understands sharing and taking turns*

pected, advise a thorough otologic and audiologic evaluation.

Classification of Decreased Hearing[21]

The deaf are those in whom the sense of hearing is nonfunctional for the ordinary purposes of life. This general group is made up of two classes based on the time the loss of hearing occurred: (1) The congenitally deaf (those born deaf) and (2) the adventitiously deaf (those born with normal hearing but in whom the sense of hearing became nonfunctional later through illness or injury).

Deafness. Hearing losses must vary from 70 to 75 decibels in the speech range to inability to distinguish more than one or two frequencies at the highest level of intensity in the better ear. This results in disability in acquiring speech and language through the sense of hearing, even when sound amplification is provided. Those whose hearing losses average 50 or more decibels in the speech range in the better ear and who had a sustained hearing loss from very early childhood are diagnosed by a hearing specialist as being deaf.

The severely hard of hearing. A minor who comes within any of the following: (1) He has a hearing loss in his better ear that is from 45 to 70 decibels in the speech range and, thus, he suffers delayed speech and language development to such an extent that it hampers his progress in a regular classroom. (2) He has a hearing loss in his better ear that averages more than 30 decibels in the speech range, the loss was sustained in babyhood or early childhood, and it has resulted in delayed speech and language development. (3) He has a hearing loss in his better ear that averages more than 30 decibels in the speech range, the loss has been diagnosed by a licensed physician and surgeon to be progressive in nature and the minor, as a result of delayed speech and hearing development, needs placement in a special day class or integrated program.

The moderately hard of hearing. A minor who: (1) has a hearing loss in the better ear of from 20 to 40 decibels in the speech range; (2) has speech or language impairment presumably associated with his hearing loss; (3) has loss interfering with his progress in a regular classroom; (4) has individual and educational needs that indicate placement in a remedial class; and (5) has been recommended by a licensed physician or surgeon, audiologist or speech teacher to receive remedial instruction.

Schools usually enroll these children in a regular classroom and give them supplementary help by a teacher specially trained to work with the hard-of-hearing. Some of these children will wear hearing aids, some will not. They may leave the classroom twice weekly to attend speech classes which include lip reading instructions. The hard-of-hearing child frequently becomes a behavior problem, and often, though not always, is educationally retarded one or two years.

Classroom environment is most important. Suggest to the child's teacher that the child be seated so that he can see the faces of his classmates with only slight turning of his head. In any event, he should always be able to see the teacher's face. He should not face direct light, for lip reading under these circumstances is almost impossible.

Family physicians should be alert to the aphasic child, the deaf mentally retarded child and the deaf cerebral palsied child. Some states require physicians to report any deaf or hard-of-hearing children under 20 years of age to the Department of Education and the local health authority. In reporting such cases the physician should give the individual's name, age at the time of examination, the date of birth, the name and address of parents or guardian.

Classes for the Deaf

Deaf children may be admitted to special day classes or schools for the deaf at 3 years. Seldom is it feasible to assign deaf children to regular classes with hearing pupils at the elementary level. The programs for hearing pupils are beyond the abilities of deaf pupils. If, however, a deaf pupil can successfully participate part time in the activities of a regular class he should have the opportunity.

Methods of Instruction

Most school systems use the oral method of instruction which includes speech reading, speech, auditory training of any residual hearing and language facility.

Agencies Serving Deaf Children

The states through their Departments of Education operate residential schools for the deaf. Departments of Education also help the handicapped become employable through their Bureaus of Vocational Rehabilitation. State Departments of Public Health through their Bureau of Crippled Children Services offer medical services to the handicapped under 21 years of age.

The larger states have many private agencies ready to aid the hard-of-hearing. Gallandet College, Washington, D. C., is the only college in the world devoted exclusively to the education of the deaf. The Volta Bureau, Washington, D.C., an information center on deafness and the education of the deaf, was founded by Alexander Graham Bell in 1887.

Types of Hearing Difficulties

Conductive hearing impairment. Pathological conditions in the outer or middle ear partially or totally obstructing the passage of sound vibrations to the inner ear produce conductive hearing losses. Causes are wax impaction, foreign objects or growths in the external auditory canal, otitis externa, otitis media, congenital malformations and some types of otosclerosis.

Perceptive hearing impairment. In this type the hearing difficulty lies in the middle ear. It results from impairment or degeneration of the sensory structures located in the inner ear. The loss is generally to high frequency sounds. Causes are meningitis, scarlet fever, measles, influenza, pneumonia, pertussis, syphilis, typhoid, diphtheria and poliomyelitis.

Psychogenic hearing difficulties. The central nervous system is the site of central hearing impairment. For instance, a child may have sustained an injury to the auditory center of the brain at birth. Tumors of the eighth nerve, degeneration of the circulatory structures in the brain, encephalitis and various brain lesions are other causes.

Defects from rock music. Teenagers have treated lightly the information that loud rock music may decrease the hearing. Family physicians have also neglected to popularize the dangers of loud music. Dey[22] presented tape recordings of a typical discotheque rock band to 15 boys for periods of 5 to 120 minutes. After hearing 2 hours of music at 100 decibels, 2 percent recovered their hearing far too slowly. At 110 decibels, 16 percent were adversely and probably permanently affected.

Instruction for the Physically Handicapped

California State Education Code Section 6802 defines a physically handicapped individual as "any minor who, by reason of a physical impairment, cannot receive the full benefit of ordinary education facilities. . . ." Children with orthopedic handicaps are included under this broad definition of physically handicapped minors.

School Instruction in Hospitals

For the purpose of school instruction any child who is confined to a hospital because of physical illness or physical conditions that make school attendance impossible or inadvisable shall be considered as being physically handicapped.

California State Education Code Section 6809 admits physically handicapped minors at the age of three years to special schools or classes for such minors.

To determine the child's medical eligibility, the administrators in charge shall secure a diagnosis and a recommendation from the family physician or medical clinic. There should also be a written release from the physician when a child is ready to return to regular school.

The information given by the physician should include the following:

–diagnosis of the case in general terms
–the general surgical plan of reconstruc-

tion (if surgery is involved in the case); what has been done and what remains to be done for the child

–points of emphasis regarding background; psychological factors that have immediate bearing on the projected care and treatment of the child

–some indication of medical prognosis as it pertains to prevention and correction of the deformity and to the nature and amount of educational and vocational help that should be provided.

Home Instruction

In some states, to be eligible for home instruction, a child must be physically unable to attend regular school because of an orthopedic handicap or because of a health impairment diagnosed by a licensed physician. The impairment is due to crippling caused by one of the following:

–cerebral palsy
–poliomyelitis
–infection such as bone and joint tuberculosis and osteomyelitis
–birth injury
–congenital anomalies such as congenital amputation, clubfoot, congenital dislocations or spina bifida
–trauma such as amputations, burns or fractures
–tumors such as bone tumors or cysts
–developmental diseases such as coxa plana or spinal osteochondritis
–other conditions such as fragile bones, muscular atrophy, muscular dystrophy, Perthes' disease, hemophilia, uncontrolled epilepsy or severe cardiac impairment.

When the condition of pregnancy makes regular school attendance impossible or inadvisable, pregnant school-age girls shall be considered physically handicapped and may be provided home instruction in some states. Base eligibility for home instruction because of pregnancy on a medical assessment. The governing board of a school district may also provide special day classes for pregnant minors.

Orthopedic Problems

As mentioned previously, children with orthopedic handicaps are included in the group of physically handicapped minors who may have special school instruction. Infant foot and leg problems were discussed earlier in this chapter. Table 3-8 lists orthopedic problems which may occur as the child grows older.

Scoliosis

The family physician is the primary medical personnel to recognize early scoliosis and to treat the nonstructural or functional variety (Table 3-9).

The *nonstructural* variety has no intrinsic spinal disease; the "C"-type curve develops secondarily to unbalanced pelvis. Balancing the pelvis causes this type of scoliosis to disappear. The *structural* "S"-

Table 3-8. Causes of Limping

Age	*Cause*
1 to 2 yr	Congenital dislocation of hip Cerebral palsy
3 to 5 yr	Monarticular synovitis following viral infections Muscular dystrophy
5 to 12 yr	Legg-Calve-Perthes disease (Fig. 3-7) (A vascular necrosis of the proxymal femoral head. The disease is self-limiting. The ossification center of the femoral head becomes necrotic and is absorbed and replaced by live bone.)
12 to 15 yr	Slipped femoral epiphysis (Fig. 3-8) (This diagnosis is frequently missed because a lateral x-ray is not taken.)
Any age	Osteomyelitis Trauma Neurological disorders Poliomyelitis Peroneal muscular atrophy Spinal deformity Rheumatoid arthritis Tumors Functional disorders

Adapted from Hastings DE, Barrington TW: Applied therapy. Ped Patient 8:323, 1966.

type scoliosis will lead to permanent spinal changes if untreated.

Examining the Spine for Scoliosis

Expose the child's back and inspect the spine while the patient is standing with his weight distributed on both feet. Mark the skin over the spinous processes. Examine the patient while standing and while bending forward touching his toes.

Inspect the level of the shoulders and the tips of the scapulas. These landmarks will be higher on the convex side and lower on the concave side of the "C" curve. Look for increased skin creases above the ilium on the concave side.

Inspect the anterior thoracic cage. The spine should be x-rayed in the standing position anteroposteriorly and laterally for anomalies of the vertebrae.

The structural scoliosis patient should be referred to an orthopedist for consultation.

Managing Strep Sore Throat and Rheumatic Fever

Strep Throat

A strep sore throat usually begins suddenly and is aggravated by swallowing. Early in the course of the disease only about 6 percent have the typical fiery red throat with palatine petechiae, a grey exudate and tender cervical lymph glands. Using these criteria the diagnosis is 90 percent accurate after 48 hours. The earlier the patient is seen, the more difficult the diagnosis. Therefore, early, when the diagnosis is most important, the diagnosis can be made only 25 percent of the time. Twenty percent of cases may be asymptomatic.

Edema of the pharyngeal tissues, especially the uvula, may cause paleness of the mucus membrane. Other findings are excoriations around the external nares and blood-tinged or purulent nasal discharge. Practically diagnostic is the appearance of a scarlet fever rash.

Epidemiological factors may be clues: (1) incidence of the disease peaking in March and April and dropping to the lowest incidence in August; (2) 25 percent of siblings between 3 and 10 years contracting the disease within 7 days after the primary case; and (3) the peak incidence between ages 5 and 10. Few infections occur under age 3.

Avoid confusing the diagnosis with infectious mononucleosis and adenovirus infections. Do a leukocyte count and a throat culture on all suspected cases. A leukocyte count above 12,000 helps differentiate strep sore throat from exudative tonsillitis or adenovirus pharyngitis. A colony count above 10 indicates a strep infection. Fifty percent of active infections will have 50 or more colonies. A colony count below 10 indicates a carrier, with or without a superimposed viral infection.

The decision to treat or await the culture report is the dilemma physicians face in treating patients with suspected strep throats. Patients with sore throats who have suggestive symptoms of strep throats should be treated as strep sore throats. Keep certain reservations in mind: If the symptoms are not diagnostic and the leukocyte count is below 10,000, the physician may wait for results of the throat culture. If the spleen is enlarged, even if the symptoms are not diagnostic, obtain a culture and leukocyte count. Treat the patient for a strep infection if the leukocyte count is up, even though the spleen is not enlarged.

Antibiotic therapy does not shorten the duration of the disease unless treatment is started during the first 24 hours. After 24 hours, therapy is to prevent complications and the transmission to others. Therapy started in the first week will reduce the incidence of complicating rheumatic fever at least 90 percent; if treatment is instituted in first 2 weeks, rheumatic fever will be reduced 70 percent.

Treatment of choice: one injection of benzathine penicillin G (Bicillin) 1,200,000 units for adults and 600,000 to 900,000 units for children. Bicillin C-R is less painful. If oral therapy is preferred, order phenoxymethylpenicillin in doses of 125 to 250 mg 3 to 4 times a day for 10 days. If erythromycin is chosen because of pencillin sensitivity, give 250 mg every 6 hr for 10 days.

Table 3-9. Causes of Scoliosis

Nonstructural type *"C" curve*	*Structural type* *"S" curve*
Unreduced congenital dislocation of hip	Congenital defects of the vertebrae
Flexion contractures of one leg	Paralytic diseases
Asymmetric growth of legs	Poliomyelitis
Poor posture	Muscular dystrophy
Standing with weight on one leg	Friedreich's ataxia
Shortening of one leg because of an old fracture	Syringomyelia
Idiopathic conditions	Idiopathic conditions

In addition, culture all contacts, and treat those with positive cultures. Up to 50 percent of siblings who come into contact with an index case acquire the infection.

COMPLICATIONS. If strep sore throat goes untreated, 6 to 10 percent of cases will develop sinusitis, acute otitis media or peritonsillar abscess. About 3 percent will develop acute rheumatic fever and a third of these latter cases will progress to rheumatic heart disease. In certain types of streptococcal infection (type 12), 10 percent will develop acute nephritis.[24,25]

Family physicians should have facilities in their office for culturing and identifying group A streptococci. Relying on commercial laboratories is impractical because of their delay in reporting.

Culturing a throat: Use two Dacron or other synthetic swabs. With the first swab clean any heavy exudate from the surface of the tonsils or the pharynx. With the second swab, bear down. The best swabs come away pink. Avoid the tongue and mouth area. In children, you may get only one chance. Rub the swab over one-sixth of a 5 percent sheep blood agar plate and later streak with a sterile wire loop. Stab the agar several times with the loop in order to demonstrate subsurface hemolysis. Drop a bacitracin disc on the plate and then incubate at 37° C for 18 to 24 hours. With a little training, the physician can learn to recognize beta hemolytic colonies, estimate the number of colonies and recognize the inhibition of their growth by the

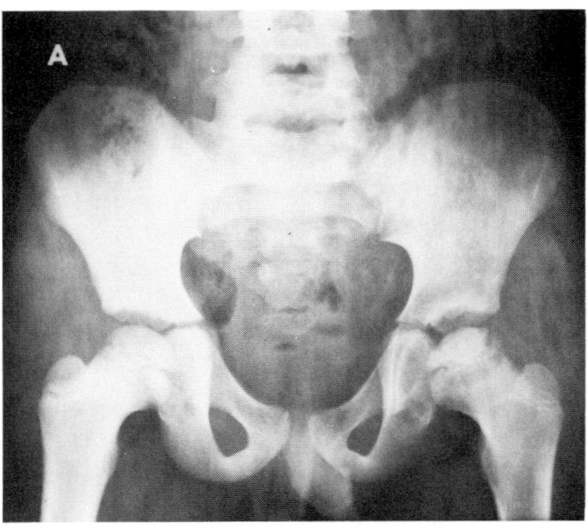

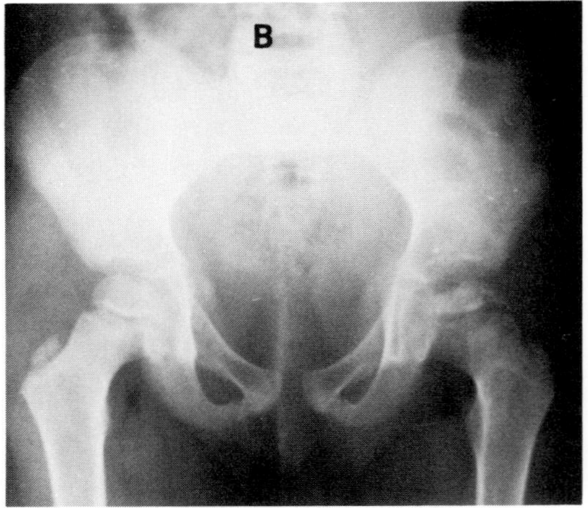

Figure 3-7. *A*, Legg-Calve-Perthes disease with osteochondritis of the femur. Note slight sclerotic and lucent areas of the left hip. This disease is found usually in males 4 to 9 years of age and begins with a pinless limp. X-ray pictures show destructive changes in the metaphyseal portion of the neck of the femur, distention of the articular capsule and thickened epiphyseal lines. *B*, Legg-Calve-Perthes disease of the left hip with osteochondrosis. Aseptic necrosis of the bone results in collapse and mushrooming of the femoral head.

bacitracin disc in the event the organism belongs to Group A. Sheep blood agar plates and bacitracin differentiation discs may be ordered from Baltimore Biological Laboratory, Baltimore, Md.; Difco Laboratories, Detroit, Mich.; Case Laboratories, Chicago, Ill.; Hyland Laboratories, Los Angeles, Calif.

For the physician concerned with the accuracy of office cultures, a recent study should put him at ease. The study reported good correlation between five private offices and a reference laboratory. Few positive streptococcus cultures were missed. Where errors were found, it was more often in the direction of overreading for streptococcus.[26]

Dependability of the ASO Titer in Determining Group A Strep Infections

Do not hesitate to use a single antistreptolysin O (ASO) titer determination on a single specimen to determine whether a patient has had a recent Group A strep infection and may be a glomerulonephritis or rheumatic fever risk.

The normal range of ASO varies with age: normal individuals 12 to 166 todd units; preschool children 85; school children 170; and adults 85. More certain evidence would be a twofold increase in the ASO titer of acute serum as compared to the patient's convalescent serum.

A high or rising titer is indicative of scarlet fever and erysipelas as well as strep pharyngitis or tonsillitis. The ASO is also directly diagnostic in rheumatic fever and glomerulonephritis. Use the ASO to detect subclinical strep infections and in the differential diagnosis of the joint pains of rheumatic fever and rheumatoid arthritis.[27]

DIAGNOSIS. In a few days following strep throat but under 4 weeks (average 19 days), the first symptoms of rheumatic fever may develop in about 3 percent of the patients with strep throat. In Jones' Guidelines for Diagnosing Rheumatic Fever two of the major criteria or one major and two minor criteria (see Table 3-10) are suggestive. To be completely valid, however, the criteria must be accompanied by evidence of a previous strep infection.

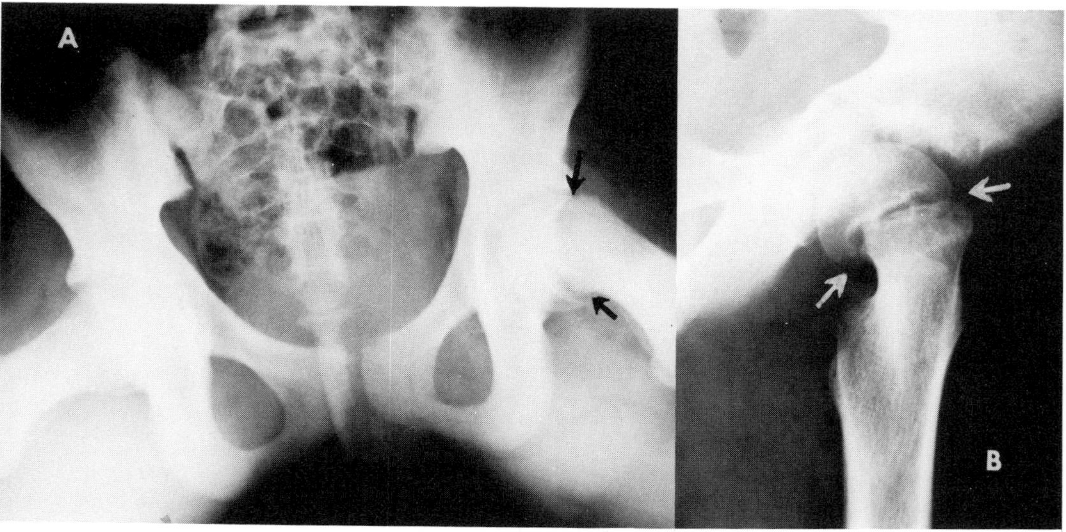

Figure 3-8. *A*, Slipped femoral epiphysis. It starts with a limp and pain during early adolescence and usually occurs in obese boys. The distinguishing feature is painful limitation of inward rotation when the thigh and the knee are both flexed. *B*, X-ray study shows the head of the femur slipped backward and downward on the neck. Surgery with pin fixation usually is necessary.

Table 3-10. Guidelines in Diagnosis of Rheumatic Fever

Major criteria	*Minor criteria*
Carditis	Previous rheumatic fever or RHD
Polyarthritis	Anthralgia
Chorea	Fever
Erythema marginatum	During the acute phase
Subcutaneous nodules	C-reactive protein
	Increased sedimentation rate
	Leukocytosis
	Prolonged PR interval on ECG
	Previous evidence of strep infection
	Increased ASO or other strep antibodies
	Positive throat culture of Group A beta hemolytic strep
	Recent scarlet fever

EVALUATING CARDITIS BY HEART MURMURS. When children sustain cardiac damage following an attack of rheumatic fever, look for mitral or aortic insufficiency. They do not have mitral or aortic stenosis because the fibrotic changes take several years to develop. The significant murmur is a basal diastolic or apical middiastolic murmur which was not previously present. A loud, long systolic murmur at the mitral area is also significant, particularly if it is transmitted from apex to left axilla or left neck. The diastolic murmur is the best evidence of cardiac damage. Do not confuse the functional systolic murmur along the left sternal border with the mitral regurgitation of RF. Do not confuse a presystolic murmur with a split first sound at apex. Do not confuse a middiastolic murmur with a third sound of a normal heart.

A prolonged PR interval electrocardiographically will occur in a third of all strep infections whether the patient develops rheumatic fever or not. Heart enlargement by x-ray study can be misleading unless the child takes a deep breath during the x-ray procedure.

INTERPRETING LABORATORY FINDINGS. An elevation of the ASO is usually above 200 todd units at least once in early rheumatic fever and, in 85 percent of the patients, the elevation represents a previous strep infection and is not specific for rheumatic fever. For a recent strep infection, a rising titer is more significant than a single reading. If ASO titer is low and rheumatic fever is suspected, order an antihyaluronidase (>128) or antistreptokinase for strep antibodies. Ninety-five percent of the cases of recent strep infections will be picked up by a combination of these tests. An increased ASO titer develops after the second week and reaches a peak in 4 to 6 weeks. The height of the titer is not related to severity of infection nor does the rate of fall parallel the course of the disease.

An antihyaluronidase titer of 1000 to 1500 follows recent strep A throat infection and will increase to 4000 with rheumatic fever.

The sedimentation rate and the leukocytes may both be increased and C-reactive protein present but none are specific for rheumatic fever. A sedimentation rate increase is a sensitive test of rheumatic activity. The rate will return to normal with adequate treatment with ACTH or salicylates. In any acute inflammation the C-reactive protein may precede the rise in the sedimentation rate and with recovery, CRP precedes the decrease in the sedimentation rate. CRP disappears when the inflammatory process is suppressed by steroids or salicylates.

Prevention of subsequent attacks. Rheumatic fever has a tendency to recur; therefore, prophylaxis is advisable. The Washington House Prophylaxis Clinic recommends a monthly injection of Bicillin (benzathene penicillin G) 1,200,000 units as being by far the most effective regimen. Because it is less painful, I use Bicillin C-R. All other programs, including oral penicillin or sulfa therapy, are far less effective.

Patients with heart disease should remain on continual prophylaxis throughout their lives. Adults with RHD found on routine examination should begin prophylaxis and remain on it for the rest of their lives. Keep patients without residual heart disease on continual prophylaxis until they are 18 and for 5 years after the last attack.[28]

Strep Impetigo and Acute Glomerulonephritis (AGN)

Strep pharyngitis is to rheumatic fever what strep impetigo is to glomerulonephritis (AGN). As the treatment of AGN is symptomatic, reliance must be placed on prevention to effectively control the disease.

Derrick and Dillon[29] recommend the following therapy for strep skin infections: Benzathine penicillin G, Bicillin or Bicillin C-R intramuscularly (under 60 lb, 600,000 U; 60 to 90 lb, 900,000 U; and over 90 lb, 1,200,000 U). Phenoxymethylpenicillin (penicillin V) orally (under 60 lb, 125 mg 3 or 4 times daily; and over 60 lb, 250 mg). Erythromycin (Enythyrocin) orally (40 mg per kg per day in four doses, up to 1 g per day). Oral penicillin or erythromycin given for at least 7 days appeared effective in clearing skin lesions and preventing AGN but are slightly less effective than intramuscular benzathine penicillin.

According to these researchers, bacitracin topical therapy and hexachlorophene scrubs only resulted in 9 and 39 percent cures respectively.

Tuberculosis

Diagnosis

The more conscious you are of tuberculosis, the more cases you will find. The skin test is still one of the first lines of defense. Base the diagnosis of pulmonary tuberculosis on a postive Mantoux reaction, acid-fast tubercle bacilli in smear and culture, and an x-ray evaluation.

The Tine, Heaf and the Mono-Vacc skin tests are all good screening agents but are not reliable for a valid diagnosis of tuberculosis. Do not use patch tests; they are too unreliable.

Overreading of a Tine test is the most common error in skin testing. Generally a positive test is a 2 mm reaction at one of 4 prong sites. But to depend on it, look for coalesence of at least two sites. If in doubt do a Mantoux test.

As a diagnostic agent the Mantoux is more reliable. To test, use intermediate PPD (purified protein derivative) 5 TUs (tuberculin units) (0.0001 mg) and give intradermally. The 5 TU strength may miss a few cases but stronger doses increase the number of false-positive reactions. A subcutaneous infection is likely to cause false-negatives. Read the reaction in 48 to 72 hours when the induration will be at its peak. Do not measure the erythema, only the induration. The reaction can be felt better than seen. An erythema of more than 10 mm without induration may mean the injection was given too deeply.

Consider an induration of 5 mm or less a negative reaction. An induration of 5 to 9 mm is a suspicious reaction. Repeat the test at a different site. In early infancy and in patients who have had close contacts with tuberculosis consider a reaction of 4 to 5 mm positive for prophylactic treatment purposes. Remember reactions of 5 to 9 mm may be caused by past immunization with BCG, an atypical mycobacteria infection or a nonspecific reaction.

If the second PPD skin test is questionable or negative, repeat the test twice at 3-month intervals. Consider an induration of more than 10 mm a positive reaction.

The routine use of second strength PPD will result in false-positives, but may be useful in patients with a granulomatious lung infection without a positive culture for tuberculosis or other mycobacteria. And yet, under these circumstances, it is better to use specific mycobacteria antigen if available. If the second strength test results in a negative test, conclude that no mycobacteria infection is present.

Before teenage, sputum examinations are unfruitful either from respiratory secretions or gastric washings. This seems to be true even when a moderate sized infiltrate is present. In teenagers, employ every means to obtain samples and, if clinically necessary, collect tracheobronchial secretions by bronchoscopy. Obtain acid-fast stained smears and cultures and occasionally guinea pig inoculations of the sputum, gastric fluid, pleural effusions, urine and pus.

Check the sedimentation rate. If increased, think of disseminated disease. A sedimentation rate is more helpful in following progress than in diagnosis. Active disseminated disease causes more monocytes (10 to 20 percent) than lymphocytes (5 to 10 percent) in the peripheral blood smear.

Early lung infiltration often is not apparent on x-ray examination. The radiographic diagnosis is made on inflammatory infiltration–soft, exudative or active. Minute calcifications are seldom noted by the radiologist but should be looked for and reported since they may be one of the first x-ray findings in latent tuberculosis. X-rays, of course, rule out a wide variety of other conditions such as bronchopneumonia, carcinoma, silicosis, histoplasmosis, blastomycosis, coccidioidomycosis, sarcoidosis and atypical pneumonia.

Chemotherapy

For the child with a positive skin test but negative x-ray findings administer INH (isoniazid) 10 to 15 mg/kg/day. For adults give 300 mg per day. Children are less likely to develop a peripheral neuropathy than adults and therefore do not need Vitamin B_6 until adolescence; then give 50 to 100 mg daily.

If the child has positive x-ray findings and a positive skin test, treat with both INH and PAS (controversial). Under the latter circumstance and with symptoms from the lung infiltrate, hospitalize the child while treating with INH and PAS. Give streptomycin, 40 mg/kg/day in complicated cases only. Seek consultation when more than INH is needed.

Continue therapy for 1 year for tuberculin-negative patients who have been exposed to tuberculosis in order to prevent their conversion to positives.

Pneumonias are treated for between 12 and 18 mo; miliaries and meningeals for 2 to 3 yr; renal tuberculosis for 2 or more yr; and bone tuberculosis for 18 mo to 2 yr.

Give children with positive skin tests who contract measles or whooping cough INH for 8 weeks. Recent converters should be treated 1 year. Anyone who has been continually exposed to an active case, whether skin test is positive or not, should receive INH for 1 year. Pregnant women with positive skin tests should be given prophylactic doses of INH from third trimester on and continued for 1 year. Many adults who have received inadequate treatment in the past or show healed adult-type tuberculosis should also receive a course of INH prophylaxis.[30]

Giving Gamma Globulin for Repeated Infections

Some children are deficient in their ability to ward off infection. Consider giving gamma globulin to these individuals. Physical abnormalities which should tip you off to the possibility of an immune deficiency state are:

- –recurrent pyogenic infection
- –recurrent and persistent otitis media
- –recurrent and persistent candidiasis
- –recurrent and prolonged viral infections
- –unusual gram-negative infections
- –interstitial pneumonia (p. carini)
- –spreading vaccinia

A preliminary check for immune deficiency might include:

- –serum gamma globulin level
- –antibody quantitation
- –antibody assay after measles to check clinical production of antibodies
- –a similar check after DPT inoculation

An interpretation of gamma globulin serum levels should be correlated with the patient's age. There are no normal serum gamma globulin levels for all ages.

More sophisticated laboratory checks occasionally needed to verify the diagnosis and to follow treatment are:

- –total lymphocyte count
- –in vitro lymphocyte growth (may be determined by requesting karyotyping and checking cell proliferation)
- –skin tests following candida and other antibody-producing diseases
- –checking skin graft rejection
- –bone marrow examination
- –lymphoid tissue examination
- –phagocytic function (NBT test)

In determining the immune deficiency state and the need for treatment, remember the following:

- –Investigate patients with Ig serum levels below 600 mg/100 m.
- –There are many sources of error in electrophoretic analysis whether done on paper or by the moving boundary technique.
- –Susceptibility to infection is not increased unless the hypogammaglobulinemia level is below 200 mg/100 ml.
- –It is impossible to raise the serum immunoglobulinemia levels to normal by giving human Ig in acceptable doses when given regularly over long periods.
- –Do not use the serum levels as a sole criterion for treatment; observe the clinical state and history and study the functioning of the white cell series and the ability to produce normal levels of isoagglutinins and antibodies to challenge antigens or recent infections.
- –To maintain adequate levels of gamma globulin, administer the protein at least once every 4 weeks.
- –Once the gamma globulin dose has been ascertained and the patient's gamma globulin rises above 100 to 150 mg percent, recheck the globulin level every 4 months.
- –A rough guide to dosage: To reach a serum level of 100 mg percent of gamma globulin, give at least 100 mg of gamma globulin per kilogram of body weight.

Childhood Sociology

Relationship Between Family and Achievement Motivation

Rosen[31] reports the ways in which family size, position in the birth order, mother's age and social class relate to the development of achievement motivation:

In *small middle class families,* the position in birth order seems to be relatively unimportant—the older and younger child in a two-child middle class family have almost identical motivation. But as the size of the family increases, achievement motivation in the oldest child becomes higher than that of the youngest child.

In *lower class families* the reverse is true: On the average the younger child has higher achievement motivation than the older child, an attitude maintained even when the size of the family increases.

Similarly the effect of the mother's age on the child's achievement motivation varies with the size of her family and social class. The achievement motivation of sons of young mothers is higher as long as the family is small. As the family size increases the motivation of sons of young mothers decreases and is surpassed by the sons of middle age and old mothers. This is particularly true in lower class families.

Relationship Between Social Class and Parental Values

Kohn[32] conducted a study to determine the relationship between social class and parental values. He believed that parents give high priority to those values that seem to them difficult to achieve and, if not achieved, would affect the child adversely. Some interpretations of his study are listed.

Parents from all classes want their children to be honest, happy, considerate, obedient and dependable.

Working class parents value honesty for their children more than middle class parents. Kohn points out this might be expected because the working class is more dependent on the honesty and trustworthiness of others than the middle class is.

Working class parents value neatness and cleanliness above the middle class parent. For the working class, neatness is more likely to assure a respectable social position.

Obedience is more valued by the working class than by the middle class who put less emphasis on conformity to authority. The middle class see obedience as somewhat inconsistent with consideraton and curiosity. The child should act appropriately, not because his parents tell him to but because he wants to.

Working class mothers place happiness second to honesty and obedience. Middle class mothers place happiness above all else even those who are ambitious for their sons.

The middle class parent puts more emphasis on self control and governing one's relationship with others. For the middle class these qualities are more likely to allow the individual to hold the social status to which he has been born.

The middle class parent values not only self control but consideration for others (again inner control)—a standard that demands he respond sympathetically to other's needs even if they be in conflict with his own.

The proportion of mothers who value curiosity rises very slowly from the working class mothers to the wives of professional men or highly educated businessmen. The value is given priority by the parents in proportion to its importance to the child's future.

Predicting Achievement Behavior

Moss and Kagan[33] studied 71 subjects from birth to 29 years of age in an attempt to correlate adult achievement behavior with personal achievement up to age 14. They report:

Striving for recognition and achievement between ages 6 to 10 correlated well with similar behavior during adulthood.

Intellectual activity rather than athletic activities for the 10 to 14 age group was positively related to achievement behavior in adulthood.

Achievement strivings during the first 4 years of school are a moderately good index to future achievement behavior during adolescence and adulthood.

Involvement in mechanical tasks for age 10 to 14 showed positive correlations with adult achievement behavior for boys but not for girls.

Maternal concern with the child's developmental progress during the first 3 years of life predicted adult achievement behavior for women but not for men.

Office IQ Testing of the Child

The Bakwin modification of the Goodenough Draw-a-Man test is the least time consuming IQ test for the determination of a child's mental age used by the family physician. Its administration and grading takes little psychological training. In fact, I seldom grade the drawings, but have children from 3 to 10 draw a man on my office record as subsequently described. Then, if later, the child has difficulty, the drawings are available and need only grading to have a record of the child's mental development. The record is as good an approximation of the child's mental age as any other test.

Give the child a sheet of paper and soft pencil. Instruct him to draw the picture of a man and to make the man as complete as possible. Do not give the child any suggestions; leave him alone, excluding parents from the test situation. Give him whatever time he demands to complete the picture.

Bakwin and associates use 28 criteria for scoring.* The 28 criteria are listed below:

Head present
Legs present
Arms present
Trunk present
Length of trunk greater than breadth
Shoulder indicated
Both arms and legs attached to trunk
Legs attached to trunk and arms to trunk at correct point
Neck present

*Reproduced from Bakwin R M, Weider A and Bakwin H: Mental testing in children. J. Pediatr. 33:384–394, 1948, with permission from author and C. V. Mosby Co., St. Louis.

Outline of neck continuous with that of head or trunk or both
Eyes present
Nose present
Mouth present
Both nose and mouth in two dimensions; two lips shown
Nostrils indicated
Hair shown
Hair on more than circumference of head, nontransparent, better than scribble
Clothing present
Two articles of clothing, nontransparent
Entire drawing with sleeves and trousers shown, free from transparency
Four or more articles of clothing definitely indicated
Costume complete without incongruities
Fingers shown
Correct number of fingers shown
Fingers in two dimensions, length greater than breadth, angle subtended not greater than 180°
Opposition of thumbs shown
Hand shown as distinct from fingers or arms
Arm joint shown (either elbow, shoulder or both)

In scoring the results, give all children the basal age of 3. Then for each four of the criteria included in the drawing, credit the child with one additional year. The total score represents the child's mental age. As an example: If the child includes eight of the criteria, two years are added to the basal age of 3 giving a sum of 5, the child's mental age.

The test can also be diagnostic in other ways, i.e. the spotting of physical defects such as blindness or neuromuscular disabilities.

Intellectually Superior Children

Mothers often ask family physicians to comment on the possibility of a child being gifted. Some understanding of intellectually superior children is necessary for a knowledgeable answer.

Psychologists do not know the factors that produce intellectually superior children. Most psychologists, however, agree that intelligence is more a matter of social engineering—a processing of human material—than the identification and training of a natural resource. Of course the quality of natural resources vary but, no matter the biological quality, the level of the final product depends on continuing social development. Mental superiority then depends on being born with a superior potential and being raised in a superior environment. Nobody knows the relative importance of these two factors. Inherited intelligence is too low in some children to allow them to develop even average mental ability; on the other hand, severe environmental impediments can present the undeveloped brilliant child from showing more than average mental ability.

With this perception in mind, the family physician may feel secure in telling the parents that their most important duties are providing a home and school environment which stimulates the enjoyment of learning; providing examples in education that their children may imitate; and providing training that produces the desire for achievement.

Among the mentally superior some are creative and some are not. A high I.Q. does not guarantee creativity. Psychologists know even less about what makes people creative than about what makes intellectually superior people. What makes a gifted or even normal child underachieve academically?[34]

- –inability of the child to use his gifts as a result of emotional conflicts caused by a poor environment
- –inability of the child to break from a limited vocational concept as a result of inadequate environmental stimulation
- –inability of the child to develop a drive or need for achievement (lack of motivation) because of a barren environment
- –failure of the child to develop a love of learning.

Recognizing Creativity in Children

Guilford[35] believes some of the traits that aid creativity and can be partially measured are:

Fluency of thought: Ideational fluency has to do with the rate with which ideas can be produced such as having the child list all the things he can think of that are solid. *Associational fluency* pertains to the completion of relationship as might be determined by listing all the words that mean the opposite of "good." *Expressional fluency* has to do with the facile construction of sentences as might be measured by writing as many four-word sentences as possible, all different, with no word used more than once.

Flexibility of thought: Spontaneous flexibility may be estimated by asking the youngster to list all the uses he can think of for a common brick. At first this test may appear to test ideational fluency as outlined above, but in this instance the examinee is scored on the number of times he changes categories (drive a nail, make baseball bases or make a tombstone rather than using one category such as build a house, build a school). *Adaptive flexibility* tests the examinees ability to change strategy, change solutions or change interpretation of a task. A short story is told to the child and he is to respond by as many appropriate titles as he can think of. The number of responses rated as clever serves as a score for originality.

The Child Who is Failing School

Physicians in general and pediatricians in particular are delinquent in their care of the educably handicapped child. The new family physician should fill this medical need, working cooperatively with the child's teacher, principal, parents and the school psychologist.

When a child is in school trouble, the physician with the aid of a psychologist should be able to diagnose the child's ailment. Furthermore, from his intimate contact with a family he should be able to initially spot the potential school failure and move to prophylactic measures.

When a school-failing child is brought to a family physician, the objective of the first examination should be to classify the child as physically, emotionally or neurologically handicapped. From these general categories, the doctor should proceed to a more specific diagnosis that will help the school plan an educational program for the child.

Causes

NORMAL INTELLIGENCE DEVIATION. This may be caused by simple idiopathic retardation or may be the result of a child of superior intelligence finding the curriculum boring and, thereby, developing unfavorable attitudes. Diagnosis is made by comparing an early developmental history to that of his brothers and sisters and by psychometric testing.

EMOTIONAL AND PSYCHIATRIC DISTURBANCES. ORGANIC. *Acute* organic disturbances are temporary mental disorders occurring in the presence of other diseases. They are deliriumlike. These include febrile diseases, drug intoxication and Sydenham's chorea.

Chronic organic disturbances may be episodes occurring in the course of a convulsive disorder or in cerebral dysarrhythmia even though there is no overt convulsion. These are epileptiform. Postencephalitic disturbances are not often found anymore. Burn encephalopathies may cause chronic disturbances following severe traumatic burns. Characteristics of these may be hyperkinesis, lack of ability to adapt to social demands and decreasing IQ. Encephalopathies following premature birth or anoxemia at birth may cause chronic disturbances. These may result in infantile general behavior or impulsive social behavior. The first clues may be that the child is small for his age and is hyperkinetic. His inability to compete causes anxiety.

Infantile anxiety. This condition develops from weak instinctual self-preservation drives and an incomplete sensory-perceptive (cortex) development at birth, all of which is slowed by a physiological anoxemia. These factors may actually threaten the life of a child so that painful tension states develop if not mothered properly. If the child is not handled properly or is misunderstood, problems may be created which could follow the child through life.

FUNCTIONAL. A prime functional disturbance is *schizophrenia*. This condition may develop slowly or start as an acute attack. It is the only psychosis that affects young people. Symptoms are:

- –lack of interest in environment and no satisfaction in ordinary events
- –preoccupation with fantasies and solitary activities
- –seclusiveness when challenged and irritability if seclusion is interrupted with striking sensitivity to being criticized
- –less physical activity than average children
- –inability to adapt to people or changes
- –inappropriate and confused speech and symbolic representation of real or imagined objects
- –misinterpretation of the acts of others

Symptoms of *psychoneurosis,* a functional disturbance, are hysteria, acute anxiety, obsessions, compulsions, phobias and abnormal behavior patterns. Neuroses are classified according to the symptoms that predominate i.e. hysterical neurosis, phobic neurosis, etc.

A youngster with a psychoneurosis develops a behavior disturbance *during adolescence with guilt feelings*. This is in contrast to a child with a primary behavior disturbance who develops his problems *early in life without guilt feelings*.

Constitutional inferiority is a neurosis in which the infant is constitutionally unable to achieve a normal or average ego. It is an inherent condition (not like primary behavior disorders, which are reactions to environmental influences).

Primary behavior disturbance. This condition develops in reaction to environmental influences. There is disharmony in family background or hostility and rejection of parent or parents nearly 100 percent of the time. A persistent behavior problem is the major complaint. Other complaints are that the child is deviating from the accepted code of morals—he is fighting, lying and stealing, has abnormal sex activities; and has consistent truancy with disobedience. Symptoms usually start at an early age (3 yr). Parents will say, "He is always bad." This is an attention-getting mechanism, or the child may be striving for power, getting revenge or demonstrating inadequacies. (In some cases symptoms of a primary behavior disorder are present from an early age but scrutiny of the history does not elicit a disturbed environment—the family is sound and other children in the same environment have developed normally. Under these circumstances the diagnosis of a primary behavior disturbance cannot be made. The alternative then is to assume that there is an inherent or constitutional inability to achieve normal development.) As the child grows older he becomes disobedient, unmanageable and disrespectful. He does not respond to punishment or show signs of guilt feelings. He has an abnormal aggressiveness to his environment (in contradistincton to schizophrenia). He has a narcissistic self-evaluation—he thinks of himself as a "big shot."

When diagnosing, rule out everything else, including feeblemindedness. Diagnosis is based on the kind of behavior problem, the early onset, the type of personality, lack of guilt and the disturbed early environment. A patient in this category may be classified as a primary behavior problem, a classification further broken down into conduct-disorder type, habit-disturbance type or a child with neurotic traits. In stating diagnosis modify by using one of these three types, depending on the symptoms exhibited by the child.

Maternal permissiveness. The child develops his behavior problems because of maternal indulgence. The mother of the child yields to the demands of the child, allowing him to break household rules relating to the discipline of time, speech, food and possessions. The indulged child is undisciplined in all of these respects. He becomes careless, destructive and insolent.

Maternal dominance. In this case, in contrast to maternal permissiveness, the mother dominates the child. Therefore, the child shows excessive shyness, anxieties, fears and unnatural submissive behavior.

PHYSICAL DISABILITIES. Various disabilities mentioned in this chapter (impaired hearing and eyesight) fall under this category. In addition there are physical abnormalities, such as cleft palate, that cause speech difficulties.

NEUROLOGICAL DISABILITIES. SPECIFIC LEARNING DISABILITIES. Under this category, a child is average or better in his schoolwork, except for one subject. He may transpose letters when spelling, he may use mirror writing when expressing himself, he may be unable to read the simplest of sentences, or he may not be able to comprehend the relationship of numbers in arithmetic. The child suffers from perceptual impairment. Ten to 15 percent of the learning disabilities are in the language area.

MINIMAL BRAIN DYSFUNCTION. In this case, in addition to perceptual-motor impairment, the child has a hyperkinetic behavior syndrome with attendant emotional overlay. (See the following section on minimal brain dysfunction.)

CONVULSION-CAUSED DISABILITIES.

HYPERKINESIA. (See later in this chapter.)

Management of Minimal Brain Dysfunction

Educators now prefer the term *minimal brain dysfunction* to the old term of minimal brain damage. In this classification are children who:

–have a history suggestive of brain damage, such as maternal rubella or exposure, Rh-negative problem, low birth weight, anoxia

–test psychologically as organically brain damaged

–have no "hard" neurological findings of brain damage, such as convulsions or cerebral palsy, but the condition is suspected because of "soft" neurological findings (described in subsequent paragraphs)

–react paradoxically to barbiturates and amphetamines

The two most important findings in determining the diagnosis are hyperkinesia and perceptual-motor impairments.

A search should be made for any prenatal, perinatal or postnatal events that would be potential causative factors of brain damage. Some are prematurity, intracranial birth hemorrhage, cerebral anoxia or infection, Rh incompatibility, head injuries, encephalitis and convulsions. It is most important to elicit the following: evidence of delayed speech and language development; evidence of delayed motor development; and a family history of reading, spelling, speech or language problem.

Routine neurological examinations and electroencephalograms do not add much to the diagnosis of the minimal brain dysfunctional child. Kenny and Clemmens[36] studied 100 children with such problems by thorough medical, psychological and electroencephalographic examinations. No significant relationship was found to any of these tests. They suggest that the diagnosis of these children was more directly related to symptoms and psychological findings than to specific medical, neurological or electroencephalographic findings.

Children are usually referred for study because of hyperkinesia or perceptual loss. Confusion exists because of the varying depth of these two symptoms and the emotional overlay that exists because of the findings. The cause of this constellation of symptoms may range from simple maturational delay to a severe brain syndrome. Of course, if "hard" neurological findings are present, the diagnosis is no longer that of minimal brain dysfunction.

"Soft" Neurological Signs

–Tics

–Nystagmus even though it fatigues

–Strabismus

–Unequal pupillary responses

–Hyperactive/unequal deep reflexes

–Fatiguing ankle clonus and Babinski

–Inability to stand on one foot ten sec by age six or inability to hop on one foot

–Inability to walk a straight line heel-to-toe or to stand heel-to-toe

–Handedness confusion or laterality

–Choreiform movement of outstretched hands

- –Intention tremor
- –Dysdiadochokinesia
- –No graphesthesia
- –Poor hand writing
- –Auditory or visual deficiencies
- –Poor verbal articulation
- –Clumsiness
- –Distractability and hyperkinesia
- –Poor motor ability to copy geometric designs
  - three-yr olds copy circles
  - four-yr olds copy crosses
  - five-yr olds copy squares
  - six-yr olds copy triangles
  - seven-yr olds copy diamonds
- –Digital awkwardness (finger-thumb appositions) with associated mirror movements in opposite hand
- –Terminal tremor on finger-to-finger or finger-to-nose testing

Perceptual Handicaps

To say that a child is perceptually handicapped is another way of saying that he has minimal brain damage *without* intellectual retardation. This damage has changed the way in which he perceives the world and the way in which he thinks about what he perceives. The term refers to an impairment in the normal processes of perception, that is, in the basic ability of all human beings to cope with and to make sense out of the environment in which they live.

The common perceptual defects are of listening (auditory or receptive aphasia), reading (dyslexia) and speaking (motive expressive aphasia).

LISTENING DEFECTS. Auditory aphasia is the inability of child to recognize what he hears.

Severe auditory verbal agnosia: The child is unable to recognize the meaning of a single word he hears. When asked to point to an object such as a comb in a group of objects, he is unable to do so although he is able to use the comb when it is presented to him.

Moderate: The child can do the above test but is unable to fully understand a simple phrase. He is not able to recognize the error in the sentence, "You eat with a knife, fork and comb."

Mild: The child is unable to understand statements containing two or three ideas although simple sentences are understood.

Minimal: The child is unable to understand long and complex statements or phrases spoken too rapidly. He will also have difficulty following directions requiring him to do three or more things in a series.

READING DEFECTS. Children with this disability are often referred to a psychiatrist because of their associated misbehavior.

Severe: Visual verbal agnosia, alexia or word blindness. The child is unable to recognize written words. If such a child is shown the written name of an object, he will be unable to point to the correct object.

Moderate: The child is able to recognize individual words but has difficulty understanding simple phrases or sentences that he reads.

Mild: Visual aphasia or dyslexia. The child has difficulty with sentences and paragraphs of more complexity and greater length with multiple ideas. The child will read key words but will omit prepositions and conjunctions.

Minimal: The child will demonstrate slowness and hesitation, rereading or reading aloud to understand. (When educators speak of dyslexia, they refer not only to specific primary dyslexia but to nonspecific secondary dyslexia as well. As the term indicates, secondary dyslexia is due to mental retardation, poor teaching, cultural deprivation and other disabilities. Educators consider that specific primary or developmental dyslexia is caused by genetic factors or brain damage.)

SPEAKING DEFECTS. These defects are termed motor or expressive aphasia.

Severe: The child is unable to call forth the specific desired word. He may be unable to utter any words, despite efforts, or may be restricted to a single word or phrase. He may utter a string of meaningless unrelated words (jargon).

Moderate: The child has difficulty selecting the exact word required and will substitute another word or phrase (paraphasia).

Mild: The child has difficulty in expressing an idea or a series of ideas in organized phrases and statements. Sentences may be incomplete, words out of order and conjunctions omitted.

Minimal: The child's defects may be manifested by slowness of speech, hesitation or transient blocks, lack of inflection or occasionally by stuttering because of difficulty finding the proper word.

Community Resources

Once the diagnosis of minimal brain dysfunction has been made and treatment instituted, the role of the physician becomes secondary to that of the home and school. Family physicians should know what community resources are available to assist the parents of these children.

Forty-two of the fifty states have parent-sponsored organizations that assist parents, such as the California Association for Neurologically Handicapped Children. The Association for Children with Learning Disabilities is a national organization similar in nature. Information can be obtained from Mrs. Robert M. Tilatson, Secretary, 2200 Brownsville Rd., Pittsburgh, Pa. 15210. A letter to "Closer Look," Office of Education, U. S. Department of Health, Education and Welfare, Washington, D. C., will obtain a list of private schools and other organizations that serve the needs of these children. The booklet, "Learning Disabilities Due to Minimal Brain Dysfunction," may be obtained from the Superintendent of Documents, U. S. Government Printing Office, Washington, D. C. 20402 at a minimal cost. The local, county or state Board of Education will provide information about special education programs within public school systems.[37]

The Hyperactive Child

Hyperactive children make up 3 to 7 percent of the pediatric age group. Symptoms are generally classified first as behavior problems and second as learning problems. Hyperactive children do poorly in school. They walk about the room, squirm at their desks, disturb their classmates and annoy their teachers. The smallest extraneous stimulus distracts the child and often triggers an emotional outburst. Symptoms are:

- –short attention span with inability to concentrate
- –overactivity and restlessness
- –distractibility by each new stimulus
- –impulsiveness (acts first, thinks later)
- –repulsing of affectionate overtures of mother by arching back and struggling

Observation of these symptoms is as definitive as any physical diagnostic signs in making the diagnosis. Diagnosis is most commonly made from these symptoms alone:

- –overexcitability, intolerance of overstimulation and easy loss of control
- –history of delay in early motor development
- –birth history suggestive of slight organic damage
- –history of convulsions
- –rate of mental development below the family average but above the mentally retarded level
- –abnormal electroencephalogram
- –history of paradoxical response to cerebral depressants

Psychological testing is often necessary and is best done by the school psychologist or referred to a private psychologist. IQ is within normal range with a disparity between verbal and performance scales as well.

DIFFERENTIAL DIAGNOSIS. The mentally retarded child will give a history of not only slow motor development but also retardation in speech and toilet training. The hyperkinetic child will be within normal range in the latter two.

A confusion of names exists but generally the following presents a clear picture: *Nonpsychotic organic brain syndrome* may be used when the physical and neurological history present hard evidence of brain damage. If the cause is known the diagnosis is clarified as *nonpsychotic organic brain syn-*

drome with trauma. If no hard neurological evidence is found, the physician is justified in making the diagnosis of *hyperkinetic reaction*. According to JAMA *Medical News* "these children suffer from a delay of physiological development of the brain."[54] If the child is hyperkinetic and also has perceptual deficiencies plus emotional overlay the diagnosis of minimal brain damage is proper.

TREATMENT. The most important help the physician can offer is making the diagnosis of hyperkinesia. This alone usually creates some optimism and starts the parents and teachers on the right track. Until the diagnosis is confirmed, teachers and parents live with the fear the child is severely brain damaged or that the child is and will remain incorrigible. Knowing that a treatable handicap exists gives hope and removes a feeling of guilt from the parents. Suggest that the child be asked to do only those chores he can perform without difficulty. Parents and siblings should maintain a friendly and helpful manner.[38]

Methylphenidate (Ritalin) 5 mg can be given a half hour before breakfast and lunch when the stomach is acid. The dosage is raised stepwise 5 mg at a time at 5 day intervals until the desired effect is obtained. Give no more than 2 mg per kg of body weight. Dextroamphetamine may be used cutting the suggested dose of Ritalin in half.

The closer the hyperkinesis symptoms are to definite brain damage, the more effective are the amphetamines. The fewer the signs of organic pathology—and here the family physician must be familiar with "soft signs" of neurologic dysfunction—the more useful is Ritalin.

Urge that the child be put in a classroom with as few distractions as possible. The teacher should rigidly organize his school work. Good behavior should be praised; criticism and punishment only increase his frustration. Teachers may use such techniques as overlearning, easy discrimination and novelty to accomplish their ends.

Too heavy an extracurricular load takes from the child's play time and interferes with adequate rest. Only the most important activities should be continued except for the unusual child who has the physical stamina and interest to manage a heavy schedule.

The child should be seen regularly by the family physician not only for dosage adjustment but also to develop a sustaining and important relationship. Remember that the least reliable informant about progress is the parent. The teacher's report and the clinical impression by the fmily physician are more significant.

Team work is the key to this multifaceted disorder. Physicians, therapists, paramedical personnel, educators, friends and relatives as well as the child himself need to cooperate.

In summary, treatment consists of combinations of drug therapy, psychotherapy, parent counseling, teacher counseling, educational management, small class size, distraction-free classroom, special educational methods and specially trained teachers.

Help for the Disturbed Child

Solicit the parents' support. Consult with them from time to time in regard to sex education, disciplinary techniques and family relationship.

Drug therapy includes:

Amphetamines in case of hyperkinesis where symptoms suggest brain damage.

Methylphenidate (Ritalin) in cases of hyperkinesis where symptoms do not appear similar to brain damage.

Thioridazine (Mellaril) in the young child who sleeps and eats poorly and is overactive.

Phenothiazines may be used symptomatically.

Imipramine (Tofranil) for enuresis after 7 or 8 yr.

Diazepam (Valium) or Oxazepam (Serax) for borderline EEG patterns. Both may cause unusual dreams.

Diphenylhydantoin (Dilantin) for definite and proven seizures.[39]

Characteristics of Underachievers

Havighurst[40] describes underachievers as those who:

- –do not like school, nor enjoy books, nor develop as good study habits as achievers
- –think of themselves as inadequate, do not develop as high aspirations and have narrower interests than do achievers
- –tend to come from low socioeconomic families, particularly if the home environment is inadequate or broken
- –do not develop popularity or leadership abilities
- –adjust poorly and do not develop vocational goals until later in life

THE TEENAGER

The termination of a protected childhood and assumption of adult responsibility causes the storms and stresses of adolescence. A life philosophy begins to develop with growing maturity. In many cases this philosophy relates to their peers rather than to parents, teachers and others of the older generation. Consequently a conflict of generations develops.

Only a rare adolescent can choose a vocational career in a final sense. An American parent of lower or middle class status usually wants his child to aim at something higher than his own calling, causing confusion in the youth. In addition, parents fail to realize that living out their own frustrated wishes through their children usually leads to their own and their children's unhappiness. Unfortunately, more often than not, occupational choices are a matter of personal accident, causing vocational misplacement and dissatisfaction in adult life.

Puberty also brings the power of reproduction, heightened sexual desire and sex consciousness. With these developments and because of the Western code of sexual morality, autoeroticism or repression and/or sublimation of sexual urges develops. These lead to further sexual deviancy, anxiety and guilt feelings.

A teenager wants to be attractive and desirable to the same and opposite sex. Therefore obtaining attractive clothing, sufficient money, and recreational freedoms cause teenage worry. In time they outgrow these concerns. In the interval, sharing their anxieties with age-mates gives some emotional relief.

Participation in school, church and community activities can release the tensions generated in these areas of heterosexual adjustment. Family physicians can go far toward alleviating these problems by personal counseling.

The Family Physician's Responsibility

If a family is in conflict, first reduce personal and family tension. The family physician as a counselor to all members of the family, and particularly to teenagers, has an opportunity to do this. One strategy is to use the periodic health examination to enlarge the counselor's role. Properly used, the physician with ingenuity can often allay conflicts and point the family in a more reasonable direction.

Use common sense when counseling teenagers; apply techniques that have been helpful in handling other people. Help the teenager become self-accepting. Give him some insight into how his parents are thinking—the parent's point of view may have escaped the youngster's attention. Glean all information possible from parents and teenager and talk to the school personnel. In any event, decide promptly whether to counsel the parents and their teenager or refer to a psychiatrist. Consulted early a psychiatrist has a much better chance of success.

Because of age, a generation gap exists between a family physician and a teenager. Recognize this gap. Don't try to bridge it with "groovy" manners nor modern ideas. You will make a big mistake if you propose being "boys together." The idea of a physician being on the same level with him and sharing experiences as equals is preposterous or even absurd to a teenager. Stay in the role of counselor, speaking frankly, sincerely and with dignity.

The most important contribution the parent can make to the child is preparing him for the responsibilities of independence. Teach parents not to build their lives so intimately around their children that they become unhappy when their children begin to show signs of independence. The family physician should point out to parents that they must prepare themselves to deal wisely with the phase of life when their children are no longer dependent upon them.

Estimating Secondary Sex Characteristics and Puberty Growth

Maturity is an ever-receding goal toward which a child begins to march at birth and continues to the end of his life. The family physician can check up on a child's maturation at any given age and determine whether or not the child is on time. Sign posts of maturity exist at age 5 as well as at 15. Physical and emotional growth can be measured at any age.

For boys the five stages of sexual maturity are as follows:

–penis, testes and scrotum are essentially the same in size and configuration as in early childhood
–noticeable enlargement of testes and penis with lightly-pigmented downy hair
–appreciable lengthening of penis and straight, coarse, pigmented hair interspersed with downy hair
–increased diameter of testes and penis with darker pubic hair
–genitalia adult in size and shape with adult pubic hair

Classify maturation in girls by breast development as follows:

–prepubertal configuration with only the papilla elevated
–areola elevated with minimal breast swelling
–breast swollen to small mound formation
–attainment of adult breast contour

A spurt in growth characterizes adolescence both in boys and girls. The growth spurt usually precedes other pubertal changes by a year or two. A delayed growth spurt indicates a delay in the onset of puberty. Girls usually begin pubertal maturation two to three years earlier than boys. Thus for several years, from approximately 10 to 13 years of age, girls tend to be taller than boys of the same age.

During the adolescent growth spurt, growth of the trunk is more rapid than growth of the legs. The later puberty occurs, the longer the period of rapid leg growth. Boys mature later than girls; therefore, men are longer-legged than women.

In puberty, boys' shoulders grow more rapidly than girls'. Pelvic diameter increases in both boys and girls, but the ratio of pelvic breadth to shoulder breadth becomes considerably greater in girls.[41]

Accelerated female maturation motivates the 13- or 14-year old to seek her companionship from 16- and 17-year old males. Many parents worry because they fear their daughters are going to be exploited sexually by "older men," whereas the girl is seeking companionship with people of her own developmental age rather than her chronological age. Such problems interfere with the relationship between parents and their children but generally represent useless anxiety based on ignorance of child development. The family physician should help relieve this type of anxiety.

Problems of Growth Retardation

The medical history is important in assessing growth patterns. Consider family growth patterns; ethnic origins; family history of diabetes mellitus, bowed legs suggesting the possibility of familial vitamin D resistant rickets. Gastrointestinal, liver or kidney disease; skeletal abnormalities; and muscle or nerve disease are factors to be considered.

During physical examination include a review of body measurements. Look for a proportionate or a disproportionate stunting as with unduly short legs. (After infancy the floor-to-pubis distance equals one half the height, and the span from middle finger to middle finger ordinarily equals the height.) If the legs are short, think of hypothyroidism, vitamin D resistant rickets and chondrodystrophy.

Evaluate secondary sex characteristics. If a male has a Hercules-type body with adult type sex hair and large penis but small testes, think of excess androgen from other sources than the testes as in the adrenogenital syndrome. A 14- or 15-year old boy with a small penis and less than 1-cm-long testes has a delayed pubescence.

Take x-rays for clues to vitamin D resistant rickets, chondrodysplasia and hypothyroidism and to evaluate growth potential by a study of the epiphysis.

Laboratory studies to rule out vitamin D poisoning and hypercalcemia, kidney disease, rickets and diabetes should include blood sugar, serum calcium, serum albumin, serum inorganic phosphorus and alkaline phosphatase.

Go one step further and attempt to rule out the more sophisticated problems of growth hormone shortages, cretinism or hypothyroidism and adrenogenital syndromes by determining growth hormone level, serum thyroid hormone (T_4 or PBI) concentrations, thyroid uptake of I^{131}, plasma cortisol and urinary 17-ketosteroids.

A few patients will need serum FSH and LH determinations, gynecography, nuclear chromatin or karyotyping for Turner's syndrome and testing for pseudohypoparathyroidism. It is best for an endocrinologist to order and interpret these tests.

A specialist should manage a patient with a shortage of growth hormone for the hormone supply is short. Most of the other correctable growth retarding endocrine problems are involved and complex. Let the endocrinologist worry about their management.[42]

Teenage Attitudes and Interests

In preadolescence he is:

- –boastful and "fantastic" in tone
- –a wishful thinker
- –lacking in modesty
- –if a boy, filled with talk of physical strength and daring exploits
- –if a girl, concerned with appearance, possessions and social status

In early adolescence his interests turn to:

- –gang activities, clubs made up of members of his own sex
- –suppression of individuality
- –if a boy, behaves aggressively, boisterously and competitively and is interested in political and social questions, personal development, possessions and pleasure
- –if a girl, is neat, docile and prim with some tomboyishness and interested in family welfare

In midadolescence there is:

- –striving for social conformity
- –an interest in parties
- –among the boys less boisterousness and an interest in social poise
- –among the girls more sophistication

In late adolescence:

- –boys become interested in social maturity, athletics and leadership
- –girls become absorbed with feminine ideals and security

Family Discipline and the Teenager's Personality Traits

A study by Peck[43] suggests that the adolescent's personality traits are closely related to the family's disciplinary pattern and emotional relationship. A family life characterized by consistency, warmth and mutual trust fostered ego strength in the adolescent. A lenient, democratic family atmosphere appeared to encourage friendliness and spontaneity in the adolescent. An autocratic, untrusting and disapproving family tended to cause hostility, dependency and an unresolved Oedipal complex.

The Impact of Mothers on the Teenager

From their studies Bayley and Schaefer[44] suggest that the mother-child relationship has a definite impact on the adolescent's personality. Mothers who were autonomy-granting and ignoring had adolescent sons who were reserved, timid and tactful. Mothers who were involved emotionally, concerned about their infant's health, and demanded excessive contact and achievement had adolescent boys who were characterized as rude, irritable, impulsive and independent. In other words, the adolescent revolt appears to be strongest in those boys whose mothers were closely interacting and involved with them as infants. Girls who were maladjusted, i.e. gloomy, sulky and hostile, more often had mothers who were hostile, controlling and punitive and made excessive contact with their daughters. Girls who were well adjusted had mothers who were autonomy-granting and loving.

The Effect of Paternal Absence on Teenage Boys

McCord and coworkers[45] have done research on the effects of an absent father in the personality development of adolescent boys. They found, if the boy was between 6 and 12 when his father left or the mother deviant (alcoholic, criminal or promiscuous) or rejecting, the adolescent boy developed feminine-aggressive behavior. Since aggressive behavior is a characteristically masculine trait, the feminine-aggressive exhibition would indicate an unstable sex role identification.

The researchers found no correlation between unusual fears in the adolescent and parental absence. Oral regression (thumb-sucking, nailbiting, excessive smoking, playing with the mouth) occurred in parental absence only if the mother was deviant or rejecting. Although intense sexual anxiety was found in 50 percent of the adolescent boys whose fathers were absent, the anxiety appeared to be more clearly related to an unstable environment.

Gang delinquency was unrelated to parental absence. In fact, this type of delinquency was higher among quarreling parents who were living together. The same conclusion was reached regarding adolescent criminality. An interesting sidelight, boys whose fathers are criminals are less apt to become criminals if accepted by their delinquent fathers than if rejected by them. Apparently paternal acceptance may operate against identification with the father if the parent is opposed to the behavior norms of the larger society.

In conclusion, McCord and fellow workers believe many adolescent problems are more likely to be related to family conflicts, rejection and deviance than to paternal absence.

Ethnic Prejudice

Wilson[46] reviewed the psychological literature and has summarized the trends as follows:

- –the level of prejudice increases as the child passes through adolescence
- –the level of prejudice stabilizes during the later ages of adolescence
- –effected or appropriate behavior becomes stabilized sometime in adolescence
- –consistency to a given ethnic group increases during adolescence

Childhood Gangs

Eisenstadt[47] maintains that our society is *achievement orientated* whereas the family is *kinship orientated.* Within the family, children are treated and status is given depending on who they are, i.e. son, daughter, eldest, youngest. Later when the child attends school and enters adult society, his status will depend more on *what* he has achieved than on *who* he is.

A child must make the transition from the family-orientated society to the larger achievement-orientated one. Therefore there is a discontinuity between the values presented to children (especially to boys) in the family and in the nonfamilial situation.

With the working father and other problems of American society, the family becomes an inadequate resource in teaching children to live outside the home. Consequently, groups of like-age children spring up; in these groups the values of the larger society which they are entering will be taught. Sponsored groups are Boy Scouts, Girl Scouts, etc., while spontaneous groups are gangs.

Gang membership during preadolescence supplements the security previously felt within the family. The adolescent takes on a new identity; consequently he must reassess himself. He extends his social sphere and becomes educated in new social techniques. He involves himself in new restrictions and patterns of obedience and conforms to new social patterns. When he voluntarily accepts restrictions the child begins to become a truly moral person.

What about the delinquent activity of some gangs? Generally, as the child matures he accepts the idea of "achievement by status." When this occurs the importance of the age group subsides and he becomes involved in activities that point him toward achieving status in our wider society.

High School Achievement

Consider the high school years a period of transition between childhood and adulthood. Hess[48] states in his study that the development of stable adult behavior continues well past high school. In fact, late adolescence and early adulthood may be a more critical period of development than adolescence. Successful performance in the early twenties is more closely related to events and experiences that occur in those years than to behavior in high school. "There seems to be a moratorium during high school, a waiting for things to happen that is abruptly broken by graduation."

Most physicians believe that high school achievement determines whether an adolescent is satisfied or dissatisfied with the high school experience. Jackson and Getzels[49] studied the school experience of students enrolled in a midwestern private school. Their conclusion appears to support the contention that "dissatisfaction with school appears to be part of a larger picture of psychological discontent, rather than a direct reflection of inefficient functioning in the classroom." There was little difference in intellectual ability and scholastic achievement between the satisfied and dissatisfied.

Girls expressed their dissatisfaction differently from boys. The girls were more likely to be self-critical, blaming themselves for their dissatisfaction. On the other hand, the boys blamed the world around them, including the adults.

Characteristics of a Male Juvenile Delinquent

Contrary to popular opinion the delinquent is likely to have the physique of an athlete. He is not undernourished and his height and weight is superior to the nondelinquent. He is masculine in bone and muscles with broad shoulders and chest and a tapering torso and narrow hips.

The delinquent is not at all the product of disease or weakness. The difference in the general health of the delinquent and nondelinquent is small. There is one physical difference, however; the handgrip of the delinquent is stronger, reflecting greater vitality. Neurologic handicaps are another significant difference between the two groups. *More nondelinquent boys have neurologic or psychoneurotic troubles than do delinquents.* The delinquent and the nondelinquent are about a stand-off as to mentality—perhaps the delinquents have a little more creative ability.

The difference that exists between the two is mainly in temperament and feeling. The delinquent lacks common sense; he finds thinking and acting in conformity with the community nearly impossible. He appears constitutionally unable to follow a methodical approach to a problem; his "social assertion" gets in the way. This social assertion is his determination to assert not his rights or his opinions but his will. He wants what he wants when he wants it, never mind what anybody else says or thinks.

Far from having feelings of insecurity or anxiety, the delinquent has no feelings of frustration nor inferiority. He does not worry about losing his job, his home or his liberty. He is an unappreciated superior being. He is self reliant, extroverted; he acts on impulse with little self control; he explodes and does not brood; he thrives on danger. The delinquent may present a charming vivacity, a liveliness of manner that makes him outshine many solid and dependable young citizens.

Too often the danger and excitement that he needs is only fulfilled by violating the law. To satisfy this craving, a delinquent will steal cars, hop trucks, keep late hours, roam the streets, drink and generally exult in destructive mischief.

Half of the delinquent boys studied by Glueck[50] were active members of gangs, organized for a definite antisocial purpose. The survey shatters the illusion that the delinquent is led into crime by bad companions. From earliest childhood he shows a preference for the company of other boys as unmanageable as himself.

Emotional Problems in Teenage Girls

Becoming an emotionally secure woman is a difficult task for most teenage girls. The girl may manifest bizarre behavior while doing so. The family physician should be able to recognize what is normal and what is abnormal behavior and give appropriate counsel.

Abnormal behavior may be recognized by two characteristics: sudden change from her usual behavior pattern and persistent adjustment difficulties in any area of her daily living. These disturbances are most likely to be found in the following areas: scholastic, social, physical and disciplinary.[51]

Scholastic: She

–begins to do poor work or fails, where previously she did well
–becomes distressed by her inability to concentrate or redoubles her study habits
–does poor school work out of proportion to her intelligence
–has a panic reaction or examination anxiety
–has marked reaction against one subject although she is a good student
–has strong antagonism to one teacher

Social: She

–feels inadequate
–relates fantasies as though they were the truth
–express ideas contrary to those of her group

Physical: She

–fatigues
–has headaches
–has dysmenorrhea

Disciplinary: She

–has behavior problems such as stealing
–fails to observe rules and laws
–is promiscuous sexually

Recognize these early signs and symptoms of emotional disturbance. Advise psychotherapy while the girl still has a flexible personality.

Referring the Teenager to a Psychiatrist

Few adolescents will accept the original offer of psychiatric counseling. Expect the following chain of events: the parents contact a family physician and arrange psychiatric counseling; the adolescent meets the psychiatrist and refuses therapy; the adolescent disappears for a variable time; finally the adolescent returns voluntarily and perhaps highly motivated for counseling.

Teenage Depression

Depression in an adolescent is frequent. It is an encouraging sign if not suffered too long nor too deeply. Bouts of teenage depression demonstrate the adolescent's ability to internalize and absorb his problems, often resulting in realigning their psychic forces into stronger and more realistic patterns. If conflict, however, depletes their self-esteem too far, symptoms of emotional breakdown appear. Depression, as known in adults, is not usually recognized until the third or fourth decade of life.

In contrast to adults, the reaction to depression in teenagers differs with the sex of the patient. The female must balance her active and passive wishes. Her passive nature demands intimacy and someone to love. Her active nature demands gratification through mastery but without exhibiting masculine competition. She must balance being and doing, pleasing and being pleased, submitting and resisting, wishing and acting. The female's self-esteem, then, is based more on passive-internal-change. She must wait to be loved, to love and to please. She must wait for a special man without too much frustration. Consequently there will be bouts of depression while she learns to handle these conflicts.

The male does not accept reality as readily as the female; he attempts to modify the world rather than himself. This he emphasizes in his action and mastery. The male reacts to threats to his self-esteem with apathy rather than depression. He protects his self-esteem by pretending that effort is not important. He substitutes passive aims for active ones, idealizing inner life at expense of outer life. This leads to "dropping-out" or drug abuse—dropping-out to avoid competition and drug use to modify reality.

When should the family physician intervene?[52] First, only if the depression occurs over a long period of time. Second, only if the teenager cannot maintain some long-term relationships, and, third, only if there is too long a delay in finding substitute gratifications.

What can the family physician do? Help the teenager understand his passivity as an attempt to maintain his self-esteem. Encourage him to engage in activities which do not threaten him. Help him understand the measure of his development and how to continue developing.

Gynecologic Problems

The physical preparation of teenage girls for later pregnancy was discussed in Chapter 2. The family physician should learn to diagnose and treat the majority of teenage gynecologic complaints also because he has known the patient and her mother over a period of years; he has their confidence and they feel comfortable with him. The mother may resent referral to a specialist who carries the aura of pregnancies and tumors.

Dysmenorrhea

The commonest gynecologic problem in adolescence is primary dysmenorrhea. Incidently, this complaint implies that the genitals probably are normal. Dysmenorrhea begins with increasing maturity since the early menstrual periods are almost invariably anovulatory.

In differential diagnosis, rule out endometriosis by careful palpatation of the internal genitalia. A history of unilateral pain, rectal pain during defecation at start of period and pain without nausea and vomiting point toward endometriosis. The finding of tender nodules in the posterior cul-de-sac will help verify the diagnosis. Other disabilities to rule out are chronic gonorrheal or nonspecific infections, tuberculosis, leukomyomas and adenomyosis.

Painful periods may begin 1 to 2 years after menstruation begins, attain a peak around age 18 and then begin to improve. Marriage relieves some of the pain and pregnancy generally cures the disability.

For severe cramps, prevent dysmenorrhea by suppressing ovulation with a combination contraceptive pill or norethynodrel 5 to 10 mg per day for 20 days starting on the fifth day of her menstrual cycle. This may be continued for 2 to 4 months. Withdraw the medication and then observe the patient for continued relief.

Golub exercise for dysmenorrhea, if done regularly, will relieve pain in about 60 percent of girls. Instruct the girl to begin the exercise the day after menstruation ceases. It will give some girls appreciable relief during the next period; others it will not help for two to three months. Tell the patient to stand with her feet 18 inches apart, knees straight, arms raised sideways at shoulder height. Next tell her to try and touch her left heel with the fingers of her right hand by bending forward at the waist and twisting to the left but without bending her knees. Tell her to stand erect again and repeat the exercise touching the right heel with the fingers of her left hand.

Abnormal Gynecologic Bleeding

Causes of abnormal gynecologic bleeding in a child are foreign body, vaginitis, rape, accident, mother's contraceptive pills, precocious puberty, bleeding defects and neoplasms such as granulosa cell tumors.

Causes of abnormal bleeding in an adolescent are dysfunctional anovulatory bleeding, contraceptive pills, pregnancy, threatened spontaneous abortion, incomplete abortion, psychogenic infection, hypothyroidism, ovarian cysts and tumors, iron deficiency, bleeding defects such as thrombocytopenic purpura and Stein-Leventhal syndrome of polycystic ovaries.

DYSFUNCTIONAL ANOVULATORY BLEEDING. Dysfunctional anovulatory bleeding accounts for 95 percent of the vaginal blood lost in teenage girls. The history of severe blood loss should be verified by a hematologic examination. If treated properly, dysfunctional bleeding will cease within 4 months. Diagnose functional bleeding by excluding other possible causes. Rule out pregnancy by checking human chorionic gonadotropin (HCG) in the urine after 40 days have elapsed since the start of the patient's last period. Take cervical scrapings for detection of the rare case of cervical cancer. A flat basal body temperature record indicates anovulatory bleeding while a characteristic ovulatory pattern indicates hypermenorrhea. Hospitalize for a D. and C. if there is need for a cervical biopsy as indicated by a positive pap smear.

Diagnose dysfunctional bleeding once systemic causes are ruled out. Start cyclical therapy. If bleeding is profuse, give Enovid 5 to 30 mg daily for 20 days. This will decrease bleeding within a few hours and stop it completely in 24 to 48 hr. After 20 days, skip 5 to 7 days and lower the dosage to 2.5 mg of Enovid-E (norethynodrel with mestranol) or Ovulen (ethynodiol diacetate with mestranol) 1 mg daily for another 20 days. Continue therapy for 3 mo or longer and follow the patient closely for 6 to 12 mo or until she resumes normal ovulatory function.

If for some reason oral medication cannot or will not be taken, resort to parenteral administration. Give Delestrogen (estradiol 17-valerate) 10 to 40 mg. (Larger doses may have to be given to the adolescent patient than to the adult). Approximately two wk later, give a booster injection of 5 to 10 mg together with 250 mg of Delalutin (hydroxyprogesterone).

If the pelvic examination is normal and the pap smear negative in the teenager, perform a D. and C. only after cyclical therapy has failed or bleeding is very profuse.

Unfortunately, women who have experienced menorrhagia in adolescence are likely to be plagued by an abnormal menstrual pattern and a diminished reproductive potential all their lives.

Amenorrhea

PRIMARY. The mean menarcheal potential age has now been set at about 12 yr of age with wide variations. Be concerned if a girl hasn't menstruated by age 15 or 16, especially if her mother menstruated at a very young age. The sequence of events are budding of breasts and the appearance of pubic hair at age 9 or 10, increased vaginal secretion and breast development to the primary mamma stage at 10 or 11 and the appearance of axillary hair and menarche at 12 or 13.

Causes of primary amenorrhea are hereditary, body build and nutritional. There also may be a delay in the developmental sequence of the secondary sex characteristics as outlined above. In a few girls who have secondary sexual development but who have not menstruated, think of the possibility of activation of the hypothalamic-pituitary-ovarian mechanism and endometrial failure to respond to the sex hormones. If there exists, however, a breast bud, estrogen is beginning to circulate. In the latter event, suspect congenital malformations of the genital tract such as imperforate hymen or internal abnormalities wherein specialty help may be needed for diagnoses.

Laboratory tests to help assess hormone production are hanging-drop preparation of urinary sediment for cornified urethral cells indicating that significant amounts of estrogen are present in the circulation; aspiration of vaginal secretions with a pipet for detecting cornified vaginal cells; and determination of pituitary and ovarian activity by giving 50 mg clomiphene citrate (Clomid) twice daily for 5 days. If low levels of pituitary-ovarian activity are present, menstruation may be triggered. If no secondary sexual characteristics are present order buccal smears. Here again, request consultation.

SECONDARY. Diagnose postmenarcheal amenorrhea whenever a year or more of amenorrhea occurs between the first two periods *or* when an amenorrhea of more than 6 months occurs during the second year after menarche. Forty periods are necessary before a girl develops her individual adult pattern.

Causes of secondary amenorrhea are stress amenorrhea sometimes called "summer," "travel" or "boarding school" amenorrhea; pregnancy; malnutrition; obesity; drastic reducing diets; and, rarely, chromophobe adenoma verified by radiographic evidence of a ballooning sella turcica.

Vaginitis

Two factors complicate the problems of leukorrhea and vaginal infections in the teenage group. The teenager will very often produce a copious amount of secretion during the years immediately after her menarche. Mothers confuse this discharge with a vaginitis. A vaginal smear taken in the office will establish the diagnosis: the absence of pus and bacteria and the presence of large masses of superficial vaginal cells indicate excessive vaginal secretion.

Vulvar spray deodorants as well as tight fitting underpants may cause an atopic vulvitis with discharge. *Bacterial:* yellowish to greenish mucopurulent and occasionally frothy discharge. *Trichomoniasis:* purulent, often watery and bubbly, frothy white to yellowish discharge. *Candidiasis:* thick, tenacious, often cheesy-white discharge. *Gonorrhea:* profuse and purulent discharge. *Diabetic vulvitis:* cheesy, curdlike discharge.

Diagnosis:[53] With a narrow 4-inch speculum, on which there is a minimum of lubrication, remove and place a drop of discharge on a slide and moisten with a drop of warm saline. Examine the wet smear under low power without a coverslip. Search for trichomonads, hyphae of fungi and pus cells. To see the fungi better add a drop of potassium hydroxide and heat. To detect Neisseria gonorrhoeae, culture on chocolate or Thayer-Martin media.

Treatment: Bacterial: have the patient insert a Furacin urethral insert in the vagina nightly for at least 1 week or until symptoms disappear. As an alternative use a triple sulfa cream. Candidiasis: treat with Mycostatin vaginal inserts at bedtime for 2 weeks. Trichomoniasis: depending on age, treat with Flagyl inserts or oral tablets.

REFERENCES

1. Swischuk LE: Respiratory distress in the newborn. *Postgrad Med* 46: 233–235, 1969.
2. Reynolds EOR: Hyaline membrane disease. *Am J Obstet Gynecol* 106: 780–797, 1970.
3. Focus on the Newborn, in Gustafson SR and Coursin DB (eds): The Pediatric Patient. Philadelphia: JB Lippincott, 1965, pp 82–85.
4. Safer breath for the newborn. *Emerg Med* 3: 83–87, 1971.
5. Diamond EF: New insights from fetology. *Med Times* 98:115–118, 1970.
6. Giunta F: Phototherapy reduces infant hyperbilirubinemia. *Postgrad Med* 46:30, 1969.
7. Preston EN: Whither the foreskin? A consideration of routine neonatal circumcision. *JAMA* 213:1853–1858, 1970.
8. Hsia DY-Y: A critical evaluation of PKU screening. *Hosp Pract* 4:101–112, 1971.
9. Miller M: Pure-tone audiometry in prenatal rubella. *Arch Otolaryngol* 94:25–29, 1971.

10. Kendall K, et al: Study of preparation of infant formulas. *Am J Dis Child* 122:224–228, 1971.
11. Hamburg L: Controlled trial of fluoride in vitamin drops for prevention of cavities in children. *Lancet* 1:441–442, 1971.
12. Fomon SJ, et al: Acceptance of unsalted strained foods by normal infants. *J Pediatr* 76:242–246, 1970.
13. McCue CN: The child with cogenital heart disease. *Med Times* 88:1414–1418, 1960.
14. Burg FD, et al: Automotive restraint devices for the pediatric patient. *Ped* 45:49, 1970.
15. Cozen LN: Orthopedic examination of the infant and child. *AFP* 4:60, 1971.
16. Kellsey DC: Bowing of the long bones in infants and childhood. *GP* 26:87–94, 1967.
17. Symposium: Pediatric foot and leg conditions: when therapy is urgent. *Patient Care* 4:124, 1970.
18. Kempe CH: Current status of immunization. *Drug Therapy* 1:45, 1971.
19. Caldwell BM, Drachman RH: Comparability of three methods of assessing the developmental level of young infants. *Ped.* 34:38, 1964.
20. A guide for vision screening in California public schools. Calif State Dept of Ed. June 1964 ed.
21. A guide to the education of the deaf in public schools of California. Calif State Dept of Ed, p 12.
22. Dey FL: Auditory fatigue and predicted permanent hearing defects from rock-and-roll music. *N Eng J Med* 282:467–470, 1970.
23. Hastings DE, Barrington TW: Applied therapy. *Ped Patient* 8:323, 1966.
24. Rammelkamp CH, Monson TP: Streptococcal infections: why it is important to diagnose and treat them quickly. *Med Time* 99:48–57, 1971.
25. When strep throat is suspected. *Infect Dis* 1:7, 1971.
26. Battle CV, Glasgow LA: Reliability of bacteriologic identification of 3 hemolytic streptococci in private offices. *Am J Dis Child* 122:134–136, 1971.
27. ASO titer on single specimen determines group A strep infections. *Infect Dis* 1:1, 1971.
28. Spagnuolo M: Prevention of rheumatic fever. *Med Times* 98: 121, 1970.
29. Derrick CW, Dillon HC: Impetigo contagioso. *AFP* 4:75, 1971.
30. Interview with Dr. Martin Rosenberg: Diagnosis and management of tuberculosis. *Ped Herald* 12: 1, 1971.
31. Family structure in achievement in motivation in Grinder RE (ed): Studies in Adolescence, ed.2. New York: Macmillan, 1969, p 199.
32. Kohn ML: Social class and parental values in Grinder RE (ed): Studies in Adolescence, ed.2. New York: Macmillan, 1969, p 187.
33. Moss HA, Kagan J: Stability of achievement and recognition seeking behavior from early childhood through adulthood in Grinder RE (ed): Studies in Adolescence, ed. 2. New York: Macmillan, 1969, p 152.
34. Havighurst RJ: Conditions productive of superior children in Grinder RE (ed): Studies in Adolescence, ed.2. New York: Macmillan, 1969, pp 501–510.
35. Guilford JP: Factors that aid and hinder creativity in Grinder RE (ed): Studies in Adolescence, ed. 2. New York: Macmillan, 1969, p 484.
36. Kenny TJ, Clemmens RL: Medical and psychological correlates in children with learning disabilities. *J Pediatr* 78:273–277, 1971.
37. Marmor J: "Normal" and "deviant" sexual behavior. *JAMA* 217:165–170, 1971.
38. Jenkins RL: Hyperkinesis: making the parents understand their child. *Med Insight* 3:48–59, 1971.
39. Goodman JD: Short-term treatment in child psychiatry. *AFP* 3:80–85, 1971.
40. Havighurst, RJ: Conditions productive of superior children in Grinder RE (ed): Studies in Adolescence, ed.2. New York: Macmillan, 1969, p 507.
41. Ames/Diagnostic No 20 (May) 1971, p 15.
42. Interview with TS Danowski reported in *Pediatr Herald* 12:1, 1971.
43. Peck RF: Family pattern correlated with adolescent personality structure in Grinder RE (ed): Studies in adolescence, ed. 2. New York: Macmillan, 1969, pp 133–140.
44. Bayley N, Schaefer ES: Maternal behavior and personality development. Data from the Berkeley Group Study in Grinder RE (ed): Studies in Adolescence, ed. 2. New York: Macmillan, 1969, pp 141–151.
45. McCord J, et al: Some effects of paternal absence on male children in Grinder RE (ed): Studies in Adolescence, ed. 2. New York: Macmillan, 1969, pp 118–132.
46. Wilson WC: The development of ethnic attitudes in adolescence in Grinder RE (ed): Studies in Adolescence, ed.2. New York: Macmillan, 1969, p 265.
47. Eisenstadt SN: From Generation to Generation. London: Routledge and Kegan Paul, 1956.
48. Hess RD: High school antecedents of young adult achievement in Grinder RE (ed): Studies in Adolescence, ed.2. New York: Macmillan, 1969, 401–414.
49. Jackson PW, Getzels JW: Psychological health classroom functioning: A study of dissatisfaction with school among adolescents in Grinder RE (ed): Studies in Adolescence, ed.2. New York: Macmillan, 1969, pp 392–400.
50. Glueck S, Gleuck E: Unraveling the threads of juvenile delinquency. Commonwealth Fund.
51. Kline CL: Recognizing emotional problems in adolescent girls. *Wisc Med J* 5:127, 1957.
52. Walters PA: When to treat and not to treat adolescent depression. *Med Insight* 3:40, 1971.
53. Huffman JW: Gynecologic examination of the teenager. *Obstet Gynecol Observer* 10:2, 1972.
54. Medical news. *JAMA* 202:28, 1967.

CHAPTER 4

Family Practice Psychiatry

Kindness makes for good public relations in dealing with *all* patients. I have observed that some of my peers have rapidly built large practices while others never developed much of a practice. I also observed that the latter displayed ill-temper and appeared unsympathetic and were inclined to argue with their patients or to resent any questioning. They forgot a fundamental truism: *be kind.*

Fortunate is the young resident who came into this world endowed with a kindly, friendly, sympathetic nature. He is even more fortunate if he realizes that he will have more success treating a patient who likes him and feels comfortable with him than he will have with a patient who feels resentful toward him.

Tame your temper. Be patient with the person who seeks your help. Listen carefully to his story and do not resent his questions; it may save you an embarrassing mistake in diagnosis.

Avoid the trap of attempting to treat your friends who have psychoneurotic problems; you cannot be objective. Refer all psychotics. The latter nearly always require the help of a psychiatrist and usually hospitalization.

Most family physicians have been told they need spend only 15 to 20 minutes a week to treat patients with psychophysiologic, autonomic and visceral disorders, anxiety, depression and conversion-obsessive neurosis and phobias. But little or no information is given to him as to exactly what he should attempt to do during this time.

Give emotional support. Help the patient realize his assets. Urge him to think positively about himself. Play down his liabilities. Reassure him about his physical condition. Give him accurate information. Relieve his anxiety and his fear of the unknown.

Allow the patient to talk; the psychiatrists call it ventilating. This will release anxiety and hostility. Listening to the patient with empathy is therapeutic in itself. Do not judge, condemn or criticize. There are times when it is wise to be silent.

If the patient has built up social and business .stress, temporarily change his environment. This will help accomplish two things: it will help establish a normal life pattern and it will take him out of social "combat." The rest need not always be in a hospital but that should be considered.

Do not be fearful of practicing psychiatry and utilizing psychiatric principles in treating your patients. Often you alone can and should treat the illness. Remember, the diagnosis and treatment of mental illness are medical problems. He is a human being who is suffering and who is, in some way, attempting to cope with problems of living. He has a right to be in a doctor's office and to receive competent medical care. He has a right to be treated with dignity and concern. Few are malingerers.

Tailor your treatment to the individual's need. Decide early whether the patient needs only one thing—advice, counseling, drugs, support or listening to. All will require insight, some require referral.

RELATING TO THE PSYCHIATRIC PATIENT

When a patient comes to your office with a minor complaint, which has been present for months or years, consider this an almost sure sign that there is a deeper, more serious problem, which is the real reason for the visit, and that the problem is most likely to be psychological.

Learn to observe accurately. Attempt to understand the patient's nonverbal communication. Every facet of the patient, including his greeting, banter, small-talk, irrelevancies, body movement and gestures, is a form of communicating with the doctor and is related in some way to the patient's health problem.

Attempt to understand the patient's personality, his defenses and his probable response to stress. Store this information for later use when the patient may be more receptive to an interpretation of his symptoms. Do not use all data at once.

Train yourself to recognize major but hidden syndromes, especially that of depression.

When you learn something new about a patient, do not react to it immediately. It is difficult to delay application of a newly discovered clinical fact. However, it is important to you to learn to consider carefully the patient's tolerance for insight.

Remember your interest and concern is beneficial in relieving the patient's pain and depression.

Do not always attempt to make the patient distinguish between organic and psychiatric disease. Do not force the patient to accept that he has no organic disease but rather a psychiatric illness. Think of the patient in toto and help the patient to think of himself in the same way.

Allow the patient to make the final decision as to the amount and depth of therapy he can accept or tolerate.

ORGANIC VS PSYCHOLOGICAL ILLNESS

Positively identifying patients with psychological illness may be one of the family physician's most difficult problems. Remember: make a positive diagnosis of a psychosis or neurosis. You are not playing fair with your patient when you run a battery of tests, declare they are all negative and, consequently, assume the patient has a psychological ailment. This is a negative diagnosis made by default.

Exclusion can help strengthen the diagnosis, but it cannot be relied upon alone. Although organic illness may appear to be ruled out by the usual diagnostic procedures, we cannot on that appearance always conclude that the patient is emotionally ill. Similarly, by excluding psychogenic disorders, we cannot definitely conclude that organic disease exists.

Your search for positive evidence of a neurosis should begin by determining how the patient has coped and is coping with anxiety (see Anxiety later in this chapter). Find out what happened when he was ill or injured. Determine how well he handled losses. Evaluation of his emotional strength during these times of stress can be a positive early finding in neurosis.

Certain characteristics of symptoms tend to denote psychogenic illness, while others indicate organic disease (Table 4-1).

If you wait for a patient or his relatives to report hallucinations, you have missed an early diagnosis of a psychosis. Probably an important early question to ask if you suspect psychosis is, "Have you had any changes in your body lately?" In this way you may elicit psychotic ideation of body members. You may be surprised at his answer. A psychotic may state his brain is rotting or a woman may think her legs are changing to men's legs. These beliefs of the patient that changes are occurring precede other more obvious findings and are a tip-off of an early psychosis.

Table 4-1. Characteristics of Symptoms

Characteristics of pain	*Organic*	*Psychogenic*
Quality	Burning, sharp, crampy, sore or catchy "It hurts."	Vague, bizarre, tingling; throbbing, irritating, nagging, numb or tight "It's hard to describe."
Location	Well localized, radiates to a well-defined course.	Poorly localized, moves around, can't put finger on it "It moves around."
Production	Generally provoked by a specific activity.	Not related to any activity "No special time."
Duration	Intermittent and decreases or increases.	Constant "It lasts all day."
Relief	Most patients find some way to get at least partial relief	Patient has found no way to obtain relief. "It just goes away."
Intensification	Aggravated by some specific activity	Not related to any activity, worse when tired "The pain is always the same."
Awakening	Commonly awakens patient from sleep	Once asleep, the patient rarely is awakened by pain

THE PATIENT WHO CANNOT ADAPT EMOTIONALLY

Identify the patient who has a guilty need to work increasingly. With this person work has been an unrecognized instrument for satisfying aggressive and erotic feelings. This could be one reason why some elderly people fail rapidly and die soon after retirement. These are the people who all through their lives had trouble adapting themselves to changes normally expectable in a life span (Table 4-2).

The person who cannot substantially renounce or modify his work pattern is also the one who had difficulty in renouncing the breast for the bottle, the bottle for the cup. He had difficulty in renouncing the pleasures of the nursery for greater responsibility of more formal schooling, the security of his parent's home for the responsibility of marriage and his own family.

One might surmise that this is the same person who cannot accept the possibility of death, for death is also another step in adaptation. The well balanced individual starts his life activity in play—a form of pleasure. Play gradually becomes work as the youngster adapts himself to reality.

Signs of Emotional Decompensation (Nervous Breakdown)

Emotional decompensation is the appearance of a mental disorder when the patient's defense mechanisms have failed to function. The person can no longer cope with stress. Signs of emotional decompensation are found in the patient who is:

–excessively quiet and disinterested
–easily discouraged or depressed
–bitter or surly
–aggressive with a chip on his shoulder
–fearful without cause
–dissatisfied with himself
–careless about his appearance and of being on time
–increasing his use of alcohol, tobacco or profanity
–suffering from psychosomatic ailments —palpitation, sweating, gastric complaints, low back pain, headaches, fatigue and dizziness
–uncooperative

Table 4-2. Transitions, Changes and Conditions That Provoke Stress

Biologic transitions	*Pathologic conditions*	*Social changes*
Birth	Severe injury	Starting, changing or leaving school
Infancy to childhood	Surgery	Moving from home to home
Adolescence	Chronic disabling illness	Changing language
Marriage	Congenital	Changing social patterns: dating, marriage, divorce, widowhood
Pregnancy and childbirth	Neoplastic	
Menopause	Degenerative	First employment
Old age	Infectious	Change of employment
	Body defects	Failure in employment
	Deafness	Retirement
	Blindness	Change in socioeconomic class level
	Deformity	

ANXIETY

Causes of anxiety are:

- –fear of being overwhelmed physically, emotionally or financially
- –fear of losing contact with loved ones (separation anxiety)
- –fear of bodily injury
- –fear of one's conscience (5- to 6-year olds)
- –fear of losing the love of one's peer group (adolescents)
- –fear of the loss of approval of one's social group

Any or all of these fears may persist, causing anxiety and depression. If a patient is unduly anxious take steps to prevent depression; if he is depressed seek out his anxieties. The train of events: the patient is threatened with the loss of an object or a loved one; this anxiety may create a feeling of anger which when turned inward may be expressed as depression.

Anxiety is a difficult feeling to live with. Rather than suffer with this distress a person unconsciously changes anxiety into physiological symptoms. This change is called *binding* or *conversion*.

Anxiety can also be bound in the symptoms of phobias, conversion symptoms and neurotic actions. The patient converts his anxiety into these symptoms and is then able to go to his physician for treatment of the physical rather than the mental symptoms. Conversion or binding is a process of great importance to the family physician.

Estimates are that 50 percent of the patients seen by physicians have some anxiety that causes discomfort (Table 4-3) that cannot be related to any physical, chemical or organic disease. The major symptoms are caused by distress in the gastrointestinal tract, but there are other forms.

A common complaint of the anxious patient is gas and belching. The chief reason for this is that his anxieties have produced the habit of swallowing. When he swallows, down goes some air. These air swallowers can puff up like balloons. Others are convinced by pain that they are having angina pectoris.

Sometimes the presenting complaint suggests the anxiety state: palpitation, choking sensations, sighing respirations and fatiguability are functional in nature. Occasionally you can tell by observing the patient—look for throbbing neck vessels, twitching, purposeless movements and flushing. All these suggest that the story being told is based upon a state of anxiety.

The rescue of a harassed patient from the grip of fear is one of the most satisfying experiences in the practice of medicine. Anxiety over a self-made diagnosis impels many patients to seek your advice. But remember the complaint made to you is never of fear, but of some symptom which the patient has sensed and upon which a fancied disease has been built. Most of these pa-

Table 4-3. Organic Reactions to Emotional-Psychological Stress

Psychologic	*Neurologic*	*Cardiorespiratory*
Anxiety states Depression Schizophrenia Neurosis	Headaches Seizures Conversion hysteria	Hypertension Angina Asthma Peripheral vascular disease
Gastrointestinal	*Genitourinary*	*Musculoskeletal*
Dysphagia Dyspepsia (ulcer) Spastic colitis Constipation Anorexia nervosa Cholecystic disease	Enuresis Frequency of voiding Dysmenorrhea Impotence Satyriasis Nymphomania	Arthritis Low back pain Shoulder-arm syndrome Torticollis

tients can be handled without reference to a psychiatrist.

A good relationship with a family doctor is the most important single factor in treating those who need no surgery or medicine. In short, you must identify the patient's anxieties and tensions and talk him out of his fears. The family physician is about the only member of the profession who is fitted to diagnose these patients. The physician must love people and be interested enough in human beings to study them.

First, do a careful history and physical examination. Learn all you can about the patient: his childhood, his school days, his working conditions and his home life. Do not hurry this process. This history-taking can continue after the initial examination. Selected tests are important. You cannot make a convincing argument that the complaint of difficulty in swallowing is due to esophageal spasm unless the esophagus has been examined. In every case explain the reason for the symptoms and the relationship of the complaints to the responsible situation. Point out such well known emotional reactions as blushing, crying, tachycardia, vomiting, diarrhea and frequent urination when under stress. In this way it is usually possible to explain to a fearful patient how the particular symptom may have arisen.

Many patients worn down by fear get hold of themselves after they have confessed to someone or talked over their troubles. These patients do not need lecturing. Show no disgust; pass no judgment. Many will return to tell you that you cured them when you showed you liked them and didn't think what they had done was unforgiveable. Listen. Be kindly, tactful and pertinent.

Don't be misled when a patient says he has no cause for worry or unhappiness; that he has nothing to tell. Later you will find, if you pursue the diagnosis, he will pour out a story of unhappiness and sorrow that caused the illness. Peculiarly enough, while you are endeavoring to get the patient's story, he or she has told it all to the patient sitting alongside him in the waiting room.

Anxiety Neurosis Vs Hysteria

Anxiety neurosis is a familial disease. When one parent is affected, nearly half the children have anxiety neurosis. Anxiety neurosis has some features in common with hysteria and the differential diagnosis is sometimes difficult (Table 4-4).

DEPRESSION

Depression of mood is a normal reaction to disappointment or loss of a valued relationship or possession. In the normal person, the mood passes quickly. A depressed mood is a common feature of the syndrome

Table 4-4. Differential Diagnosis in Anxiety Neurosis Vs Hysteria

	Anxiety neurosis	*Hysteria*
Sex	More common in females 2:1	Almost exclusively women
Age of onset	Can be diagnosed in early 20's	Can be diagnosed in early 20's
Symptoms in organ systems	May involve several systems but has a stereotyped pattern	Involvement of several organ systems
Other symptoms	Symptoms referrable to the autonomic nervous system: palpitation, tachycardia, rapid and shallow breathing, dizziness and tremor. Concern about a life-threatening ailment or death. Phobias are common	Complicated medical history and polysurgery. Conversion symptoms such as amnesia, blindness and paralysis common but not universal. Talkative, cheerful or hostile. History is a better guide than immediate clinical impression
Response to symptoms	Physical symptoms accompanied by fear; seldom seen in emergencies; see fewer doctors; have less surgery	Petulance, irritation or indifference. Dramatic attacks; often seen in emergencies; see many doctors; have more treatment and surgery
Attacks	Definite onset and spontaneous termination	Polysymptomatic; does not change or worsen
Between attacks	Relatively asymptomatic except for fatigue and lack of stamina	Constant marital and domestic trouble; miss work frequently

but may be obscured by other symptoms if not specifically inquired into.

Depression is associated with the following:

- –self-deprecation and remorsefulness about inconsequential acts of the past
- –concern about death or religion
- –obsessions, repetitive thoughts or impulses
- –vegetative symptoms of anorexia, loss of weight and persistent insomnia
- –thoughts of suicide
- –radical changes in life
- –mania (does not occur often but when it does it is pathognomonic of depression)
- –family history of depression, mania or alcoholism
- –physical complaints

In one study, the chief complaint in half the patients was constipation, spells, headache, blurred vision, assorted pains, and paresthesias. The physical symptoms disappear as the depression abates. Until then, nothing relieves the physical complaints.

The first attack of depression may occur at any age of life. Half the patients are seen by a doctor during their first attack. Uncomplicated depression has a high rate of spontaneous remission. Most recover whether treated or not.

Depressives are plagued by poor concentration, irritability, slow thinking and fear of losing their minds. Physically they are unkept, untidy, and have immobile facies and a tremor of the outstretched hand. They show poor judgement, resigning from jobs, selling their homes and leaving their spouses.

Complications of depression are suicide, alcoholism, and disruption of personal, social and financial lives. Fifty percent have suicidal thoughts and 15 percent die by suicide. The classical patient with depression who has suicidal ideas should be hospitalized. A psychiatrist is often needed.

Antidepressive medication and electroconvulsive therapy shorten the depression and relieves symptoms in almost all patients.

Legal Risks

Antidepressants have made it possible to treat more depressed patients on an outpatient basis. Consequently, more family physicians are doing so, increasing their legal and ethical responsibilities.

Make the diagnosis of depression after a careful history and physical examination. Diagnosis can be made on the commonly accepted symptoms of weeping, weight loss, insomnia or slow speech.

Organize and plot a therapeutic course for several weeks ahead, including frequent office visits. Document in writing the suggested visits both in your records and in a memo to the patient.

If the patient is suicidal, notify your office nurses, your answering service and other physicians who may be covering for you of the patient's tendency. Pass along explicit instructions.

Do not prescribe more than a dangerous dose of any medication (Table 4-5), and mark each prescription nonrefillable.

Be on the alert for the cardinal clues to impending suicide (see following). Do not hesitate to directly ask the patient if he has such thoughts.

Refer severe psychotics, the complicated neurotic and the severely depressed child. If parents and family refuse to cooperate, withdraw from the case after giving written notice to those involved. A reasonable date should be set for your withdrawal, allowing reasonable time for employing other care.

Legal risks that may develop follow:

- –failure to diagnose
- –failure to recognize organic disease in the depressed
- –failure to seek consultation after a reasonable therapeutic trial
- –failure to keep the family advised of the danger
- –failure to be available
- –failure to be prudent in ordering drugs, i.e. too heavy dose, too many pills.

Recognizing the Suicidal Patient

Be constantly alert to signs of a suicidal patient. Characteristics of a patient who is contemplating suicide are that he:

- –feels lonely and isolated
- –believes his problems are overwhelming
- –feels powerless to change his situation
- –overestimates his problems
- –underestimates possible solutions
- –believes suicide his only alternative

Warning clues for potential suicide are a patient who:

- –makes any attempt at suicide no matter how minor
- –is disoriented, dazed, preoccupied, or having hallucinations
- –claims he would be better off dead or that others would be better off with him dead
- –becomes agitated upon being informed of the need for a tissue biopsy
- –is hospitalized but attempts to avoid tests
- –becomes upset each time his relatives visit him
- –begins to give away his prized possessions
- –does not talk to anyone
- –sleeps most of the day
- –consults a lawyer and puts his affairs in order
- –makes funeral arrangements

Table 4-5. Guide For Prescriptions of Antidepressants in Suicidal Patients

Antidepressant	*Availability*	*Dosage*	*Prescription (no more than)*
Elavil (amitriptyline)	10, 25, and 50 mg tablets	25 mg q.i.d.	40 tablets (10-day supply)
Norpramin (desipramine)	25 and 50 mg tablets	25 mg q.i.d.	40 tablets (10-day supply)
Tofranil (imipramine)	10, 25, and 50 mg tablets	25 mg q.i.d.	44 tablets (11-day supply)
Aventyl (nortriptyline)	10 and 25 mg tablets	60 mg daily	(15-day supply)
Marplan (isocarboxazid)	10 mg tablets	10 mg b.i.d.	24 tablets (12-day supply)
Niamid (nialamide)	25 mg tablets	25 mg t.i.d.	36 tablets (12-day supply)
Nardil (phenelzine)	15 mg tablets	15 mg t.i.d.	30 tablets (10-day supply)
Parnate (tranylcypromine)	10 mg tablets	10 mg b.i.d.	24 tablets (12-day supply)

- –has been advised he will need surgery that will result in a change in his body structure
- –has been informed he has a terminal illness
- –has given birth to a stillborn or an infant with congenital malformations
- –suffers the loss of a close friend or relative
- –questions how many sleeping pills would put him to sleep forever
- –thinks his family will be better off with his insurance

Remember the patient is ambivalent: on the one hand wishing to die and on the other hoping to be rescued. This ambivalence is what enables intervention. If you are suspicious of a potential suicide make frequent contact with the patient. Suicide is seldom attempted when others are present. The nurse is helpful in situations like this. Inform the nursing staff and the patient's family of your suspicions.

Allow the patient to talk about his feelings. He gains some relief by talking about his desperation. Help the patient find alternative solutions to his problems.

Remember:

- –Of 10 people who commit suicide, 8 will have given definite warnings.
- –Patients who are suicidal are so for only a short time; they are not suicidal forever.
- –Most suicides occur within 3 months of improvement. Be vigilant during this time.
- –Suicide does not run in families.
- –Suicide is not exclusively a disease of any class of people.
- –Others than the depressed or insane commit suicide.
- –Suicide is preventable in most cases.

WHEN THE SICK OR ELDERLY BECOME CONFUSED

Watch for the onset of confusion and disorganization in your elderly patients, even if they have minor ailments. Be on the alert for confusion and disorganization in patients who:

- –have previously been psychotic and have developed an illness
- –are toxic from alcohol or drugs
- –have metabolic or electrolyte disorders
- –are immobilized
- –have any major or life-threatening ailment

Give either antianxiety or antipsychotic drugs (Table 4-6) depending on the situation. Antianxiety drugs may cause confusion in some patients.

Antianxiety Drugs

Valium (diazepam) tablets: 2, 5 and 10 mg. Dosage 5 to 60 mg per day divided into 4 doses daily.

Librium (chlordiazepoxide) capsules: 5, 10 and 25 mg. Dosage 15 to 300 mg per day divided into 3 or 4 doses daily.

Miltown (meprobamate) tablets: 200 and 400 mg. Dosage 800 to 3200 mg divided into 3 or 4 doses daily.

Serax (oxazepam) capsules: 10, 15 and 30 mg. Dosage 30 to 90 mg daily divided into 3 to 4 doses daily.

Antipsychotic drugs

Trilifon (perphenazine) tablets: 2, 4, 8, and 16 mg. Start with 1 mg t.i.d. and increase 2 to 3 mg daily until improvement occurs. Little sedation. May produce parkinsonism. Potentiates sedatives and narcotics.

Stelazine (trifluoperazine) tablets: 1, 2 and 5 mg. Dosage 6 to 64 mg daily. Description as above but has a narrow therapeutic-toxic range.

Thorazine (chlorpromazine) tablets: 10, 25, 50 and 100 mg. Dosage: 25 to 400 mg daily divided into 2 to 4 doses. More sedating than those listed above. Good antipsychotic. Usually can start with 10 to 25 mg 2 to 4 times daily. Doses of 1000 to 2000 daily have been used in hospitalized psychiatric patients.

Haldol (haloperidol) tablets: 0.5, 1 and 2 mg. Dosage 2 to 20 mg daily divided into 2 or

3 doses daily. Nonphenothiazine. Good antipsychotic but early and severe parkinsonism occurs.

THE TERMINALLY ILL

To the terminally ill patient and to some physicians, cancer is a death sentence. Consequently the word is seldom mentioned, maybe not at all. Eighty percent of the patients know and accede to this conspiracy of silence. You should give some thought as to why this is so. There are two possibilities —to protect the patient from an awareness of death *or* to protect you, the physician, from the need to defend yourself emotionally. The latter may be the cause of this silence—the emotional sustenance of the patient is more than you can give. And since, in this circumstance, your best defense is to avoid the patient, you keep an emotional and even physical distance between you and the patient.

But you are a physician; your purpose in life is to heal and comfort the sick. Do not abandon the patient; attempt to identify with him.

If you can get over that first hurdle you will learn the patient wants to talk about many things. A quiet discussion of his thoughts and fears will be good for both of you. Most important you will find that the patient's greatest fear is that he will be abandoned, that he will be left to die alone, perhaps during the night. Consequently, he develops an insomnia because he is fearful he may not awaken.

Under these circumstances, how does the patient decide he is being abandoned? Generally by your interest and actions. Are your visits becoming less frequent? Are you spending less and less time with him when you do visit? Do you avoid words of substance, speaking in hollow words and phrases? To the patient this spells abandonment, and you are adding to the patient's despair rather than helping him through the greatest fright of his life.

Abandonment is also in your failure to touch the patient. To the dying his body is disgusting and repulsive as though it were already dead. He believes he is offensive to those about him. Do not be afraid to touch the patient, to hold a hand, anything to let him know that he is not loathsome. He will take heart when he knows you are not afraid of him, and he can still be appreciated as a flesh-and-blood person.

RECOGNIZING THE EMOTIONALLY DISTURBED CHILD

You may need help in evaluating childhood psychiatric problems if the child is under 6 years of age. The assessment of emotional disturbances is difficult because of the lack of communication. After the child is 6 years old, you may be able to evaluate his emotional state yourself.

Observe the child carefully. Does he have the physical stigmata of anxiety? Ask the child to leave his parents and enter a consultation room with you. Try to persuade him at least three times. The inability to leave the parent after six, implies immaturity or emotional disturbance.

Ask the child if there is anything wrong with him. If he indicates he is "bad" or that others "pick on him," ask him to tell you more about it. Evaluate his train of thought. Is it logical or illogical?

If he hesitates to tell you about himself, ask him to tell you about his best friend. In doing so, he will probably be telling more about himself than his friend.

Do not hesitate to ask him if there is trouble in his family. Again evaluate his logic.

Ask him what he is going to do when he grows up. Failure to get an answer indicates immaturity; he is probably saying he wants to remain a baby.

Be suspicious of schizoid tendencies in a passive, isolated child who wants to be an explorer or some other unusual pursuit. A child who appears mature and confident, who wants to be a fireman like his uncle, probably has good identification.

Assess his aggressiveness by asking whether he fights a lot. Checking into his actions during a fight may give you some idea whether his aggressiveness is controlled and integrated or primitive.

To evaluate his psychosexual maturity ask the child if he knows where babies come from. A refusal to answer or an unrealistic answer at age 10 or 12 suggests immaturity. Then ask a boy whether he likes girls (the opposite with girls). Follow-up by asking whether he intends to be married.

By evaluating the child's answers to such questions you will be able to assess his aggressiveness, his maturity, his identification and his psychosexual development. Take no more than 10 to 15 minutes for this examination.

If he or she is grossly immature and fails in one of the other above four areas, a referral to a psychiatrist is in order. If the child's failures are only mild, you can probably counsel the child and his parents while further evaluating the family.

CHAPTER 5

Surgical Principles and Emergencies

THE OPERATING ROOM

Who's Who

For all practical and legal purposes the *surgeon* assumes full responsibility for all acts of medical/surgical treatment in the OR. Hospital employees in the OR act under the surgeon's direction.

The *scrub nurse* (who may or may not be a nurse) scrubs, puts on her sterile gown and gloves and enters the sterile field. Thereafter she confines herself to the limited areas covered by sterile drapes. She arranges instruments and supplies, opens and prepares sutures, provides instruments, and assists the surgeon as needed.

The *circulating nurse* is outside the sterile field. She prepares the patient for surgery, takes care of his needs, preps the operative site, and watches for breaks in aseptic technique. She serves as liaison between OR personnel and other hospital personnel. The circulating nurse may be the more experienced nurse and actually supervises the beginning scrub nurse.

The *anesthesiologist* generally plans and administers the appropriate anesthesia. He checks the patient the night before surgery and sometimes plans jointly with the surgeon the conduct of the operation.

Prevention of Accidents

The family physician may not often be in charge of the operating room or even be in the position to change the traditional operating room techniques. But whenever he is in the room, he should be on the alert for breaks in aseptic technique and for hazards to the patient.

Faulty equipment is one source of injury to the unconscious patient. Whenever anesthetic machines appear or act faulty, suggest that it be quarantined until checked out for dependability. In choosing gas machines, purchase equipment which, if it fails, does so in a safe condition, i.e. turns off the anesthetic, blows a whistle. Discard equipment that appears to be nearly worn out. During surgery is no time for equipment failure.

Burns of many varieties are frequent sources of injury. These injuries may come from lights and even from application of ice for cooling. The low heat from electrical equipment or a heating blanket that doesn't exceed 37° may burn the patient by a slow accumulative cooking effect. Be wary of any electrical equipment attaching the Bovie to the electrocardiograph. Remember two points about the Bovie: if the Bovie does not appear to be working properly do not ask the nurse to turn it up until all connections have been checked; secondly, if the nurses have connected two electrodes for your convenience, investigate before turning the machine on, where the second electrode is lying and whether it may be touching a wet towel or drape.

A serious burn can be caused by an inadvertent intra-arterial injection of an anesthetic or other chemical agent. Cannulas, needles and intravenous catheters are often inserted into the back of the hand or wrist and covered by the drapes only to disclose a grossly deformed hand when it is finally uncovered.

Injuries also result from poor choice of endotrachial tubes either in sizes, lengths, or in faulty or worn tubes. Tubes which are too small may clot with mucus and blood. As time passes the gases may tend to solidify the mucus, causing an obstruction. On the other hand, a tube that is too large may physically injure the larynx or trachea. Select low pressure cuffs whenever possible. When choosing disposable endotracheal tubes, over-inflate the cuffs with 30–40 ml of air or water before using. After insertion into the trachea, only 3–4 ml of pressure may be necessary to seal the tube.

Prevent any trauma to the patient. Watch for masks that are too tight over the eyes or cause abrasions to the cornea. Tape eyes shut with nonresidue tape. Gently pull the tape off when finished. If the eyes cannot be taped shut, install some eye emollient at the start of the operation. If a nasal tube is being used, inspect for pressure about the ala nasi. The tubes should lay downward over the lip to prevent pressure ulceration about the nose.

Other reported types of trauma to the anesthetized patient include the vigorous use of the Stryker saw. The patient obviously is unable to complain of the heat generated or the pressure exerted while the surgeon is removing a cast. All kinds of compression trauma have been reported. The radial, median, ulnar, peroneal and lateral femoral cutaneous nerves have been injured by pressure from the operating table, the Mayo stand and other operating room equipment.

Proper Method of Gowning

Shake out a folded gown and hold it by the inside lining. Open the gown from the inside in such a fashion the hands and arms slip into the sleeves. Work your arms down through the sleeves, being careful not to touch unsterile equipment, especially overhead equipment. Someone will pull the gown over your shoulders and tie it from behind.

Sutures and Ligatures

Swaged sutures are sutures with an appropriate needle attached. The needle and suture are of the same diameter and their fusion point forms an unbroken line. Advantages are they do not unthread, they can be discarded, they do not need to be threaded and the surgeon does not need to identify both suture and needle.

Eyed needles, however, are still in widespread use and come in multiple sizes and shapes. They may be recleaned and reused. Obviously, they must be threaded at each using.

The body's tissue responds to any suture (Table 5-1) or ligature as though it were a foreign body. An absorbable (temporary) suture is attacked and broken down by tissue enzymes and is eventually dissolved and digested. Tissue enzymes cannot dissolve a nonabsorbable (permanent) suture, but act to encapsulate or wall off the suture.

Handling Absorbable Sutures

Do not soak or autoclave absorbable sutures. Do not store them near stoves or radiators. If cut strands are stored beneath uncovered sterile Mayo tray, be sure not to pull them across the tray edge which may be sharp or rough.

Table 5-1. Sutures

Absorbable	*Non-absorbable*
Surgical gut (catgut)	Surgical silk
Plain	Surgical cotton
Chromic	Stainless steel wire
Collagen	Silver
Plain	Linen
Chromic	Dermal
Fascia lata strips	Synthetics
Cargile membrane	Nylon
	Polyester fiber
	Polyethylene
	Polypropylene

If strands dry out before needed, have them dipped momentarily into tepid (not hot) water to restore pliability. Straighten strands with a gentle pull; do not weaken strands by hard pulls. Avoid crushing them in instruments. Check needle eyes for rough inner edges which may damage strands.

Handling Nonabsorbable Sutures

Black braided silk and dermal: Dry strands are stronger than wet strands; therefore, store strands in dry towels. *Cotton and linen:* Wet strands are stronger than dry strands; therefore, moisten strands prior to use. *Stainless steel wire:* Avoid kinks and bends. *Polyester fiber:* Use wet or dry. *Nylon:* To straighten kinks or bends, caress nylon strands between gloved fingers a few times.

Aphorisms

OB-GYN surgeons seem to prefer surgical gut for all layers except the skin. Orthopedic surgeons use more surgical silk, stainless steel and dermal sutures and less surgical gut. Plastic surgeons generally prefer synthetic materials such as nylon and polyester fiber because of their minimal tissue reaction characteristics. The majority of neurosurgeons prefer surgical silk.

Generally speaking, synthetic sutures have very smooth surfaces and special care must be taken to tie the knot securely. Synthetic materials have a greater tendency to slip than surgical gut, silk or cotton.

The ends of surgical gut are cut relatively long—about 6 mm from the knot. Silk and cotton ends are cut close to the knot—about 3 mm—to minimize the amount of foreign material left in the wound.

Do not use nonabsorbable sutures in the presence of active infection since bacteria become harbored in the interstices and the suture acts as a continual feeder of the infective organisms.

Use nonabsorbable sutures on all large arteries, whether the field is sterile or not. Silk is preferred to surgical gut for bad traumatic wounds after debridement.

Suture Technique

Handle tissue gently and minimize trauma by instruments (Fig. 5-1). Obtain meticulous hemostasis and plan precise approximation.

Use the least amount of and the smallest size of suture consistent with holding power. Placement of two fine sutures close together will cause less reaction than one large suture. Interrupted sutures are generally considered preferable to continuous.

Thread needle from inside curve of needle while held in needle holder but be careful not to puncture glove. Contrary to the conventional way, thread needle eye over end of strand unless strand is limp. Pull short end of strand 2 to 3 in through the needle eye. For deep suturing, make the short end about 4 in long.

Pass the handles of the needle holder toward the surgeon with the needle pointing toward his thumb. Return the needle in the same way.

Keeping track of needles is best done on a one-to-one basis—exchanging one empty needle for a needle with suture.

Knot Tying

Knot tying is a detail in the complex art and science of surgery that warrants thorough mastery.

Attempt to make the knots small but firm. Cut "whiskers" short. Do not use excessive tension when tying a knot. Excessive

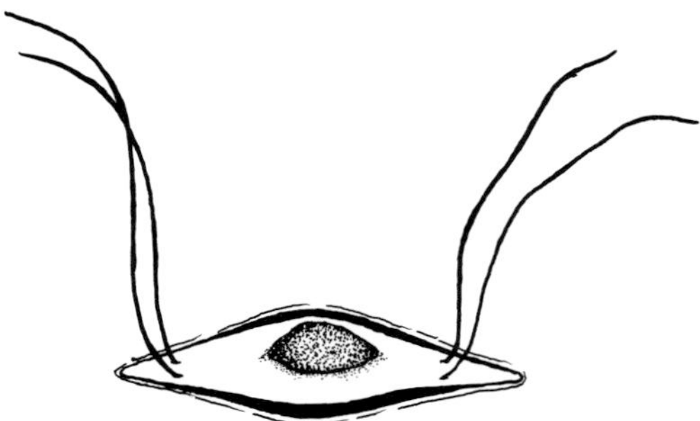

Figure 5-1. An old method of excision of small skin tumors. The two sutures avoid excessive use of thumb forceps and clamps but allow for all needed manipulation.

tension strangulates tissue and weakens the suture. Tie sutures for hemostasis tighter than for tissues. Extra ties do not add strength to a poorly tied knot but do add bulk.

Do not use granny knots. Use double square knots when tying nylon.

Surgical Scrub

Preliminary wash (Time: 1 min). Wet hands and forearms and wash well with 3 to 4 drops of soap. Clean nails with nail file. Rinse hands and forearm.

Surgical scrub (Time: 5 min). Select scrub brush. Place 3 to 4 drops of soap (see below) in palm. Start scrubbing the little finger and continue scrubbing all sides; repeat on all fingers. Continue by scrubbing palm, back and sides of hand. Repeat procedure on the other hand. Scrub forearm up to 1 in above the elbow; then return to other arm and do the same.

Rinse thoroughly from fingertips to elbows. Keep elbows flexed and hands up, allowing water to drain from clean area to dirty. Repeat scrub. Rinse and allow a slight coat of soap to remain. Rinse brush and drop in basin. Drain hands and forearms. With hands up, back through door into operating room.

Recent research indicates that hexachlorophene is more effective than iodine as a scrubbing agent. Iodine preparations produced a greater immediate reduction in the bacterial count but, as a practical matter, lost this advantage after 45 to 60 min under operative conditions with the surgeon wearing gloves. In fact, the bacterial count inside the gloves following an iodine scrub was higher than the count following hexachlorophene agent after 1 hr.

Drying hands, arms and elbows. Remove top towel of pack by grasping center of towel. Dry one hand to the elbow with half the towel. With the opposite end of towel, dry other hand ending at the elbow. Keep the towel away from your body at all times and do not go back over previously dried areas. Spread towel and discard.

RESUSCITATION

First Steps in an Emergency

Immediate action is a requisite. Roll patient into a supine position and tilt the patient's head back until the anterior neck structures are stretched (Fig. 5-2A). This generally lifts the tongue off the posterior pharyngeal wall. Push the lower teeth ahead of the upper ones by pressure on the angle of the mandible.

Inflate the lungs with positive pressure. Clearing the airway with exhaled air is more important than oxygen administration. This may be done by mouth-to-mouth resuscitation, mouth-to-gadget breathing or bag-mask. Of the latter, the Laerdal RFB II unit is first choice; the Puritan unit second choice; and the Ambu unit third choice.

If you are alone with the patient, exhaled air will be the only source of positive pressure because squeezing a bag will be impossible. The solution: take the bag off the mask, seal the mask over the patient's nose and mouth, and blow into the mask. If the lungs fill, ventilate about five times.

Palpate the carotid pulse (Fig. 5-2B). If no pulse is felt, do external cardiac massage 15 compressions at 1 second intervals and then two lung inflations. Continue this pattern.

In the meantime, start to clear the airway. Put a pillow under the patient's shoulders. Clearing the mouth may be difficult because the patient may have his teeth clenched. If so, push the lower teeth down with the thumb while pulling the maxillae up with the index finger of the opposite hand (Fig. 5-2C). Protect the patient's lips.

Free one hand for handling a suction tip or manually removing food or other objects from the mouth (Fig. 5-2D). Cross the thumb and index finger of one hand, pressing down with the thumb while anchoring the upper jaw with the index finger. Occasionally you will need to insert the tip of your index finger behind the last molar to pry the mouth open. Portable suction equipment (Fig. 5-2E) is available but must produce a negative pressure of 300 mm Hg when occluded and a flow of at least 30 L/min when open. If the patient's jaw remains clenched, pull the

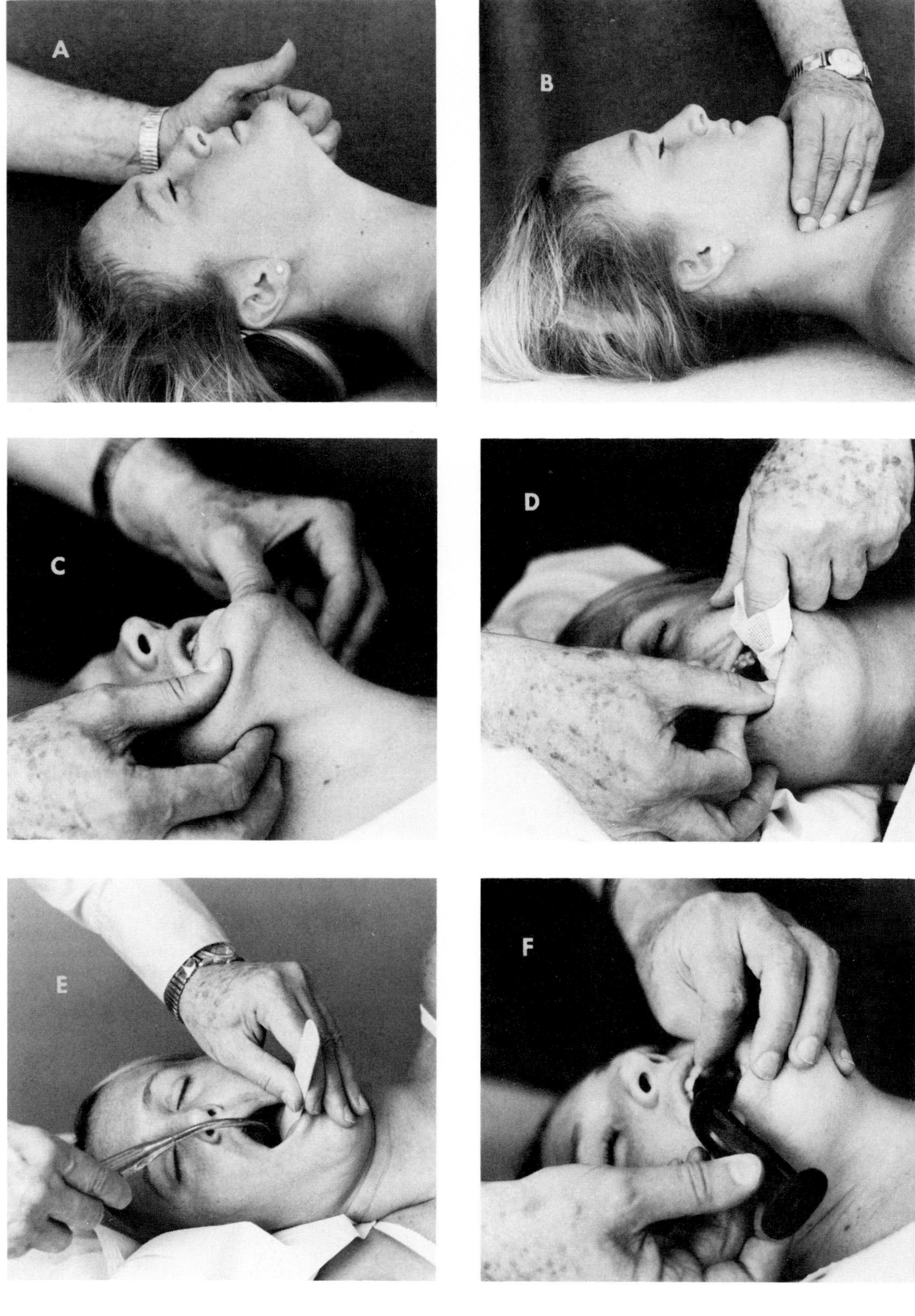
A
B
C
D
E
F

cheek back, put your thumb or index finger on the gum behind the last molar and push down hard.

If one is available, insert an airway in the usual fashion (Fig. 5-2F). The crossed fingers again can be used to open the mouth. Do not push the tongue back into the throat. Introduce the airway along the roof of the hard palate. The insertion is easier if the tongue is held forward with a tongue blade or the fingers. In the case of a convulsive patient with trismus, keep the airway open with a nasopharyngeal tube.

Continue ventilating the patient by whatever method has been successfully established. This is more important than intubating or doing a tracheotomy. If air flows through the esophagus into the stomach, deflate the patient's abdomen by direct pressure with a hand over the epigastrium.

Stay with the patient, keeping his head tilted back and his airway open. Continue assisting his breathing until arrival at an emergency room or hospital where more help will be available. If oxygen is handy, attach it to the bag mask or run it under the edge of the mask. At this point, give specific medications for asthma, epinephrine, etc. Relieve bronchospasm quickly or correct the low pH with sodium bicarbonate.

Intubation

When

If the above steps to ventilate the patient fail, think of intubating the patient. Aspiration of gastrointestinal contents and excessive tracheobronchial secretions are common reasons for ventilatory failure. Watch for insidious signs of respiratory failure: sudden changes in respiratory rate, rib retraction and flaring nares. An increasing pulse rate of 15 or more beats in 30 minutes and cyanosis indicate that resuscitation is unsuccessful.

If you are inexperienced in intubation the chances for a successful operation are poor in an emergency situation. But once in the hospital, if continued artificial respiration appears to be necessary as in coma or paralysis, intubation is a wise course.

Almost always intubate for a cardiac arrest. If arrest should recur or a dangerous arrhythmia arise, a patient already intubated has the best chance of survival. Attention then can be focused on aspirating, ventilating and monitoring blood gases.

An arterial puncture and blood gas study helps guide treatment. A rough guide to follow is the 50/50 rule. A P_{CO_2} greater than 50 with a P_{O_2} less than 50 indicates the need for artificial ventilation or more effective ventilation.

How

Learn the technique on the anesthetized patient. Select a straight or curved blade laryngoscope, whichever is easiest to handle.

Sit or stand above the patient's head. Properly position the patient's head. Pulling his head back over a pillow or stretching the anterior neck structures is poor technique. Attain the best position, peculiarly enough, by pushing the top of the head down toward the shoulders while the head is tilted back. This maneuver actually relaxes the anterior neck muscles. The head, not the shoulders, should be on a small pillow.

Open the patient's mouth with your fingers. Introduce the blade of the laryngoscope on the right side of the patient's mouth, pushing the tongue to the left. Tip the blade anteriorly until the epiglottis comes into view. Slide the tip of the blade over the

Figure 5-2. Emergency action in airway obstruction. *A*, Tilt the patient's head back, stretching the anterior neck muscles. *B*, Palpate for the carotid pulse. *C*, Lift the jaw forward so that the lower teeth are in front of the upper teeth. Lift by pulling up on the rami of the mandible. With the fingers under the mandible, the thumbs are free to hold a mask or a bag to help in giving artificial ventilation. *D*, Cross the thumb and index finger for leverage in opening the mouth. Considerable mucus and vomitus may be cleaned from the mouth and pharynx by a finger swathed in gauze. *E*, A more effective method of clearing the pharynx is with a suction unit. *F*, When the airway is clear, insert a pharyngeal tube.

base of the tongue into the space between the epiglottis and the base of the tongue while pulling the tongue forward.

Observe the pale yellow vocal cords between the epiglottis in front and the arytenoid cartilages behind. The opening of the larynx is vertical; the opening of the esophagus is horizontal. When the vocal cords are visualized, slide the tube along the right side of the mouth behind the epiglottis into the triangular space between the vocal cords. If the cords are shut wait until the patient takes a breath. When the cords separate, then slide the tube through the opening. If the tube is too large or too small, take it out. Ventilate the patient a few times and try again with a more suitable size. Allow 1 minute to intube. If that time is insufficient, remove the scope, reposition the patient and ventilate. Then try again.

After the insertion, check the tube to be certain it is in the trachea and not the esophagus. Beginners may push the tube too far and actually enter a bronchus. To verify the placement for long term therapy, confirm the position by an x-ray.

Put a bite block or rolled gauze between the teeth to prevent biting the tube. Inflate the endotracheal tube cuff through the pilot tube with a syringe and lock. Apply pressure to the lungs with bag or machinery and listen for air leakage. Do not inflate the cuff more than eough to stop the sound of air percolating. With adhesive, tape the bite block and tube in place.

Size of endotracheal tube: The outside diameter of tubes range from 3.0 to 12.0 mm. Use the 3.0 mm for premature babies. For children between ages 1 and 3, use a tube with an outside diameter of 4.5 mm. Beginning at about 8 years, use a 6 mm cuffed tube. Women take an 8 to 11 cuffed tube while men take a size somewhere between 9 to 12 mm. Select a tube that will fit snugly into the patient's nostril or about the size of his little finger.

Tracheotomy

When

In the acute emergency, intubation is always preferred to tracheotomy. Think of a tracheotomy as complementary to intubation: as a procedure preceding tracheotomy or as a part of the tracheotomy.

Do a tracheotomy on the patient who will need intubation more than 3 to 4 days. Do a tracheotomy earlier than 3 to 4 days if the patient needs to talk or is frightened because he cannot talk. Do a tracheotomy on patients with head injuries who tend to cough up "buck." Avoid a tracheotomy in children under 3 years of age.

Secretions can be aspirated more effectively by tracheotomy. Tracheotomy care takes less meticulous nursing. Laryngeal stenosis and superinfections are more common with endotracheal tubes than with tracheotomies. Laryngeal stenosis is probably the most difficult complication to treat.

How

If at all possible do a tracheotomy in the hospital using routine OR techniques, prepping and draping as usual. Keep the patient's face visible. Plan on leaving in or inserting an endotracheal tube for the tracheotomy. This will provide effective ventilation and oxygenation throughout the procedure.

A general anesthesia by an anesthesiologist is preferable. If an anesthesiologist is not available do a local block with 0.5 percent lidocaine and 1:200,000 epinephrine infiltrating the tissues along the line of the proposed incision.

Place a pillow under the patient's shoulders and pull his head back, stretching the anterior muscles of the neck. Make a 5 cm skin incision downward from the cricoid cartilage over the first two or three tracheal rings. Clamp and tie any bleeders as they occur to prevent the aspiration of blood when the trachea is opened. Continue by blunt and sharp dissection through the superficial tissues down to the trachea. Clamp, divide and ligate the thyroid isthmus.

With the tip of the index finger identify the first tracheal ring. Incise and remove the pretracheal fascia. Draw the endotracheal tube back, being careful to keep it well within the larynx. Stabilize the trachea with a tracheal hook. Hook the trachea on one side to avoid interfering with the tracheal incision. Make an inverted V-shaped incision through the second and third tracheal rings. Turn the tracheal flap downward and stitch the top of the inverted V to the skin. Use a Trousseau dilator to spread the tracheal opening.

Choose and insert a tracheostomy tube. The tube should fill the trachea but move in and out easily. Check the tube's position relieving any pressure on the anterior or posterior walls of the trachea. When once in place, inflate the cuff. If needed the tracheostomy tube can be connected to ventilation equipment and the endotracheal tube withdrawn.

Close the skin wound loosely around the tube. Secure the tube by encircling the patient's neck with umbilical tape and tying in a square knot. Slit a square of lint free gauze half through and apply as a dressing around the tube and under the flange.

Predicting Survival after Cardiac Resuscitation

An electroencephalogram can be used to predict survival or death after cardiac resuscitation with nearly 100 percent accuracy. Such findings as paroxysmal activity, consistent low amplitude and episodic reductions in amplitude are signs of a poor prognosis. Readings are most valuable if taken before the patient regains consciousness when the outcome of the cardiac arrest is in doubt. The slower the repetition rate, the more grave the prognosis.

Medicolegal Implications

Liability in cardiac arrest cases depends on two factors: whether action was taken soon enough to prevent brain damage or death and whether the cardiac arrest arose because of negligence on the part of the physician.

In regard to the latter, liability may be established if the patient's preoperative condition is such that the procedure should be delayed. And secondly, although the preoperative condition does not contraindicate surgery, the improper administration of anesthesia or other procedures that precipitate emergency may be viewed as negligent.

In regard to whether prompt action was taken, courts have stated that if a surgeon in a special field (such as an ophthalmologist) does not know how to cope with cardiac arrest, he should have a surgeon standing by who does. It appears that the only practical course for all physicians doing surgery or giving anesthesia is to be knowledgeable regarding procedures to perform in case of cardiac arrest. The surgeon or anesthesiologist cannot wait for someone else to come to his rescue. If response is immediate, there is no liability, even if his actions did not result in success.

SHOCK

Signs and Symptoms

The skin becomes pale, grayish or slightly cyanotic and moist and sweaty. This pallor may turn into violaceous skin mottling in dependent areas of the body. The nail beds and ear lobes become a dusky color. The patient may be anxious and restless. With unfavorable progress, he becomes dull and apathetic with lessened sensitivity to pain.

Quick Clinical Assessment of Potential Shock

Take the patient's blood pressure and pulse rate while he is lying at rest in the supine position on a bed or examining table. Then repeat the examination one minute after the patient raises his head and trunk to a sitting position.

If blood loss is small, less than 500 ml, there should be no change in the blood pressure reading, but the pulse may accelerate 20 to 25 beats per minute.

If the blood loss is about 1000 ml, the pulse will accelerate 30+ beats per minute. The diastolic blood pressure may increase 30 mm.

If the blood loss is about 1500 ml, the pulse may drop as low as 20 beats per minute and the patient may faint.

The body will compensate for losses of blood up to about 750 ml but beyond that point the circulation is compromised and symptoms appear.

Treatment

Ventilation

Suspect respiratory failure whenever the patient's respiration is shallow, labored or his breath sounds diminished.

Verify the diagnosis by determining pH, PCO_2 (arterial carbon dioxide pressure) and PO_2 (oxygen tension) on arterial blood. Obtain arterial blood by an arterial puncture or through an intra-arterial monitoring catheter (see later in this chapter). Intra-arterial monitoring provides for serial sampling of arterial blood gases in patients with respiratory insufficiency as well as continuing direct measurement of arterial blood pressure.

Weil proposes the following guidelines: "When pH is less than 7.35 units and PCO_2 exceeds 46 mm Hg, the patient has respiratory acidosis. For practical purposes, when the PO_2 in arterial blood is less than 70 mm Hg (93% saturation), oxygen exchange is defective."[1]

Treat respiratory acidosis by clearing the airway and if necessary by mechanical ventilation. Increase the humidified oxygen concentration to 40 percent if needed to raise the PO_2 of arterial blood to 70 percent or more.

Infusion

Insert a central venous catheter and connect a manometer (see later in this chapter).

Start with 1000 ml of lactated Ringer's solution and give in 30 min. Then the rate of flow can be adjusted to 15 or 20 ml/min until shock abates or central venous pressure (CVP) increases to a nonpermissive level. If anemia is a factor in causing the shock, use whole blood to expand the blood volume.

If shock is deep start intravenous lines at least in two extremities with one line in an upper extremity. Lactated Ringer's (Hartman) solution is accepted as being preferable to glucose in water or saline. Glucose-water solutions do not effectively increase the plasma volume because it is rapidly distributed throughout the total body water. Lactated Ringer's is superior to saline for acute resuscitation since it does not contain excess chloride ions as does saline.

Insert a urethral catheter and measure urinary flow.

If doubt exists as to blood volume and the CVP is questionable, measure the blood volume by either the radioisotropic or dye dilution method. Many hospitals are not equipped to measure cardiac output and plasma volume. Most physicians depend on the CVP as a guide for fluid repletions. Be guided also by blood pressure, mental status of the patient and the rate of urine flow. Although CVP measurement does not directly measure hypovolemia, it does indicate whether the volume of blood returning to the heart can be received and ejected by the right ventricle. (Normal CVP is 30 to 100 mm H_2O. Borderline CVP is 120 to 200 mm H_2O indicating myocardial incompetence.)

Be alert to the failure of CVP measurements as a guideline in fluid repletion. Occasionally the CVP is increased to levels above 110 mm of H_2O after massive blood or fluid loss in elderly patients who have limited cardiac reserve. The pathophysiology: reduction in blood volume decreases venous return; low venous return causes a fall in cardiac output and blood pressure which in turn reduces blood supply to coronary arteries. The end result is a decrease in the contractile power of the heart muscle and the CVP rises. In this instance,volume repletion will relieve shock.

Weil[1] points out there is still another way to assess blood volume and cardiac function—fluid challenge. Establish the mean CVP over a 10 min observation interval. Administer 200 ml of intravenous fluid, saline glucose or Ringer's in 10 min. Then again observe the CVP for 10 min. Discontinue the infusion if the CVP increases more than 50 mm of H_2O. On the other hand, if the CVP does not increase more than 20 mm or decreases, given another 200 ml of fluid during the subsequent 10 min. Alternately infuse 10 min and observe 10 min. Whenever the CVP pressure increases more than 50 mm, the infusion should be discontinued. A CVP above 160 mm of water indicates cardiac failure.

As the CVP approaches 200, consider two other measures: phlebotomy and/or digoxin. The phlebotomy could be used to reverse the effects of the infusion. Attach a vacuum bottle to the CVP catheter for the ready performance of a phlebotomy. Use digoxin 0.75 to 1 mg intravenously to increase cardiac efficiency if the patient has not been previously treated with digitalis. If necessary give up to four additional injections of 0.25 mg at 30 min to 2 hr intervals. Clinical judgment and electrocardiographic monitoring for arrythmias, bradycardia or tachycardia will determine the need for further digoxin administration.

Vasoactive Agents

If shock persists after the infusion of electrolyte solution or blood or both in amounts which elevate the CVP, try a vasopressor such as Levophed or Aramine. If an elevation of the systolic blood pressure to 90 mm Hg increases urinary flow to a normal ≥ 40 ml/hour, continue intravenous volume expansion to maintain normal CVP, and titrate the flow of the vasopressor to maintain the blood pressure at 80 to 90 mm Hg.

If shock continues in the presence of a normal or high CVP, which precludes further volume expansion, or in those with persistent tachycardia (<140 beats/min), which precludes giving Isuprel hydrochloride, try Dibenzyline.

Seldinger Technique for Measuring CVP

Connect the electrocardiogram to the patient for monitoring. Suspend a solution of blood on a bedside IV pole. Close flow control clamp. Hang the manometer on the pole with its stopcock at the level of the heart. Remove the protector from the stopcock and connect the administration set.

Turn stopcock handle toward the extension tube. Slowly open the administration flow control flow and fill the manometer half full. Do not overfill. Close the flow control clamp and turn the stopcock handle toward the manometer. Attach a sterile Cournand needle, open flow control clamp to expel air in tubing and close clamp.

Choose the tapered polyethylene catheter to be used. Estimate the distance from the needle site to the right atrium on the surface of the patient's body. Connect the external end of the catheter to the manometer. Then fill the entire catheter-manometer system with saline solution up to the 10 cm mark on the manometer. This will enable the observer to watch deflections in the saline column during insertion.

Insert the Cournand needle into a suitable vein, preferably the medial basilic when present. Withdraw the cannula and insert a Teflon guide wire into the vein. Then remove the Cournand needle. Be sure the needle has a smooth heel so the guide is not cut when the needle is withdrawn. Then advance a large tapered polyethylene catheter over the Teflon guide through the vein into the superior vena cava or the right atrium.

If no vein can be entered percutaneously do a "cut down." Use strict aseptic technique. Use a site 2 cm lateral and 2 cm cephalad to the superior edge of the medial epicondyle of the humerus. Make a transverse incision to each side of this point. Bluntly dissect out the vein and tie the vein with a 4-0 silk suture. Insert the catheter cephalad to the suture by the Seldinger method or nick the vein with small tissue scissors and insert the catheter directly.

When the catheter enters the thorax, observe an inspiratory fall and expiratory rise in venous pressure. Advance the tip through the superior vena cava into the right atrium and even the right ventricle. When the catheter touches the right atrium or ventricle, aberrant impulses may occur. Withdraw the catheter, if the electrocardiographic tracing shows a ventricular dysrhythmia or a marked supraventricular tachycardia.

An abrupt rise in pressure and pulsation of the saline column indicates that the catheter is in the right ventricle. Withdraw the catheter to a point just proximal to the tricuspid valve and the pressure drops about 100 mm H_2O and the prominent ventricular pulse action disappears. Withdraw the catheter another 3 to 5 cm to a point near the junction of the superior vena cava and right atrium. Secure the catheter at this point by tying the vein over the catheter with plain-000 gut.

If blood is not easily withdrawn think of the possibility of wedging in the jugular vein or obstruction due to thrombosis in the vein or compression from without.

To assure proper placement when there is doubt, fill the catheter with Hypaque-M. Two ml of dye is enough to completely fill the catheter. Order a portable chest x-ray and look for the catheter's shadow. Aspirate the dye following the examination.

For central venous pressure monitoring, have the patient lying supine with bottom of stopcock at the level of the right atrium. Measure venous pressure intermittently by turning stopcock handle towards the administration set and read the fluid level in the manometer. If fluid level rises toward the top of the manometer, turn the handle towards the manometer before the fluid level reaches the air filter. Measure venous pressure continuously by turning the handle so it points to the bottom of the stopcock.

Hazards of CVP Monitoring

Consider the following disadvantages before instituting CVP monitoring:

- –Clotting of the apparatus and the time consuming measures needed to prevent it.
- –Venous thrombosis plus danger of septic pulmonary emboli.
- –Contamination by manometer overflow resulting in staphylococcal bacterial endocarditis and septic emboli.
- –Inaccurate and misleading readings by paramedical personnel incapable of operating technical devices.
- –Confusion about the interpretation of readings, i.e. the latency of changes in pressure in pulmonary edema.
- –Dependency on CVP measurements, causing delay in observing clinical signs of increasing venous pressure, i.e. bulging external jugular or sublingual veins.

The physician should ask himself whether the information to be obtained justifies the exposure of his patient to these hazards of long-term monitoring. Most hazards are averted by short-term employment.[2]

Placing Intra-Arterial Catheters for Monitoring Blood Gases

An intra-arterial monitoring catheter is a small plastic tube that is passed through the skin into the lumen of the femoral artery. These catheters have two major applications: the collection of arterial blood samples for measurement of blood volume, central hematocrit, blood gases and electrolytes; and the direct measurement of arterial blood pressure.

Consider intra-arterial monitoring for:

- –blood pressure determination in patients with sustained hypotension or low blood volume and when the blood pressure is difficult to measure by the cuff method
- –blood pressure during the administration of rapid-acting hypertensive or hypotensive drugs
- –in research when more precision is needed in pressure readings than can be obtained from the cuff method
- –for serial sampling of arterial blood, as in patients with respiratory failure or other disorders which may alter arterial blood gases

Insert an intra-arterial catheter by precutaneous technique. Usually a "cut down" is not necessary. Locate the site for puncture over the point of maximal femoral impulse close to the inguinal ligament. Lightly infiltrate the area with 2 percent lidocaine through a 25 gauge needle.

Pass an 18-gauge thin-wall Cournand arterial needle through the skin into the underlying femoral artery close to the inguinal ligament. For insertion, point the needle 45° cephalad. (The Cournand needle is made by Becton-Dickinson Co.) An alternative needle is the Potts-Cournand 18-gauge needle. Both are disposable.

Remove the stylette and adjust the position of the cannula by slowly withdrawing it. When the tip of the needle is properly positioned in the artery, blood will spurt from the needle in unison with the pulse.

Introduce a flexible stainless steel guide wire into the cannula and pass it several cm into the artery. (The guide wire is a fixed core wire with a 3 cm flexible tip, diameter 0.035 in, length 70 cm, and available from the V. S. Catheter and Instrument Co.)

Remove the cannula leaving the wire in place. Apply local pressure to prevent bleeding. Pass the intra-arterial monitoring catheter over the wire, through the skin and into the lumen of the artery. ("Formocath" Polyethylene catheter by Becton-Dickinson Co. The internal diameter is 0.045; the outside 0.062. The catheter can be gas or cold sterilized. The tip of each catheter is tapered over steam, with a 0.025 guide wire inside.)

Release local pressure. Withdraw the guide wire and leave the catheter in the lumen of the artery. Fasten the catheter securely to the skin. Withdraw the first sample of blood for laboratory testing into a heparinized syringe and leave the catheter flushed free of blood and full of heparinized saline.

The major complication encountered during precutaneous insertion is subcutaneous bleeding with hematoma formation. Bleeding may occur when the Cournand needle is withdrawn over the guide wire, but direct pressure over the puncture site until the catheter is inserted will minimize this hazard. Bleeding may occur when the catheter is withdrawn. Again pressure over the wound for 5 to 10 min will minimize this complication.

Watch for the complications during monitoring.

The catheter will stop functioning if there is clotting of blood within the catheter. To prevent this complication, flush the catheter with weakly-heparinized saline routinely every half hour.

Occasionally the catheter stops functioning because it becomes kinked against the arterial wall.

The site of the insertion should be examined regularly for slippage of the catheter or local swelling. Hematomas may form rapidly. Check all components of the system regularly, such as the site of insertion, the catheter, the dressing and the tubing and all components.

Do not introduce clots or air bubbles into the system.

The family physician will not often need to monitor the arterial blood pressure by this method. Intra-arterial blood pressure monitoring is more of a research tool and the equipment is complicated. But the repeated sampling of arterial blood is often required in the management of patients with serious respiratory problems. Intra-arterial monitoring is especially useful in management of patients on controlled ventilation.

Three syringes are required for the sampling of blood from an intra-arterial catheter. Use the first syringe to withdraw the heparinized saline that is in the catheter. This heparinized saline has prevented blood from clotting in the catheter. The volume in the catheter is small and arterial blood soon follows the saline into the syringe. This mixture of saline and blood is unsuitable for laboratory testing.

The second syringe is used to sample the arterial blood. (Apply this technique for the collection of a single sample of arterial blood using an ordinary syringe and a 20-gauge needle.) Prepare the syringe by rinsing it with a small amount of concentrated heparin. Expel the heparin upward so that heparin will remain in the tip of the syringe and eliminate any trapped air. The small amount of heparin remaining will coat the walls and tip of the syringe and keep the blood sample from clotting. If too much heparin remains in the sample needle, the blood sample will be diluted and give a false high PO_2 reading.

The sample of blood should be drawn bubble-free and then capped, iced and sent to laboratory to be analyzed *immediately* since arterial blood gas tension can change rapidly in the sampling syringe. After using the second syringe, arterial blood remains in the catheter.

The third syringe contains normal saline that has been heparinized with one unit per ml. A small amount of blood is withdrawn into the syringe to be sure the catheter is still working and to aspirate any clots that may have formed. Inject the flush solution into the catheter; several ml are needed to thoroughly remove blood from the catheter and leave it filled with heparinized saline.

Measuring Intravascular Volume

The indicator dilution technique is dependable for measurement of blood volume. The physician has a choice of three tests: radio-iodinated serum albumin I^{131} (Risa); a nonradioactive tracer, Evans blue (T-1824); or red blood cells of the recipient tagged with radioactive chromium. The technician injects a tracer into a vein. Blood samples are then collected from the opposite arm at 15, 25 and 35 min. The whole test must be done with technical proficiency and care. Do not administer radioisotropes to children or pregnant women. In the presence of active bleeding, the isotrope is lost via the bleeding site and a false value will be produced.

Normal plasma volume ranges from 35 to 43 ml/kg of body weight (16 to 20 ml/lb) for women and from 38 to 47 ml/kg (17 to 21 ml/lb) body weight for men.

Determination of red blood cell mass in conjunction with measurement of plasma volume permits definition of body hematocrit levels. From a practical point of view, base treatment on plasma volume and central volume hematocrit. Gauge the use of whole blood, red blood cells or plasma on serial changes in the central venous hematocrit level.

In summary, the blood volume determination may be useful to plan the most appropriate blood component for replacement therapy. For instance, normal total blood volume and decreased red cell mass indicates the need for packed red cell transfusion.

Use the volume determination to follow the clinical course. Immediately after acute severe hemorrhage, the hemoglobin concentration, hematocrit value and red blood cells may be normal and not indicate the severity of blood loss whereas appropriate measurements will show decreased blood volume, plasma volume and red cell mass.

A family physician can, therefore, alert the surgeon to unexpected blood losses. He can also state the need for replacement of the appropriate blood component which may vary with the surgical procedure. Example: in thoracoplasty the blood loss may be 900 ml representing approximately equal red cells and plasma losses. In gastrectomy, the blood loss may be 1800 ml representing a red cell loss of 400 ml and a plasma loss of 1400 ml.

Bacterial Shock

Infrequently bacterial shock is superceded only by the shock of hemorrhage and myocardial infarction. The most common offending organisms are gram-negative bacteria. Gram-negative bacteremia results in a 40 percent mortality and gram-negative shock raises the mortality to 50 to 80 percent.

In a child gram-negative shock usually starts by an abrupt elevation in temperature. If shock is profound the temperature may be normal or even subnormal. This onset is usually followed by varying degrees of tachypnea with respiratory alkalosis, tachycardia, oliguria and mental depression.

Basic treatment includes the general measures outlined for shock plus the control of infection by antimicrobial agents and/or surgical drainage. Before starting any antibiotic therapy, cultures of blood, urine and any exudate should be collected for bacterial identification and sensitivity studies.

Use aseptic technique for the blood culture venipuncture. Scrupulous care must be taken to avoid contamination. Draw samples several times during the 24-hr period. The blood obtained should be cultured immediately, utilizing media and methods suitable for both anaerobic and aerobic organisms.

The events of septicemia may be rapid ones, and it is rarely possible to await the results of culture studies before beginning treatment. In this connection, keen observation and a detailed knowledge of the events preceding the septicemia are of value.

Responsible organisms in order of frequency are usually considered to be: Escherichia coli, Proteus, Aerobacter, Pseudomonas and Paracolon.

Before bacteriological studies are completed, give Kanamycin sulfate and colistimethate sodium. This will cover about 95 percent of organisms involved in bacterial shock. Give Kanamycin and chloramphenicol if it is reasonable to suspect that the shock is not due to Pseudomonas, which is more often associated with burns, hematologic disease or IV catheters.

The following rules are helpful:

- –Shock associated with infection from an indwelling catheter—suspect Staph
- –Shock associated with infection from prolonged IPPB—suspect Klebsiella
- –Shock associated with GU infection —suspect E. coli
- –Shock associated with skin lesions —suspect Pseudomonas or Staph
- –Shock associated with renal stones, alkaline urine and hospital exposure —suspect Proteus

In addition to the usual shock therapy, urine volume and blood urea nitrogen should be determined frequently and the antibiotic dosage modified in accord with the degree of renal failure present.

Remember with gram-negative shock there is decreased cardiac output, altered peripheral resistance and poor venous return. Infusions can be life saving, although 5 or more L may be required before the arterial blood pressure increases.

In bacterial shock consideration should be given to steroid therapy. General consensus suggests that steroids may or may not be helpful, but are not likely to be dangerous. If steroids are chosen, give massive doses—500 to 6,000 mg hydrocortisone or its equivalent.

TRANSFUSIONS

The family physician generally depends on the ability and integrity of a laboratory technician when he orders blood for transfusion. The doctor who administers a transfusion, however, without securing a complete report of the laboratory results is responsible for any reaction that may occur. If he asks the laboratory to short cut its normal procedure in selecting blood, he certainly shares heavily the responsibility of untoward results.

Emergency Transfusions

Use emergency transfusions only in situations where delay might jeopardize life. Hospital blood banks have classified emergency transfusion as *extreme emergency* and *emergency*.

In the case of an extreme emergency, there is a mutual understanding that no time for blood grouping or Rh determination exists. Consequently the laboratory will make one of two choices and deliver either Group O (preferably Rh-negative) with 70 percent of the plasma removed or Group O, free of hemolytic anti-A and anti-B.

See that a routine and an emergency slide crossmatch is done on all blood given out in extreme emergency after the patient's blood specimen is obtained. Try to obtain the sample before starting the transfusion or at the same time. Never collect the blood for typing from the same vein in which an infusion is being given.

A healthy person can lose more than 40 percent, or about 2 L, of his blood before developing irreversible hypotension. A patient can lose half this amount acutely without serious effect. The loss of 500 ml is inconsequential.

When time is available, determine specific blood group by a crossmatch on freshly drawn blood even though the patient has received nonspecific blood.

In emergency or extreme emergency the physician or his representative must sign before blood is released (AABB Standards).

If at all possible, have an Rh determination in all transfusions to avoid the use of Rh-positive blood in Rh-negative recipients. From a practical standpoint, this is not always feasible. When only one transfusion is to be given, the Rh factor is of no importance *except* during pregnancy or in women who are likely to become pregnant in the future.

In the emergency class allow 15 minutes for testing after the blood bank receives the patient's blood. In this event the technician will do the following: determine blood group and Rh factor, crossmatch and spin read for ABO incompatibilities, make an emergency slide crossmatch converted to Coombs for atypical antibodies other than ABO and remove 70 percent of the plasma in the event group A or B must be given to an AB patient because of lack of proper type.

Transfusion Reactions*

Reactions to blood transfusions occur in 2 to 10 percent of all recipients (Table 5-2). Baker[3] classifies types of reactions as allergic (46 percent), febrile (44 percent) and hemolytic (10 percent).

The most common symptoms of allergic transfusion reaction are itching, erythema, urticaria, chills and fever. Reduce the incidence of allergic symptoms by the use of an antihistamine (Benadryl 50 mg) given intramuscularly before the transfusion. Antihistamines are given routinely in many centers and are mandatory in patients with a strong history of allergy. Do not add the antihistamine to the container of blood.

Generally it is best to continue transfusions even though itching and minor allergic symptoms occur. However, if a reaction starts with fever and chills and no itching or urticaria is detected, discontinue the transfusion. Allergic reactions seldom appear before 300 ml are given or the equivalent volume of packed cells or plasma.

For more serious reactions such as laryngeal edema or bronchospasm, consider steroid administration and/or epinephrine or IV hydrocortisone.

Febrile reactions also generally occur after 300 ml or more blood has been given and as late as 24 hr after transfusion. The fever may be trivial or as high as 104°. Chills are associated with high fever. Transfusions of incompatible leukocytes are the common cause of febrile transfusion reactions, but the causes are complex and undetermined.

Avoid some of the trouble by administering leukocyte-poor blood. A simple, efficient method: invert a plastic bag of blood for 24 hr or more, allowing a buffy coat to form. Then drain the bulk of the packed red cells into a transfer pack without disturbing the buffy coat and the plasma that remains in the original bag. This will remove 85 to 90 percent of leukocytes.

Contaminated blood may also cause transfusion reactions. Recognize bacteria in blood by a dark brown supernatant plasma. Never administer such blood.

Hemolytic transfusion reaction occurs in response to the destruction of the donor's red cells by the specific isoantibodies in the recipient. Recognize these reactions by chills, fever, tachycardia, dyspnea, chest and *flank* pain.

Stop the transfusion immediately. Return the donor's and the patient's blood to the laboratory for crosschecking. Check the recipient's serum and urine for free hemoglobin. Administer diuretics, such as mannitol and ethacrynic acid. Alkalinize the urine by administering at least 88 mEq/l of bicarbonate to decrease the precipitates of acid heme in the renal tubules. Treat shock. Steroids are of dubious value.

Follow any suspected or confirmed transfusion reaction. Monitor the patient's serum and urinary bilirubin for 3 to 4 days. If the patient develops oliguria or anuresis, give fluids and electrolytes as needed. If renal failure threatens, peritoneal lavage may help.

The most effective treatment is prevention. This consists of:

- –withholding transfusions of whole blood or red cells unless absolutely necessary
- –doublechecking all identifying characteristics of each unit of blood to be given
- –checking the recipient's identity by name and hospital number
- –watching the patient closely for signs of reaction during the first 100 ml of infusion.

*Adapted from Baker RJ, et al: Transfusion reaction: A reappraisal of surgical incidence and significance. Ann Surg 169:684–693, 1969, with permission.

Table 5-2. Mechanisms of Transfusion Reactions

Mechanical	*Hypersensitivity*	*Transmission of agent from donor to recipient*
Air embolus	Rhinitis	Hepatitis
Circulatory overload	Urticaria	Malaria
Extravasation	Angioneurotic edema	Syphilis
	Laryngeal edema	
	Serum sickness	
	Pulmonary hives	

Contamination	*Immunologic*
Bacterial pyrogen	Intravascular hemolysis
Bacteria	Febrile
	Leukocyte
	Platelet

Adapted from Krevans JR: Transfusion reactions in Conn HF, Conn Jr, RB (eds): Current Diagnosis. Philadelphia: W. B. Saunders Co., 1968, p. 327.

Blood Fractions

Whole Blood Vs Packed Red Blood Cells

When contemplating a blood transfusion think first of packed red blood cells as primary consideration rather than whole blood. Administer whole blood primarily for blood loss sufficient to cause hypovolemic shock. Eighty percent of all patients needing blood can probably be treated to greater advantage with sedimented red cells.

The pathophysiology of several disease states may be complicated by whole blood, i.e. cardiac decompensation, hepatic cirrhosis, uremia, acute burns and the anemia associated with bone marrow failure. This is true also of the debilitated, the aged and the patient of small size.

Red blood cells are the only blood component that can increase the oxygen-carrying capacity of the patient's circulation. Plasma proteins, platelets, electrolytes, leukocytes, coagulation factors and wastes are all unnecessary by-products given the patient when whole blood is used to increase the oxygen-carrying capacity of the blood. In most cases preoperative anemia and surgical blood loss can best be treated with packed red blood cells and/or balanced salt solutions.

Packed red blood cells are prepared by removing two thirds of the plasma-anticoagulant solution from a unit of citrated whole blood.

By using packed red blood cells the physician avoids hypervolemia and circulatory overload, excess metabolic load, exposure to antigens and exposure to infectious agents.

Whole blood contains four times as much potassium and ammonium as packed red cells and threatens both patients with renal or hepatic dysfunction and the catabolic postoperative patient. White blood cells, platelets and plasma proteins, specifically immunoglobulins, are antigens and can induce uncomfortable or even life-threatening reactions with repeated transfusions. Hepatitis is of greatest concern; the incidence of hepatitis is reportedly lower after packed red cells than after whole blood.

Use of packed cells results in more efficient use of a unit of blood collected from a donor. Instead of benefiting 1 patient, 6 or 7 patients may be treated. Last of all, and on the positive side, a more rapid rise occurs in the recipient's hematocrit (Table 5-3).

Table 5-3. Average Rise in Hematocrit* after Infusion of One Unit of Packed Red Blood Cells (Hematocrit 65%–70%—30 ml Content)

Body Weight		*Males*		*Females*	
Pounds	*Kilograms*	*Blood Volume*	*Rise in Hematocrit*	*Blood Volume*	*Rise in Hematocrit*
44	20	1,350	6.6	1,260	7.0
66	30	2,025	4.6	1,890	5.0
88	40	2,700	3.6	2,520	3.9
110	50	3,375	3.0	3,150	3.2
132	60	4,050	2.6	3,780	2.7
154	70	4,725	2.2	4,410	2.3
176	80	5,400	2.0	5,040	2.0
198	90	6,075	1.7	5,670	1.8
220	100	6,750	1.5	6,300	1.6

Reprinted from Physician's Handbook of Blood Component Therapy, Amer. Assoc. of Blood Banks, Chicago, 1969, p. 6, with permission.

*Assuming patient's pre-transfusion hematocrit is 30%

The AABB gives the following example: "A patient with a hematocrit of 20 percent and a blood volume of 4,600 ml who is infused with one unit of whole blood would have blood volume increased to 5,117 ml and the hematocrit to 21.9 percent while infusion of one unit of packed red blood cells would elevate the blood volume to 4,900 ml and the hematocrit to 22.8 percent."[17]

For red blood cell transfusion the patient and donor should be typed for ABO and Rh. See that a 45 to 60 min compatibility test for antibodies is run.

If cells are heavily packed and do not flow well, dilute them with 0.9 percent normal saline, using a Y connection for the saline.

Who would receive one unit of blood? Probably no one except a baby in hemorrhagic distress. If a patient needs one unit of whole blood that patient probably needs multiple transfusions. Very little good can be done unless the blood's function is increased by at least 20 percent. Only if the patient's hemoglobin is 6 g percent can the hemoglobin be increased by 20 percent. If the patient needs blood volume, no single unit of blood will raise the volume 20 percent.

In 10 percent of surgical cases, the patient may come to surgery with an anemia for which there is no time for treatment. Under these circumstances a unit of packed cells may be indicated.

A single unit or less of red blood cells may be needed for a child who requires less because of his size and blood volume. The usual amount is 10 ml/kg per transfusion.

The patient with cardiac disease and anemia may improve with one unit of red cells given 24 hr apart to prevent overloading his circulation.

And last of all, the patient with a hemoglobin of less than 6 g will show significant improvement with one unit of packed red cells.

During surgery many medical centers are now replacing one unit of blood loss with 2 to 3 L of balanced saline with no untoward effect even with hemoglobins as low as 8 g. The volume replacement appears to be more beneficial than raising the hemoglobin level of 8.5 to 9 or 9.25 with one unit of whole blood. For elective surgery, prepare the patient with iron therapy during the preceding 3 to 4 weeks.

A wise course is to determine blood replacement for chronic anemia by clinical judgment rather than by an arbitrary hemoglobin level. For instance, if a patient became anemic very slowly, that patient can tolerate low levels without undue symptoms; a chronic cardiac patient may not tolerate even slight lowering of the hemoglobin without symptoms.

Determining the amount of blood replacement is necessary. Determine blood volume (see earlier in this chapter). Compare the patient's blood volume with the normal values as calculated in Table 5-4.

Table 5-4. Normal Values for Blood Volume (ml)

Women:	Body weight kg X 63	= total blood volume
Men:	Body weight kg X 67.5	= total blood volume

Reprinted from Transfusion 3:315, 1963, with permission.

Platelets

Bleeding patients with thrombocytopenia need platelets. Consider the case as serious if platelets fall to 10,000/cu mm of blood.

Consider prophylactic platelet infusion for:

- –patients with a *temporary* platelet depletion from acute leukemia or chemotherapy (chronic blood dyscrasias are not benefited)
- –patients of impending surgery with platelet counts between 30,000 and 100,000 per cu mm (this situation calls for a platelet count of at least 100,000)
- –patients with ecchymosis, petechial or gingival bleeding, hematuria, melena or internal bleeding with platelets below 100,000

Calculating of platelet dosage: One unit of platelets will raise the count 15,000/cu mm.

$$\frac{\text{Desired level} - \text{initial level}}{\text{Increment per unit (15,000)}} = \text{Units to be infused}$$

Platelet concentrates are the blood fraction of choice. One hundred and fifty ml will supply the same quantity of platelets as 3 units of fresh whole blood or 1,320 ml of platelet rich plasma.

Platelets must be transfused through a nonwettable infusion set that contains an 80-micron mesh nonwettable filter and a nonwettable needle.

Single Donor Plasma

The pooling of plasma increases the risk of hepatitis contamination and is being discouraged. Use single donor plasma for expansion of blood volume in shock due to plasma loss. This occurs in burns, peritoneal injuries, acute pancreatitis, mesenteric thrombosis and in initial treatment of shock resulting from hemorrhage while blood is being crossmatched. The suggested dose is 250 to 300 ml in an adult, followed by a similar dose in 30 minutes if necessary.

Check the hematocrit for anemia. If anemia is present, administer packed red blood cells.

Single Donor Fresh Frozen Plasma (Fresh Frozen Lyophilized Plasma and Single Donor Fresh Plasma)

Use these plasma components for the treatment of clotting factor deficiencies when specific concentrates are not available or when the factor deficiency has not been found. These components contain all clotting factors except platelets.

Give in amounts necessary to control bleeding. Clinical response is a good indicator of successful treatment. In some instances specific assays may help guide treatment.

Again these patients may need packed red blood cells. Seek consultation. This component carries a high risk of hepatitis.

Single Donor Factor VIII

Rich cryoprecipitate is mentioned for completeness. Use this factor to treat hemophilia. Seek consultation for review of diagnosis and methods of administration.

Factor VIII plasma is stored in frozen state (–20° C). Therefore it can be stored for future use. If this fraction were salvaged from most blood donated, there would be an adequate supply to treat all hemophilic patients. Insufficient quantity is its major drawback.

Roughly one bag of cryoprecipitate per 12 kg of body weight every 12 hours will maintain patients. The original priming dose should be twice the amount. Give group specific fraction for ABO blood to avoid red cell hemolysis.

Factor II–VII–IX–X Complex

This combination is now available and is used in the treatment of Christmas disease and some cases of severe liver disease with hemorrhagic tendency. Seek consultation before using it. It also has a high risk of transmitting hepatitis.

Albumin and Plasma Protein Fraction

Albumin is available in a 5 percent buffered saline solution or a 25 percent salt-poor form.

Plasma protein fraction is a commercial preparation containing most of the albumin plus the alpha and beta globulins of whole plasma. These preparations have been heated to 60° C for 10 hours to inactivate the hepatitis agent.

Commercial preparations available are Plasmanate (Cutter Labs, Berkeley, California), Plasmatein (Courtland Labs, North Chicago, Illinois), Plasma Protein Fraction (Hyland Labs, Costa Mesa, California).

Use these fractions interchangeably. Consider their use to combat liquid and sodium losses and to prevent hemoconcentration in burns if plasma is not available.

These are plasma volume expanders. Use whenever plasma is indicated to restore or maintain volume in a patient with hypovolemia without acute blood loss.

Treat hypoproteinemia with 25 percent (salt-poor) albumin. Do not exceed 2 to 3 ml per minute infusion rate; nor more than 5 to 10 ml per minute for the 5 percent albumin fraction. The total dose is generally conceded to be about 1 ml per pound of body weight per day until the desired response is obtained. For hypertensive or decompensating patients, add 1 volume 25 percent albumin to 1½ volume of 10 percent glucose and infuse by continuous drip at the rate of 100 ml per hour.

Check the CVP initially and during administration. Happily these fractions do not carry hepatitis.

To prevent or treat cerebral edema, give 25 percent albumin. Do not overtreat because 1 g of albumin can pull approximately 15 to 20 ml of fluid into the vascular tree. Twenty-five g of albumin can increase the fluid volume by about 500 ml.

Dextran as a Plasma Substitute

Dextran is not a plasma fraction but is mentioned because of its frequent use in an emergency as a plasma substitute. Recently Dextran has been advocated as a therapeutic and prophylactic agent for cases of thrombophlebitis and purpura fulminans.

Obviously Dextran is free of the hepatitis virus. A disadvantage is that in large amounts Dextran interferes with crossmatching if needed later. In rare cases Dextran is reported to cause allergic reactions and to increase bleeding tendency.

Fibrinogen

This is used for specific replacement therapy when bleeding is due to lack of fibrinogen as in congenital or acquired hypofibrinogenemia. Hemorrhage may follow a fibrinogen level lower than 100 percent.

Hypofibrinogenemia associated with intravascular coagulation may be the family physician's only contact with this problem.

Intravascular clotting is seen with the following:

- –obstetrical complications such as premature separation of placenta, retention of dead fetus or amniotic fluid embolism
- –extensive surgery
- –septicemias, particularly with the meningococcemias
- –malignancies (prostate, lung, stomach, colon, ovaries or pancreas)
- –granulocytic leukemias
- –hemolytic transfusion reactions

–giant hemangioma syndrome
–purpura fulminans
–snake bite
–extensive trauma

The use of fibrinogen is controversial. Twenty-five to 30 percent of patients receiving fibrinogen develop hepatitis. Seek consultation. Remember cryoprecipitate contains a significant amount of fibrinogen and is a satisfactory substitute if given in adequate quantity.

Immune Serum Globulin and Specific Immunoglobulins

Immune serum globulin contains the gamma globular fraction of pooled human plasma and contains infectious disease antibodies to which the general population has been exposed.

If the serum has been checked for specific antibodies, it will be termed specific (i.e. tetanus immune globulin). Give immune serum globulin in cases of gammaglobulinemia or hypoglobulinemia (see Chapter 3 for indications). Dosage: 0.25 to 0.50 ml of serum/pound of body weight at 2 to 4 weekly intervals IM.

Measles: modification, 0.1 ml/pound of body weight and for prevention, 0.2 ml/pound IM given within 6 days after exposure.

Polio: If not immunized or immunization uncertain, give 0.14 ml/pound IM as soon after exposure as possible.

Infectious hepatitis exposure: For family members and other intimate contacts, give 0.01 or 0.02 ml/pound of body weight. For continued exposure give 0.05 ml/pound every 3 to 6 mo IM.

Rho (D) factor: Rho (D) immune globulin is indicated for the active maternal immunization to the Rho (D) factor. (See Chapter 3 for indications.)

Commercial laboratories have prepared immune serums from hyperimmunized persons. They are free of risk of hepatitis transmission. Available are human tetanus, pertussis, mumps, and vaccinia immune globulins.

Tetanus immune globulin: For prevention in the nonimmunized give 250 units IM. For children, 2 units/pound of body weight.

Pertussis immune globulin: For prevention, give 1.5 ml IM dose as soon after exposure as possible. If longer than a week after exposure, double the dose. For the child already coughing, give 1.5 ml every day or two until evidence of improvement.

Mumps immune globulin: For prevention, particularly in adults, give 1.5 ml up to 90 pounds, two 1.5 ml vials for 90 to 150 pounds and one 4.5 ml vial for persons over 140 pounds, within 1 week of exposure. Give IM. Increase the dose if more than 1 week has elapsed since exposure. Mumps immune globulin may also be used for treatment if given as soon as possible.

Vaccinia immune globulin: Use for prevention or modification of smallpox. The serum may also be useful in treatment of complications of smallpox vaccination, i.e. vaccinia implants, vaccinia necrosum and generalized vaccinia. Seek consultation.

Prevention of Transfusion Abuse

The American Medical Association's Committee on Blood[5] believes the hospital staff represented by a transfusion committee should study, continually monitor and document the use of blood and its fractions for transfusion. Family physicians should back this stand and volunteer to serve on such committees. Committee activities include

–insuring the adequacy, quality and safety of blood
–reviewing records of all transfusions and transfusion reactions
–reviewing all instances of transmissable disease, including hepatitis
–reviewing questionable blood use such as single units
–identifying unnecessary wastes
–carrying on continuing staff education on proper use of blood fractions
–assisting in obtaining replacement donors and donor recruitment

BLOOD COAGULATION PROBLEMS

Unless the family physician treats an unusual number of blood coagulation problems he will not be competent to diagnose the more complicated and rarer hemorrhagic diseases. The nomenclature is jumbled, the etiological factors are obscure and the pathophysiology is vague.

Family physicians should understand the principles of hemostasis. They should be able to screen for the defects in each of the four stages of blood coagulation and institute emergency treatment for acute bleeding problems.

A classification of nomenclature is the first step in understanding the coagulation process (Table 5-5). Without understanding terms, a physician cannot make a useful search of the literature. The Committee on Nomenclature for Blood Coagulation of the International Hematology Congress suggests the following:

Table 5-5.

Factors	Synonyms*
I	Fibrinogen
II	Prothrombin
III	Thromboplastin (tissue)
IV	Calcium
V	Proaccelerin, labile factor
VI	No longer used
VII	Serum prothrombin conversion accelerator (SPCA), stable factor
VIII	Antihemophilic factors (AHF)
IX	Christmas factor, plasma thromboplastin component (PTC)
X	Stuart factor, Stuart-Prower Factor
XI	Plasma thromboplastin antecedent (PTA)
XII	Hageman factor
XIII	Fibrin stabilizing factor (FSF)
Profibrinolysin	Plasminogen
Fibrinolysin	Plasmin

*Hematologists call the first four factors by either name or number.

Coagulation

Stage 1 (Formation of thromboplastin). Clotting occurs when the platelet factor is released to react with Factors VIII and IX in the presence of Factors V, X, XI, XII and calcium to form plasma thromboplastin (intrinsic thromboplastin). This reaction usually requires 3 to 5 min. Ninety percent of clotting abnormalities occur in this stage.

Stage 2 (Conversion of prothrombin to thrombin by thromboplastin). Note: Besides the intrinsic plasma thromboplastin of stage 1, additional thromboplastin comes from the surrounding tissue. This additional supply is called the extrinsic thromboplastin. Therefore two sources of thromboplastin spark the conversion of inactive prothrombin to thrombin in the presence of Factors V, VII, X and calcium. The intrinsic plasma thromboplastin will convert prothrombin into thrombin in 8 to 15 sec. The extrinsic tissue thromboplastin converts prothrombin into thrombin in 12 to 15 sec. For proper clotting, both intrinsic and extrinsic systems are needed. A Factor VII deficiency (not required in the intrinsic system) causes bleeding as does a deficiency of Factor VIII (not required in the extrinsic system). Stage 2 is the thrombin phase of coagulation.

Stage 3 (Fibrinogen is converted to fibrin by thrombin). The thrombin produced in stages 1 and 2 now converts fibrinogen to fibrin and with the help of calcium and Factor XIII the fibrin changes into a stabilized form. This is the fibrin phase of coagulation and takes less than 1 sec. During these three stages a visible clot occurs.

Stage 4 (Lytic action of plasmin [fibrinolysin] on fibrin). The presence of free plasmin in more than trace amounts is abnormal.

Hemorrhagic Disorders[6,7] (Table 5-6)

Thrombocytopenia is the commonest cause of generalized bleeding disorders. Too few platelets can reflect a decrease in their production, an increase in their destruction or a combination of both mechanisms. The diagnosis of thrombocytopenia is easily made. But the differential of its cause—obviously all important to proper management—can be difficult.

Thrombocytopenia purpura is a deficiency of platelets either in numbers or function. Lack of any other factors (except calcium, which is never so deficient as to interfere with coagulation) leads to the hemophilia-like disorders. Secondary thrombocytopenias are due to a definable exogenous agent or underlying disease.

Table 5-6. Causes of Hemorrhagic Disorders

I. Platelet disorders (thrombocytopenias)
  A. Decreased production
    1. Bone marrow replacement
      a. Leukemias and other malignancies
      b. Fibrosis and sclerosis
      c. Lipoidosis
    2. Bone marrow aplasia
      a. Radiopathic drug-induced
      b. Ionizing radiation
      c. Chemotherapeutic agents
    3. Drugs
      a. Thiazides
      b. Estrogen
      c. Ethanol
  B. Increased destruction
    1. Physical and chemical agents
      a. Drugs, chemicals and foods
      b. Post-transfusion
      c. Collagen vascular diseases
      d. Lymphomas and carcinomas
    2. Post-infection
      a. Rubella, varicella or mumps
      b. Vaccination
    3. Bacteremia and viremia
    4. Splenomegaly
    5. Extensive burns, heat stroke
    6. Congestive heart failure
    7. Premenstrual thrombocytopenia
    8. Extensive burns, heat stroke
    9. Massive exchange transfusions
    10. Postpartum thrombocytopenia
    11. Hereditary (Aldrich syndrome)

II. Coagulation disorders
  A. Defective thromboplastin formation
    1. Hemophilia A, classic, Factor VIII deficiency
    2. Hemophilia B, Christmas, Factor IX deficiency
    3. Factor XI (PTA) deficiency
    4. Von Willebrand's disease
  B. Defective rate or amount of thrombin formation
    1. Vitamin K deficiency
      a. Liver disease
      b. Biliary obstruction
      c. Malabsorption syndromes
      d. Anticoagulant therapy
    2. Congenital deficiencies of Factor II, V, VII, and X
  C. Decreased fibrinogen resulting from intravascular clotting and/or fibrinolysis
    1. Obstetric abnormalities
      a. Amniotic fluid embolism
      b. Premature separation of placenta
      c. Retention of dead fetus
    2. Congenital deficiency Factor XIII
      a. Congenital afibrinogenemia
      b. Hypofibrinogenemia
    3. Neoplasms
    4. Transfusions
    5. Gram-negative septicemia and meningococcemia
  D. Circulating anticoagulants
    1. Heparin therapy
    2. Dysproteinemias
    3. SLE
    4. Postpartum state
    5. Some cases of hemophilia
III. Vascular disorders
  A. Congenital
  B. Acquired
    1. Infections
    2. Immunologic reactions
      a. Allergies
      b. Drug sensitivity
    3. Metabolic conditions (scurvy, uremia, polycythemia vera or diabetes mellitus)
    4. Drugs and chemicals
    5. Dermatologic conditions
    6. Systemic disorders
IV. Connective tissue disorders
  A. Congenital
  B. Acquired

Adapted from Harrington WJ: Differential diagnoses and management of thrombocytopenia. Medical Times 99:54, 1971.

Screening tests

History. The history gives the most important clues. Suspect a coagulation disorder if excessive bleeding occurred from the umbilical cord at birth or after trauma, surgery or dental extractions.

Physical examination. This may give a clue. Investigate for a hemorrhagic disorder whenever there is epistaxis, bleeding from the gums, multiple epistaxis, purpura or ecchymosis.

Hemogram. A hemogram or complete blood count is important since coagulation disorders often accompany blood dyscrasias, leukemia, polycythemia or multiple myeloma.

Tourniquet test. The Rumpel-Leede test is often positive in scurvy, allergic purpura, thrombocytopenia or thrombocytopathy. Normal: 0 to 20 petechia in a circle 3 cm in diameter below the bend of the elbow after inflating the blood pressure cuff to 90 mm mercury for 5 min.

Ivy bleeding time. Test for vascular and platelet function with this method. Bleeding time is a measurement of the time required for bleeding to stop after injury to superficial blood vessels. It may be prolonged in vascular disorders. Normal: 1 to 9 min.

Platelet estimation. Evaluate the number of platelets. Platelets are present in normal numbers in all conditions except thrombocytopenia. Normal range: 150,000 to 400,000.

Activated partial thromboplastin time (PTT) and/or thromboplastin generation. These are procedures to evaluate Stage I deficiencies (Factors V, VIII, IX, X, XI and XII). The activated PTT has recently replaced the cruder Lee and White clotting time because of its increased sensitivity. This test screens for all factors needed for thromboplastin formation except Factor VII. Normals less than 45 sec. Note regarding Lee and White coagulation test (replaced by PTT): The test's greatest disadvantage is its insensitivity to moderate bleeding disorders; the coagulation test may not be effected until specific coagulation factors fall below 1 to 2 percent of normal. Hemophiliacs will lose 78 percent of their normal antihemophilia globulin before being detected by the coagulation time. Use the Lee and White coagulation time as a guide to heparin therapy and not as a routine check for coagulation defects.

One-stage prothrombin time. Evaluate stages 2 and 3 (deficiencies of Factors I, II, V, VII and X) with this method. Consequently the prothrombin time measures all factors involved in stage 2 and 3 coagulation mechanism. The prothrombin time will commonly be prolonged in vitamin K deficiency, coumadin therapy and severe liver disease. Factor V (parahemophilia) deficiency also causes a prolonged prothrombin time and congenital hypoprothrombinemia. This can be diagnosed by a Factor V assay.

Clot retraction time. This is dependent on platelet number and their functions, the quality of fibrinogen and the packed cell volume. Clot retraction and the expression of serum from the clot are poor in thrombocytopenia.

Euglobulin lysis time or clot lysis. The most effective test, this checks the fibrinolysis of stage 4. This tests for the activation of the fibrinolytic system. The test may be abnormal in shock as a result of hemorrhage, carcinoma or the intravascular coagulation syndrome. In the last condition the platelets will also be low and the prothrombin time prolonged.

To determine which specific factors are deficit use a *four-part system.* The hospital laboratory technologist will understand what is meant by the four-part system. The procedure is helpful as a supplementary test to the thromboplastin generation test. First do an activated PTT on the patient's plasma. When the PTT is prolonged, three corrective tests are performed on the plasma.

The technologist attempts to correct the deficiency by adding Factors VIII and IX. If the correction is successful then a Factor V or VII deficiency would be indicated. If the prothrombin time was also prolonged, the deficiency could be assumed to be Factor V; a normal prothrombin time would indicate a Factor VIII defect.

Now the technologist adds Factors VII, IX and X. If the PTT time is corrected, a Factor IX or X deficiency is assumed. Again the prothrombin time helps to differentiate: a prolonged prothrombin time would indicate a Factor X deficiency; a normal prothrombin time, a IX deficiency. A correction by the addition of all the factors in both additions would suggest a Factor XI deficiency. A family physician will probably need help on interpreting this four-part system.

Unless the family physician wants to make an extensive study of the rarer diseases and tests, these studies are about as far as he can usefully go towards a diagnosis.

Treatment

If bleeding has resulted from an abnormality in platelets, either in their number or in their function, administer fresh platelets.

Counterindications to the transfusion of platelets are the following:

- if early marrow recovery after chemotherapy or radiation is expected
- in neonatal thrombocytopenia use only maternal platelets
- premature platelet transfusion in chronic disease because of the danger of isoimmunization, rendering platelet administration useless later in the disease
- transient thrombocytopenia from exogenous agents, i.e. in quinine depression, recovery can be expected within a week.

Obtain platelets from fresh whole blood collected in siliconized or plastic containers, or from platelet rich plasma or commercial concentrates. The administration of platelets will not be necessary if the platelet count is above 100,000. A 25 ml unit usually contains 70 to 80 percent of the platelets found in a unit of blood. In general, give 5 units.

Take a platelet count 1 hour post transfusion and if needed give additional platelets. Platelets are of value up to 24 hours from the time of donation. Remember, platelets are never given to treat a low platelet count but only for the hemorrhagic emergency.

Steroids will benefit the patient with the purpura of thrombocytopenia. Give 15 to 20 mg daily. Try prednisone in semi-emergencies. In the event, however, of intracranial hemorrhage or other life-threatening emergencies, do not depend on platelets or steroids. An emergency splenectomy is the treatment of choice.

Splenectomy remains the most effective procedure for treatment of idiopathic thrombocytopenia in adults and carries little risk despite profound bleeding. The operation will cure approximately 75 percent of the patients. Steroids will hold the disease in remission for the other 25 percent.

Do not fail to treat the specific causes of thrombocytopenia as outlined earlier.

Investigate a patient with a normal prothrombin time and an abnormally long PTT for hemophilia A and B (deficiency of Factors VIII and XI respectively). Ask the laboratory technologist to find whether the abnormal thromboplastin generation test can be corrected by absorbed plasma. The plasma corrects TGT in hemophilia A; the plasma remains uncorrected in hemophilia B. Again, in hemophilia A an assay of Factor VIII of less than 2 percent indicates a classical hemophilia; less than 3 percent, a moderate hemophilia; and less than 16 percent, a mild hemophilia.

Delay surgery and dental extractions in suspected cases of hemophilia. Refer the patient to a hematologist for verification of the diagnosis.

Antihemophilic factors concentrate (Hemofil) is now on the market for treatment of Hemophilia A. Konyne or Factor IX concentrate will supply the deficient factor in Hemophilia B or Christmas disease. Cryoprecipitated human plasma for treatment of Hemophilia A and von Willebrand's disease is now available. Give 10 units initially and follow with 5 units every 12 hr. The volume of each unit is 10 ml. Twenty ml will restore the antihemophilic globulin from a pint of plasma. Until bleeding stops give enough AHG intravenously daily to maintain at least 20 to 30 percent of a normal level.

The cryoprecipitated plasma can be stored frozen; consequently, encourage hemophiliacs to come for treatment when bleeding starts. Admit patients with hemophilia to the hospital for dental extractions or surgery and administer AHG before and after the operation. Pack tooth sockets lightly with thrombin preparations or Russell viper venom (Stypven).

Abnormalities in prothrombin time in patients with a normal PTT and thrombin time are due to deficiencies of vitamin K-dependent factors, especially Factor VII. Use vitamin K to correct this deficiency.

Vitamin K is present in a number of foods, and certain bacteria in the intestines produce more vitamin K. In the liver vitamin K changes to prothrombin. The absence of bile salts inhibits the absorption of vitamin; consequently, a clinical prothrombin deficiency develops in two classes of patients: newborn babies in whose intestines the vitamin

K-forming organisms have not become established (hemorrhagic disease of newborn) and patients with obstructive jaundice whose intestines contain no bile salts. Prevent the former by giving vitamin K, 5 mg IM daily for a few days before delivery. Patients with obstructive jaundice should receive similar treatment in preparation for surgery to prevent serious hemorrhage.

Specific coagulation factor deficiencies are not rare. Correct these deficiencies by fresh whole blood, fresh frozen plasma or by protein fractions. A hematologist may detect these factors by a study of the PTT, prothrombin time, thrombin time, and analysis for individual coagulation factors.

Detect anticoagulants by the prolongation of all plasma screening tests and the failure of normal plasma to correct the defect. Heparin may be the culprit if the coagulation defect can be corrected in the test tube by protamine sulfate.

Detect fibrinolysis by whole blood clot lysis, euglobulin clot lysis time, plasminogen determination and screening tests.

Keep the defibrination syndrome or intravascular coagulation syndrome in mind when studying coagulation disorders. Suspect the syndrome if the fibrinogen is low or absent, the platelets decreased and the prothrombin time prolonged. The syndrome usually responds to heparin and fibrinogen. Seek the help of a hematologist before giving the heparin to patients with afibrinogen or the defibrination syndrome. Give fibrinogen for either condition. Fibrinogen also has high concentrations of the antihemophilic factors and may be of value when the concentrates are not available.

Bleeding occurs if the fibrinogen level falls below 100 mg percent. Hypofibrinogenemia may be congenital but more commonly follows disseminated intravascular clotting from amniotic fluid embolism, extensive surgery, hemolytic blood reactions or fibrinolysis following trauma or surgery to the prostate, lungs or stomach.

Give at least 4 g initially and follow by amounts sufficient to keep the fibrinogen level above 100 mg percent.

Ionized calcium is a vital ingredient of the coagulation process. Give the patient calcium chloride or calcium gluconate whenever multiple transfusions with large amounts of citrate have been given or when there is liver damage and citrate detoxification is questionable.

OFFICE CARE OF WOUNDS AND LACERATIONS

The Office Operating Room

Preparation of the OR

The furniture of the room should be washable. Clean the room frequently with hot water and strong soap or a detergent. Rinse well. In the selection of the ceiling, wall and floor coverings, choose materials that are easily cleaned.

Miscellaneous Equipment

Miscellaneous equipment needed in the OR follows:

–Iodoform packing for abscess cavities
–razor
–#15 scalpel blade for excisions
–disposable gloves
–Q-tips
–Ethicon 5-0 nylon chromostat needle with attached suture
–disposable syringe with needles of varying sizes
–2x2 and 4x4 sterile gauze squares
–2- and 4-inch Kling bandages
–Telfa pads
–regular and paper adhesive
–tincture of benzoin
–Vaseline- or furacin-impregnated gauze
–plastic or collodion spray dressing
–Steri-strip closure strips
–Betadine (the best antiseptic) or 1 percent aqueous Zephrian (replace Zephrian monthly because of colonization)
–hydrogen peroxide
–normal saline for irrigation
–tape remover (ether or benzine)
–Betadine, Bacimycin or Neosporin ointment
–pHisoHex for surgical scrub
–G-11 soap for open surfaces

–Xylocaine ½ or 1 percent for local anesthesia
–Xylocaine 0.5 percent with epinephrine (1:200,000) (You may use up to 1 ml/kg of the latter; do not use on fingers)
–silver nitrate sticks
–alcohol
–ethyl chloride spray

The following instruments are needed on the suture tray:

–large smooth forceps for prepping the area
–large scissors for cutting dressings
–curved and straight hemostats for picking up bleeders
–small toothed forceps for tissue manipulation
–small curved sharp scissors for debridement of ragged wounds
–small straight sharp scissors for removing sutures
–large curved clamp for picking up things and aiding in the application of the dressing
–an ear syringe for saline irrigation of the recesses of a wound
–a needle holder

Care of Office Instruments

Sterilize stainless steel instruments in distilled water or steam generated from it. If distilled water is not available, boil in water that is alkaline. Sklar Stir-tabs are convenient for this purpose. Dry all residual moisture from instruments after sterilization, especially from lock areas and crevices.

The Sklar Manufacturing Company has prepared a lubricant, Sklarol, for the locks of hemostats and other box lock instruments. A drop or two will prevent binding.

Because of the water in alcohol, instruments immersed in it for long periods may spot or discolor. Adding a little soda will minimize this.

Do not expose stainless steel for more than 4 hours to any of the following: aluminum chloride, barium chloride, bichloride of mercury, carbolic acid, chlorinated lime, citric acid, Dakin's Solution, ferrous chloride, Lysol, mercuric chloride, mercury salts, phenol, potassium permanganate, potassium thiocyanate, sodium hypochlorite, stannous chloride or tartaric acid.

If instruments do come in contact with the above, clean well after use. Avoid iodine, hydrochloric acid, sulfuric acid, ferric chloride and aqua regia.

Course of Care

Functional Evaluation

Inspect the extremity distal to the wound. A physical examination should be made before all the first aid bandages are removed. Start by counting the pulse in the area and proceed to a functional check of the muscles and tendons of the part. Most of this inspection can be made without uncovering the wound. Check the 5 p's: paresthesia, pain, pallor, paresis and pulselessness. Failure to conduct a thorough evaluation before treating an injured hand is *prima facie* evidence of negligence.

OBSERVE AND RECORD. It is important that you keep careful and thorough records. Observe and record:

–type of injury
–where and how the injury occurred
–injury to the major or minor hand
–previous injuries to the extremity
–any systemic disease or previous surgery
–patient's description of the injury (chief complaint)

Examine and record:

–site of injury
–condition of all joints of the extremity
–type of injury
–loss of function
–tendon injury
–sensation to pin prick
–vascular and skin condition
–amount of swelling

Check and record: radial nerve function by voluntary wrist extension, extension of the metacarpophalangeal joints of the fingers and extension of the terminal phalanx of the thumb with the thumb adducted; ulnar nerve function by having the patient adduct and abduct his index and little fingers or by checking for a sensory deficiency in the little finger; and median nerve function by testing for sensory deficiency in the palmar surface of the terminal phalanx of the index finger.[8]

CONSENT. You will never make a mistake by obtaining a Consent to Operation form from your patient. At times this seems superfluous but it is a good habit for your staff to anticipate.

Procedure

WASHING. The oldest simplest and single most important means of preventing the spread of infection is handwashing. To wash properly: remove jewelry, use a germicidal soap or detergent, scrub well for 2 to 3 minutes and rinse thoroughly. (Three minutes are sufficient if you use hexachlorophene several times during the day for handwashing.) While rinsing your hands, keep the water running from the washed areas to the unwashed. Clean the nails with an orange stick. Turn the water off with the elbow or by using a foot control.

ANESTHESIA. The best technique in administering anesthesia is to block a digital or regional nerve or infiltrate locally with 1 percent carbocaine or 0.5 percent Xylocaine for body injuries. Do not use epinephrine in the hand or fingers because of vasospasm and possible circulatory damage. Wait 10 minutes before beginning to scrub the wound.

Most operators prefer Xylocaine with epinephrine for local anesthesia about the face. Whether the doctor uses 1 or 2 percent solution depends on how much anesthesia will be needed. When a large quantity is needed, even a ½ percent solution is in order. If the injection is likely to distort landmarks such as the vermillion border, mark the margins with a puncture mark or a skin dye before injecting the anesthetic solution.

SCRUBBING THE WOUND. First shave about the wound, but never shave off the eyebrows. If the wound is 3 hours old, preliminary scrubbing is essential. Scrub with a scrub brush and saline or hexachlorophene; Zephiran and iodine cause tissue damage. The purpose of the scrub is to disrupt the coagulum, which forms over an exposed wound, so an antibiotic has access to the injured cells and bacteria. Scrub thoroughly; don't hurry the scrubbing process. If the wound is dirty, scrub for 10 minutes and use copious amounts of sterile saline to rinse.

PREPARING THE PATIENT'S SKIN. Cleanse the surrounding area with ether, apply 3½ percent tincture of iodine and rinse with isopropyl alcohol. Don't skimp on the area prepared; if possible prepare the skin for 12 inches around the wound.

ANTIBIOTICS. Systemic antibiotics are more effective than topical application according to a study by Edlich and Wagensteen.[9] They present evidence that presurgical administration of an antibiotic is more effective than when given postsurgically.

A legal note regarding the use of injectable penicillin: allergic reactions to penicillin provoke a large number of malpractice suits. The outcome, in most instances, hinges on whether the family physician knew or determined whether the patient was or was not allergic to penicillin. Some difficulties can be avoided by recording the following on the patient's chart: "Patient denies previous allergy to penicillin," and then recording the details of the injection.

USE OF GLOVES. Good surgical technique still requires that the operator and his assistant wear gloves for minor surgery. If a patient sued because of wound infection and the physician had not worn gloves, he might have difficulty proving that due precautions had been taken and that usual practices had been employed. No patient ever has sterile skin and no physician ever has sterile hands, no matter how long he scrubs or with what solution he rinses. Scrubbing, after all, only gives a clean skin and has little effect on the hair follicles, sweat glands, oil glands or even the deep creases and folds. The hands are the cleanest immediately after scrubbing and become progressively dirty. As time passes bacteria emerge from gland orifices. If the hands are inside the glove, the outside of the glove is still sterile. The weight of opinion would appear to be against doing even minor office surgery without gloves.[10]

DRAPING THE SITE. Drape the wound site to keep a sterile field. Sutures should never be long enough to dangle onto an unsterile field.

INSPECTION AND DEBRIDEMENT. Debridement is essential except for superficial lacerations of the skin and subcutaneous tissues. Avoid disfigurement by conservative debridement of wounds of the face and hands. In other areas, however, trim ragged edges and excise contaminated tissue. Extensively excise damaged and devitalized muscle. Repair muscle by reapproximating the fascia surrounding the muscle mass. Drain any space made by a major muscle resection with a soft rubber or polyethylene tube and culture the discharge regularly.

Consider the wound—how it was caused, where it is located and what tissues have been affected. (A caution: know your own capabilities and refer when you have reached your limit.) For care of wounds of specific areas of the body see the section so titled later in this chapter.

If primary facial repair must be delayed because of the patient's general condition, wash up the wound, apply a sterile moist compress with a little pressure and give an antibiotic. With these precautions the operator may delay primary repair for 8 to 10 hours.

Repair human and dog bites in the usual fashion after debridement. Antibiotics have eliminated the old open wound method of care.

As a general rule, tie off an unnamed artery or vein. Repair larger vessels such as the femoral, popliteal and brachial arteries. The best way to control hemorrhage is by simple, direct, external compression. Tourniquets, blind clamps and mass ligatures are out.

Suspect arterial injury when a penetrating wound lies over the route of a major artery and when a closed injury displays a rapidly increasing hematoma. Look for these signs: distal arterial insufficiency, absent pulses, pallor, patchy cyanosis, coldness, paresthesia, loss of feeling, paralysis or ischemic pain. If signs of arterial insufficiency continue for more than 2 hours, have the wound explored.

Dispose of all dressings and tissues contaminated by body discharges in impervious bags. Close, seal and burn the bags. Never reuse disposable bags.[11]

CLOSING THE WOUND. For primary single-layer closure of the scalp, use monofilament nylon (3-0) or stainless steel (5-0) sutures. For facial repairs, use an absorbable subcuticular (4-0) chronic suture for wound approximation and 5-0 nylon for cosmetic alignment. Remove the nylon sutures after 48 hours and replace with adhesive butterfly tapes. For a fibrous layer, use nonabsorbable silk or synthetic 3-0 or 4-0 sutures; for the fatty layer, absorbable chromated gut treated to resist absorption for as long as 14 to 21 days; and for skin closure, fine nonabsorbable 4-0 nylon or 5-0 stainless steel. The strength of the repair comes from the sutures in the fibrous layer. The sutures in the fatty layer merely close the dead space. Accurate approximation of tissues is the key for good cosmetic results.

Family physicians could give more thought to the use of multiple rayon filaments (Steri-strip skin closures) distributed by the surgical services of the 3M Company. These are handy for the closure of small wounds about the face, but some surgeons are now using them for major surgical wounds and lacerations. In my own practice, I've limited their use to smaller wounds, especially when I wish to avoid puncture scars and stitch abscesses. An added inducement is their use in children who are uncooperative with placement of sutures or in their removal.

Steri-Strips stay on wet draining wounds satisfactorily. They are advertised as being hypoallergenic. Use Steri-Strips when removing primary sutures early for cosmetic reasons.

Application is easy. Dry the skin edges and place the first strip in the mid wound area, pulling the edges together. Working out both ways on the wound, place other strips ¼ to ½ in apart until the wound is solidly closed. Complete the closure with additional strips parallel to the wound to give added protection and strength.

SPLINTING. Healing is facilitated by simple, relaxed positioning and splinting of the injured part. Remember to elevate the extremity to heart level.

TETANUS PROPHYLAXIS. Inject a booster dose of tetanus toxoid or if the patient has not been actively immunized, give human tetanus antitoxin. There are numerous cases wherein physicians have been charged with negligence in the care of a wound and the failure to administer tetanus antitoxin. If the patient claims to have had proper boosters for tetanus, you are entitled to rely on the patient's statement. Be sure to document the reason for nonadministration, however.

Your failure to administer a scratch test before giving a full dose of tetanus antitoxin will create liability. Proper testing requires the observation of the sensitivity test for 15 to 30 minutes before giving the antitoxin. If the scratch test does not indicate a positive reaction, you will not be held negligent, even if the patient has a reaction to the antitoxin. Be sure to document in writing all test results.

RECORD. Record everything that was done. Record whether the repair was done in the hospital or office, the findings, what was done, dressings used, whether tetanus was administered, x-ray and laboratory findings, follow-up care and plans for future reconstruction including stages and alternatives.

The family physician who works full or part time in an emergency room must remember that:

- –the physician is responsible for the patient until the patient is transferred to a hospital or to the care of another physician.
- –the patient is entitled to an adequate examination
- –the physician will be held to the same standard of diagnosis and treatment as in all medical practice
- –any negligence must worsen the patient's condition to be actionable.

Care of Specific Areas of the Body

Repair joint injuries in the hospital and within 4 to 6 hours. Remove all foreign matter and irrigate all contamination from the joint.

Torso

In lacerations to the torso, examine for associated deep injuries. Blunt trauma may be associated with hidden injuries. Consider hospitalization for 24 to 48 hours in suspiciously dangerous wounds, surgically repaired or not. Wounds resulting from high-velocity missiles are usually jobs for surgeons. All penetrating wounds require painstaking evaluation with x-ray study and other indicated techniques.

Head

All patients with head wounds (face or scalp) should have a neurological examination to rule out skull fractures and brain injuries. If indicated, obtain x-ray pictures before any surgical repair. Experienced physicians should repair injuries involving the eyelids, the parotid gland and its duct, the facial nerve, the lips or the ear.

In deep injuries of the anterior triangle of the neck, the physician will need all the help he can get—x-rays, perhaps carotid angiography, direct laryngoscopy and a tracheostomy.

FACIAL INJURIES. Perform a physical examination of the face. With injuries of the forehead or eyebrow examine for an area of anesthesia. Anesthesia above the injuries indicates damage to the supratrochlear cr supraorbital nerves. Inability to lift the upper eyelid suggests a levator muscle injury. Repair injuries to the lacrimal duct, levator muscle or tarsal plate in a hospital operating room, unless the office OR is unusually well equipped.

With injuries in the preauricular area, check for injury to the parotid gland and its duct and to the facial nerve. Have the patient move his eyebrow, close his eyelid, smile or pucker his lips.

Learn to palpate the bony ridges of the face with both hands palpating both sides of the face at once. Palpate the ridges about the eye for tenderness, displacement, stop-offs and crepitation. Put both fingers in the patient's ear canal and have him open and close his mouth to examine for injury to the condylar head of the mandible. Continue examining along the edge of the mandible to the chin. Palpate inside the mouth for fractures of the maxilla, teeth and mandible. Shake the teeth for any looseness. While the patient opens and closes his mouth, observe the teeth for malocclusion, deviation and crossbite.

Examine the nose externally and internally by observation and palpation. Skillful physical examination is more accurate in assessing nasal injuries than is an x-ray examination. Reduce septal displacements as soon as possible, at least within 24 hours.

Do not forget to palpate for injury to the maxillary-zygomatic or molar area. A fracture in these parts is usually through the foramen from which the infraorbital nerve exits.

Severe ecchymosis of the eyelids following blunt trauma without any evidence of fracture on examination should suggest a fracture of the orbital floor. X-ray examination can readily detect this fracture.

Treat fractures of the zygomatic arch and the maxilla conservatively, i.e. antibiotics, fluid diet for 2 weeks to avoid chewing and displacement of bony fragments, and restraint in blowing the nose to avoid forcing infection into the sinuses and soft tissues.

To repair facial lacerations, proper equipment is essential. Have small instruments available. Use skin hooks where possible to avoid traumatizing more tissue. Slant the edges of the wound by trimming so the sutures produce slight eversion when tied. This trick will produce a flat scar rather than a depressed one. Undermine the skin particularly if necessary to overcome tension when closing the wound.

Place subcuticular sutures with an atraumatic needle and bury the knot. Use 5-0 white nylon or 5-0 plain or chromic sutures. Do not squeeze or pinch the skin. Use the forceps as a hook only. Do not use subcuticular sutures where the skin is thin as on the eyelids.

Placing the subcuticular sutures should relieve the tension and approximate the edges. Then place the skin sutures. Use suture material as fine as possible (5 or 6-0 nylon) and place ⅛ inch apart. Be meticulous about bringing all the landmarks together accurately such as the vermillion border of the lips, the edges of the eyebrow and the nasal alar rim.

Hand and Wrist

Refer patients with flexor tendon injuries of the hand and wrist to a hand surgeon. If none is available, clean and close the wound. Apply a pressure dressing, elevate the hand to heart level and maintain the affected joints in 45° partial flexion to prevent edema and stiffness. Lacerations with tendon injuries may be repaired by a hand surgeon within 6 hours if not probed and contaminated. The other alternative: close the skin with simple interrupted sutures (4-0 or 5-0) wire or synthetic. Keep dressed for 6 days changing every 2 days. Check for infection regularly, daily if necessary. Flex the joints 2 to 3 times a day. Continue until secondary tendon repair can be done.

Repair lacerations of the extensor tendons at the wrist by primary tenorrhaphy using 3-0 or 4-0 stainless steel wire. Splint the wrist in extension for about 4 weeks. Keep fingers free for exercise.

Repair lacerations of extensor tendons over the back of the hand by simple suturing using 4-0 or 5-0 wire or silk. Again splint in extension for 3 to 4 weeks.

In extensor tendon injuries proximal to the proximal interphalangeal joint, splint the finger in extension.

In extensor tendon injury distal to the the proximal interphalangeal joint, splint with the proximal interphalangeal joint flexed 45° and the distal interphalangeal joint in full extension for 4 to 6 weeks.

In extension tendon injuries to the extensor mechanism of the finger over the digits, splint the distal interphalangeal joint in extension.

Do not attempt to repair flexor tendons of the fingers or wrist unless skilled in such surgery. Treat by simple closure and flexion splinting for 3 weeks.[12]

FINGERTIP INJURIES. The initial examination should include x-rays to rule out foreign bodies and fractures. Blocking the digital nerves at the proximal finger crease will produce anesthesia distal to the middle joint. Inject 2 or 4 ml of 1 percent lidocaine *without* epinephrine at each corner of the volar aspect of the first phalangeal joint.

When anesthesia is complete scrub the patient's hand and forearm. Change gloves and wrap the finger with a Penrose starting at the tip and stopping at the base of the finger. Anchor with a hemostat. This should remove blood from the finger. Unwrap the Penrose from the tip to expose the wound for repair.

Perform debridement and if possible close the laceration with 5-0 nylon suture. Repair the nail bed with 5-0 plain catgut sutures.

If a split thickness graft is needed, take tissue from the inner aspect of the wrist. Make a wheal with lidocaine and shave off the needed skin with a #10 blade. If a full thickness graft is needed, excise tissue from the flexor surface of the wrist and primarily close the resulting elliptical defect.[13]

INJECTION SITES

Injection sites are indicated in Figures 5-3, 5-4 and 5-5.

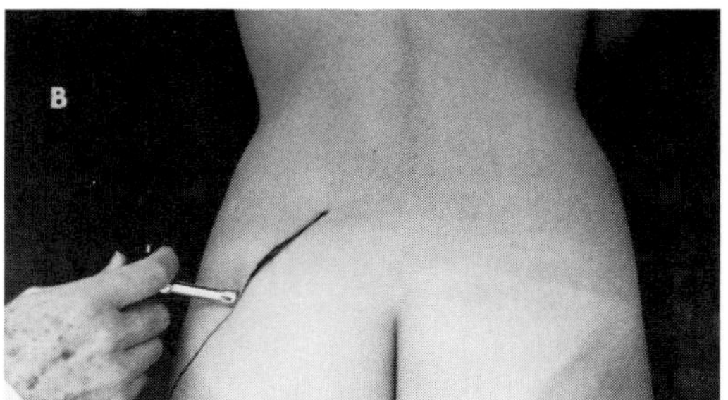

Figure 5-3. Gluteus medius injection site. Draw an imaginary line between the posterior superior iliac spine and the greater trochanter of the femur. Inject above and outside the diagonal line.

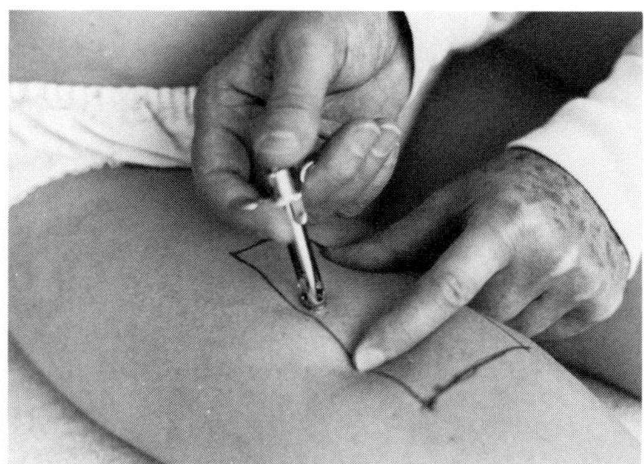

Figure 5-4. Vastus lateralis injection site. Imagine a rectangle bounded proximally a hand's breadth below the greater trochanter and distally a hand's breadth above the knee.

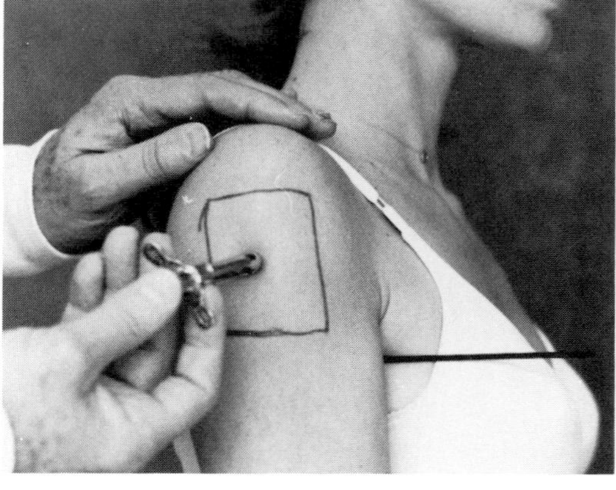

Figure 5-5. Mid-deltoid injection site. Imagine a rectangle bounded above by the lower edge of the acromion and below by the level of the armpit. The area is small and cannot tolerate repeated or large injections.

REACTIONS TO LOCAL ANESTHETICS

Psychological reaction. The symptom of this is a feeling of faintness but a slow pulse. To treat:

- discontinue injecting the anesthetic
- have the patient sniff an ampule of aromatic ammonia
- help the patient lie down
- inject ephedrine 10 to 15 mg IM if needed

Wheezing. Symptoms are wheezing, bronchospasm and hypotension. To treat:

–elevate the patient's feet
–use a medihaler-epi or Bronkometer
–administer oxygen
–inject epinephrine 0.2 to 1 ml of a 1:1000 solution SC or IM
–inject Benadryl 25 to 50 mg IV

Histaminic reaction. Symptoms are urticaria, itching or skin rash. To treat:

–inject Benadryl 10 to 15 mg IM or IV
–inject epinephrine 0.2 to 1 ml of a 1:1000 solution SC or IM
–follow up with oral antihistamines

Epinephrine reaction. Symptoms are tremor and tachycardia, pallor and cold and clammy skin. To treat:

–apply a tourniquet proximal to the injection site
–give oxygen if shock occurs
–inject Seconal 100 mg IM for tremor and tachycardia

Minor toxic systemic reaction. Symptoms are slurred speech, teeth grinding and increased blood pressure. To treat:

–discontinue administration of drug
–apply a tourniquet
–elevate the feet

Toxic systemic reaction. For muscle twitching start IV glucose to dilute the anesthetic and give Pentothal 25 to 75 mg IV.

For cyanosis, give oxygen.

For hypotension with a slow pulse, give ephedrine 20 to 25 mg IM.

For hypotension with a fast pulse, give phenylephrine 1 to 2 mg IM.

For weak or absent pulse, apnea, gasping or rapid shallow respiration, clear the airway and start resuscitation mouth-to-mouth and phone for an ambulance.

For absent carotid pulse, start closed chest cardiac massage. Inject epinephrine, 0.1 to 0.2 ml of a 1:1000 solution, directly into the heart and give sodium bicarbonate, 50 ml ampule IV.

TREATMENT OF INSECT STING ALLERGY

Most insect stings are treated by family physicians and the physician should be prepared to give preventive therapy. Most patients require no emergency treatment except the removal of the sting sac. The treatment of the allergic patient, however, requires prompt and knowledgeable treatment. Yellow jackets and honey bees account for about 75 percent of the stings.

Remove the sting sac. Apply a tourniquet above the sting if on an extremity. Administer epinephrine, 0.3 ml subcutaneously of a 1:1000 dilution for a moderate case. Use larger amounts if indicated. If an injection is not practical, have the patient carry a nebulizer and, upon being stung, take six inhalations rather than the usual three given to asthmatic patients. Later use antihistamines for itching, prednisone for hives or wheezing and oxygen if indicated. As preventive therapy, consider weekly hyposensitizing injections. Start with the weakest dilution to give a positive skin test and gradually work up to the maximum of 0.25 ml of a 1:10 dilution as tolerated. Then administer monthly boosters.[14]

INTRAVENOUS REGIONAL ANESTHESIA

Intravenous regional anesthesia has been attempted several times in this century, but not until the development of mepivacaine hydrochloride has it been a successful method of local anesthesia. Costly and Lorhan[15] have now used the method several hundred times and report the following technique.

Insert a #21 scalp-vein needle into a vein distal to the injury and secure. Exsanguinate the injured extremity with an Esmarch bandage. Apply a pneumatic tourniquet as proximal to the body as the arm or leg will permit. Inflate to 250 mm Hg. Slowly remove the Esmarch bandage. Inject a test dose of 5 ml of solution (30 mg) and wait 3 minutes. If no adverse reaction, inject the entire dose rapidly. Anesthesia is immediate.

If the arm or leg is injured precluding the Esmarch bandage, raise the arm for 3 minutes with the artery digitally compressed. When the arm is bloodless, inflate the proximal tourniquet. Apply a second pneumatic tourniquet just distal to the first but still distal to the operative site. Inflate to 250 mm of Hg, and remove the first tourniquet. Place webroll under the tourniquet to protect the skin. Remove needle and prepare operative site for surgery or manipulation.

If the tourniquet is on over 30 minutes, deflate the cuff at the end of the operation. If the tourniquet is on less than 30 minutes, deflate the cuff for 10 seconds, reinflate for 3 minutes and then deflate and remove. The authors warn against the use of any anesthesia containing preservatives such as methylparaben or benzyl alcohol.

TO OPERATE OR NOT TO OPERATE

The family physician who refers some of his surgery to surgeons, must give careful consideration as to the most expeditious time to refer. If there is damage to the patient, an unreasonable delay may bring the charge of malpractice. Consider the following guidelines.

If under certain circumstances a "wait and see" attitude will be considered unjustified by your peers, then a cause for negligence exists and a determination by a jury most likely will be made.

Generally, a judgement to delay or refrain from performing surgery will be respected as long as the judgement is a considered one and does not violate principles of the standard of care required. The patient must prove negligence by expert testimony.

Delaying surgery because of some nonmedical reason such as finances could establish negligence.

If the patient refuses or delays accepting your advice, no negligence exists, even if damage to the patient later occurs.

You may be held negligent if, while dealing with a condition that could require emergency surgery, you do not institute tests to detect the condition.

A general rule: As long as the delay occurs under circumstances where a reasonable physician would do the same thing, no negligence is present even if damage results.

Liability for Unnecessary Surgery

If your decision to advise surgery is based on careful consideration and reasonable evidence and tests, a misdiagnosis is not negligent. Be sure that reasonable tests are made to confirm your diagnosis.

Unnecessary surgery can be actionable if an expert witness testifies that even if no harm was done the surgery was truly unnecessary. A jury is likely to give fairly large awards for the pain and anguish.

Actually more suits are started for failure to operate when surgery is indicated than for operating unnecessarily.

ABDOMINAL TRAUMA

Trauma is the number one cause of death in persons from 5 to 25 years of age. Abdominal trauma is the third ranking cause of death in the total population followed by cardiovascular diseases and cancer. The organ most frequently injured is the spleen, followed by the liver, kidney and bowel.

The treatment of penetrating wounds of the abdominal wall is clear. Consider every wound that conceivably could have penetrated into the abdominal cavity as having done so until disproven by operation.

Nonpenetrating wounds are more complex. An unexpected blow on the relaxed abdomen is the most common cause of serious internal injuries.

Diagnosis

Early recognition of the injury and immediate surgical repair are essential. Take a careful history inquiring into:

- events preceding accident
- speed of car and type of injury
- time and place of injury
- location, duration and kind of pain
- ingestion of alcohol, coumadin, steroids, etc.
- vomiting

–whether the patient can urinate or not and if blood is present

Perform a screening physical examination, including a check for associated injuries; inspection for open wounds and bleeding, shock, pallor and type of respiration; check for pulse, local tenderness, rigidity and muscle spasm or guarding; and auscultation of the abdomen for peristalsis.

If the first examination does not confirm the presence of an acute abdominal injury and doubts exist, repeat examinations by the same examiner at 20 min intervals until the diagnosis is clear. Remember, too, the first examination may be unreliable in the presence of shock or if the laceration is plugged by a clot, omentum or adhesions or if other major injuries have occurred. Some abdominal organs which have sustained injury may rupture later.

Resist the urge to probe or irrigate abdominal wounds unless in the OR.

Laboratory Checks

When in doubt, surgery is not to be postponed awaiting laboratory results except for the routine. The following laboratory checks should be made: serial hematocrit and white blood counts; serum amylase; urine diastase; urinalysis for hematuria. Order a scout x-ray film of the abdomen checking for air, distended loops of small bowel, fractures, and soft tissue shadows of liver, spleen, kidneys and of the psoas muscle. Also have a chest upright left lateral decubitus taken for determination of an elevated diaphragm, fractured ribs, pneumoperitoneum or loops of bowel in the chest. Consider other x-rays such as intravenous pyelogram, cystogram, gastrografin upper gastrointestinal series and catheter injection of abdominal wounds. Inject gastrografin through a tube to detect a ruptured diaphragm. Use the same substance to help differentiate an injured duodenum from a pancreatitis—an important differentiation.

Last of all, consider an abdominal paracentesis, a four-quadrant tap if necessary, checking for blood, gastrointestinal contents, bile, urine or pancreatic enzymes.

Treatment

These injuries are emergencies and the decision to operate is based on clinical judgment after the history and physical examination.

The first consideration should be the management of shock. Include the insertion of a nasogastric tube and catheter drainage. Begin antibiotics early.

The *spleen* is the most frequently injured abdominal organ following blunt trauma to the abdomen. Selective arteriography and scans may help verify the injury. A splenectomy is imperative.

A ruptured *liver* requires surgical repair to control hemorrhage, to remove all nonviable tissue and to provide proper drainage of liver and bile ducts when needed. One word about blunt trauma to the bile ducts: There may be an interval of 3 to 4 days following injury before ascites or icterus occurs. An abdominal tap may strike free bile in the peritoneal cavity. Rarely is a subtotal hepatectomy required. Usually the control of hemorrhage is by employment of mattress sutures with the judicious use of Oxycel or Gelfoam plus ligation of appropriate arteries.

Genitourinary tract injuries are common, especially in children. The most important signs and symptoms are flank pain, hematuria, and a costovertebral angle tumor. Verify the diagnosis by an intravenous pyelogram. If visualization of the urinary tract is missing, request a retrograde study by an urologist. Conservative treatment is the rule. Occasionally a nephrectomy will be needed. Close bladder perforations. Consider suprapubic cystostomy and catheter drainage.

Do not fail to recognize *pancreatic* injuries following trauma. If associated with splenic, duodenal or retroperitoneal injuries, pancreatic injuries are difficult to recognize unless the physician has the foresight to order a serum amylase. Surgery consists of hemorrhage control and drainage. Conservative debridement and occasional subtotal pancreatectomy are measures of choice. Most important is the control of pancreatic secretions by wide sump drainage. At least 50 percent of these patients have associated injuries to the retroperitoneal area. Complications include the formation of a pseudocyst, infection, fistula formation and gastrointestinal bleeding.

The second and third portion of the *duodenum* are the most common sites of rupture of the intestine. Making a preoperative diagnosis is vexing. The injury occurs during traumatic violence, as in a steering wheel injury when the duodenum becomes "fractured" by pressure over the rigid spine. Two unlikely findings may draw the alert physician to the injury. They are testicular pain and retroperitoneal emphysema. Occasionally a Hypaque UGI series will confirm the suspicion. Surgery should include debridement of lacerated edges, closure, drainage and possibly a jejunal patch. Establish adequate drainage and decompress internally. Repair most duodenal lacerations by simple sutures. The most common postoperative complications are fistula formation and pancreatitis.

Eight percent of *small bowel* trauma occurs between the duodenojejunal and the terminal ileum. Be on guard for an associated mesenteric injury. The peritonitis that follows bowel perforation may be both chemical and bacterial. Surgery consists in simple closure and occasionally a resection and anastomosis.

Injuries to the *colon* occur following medical instrumentation and surgery as well as from accidents. Base the diagnosis on the results of an anal digital examination and sigmoidoscopy. Make AP and lateral decubitus x-rays studies. The surgeon will choose definitive treatment from a wide choice of surgical procedures such as primary closure with or without colostomy, exteriorization, resection with colostomy or resection with anastomosis. Drain the area and give the patient massive doses of antibiotics.

Penetrating *stomach* injuries are nearly always associated with injuries of nearby tissues and with a high percentage of pleural injuries. The diagnosis is seldom a problem because of the ease of finding bloody aspirate in the nasogastric tube. Surgical treatment consists of debridement and primary closure and occasionally a subtotal gastric resection.

Prevention of Infection in Gunshot Wounds

Start antibiotics within 30 to 60 minutes following the injury. Antibiotics started later increase the incidence of infection four times.

Start penicillin with the first intravenous infusion by adding aqueous penicillin, 1,000,000 units to the infusion. Continue with 3,000,000 units for 3 to 5 days following surgery.

Start tetracycline 250 mg with the first intravenous infusion but drip this drug in as an IV piggyback. Continue tetracycline 3 to 5 days postoperatively as with the penicillin.

Skillful early debridement is as essential as antibiotics in preventing later infection. Repair all injured organs and close all penetrating wounds of the GI tract.

Culture all drainage sites in preparation for later antibiotic selection.

Tapping a Belly

Choose a puncture site: Select a site in the lower quadrants but avoid abdominal scars. Be sure the bladder is empty. Avoid the inferior epigastric arteries by outlining the border of Hesselbach's triangle. Draw a line from the umbilicus to a point midway between the anterior superior iliac spine and the symphysis pubis. The line marks the lateral boundary of Hesselbach's triangle. Stay away from this landmark.

Puncture technique: Prepare the site with Betadine solution. Raise a skin wheal with 1 percent Xylocaine. Infiltrate to the peritoneum. Introduce a 18- or 20-gauge spinal needle with stylus in place perpendicularly into the peritoneum. The needle penetrates the peritoneum with a kind of snap. Leave the needle in place and replace the stylus with a 10 ml syringe.

Search for abdominal fluid: Apply gentle negative pressure by raising the plunger. If fluid fills the syringe, nothing more need be done. If no fluid is found, advance the needle slowly while maintaining gentle suction. Rotate or angulate the needle as indicated. If no fluid is found, simply remove the needle while maintaining gentle suction.

Note: Experimental attempts to puncture loops of exposed bowel with a lumbar needle have proved fruitless unless the bowel was held firmly as by adhesions. Further, intestinal loops punctured by an 18- and 20-gauge needle don't leak until high internal pressures are reached, something on the order of 260 to 350 mm mercury.

Diagnostic peritoneal lavage, in some quarters, is replacing the classic four-quadrant paracentesis in an attempt to detect hemorrhage following blunt trauma to the abdomen. The suggested technique for this follows: Select a low midline abdominal site avoiding organs and previous incisions. Be sure the bladder is empty. Prep the area and infiltrate with 1 or 2 percent Xylocaine with epinephrine, the latter for hemostatic effect. Exclude patients who have had previous surgery. Incise the skin and subcutaneous tissues to the peritoneum in the midline. Introduce a peritoneal dialysis catheter with multiple side holes plus the stylet through the peritoneum but directed away from the midline to avoid the shallow cavity over the vertebrae. A trocar is not always needed. As the catheter or trocar pierces the peritoneum, have the patient tense his abdominal muscle; thus the piercing of the peritonium can be better felt. Infuse 1 L of saline or Ringer's lactate into the abdomen (300 to 500 ml in children). Rotate the patient from side to side. Withdraw the lavage gravitationally by lowering the infusion bottle to the floor.

Results: Consider the return of bloody fluid a positive test. Examine further under the microscope for erythrocytes, white blood cells, bacteria, meat and vegetable fibers. This fluid also can be checked for amylase and bile. Gross blood or erythrocytes greater than 100,000 per ml indicates intraperitoneal bleeding; a white blood cell count above 500 per ml or bacteria, an inflammatory reaction.

CHEST INJURIES

Of 50,000 automobile deaths, 25 percent were caused by thoracic injuries. In another 50 percent, chest injuries were a major factor in deaths.

Considerations

In an emergency inspect and quickly evaluate for dyspnea, color of skin, level of mental status and the presence of dilated neck veins and peripheral veins. Coughing, crowing or choking may indicate airway obstruction by a foreign body. Help the patient into a head-down position and strike him on the back between the shoulder blades. Occasionally compression of the abdomen while the patient is in this position will force air out of the lungs and hopefully dislodge any foreign body.

The paradoxic movement of flail chest should lead you to suspect subcutaneous emphysema or a displaced trachea. Other symptoms are hyperresonance on percussion, tactile frematus on palpation and breath sounds on auscultation.

First steps in treatment: Start an intravenous infusion. Order an x-ray of the chest for pneumothorax and hemothorax. If the patient is cyanotic and tachypneic, intubate and give positive pressure respiration. Occasionally 100 percent oxygen may be needed for a short time. Do a tracheotomy if the patient will need positive pressure ventilation for more than 5 to 7 days. Some patients will not oxygenate their blood well. To assess the severity of any shunting, monitor the arterial blood gases. Have the patient breath 100 percent oxygen for 20 minutes. If the patient cannot raise his pO_2 above 80 to 100 mm of mercury, he has a significant pulmonary shunt and will require positive pressure ventilation for several days.

The most common problems are pneumothorax (Fig. 5-6) and hemothorax. Decide early whether intercostal tube drainage will be necessary.

The next most common problem is heart contusion. Check the status of the heart muscle with the electrocardiogram. Contusion will appear similar to myocardial infarction. Treat with bed rest.

Examine the patient frequently for ruptured papillary muscle, rupture of the ven-

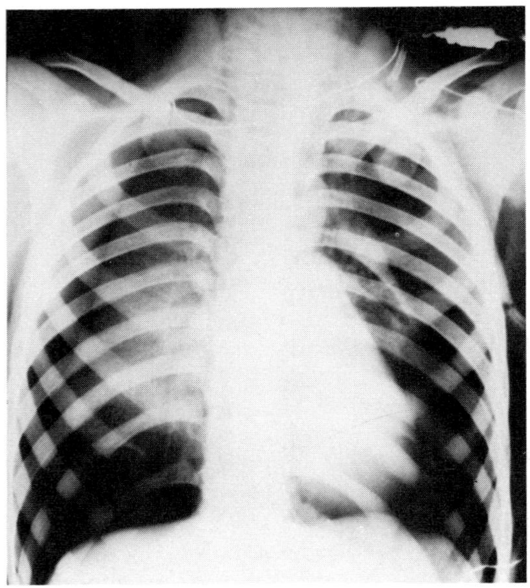

Figure 5-6. Bilateral pneumothorax in a patient who suffered a skull fracture.

tricular septum, rupture of the aortic valve and cardiac tamponade.

Sixteen percent of patients who die following an automobile accident have a fracture of the aorta. Virtually all patients with a fracture of the aorta die, but approximately 15 percent of them will survive long enough for reparative surgery. Check the femoral pulses and compare the blood pressure of the upper and lower extremities. If anuria occurs with a normal blood pressure, seek consultation with a cardiac surgeon.

Pneumothorax

Pneumothorax occurs when air enters the pleural space by penetration of the chest wall, laceration of the lung, perforation of bronchus or trachea, tear of lung by indriven rib fragment (Fig. 5-7) or rupture of alveoli secondary to blunt trauma or straining.

Open Pneumothorax

In this condition there is communication between the pleural cavity and the atmosphere (Fig. 5-8). The opening may be in the lung or the chest wall. As air enters the pleural cavity the pleura's negative pressure is diminished, the lung collapses and the mediastinum compresses the opposite lung, impairing ventilation and venous return. The mediastinum shifts to the affected side, creating a side-to-side shift (flutter) of the mediastinum and further reducing venous return.

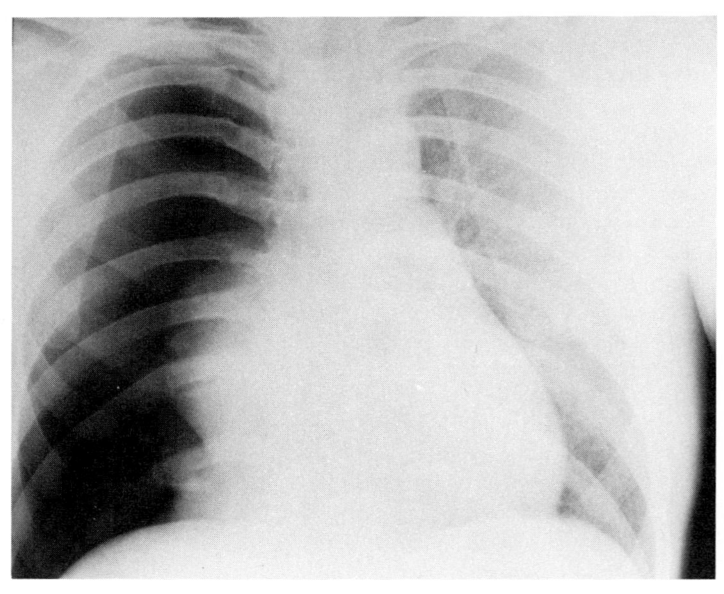

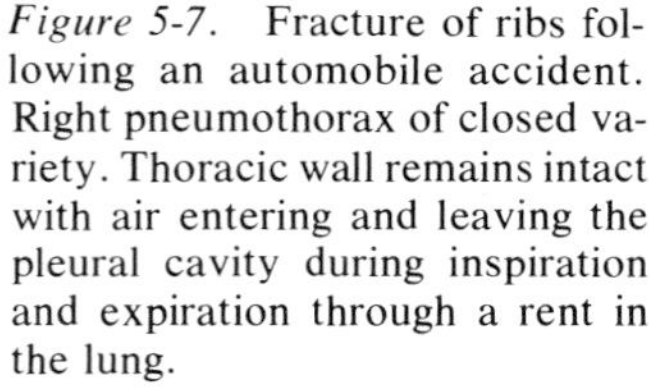

Figure 5-7. Fracture of ribs following an automobile accident. Right pneumothorax of closed variety. Thoracic wall remains intact with air entering and leaving the pleural cavity during inspiration and expiration through a rent in the lung.

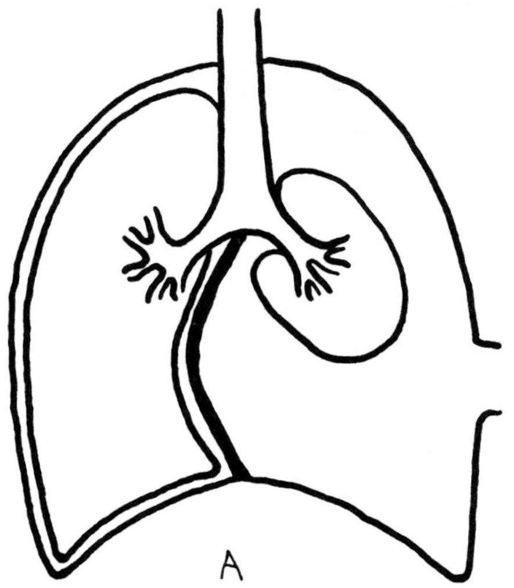

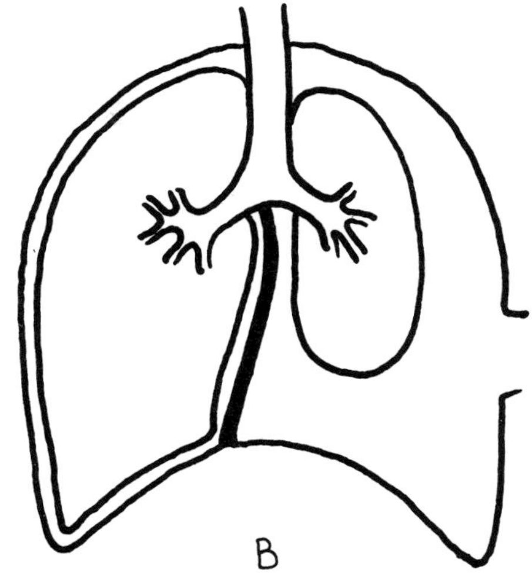

Figure 5-8. Mechanism of open pneumothorax. *A*, On inspiration the homolateral lung collapses because air is sucked through the opening into the pleural cavity and the contralateral lung collapses because the mediastinum is sucked over. *B*, At the end of expiration the reduction in chest size forces air out through the opening. Compression in the contralateral lung forces air out the opening and pushes over the mediastinum.

Symptoms and signs are:

- –sudden chest pain
- –dyspnea
- –air entering pleural cavity on inspiration
- –air leaving the pleural cavity on expiration
- –on the affected side, movement of the chest wall is diminished, the percussion note hyperresonant and breath sounds decreased

Treatment. Cover the open wound with a hand, the patient's arm or with vaseline gauze to stop the sucking of air in and out of the pleural cavity (Fig. 5-9).

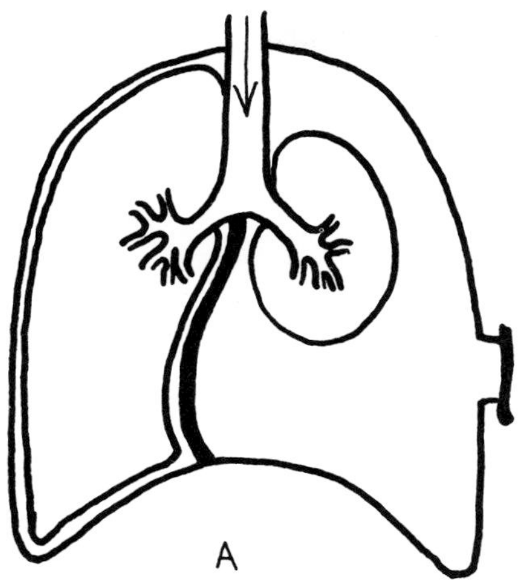

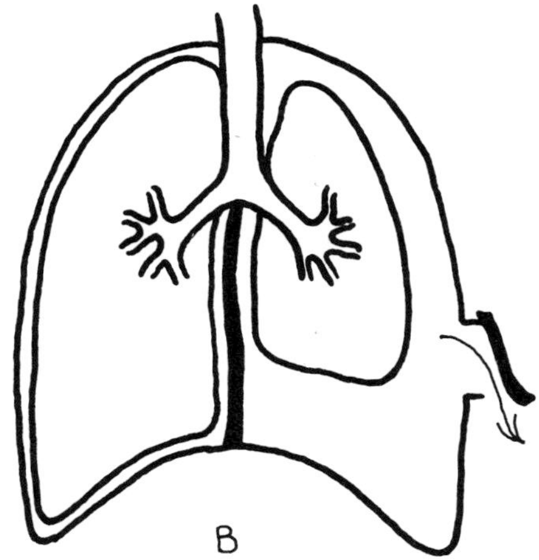

Figure 5-9. Treatment of open pneumothorax. *A*, Place a rubber dam over the opening. On inspiration, the rubber dam is pulled firmly to the chest wall, stopping air from entering the pleural cavity. *B*, During expiration the dam allows air to escape from the pleural cavity. After a few respirations, the pneumothorax will be overcome.

As an emergency measure, with the wound open, ask the patient to cough or force the air out of his lungs; then quickly close the wound as he inspires again. Have the patient repeat this a few times, some re-expansion of the lungs will occur.

As soon as possible institute tube drainage of the thorax. The technique is simple. Make a small emergency incision in the second or third interspace at the midclavicular line with any instrument at hand. After the skin is incised, push a hemostat into the pleura. When a channel is opened, push a tube into the pleural cavity. Attach the tube to an under-water-seal suction.

Tension Pneumothorax

In this variety of pneumothorax, the opening in the lung, bronchus or chest wall acts as a valve to allow air to enter the pleural cavity on inspiration but not to escape dur-

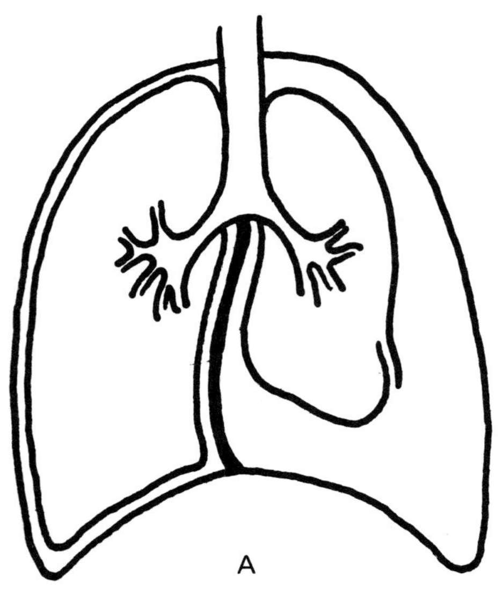

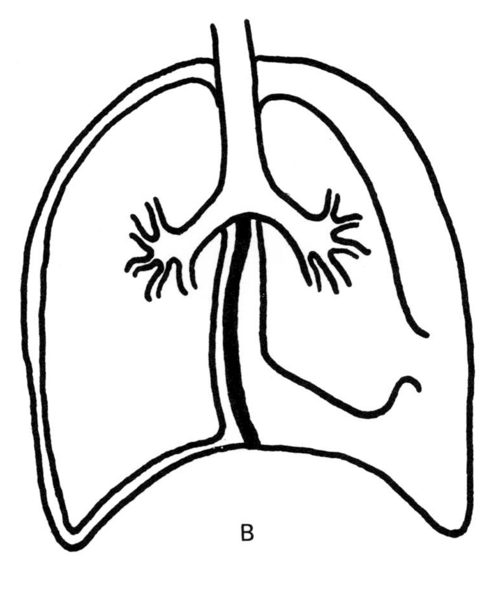

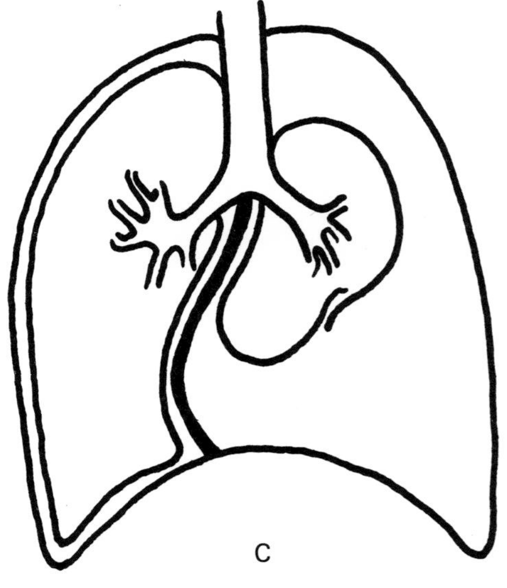

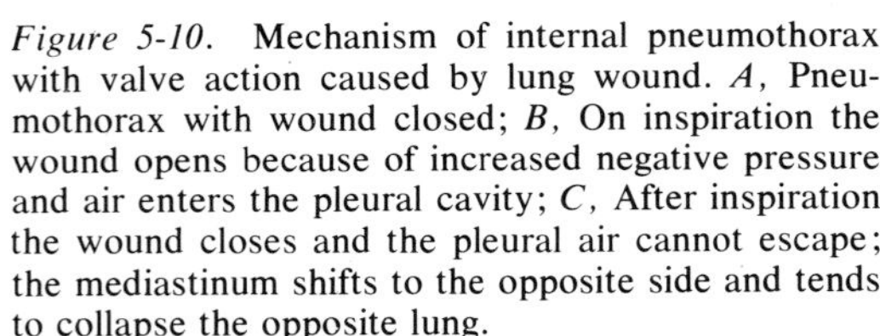

Figure 5-10. Mechanism of internal pneumothorax with valve action caused by lung wound. *A*, Pneumothorax with wound closed; *B*, On inspiration the wound opens because of increased negative pressure and air enters the pleural cavity; *C*, After inspiration the wound closes and the pleural air cannot escape; the mediastinum shifts to the opposite side and tends to collapse the opposite lung.

ing expiration (Fig. 5-10); consequently, as the pressure builds up the affected lung collapses, the mediastinum shifts and compresses the opposite lung. The depressed respiration and diminished venous return will cause the most lethal pulmonary distress (Fig. 5-11).

Symptoms and signs are:

- –cyanosis
- –extreme air hunger
- –hypoxia with its resulting agitation
- –trachea deviated toward the uninjured side
- –hyperresonance of the affected side

The quickest way to verify the diagnosis of tension pneumothorax is by aspiration. Insert into the pleural cavity through any interspace a 17- or 18-gauge needle attached to a moistened 10 ml syringe. If there is increased pleural pressure, the plunger will be pushed outward.

Treatment. Relieve the intrapleural pressure by opening the chest preferably in the second or third interspace in the midclavicular line. This may be done with any sharp instrument, such as a nail file or screw driver in an emergency.

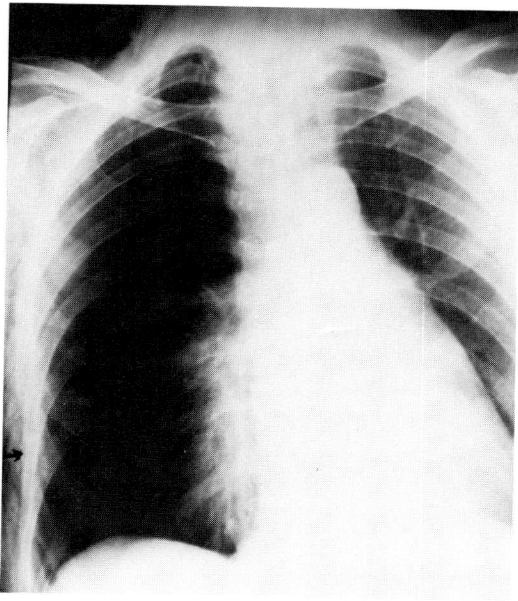

Figure 5-11. Fracture of seventh rib on right with tension pneumothorax and subcutaneous emphysema.

Better still relieve the pressure by inserting a 14- to 16-gauge needle into the pleural cavity. Tie a *perforated* rubber finger cot or condom on the hub of the needle for a flutter valve.

Again the treatment of choice is underwater-seal drainage. Suspect injury to the trachea or bronchus if air continues to leak into the pleura. In this event, the suspicion should be verified by bronchoscopy and the injury surgically repaired.

Spontaneous Pneumothorax

The commonest cause of spontaneous pneumothorax is the rupture of a small vesicle under the visceral pleura, which allows air to pass from the lung to the pleural space. Spontaneous pneumothorax is most common in young men, and in 10 to 20 percent of the patients it recurs, sometimes repeatedly.

Symptoms and signs are:

- –sudden pain in the side of the chest
- –dyspnea
- –decreased respiratory excursion on the affected side
- –mediastinal shift toward the healthy lung
- –decreased tactile fremitus
- –hyperresonant percussion
- –decreased breath sounds

Some patients fall into shock early; others show little systemic effect. X-ray studies reveal air in pleural cavity. There is rarely any evidence of lung disease.

Treatment. If seen early, hospitalize the patient for observation to avoid the small but definite chance of a complicating tension pneumothorax. If seen later, allow the patient to rest at home for a few days until x-ray pictures show expansion of the lungs.

If the patient is distressed or dyspneic, check the pressure in the pleural cavity by inserting a needle on a moist syringe into the thorax. If a tension pneumothorax had developed, the plunger will move out.

In this event the normally negative pressure of the thorax has become positive. Insert a tube or soft rubber catheter through an intercostal space. Place the distal end of the tube in an under-water-seal. Instruct the patient to cough gently. This will expel the air from the pneumothorax and expansion of the lung will take place.

Hemothorax

The pathophysiology and the treatment will vary depending on the amount of blood in the pleural cavity. If the quantity of blood is less than 350 ml, classify the hemothorax as minimal. The only positive sign is an obliteration of the costophrenic angle on x-ray examination. No treatment is necessary because the blood will reabsorb in 10 to 14 days. Observe the patient for further bleeding.

If the quantity of blood in the pleural cavity is approximately 1500 ml the patient will be breathless and he will have the usual physical signs of fluid in the thorax. X-ray examination in the upright position will show a shadow curving laterally upward on the involved side. If the patient is x-rayed in the supine position, the blood may be overlooked because the amount will only cast a light diffused shadow. Classify this as a moderate hemothorax. Confirm the diagnosis by needle aspiration.

Tube drainage is the treatment of choice but thoracentesis may be done as an emergency measure and may yield 500 ml of blood. Until tube drainage is instituted, do a thoracentesis every 6 hours. For both procedures, enter the thorax through the fifth or sixth interspace in the midaxillary line. Bleeding will nearly always stop. Consider an exploratory thoracostomy only if bleeding continues rapidly.

A massive hemothorax usually is the result of bleeding from high-pressure vessels such as the intercostal or internal mammary arteries.

Signs and symptoms are:

- severe pain in the chest
- cyanosis from compression of lungs
- engorgement of neck veins
- displaced trachea to the contralateral side at the level of the suprasternal notch
- dullness, decreased breath sounds and limited respiratory excursions on the injured side
- shock from the loss of blood

Treatment. Immediately begin replacing blood. Use bank blood and consider autotransfusion if there has not been an injury to the trachea, bronchus or any hollow organ which would contaminate the blood.

As quickly as possible begin removing blood from the pleural cavity either by needle and syringe or, if equipment is available, by large bore (34 or 36) tube connected to continuous under-water-seal suction. Use the three-bottle system. There are disposable units available for this purpose.

Seek consultation for prompt exploratory surgery in massive hemothorax.

Flail Chest

Flail chest is paradoxical respiratory movements of a portion of the chest wall resulting from double fractures of three or more ribs or the fracture of several ribs plus costochondral separation or severe sternal fractures. The separated portion of the chest wall moves in the opposite direction to the rest of the thorax. The seriousness of the handicap depends on the number of ribs involved and whether the injury is bilateral or not.

As the thorax expands, the injured ribs sink in. On exhalation, the injured ribs pouch out. The changes in the air pressure within the pleural cavity causes the mediastinum to shift from side to side (mediastinal flutter) and interferes with the physiological intake and output of air. Air may only shift from side to side within the bronchial tree. The return of venous blood to the heart is also impeded. Flail may not appear early but only later when secretions accumulate in the bronchial tree and the patient must breathe more forcibly to maintain respiratory function. The harder the patient fights for breath, the greater the flail as a result of the greater pressures created in the thorax. Approximately 35 percent of patients with crushed chests have no thoracic wall abnormality when initially seen but develop a flail chest subsequently.

Treatment. Use first aid measures to prevent a potential flail or to treat minor amounts of flail. Apply external compression. Improve the patient's ability to cough up secretions by giving pain relief, preferably by intercostal nerve blocks. Manually support the injured side while having the patient cough. Position the patient on the affected side. Strap the chest circumferential with adhesive and a rolled pad over the flail. Remember external compression is only a temporary expedient and if continued or applied too vigorously may impair ventilation and the cough reflex predisposing to atelectasis and pneumonia.

Traction of the chest wall can be maintained by connection to a Balkan frame. Grasp ribs with towel clip with or without local anesthesia or sterile technique depending on the emergency and pass a stainless steel wire around the ribs. This is easy if a large curved needle swaged onto the wire is available. Grasp the sternum with a uterine tenaculum with the blades inserted through small incisions on each side of the sternum. A Kirschner wire passed behind the sternum is the best method of sternal traction and avoids infection, necrosis, pneumothorax or hemothorax.

Seek consultation for possible surgical fixation for flail chest complicated by intrathoracic injuries requiring thoracotomy, for anteriolateral flail with rib displacement or if there is no evidence of flail improvement with assisted ventilation after 2 weeks.

Treatment includes positive pressure breathing. For patients in respiratory distress with a severe flail chest, immediately intubate or do a tracheostomy and mechanically assist their breathing. Any less measure may prove fatal. Do not start positive pressure breathing until blood or air has been removed from the pleural cavity by intercostal tube drainage. Air in the pleural cavity from a lacerated lung can quickly be converted into a tension pneumothorax by positive pressure breathing. Set the pressure at the lowest level that produces adequate ventilation, usually between 15 and 20 cm of water. This will keep venous blood return to the heart at near physiological levels. Use room air or low oxygen percentage to assist ventilation. Occasionally 60 percent or more oxygen may be needed but for only short intervals.

Rib Fractures

Family physicians take rib fractures too lightly, especially in the elderly. About one third of the patients with rib fractures also have pneumohemothorax, one fourth have pneumothorax and approximately one fifth have hemothorax.

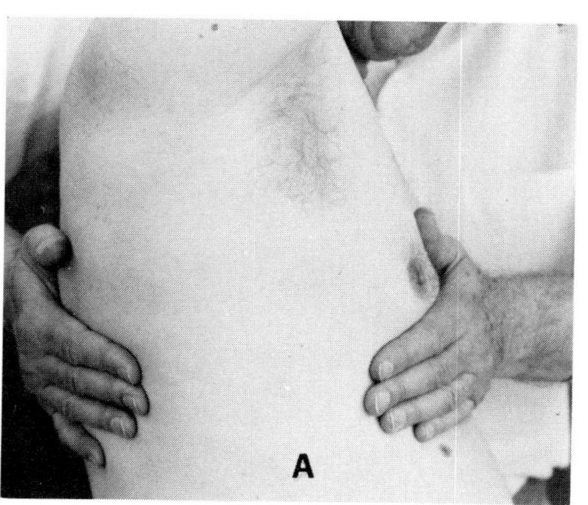

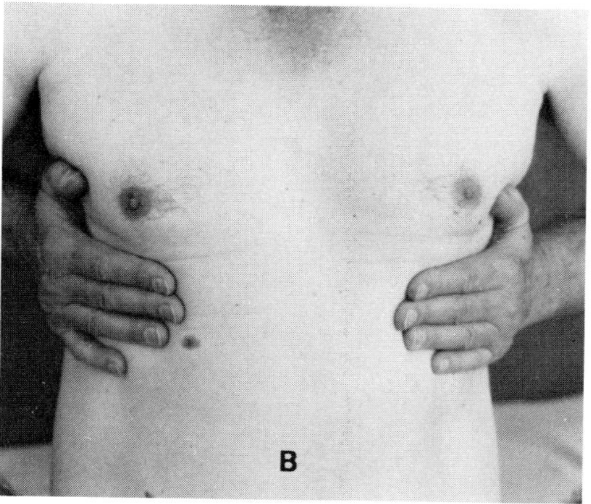

Figure 5-12. *A*, Test for lateral chest wall rib fracture. Anteroposterior pressure on chest causes pain at fracture site when the fracture is located on the lateral chest wall. *B*, Compression test for rib fracture. Pressure on the lateral chest wall causes pain in the chest if fractures of the ribs or cartilages of the anterior or posterior walls exist.

If by physical (Fig. 5-12) and x-ray examination no complication can be found, the treatment of rib fractures centers around pain relief.

Chest strapping has fallen into some disrepute. But on young and healthy patients, strapping may be sufficient, keeping in mind that it limits ventilation and may induce atelectasis and pneumonia.

Occasionally local infiltration of an anesthetic into the fracture site may give relief, but it is usually short acting and undependable.

Paravertebral block, injected close to the vertebrae, produces anesthesia but because of frequent systemic reactions the procedure has never become popular.

The most effective and least dangerous method of pain control is by intercostal nerve block, preferably near the angle of the rib. The technique is simple. Use a 25-gauge needle on a 5 ml syringe. First raise a wheal on the skin near the lower border of the injured rib. Then introduce the needle perpendicularly through the skin to the edge of the rib. Withdraw the needle slightly and then slip it under the lower border of the rib advancing the needle about 4 mm within the intercostal space. Aspirate for blood and if none is found inject about 5 ml of the chosen anesthetic. If pain relief is insufficient, inject the rib above or below. Usually one or two injections are sufficient.

Cardiac Tamponade

Usually small puncture wounds in the chest about the heart do not cause sudden death but they may cause cardiac tamponade. After this type of injury the inelastic pericardium may fill with blood. Patients do not tolerate more than 150 to 200 ml of blood in the pericardium. That amount can cause shock and death.

Signs are:

–puncture wounds about the chest
–falling or absent blood pressure
–chest pain
–dyspnea *but not orthopnea*
–shock with anxiety and ashen color
–tachycardia and pulsus paradoxus
–jugular venous distention
–abnormal pulsations of the internal jugular veins along the medial border of the sternomastoid (may be the only clue)
–muffled heart sounds
–absent precordial impulse
–shock out of proportion to the severity of the wound
–blood in pericardium

Central venous pressure measurements usually will settle the diagnosis.

Treatment. Aspirate the pericardium immediately. Even the aspiration of 15 to 20 ml may save the patient's life. Help the patient into a semi-Fowler position. This allows the blood to accumulate in a dependent portion of the pericardial sac. Use a 16- to 18-gauge, 3-in needle. Insert the needle upward and slightly lateralward through the skin and subcutaneous tissues beginning just left of the xiphoid process. Advance the needle until blood can be aspirated or until the needle touches the heart wall. The depth of the insertion is usually about 4 cm. When the heart wall is touched, a scraping sensation can be felt as the myocardium moves across the needle point.

If time permits, do pericardiocentesis in the operating room with electrocardiographic monitoring.

Observe the patient for recurrent bleeding, which may occur in minutes or after a few days. Because of this uncertainty, consult a chest surgeon regarding the advisability of a thoracostomy with cardiac repair.

Skillful surgical exploration is likely to entail less risk and provide a larger salvage than repeated pericardiocentesis.

MASSIVE GI BLEEDING

Today most GI bleeding emergencies are treated in a hospital. However family physicians generally write the first hospital orders. Your early treatment of the case may well determine whether the patient lives or dies.

Hospital Orders Pending Consultation

Absolute bed rest. If the patient is in shock, keep his head lowered.

Give nothing by mouth. Feeding a patient to stop bleeding is dangerous.

Start IV infusion with lactated Ringer's solution 1000 ml every 6 hr. Use a 15-gauge needle or, better still, a 16-gauge plastic central venous catheter.

Insert nasogastric tube, large bore (18 French) and connect to constant suction. Aspiration of frank blood or 4 plus guaiac is evidence of bleeding above the ligament of Treitz, i.e. esophagus, stomach or duodenum. Leave the tube in place 24 to 48 hr to monitor continued or recurrent bleeding. Irrigate the stomach with iced saline from time to time.

Type and crossmatch 4 units of blood and keep 4 units available at all times. As each unit of blood is administered add another unit to the 4 reserve units.

Record pulse and blood pressure every 30 to 60 min (every 15 min if in shock) and hemoglobin and hematocrit every 3 to 6 hr. Remember that in fast bleeding the extent of blood loss may not be indicated by the hemoglobin level. The clinical condition, particularly the pulse rate, is as good an indicator as the hematocrit.

Record intake and output. Record the character of all stools, vomitus and products of gastric suction. Install a polycatheter if patient is in shock. A urinary output of 25 ml/hour indicates satisfactory volume replacement.

Phenobarbital 100 to 200 mg IM stat and repeat every 2 to 6 hours PRN. Do not oversedate. Avoid sedation in elderly or the diabetic.

Dramamine 25 to 50 mg IM every 6 hr PRN for nausea. Avoid Vistaril, Atarax, Compazine and other phenothiazines which are hypotensive in nature.

Do the following: platelet count, prothrombin time, partial thromboplastin time, serum creatinine and blood urea nitrogen. If patient is over 40 years of age, order an EKG. If history suggests liver disease, order a liver panel including bilirubin, serum protein, alkaline phosphatase and glutamic oxalacetic transaminase.

Start GI bleeding record (flow sheet). Horizontal columns should record time of day and vertical columns record hematocrit, blood pressure, pulse, blood recovered and blood or cells given. Record blood units given by numbers to identify the number of units given.

CVP Monitoring

Advantages of CVP monitoring are:

- –prevention of undertransfusing by maintaining CVP above 5 cm of water
- –prevention of overtransfusion by limiting CVP to 12 cm water
- –signaling of early recurrence of bleeding before alterations in vital signs occur.

Disadvantages of CVP monitoring are:

- –pneumothorax, hemothorax and thrombosis of the vein
- –misplacement, poor functioning and undependable results
- –qualified personnel are needed for monitoring

There are alternatives to CVP monitoring. In the average healthy patient, observe how high the column of blood distends the external jugular vein. This observation may be as accurate as CVP monitoring. Monitor the pulse rate to determine the adequacy of volume replacement. If there is no nurse to monitor the pulse, stay at patient's bedside and do so yourself.

If the patient is in shock switch to whole blood as soon as available. Whole blood should also be used if the tilt test is positive or if the hemoglobin is 7.5 g or below or the hematocrit below 30. As a general rule, continue transfusing until the hematocrit is 35 to 40 or the hemoglobin 10 to 11. In fast bleeding this may not be possible. Repeat the tilt test from time to time to determine blood volume. Consider packed red blood cells for the elderly or those with cardiac problems.

Other elective orders might include neomycin sulfate 1 g every 4 hr to reduce intestinal flora or vitamin K_1, 25 mg IV to correct prothrombin deficiency.

Call for surgical consultation.

Diagnosis

Diagnosis of massive GI bleeding may be impossible to make for various reasons. The patient may be too sick to give a history, he may die in the first few hours or days and hemorrhage may be the first sign of illness in an otherwise healthy person. Laboratory examinations on a bleeding patient seldom are diagnostic: blood clots can simulate filling defects, small polyps can be missed, bleeding from a Meckel's diverticulum can be almost impossible to prove and some patients with one known clinical condition may be bleeding from another.

History Important

Clearly establish the source, amount and duration of bleeding not only for the immediate episode but for any previous GI hemorrhages. With previously known GI tract lesions, 40 percent of the patients bleed from a different lesion. In addition to the main cause of bleeding, 50 percent of the patients have an additional lesion that could cause hemorrhage.

Question the patient for symptoms of a duodenal or gastric ulcer. Has the patient had a burning, boring, aching or gnawing hunger pain? Is it relieved by food, alkalis or vomiting? Does the pain have periodicity (the most reliable symptom of a duodenal ulcer)? Where does the pain radiate (to the back as in a posterior penetrating ulcer, or to the right quadrant as in anterior perforation)? Does food aggravate the pain? If so, think of a gastric ulcer. If food relieves, think of a duodenal ulcer.

Question the patient further regarding rhythmaticity of the pain:

food, comfort, pain=duodenal ulcer
food, comfort, pain, comfort=gastric ulcer

Find out if there has been a change in the nature of the pain recently. Sudden changes in ulcer symptoms indicate complications. Perforation of an ulcer commonly occurs on the anterior wall of the duodenum; profuse hemorrhage usually comes from the posterior wall.

Avoid two traps: the historical evidence of an ulcer does not preclude bleeding from another site and bleeding may come from an asymptomatic ulcer.

Have the patient describe the color of the blood whether in the vomitus or in the feces. Vomiting of bright red blood may signify the rapid bleeding of a Mallory-Weiss syndrome or the bleeding of ruptured esophageal varices. Coffee grounds vomitus indicates bleeding from the upper GI tract. On the other hand, black stools (melena), are most frequently old blood from the upper GI tract, while bright red blood in the stools may be blood from hemorrhoids or other points in the lower GI tract.

Another important item is the medication history. Has the patient been on anticoagulants? Ingesting large amounts of Aspirin? Taking steroids, indomethacin, reserpine or phenylbutazone? Any stigmata of cirrhosis, with or without the history of alcoholism, makes the diagnosis of varices likely.

Don't overlook the history of a weight loss that might be a tip-off to a malignancy, nor the recurrent cramps and diarrhea of ulcerative colitis and Crohn's disease.

The knowledge and treatment of associated diseases may make the difference between the success or failure of bleeding control. Watch for myocardial infarction in cardiac patients who suffer shock while bleeding. MI may be hard to detect during the confusion of the treatment of shock. Patients with congestive heart failure will need CVP monitoring. Renal and pulmonary diseases also increase the risk of dying from GI bleeding.

The most frequent sites of bleeding are indicated in Figure 5-13.

Examination

Limit the physical examination when the patient is actively bleeding to assessing the patient's cardiovascular status and his mentation. Abdominal examination usually proves fruitless in GI bleeding unless a tumor is present. A few findings may suggest peptic ulcer disease. These findings are tenderness in the midline, superficial epigastric tenderness, Mendel's sign such as

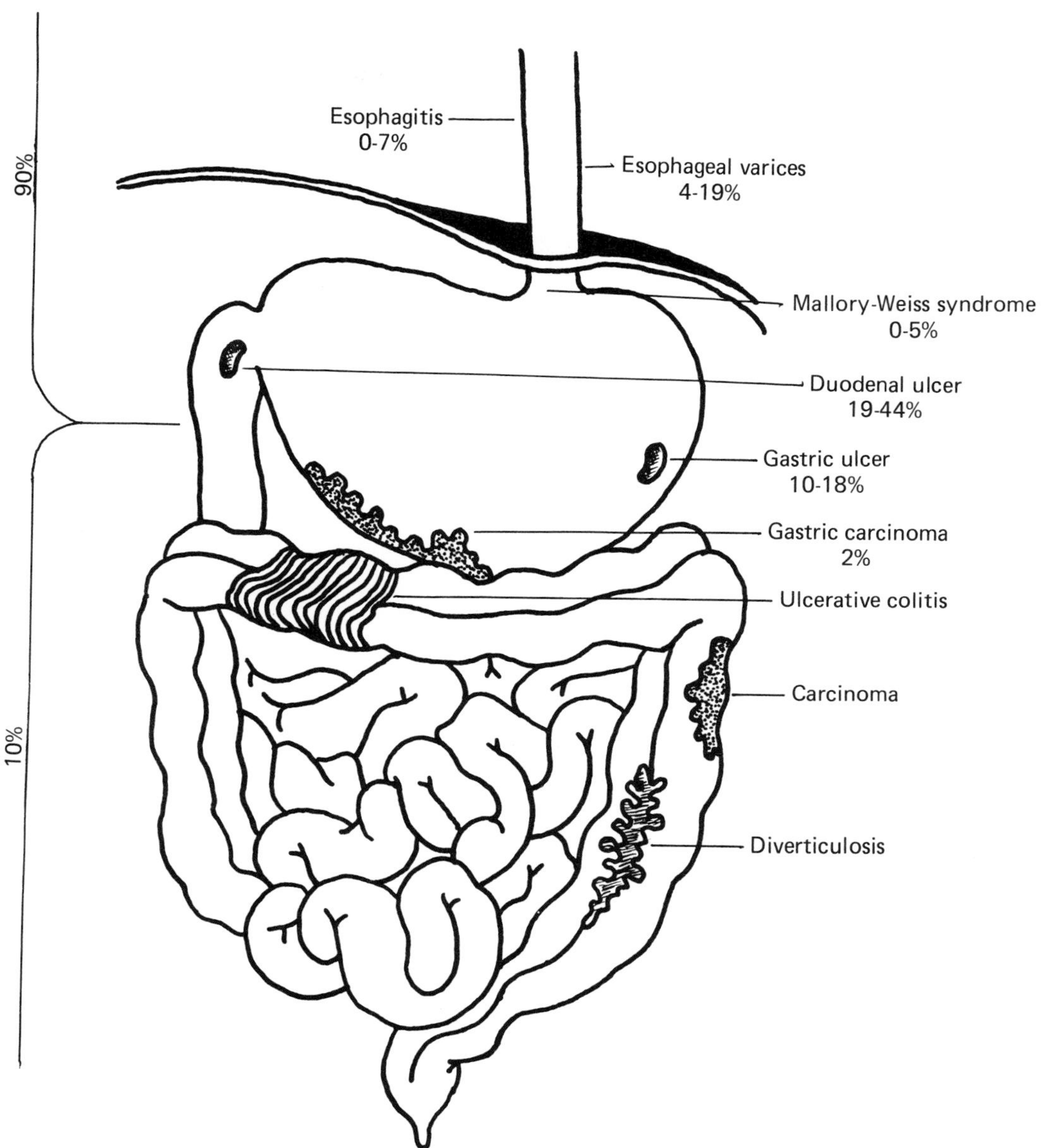

Figure 5-13. Common causes of GI bleeding.

localized tenderness to percussion and localized epigastric hypothermia. Notice that the patient points to the painful site with a finger rather than with the hand.

To help with the differential diagnosis do a digital rectal examination and check any stool for blood. If the patient is a woman do a bimanual pelvic examination and, in the case of a man, do a rectoabdominal in search of the telltale mass of colonic diverticulitis.

Follow the digital examination with first the anoscopic and finally the sigmoidscopic check. Do the sigmoidscopic anytime and anywhere with the patient prepared or unprepared. The examination can be done in a hospital bed either with the patient in knee-chest position or in the Sims position, depending on the patient's condition. Even without preparatory enemas, clues to the cause of bleeding can sometimes be found.

Don't forget to inspect the anus for hemorrhoids, the most common cause of bleeding in patients with lower GI hemorrhage. The blood from bleeding hemorrhoids is usually bright red and will squirt into the toilet water. Contrary to popular opinion, hemorrhoids can cause serious bleeding with the patient's hemoglobin dropping to 4 or 5 g. Follow-up with a barium enema x-ray study.

During GI bleeding the decision as to when to order an upper GI series of x-ray studies is always perplexing. A general working rule: order x-rays early if the patient's condition permits. Diagnostic x-ray pictures are difficult to obtain during active bleeding. Clots can obliterate the mucosal pattern and, with blood transfusions running, free manipulation of the patient is hindered.

If medical treatment appears successful, delay the x-ray examination several days or until the patient is comfortable and his vital signs are stable. At this time the radiologist can do a more thorough study. But, early examination may help differentiate between bleeding esophageal varices and duodenal ulcer. And this could determine the site of the surgical incision.

Under the circumstances, ulcer craters may not be seen more than 50 percent of the time but duodenal deformity is significant. Gastric ulcers, when present, are seen 90 percent of the time.

Following a negative GI series, order an endoscopic examination. Endoscopy is especially helpful in identifying mucosal tears from vomiting, bleeding gastritis and stress ulcers. The examination may help differentiate the bleeding from peptic ulcer and varices or any other upper GI bleeding diseases. Suggest esophagoscopy first and then gastroscopy. These examinations should be done by a physician who is experienced in the procedures. The reports will be no better than the mind and eye of the observer.

If the diagnosis is still in doubt and if the service is available, consider angiographic radioactive studies to localize the bleeding point.

Surgery

Indications for Surgery

The outcome of GI bleeding depends more on constant observation and a knowledge of the rate of bleeding than any other factor.

The patient's course and response to hospitalization and treatment are the best guides to the decision for or against an operation.

Surgery should be considered when:

- –shock develops
- –blood loss reduces the circulating red cell mass to less than 40 percent of normal
- –there is a need for more than 3 L of blood within the first 24 hr
- –bleeding persists after 48 hr
- –rebleeding starts during the same hospital admission
- –a patient requires 500 ml every 8 hr after initial blood replacement
- –the patient who has had two or three bleeding episodes from a known source starts bleeding again.

Even with these guidelines, the time for surgery will vary with the patient's age, the cause of the bleeding, the amount of blood available for transfusion and the associated diseases. For example:

- –do earlier surgery in the elderly patient (They are better able to tolerate surgery than they are able to withstand the cerebral, cardiac and renal damage associated with severe bleeding.)
- –attempt longer medical control of bleeding in the young and healthy
- –do surgery earlier when either blood type or supply is limited for repeated transfusions
- –do surgery for a gastric ulcer earlier than for a duodenal ulcer
- –delay surgery for the patient bleeding from diverticulosis.
- –the patient's risk increases whenever there is an associated liver disease

Surgical Treatment for Upper GI Bleeding

Once the cause of the bleeding has been determined or all diagnostic tests have been done plan a definitive treatment program. Factors that will influence the surgeon's choice of treatment are the amount and rate of bleeding, the nature of the bleeding lesion, the age of the patient and associated diseases.

In the critically ill patient, the operative objective is to control the hemorrhage. A longitudinal incision centered over the pylorus is made. After the abdomen is opened, external inspection or palpation of the proximal duodenum usually confirms the presence of an ulcer. The surgeon will visualize the bleeding point, and ligate the vessel with No. 00 nonabsorbable (silk or cotton) sutures using the double bite or the figure-of-eight technique. If the tissue about the bleeding point is friable and hard to suture, the surgeon can solve the problem by excising a portion of the rectus muscle and tying it over the area as a tampon. The linear pyloric incision is then closed transversely, completing a pyloroplasty (Fig. 5-14).

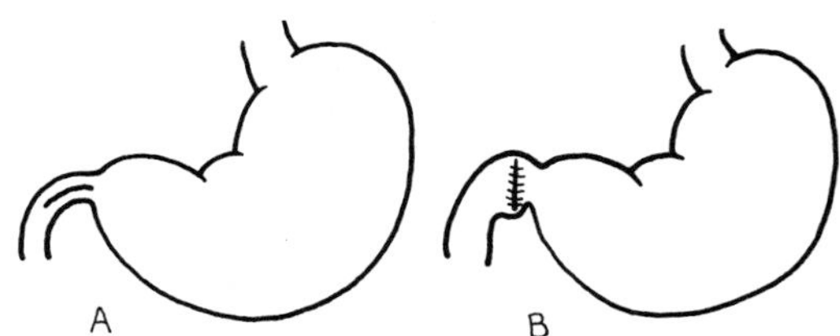

Figure 5-14. Pyloroplasty. The Heineke-Mikulicz requires, *A*, incising the pylorus longitudinally and, *B*, closing the wound transversely, thus enlarging the lumen.

If a bleeding point is not seen in the pyloric area a truncal vagotomy is done. Two or more trunks must be found and sectioned; otherwise the beneficial effects of the vagotomy will be lost. If the bleeding appears to be coming from a proximal location, a second gastrotomy is done, allowing inspection of the entire gastric mucosa.

With the less critically ill patient, the surgeon may choose one of several types of resections (Fig. 5-15). For a lone gastric ulcer a 50 percent distal gastric resection designed to include the ulcer is recommended. The morbidity and mortality rates are low when the operation is done electively. Long term ulcer recurrences are more frequent after vagotomy and drainage (pyloroplasty or gastroenterostomy) than with subtotal resection. One report puts the figure as high as 38 percent in cases followed

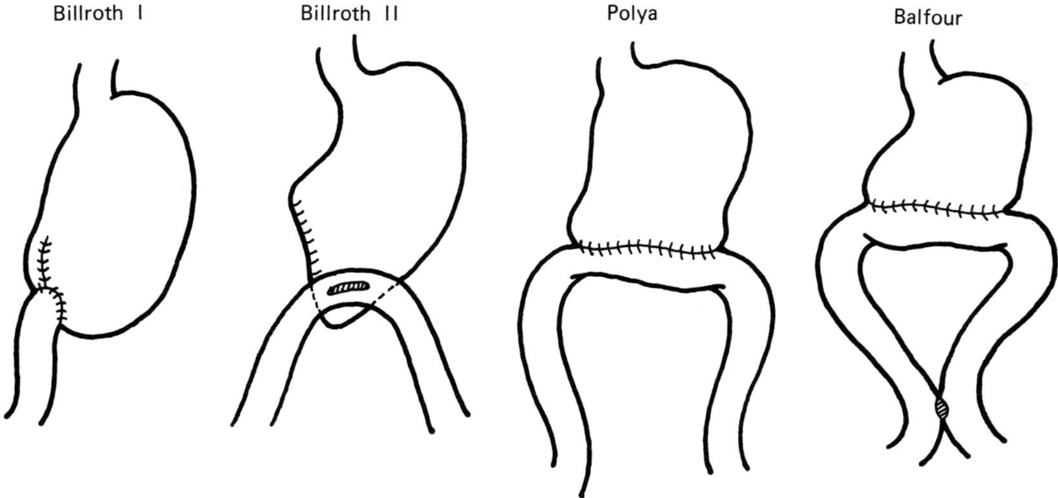

Figure 5-15. Billroth I, gastroduodenostomy following subtotal gastric resection. Types of gastrojejunostomy following gastric resection: Billroth II, Polya and Balfour modifications.

5 years or more. Most surgeons now resect when the patient's condition is noncritical but use the simpler and faster vagotomy, drainage and suturing under critical conditions.

A vagotomy and pyloroplasty is highly effective for hemorrhagic gastritis. When a Mallory-Weiss laceration has occurred, the wound is simply sutured with running gut through the gastrotomy incision.

Stress ulcers present the most difficult surgical problem. They tend to be multiple (reported to be as many as 200 in one stomach). A survival rate of 30 to 40 percent is the best that can be expected from surgery no matter what innovative procedures the surgeon chooses.

Postgastrectomy Complications

Family physicians observe and treat postgastrectomy complications more frequently than the surgeons who perform the surgery. Some postgastrectomy complications are easily identified while other complications are insidious and may occur 1 to 2 years following surgery.

The results of surgery are excellent or good in 75 to 85 percent of the patients, but varying degrees of malnutrition and unpleasant symptoms may occur. Subtotal gastrectomy results in more symptoms than vagotomy combined with pyloroplasty or gastroenterostomy (Fig. 5-16).

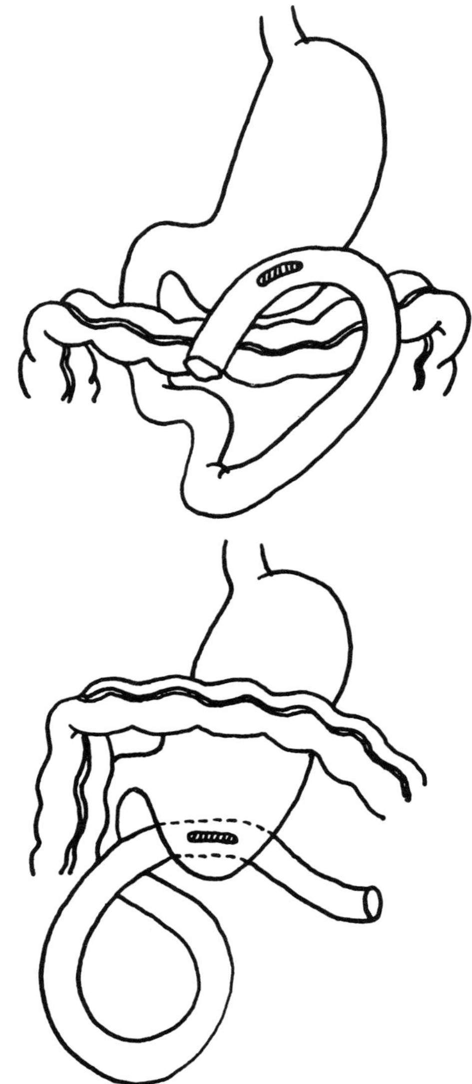

Figure 5-16. Two types of gastroenterostomies: *A*, Anterior; *B*, Posterior.

DUMPING SYNDROME. Symptoms start either during a meal or within half an hour. The distress is described by the patient as a sensation of abdominal fullness, rolling or churning, nausea, palpitations, dizziness and faintness. These symptoms gradually subside and the patient is left weak and exhausted for a couple of hours. The syndrome occurs in up to 70 percent of post-subtotal gastrectomy patients.

Symptoms may be categorized into two groups: those which result from rapid jettisoning of stomach contents into the small intestine and those resulting from hemodynamic changes. The symptoms are uncomfortable enough to make the patient question whether life was better before or after the surgery.

The causes of the symptoms are poorly understood. Most authorities agree they probably result from excessive stimulation of the jejunum by large meals, iced water, or sweet foods and drinks. The problem, however, is more than precipitatious emptying of the stomach into the jejunum; rather it involves adequate handling of the glucose load. The physiological changes which occur are decreased plasma volume, decreased serum potassium, rapid and prolonged alimentary hyperglycemia and increased blood and urine serotonin.

Serotonin is released in great quantity (64 percent increase) from the intestinal tract into the circulatory system during the dumping syndrome. There appears to be no correlation between the type of gastrectomy and serotonin changes or symptoms.

For treatment, suggest dry meals, high in proteins and poor in carbohydrates. If this is insufficient, administer sodium tolbutamide (Orinase) 0.25 to 1.0 g 10 to 30 min before meals to help prevent attacks. But in severe cases digestion is so unpleasant that many patients end up nutritionally disabled. Occasionally some type of surgical revision of the first operation becomes necessary.[16]

Another type of dumping syndrome is the *late hypoglycemic attack*. In this case the symptoms are the result of functional postprandial hyperinsulinism. Patients who suffer these attacks generally have been unstable and may have suffered similar attacks previous to the gastrectomy. To verify the diagnosis, check a 2-hr postprandial blood sugar for hypoglycemia.

An oral glucose tolerance test may be instructive in understanding this syndrome. The curve rises to 200 to 300 mg/100 ml within 30 min after the oral administration of glucose. This is followed by a rapid fall in the next hour to hypoglycemic levels when symptoms occur. Reassure and advise the patient to eat small frequent meals with a low carbohydrate content.

Often overlooked is the *atypical dumping syndrome*. Weakness and exhaustion after meals are the most common symptoms. Sleepiness, drowsiness, yawning, apathy, falling asleep and restlessness are more frequent after test meals of hypertonic glucose than after regular meals. Belching and vomiting, commonly regarded as components of the dumping syndrome, are, in fact, symptoms of the small stomach syndrome or the afferent loop syndrome. Most "dumpers" are unable to vomit.

WEIGHT LOSS. Following a gastrectomy, the majority of the patients will lose weight but finally level off at a lower plateau. This weight loss is difficult to regain, and is probably the result of inadequate food intake plus a stomach inadequate to hold large amounts of food.

STEATORRHEA. A few patients will develop steatorrhea, resulting in part from poor mixing of food with pancreatic juice and a bacteriologic contamination of the small bowel, which under ordinary circumstances is sterile.

IRON DEFICIENCY ANEMIA. This develops in about 20 to 30 percent of the patients following subtotal gastrectomy. It requires iron therapy.

VITAMIN B_{12} DEFICIENCY AND FOLIC ACID ANEMIA. These are unlikely following subtotal gastrectomy but must be guarded against following a total gastrectomy. Total gastrectomy removes the organ of intrinsic factor secretion.

RECURRENT MARGINAL ULCERS. Ulcers are not uncommon. They may or may not bleed again.

PULMONARY TUBERCULOSIS. For some unexplained reason a higher incidence of pulmonary tuberculosis occurs after gastrectomy.

Prevention of Bleeding in an Ulcer Patient

Family physicians should be able to identify the ulcer prone patient. Look for the following characteristics:

- –emotional immaturity
- –dependency but his dependency masked by external vigor.
- –depression and anger when his needs are not gratified.
- –occasionally an effeminate-appearing, thin young man.

To verify suspicions order a serum pepsinogen. If the patient is found to be a hypersecretor, teach him to live within his emotional bounds. Hospitalize the patient whenever he shows signs of stress and frustration. With this approach he may learn to handle his emotions, reduce gastric secretions and prevent gastric bleeding.

TONSILLECTOMY AND ADENOIDECTOMY

Rarely perform the combined operation before the age of 4 and, as a general rule, do not do a tonsillectomy under 2. Although tonsillectomies with or without adenoidectomies are the most frequent surgical operation performed in the United States, about 1 child out of 1000 dies from its performance and 15 develop serious complications.

Indications for surgery are:

–airway obstruction (operate before alveolar hypoventilation, carbon dioxide retention and cor pulmonale develop
–persistent and uncontrollable heavy snoring and mouth breathing
–chronic or recurring otitis media with or without hearing loss (there are those who suggest an adenoidectomy sufficient in this case)
–dysphagia, recurrent tonsillitis and unilateral hypertrophy indicating the possibility of a tumor

The effect of a tonsillectomy and/or adenoidectomy on immunoglobulins isn't entirely settled. However, immunoglobulins are not believed to be affected in any permanent way or, if affected, in no great quantity because only IgA is excreted in the tonsils and in small quantities compared to the quantities secreted from the entire gastrointestinal tract.

Consequently there is no conclusive evidence that a tonsillectomy and an adenoidectomy have a general or systemic effect on the immunoglobulins. Likewise there is no conclusive evidence that infections or metabolic or neoplastic diseases are more common after the operation.

REFERENCES

1. Weil MH, Shubin H: The "VIP" approach to the bedside management of shock. *JAMA* 209:337, 1969.
2. Gorday E: The CVP measurement. *Med Counterpoint* 3:42, 1971
3. Baker RJ, et al: Transfusion reaction: a reappraisal of surgical incidence and significance. *Ann Surg* 169:684–693, 1969
4. Krevans JR: Transfusion reactions in Conn HF, Conn, Jr, RB (eds): Current Diagnosis. Philadelphia: Saunders, 1968, p. 327.
5. Guide for Hospital Committees on Transfusions. Pamphlet by the AMA.
6. Harrington WJ: Differential diagnosis and management of thrombocytopenias. *Med Times* 99:54–66, 1971.
7. Holvey DN (ed): The Merck Manual of Diagnosis and Therapy, ed. 12. Rahway, NJ: Merck Sharp & Dohme Research Laboratories, 1972, pp 287–300.
8. Symposium: Legal risks in managing hand injuries. *Patient Care* 2:71, 1968.
9. Edlich R, et al: Studies in the management of the contaminated wound. *Am J Surg* 121:668, 1971.
10. Sterile gloves and minor surgery. Questions and Answers. *JAMA* 166:1107, 1958.
11. Heckinger RF: Asepsis in the office. *Emerg Med* 3:202–208, 1971.
12. Symposium: Managing wounds of the hand. *Patient Care* 2–51, 1968.
13. Horner R, Brallier F: Pointers on injured fingertips. *Emerg Med* 2:64, 1970.
14. Barr SE: Prompt help is needed for insect sting allergy. *JAMA* 225:365, 1973.
15. Costly DO, Lorhan PH: Intravenous regional anesthesia. *Arch Surg*. 103:34, 1971.
16. Stahlgren LH: The dumping syndrome: A study of its hemodynamics. *Hosp Practice* 5:59, 1970.
17. Physician's Handbook of Blood Component Therapy. Amer Assoc of Blood Banks, Chicago, 1969, p. 6.

GENERAL STUDY AIDS

Lewis CM, Weil M: Hemodynamic spectrum of vasopressor and vasodilator drugs. *JAMA* 208: 1391–1398, 1969.
Barnett JA, Sanford JP: Bacterial Shock. *JAMA* 209: 1514–1517, 1969
Weil MH, et al: Fluid repletion in circulatory shock: central venous pressure and other practical guides. *JAMA* 192:668–674, 1965.
Kaufman RM: Transfusion reactios. *AF/GP* 1:65, 1970.
Chaplin, Jr, H: Packed red blood cells. *N Eng J Med* 218:367, 1969.

Am Assoc Of Blood Banks: Physician's Handbook of Blood Component Therapy. Chicago, Illinois, 1969.

Sirridge MS: Medical Technology Philadelphia: Lea and Febiger, 1967, pp 66–71.

Quick HJ: Detection and diagnosis of hemorrhagic states. *JAMA* 197:138, 1966.

Gans H: Diagnosis and management of hemorrhagic diseases. *GP* 37:130–139, 1968.

Wallach J: Interpretation of Diagnostic Tests: A Handbook Synopsis of Laboratory Medicine. Boston: (Little, Brown and Co) 1970, pp 242–252.

Westermann MP: The common hemoglobinopathies. *AF/GF* 2:87–94, 1970.

Editorial: Hemophilia Prophylaxis. *JAMA* 212:2256, 1970.

Huse WM: Chest injuries: what you *must* know. *Res/Int Consult* 2:53–56, 1973.

Zollinger RM, Nick WV: Upper gastrointestinal tract hemorrhage. *JAMA* 212:225, 1970.

Nagel CB: Surgical management of massive hemorrhage from the stomach and duodenum. *AFP/GP* 1:85–92, 1970.

CHAPTER 6

Fracture and Trauma

LEGAL LIABILITY IN FRACTURE CASES

A physician must have a reasonable standard of skill and he is obligated to use that skill in treating his patients. In addition to knowledge of treatment of specific parts he must possess a knowledge of the circulatory and inflammatory complications associated with the injuries he treats; he must deal with them promptly and efficiently. He is *obligated* to investigate repeated complaints that could be associated with complications. He is expected to follow up acute treatment at proper intervals or provide a substitute when he is away.

The patient must recognize that the doctor does not guarantee his treatment. He is not responsible for a mistake, an error in judgment or for a bad result as long as he uses the requisite degree of skill and care. The patient is *obligated* to follow the physician's orders. If he does not (contributory negligence) he will be unable to recover damages from the doctor. In most tight-cast court cases, the court will not allow the patient to recover damages unless expert medical testimony is presented on the patient's behalf.

EVALUATING NERVE AND VASCULAR INJURY TO THE HAND AND FOOT

Tests for Nerve Injuries

Median Nerve Injury

The ability to touch the tip of the thumb to the tip of the little finger indicates normal motor function of the median nerve. Therefore, injury to the median nerve or its motor branch results in inability to oppose the thumb and the little finger.

In Ochsner's test for median nerve paralysis the patient can clasp his hands, but cannot flex the index finger on the paralyzed side when the innervation of the flexor digitorum sublimis has been injured below the antecubital fossa.

Paralysis of the abductor pollicis brevis prevents full range of thumb abduction. In this test have the patient raise his hands in front of him and have him attempt to touch the tips of the index finger and the abducted thumb to the corresponding fingers of the other hand. This is called Wartenberg's sign or the Oriental prayer sign.

Loss of pin prick sensitivity in the palmar tips of the index and little finger indicates major nerve injuries to the median and ulnar nerves respectively. Even if the patient appreciates pin prick and normal sensation he may have a loss of two-point discrimination or gnosis in lesser injuries than full severance of the median nerve. If this function is lost the patient is unable to differentiate between small objects. Weber's two-point discrimination test uses a bent paper clip for tactile gnosis. The examiner attempts to find the point distance at which the patient perceives two points rather than one. The test requires the blunt ends of the paper clips be used and the skin be lightly touched simultaneously by both prongs. Normals: 2 to 4 mm or pulp of index finger; 3 to 5 mm on the little finger; 6 to 12 mm on extension aspects of the hand. This evaluates the ability of the fingers to "see" (gnosis).

Look for thenar eminence atrophy in long-standing cases of median nerve damage. Thenar atrophy also occurs in long-standing cases of carpal tunnel syndrome.

For a final evaluation of total hand function have the patient perform the pick-up test. This test is a valuable method in determining the practical worth of the hand and assessing injury to the median nerve. The patient is asked to pick up various small objects, name them and put them into a small box. This is done first with the good hand with eyes closed and then with the injured hand. If he fails to perform, have the patient repeat the test with the eyes open. Grade the performance in quickness and accuracy.

Ulnar Nerve Injury

Test the integrity of the ulnar nerve to the dorsal interossei by having the patient fan his hand out, fully extending it in abduction. If the patient cannot extend his ring or little finger, he has ulnar nerve paralysis. This deformity also occurs in syringomyelia. It is called preacher's hand or benediction hand.

Test ulnar nerve integrity to the volar interossei by the paper-pulling test. In this test, the patient holds a piece of paper between his fingers while the examiner attempts to pull the paper free, thus testing the strength of the adductors. In the adductor pollicis test for ulnar nerve paralysis have the patient grasp a small magazine between his thumbs and index fingers. Have him attempt to pull the paper apart. The thumb flexes at the I-P joint as a result of an inadequate adductor.

The ulnar nerve is most vulnerable near the elbow where it curves posteriorly around the medial epicondyle. Injury here results in adductor weakness of the fingers.

Localized atrophy of the hypothenar eminence suggests an old ulnar nerve injury.

Radial Nerve Injury

The normal ability to extend the thumb and fingers excludes injury to the radial nerve. Therefore, check for damage by having the patient extend his fingers and thumb.

The radial nerve spirals around the humerus where it is exposed to injury from fractures of the shaft. Damage to the innervation of the extensor carpi radialis longus produces wrist drop. Always check for wrist drop. Causes of this condition are lead, arsenic and alcohol poisoning and poliomyelitis as well as trauma.

Tibial and Peroneal Nerve Injury

Footdrop indicates common peroneal nerve paralysis. However, dorsiflexion of the great toe excludes lesions of the common peroneal nerve.

If sensation is lost in the web between the great and second toes an injury to the tibial nerve is indicated.

Unless there are counterindications, always immobilize the hand in the position of function with the wrist slightly dorsiflexed and the index and middle fingertips touching the thumb pulp in the writing position.

The hand assumes this functional position during deep-seated infections.

Check Arterial Circulation of the Legs

The arteries of the leg are the dorsal, posterior tibial, popliteal and femoral.

When a peripheral artery pulse is decreased look for:

- –thrombosis associated with collagen diseases, i.e. lupus, or with the arteritides whether allergic, inflammatory or incidental to a general infectious disease (typhus); arteriosclerosis with or without aneurysm; Buerger's disease; following cannulation, arteriography or monitoring (some loss of pulse in 30 percent of the patients); following accidental or surgical trauma to bones and soft tissue
- –embolism as a complication of heart disease, i.e. rheumatic heart disease as well as coronary heart disease (only 25 percent of cardiac emboli are associated with auricular fibrillation); heparin-loosened clot
- –spasm of artery following trauma and diseases of the CNS

–lessened blood flow by decreased blood pressure as in shock
–lessened blood flow by effect of drug therapy on caliber of the arterioles
–frostbite

Remember:

–Do not depend on palpation alone when determining whether a peripheral pulse is present. Check with an oscillometer.
–Muscle tissue will die within 4 hr of near total ischemia.
–Ischemia of 24 hr will result in a "hard" contracture and a flail joint.[1]

X-RAY STUDIES IN FRACTURE AND TRAUMA

Family physicians whether working with a radiologist or not should keep a few rules in mind when employing radiographs in traumatic work. Learn what the standard views are for specific anatomical locations, i.e. anteroposterior, lateral and oblique. Order these standard views before requesting special ones.

Confusion in interpreting epiphyseal injuries occurs with radiologists as well as with family physicians. Resolve this confusion by x-raying the opposite healthy joint.

If a radiologist interprets the x-ray plates, he should form an opinion on whether there is shortening of the extremity and how much, whether the alignment as to joints and weight bearing are satisfactory, whether there is any torsion of the fragments and whether opposition is satisfactory and if not to what degree it is off. The physician may also be able to infer whether soft tissue is injured or caught in the fracture fragments and to what degree the cartilage or periosteum has been injured.

In order to determine the diagnosis and extent of injury, x-ray pictures should be taken before manipulating the parts and again after reduction and/or after immobilization. Usually the next x-ray picture is taken approximately 1 week later to check the efficacy of the immobilization. If the position of the fragments is good, no more x-rays need be taken for 6 to 8 weeks and then to verify callus formation (Fig. 6-1). If the cast or traction has had to be changed, follow such manipulation with an x-ray study. Last of all, check an x-ray picture before dismissing the patient.

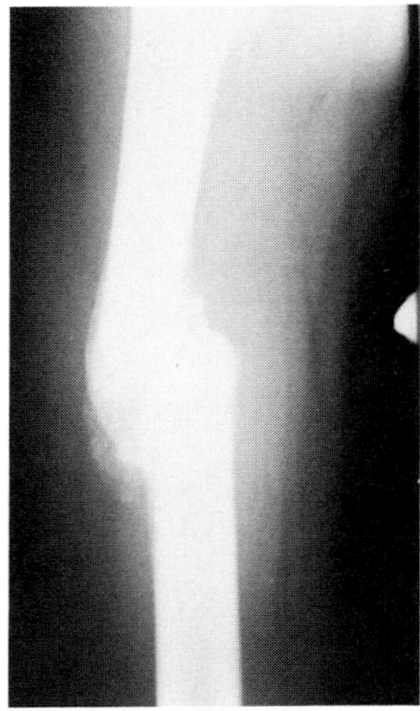

Figure 6-1. Fractured femur with callus formation.

The radiographic appearance can be helpful in assessing the stage of fracture healing. Look for:

–swelling and hematoma around the fracture
–developing osteoporosis adjacent to fracture site plus organization of the hematoma and formation of fibrous callus
–deposition of calcium in primary callus, visualized in periosteal and interosseal regions
–increasing density of primary interosseal bony callus
–decreasing periosteal callus as interosseal callus increases
–gradual reformation of bony trabecular and bony contour (Fig. 6-2)

X-rays may show the early changes of traumatic myositis ossificians, a late complication of soft tissue injury.

USING PLASTER

Saturate plaster bandages with room temperature water (70 to 75° F). This tem-

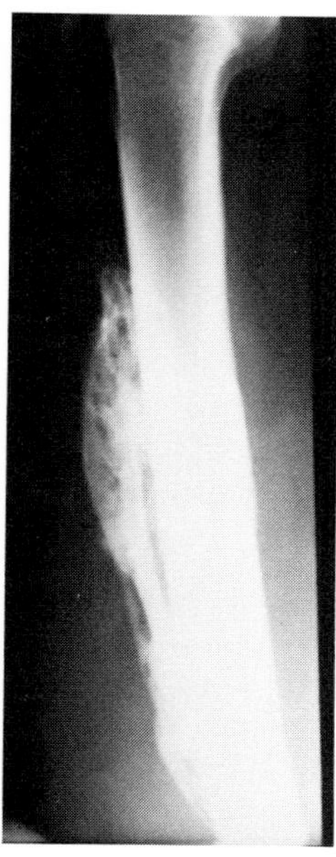

Figure 6-2. Myositis ossificans; muscle calcification following an old football injury.

perature will not chill the patient nor will it cause the generation of excessive heat or loosen the bond between the plaster and fabric. Immerse the bandage loosely in water in a vertical position for 5 seconds. By that time the bandage should stop bubbling. Keep your thumb under the loose end of the bandage. This will eliminate searching for the end of the roll.

Warm water hastens setting; cool water slows. All foreign substances, including salt, have a weakening influence on cast strength. Squeeze excess water from the wet roll. The less water left in the roll, the quicker the cast will dry and become strong.

The time between immersion and firmness is called the setting time. Fast setting is from 5 to 8 minutes, extra fast 2 to 4 minutes. This is modified by the room temperature, humidity, foreign substances and thickness of the cast.

Plaster casts should be no thicker than necessary for the strength needed. Thin casts are more comfortable for the patient and may aid recovery because of freer ambulation. Thick casts create heat, dry slowly, cloud recheck x-ray films and are difficult to remove. When making reinforcement splints use no more than 5 to 8 plies.

In applying the plaster, rub each turn of bandage into the layers below to form a solid, well fused cast. Excessive molding or bending while the cast is drying will result in a weak and flabby cast.

INJURIES TO THE UPPER EXTREMITIES

Obtain a detailed history of the injury. The type of injury may well save time and expense and allow the physician to zero in on the most likely injuries. The patient's description of the exact area of pain as well as the area of disuse is important. Record the details of the history on the patient's chart.

Resistant active testing is the most fruitful physical examination procedure. The best overall maneuver to detect serious injury or fracture of the upper extremity is, first, to have the patient extend the entire arm. Then the examiner should grasp the extended hand, as in a handshake, and have the patient squeeze. A patient with a fractured radius will be unable to squeeze the examiner's hand. The examiner attempts to pronate and supinate the arm while the patient resists. If the patient is able to resist these turning and twisting movements he has no fracture of the hand, forearm, arm, clavicle or scapula. The opposite is true in a fracture. A serious sprain will give a positive test.

Differentiate between strains and sprains. A *strain* results from stretching ligaments and tendons of a joint beyond their natural limits. These injuries may not start hurting until hours later or during the night or even the next morning because of swelling and stiffness. A *sprain* is an immediate tearing of ligaments or tissues and causes immediate pain and disability.

A common injury is that of a person falling on his outstretched hand. When this happens look for the common Colles' fracture, semilunar dislocation, navicular fracture, Monteggia fracture, fracture of the head of the radius, posterior dislocation of the elbow, supracondylar fracture of the elbow, fracture of the shaft of the humerus, bruise of the head of the humerus, clavicle fracture or subcoracoid dislocation.

Dislocation of the Semilunar

The great majority of these dislocations, with or without fractures, are the result of a fall on the extended hand. The hand is pushed violently backward and the semilunar bone pops forward. When the hand is returned to its normal position, the semilunar bone remains forward out of place, the distal articular surface facing directly forward (Fig. 6-3).

The patient may believe he has only a swollen wrist and may continue to work. There is swelling, stiffness and pain. Pressure on the median nerve causes tingling and numbness. On examination, a prominence on the front of the wrist can be seen and palpated.

Reduction under general anesthesia is necessary, even if the dislocation has been unrecognized for days. If the family physician has never reduced a semilunar he should call an orthopedic consultant.

Dislocations of the Head of the Humerus

The most common dislocation of the humerus is the anterior or subcoracoid variety (Fig. 6-4). The second most common is the downward or subglenoid type. Quick shoulder dislocation with a spontaneous reduction, a common sports injury, is frequently misdiagnosed.

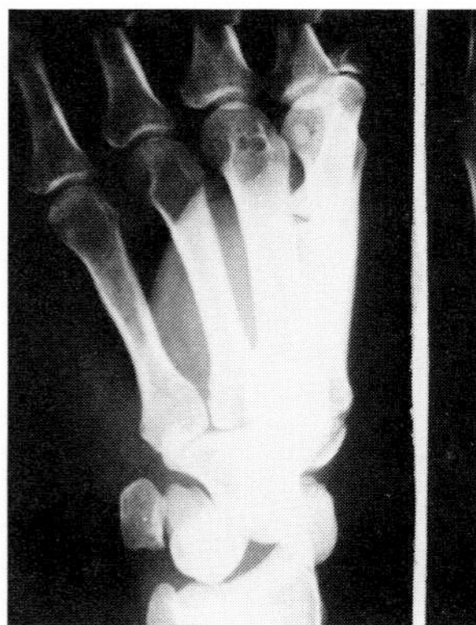

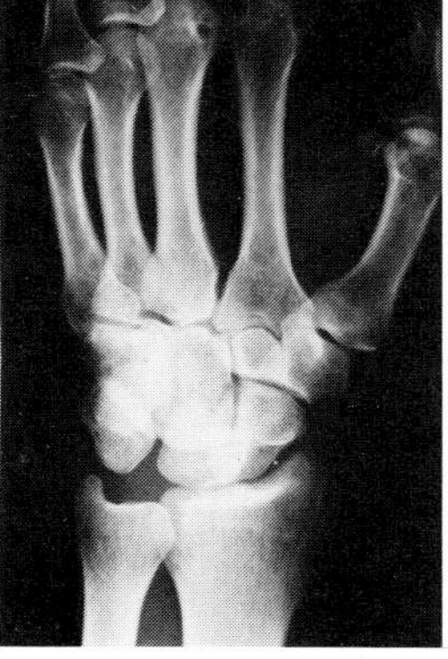

Figure 6-3. Dislocation of the perilunate with lunate in place.

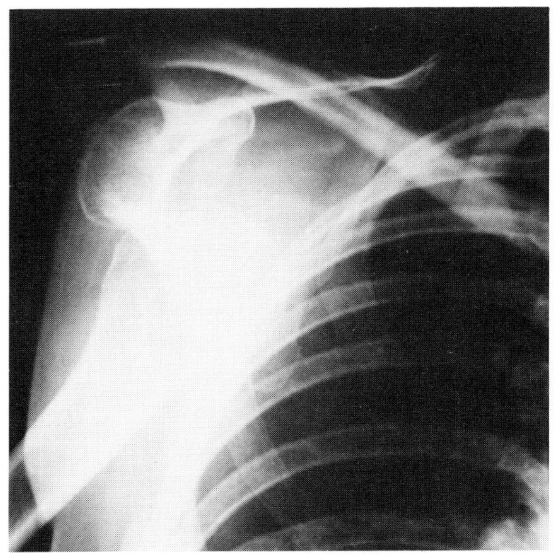

Figure 6-4. Anterior dislocation of the shoulder.

To understand the mechanism of action, remember the arm can be elevated until the humerus infringes on the point of the acromion. This position is the mechanical limit of the joint. When violent force is applied to the arm in this position, as in football tackling, the acromion is likely to act as a fulcrum prying the head of the humerus through the weak inferior or anterior part of the joint capsule. After the head of the humerus has broken through the capsule and the arm again falls to the patient's side the head of the humerus comes to rest in one of several positions, thus determining the type of dislocation (Fig. 6-5).

If the head is found directly below the glenoid fossa the dislocation is termed an inferior or subglenoid type. If the head is found below the coracoid process the dislocation is of the anterior or subcoracoid variety. If the head is pushed further medially and rests under the clavicle it is of the subclavicular type. Rarely does the humeral head rest posterior to the glenoid; this is the backward or subspinous type. Not only is the backward dislocation a rare occurrence but also it is frequently misdiagnosed, par-

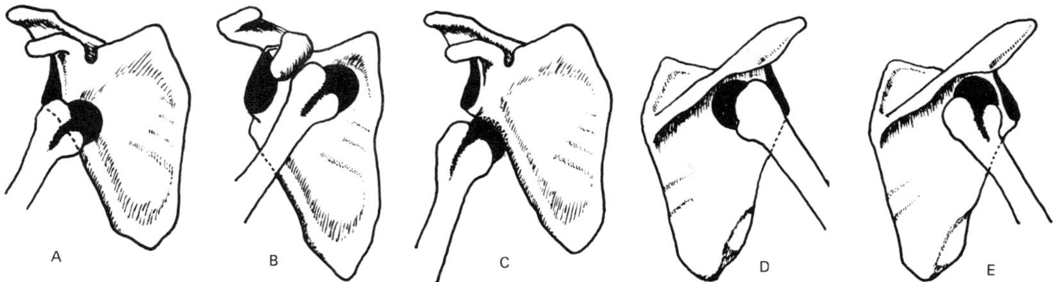

Figure 6-5. Types of shoulder dislocations: *A*, Subcoracoid (anterior); *B*, Subclavicular (anterior); *C*, Subglenoid (inferior); *D*, Subspinous (posterior); and *E*, Subacromial (posterior).

ticularly when complete reliance is placed on an anteroposterior x-ray.

Diagnosis

The patient carries his arm away from his body in the dislocation.

With the patient undressed look for a flattening of the deltoid area of the arm (the ruler test of Hamilton). Ordinarily the bulge of the deltoid prevents a ruler from touching the acromial tip and the lateral epicondyle of the elbow simultaneously. After a dislocation, the head of the humerus along with the deltoid sinks in, allowing the ruler to touch both prominences simultaneously (Fig. 6-6). The test is also positive in a medial displacement following a fracture of the humeral head.

Notice the increased girth of the shoulder joint (Fig. 6-7). Verify by measuring the joint by slipping a tape measure through the axilla and bringing it up over the acromial tip (Calloway's test).

Ask the patient to place the hand of his injured arm on the opposite shoulder (Duga's test). The test indicates a fracture if he is unable to do so.

Attempt to palpate the humeral head in the axilla beneath the glenoid, below the coracoid or in a posterior position. Measure the arm for increased distance from the acromion to the joint of the elbow.

Order x-ray studies to verify diagnosis. Generally a neutral anteroposterior view is enough to make the diagnosis. If a better view of the glenoid process is needed, order an x-ray picture with the opposite shoulder elevated 45°.

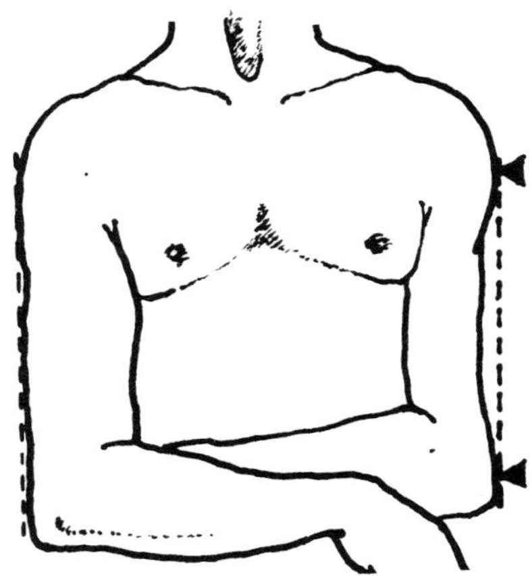

Figure 6-6. The rule test for fracture of the humeral neck or anterior dislocation of the humeral head.

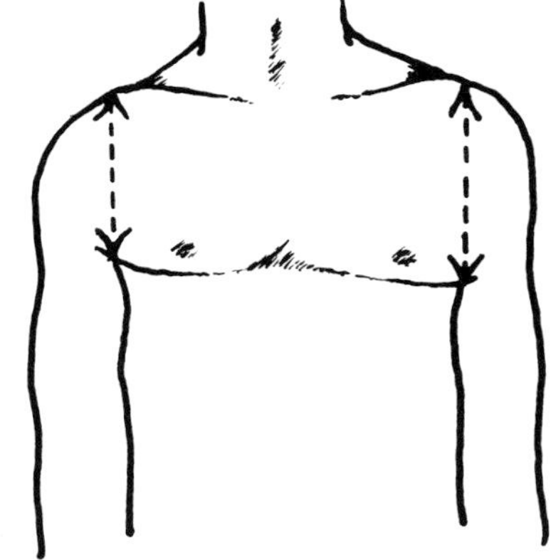

Figure 6-7. Increased girth of the shoulder indicates an anterior dislocation of the humeral head.

Check for motor, sensory and vascular changes and note any abnormalities. Palpate the pulse in the arm and wrist to detect compression of the axillary vessels. Damage to the axillary nerve may cause paralysis and atrophy of the deltoid muscle. Check for injury to the brachial plexus.

During the violence of the injury and as the head of the humerus slips under the glenoid, two bony injuries can occur: the greater tuberosity of the humerus becomes shirred off and/or the lower lip of the glenoid fossa chips off. If the violence is great, the neck of the humerus may break.

Whenever the patient complains of pain or a sense of danger on forced abduction and external rotation of the arm, consider the possibility of a dislocation that has spontaneously reduced.

Treatment

Try reducing an uncomplicated anterior dislocation by the straight pull method (Fig. 6-8). Have the patient lie prone on an examining table with the injured arm hanging freely over the side of the table. When once in position have her hold a 5 lb weight until reduction occurs. A general analgesia such as intravenous Valium and/or Demerol may produce satisfactory relaxation.

If simpler methods fail, reduce by the Kocher's maneuver (Fig. 6-9). First grasp the patient's arm at the wrist and elbow. Flex the elbow to 90°. Move the elbow against the chest. Externally rotate the wrist. Holding this position, pull on the elbow while moving it slowly toward the midline of the body. Reduction may occur at this point. If not, when the elbow is as far medially as it will go, push the wrist slowly toward the healthy shoulder until the hand rests on the acromion.

Cooper's (Hippocratic) method results in a satisfactory reduction in uncomplicated downward dislocations (Fig. 6-10). Help the patient into a supine position. Take your shoe off and, while resting against the side of the examining table, place your heel in the patient's axilla. Steady the patient's arm by holding the wrist. Maneuver your heel into the axilla until it is wedged between the chest wall and the upper end of the humerus. While pulling the extended arm, move it slowly toward the body, allowing the heel to act as a fulcrum prying the head of the humerus outward. At this point reduction may occur. If not, gently rotate the arm outward.

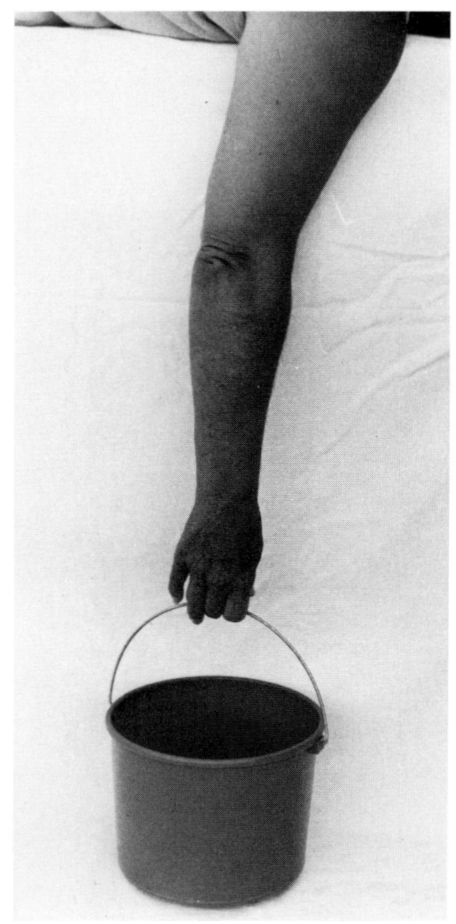

Figure 6-8. Straight pull method for reducing an uncomplicated anterior dislocation of the shoulder. The pail should have at least 5 lb of weight.

After the first dislocation, immobilize the shoulder 3 to 6 weeks in a plaster Velpeau. Surgical correction is not usually done unless dislocation recurs. The arm may also be taped. Flex the elbow to 90° and loop the tape around the proximal ulna and the shoulder, forcing the head of the humerus against the acromion as is done in an acro-

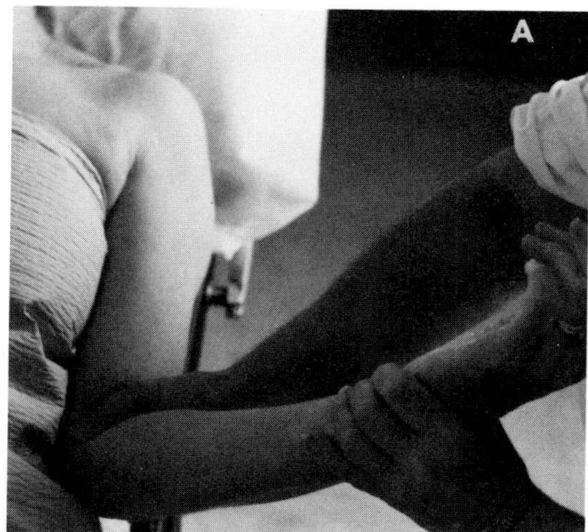

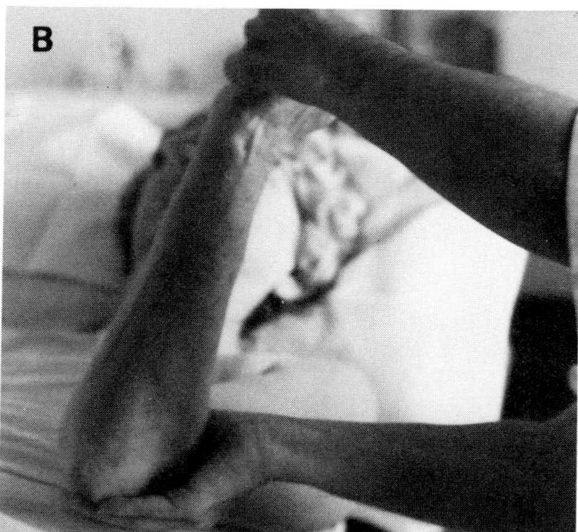

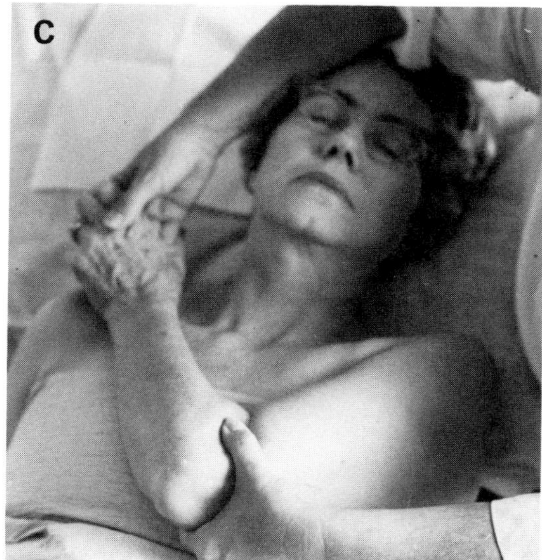

Figure 6-9. Kocher's method of reducing anterior shoulder dislocations. *A*, Grasp the patient's wrist in one hand, hold the elbow with the other and flex the forearm to a right angle, holding her elbow against her chest. Bring the wrist slowly outward until the arm is in full external rotation. *B*, Make traction on the elbow as it is brought forward and inward toward the midline. Maintain external rotation while proceeding. *C*, If reduction has not occurred the wrist is brought inward until the hand rests on the opposite shoulder.

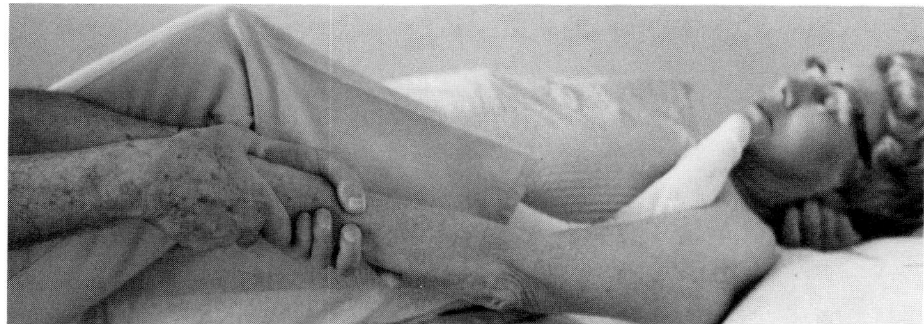

Figure 6-10. Reduction of a dislocation of the head of the humerus by Cooper's method. The physician's heel lies between the patient's chest wall and the upper end of the humerus and acts as a fulcrum. Make traction on the arm while bringing the arm close to the body, forcing the head of the humerus outward. If the head does not slip in, gentle outward rotation of the arm may help.

mioclavicular separation (see following pages). Place a thin pad in the patient's axilla. Keep the arm flexed in a sling and swathe. Most important, keep the patient's arm at her side. Exercise the hand and forearm immediately. In older patients, gently move the shoulder from time to time to prevent stiffness. After 3 weeks remove the taping but continue the sling. Begin active use of the arm but do not allow the patient to elevate the arm above 60° for 5 to 6 weeks. Then gradually begin full motion.

Do nothing special for a fracture of the inferior lip of the glenoid. Similarly, fractures of the greater tuberosity do not need special treatment if the fragments are in good position.

If the tuberosity, however, has been retracted by the supraspinatus, request consultation. The arm will need elevation and immobilization by a hand-on-the-head position. If this position does not reduce the fracture, open reduction will be necessary. If the bursa has sustained extensive damage, expect an unusually long convalescence. Deltoid muscle weakness indicates brachial plexus or circumflex nerve damage. In this event, again request a consultation for the arm will need immobilization in an abducted position for 3 to 10 weeks or until the symptoms subside.

Rehabilitation Exercises: Order hand and forearm exercises while the arm is still immobilized. Then in about 2 weeks or when any cast or sling halter is removed order the following graded exercises. Have the patient purchase or rent certain gymnasium equipment. Doctors who treat frequent traumatic cases keep rehabilitation equipment in their office for loan to patients.

For shoulder exercises a wall pulley, a cord with a handle and a bucket with weights from 1¼ to 15 lb, are necessary. Place the pulley on the wall, loop the rope through the pulley and, on the distal end of the rope, tie the appropriate weight. Seat the patient in a chair at right angles to the wall. Ask the patient to fully extend his arm and pull the weight up and then let it slowly descend.

Acromioclavicular Dislocation

Acromioclavicular (AC) dislocations (Fig. 6-11) are a frequent injury in contact sports. Any violent force which pushes the acromion downward and inward may shear first the acromioclavicular ligament and, with sufficient force, also the coracoclavicular ligament. The first causes an incomplete subluxation, the second a complete dislocation.

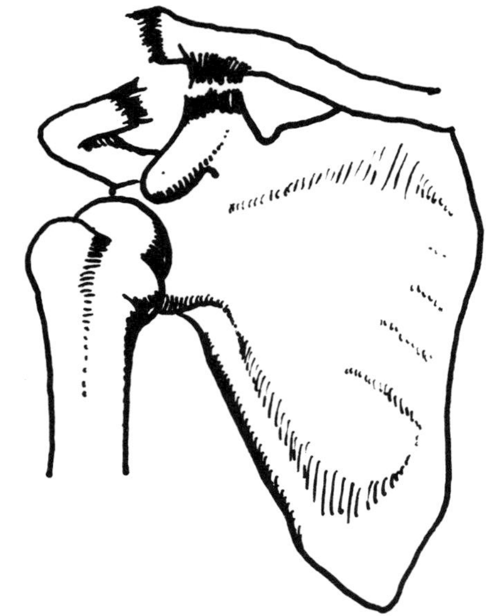

Figure 6-11. Acromioclavicular dislocation. Complete dislocation with all ligaments torn. If the coracoclavicular and acromioclavicular ligaments are intact the dislocation may be incomplete.

A firm diagnosis is essential. Treatment depends on the severity of the sprain. For minor sprain of the ligaments, apply an ice bag for 36 to 48 hours and follow up with heat. Occasionally a sling may be necessary.

For moderate sprains where laxity is present with pain and tenderness order more specific treatment. Order an x-ray film with the patient standing with his back to the cassette and holding weights in each hand. Search the x-ray films for an associated clavicular fracture. Films should include both shoulders for comparison. A companion film of the uninjured shoulder may help a puzzled radiologist arrive at a dependable diagnosis. Generally the outer end of the clavicle rides a little higher than the acromion. Usually only the acromioclavicular ligament is sprained.

Obtain reduction by outward-backward traction of the shoulder while pressing down on the outer end of the clavicle. A Kenny-Howard sling-halter applied while holding reduction may be sufficient immobilization if it is tightened up every few days.

Adhesive taping may work as well. Three pads are necessary, a thick 2 in pad for the axilla, a 1 in thick, 3 in square felt pad for the lateral third of the clavicle and another felt pad for the undersurface of the forearm. First flex the forearm. Start a 2 in adhesive tape low on the midline of the back, bring it up and over the pad on the clavicle and down the anterior surface of the arm. As the tape is looped under the forearm, exert enough pull to hold the clavicle in place. Continue the tape up the back of the arm, over the shoulder and down onto the chest.

Apply a wrist sling to keep the forearm flexed 90° and a muslin bandage swath to keep the arm close to the chest. With the 2 in pad in the axilla acting as a fulcrum, the shoulder tip is pulled outward, lessening the possibility of a recurrence of the subluxation. Continue immobilization for 3 to 4 weeks.

Start hand, wrist and forearm exercises early.

Complete dislocation is the rule in severe sprains. The displacement is more prominent than with moderate sprains and the patient is unable to use his arm. Both the acromioclavicular and the coracoclavicular ligaments are ruptured. Palpate for the deformity, which is usually obvious. The distal end of the clavicle may be movable on the acromion. Have the patient place the hand of the injured shoulder on the opposite shoulder and lean forward. While in this position, press the distal end of the clavicle in and sense the spring downward as the clavicle becomes reduced.

Consider another method to detect separation: Place one hand, preferably the left, on the acromion. With the right hand push the humerus upward. Palpate for the laxity of a separation with the left hand (Fig. 6-12).

A consultant should help make the decision whether to treat as outlined under a moderate sprain or to reduce surgically, repair the ligaments and immobilize until healed.

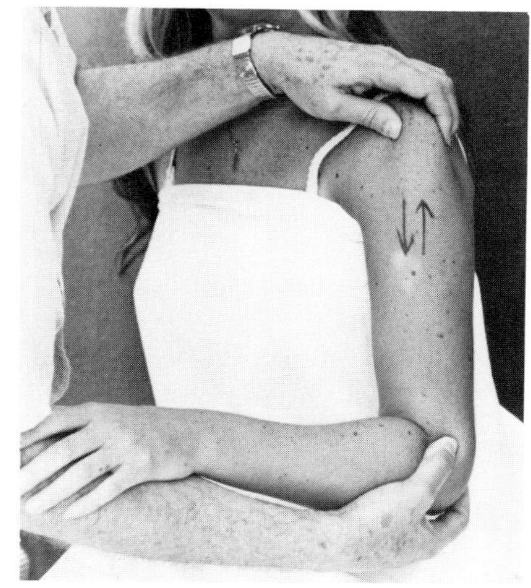

Figure 6-12. Testing for acromioclavicular separation.

Fractures of the Clavicle

Fracture of the clavicle is the most frequent fracture of infants and children (Fig. 6-13). The injury commonly occurs at the clavicle's weakest spot—the middle third.

After a fracture, the patient carries himself in a characteristic posture—head forward and inclined to the injured side and cradling the injured elbow in his uninjured hand. Inspection, palpation and x-ray studies verify the diagnosis and the severity of the dislocation (Fig. 6-14).

Apply a soft figure-of-eight bandage if the fracture is in the middle third without any great displacement.

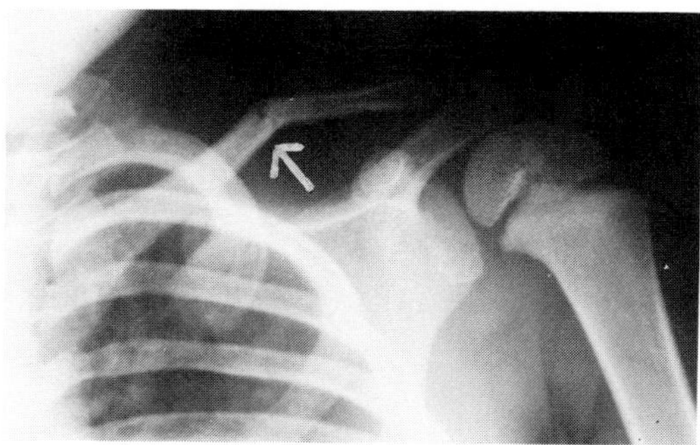

Figure 6-13. Fractured clavicle.

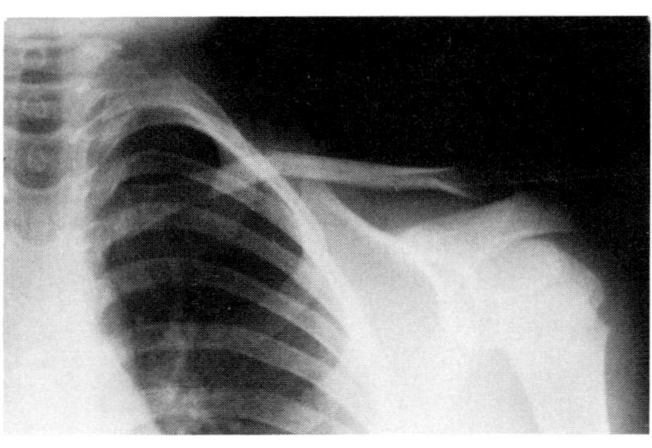

Figure 6-14. Fracture of the left clavicle. Clavicular fractures are best viewed by a special anteroposterior view of the clavicle. With the patient supine the x-ray head focuses on the clavicle from a 15° inferior position.

For the figure-of-eight select 5 yd of flannel or muslin bandage, 2 to 4 in wide. Also needed are three felt or cotton pads 6 by 8 in depending on the patient's size for protection of the axillae and scapulae. Place the pads. While an assistant holds the injured shoulder up and back, apply the figure-of-eight bandage, pinning in back with a safety pin. The two anterior shoulder loops can be prevented from slipping by pinning a short piece of the bandage across the chest, anchoring the loops.

If there is considerable displacement, attempt reduction by pulling the shoulders upward and backward. An assistant may help by placing his knee between the patient's scapulae while pulling the shoulder backward and upward. No anesthetic is required if done gently. When needed, infiltrate 10 ml of Xylocaine plus 150 turbidity units of hyaluronidase into the hematoma. If no assistant is present, help the patient into a supine position. Place a 6 x 12 in sandbag between his shoulder and then press the shoulders down toward the examining table. In either of these positions, manipulate the fragments into position. Apply a Billington yoke for immobilization. Maintain immobilization for 6 to 8 weeks.

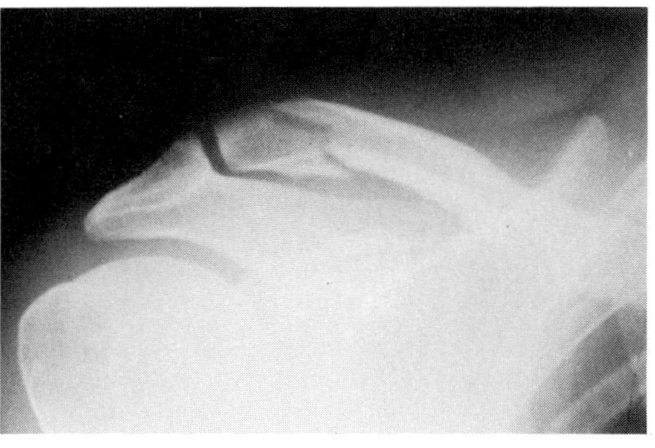

Figure 6-15. Fracture of the outer third of the clavicle.

Treat fractures of the outer third of the clavicle (Fig. 6-15) with a figure-of-eight bandage unless it appears the coracoclavicular ligament is ruptured. In this event have the patient wear a Kenny-Howard sling-halter for 6 to 8 weeks.

Approximately 200 devices have been manufactured to immobilize clavicular fractures. Few have been entirely satisfactory. With fairly good approximation of the fragments, anticipate excellent functional results. Expect a subcutaneous callus, which may be seen and felt for sometime but eventually fades away. Even with poor approximation anticipate good functional results; cosmetically the result is variable.

Fracture of the distal end of the clavicle often results in nonunion, especially if the coracoclavicular ligament is ruptured. In rare instances, nonunion causes persistent pain with symptoms of brachial plexus pressure. Refer the patient to an orthopedist for surgical repair.

Fractures of the Head and Neck of the Humerus

In the upper extremity, fracture of the shoulder is next in frequency to the Colles' fracture. They are caused by falls on the hand and arm or by direct violence to the arm. The patient will complain of pain in the shoulder after a fall or blow.

To establish a diagnosis, first tap the flexed elbow (pain in the humerus suggests a fracture). Grasp the head of the humerus from above the acromion and, with the other hand, rotate the flexed forearm. Suspect a fracture if the head of the humerus does not rotate. Inspect the lateral profile closely for angulation. Make the ruler test of Hamilton;

if considerable displacement is present the test will be positive. Measure the distance from acromial tip to the epicondyle on both sides (Figs. 6-16) (the arm with the impacted fracture will be shorter).

When a fracture is suspected, immobilize the arm with a sling and a swath dressing until treatment can be started.

X-ray studies (Figs. 6-17, 6-18, 6-19 and 6-20) will determine treatment. In addition to AP and lateral x-ray films, consider an oblique axillary view if pain and spasm make it impractical to pose the extremity for a proper axillary view. Occasionally a stereo film can be helpful.

If no displacement has occurred, only immobilization and protection will be necessary. Use the following criteria to decide if displacement is significant: If the victim is young, an angulation of 10 to 15° and no

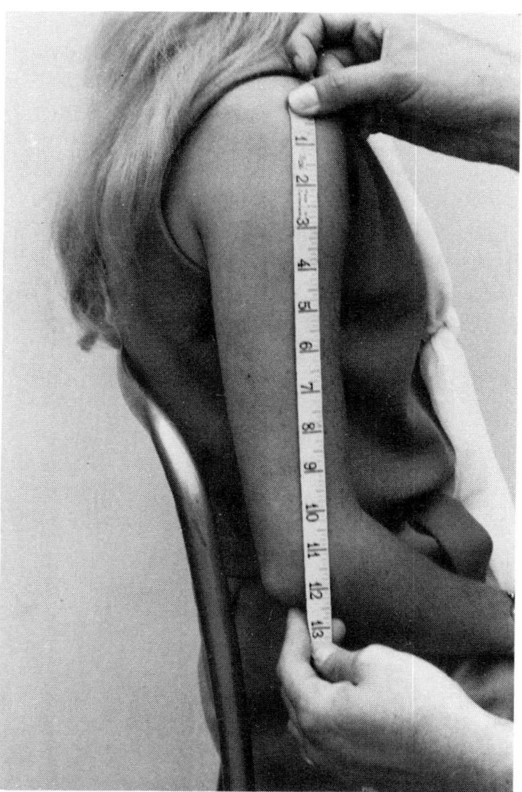

Figure 6-16. Evaluate the length of the humerus to determine overriding fractures of the shaft or fracture-dislocations of the head.

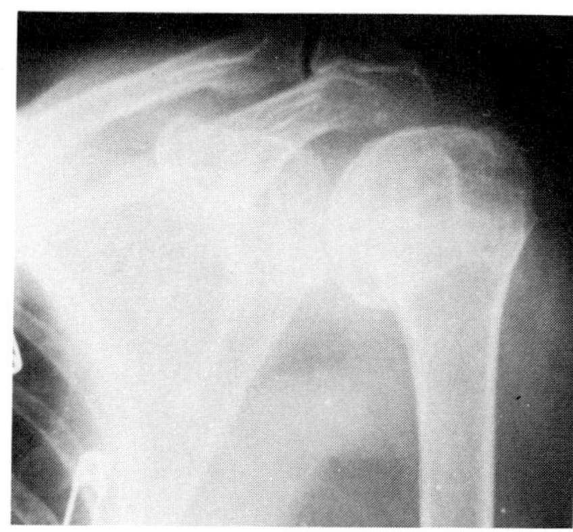

Figure 6-17. Impacted fracture of the surgical neck of the left humerus.

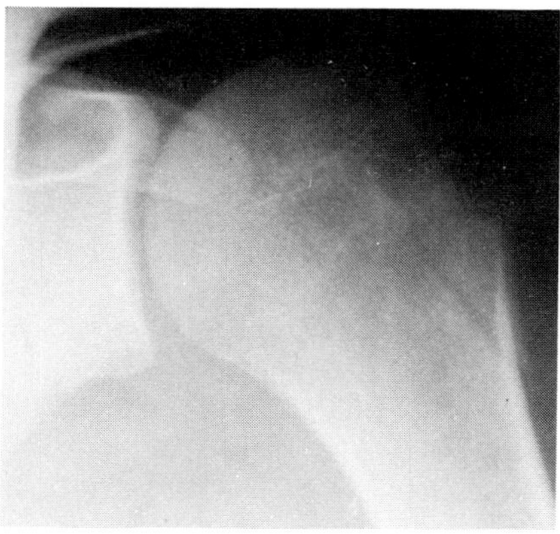

Figure 6-18. Fracture of the greater tuberosity in good position.

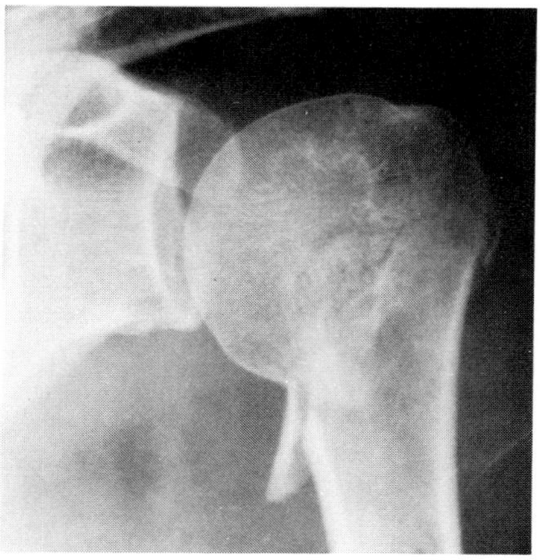

Figure 6-19. Fracture of the anatomic neck of the humerus.

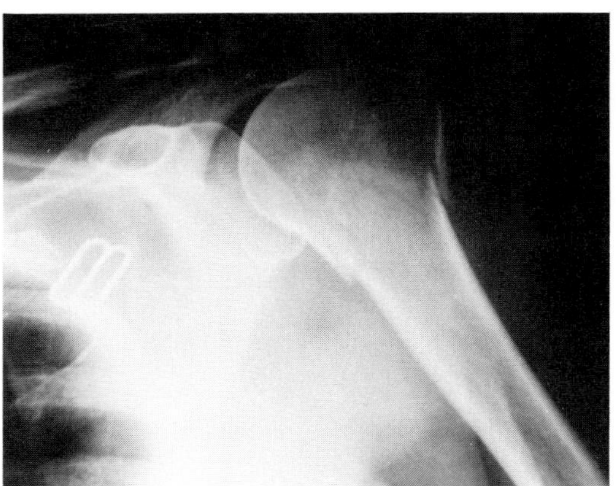

Figure 6-20. Fracture of the head of the humerus without serious displacement.

more than a third sidewise displacement is allowable. In the older person with a possible impaction, allow a 30 to 45° angulation and no more than a two-thirds sidewise displacement. If the patient is elderly and meets the above criteria, add an axillary pad and continue treatment with the first aid dressing or with a light circular hanging cast (Fig. 6-21) and body or neck swath.

To prepare an axillary pad select a piece of sheet cotton, 20 x 8 in. Bisect it with a strip of bandage long enough to encircle the patient's neck. Fold the cotton over the bandage, making the pad 10 x 8 in. Wrap it in gauze, powder it and place it high in axilla. Fasten in place by encircling the neck with the gauze bandage and tie. Finish with a wrist sling and a body swath about the chest.

Start exercising the hand and forearm immediately. X-ray in 1 week to verify satisfactory reduction. In 2 weeks replace the initial bandage with a simple triangular sling and start stooping exercises, wherein the patient stoops forward and allows the arm to dangle in circles.

Callus usually is felt in 4 to 5 weeks when the sling or cast may be removed and light ordinary activities resumed. Have the patient wait another month before resuming heavy pulling, pushing or twisting.

With children, in the event the fracture was transverse and the fragments displaced or comminuted or the greater tuberosity extensively avulsed, request consultation or proceed with manipulation and application of a spica cast with the arm abducted and externally rotated. Extend and abduct the arm while making traction as illustrated, then externally rotate the hand 90°. Immobilize in a spica cast with the forearm flexed 90° for 6 weeks.

Remember that in children with open epiphysis (Fig. 6-22) there exists a tremendous capacity to remold. If there is any semblance of reasonable alignment, the capacity to heal and remold is great and a complex

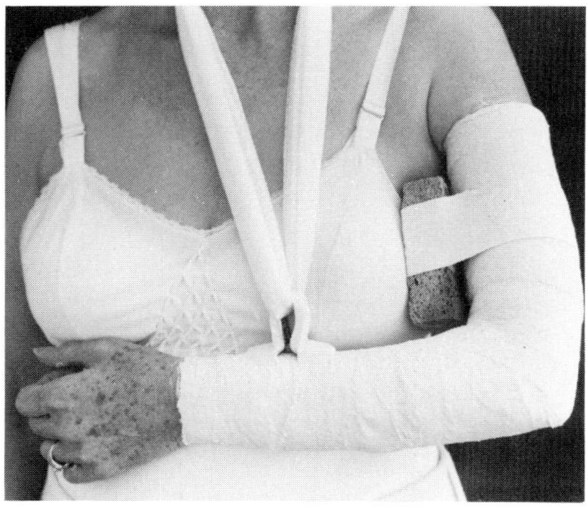

Figure 6-21. Hanging cast for fractures of the shaft of the humerus.

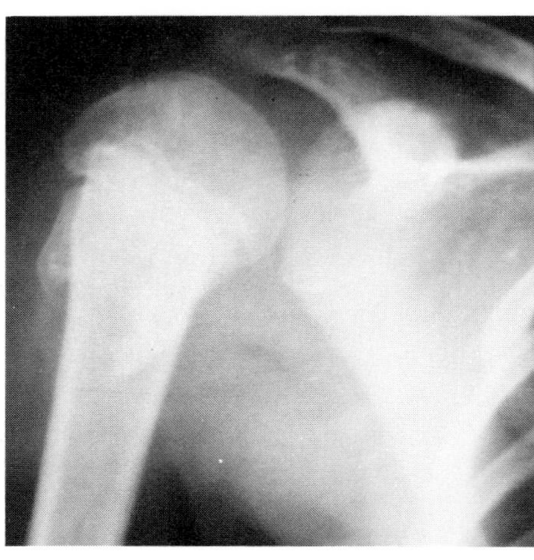

Figure 6-22. Fracture of the neck of the humerus with some epiphyseal separation.

program is not necessary. Attempt to manipulate with or without anesthesia and immobilize the shoulder by sling and swath.[2]

Limit physical activity with this injury until full motion has been obtained in the elbow and adequate x-ray evidence of healing is noted.

Deltoid paralysis may occur following injury to the circumflex or axillary nerve or even the brachial plexus. Or there may be a decreased blood supply resulting from injury to the axillary blood vessels. The biceps tendon may rupture and additional associated fractures and soft tissue injuries may occur.

In most cases there is some limitation of mobility for months. To minimize this, continue an active physical therapy program, such as active-passive abduction and rotary exercise, including performance of the active wheel-and-wall climbing exercises.

Fractures of the Shaft of the Humerus

Fractures of the shaft of the humerus follow falls on the hand and forearm or direct or muscular violence during wrestling or throwing a ball. The upper arm is useless and painful. The patient holds the injured arm by the opposite hand.

To establish diagnosis, inspect the arm for angulation deformity and gently palpate the shaft of the humerus along its medial and lateral aspects for local swelling and tenderness. If still in doubt, very carefully abduct the elbow while holding the proximal shaft with the other hand. Crepitus and mobility can be felt unless there is muscle tissue wedged between the fragments. Evaluate the radial pulse and test for radial nerve injury: have the patient pronate the forearm and flex the elbow while you observe for wrist drop. Anesthesia on the radial dorsum of the hand is evidence of sensory loss of the radial nerve (Fig. 6-23).

In the uninjured arm, the external epicondyle lies in the same plane as the greater tuberosity. With loss of these landmarks, rotary displacement has occurred.

First aid includes an axillary pad, sling and swath.

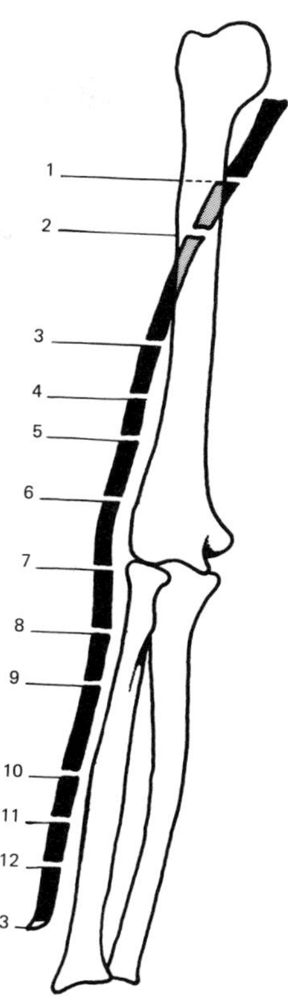

Figure 6-23. The radial nerve with the muscles it serves: *1*, Long head, medial head and lateral head of triceps; *2*, Brachioradialis; *3*, Extensor carpi radialis longus; *4*, Extensor carpi radialis brevis; *5*, Supinator; *6*, Aconeus; *7*, Extensor digitorum; *8*, Extensor digiti minimi; *9*, Extensor carpi ulnaris; *10*, Abductor pollicis longus; *11*, Extensor pollicis longus; *12*, Extensor pollicis brevis; *13*, Extensor indicis.

Even with the fragments in good position, a light well-padded spica cast is the most effective treatment. Fewer deformities and complications occur with this cast.

Favor a spica in children but give consideration to a Valpeau's dressing, a lightweight hanging arm cast, or swath and sling.

Eight to ten weeks of immobilization appears to be the safe rule and, if callus is unsufficient at the end of 2 weeks, continue immobilization with an axillary pad, sling and swath dressing. Heat, massage, continuous elbow action and stooping exercises of the shoulder are started. Do not allow active use of the arm until reasonably solid union is demonstrated.

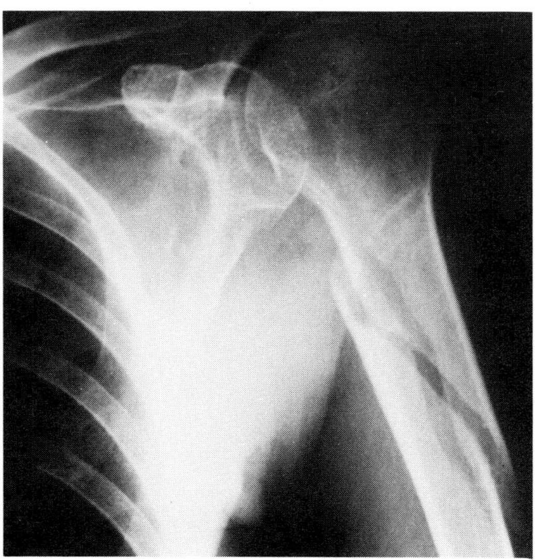

Figure 6-24. Fracture of the proximal shaft of the humerus in good position. This is a suitable case for a hanging cast.

The hanging cast has been used for years and may still be considered for the elderly with incomplete fractures or fractures of the proximal humerus in good position (Fig. 6-24). The one advantage of the hanging cast is that it allows earlier movement of the arm and consequently less stiffness and pain during the rehabilitation period.

Some orthopedists use a hanging cast to treat fractures of the humerus at any level —from the anatomical neck to the supracondylar area and occasionally even for fractures of the condyles.

Unless the family physician is experienced in treating transverse fractures of the humerus in bad position and can apply abduction casts, he should seek consultation. The same may be said for the oblique and comminuted fractures of the humerus.

Transverse fractures of the shaft of the humerus unite slowly. Delayed or nonunion is not rare. Interposed muscle between the fragments may prevent reduction and require surgery. Suspect this complication when crepitus cannot be felt. Fractures in the lower third of the shaft frequently angulate because of the imbalance between the biceps and the pronators. The amount of pronation-supination of the forearm demands close discrimination.

Injury to the radial (musculospiral) nerve is always a possibility. Remember the nerve lies in direct contact with the bone as it winds around the middle third of the humerus.

Fractures about the Elbow

Falls on the extended or flexed elbow may cause fractures about the elbow (Fig. 6-25). In adults, fractures in and about the elbow frequently cause impaired function in addition to pain. In children, troublesome complications include vascular and neurological complications as well as valgus and varus deformities. Consider referral.

There may be early complications. Look for impaired arterial circulation with diminishing radial pulse and impaired venous return with increasing cyanosis and edema. No matter how uncomplicated the fracture, check the radial pulse following immobilization. Any cast that interferes with the circulation should be removed even if reduction of fragments is sacrificed. Occasionally elevation of the arm will increase circulation.

Causes of Volkmann's ischemic contracture are tissue tension due to swelling or hemorrhage, rupture of the brachial artery with pressure of hematoma, pressure of bone fragments on the brachial or other major arteries or constriction of circulation following the application of tight dressings or tight casts.

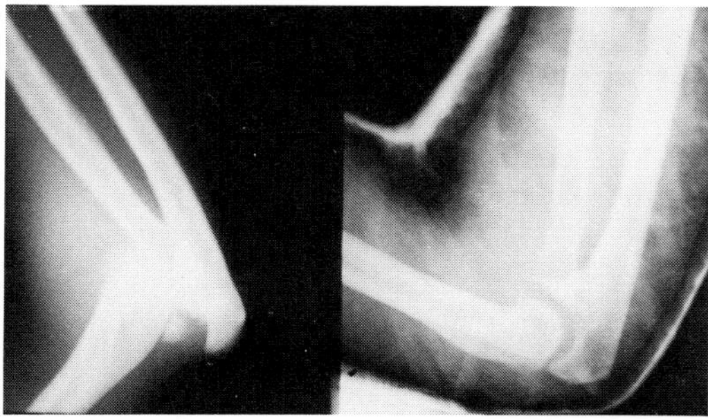

Figure 6-25. Pre- and postreduction views of fracture-dislocation of the right elbow (posterior dislocation). Elbow is hyperextended with traction and then the elbow is flexed for reduction while posterior traction is made on humerus.

Early signs of Volkmann's contracture are:

–burning pain in hand and forearm
–tingling and numbness of hands and fingers
–weakness or paralysis of flexor muscles of hand
–extension of fingers causes pain
–decrease of radial pulse
–loss of color in the hand
–after 48 hr pain decreases and the typical contractures and atrophies appear (wrist flexes; knuckles hyperextend; fingers flex; skin, hand and fingers atrophy; hand becomes hypersensitive to cold; and the fingernails may curve)

Injury to the radial nerve at the elbow causes wrist drop and hyperthesia over the dorsum of the first and second metacarpal. Injuries to the ulnar nerve cause weakness in thumb adduction and adduction of the fourth and fifth fingers. Sensory disturbances occur in the fifth finger, the lateral side of the fourth and the ulnar side of wrist and hand. Check for injuries to the median nerve by testing for weakness on flexing the fingers and thumb, paresthesias and numbness in the radial palm and in the area supplied by the median nerve.

After treatment and without any radiologic evidence of damage, the patient may not be able to fully extend the elbow, either temporarily or permanently. This may follow poor reduction but also may occur without any dereliction on the physician's part. The physician has little control over the development of joint fibrosis and myositis ossificans.

In supracondylar fractures (Figs. 6-26 and 6-27) constant care must be exercised in reducing sidewise or rotary motion. Permanent deformities in the carrying angle of the arm is the most common complication of supracondylar fractures. Another complication interfering with good results in children is fractures or separations of the epiphysis. The results will depend on what was damaged and at what age the damage occurred (Fig. 6-28).

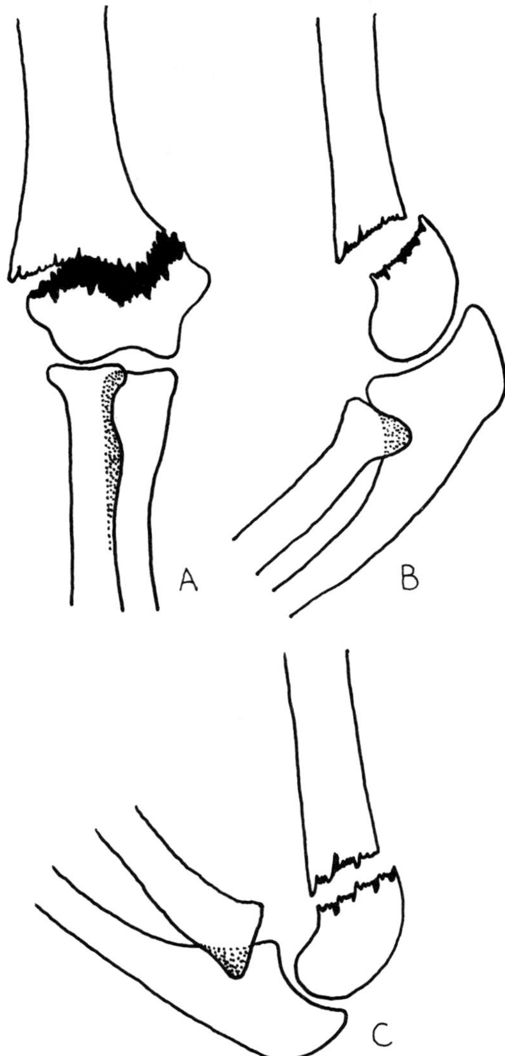

Figure 6-26. Supracondylar fracture of humerus: *A*, AP view; *B*, Lateral view; *C*, Fracture reduced and fixed with the elbow in flexion.

Some elbow landmarks to aid in diagnosis (Fig. 6-29): When the elbow is extended the olecranon process lies in a straight line between the medial and lateral epicondyles. In flexion, the olecranon process moves downward creating an equilateral triangle between the three bony prominences.

The normal deviation of the forearm from the arm is 10° lateral. In cubitus varus, the deviation is less than 10°, and in cubitus

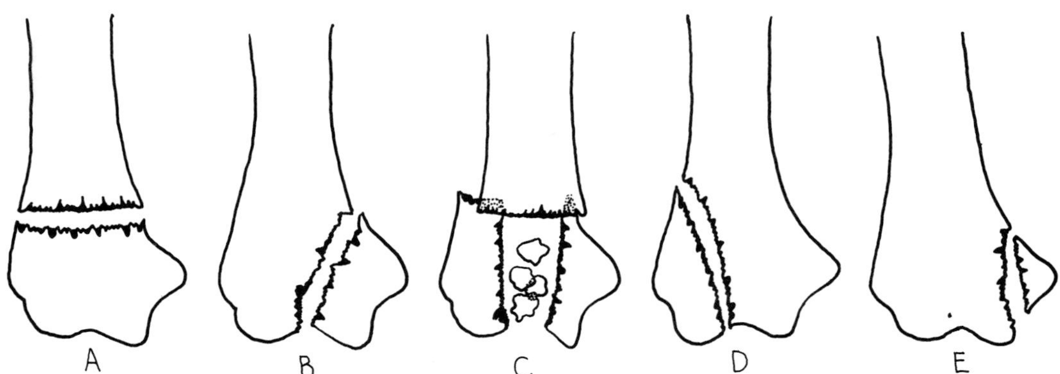

Figure 6-27. Variety of fracture lines at distal end of humerus: *A*, Supracondylar fracture without displacement; *B*, Oblique epicondylar fracture; *C*, Comminuted "T" fracture; *D*, Oblique epicondylar fracture; *E*, Epicondylar fracture.

valgus the deviation is more than 10° (Fig. 6-30). (Valgus means out; varus in.)

Apply an elastic pressure bandage about the elbow as first aid treatment. Immobilize in an internal right-angled splint and have the patient elevate his arm when not walking. Pack with an ice bag.

Unless a family physician is skilled and accomplished, it is best that he refer most elbow fractures to an orthopedist. One exception is the treatment of uncomplicated elbow fractures in good position. The treatment is simple when there are no vascular or neurological complications and the fragments have not been displaced. Some kind of an internal right-angled splint and wrist sling is all that is required. For a safe approach, apply two plaster splints. Fasten in place with roller gauze. When the swelling subsides trim the gauze off and add circular plaster, converting the splints into a cast. If no swelling is anticipated apply plaster about the splints while they are still soft and wet.

For young children use the horse-collar dressing in the flexed position instead of the splint and cast. Prepare the sling by cutting one piece of rubber tubing long enough to

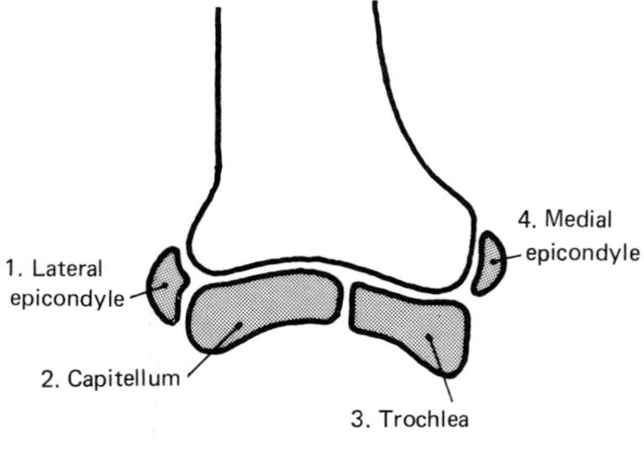

	Time of Appearance	Fusion of the Epiphysis
Fuse together at 14 yr	1. 13 yr 2. 11 mo - 3 yr 3. 9 yr	16-17 yr
	4. 5-6 yr	18 yr

Figure 6-28. The epiphysis at the lower end of the humerus, indicating appearance and fusion.

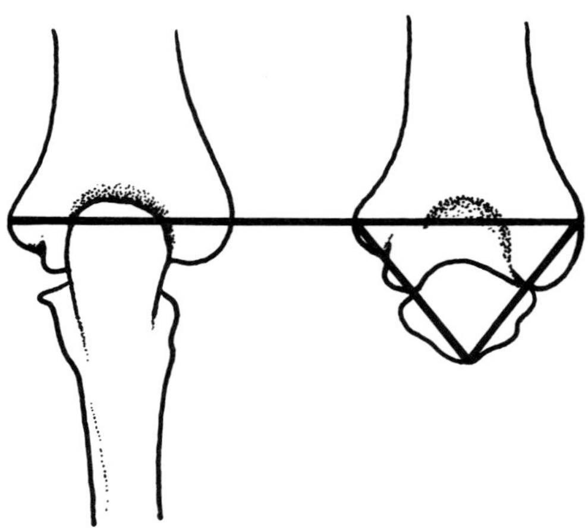

Figure 6-29. Posterior aspect of the elbow. When the elbow is flexed the epicondyles and tip of the olecranon make a triangle; when the elbow is extended the tip of the olecranon and the epicondyles make a straight line.

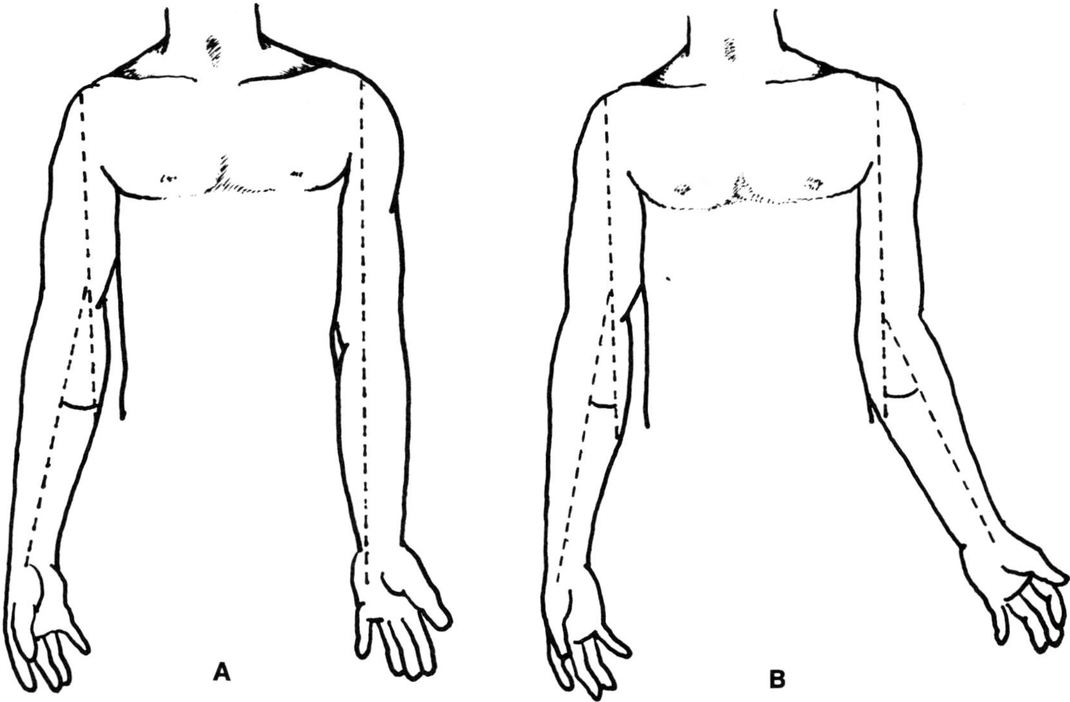

Figure 6-30. *A*, Normal (5° to 10°) and lost carrying angle (cubitus varus) of the forearm; *B*, Normal and abnormal carrying angle with the forearm forced more than 10° lateralward (cubitus valgus).

encircle the child's neck and one piece to encircle the wrist of the injured arm. Roller bandage is threaded through the lumen of the rubber tubes. The larger tube is then fitted about the child's neck and the smaller about the wrist. Tie the bandage short holding the elbow in flexion.

The orthopedist may choose one of several methods of treatment for fractures:

In children, Dunlap's traction or a modified Dunlap's until swelling subsides in 5 to 6 days, then immobilized in flexion.

Manipulation and immobilization for supracondylar and transcondylar fracture, for some trochlear and capitellar fractures and simple epicondylar fractures.

Hospitalization and continuous traction for threatened arterial shut-down, for severe swelling and bleb formation, for comminuted fractures with displacement and for complicated trochlear and capitellar fractures. Continuous traction becomes the method of choice when manipulation fails or the fragments cannot be held by splinting or vascular problems follow immobilization.

Hospitalization and open reduction for compound fractures or when the radial pulse does not return after 30 min in traction. Open reduction is the method of choice for certain Y, T, trochlear, capitellar, epicondylar or supracondylar fractures that are irreducible. Condyle fractures with rotation usually require open reduction after proper preparation. Diagnosis usually requires x-raying both elbows for comparison.

Considering the complications and the various methods of treatment, I advise family physicians to refer elbow injuries to an orthopedist colleague.

Fractures of Both Bones of the Forearm

Fractures of both bones of the forearm may be the result of either direct or indirect violence. There is a wide variety of fractures: transverse, oblique and comminuted.

When the violence is direct and severe, a transverse fracture at about the same level in both bones usually takes place. When the violence is indirect and associated with torsion, the fracture lines are usually oblique and the fracture of the bones may take place at widely different levels.

Recognize the fracture sites by the local swelling and tenderness or by palpable irregularity of the bones. Check carefully for multiple fractures. X-rays are essential for the accurate determination of all fragments.

Immobilize the arm from knuckles to the axilla on an internal well-padded right-angled splint. Protect the back of the forearm with an additional splint. Bandage all in place and put the arm in a triangular sling for first aid. Have the patient keep the arm elevated and apply ice bags.

Fractures are in good position if the interosseous space is not narrowed, if no unusual angulation is present and if one half to one third of the ends are in stable opposition.

When the radius is fractured in the upper third fix the forearm in full supination. If the fracture is in the lower third, put the arm in moderate pronation, flex the forearm to 90° and apply molded plaster splints from the knuckles to the axilla. If swelling is anticipated, bind the splints with bandage and adhesive, which can be removed in 4 to 5 days, and convert the splints into a cast by applying circular plaster. If there is no substantial swelling, complete the cast at the first setting.

Place the arm in a triangular sling. Keep it elevated and at rest. Exercise fingers and shoulders from the beginning. Take x-ray pictures after the cast is completed and 1 week later. In a few days have the patient discard the sling and start active use. Immobilize children's fractures for 4 to 6 weeks and adult's fractures for at least 6 weeks. Check x-ray films and palpate at the end of these periods for callus and union. If union is solid, do not immobilize further. If little callus has formed, apply an unpadded cast for 4 more weeks.

Greenstick Fractures with Angulation

If there is little or no swelling and the interosseous space is normal, apply the cast from knuckles to axilla, placing a felt pad over the angulation before casting. When the cast has set, cut a wedge out of the cast at the point of the angulation. Then merely cut the cast on the opposite side of the forearm. Correct the angulation by closing the wedge and apply a few rounds of plaster to wedge the cast at the new angle.

One can also attempt to manipulate the angulation by pressing the thumbs into the interosseous space and overcorrecting the angulation. Do not grasp the forearm by the hands or the bones will be forced into the interosseous space, complicating the procedure.

Approach fractures with displacement cautiously. The secret is a good anesthesia, preferably a general anesthetic that will give total relaxation of muscles. Do not attempt local infiltration for no hematoma, an essential for good anesthesia, is present. Morphine sulfate gives far better relaxation. Secondly, an assistant may help apply strong traction and countertraction and this way you may pull the fragments into apposition. X-ray. If apposition is poor, continue traction and countertraction until the position is satisfactory. Apply a knuckles-to-axilla cast as described. It is absurd to immobilize fractures of this type with short splints, which do not prevent motion between the radius and ulna nor motion of the elbow.

Nonunion most frequently results from incomplete immobilization or too short duration of immobilization. Adults may need immobilization as long as 3 months.

Unstable, oblique or comminuted fractures of the forearm or reductions that tend to displace in the cast require operative reduction. Seek consultation.

Fractures of the Wrist and Hand

Colles' Fracture

Do not call all fractures of the wrist Colles' fractures. The term identifies only the anatomical area injured. Modify the term by anatomically describing the fracture, stating its location, direction of fracture lines, exact displacement and degree of comminution. Even more inaccurate is the habit of speaking of noncomminuted wrist fractures as "simple" Colles' fractures. There are no simple fractures of the wrist.

Dorsiflexion fractures of the lower end of the radius with or without a fracture of the ulnar styloid is the most common fracture in adults. The radius is fractured within 1 in of its distal end. In about 50 percent of the cases a concomitant fracture of the ulnar styloid process also occurs.

The cause of this fracture is a fall forward on the dorsiflexed hand. The wrist needs to be flexed and pronated in order to give way. Often when a person is drunk there is no righting reflex. When he falls without this reflex, there is no fixing nor pronation and consequently no injury.

While making a diagnosis check for the silver-fork deformity. Lay the pronated arm on the examining table and observe its resemblance to the outline of a silver fork lying horizontally with the tines pointing downward (Fig. 6-31).

To differentiate swelling from a fracture, palpate the volar aspect of the radius and compare with uninjured side for a loss of the normal convexity below the fracture. Palpation of the radius from Lister's tubercle up gives the same information as a lateral x-ray picture of the bone. Palpation of radius from the anatomical snuffbox up is similar to the findings of an AP x-ray film of the wrist.

Check x-rays for loss of the normal angles of articulation (Figs. 6-32).

The styloid process of the radius is 1 cm longer than the ulnar styloid; consequently, the angle of articulation is not at right angles to the shaft of the radius but is inclined about 25° toward the ulnar side. In the lateral view, the articular surface is inclined volarward 15°.

Evaluate the fracture. Is it a greenstick fracture without displacement? Is there marked impaction? Overriding? Comminution? Is there subluxation of the radioulnar joint? Look for associated fractures of the radial styloid, the navicular or other hand bones. Inspect for a lateral shifting of the hand from the long axis of the radius and check for epiphyseal separation.

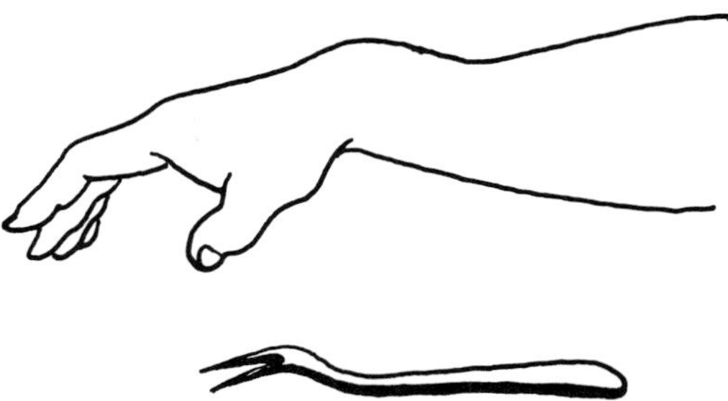

Figure 6-31. Silver-fork deformity of Colles' fracture.

Apply a temporary padded wooden splint to the dorsal aspect of the arm as soon as possible to prevent swelling and trauma. This splint should extend from the knuckles to the elbow with the hand in midposition of rotation and flexion. Cover with a firm bandage and have the patient carry the arm in a sling. Apply ice bags.

Order x-ray pictures and determine the exact diagnosis. If the fracture fragments are in good position apply two plaster splints, one posterior over the dorsal aspect of the hand and forearm from the knuckles to the elbow and the other anterior over the

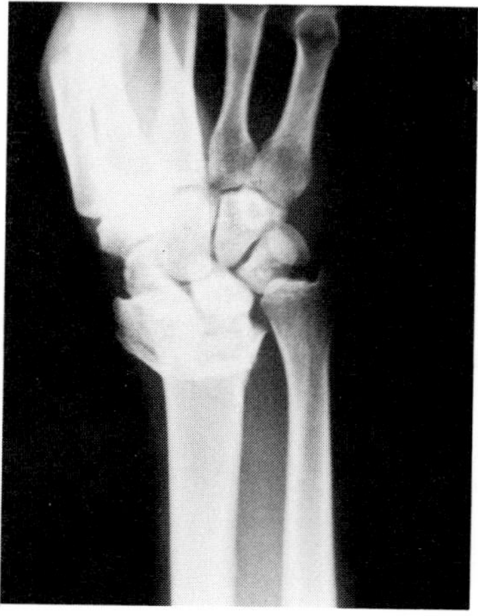

Figure 6-32. Colles' fracture. Notice that the distal ends of the radius and ulna are nearly horizontal. (The radius extends 1 to 1.5 cm past the styloid of the ulna in an uninjured wrist.)

volar aspect of the forearm from the fracture site to just below the elbow.

Treat the distal end of the volar splint in one of two ways: (1) end the splint at the wrist or even proximal to the fracture and continue immobilization of the hand with tape and gauze or (2) extend the splint onto the volar aspect of the hand, molding it about the thenar and hyperthenar eminences. Do not extend the plaster between the thumb and index finger. Be sure the wrist is immobilized in ulnar deviation and in a slightly flexed position.

Bandage the splints into place and recheck x-rays. If the position is satisfactory leave the splints in position until the swelling has subsided and then complete the cast with circular plaster gauze. If no edema is anticipated, complete the immobilization with the immediate application of circular plaster gauze.

Some general principles of casting and immediate care of a Colles' fracture are:

- –do not immobilize the wrist in hyperflexion
- –do not immobilize joints that do not need immobilization (allow movement of thumb and fingers)
- –prevent or reduce swelling in the hand or fingers by keeping the wrist elevated above the elbow until swelling subsides (Do not hesitate to cut or remove the cast if in doubt.)
- –have the patient move all the arm joints at least three times daily. The patient should continue use of the fingers.

Remove the cast in 4 to 6 weeks. Do not remove the cast early for physical therapy. The best form of therapy is active use and this can be done while the wrist is protected by the cast. After removal of the cast order hot soaks and activity. This will restore the wrist to full function and strength.

COLLES' FRACTURE WITH DISPLACEMENT OF FRAGMENTS. Study the anteroposterior x-ray views carefully for presence and degree of radial shifting of the hand, angle of articulation, shortening of the radius, fracture of the ulnar styloid and disturbance of the radioulnar joint. Check the lateral view for an abnormal articulation angle, the degree of impaction and loss of substance.

Not all fractures of the wrist can be reduced and immobilized by closed manipulation and casting. In unstable radial fractures, an orthopedist may need to insert Kirschner's wires transversely through the bases of the index, middle and ring metacarpals and through the proximal ulna and incorporate the wires into a cast to maintain traction and reduction.

Reduction under general anesthesia is the treatment of choice and is essential in children with a total dorsal displacement of the lower sixth of the radius. In many, however, local infiltration of 1 percent Xylocaine will suffice. Infiltrate about 10 ml into the dorsal side of the fracture and 3 to 4 ml in and about the ulnar styloid. Wait 10 min before beginning reduction.

Help the patient into a prone position on the operating table. While an assistant applies countertraction to the forearm, grasp the patient's thumb in one hand and his second, third and fourth fingers with the other and make firm traction for a couple of minutes. When muscle contraction shows signs of relaxing, take the patient's hand as though shaking hands and break up any impaction, if present. Do this by forcing the hand backward while making traction and countertraction. Use the thumb of the free hand to aid disimpaction by pressing distally on the dorsal fragment. Complete the reduction by seizing the forearm with both hands and with one thumb above and one below the fracture press the distal fragment toward the flexor side. Flexing the hand while pulling into ulnar deviation allows the tendons to help reduce and maintain reduction.

While the wrist is still in traction, apply a plaster cast or splints similarly to and with the same precautions as for the undisplaced Colles' fracture. Discontinue traction after the plaster hardens. If the fracture is severely comminuted, run the cast above the elbow. Recheck the x-rays. The bones and their angles of articulation should be approximately normal.

Warn the patient to report any vascular problems such as sensations of pins and needles, coldness, blueness or numbness. Keep the hand elevated above the elbow for a few days. Ice bags help to control swelling and pain. Examine the cast and hand the following day. If evidence of circulatory deficiency appears, split the cast or loosen the splints. If appropriate, do not convert the splints to a full circular cast until the swelling subsides in 3 to 5 days. Recheck films in 1 and 3 weeks.

Epiphyseal dislocations in children are special dorsiflexion fractures, often misdiagnosed on the original x-ray studies.

Other Fractures and Dislocations about the Wrist and Hand

DISLOCATION OF THE RADIOULNAR JOINT. Apply a tight binding that presses the ulna against the radius for 3 to 4 weeks. If pain continues, cast for 4 weeks. If these methods fail, consider referral for open fixation.

ISOLATED FRACTURE OF THE ULNAR STYLOID. Treat many of these fractures by immobilizing the hand for a short time or infiltrate with Xylocaine and allow restricted movement.

FRACTURE OF THE DORSAL LIP OF DISTAL RADIUS. Reduce by traction and manipulation. Immobilize in moderate flexion and extreme ulnar deviation for 6 weeks. Recheck x-rays frequently because reduction often fails. Watch for dorsal dislocation of the carpal bones. Recurrent displacement requires the treatment of an orthopedist.

FRACTURE OF THE PALMAR LIP OF THE DISTAL RADIUS. This fracture is opposite in cause and damage to the dorsal lip fracture. Watch for palmar dislocation of the carpus. To reduce, apply traction and immobilize in dorsiflexion and ulnar deviation.

SMITH'S FRACTURE OR PALMAR-FLEXION FRACTURE. Like Colles' fracture, this is a break of the distal end of the radius but displaced volarward in contrast to the dorsal displacement of Colles'. The deformity resembles a horizontally placed silver fork with its tines pointing upward (Fig. 6-33). Displacements are often identified by the sound and feel of a mushy crepitus. Reduction is sometimes difficult. If the epiphysis is fractured, disturbances of bone growth may ensue. The treatment is basically similar to the Colles' fracture but it is better to refer the patient to an orthopedist.

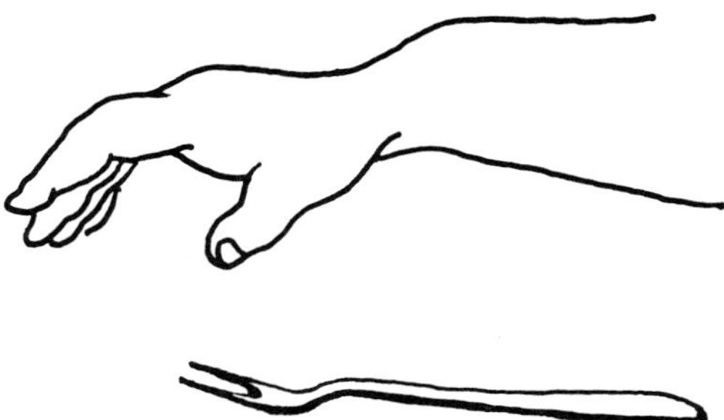

Figure 6-33. Smith's fracture (reversed silver-fork deformity, reversed Colles').

Treatment follows the same principles as suggested for Colles' fracture. More difficulty is encountered in reduction and in preventing recurrences of dislocation. Greater traction is needed for reduction. For manipulating the fragments, place the thumbs on the flexor sides of the fracture and press toward the dorsum, the reverse motions made in reducing Colles' fracture. If unexperienced in this reduction, refer to an orthopedist.

FRACTURE OF THE NAVICULAR. A fracture of the navicular is often misdiagnosed as a wrist sprain. It is the most common fracture of the carpal bones (Fig. 6-34)

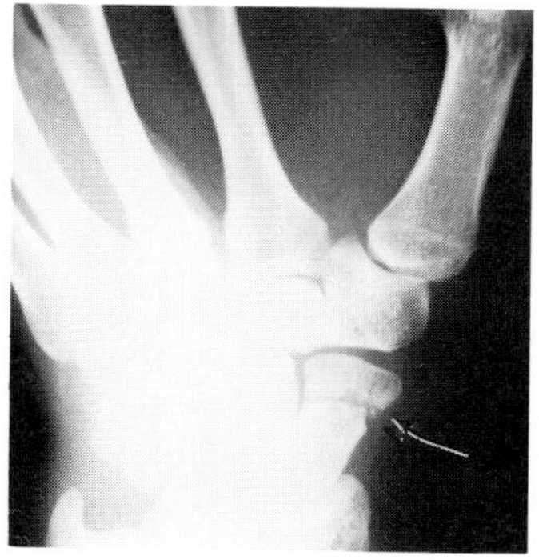

Figure 6-34. Fracture of the navicular.

and occurs after a fall on the outstretched hand. The symptoms are pain on flexion and extending the wrist plus tenderness in the anatomic snuffbox. Extension of the thumb accentuates the borders of the snuffbox, a triangular hollow at the base of the thumb. Palpate the radial pulse and the radial styloid process at the base of the snuffbox. Compare the tenderness and position with the navicular of the opposite hand.

The first x-ray films made are often negative for fracture. When suspicious of a navicular fracture, do not be satisfied with the usual anteroposterior and lateral views. Order an oblique view of the wrist and a special navicular view.

If no fracture line can be seen but there is tenderness in the snuffbox, treat as though a navicular fracture existed. Immobilize the wrist with the hand in slight dorsiflexion and radial deviation with a circular plaster cast over stockinette. Begin the cast at the elbow and extend to the metacarpophalangeal joints of the second to the fifth fingers and to the interphalangeal joint of the thumb with the latter in a slightly adducted position.

Remove the cast and recheck x-rays in 4 days. By then a fracture line will show clearly because of resorption of bone about the fracture. When a fracture has been verified, continue immobilization 8 to 10 weeks or until there is definite x-ray evidence of healing even if it takes 6 months.

Nonunion (Fig. 6-35) had best be handled by an orthopedist. The family physician's job is to *recognize* the fracture and immobilize early. Frequent x-ray rechecks are indispensable to proper follow-up.

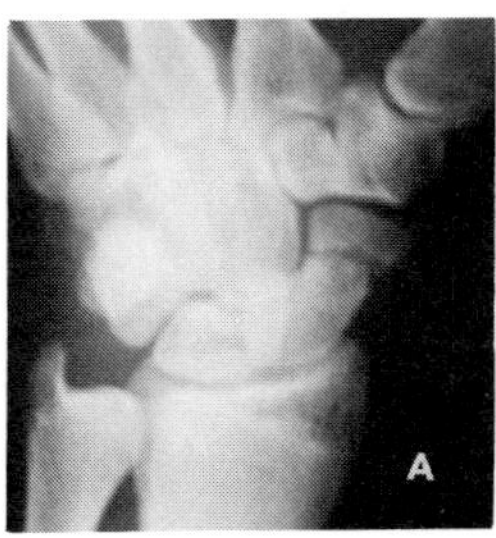

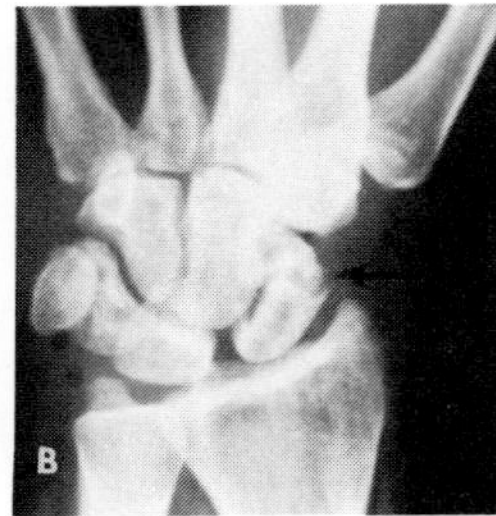

Figure 6-35. Fractures with nonunion of the navicular.

Nonunion is due to inadequate immobilization or aseptic necrosis following interference with the bone's blood supply.

BENNETT FRACTURE-DISLOCATION. To an inexperienced family physician this may appear as a simple chip fracture of the proximal end of the first metacarpal. The fracture is nearly always associated with a dislocation that may be so small as to be almost undetectable.

The fracture usually occurs after a blow to the dorsum of the thumb or a fall on the abducted digit. Remember any injury that results in interference with the wide motion of the thumb by chronic dislocation or arthritis is a major disability.

Recognize Bennett's fracture by the acute tenderness and swelling over the proximal end of the first metacarpal. If considerable dislocation exists, a distinct deformity can be palpated.

For first aid, apply a well padded wooden splint to the dorsum of the thumb. The splint should be 8 to 10 in long and twice as wide below as above. Fix the thumb and wrist to splint with adhesive and cover with an elastic bandage. Apply ice.

In an emergency a major dislocation can be reduced by exerting traction on the thumb, while pushing the proximal end of the metacarpal into place and bringing the distal end of the bone into full abduction. Immobilize in an unpadded gauntlet cast with the thumb abducted. X-ray immediately and if the position is not perfect, remove the cast and try again or refer to an orthopedist.

A word of advice: Bennett's fracture-dislocation nearly always needs Kirschner wire fixation and open reduction. Generally a family physician is wise to refer these fractures at once.

DISLOCATION OF THE METACARPOPHALANGEAL JOINT OF THE THUMB. A blow on the hyperextended thumb may result in a dislocation of its prominent metacarpophalangeal joint. The deformity is obvious. The proximal phalanx is dislocated anteriorly and the head of the metacarpal posteriorly. The anterior aspect of the capsule is usually torn.

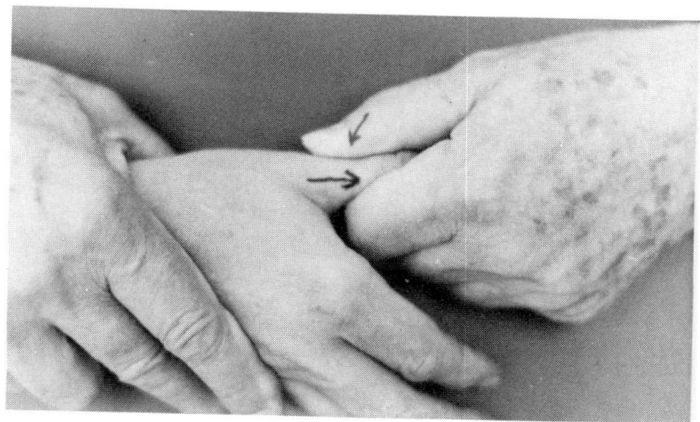

Figure 6-36. Treatment of dislocation of the thumb. Reduce metacarpophalangeal joint by traction on the markedly abducted thumb while making pressure against the base of the proximal phalanx.

To treat (Fig. 6-36), grasp the patient's thumb so that pressure can be made over the base of the dislocated proximal phalanx with the ball of your thumb. Make traction and abduct the thumb while pressing the dislocated phalanx into position. Then flex the thumb while holding the phalanx in position. Immobilize in a neutral position for 3 weeks in a short plaster cast extending from the wrist to the distal phalanx.

If difficulty in reduction occurs, think of the possibility of a button hole tear in the anterior capsule through which the head of the metacarpal bone has slipped and been entrapped. No amount of traction or manipulation in such cases will allow the head to be replaced in its normal position because the button hole in the capsule prevents it. By simple operative approach the capsule can be released and complete reduction obtained.

METACARPAL FRACTURES. Fractures of the metacarpal bones are common, especially fractures of the fifth metacarpal known as the boxer's fracture. A blow directed upward through the knuckles such as fighters sustain or a blow on the dorsum of the hand causes metacarpal fractures.

Metacarpal fractures are not usually accompanied by much displacement and need only immobilization. If posterior angulation exists, manipulate and extend the distal fragment by thumb pressure on the volar aspect of the metacarpal; this will reduce the fracture. For anesthetic use local infiltration with Xylocaine.

Generally with fractures of the metacarpals that do not tend to displace, simply placing a bandage roll in the patient's hand and flexing his fingers around it will maintain reduction. In the elderly, sustained tight flexion of the fingers may cause contractures. Actually an unpadded cast is better because it fixes the fragments securely and prevents use of the uninjured fingers. Extend the cast from the wrist to the base of the flexed first phalanx of the injured finger. Allow freedom of all uninjured digits. Mold the cast to hold the distal fragment upward and the proximal fragment downward. Continue immobilization for 3 to 4 weeks; then begin active motion even though no x-ray evidence of callus exists.

When there is considerable displacement and the fracture line is oblique, expect difficulty in reduction and immobilization. In this event refer to an orthopedist for skeletal traction or internal fixation.

FRACTURES OF THE PHALANGES. Suspect fractures of the phalanges by the swelling and local tenderness of the finger. Tapping on the end of the finger causes pain at the site of the fracture. Smaller fractures cannot always be found without x-ray studies.

Check for rotational deformity if a phalanx has a complete fracture or there is overriding. Do this by having the patient extend and flex the fingers of his hand (Fig. 6-37). Normally in extension the fingers spread apart but in flexion they pull together in the palm. If there is rotational deformity of a finger the injured finger will override or underride the adjoining digit during flexion. Correct the deformity by manipulating the

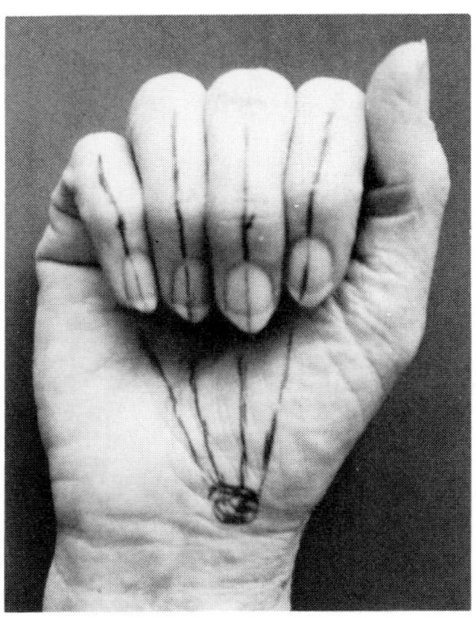

Figure 6-37. Check for rotational deformities of the proximal or middle phalanges following fractures by asking the patient to flex her fingers. When in normal position the fingers will crowd together and all point toward the styloid process. If rotational deformity is present the injured finger will be under or over its neighbor. Keep this in mind when immobilizing fractured fingers.

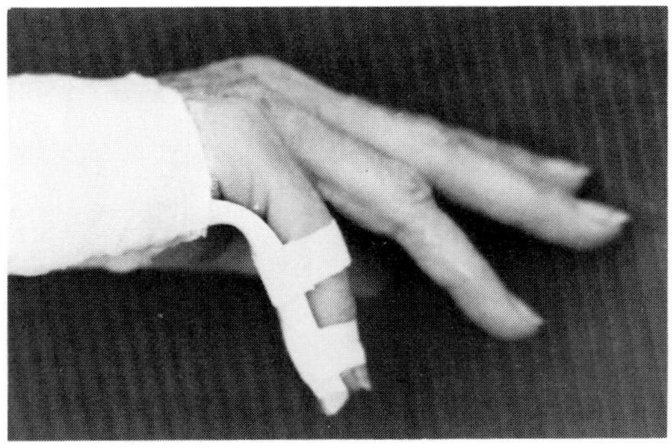

Figure 6-38. Immobilization following fracture of the proximal phalanx. The MP joint is immobilized in flexion and the PIP joint in extension.

finger tip into proper position before taping or casting.

In all phalangeal fractures that involve joints inspect the x-rays carefully for minute dislocations. Resort to open surgery if needed to get anatomical reduction of joint fractures. Do not hesitate to compare the x-ray shadow with its uninjured companion if in doubt as to displacement or joint injury.

First aid treatment is immobilization of the finger on a well padded wood splint applied to the dorsum of the finger and hand from the wrist to the end of the finger and secured with adhesive tape.

Take x-ray pictures and decide on treatment. Correct the volar angulation by flexing the finger; flex the metacarpophalangeal joint approximately 45° and the proximal interphalangeal joint as far as possible without interfering with the circulation. Immobilize in a plaster cast from the wrist to and including the injured digit.

Another treatment which allows better observation of the injured finger, is to apply a plaster wristlet in which a metal splint is incorporated. Bend the metal splint so as to immobilize the finger in proper flexion and tape the finger to the splint (Fig. 6-38). Caution: do not immobilize in extension on a tongue blade. Recheck x-rays are essential because, although the finger is immobilized, the proximal phalanx has a tendency to angulate.

The base of the middle phalanx on its dorsal and lateral surfaces is the most frequently fractured area of the fingers (Fig. 6-39). Fortunately, fractures of the middle phalanx are fairly stable. Consequently, immobilization of the distal and proximal joints in a finger splint is usually adequate.

The fracture may be angulated either posteriorly or anteriorly, depending on whether the fracture occurs distally or proximally to the insertion of the flexor sublimis. If the fracture is angulated volarward,

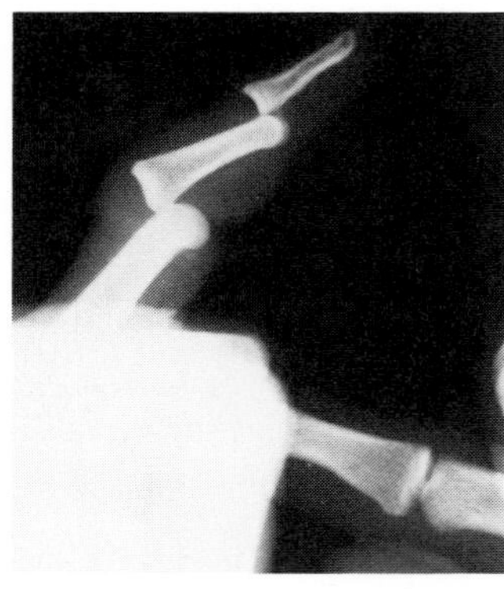

Figure 6-39. Dislocations of the DTP and PTP joint.

reduction is best done by immobilizing the finger in flexion. If the fracture is angulated dorsalward, fix the finger in extension. Again a small plaster wristlet extending over the injured finger is preferable to a tongue blade.

Rarely are the fracture fragments greatly displaced in the distal phalanx. If the joint is not involved in a major way (more than 50 percent of the joint surface) simple immobilization in a metal or wooden splint for 2 weeks is sufficient. If 50 percent or more of the articular surface is involved advise open reduction to prevent subluxation (Fig. 6-40).

Occasionally the extensor tendon is pulled loose from its moorings on the distal phalanx. If this is complete the patient will be unable to extend the distal joint, causing a mallet finger. If the flexion is less than 30° the deformity is of no consequence except to the most fastidious woman. If the flexion is more than 30° advise open repair.

Dislocation of finger joints usually follows hyperextension. The distal bond rests on the dorsum of the proximal (Fig. 6-41). These dislocations can often be reduced by traction without anesthesia. If traction fails think of possible buttonhole dislocation.

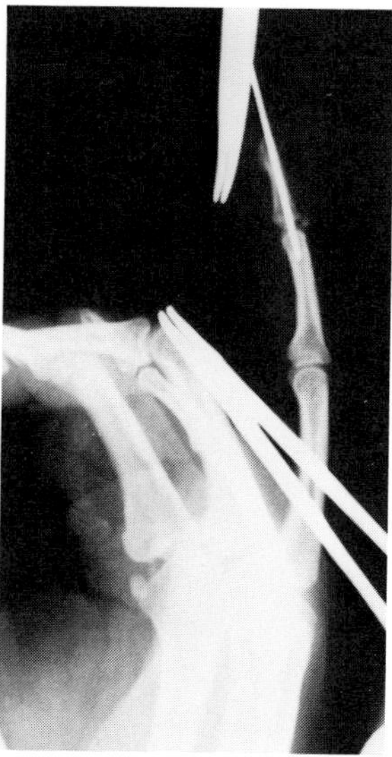

Figure 6-40. Internal fixation of the distal phalanx by a pin through the distal into the middle phalanx.

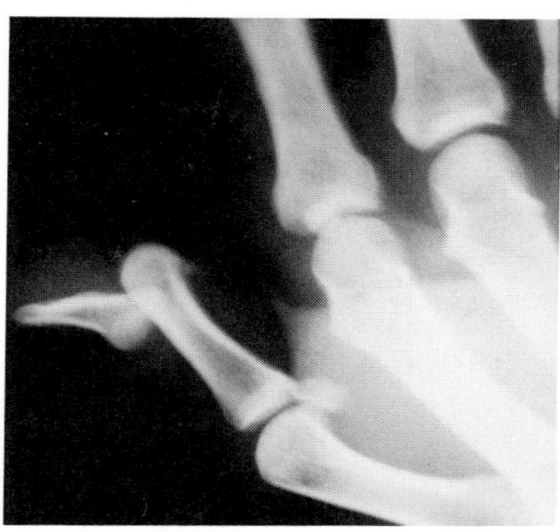

Figure 6-41. Dislocation of finger joints with the distal bone resting on the dorsum of the proximal.

Baseball finger results from a violent backward dislocation of the terminal phalanx onto the dorsum of the middle phalanx. To tape such a finger cleanse the finger and paint with tincture of benzoin; use two 5 in lengths of ½ in adhesive tape and anchor one end of the tape to the finger-pad near the distal end of the finger, bringing the free end of the tape around the finger and crossing it over the proximal nail; continue taping along the proximal phalangeal joint side of the finger; finish the splinting by again crossing over the finger near the base of the proximal phalanx. Do the same on the opposite side of the finger.

The object is to immobilize the distal interphalangeal joint in moderate extension and the proximal joint in 60° flexion. Continue the splinting, renewing the tape when needed, for 4 to 6 weeks.[3]

FINGERTIP INJURIES. Closing doors on a finger often causes fingertip injuries resulting in denuded bone, lost tissue and macerated structures of the finger. Do not shorten or excise bone in order to have enough skin to close the wound. If finger length must be sacrificed do so later after skin grafts or flaps have been tried. Suture into place any tissue fragments which are connected in any way to the stump. Use skin that has been avulsed as a free graft. Before applying the skin as a graft, remove all fat and subcutaneous tissue. Generally allow no hand or finger wounds to granulate in.

Either undermine the edges of small wounds and close by first intention or excise avascular tissue and apply skin grafts or pedicle flaps.

Severed fingers cannot be replaced successfully.

Hand and Finger Rehabilitation

One of the best hand and finger exercises I have seen is the Hand Helper marketed by Medder. The device can be adjusted to exercise one finger, two fingers or the entire hand. Tension can be graduated by adding or removing silicone rubber bands. It is small enough to be carried about in a pocket or purse.

INJURIES TO THE LOWER EXTREMITIES

A quick evaluation of injuries (Fig. 6-42) to the pelvis, hip, knee and ankle can be made by having the patient straight leg raise, first actively and then against resistance. Then, while still resisting, have her attempt to rotate her foot and leg first inward and then outward. Finally ask her to squeeze a fist held between her knees. This will cause pelvic pain because the adductors are attached to the pelvis. If a patient is drunk just twist his legs and feet back and forth and watch his face.

Fractures and Dislocations of the Hip

Examine for suspected hip fractures with the patient in supine position. Face the patient and place your thumbs upon the patient's anterior superior iliac spines. The fingers naturally encircle the greater tuberosities and small disparities between the two sides are readily noticeable.

Now with the thumb follow the inguinal ligament medially until the pulsating femoral artery is felt. To palpate the small portion of the extracapular femoral head, position the thumb below the inquinal ligament and lateral to the femoral artery. Now rock the femur gently, palpating for crepitus. If no movement of the head is felt consider fracture of the neck. If no head is felt suspect dislocation.

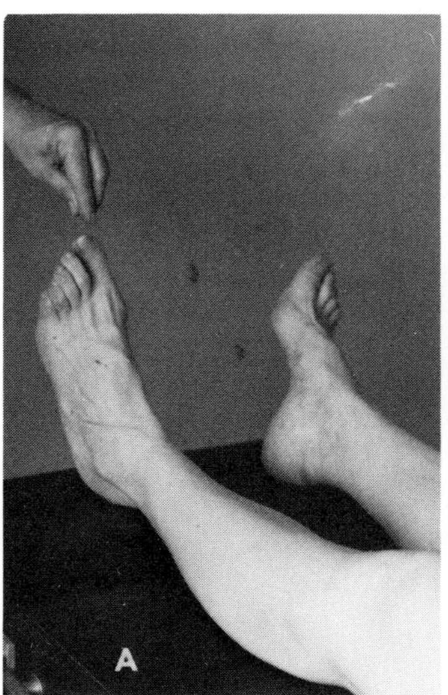

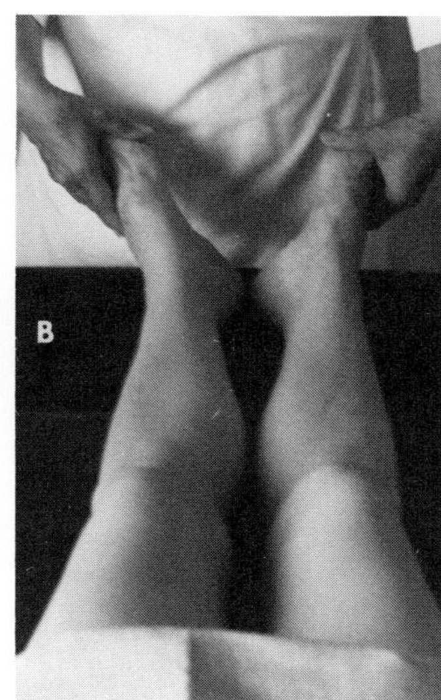

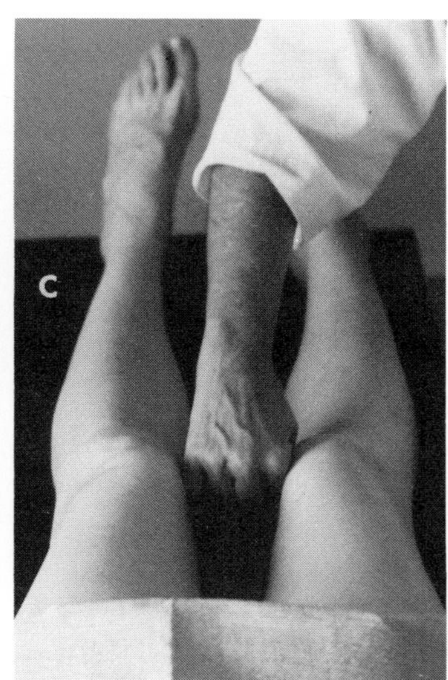

Figure 6-42. Examination of the lower extremities for fractures and dislocations of the hips, thighs and legs. *A*, Ask the patient to lift her leg and touch your hand. If the patient can lift her leg request that she lift against resistance. *B*, Rotate the feet outward and ask that they be rotated inward against resistance. Then rotate her feet inward and ask that she rotate her feet outward against resistance. *C*, Place your fist between the patient's knees and ask her to squeeze her knees together.

Classify fractures of the hip as intracapsular (fractures through the anatomical neck) or extracapsular (intertrochanteric fractures). The gravity of the problem and the treatment of these two injuries vary considerably. Fractures of the neck of the femur (the intracapsular type) are the most serious (Fig. 6-43).

If the fracture is extracapsular or intertrochanteric the femur usually lies in an abnormal outward rotation of about 90° (Fig. 6-44). Further inspection reveals a shortening of the leg. When the fracture is intracapsular, the capsule restrains abnormal rotation to 45° or less. If the patient can lift the foot from the bed the fracture is probably impacted. In some instances, when the impaction is solid, the patient can walk on his leg. As a further test rock the femur or the foot from side to side. Do this manipulation first: if it causes pain other more painful testing maneuvers are unnecessary.

With fractures of the hip the leg is in extension. In dislocations, however, there is a typical deformity of flexion that is not difficult to recognize (Fig. 6-45). In a posterior dislocation the involved leg appears shortened. It is held in moderate flexion, adducted and internally rotated with the knee resting on the well leg. Severe pain is caused by any movement. In an anterior dislocation the hip falls into flexion, abduction and external rotation. A dislocated hip may be unrecognized if associated with a fracture. In this circumstance poke the thumbs of the examining hands into the gluteal mass and palpate for the dislocated femoral head. The four types of dislocation are named after the area in which the head comes to rest —posterior, obturator, pubic and ischial.

Hip fractures are grave injuries from the standpoint of life. Shock, emboli and other complications are frequent. These fractures most often occur in the elderly when the general resistance and the will to live is low. Intracapsular fractures are common, especially in the aged. Before 50 they are uncommon. Falling on the greater trochanter is the usual cause. Nonunion is the most frequent major complication.

The fracture can easily cut off the blood supply to the femoral head and, subsequently, it acts as a foreign body in the capsule. Open fixation by pinning is the treatment of choice. The procedure should be done by someone trained in the latest techniques.

A word about impacted fractures of the neck. The good results, which occasionally occur in impacted fractures of the neck when little or nothing is done, can be explained by the fact that the impaction leaves

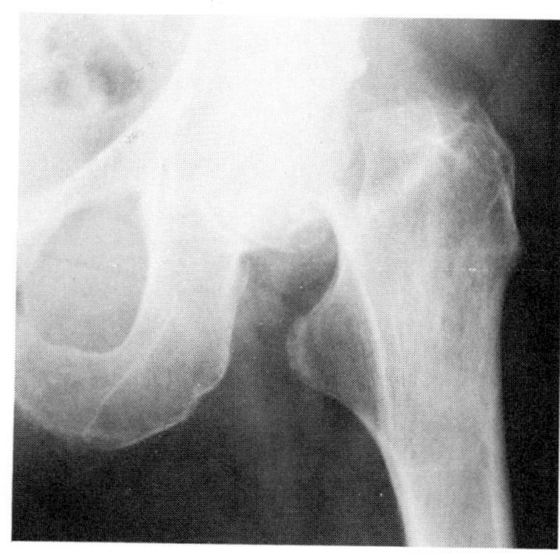

Figure 6-43. Subcapital fracture of the left femoral neck (basocervical).

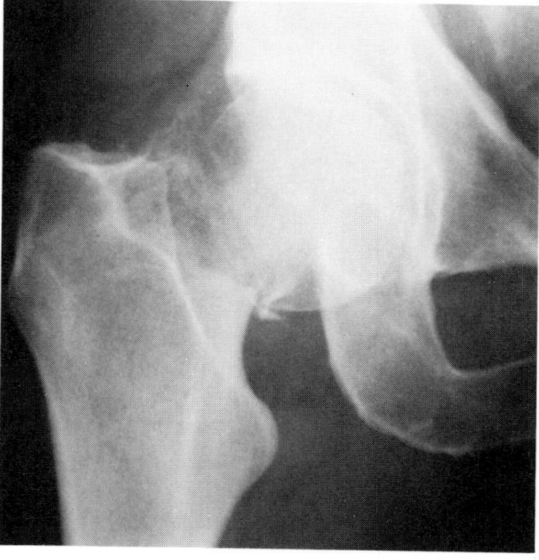

Figure 6-44. Fracture of the femoral neck. Notice the prominence of the lesser trochanter caused by some external rotation of the lower extremity.

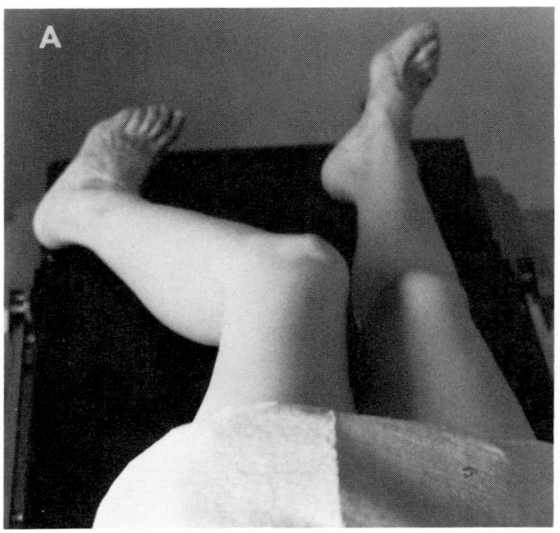

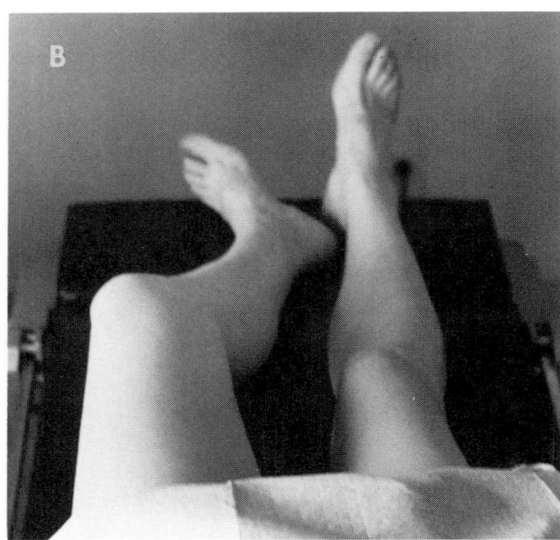

Figure 6-45. *A*, Posterior dislocation of the hip; *B*, Anterior dislocation of the hip.

the blood supply intact. A rule to remember is, "Never break up the impaction." Be sure it is impacted, however.

Intertrochanteric fractures occur at the same age period as fractures of the neck and with about the same frequency. The line of fracture runs through the greater trochanter toward the region of the lesser. They are serious injuries but treated by most methods all unite. If treated indifferently, they unite with deformity.

Dislocation of the hip is not an infrequent occurrence. Violence to the widely abducted or adducted leg is the usual cause. The dislocated head usually falls into a superior and posterior position in respect to the acetabulum. The patient will need an anesthetic and/or a proper dose of anactine while reduction is made. Stand astride the patient's pelvis, facing his feet, and flex his thigh and knee. Grasp his leg with your forearms beneath the knee. Place your unshod foot on the patient's pubis and make powerful traction and countertraction. Rotate the leg counterclockwise if the dislocation has been posterior. This is usually sufficient to pull the head directly over the rim into the acetabulum. With the use of anactine the reduction becomes simpler than it sounds.

Frequently, Bigelow's maneuver is successful. In this instance, flex and abduct the patient's thigh over his abdomen. Second, abduct the thigh while the hip and knee remain flexed (counterclockwise movement). Then while holding the foot in abduction, slowly extend the hip and knee. Last of all, by adduction and internal rotation, bring the injured leg parallel to the uninjured leg.

Reduce anterior dislocations by a reverse Bigelow maneuver: the flexed hip is adducted (clockwise movement) and brought to a neutral position in extension. Usually the operator hears a loud click as the head pops back into the acetabulum.

Immobilize in 6 to 8 lb traction with Buck's extension on a Thomas splint. Begin active motion in 4 weeks. Have the patient start crutch walking in 6 weeks. Weight bearing should not begin until there is good radiographic evidence of a viable and transformed head. After a careful study of the x-ray have an orthopedist help make a decision on when the patient should bear weight.

Complications of hip dislocations are aseptic necrosis, fractures of the acetabulum that require open reduction, injury to the sciatic nerve (always check nerve function before and after reduction) and myositis ossificans of the capsule, causing great loss in motion.

Fractures of the Shaft of the Femur

Femoral shaft fractures occur most frequently after falls, direct violence and automobile accidents.

The family physician's most important responsibility centers around the emergency care of the fracture. As much as 2 L of blood may accumulate in the soft tissue of the thigh. Mild to dangerous shock accompanies these fractures and great damage can be done if the fracture is improperly handled.

Do not move these patients until splinted, preferably with a Thomas splint applied over the trousers. If no Thomas splint is available bandage in place a splint that reaches from the axilla to the foot. If this is impossible, bandage both legs together. These patients are ambulance cases and should not be moved until a stretcher and ambulance is available.

Considering possible complications, these fractures are best treated by an orthopedist. For infants up to age 3 or less than 50 lb, Bryant's traction is the best treatment. Include both legs in the overhead traction. The infant should be lifted by the suspension until no weight is borne on the back of the sacrum. One should be careful that the skin of the foot and heel remain exposed. After 4 to 6 weeks, replace traction with a spica cast. These patients should be watched carefully for circulatory deficiencies that lead to ischemic fibrosis or gangrene. Union is adequate in 3 months.

Fractures in children and young adults continue to be best treated by Russell's traction or balanced suspension. Orthopedists generally believe that balanced suspension is preferable to Russell's traction.

In any event, the parents should never be promised the legs will be exactly equal. During the first post-fracture year the leg may be a quarter inch longer or shorter than the uninjured leg. This is an acceptable figure. At the end of a year, extremity length is usually near equal.

Consider all the common fracture sites (Fig. 6-46) following injuries to the upper leg.

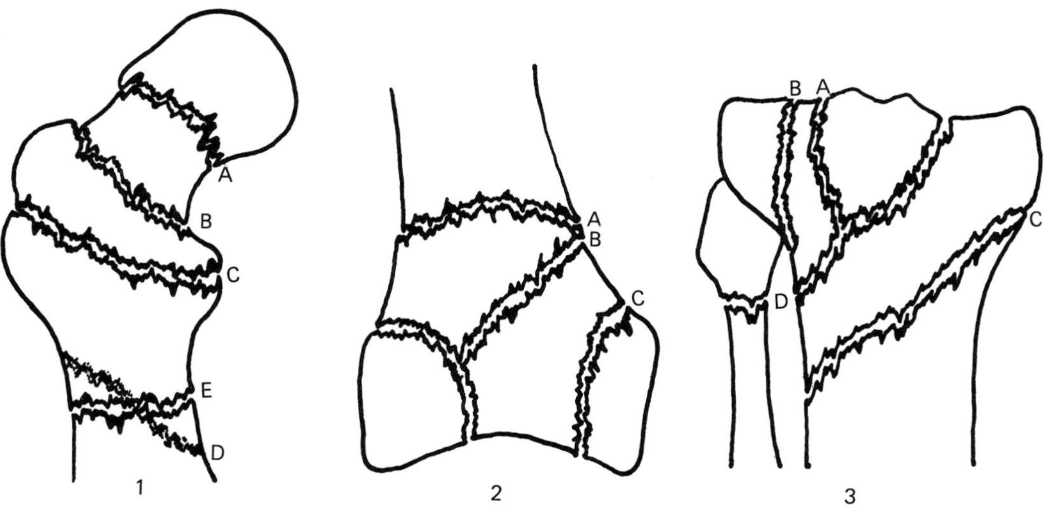

Figure 6-46. Common fracture lines: *1*, Upper extremity of femur: *A*, Subcapital fracture of neck of femur; *B*, Fracture through base of neck; *C*, Petrochanteric fracture; *D*, Oblique subtrochanteric; *E*, Transverse subtrochanteric.

2, Distal extremity of femur: *A*, Supracondylar fracture of femkur; *B*, Intercondylar Y-fracture; *C*, Medial condylar fracture.

3, Proximal extremity of the tibia and fibula: *A*, Intercondylar Y-fracture of tibia; *B*, Fracture of lateral condyle; *C*, Infracondylar fracture of tibia; *D*, Fracture of neck of fibula.

Injuries about the Knee Joint

Knee injuries are the most common injury in athletics, accounting for approximately 35 percent of all athletic injuries. The elderly and the obese are frequent victims of knee cartilage injuries often mistaken for degenerative joint disease.

As an anatomic review, on the medial aspect of the knee is the medial collateral ligament. It extends from the femoral condyle and attaches to the inferior and posterior margin of the tibia. On the lateral aspect of the knee the lateral collateral ligament extends from the lateral epicondyle of the femur to the head of the fibula.

Within the joint are two ligaments—the anterior cruciate and the posterior cruciate. They prevent backward and forward displacement of the femur on the tibia.

Also within the joint are the menisci, located on the tibial plateau between the condyles of the tibia and femur. The medial meniscus is semilunar in outline and is shaped like a "C." The lateral cartilage is more circular and appears as an "O." The menisci spread the synovial fluid over the articular surfaces and act as shock absorbers.

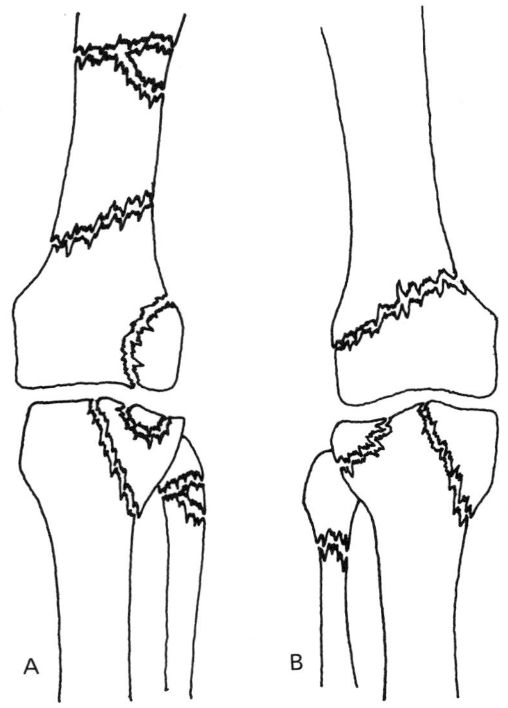

Figure 6-47. *A*, Fractures associated with rupture of the medial ligament; *B*, Fractures associated with rupture of the lateral ligament of the knee.

Ligament Injuries

A minor twisting strain with the knee in flexion results in a partial tear of the medial collateral ligament. Fractures of the tibia or femur may cause rupture of the ligaments (Figs. 6-47 and 6-48).

Violent abduction of the leg with the knee extended may cause the *unhappy triad*—a tearing of the medial collateral and, if the force continues, tearing of the anterior cruciate ligament and the medial meniscus. The tear in the ligament may occur anywhere in its length. It may be slight or complete and at the femoral end it may pull away a portion of the periosteum.

Tenderness over the femoral attachment of the medial collateral ligament indicates a partial tear of the ligament. When a complete tear is suspected palpate for tenderness first over the joint line and then check the tibial or femoral attachments.

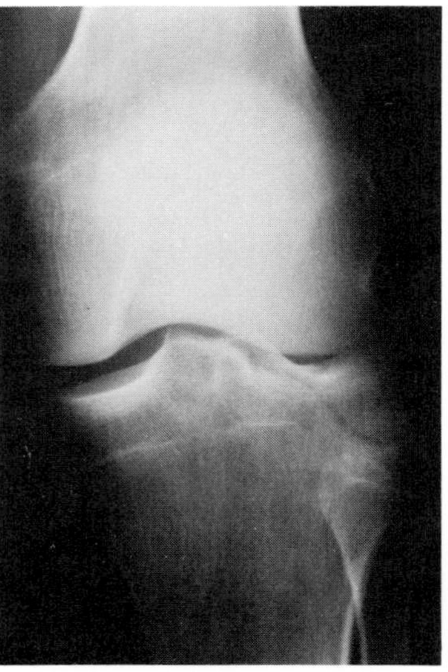

Figure 6-48. Fracture of the lateral tibial plateau with tear of the medial collateral ligament.

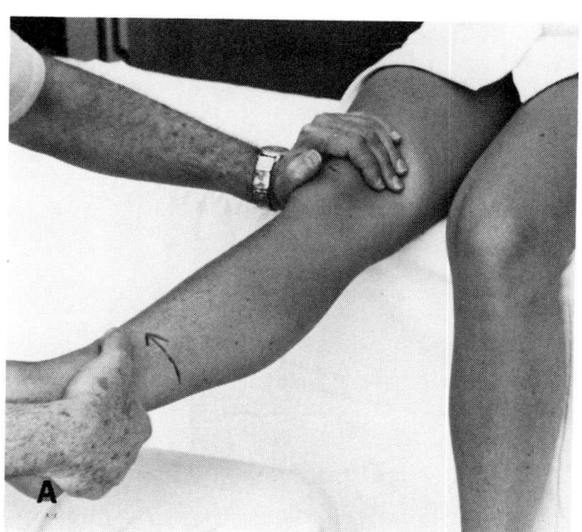

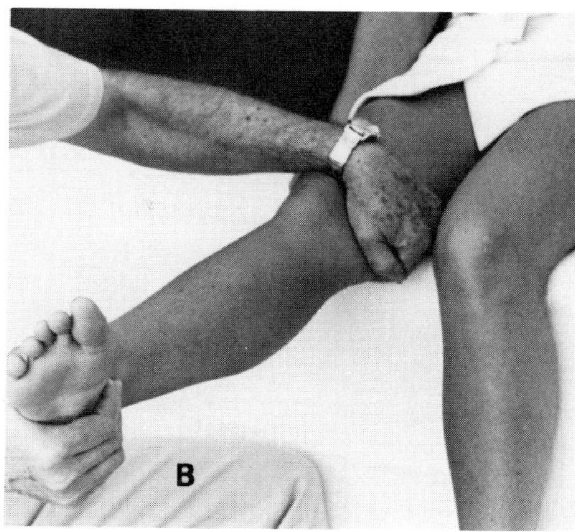

Figure 6-49. *A*, Abduction stress test for medial collateral ligament tear. The abduction test should be done with the knee fully extended and again flexed 30°. *B*, The adduction test for a tear of the lateral collateral ligament or lateral meniscus. If, while the knee is under stress, the tenderness is directly over the joint suspect meniscus injury; if over a ligamentous attachment suspect a ligament injury under the painful site.

Inspect for swelling and tenderness over the medial femoral condyle and palpate for tenderness in the same area. The abduction test for medial ligament injury is shown in Figure 6-49A and the adduction test for lateral collateral ligament tear or meniscus injury is illustrated in Figure 6-49B. Also perform the drawer test for cruciate ligament injury.

Treatment of sprains requires protection from further injury until local reaction has subsided. Apply ice packs and aspirate joint fluid or blood if necessary (see Chapter 7). Examine and x-ray to evaluate the extent of tearing and instability.

Wrap in compression dressing to minimize swelling (Fig. 6-50). Apply an elastic adhesive bandage from 4½ in below the patella to 4½ in above it. Select two rubber pads approximately 8 in long, 2 in wide and ¼ in thick. Place them longitudinally on each side of the patella and continue to wrap the bandage over them.

Early surgical repair is the treatment for complete rupture of the ligaments of the knee. Consequently, the decision of whether to operate or treat conservatively must be made early. The difficult decision is in differentiating a torn meniscus, which may be treated conservatively, and a ruptured ligament, which should be repaired early. If in doubt, call an orthopedic surgeon. If conservative treatment is chosen, the knee should be immobilized by a cotton cast, plaster splints or cylinder cast until symptoms subside and healing occurs.

Follow up with proper rehabilitation to regain muscle strength before strenuous activities are begun.

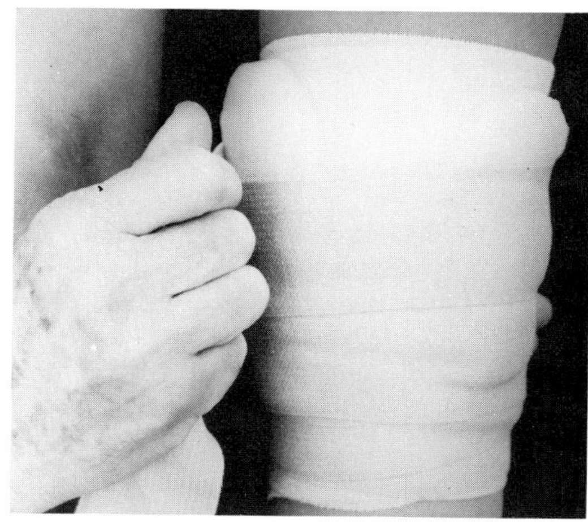

Figure 6-50. Pressure dressing for the knee.

Early activity reduces the rate of muscular atrophy, which may be found as early as the second post-injury day. Without rehabilitative exercise, orthopedists claim that muscular atrophy may proceed at the rate of 3 percent per day.

Start with straight-leg raising or, in the event the patient is an athlete, begin whirlpool bathing as quickly after the accident as possible. Instruct the patient to raise and hold the leg 10 to 15 seconds. Repeat five times in two sets four times daily. If straight-leg raising is too strenuous for the older patient, instruct him to straighten out both legs while sitting in a chair or lying in bed. When his legs are extended, have him tighten the thigh muscles by pressing the underside of his knee down against the bed. As muscle strength picks up have the patient place his hand under his knee and press down, contracting the thigh muscles and elevating the heel slightly. Repeat for 5 minutes every hour.

While the patient is in the same position with legs extended before him, have him point his big toe toward his knee without allowing the knee to move. This should be done 5 minutes every hour. Discontinue straight-leg raising when the knee is free of pain.

Have the patient exercise the knee and strengthen thigh muscles by raising his leg while sitting on a table. Determine the range of motion by what can be done without pain. Emphasize the importance of complete knee extension. Extend the leg at the knee joint ten times or in two sets of five times. Flex the leg to 90° at the knee joint the same number of times. If the leg does not fully extend, have the patient place a man's belt about his ankle and thus help the leg to full extension. Repeat four times daily until the muscles can fully extend the leg.

When the patient can raise his leg 2 to 4 times a day to full extension without assistance start him on weight lifting by having him hold 1½ lb for 6 sec with his leg fully extended. Repeat 10 times once daily adding weight as tolerated.

If these exercises cause no swelling nor soreness have the patient proceed to lifting weights from the hanging flexed position of the knee to full extension holding for the count of two. The maximum load is determined by the number of pounds the patient can lift 10 times. Have him start the set of exercises by lifting one fourth the maximum load 10 times. After a rest, he should lift half the maximum load 10 times and finally the full load 10 times. Have him determine his maximum load each 7 days until he reaches 50 to 75 lb.

If the patient is an athlete instruct him in crutch running for general conditioning. The nonathlete may use the exercise bicycle, swim or perform arm and trunk exercises or weight lifting to the point of breathlessness.

Have the patient begin weight bearing when he can lift a 10 lb weight 50 times, when he can fully extend his leg, when there is no evidence of swelling and when x-ray studies confirm healing.

Marcus Stewart uses the following criterion for postmeniscectomy activity. The patient may walk when he is able to lift a 10 lb weight 50 times. This may be in 3 days or 3 weeks. The high school athlete cannot return to full activity until he is able to lift 25 lb 50 times and the college athlete when he can lift 50 lb 50 times.

Finally, to give strength and confidence to the patient, have him step up 40 times on a 20-in stool, alternating legs and straightening both legs each time.

To take stress x-ray pictures of the knee joints, have the patient lie down with legs extended and place a pillow between his knees. Bring his ankles together and take an anteroposterior x-ray picture of both knees. A widening of the outer or lateral joint space indicates the external lateral ligaments are ruptured.

Put the pillow between the patient's ankles and force the patient's knees together to x-ray again. A widening of the inner or medial aspect of the knee demonstrates medial ligament damage.

Injured Menisci

Injuries to the menisci are the most common derangements of the knee joint. The medial meniscus is more frequently injured than the external. The injury is most likely to

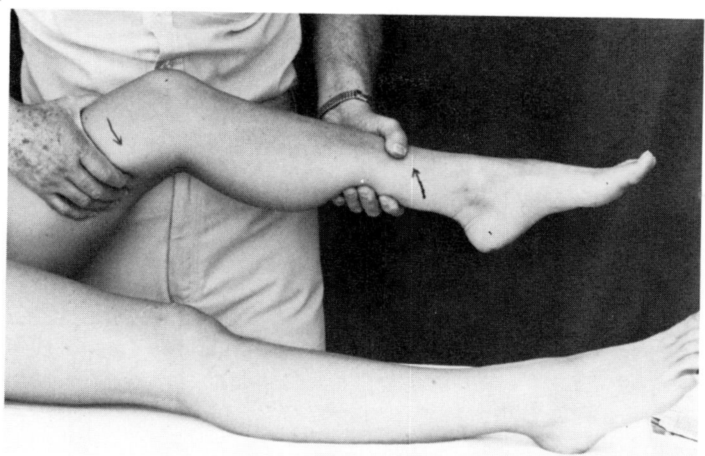

Figure 6-51. Test for knee locking. Check for complete extension and flexion. If the patient cannot fully extend her leg the chances are that she has a displaced meniscal tear. Loose bodies can also cause locking.

occur when the weight-bearing knee is flexed and the femur is internally rotated on the tibia while the foot is fixed. The same forces can rupture the internal collateral ligament. When a portion of the meniscus slips between the femur and the tibia, the knee locks and cannot be fully extended (Fig. 6-51).

Suspect meniscus injury rather than ligament injury if the pain is worse during the day and if the knee is less painful while walking down stairs.

With an acute injury the patient frequently complains of "something snapping" followed by severe pain and occasionally a locking. The diagnosis is simple if the knee is locked. When the knee becomes chronically deranged the locking may occur with the slightest provocation and the patient with the aid of friends may learn to unlock his knee. When the knee does not actually lock, the patient may be able to flex the leg but cannot extend it further than 150° to 160°. Remember locking occurs in only about 25 percent of the cases. The most common sign is tenderness over the tibial collateral ligament at the joint line when the knee is flexed.

Two tests will help confirm the suspected diagnosis of a meniscus injury, the McMurray and the Apley tests. To do the McMurray test (Fig. 6-52) place the patient in a

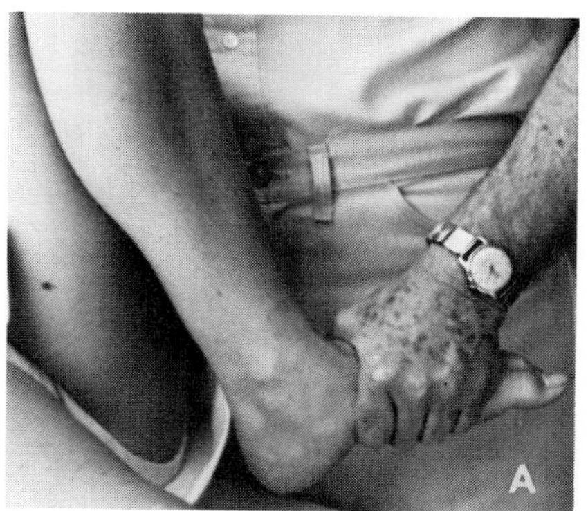

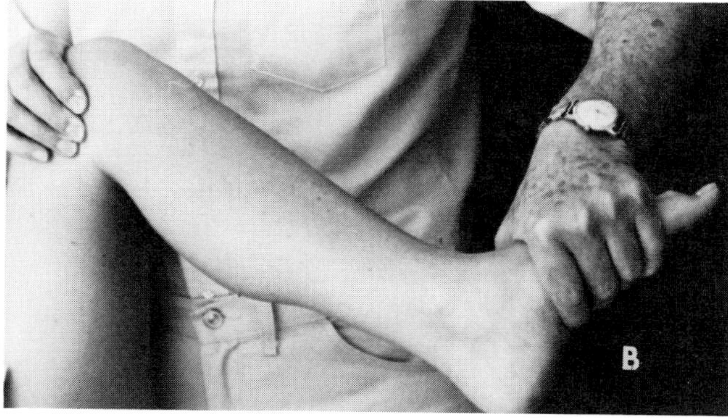

Figure 6-52. McMurray test for meniscus injury. *A*, Place the patient in supine position. Flex her knee until her heel is flush with her buttocks. Place the fingers of your right hand on the knee around the joint lines. Externally rotate her foot with your other hand. *B*, Hold your hands in the same position while the patient's leg is extended. Suspect a medial meniscus tear if a clock or abnormal motion with pain in the knee occurs. Check the lateral meniscus by performing the same test while the foot is internally rotated.

supine position. Flex her leg until her heel touches her buttocks. Place the fingers of your right hand on her knee around the joint line. Externally rotate her foot with your opposite hand. To test the posterior half of the medial meniscus continue holding her foot in lateral rotation and extend her knee while feeling and listening for a click. Clicking, pain or laxity indicates a medial meniscus tear. When looking for a lateral meniscus tear do the same maneuver but internally rotate the foot.

The Apley test actually involves several maneuvers (Figs. 6-53), some of which should cause pain. A positive Apley is more dependable than the McMurray test. Turn the patient over into a prone position. While the patient is lying with legs extended invert her foot and flex her leg to 90°. Repeat the maneuver while everting her foot. Pain is elicited if the test is positive for a meniscus tear. Continue the test by flexing her leg to 90° and forcefully rotating her foot in both ways. This is done to rule out a ligament tear or a rotational strain. Now press down on the foot and rotate again. If pain occurs in outward rotation, suspect an injury to the medial meniscus. To finish the test have an as-

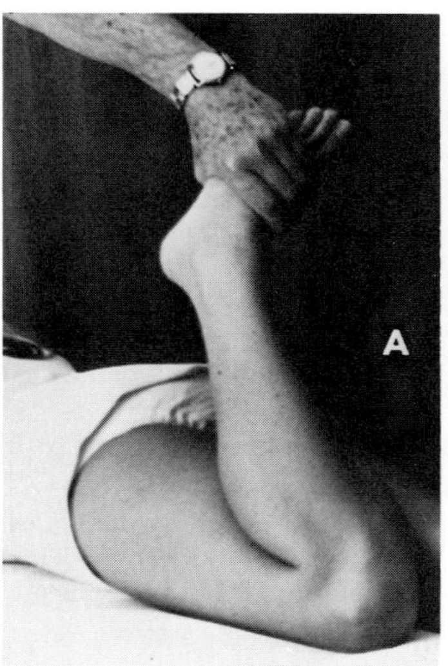

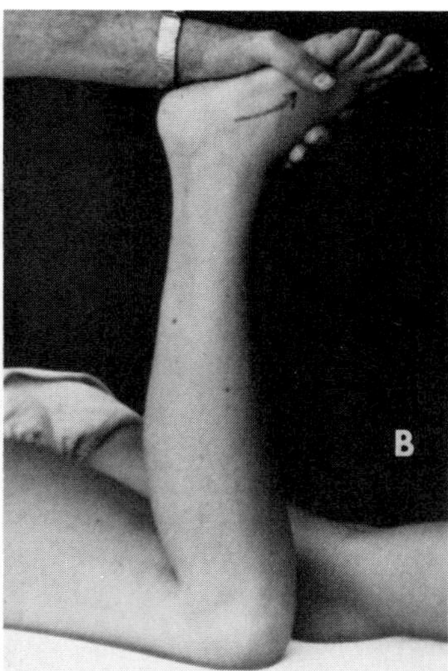

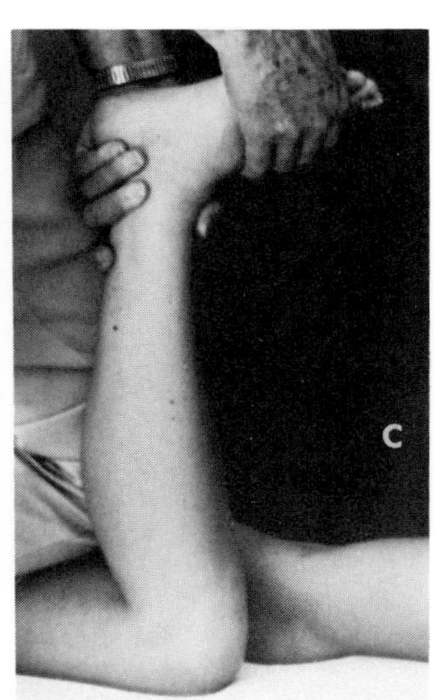

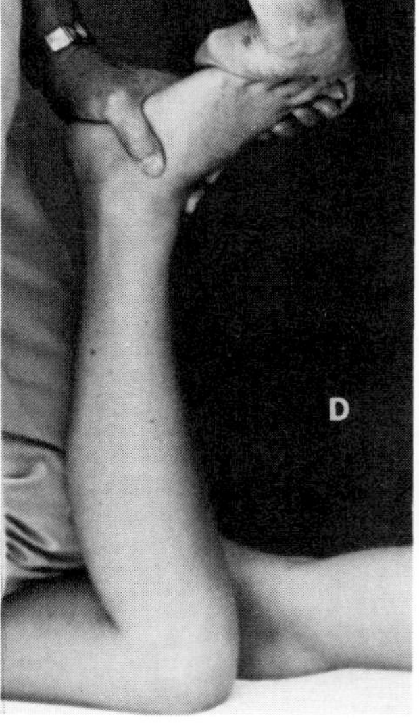

Figure 6-53. Apley test for meniscus injury. *A*, Place the patient in the prone position. Invert her foot and flex her knee past 90°. Repeat the test with her foot in eversion. Pain is elicited if the test is positive for a meniscus tear. *B*, With the patient in the same position flex her knee to 90°. Quickly rotate the foot internally and externally. This is done to rule out a ligament tear or a rotational strain. *C*, Continue the Apley test by fixing the patient's thigh to the examining table with your knee. Test her knee joint by lifting up on her ankle while rotating internally and externally. *D*, Press down on her leg while again rotating her knee internally and externally.

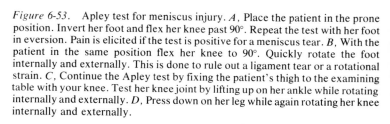

sistant fix the patient's thigh to the examining table and then, while her leg is still flexed 90°, pull up on the foot and again rotate both ways. If pain occurs while the foot is laterally rotated suspect an injury to the tibial collateral ligament. Apley's tests are positive for lateral meniscus tear when the maneuvers are reversed by inward rotation of the foot.

Pressure on the foot in the Apley test position (Fig. 6-54) increases pain in knee cartilage tears.

This is a good time to check the cruciate ligaments also. Instruct the patient to lie in the supine position with his knees flexed 90° and feet flat on the table. Grasp the leg below the knee with both hands and alternately push and pull the leg backwards and forwards. Suspect a torn posterior cruciate ligament with excessive posterior mobility and a torn anterior cruciate ligament with excessive anterior mobility (Fig. 6-55).

Another test, the Childress' duck-waddle, is a strenuous test but applicable to testing athletes. Have the patient squat and waddle on his toes, swinging from side to side. He will be unable to completely flex his legs and pain or clicking will occur if there is rupture of the posterior horn of the medial meniscus.

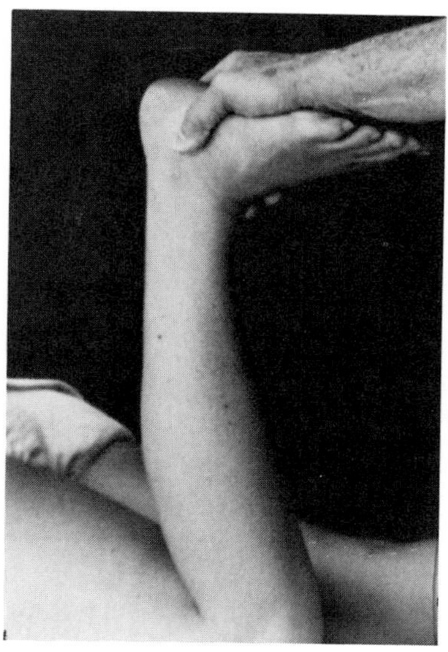

Figure 6-54. Pressure on the foot increases pain in knee cartilage tears.

A suspected meniscus tear should be verified by conventional x-rays as well as double contrast arthrogram. This is possible because torn menisci can be treated conservatively, delaying surgery until a final evaluation is made several weeks or months later.

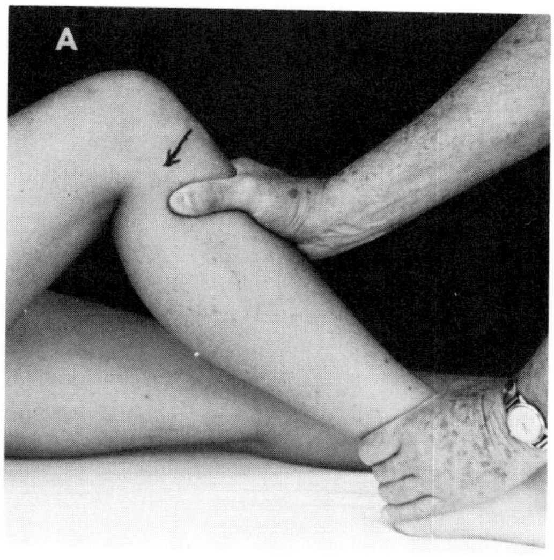

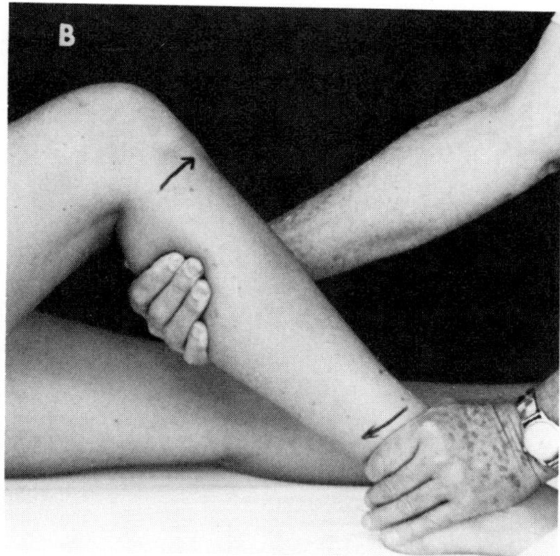

Figure 6-55. *A*, Testing for a posterior cruciate ligament tear; *B*, Testing for an anterior cruciate ligament tear.

In treatment aspirate any effusion present. Anesthetize the local points of tenderness with 1 percent Xylocaine. Occasionally a general anesthesia may be necessary.

Allow the leg to hang over the end of the table. Pull down on the ankle and, while abducting and externally rotating the leg, rapidly extend it. When the meniscus is reduced the leg can be fully extended. Immobilize the joint for 4 to 6 weeks with a cast or a gelatin boot plus a posterior plaster splint. Wedge the heel up $^1/_8$ to $^5/_{16}$ of an inch and allow the patient to walk on the leg.

Surgery is advisable if the diagnosis of a meniscus injury with displacement with or without locking is confirmed. Advise rehabilitation exercises as for ligament tears, mentioned previously.

Fractures of the Patella

Order an x-ray of the knee and search first for a simple fissure or stellate fracture without displacement and secondly for a patellar fracture with displacement.

If there is more than a 2 to 3 mm separation of patellar fragments consider hospitalization and surgical repair (Fig. 6-56). Ordinarily open repair should be done by an orthopedic surgeon, because not only may the patella need encircling wire but also the medial and lateral capsule may need catgut repair.

If there is no separation of fragments but only an undisplaced line or stellate fracture, apply a pressure dressing, splint, aspirate and elevate until swelling subsides. Apply a cylinder cast for 4 to 6 weeks. Rehabilitative physical therapy with heat, massage, isometric exercises and flexion and extension will hasten recovery.

Dislocation of the Patella

To reduce a dislocated patella, have an assistant raise the hyperextended knee, flexing the thigh on the abdomen. This maneuver will relax the quadriceps and allow reduction of the patella by simple pressure in the appropriate direction. Immobilize with a posterior splint and apply

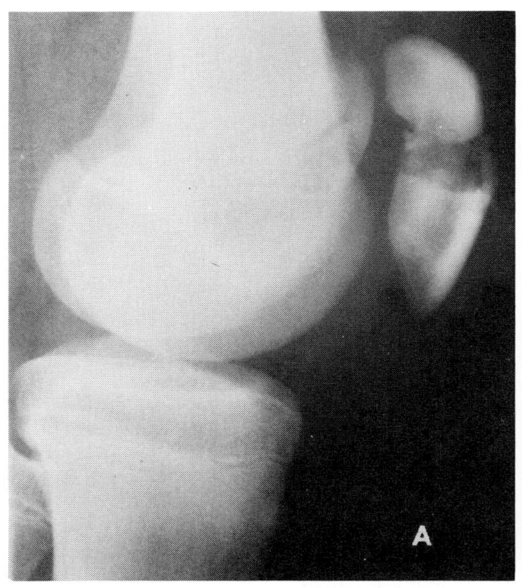

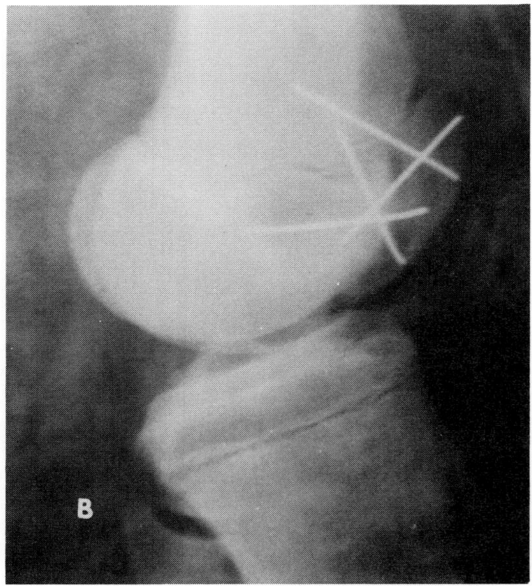

Figure 6-56. *A*, Fractures of the patellar and lower femur. Patellar fragments separated more than 3 mm will need surgical repair. *B*, Fracture of the articular surface of the femur immobilized by pins. This comminuted fracture has been surgically excised and the tendons repaired.

a pressure dressing and ice bags. Allow the patient to walk immediately but continue the use of the posterior splint for 4 weeks.

Fractures of the Tibial Tuberosities

X-ray examination may show either or both tibial tuberosities broken (Fig. 6-57). Clinical examination may indicate other disarrangements of the knee, particularly a rupture of the opposing lateral ligament.

Institute emergency treatment while awaiting x-ray study. This includes aspiration, pressure dressings, splint, elevation and ice bags. Two important points to remember: Examine for and record the results of any peroneal nerve injury. Can the patient dorsiflex the big toe? Is there anesthesia of the dorsum of the foot or lateral ankle?

Take x-rays with precision. Obtain a true anteroposterior view. Place the legs and feet exactly parallel to each other in the long axis of the body and include in the picture a considerable length of the tibia and femur. If the amount of displacement of the fragment is still questionable, obtain an x-ray of the good knee for comparison.

Fractures of both tuberosities of the tibia are rather serious. Hospitalization and speciality care is indicated unless the family physician is experienced in their treatment.

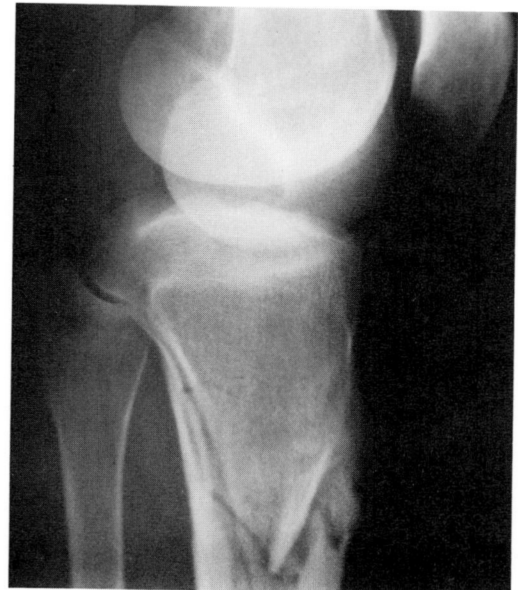

Figure 6-57. Crushing fracture of proximal end of the tibia. Consideration should be given to accurate reduction and fixation with threaded pins.

Reduce the fragment to a near-perfect position (Figs. 6-58 and 6-59). For fractures

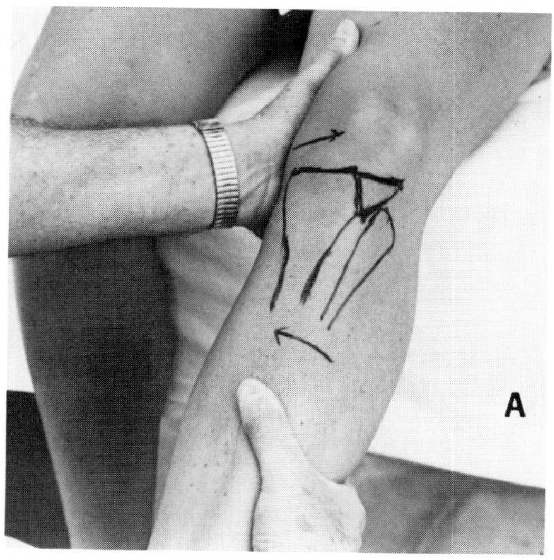

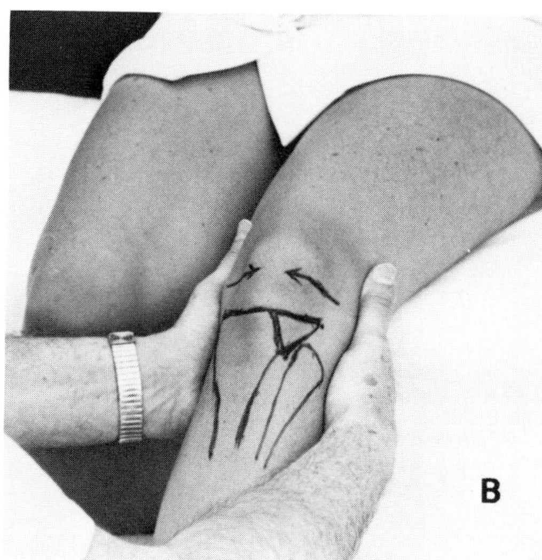

Figure 6-58. Correction of displacement of the outer tuberosity of the tibia (see Fig. 6-59). *A*, Forced adduction of the leg corrects the downward displacement of the tuberosity and, *B*, lateral compression helps correct the widening.

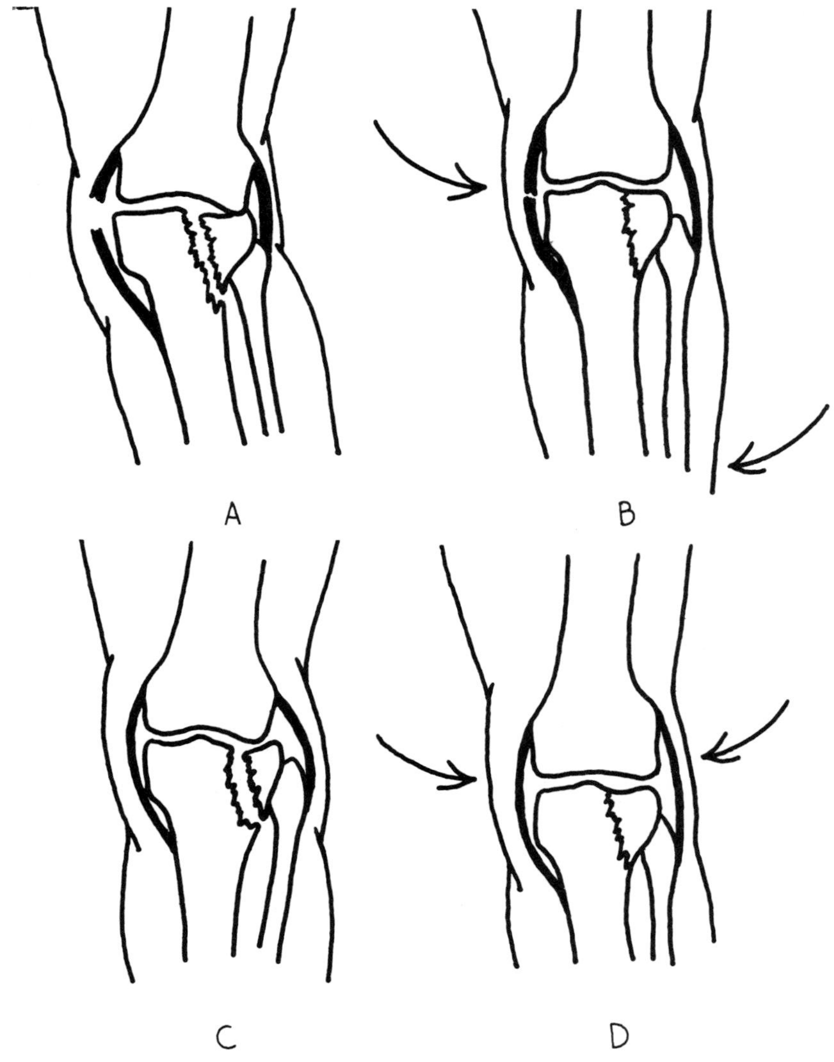

Figure 6-59. *A*, Displacement of the outer tuberosity of the tibia; *B*, Forced adduction of the leg with counterpressure on the inner knee corrects the downward displacement of the tuberosity; *C*, Displacement; *D*, Lateral compression with the palms of the hand corrects the widening (see Fig. 6-58). Orthopedists have been known to use a wood vice to correct the widening.

of the lateral tuberosity place the palm of one hand on the medial aspect of the knee for counterpressure. Grasp the leg below the calf with the opposite hand and adduct the leg. Pay little heed to an associated fracture of the head of the fibula. Concentrate on a near perfect apposition of the tibial tuberosity. Reverse the maneuver if the medial tuberosity is broken. Plaster splint and cast the leg from the ankle to midthigh for 8 to 10 weeks. If this simple maneuver does not reduce the tuberosity it is probably displaced downward and impacted. Reduction may be difficult in this case. Hospitalize the patient and seek orthopedic consultation. In adults open reduction with elevation of the fragment and fixation with screws and bolts may be necessary.

If reduction is satisfactory apply a walking iron or heel. The patient should use

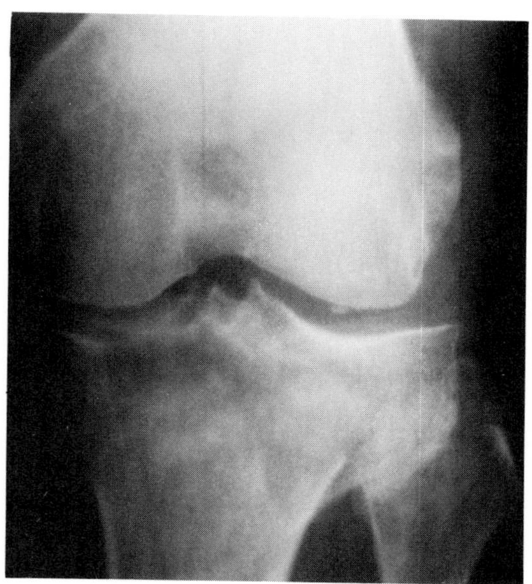

Figure 6-60. Fracture of the lateral plateau. If depressed, these fractures are best treated by open reduction, accurate alignment of joint surfaces, fixation by threaded pins or screws and removal of displaced semilunar cartilages or repair of torn cruciate ligaments.

crutches for walking but use the leg as much as possible. Recheck x-rays in a week. Good results can be anticipated with rehabilitative exercises. In many instances it is wise to have the patient use a pick-up walker for 2 to 3 months.

Warn the patient about the intra-articular nature of the fracture, i.e., ensuing traumatic arthritis and the relaxing of supports about the knee. Remember the soft tissue injury may be as important, or more so, than the fracture.

Consider open reduction with screw or metal fixation (Fig. 6-60) in long oblique fractures that appear vulnerable to slipping.

Bursitis about the Knee

Four bursae of clinical importance surround the knee joint. The largest bursa, the infrapatellar, lies between the quadriceps tendon and the femur. The smallest bursa lies between the patellar ligament and the infrapatellar fat pad. The most prominent lies between the skin and patella. The fourth lies between the skin and the tibial tuberosity.

Trauma or disease may cause the bursae to fill with synovial fluid, blood or pus. Effusion in the infrapatellar bursa causes a horseshoe-appearing swelling about the patella. This bursa is continuous with the knee joint.

To examine for joint effusion, lay one hand over the suprapatellar area with the fingers encircling the patella and push gently against the swelling while the index finger of the other hand pushes the patella downward. If sufficient fluid is present in the joint the patella will suddenly strike the femur causing a palpable click. Detect small amounts of fluid by compressing the fluid from one of the hollows about the patellar ligament. Free the hollow and watch it fill with fluid.

Be on the alert for the following diseases of the bursae:

–infrapatellar bursitis (clergyman's knee) to be distinguished from liposynovitis infrapatellaris (Hoffa's disease)
–morrant Baker's cyst (popliteal cyst) in midline of the popliteal space
–semimembranous bursitis in the medial popliteal space
–anserine bursitis as a fluctuant swelling on the medial aspect of the knee

Do not confuse the following diseases with bursitis:

–popliteal aneurysm
–neuromyxofibroma with its characteristic pain radiating down into the foot
–popliteal abscess
–rupture of the rectus femoris muscle with loss of muscle mass in the suprapatellar area
–rupture of the patellar ligament with an upward shift of the patella
–chrondromalacia patellae with degeneration of the articular surface of the patella (pressing the patella against the condyles causes tenderness)

Knee Joint "Mice"

Loose bodies in the knee joint cause recurrent pain, effusions and locking. Diagnose by x-ray examination, which may show shadows suggestive of chips of bone, an osteophyte from osteoarthritis or a flake of bone from osteochondritis dissecans.

Fractures and Injuries to the Leg

March Gangrene

March gangrene is an ischemic necrosis of the anterior leg muscles. The condition is overlooked by family physicians and orthopedists alike. Any physician treating athletes should keep the possibility of ischemic necrosis in mind. The symptoms begin several hours after vigorous exercise of the legs as that undertaken during a football game. The patient complains of stiffness and pain. Inspect the muscles in the anterior tibial muscular compartment for swelling, tenderness and warmth. Act promptly. Gangrene with atrophy will result if the fascial sheath holding the muscles is not incised.

Fracture of the Shaft of the Tibia

Take x-rays to confirm the type and extent of the fracture but finding localized tenderness along the easily palpable tibial ridge and pain at the site of the injury on percussion of the heel are highly suggestive of a fracture. Roll a pencil over the tibial ridge to detect the exact location of the fracture.

Treat undisplaced fractures of the tibia, whether of the transverse, oblique or slightly comminuted types, on an outpatient basis. But in long oblique fractures that appear vulnerable to slipping, consider screw or metal fixation in open reduction. Fractures in the upper half, particularly the upper third, of the tibia heal rapidly in 6 to 8 weeks. Search carefully for evidence of an actual or threatened compound fracture. If suspected, hospitalize and seek consultation. Hospitalize also for much soft tissue injury or if the circulation seems impaired. Adjust any minor displacement by traction and local pressure. Immobilize with a plaster cylinder cast from the foot to the upper thigh. Avoid angulation or rotation by checking leg alignment. A string anchored at the anterosuperior spine and running down, bisecting the patella, should end between the great and second toe. In children look for an associated epiphyseal injury or separation.

Recheck the x-rays. If minor angulation persists cut a wedge out of the appropriate side of the cast at the level of the fracture (Fig. 6-61). Cut the opposite side of the cast so that the angulation can be corrected. Reinforce with fresh plaster, but be careful because some skin is irritated by plaster.

A stress fracture of the tibia is an incomplete fracture and results from repeated strenuous use of the leg. The fracture is frequently overlooked for the pain may resemble claudication coming on with the exercise

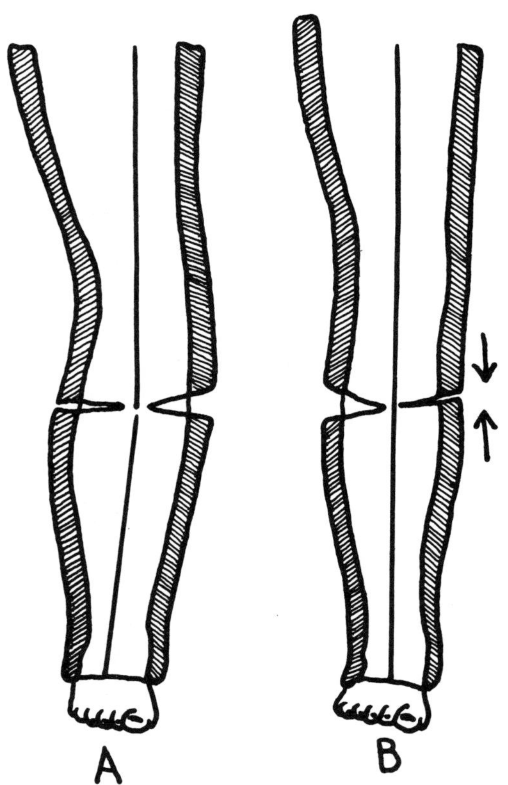

Figure 6-61. Wedging a cast. *A*, If the lower leg is set in an exaggerated lateral position, *B*, remove a wedge from the cast and readjust the angle.

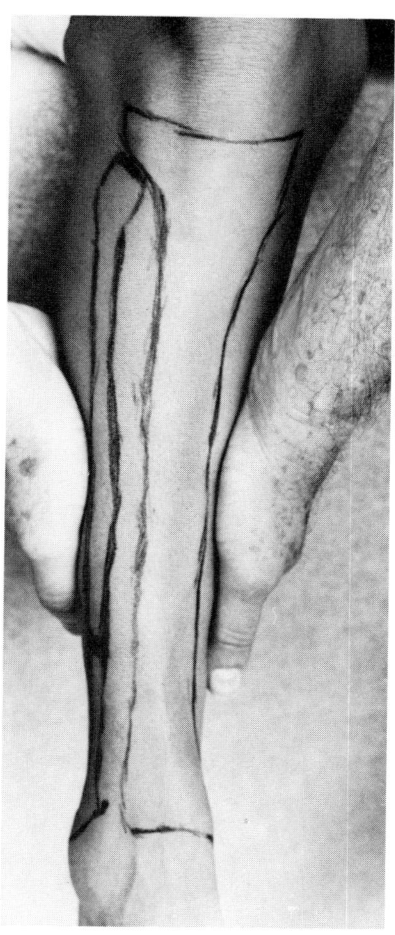

Figure 6-62. Fractures of the lower third of the fibula are best detected by squeezing the tibia against the fibula.

of walking and is dull aching in nature. To diagnose, spring the tibia by grasping the tibia at both ends and pull against your knee as one would break light kindling. X-rays are frequently negative.

With displacement, adults frequently need the fracture site infiltrated with 1 percent Xylocaine. In youngsters with displacement, a general anesthetic will probably be necessary. These are best cared for by a specialist.

Immobilize with a plaster cast 8 to 10 weeks for children and 10 to 16 weeks for adults.

Occasionally recheck position by x-ray. Keep the cast on until callus is demonstrated.

Fracture of the Shaft of the Fibula

Fractures of the fibula are often overlooked because the patient can walk. Generally an examiner can compress the fibula against the tibia and feel the fibula spring back (Fig. 6-62). In complete fracture the spring is lost and the maneuver causes pain at the fracture site.

Reduction and casting is seldom necessary. Occasionally inversion of the foot while the knee is flexed will improve the position. Watch for peroneal nerve injury.

A gelatin boot for 4 weeks will alleviate some pain and repeated infiltration of 1 percent Xylocaine will also prove helpful.

Fractures of the neck of the fibula do not uniformly do well. Request consultation if in doubt. Otherwise the prognosis is excellent.

Fractures of the Shafts of Both Bones of the Leg

This injury is the most common cause of a compound fracture of the leg (Fig. 6-63). When the fracture is complete the foot is turned outward in obvious deformity. Do

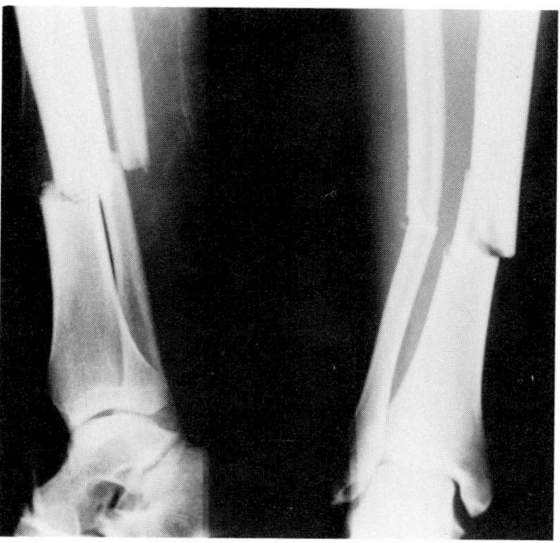

Figure 6-63. Fractures of the lower third of the tibia and fibula.

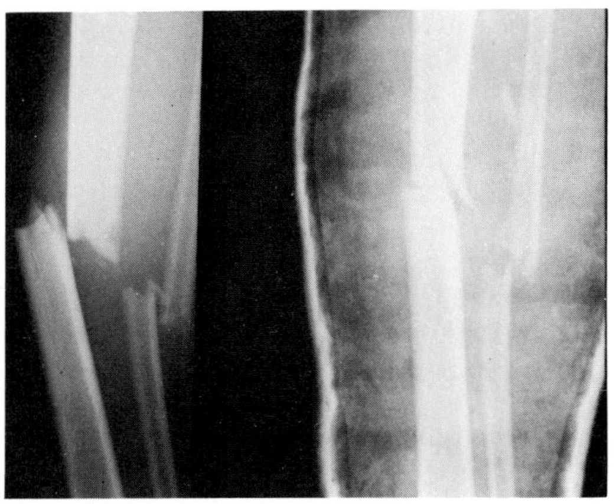

Figure 6-64. Fractures of the tibia and fibula *Left*, before and, *Right*, after reduction.

not manipulate until the arterial pulse is checked. Hospitalize and request consultation.

Fractures of both bones in the upper and middle third in good position may be immobilized in a circular cast for 10 to 12 weeks. Check the position frequently by x-rays (Fig. 6-64). Use the same treatment principles as previously outlined for fracture of the shaft of the tibia.

Fractures and Injuries to the Ankle

Inspect the ankle as early as possible. The anatomic landmarks are more visible and the points of tenderness more accurately

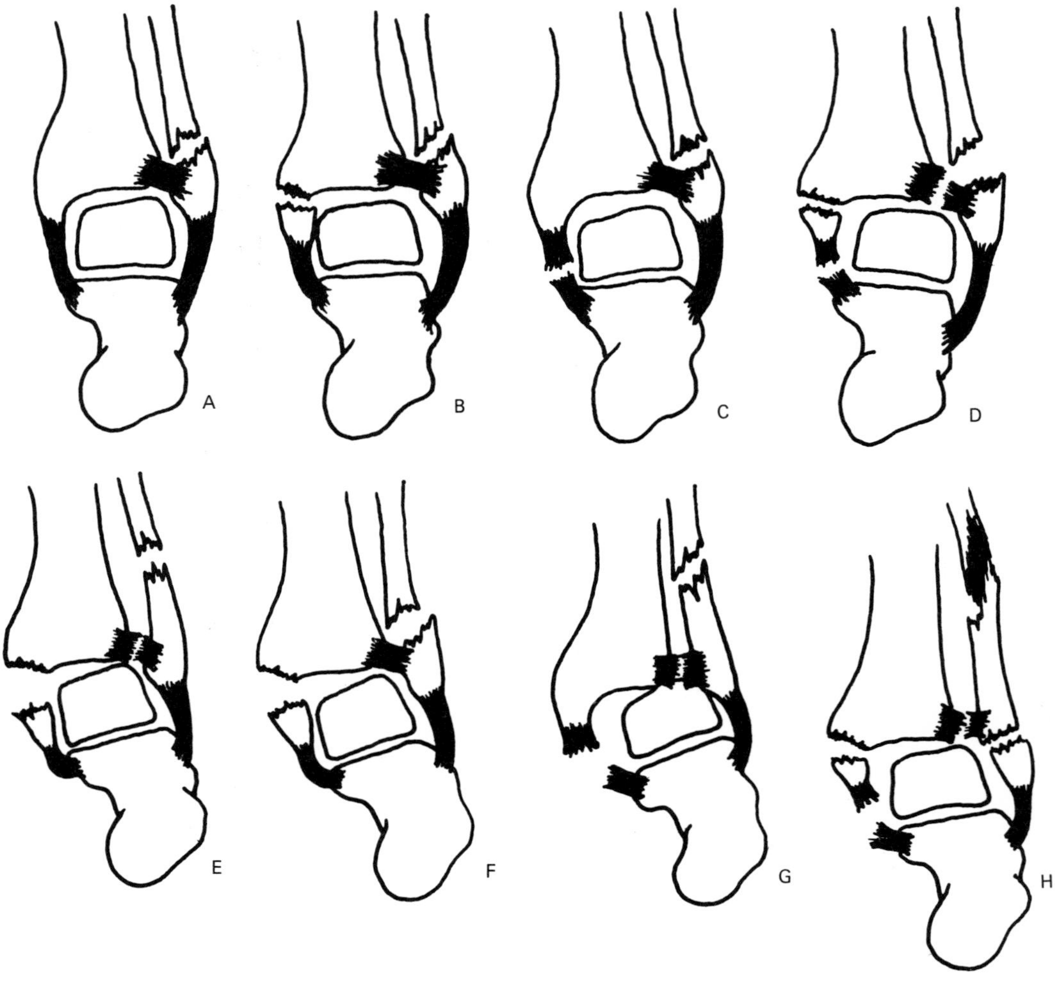

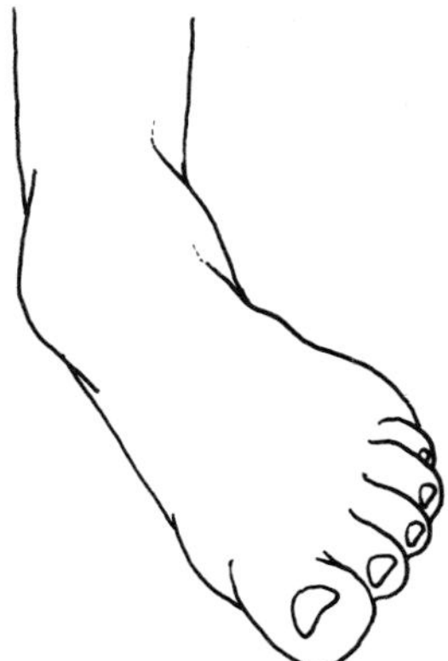

Figure 6-66. Fracture with foot thrust forward. Also called abduction, Pott's and eversion-external rotation fracture.

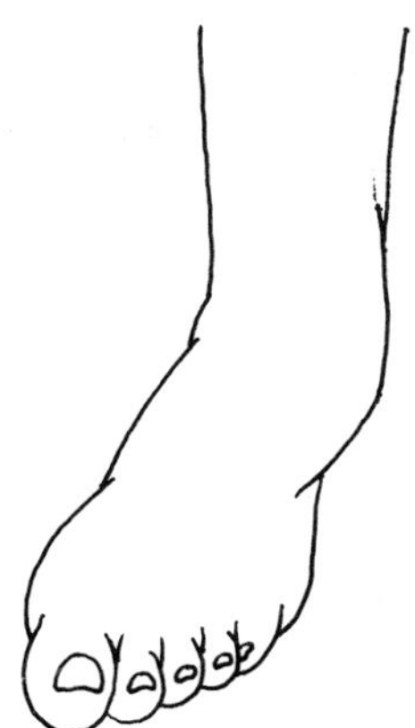

Figure 6-67. Fracture with inward dislocation of the foot. Also called reversed Pott's, inversion-internal rotation and adduction fracture.

palpated before swelling and internal bleeding occurs.

If possible determine how the injury occurred. Was the injury caused by eversion-external rotation of the foot, inversion-internal rotation of the foot, forward or backward thrust against the articular surface of the tibia or upward thrust against the articular surface of the tibia?

Knowing the nature of the force that caused the injury will help the examiner establish the type of disarrangement or fracture (Fig. 6-65). Injuries of eversion-external rotation are caused by forcible eversion or abduction of the foot and external rotation when the long axis of the talus is violently twisted about on its vertical axis, wedging the malleoli apart.

The major strain is on the internal lateral ligament or the internal malleolus. If the internal lateral ligament holds, then the internal malleolus may be broken off transversely. If the force continues the talus and foot will jam against the external malleolus, first rupturing the tibiofibular ligament and then breaking the external malleolus and even the shaft of the fibula somewhere proximal to the ankle. If the tibiofibular ligament holds, a fracture at the base of the external malleolus occurs. With this injury the foot is displaced outward (Fig. 6-66) and is commonly referred to as an abduction fracture. On x-ray study the talus and all broken parts tend to move laterally. The patient cannot walk or stand.

Injuries of the inversion-internal rotation type (Fig. 6-67) are caused by forces opposite to the eversion-external rotation forces, i.e. the foot is turned in, the talus again is turned on its vertical axis but inward wedging forces the malleoli apart. The strain falls on the tibiofibular and the external lateral ligaments and may fracture the external malleolus at the level of the upper border of the talus.

Figure 6-65. A, Eversion-external rotation (adduction) fractures; *B,* Fracture of fibula with fracture of the inner malleolus (bimalleoli); *C,* Fracture of fibula with tear of the internal lateral ligament; *D,* Fracture of fibula, tip of tibia, tearing of tibiofibular ligament and sometimes the interal lateral ligament; *E,* Fractures of internal malleolus and fibula with rupture of the tibiofibular ligament and lateral displacement of the talus; *F,* Fractures of internal and external malleoli and lateral displacement of talus with tibiofibular ligament intact; *G,* Fracture of lower third of the fibula with rupture of the internal lateral and tibiofibular ligaments and lateral displacement of the talus; *H,* Fractures of fibula and internal malleolus with rupture of the tibiofibular ligament and lateral displacement of the talus.

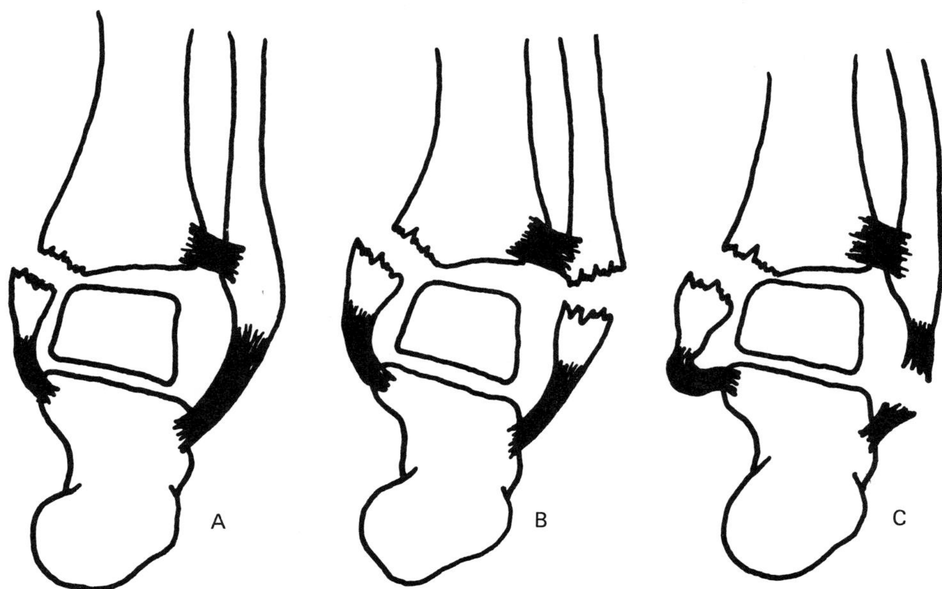

Figure 6-68. Inversion-internal rotation (abduction) fractures. *A*, Simple fracture of internal malleolus; *B*, Fracture of both malleoli; *C*, Fracture of internal malleolus and rupture of external lateral ligament.

Then if the force continues the talus impinges against the internal malleolus, breaking it vertically (Fig. 6-68). When the foot is displaced inward the fracture is referred to as the adduction or bimalleolar fracture.

Injuries by forward or backward thrust against the tibia: If force is applied while the foot is dorsiflexed (Fig. 6-69), the anterior margin of the tibia may be broken off and the foot dislocated forward (Fig. 6-70).

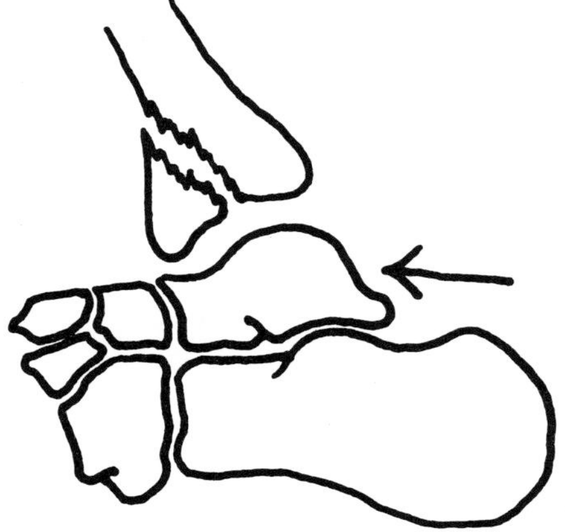

Figure 6-69. Fracture of the anterior margin of the tibial articular surface caused by excessive dorsiflexion, a violent forward thrust of the foot or a fall on the foot.

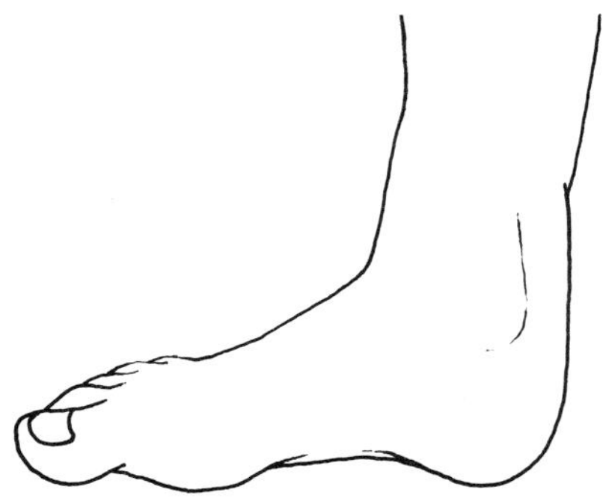

Figure 6-70. Fracture with anterior dislocation of the foot.

If force is applied while the foot is plantar-flexed, the posterior margin of the tibia breaks off and the foot is dislocated backward (Figs. 6-71 and 6-72). If force has been sufficient both the medial and lateral malleoli are broken. This is often called the trimalleolar fracture. The backward dislocation of the foot with the posterior fracture of the tibia is often associated with the eversion-external rotation type injury.

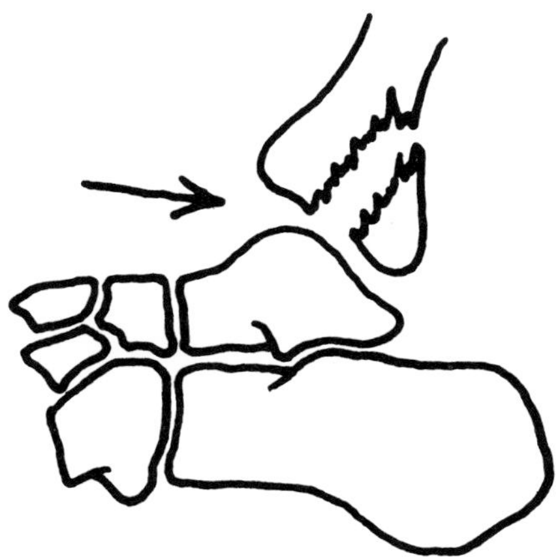

Figure 6-71. Fracture of the posterior margin of the tibia! articular surface with posterior dislocation of the foot. This is caused by a backward thrust on the foot or excessive external rotation. It is often associated with abduction fractures.

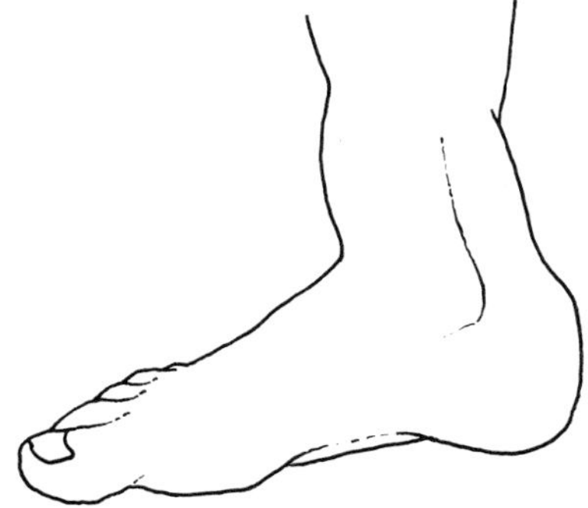

Figure 6-72. Cotton's fracture, fracture with backward dislocation of the foot.

A rare fracture occurs following abrupt upward thrust against the articular surface of the tibia. It is referred to as the compression type fracture. The talus is driven up between the fibula and tibia, crushing or splintering the articular surface of the tibia (Fig. 6-73).

In your initial examination look for deformity, swelling, ecchymosis or bleb formation, acute points of tenderness and increased joint laxity or mobility.

Characteristic deformity indicating foot displacement may be visible before swelling occurs. Lateral, anterior or posterior displacement of the foot indicates disruption of the joint.

Search for tenderness. Palpate the outer malleolus. If there is point tenderness of the malleolus, suspect a fracture. If the point tenderness is below the malleolus suspect a sprain of the external lateral ligament. In general, tenderness over the external and internal lateral ligaments or the tibiofibular indicates sprain or rupture of these ligaments. Check the entire fibula for point tenderness and the space anterior to the Achilles tendon (Fig. 6-74). Squeeze the tibia and fibula in the calf area to elicit pain in the lower fibula. If compression of the calf causes pain in the ankle suspect a fracture in the lower fibula.

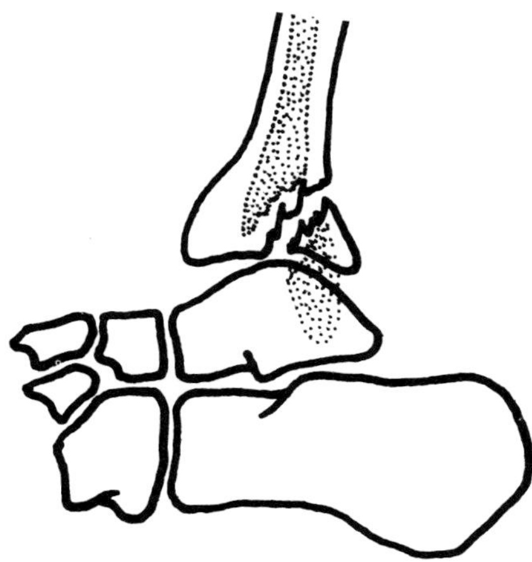

Figure 6-73. A complicated fracture of the posterior margin of the tibial articular surface plus a fracture-dislocation of the fibula.

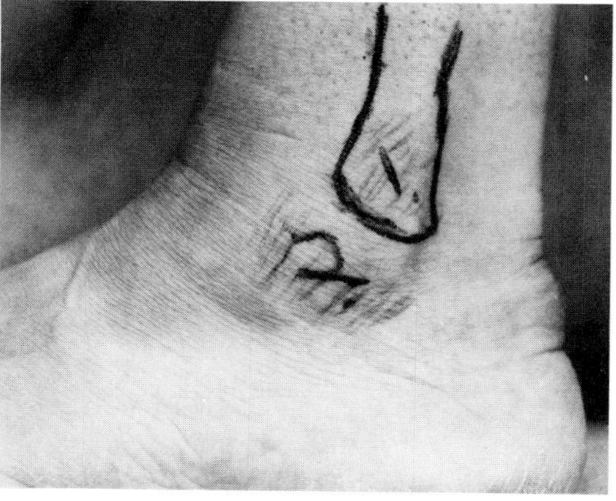

Figure 6-74. Injuries to the ankle: *1*, Tenderness over the distal end of the fibula suggests fracture; *2*, Tenderness distal to the fibula suggests ligamentous sprain or strain.

Grasp the heel and press gently but firmly medially and laterally. Compare the mobility with the uninjured foot. X-ray films may be unreliable if the joint is not manipulated to the point of maximum pain and dislocation. If still in doubt test for increased mobility under local anesthesia (5 to 10 ml of 1 percent Xylocaine in each side) and again check anteroposterior x-ray views in forced eversion and inversion. Check all suspicious laxity again if and when the patient is anesthetized. Push the foot backward and forward medially and laterally using the ankle as a fulcrum. If the above maneuvers reveal any dislocations, a simple cast is insufficient. Consult an orthopedist regarding stabilization measures.

X-ray films should be inspected for fractures of the malleoli, disruption of the articular surface of the tibia, separation of the tibia from the fibula and displacement of the talus. The articular surface of the talus lies anatomically exactly below the articular surface of the tibia and fits nicely between the malleoli. When in doubt about displacement compare the x-ray picture with one taken of the uninjured ankle.

Remove the shoe for emergency treatment. Leave the tape on if the victim is a football player. Apply ice preferably within 30 seconds. If needed continue cold therapy for 48 hours. If the ankle is to be splinted, pack ice in and about the splint. Do not attempt to reduce the ankle on a football field or other inconvenient place. Wrap the foot, ankle and leg with an elastic bandage to reduce swelling.

Immobilize the ankle for transportation. If no commercial splints are available, immobilization can be obtained by strapping two padded boards to the sides of the legs (Fig. 6-75A). The splints should reach from the heel to the knee. Keep the foot from dangling by strapping the foot to the splints with a figure-of-eight dressing. In an emergency a pillow splint can be used (Fig. 6-75B).

Use a local or, if needed, a general anesthetic for reduction. Flex legs on thigh during reduction to relax the calf muscles.

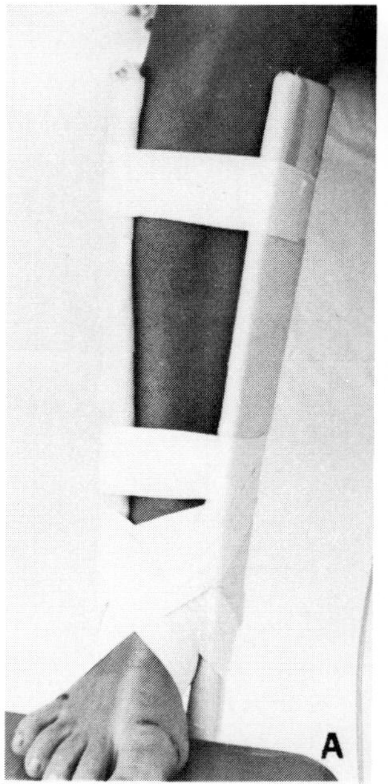

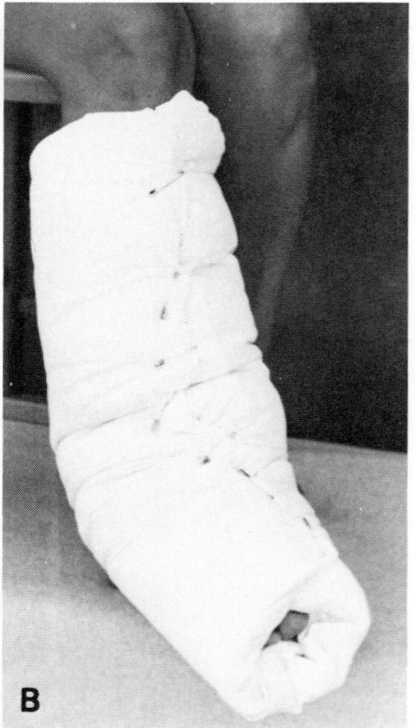

Figure 6-75. *A*, Application of wooden splints for first-aid treatment of ankle fracture. The pressure dressing has been omitted for clarity. *B*, Use a pillow splint for immobilizing the ankle and foot.

Fracture of Either Malleoli in Good Position and Without Torn Ligaments

Support a fracture of this type with pressure dressings with firm adhesive strapping, an elastic adhesive bandage or a gelatin boot. If the fracture is slight such as a fissure fracture an injection of a few ml of 1 percent Xylocaine at intervals of 2 days may keep the patient comfortable. Within 3 to 4 days the patient should be able to walk without pain. Reapply the dressing when it becomes loose. Replace with an elastic ankle support in 3 to 4 weeks.

If the fracture is comminuted or displacement appears likely, immobilize with a padded cast as soon as the swelling subsides.

Fractures of Both Malleoli in Good Position with a Fracture of the Tibia in Good Position

Apply an unpadded cast for 6 to 8 weeks for these fractures. Follow with a gelatin boot for another 4 weeks. For best results wedge up the heel $^1/_8$ to $^3/_{16}$ of an in and wear an elastic ankle support for 3 to 6 months.

Fracture of Eversion-External Rotation with Displacement

Plan immediate reduction of these fractures, also known as Pott's fracture or abduction fracture (Fig. 6-76). Inject 10 ml of 1 percent Xylocaine for local anesthesia in each fracture site and wait 10 to 15 min before attempting reduction. If the patient cooperates poorly administer a general anesthetic.

Allow the patient's leg to hang over the edge of the operating table with the knee flexed. Grasp the inner side of the leg above the ankle with one hand and with the other press firmly inward on the heel and outer malleolus.

Apply two 4 to 6 in plaster splints, one on each side of the leg, reaching from the knee down the leg and across the sole of the foot. Keep the foot at right angles, but not inverted or everted. Bind the two splints together with gauze. Mold the plaster about the heel and outer malleolus until the plaster dries. Mold into adduction, overcorrecting. Wrap the splints in an elastic bandage from toes to knee.

Check x-ray pictures and, if reduction is unsatisfactory, repeat reduction. If reduction is satisfactory keep the leg elevated and the ankle under ice for 24 to 48 hr. Remove the bandages when the swelling has subsided. Do not disturb the splints unless they do not fit well. Otherwise wrap the leg with wet plaster bandages. If the splints need changing do so and reapply the splints with the same heel pressure as when the first splints were applied. Add a walking heel or iron and maintain the cast for 6 to 8 wk. Allow the patient to walk without crutches.

Replace the cast with a gelatin boot from the toes to the knee and wedge up the medial side of the heel $^1/_8$ to $^3/_{16}$ of an inch.

In some instances the eversion-external rotation fracture is associated with a fracture of the posterior margin of the tibial articular surface with posterior dislocation of the foot.

Start reduction by pulling the foot forward and, while dorsiflexing, reduce the lateral

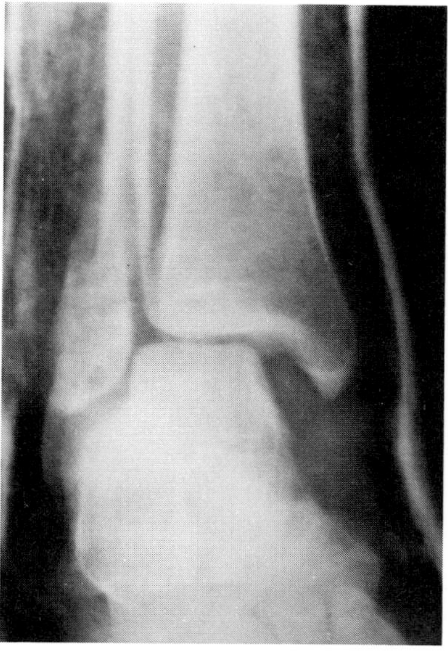

Figure 6-76. Abduction fracture of ankle with laceration of internal lateral ligament, separation of articulation of tibia and fibula, lateral displacement of talus, fracture of lower third of the fibula and laceration of tibiofibular ligament.

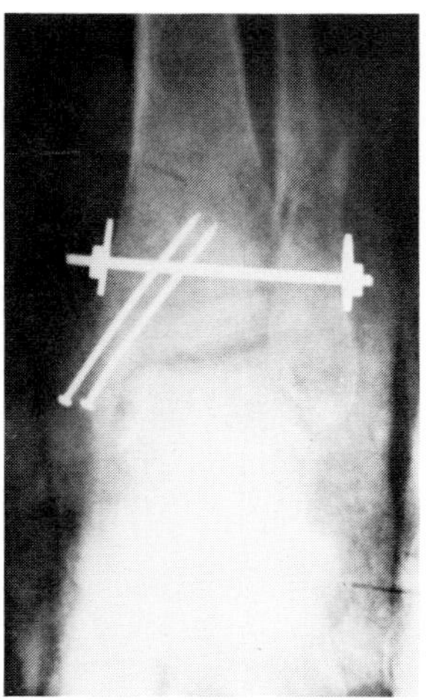

Figure 6-77. Ankle fracture. The ankle remained unsatisfactory until the joint was stabilized with a through-and-through screw.

displacement as in the simpler eversion-external rotation fractures and apply the lateral splints. Have an assistant hold the ankle's position while the cast is drying. Keep pressure on the lateral malleolus while the assistant holds the foot forward and dorsiflexed. Convert the splints into a cast when the swelling has subsided and keep the ankle casted for 8 to 10 wk.

Again in these abduction fractures the external malleolus may be displaced outward, the intermalleolar space widened but no fracture of the inner malleolus found. Suspect rupture of the internal lateral and the tibiofibular ligaments. To verify the suspicion, take x-rays while the foot is forcibly everted. Reduce the cast as in all eversion-external rotation fractures.

Fractures with Displacement of the Malleoli and/or the Talus

These are serious injuries and great disability may result if the most accurate reduction is not obtained (Fig. 6-77). Hospitalize and seek orthopedic consultation.

Fracture of Inversion-Internal Rotation

Adduction fractures are characterized by a fracture of the internal malleolus and possibly another in the fibula below the level of the ankle joint. The malleoli and the talus are displaced toward the inner side. Contrary to the abduction fractures, a serious ligament tear can be suspected when the outer malleolus shows no fracture but the intermalleolar space is widened. To check for this, force the foot into inversion and x-ray.

Treat these fractures similarly to the eversion-external rotation fractures except the manipulations are reversed. Force the heel and inner malleolus outward. Do not

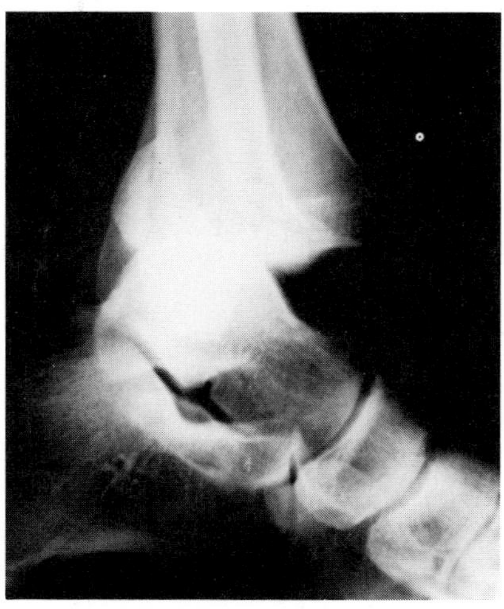

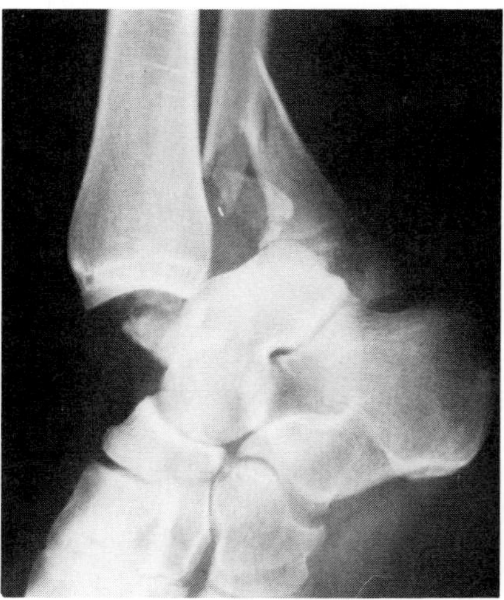

Figure 6-78. Fractures with posterior dislocations of the ankles. These displacements can be reduced but reduction can be maintained only with difficulty. Open surgery is often required.

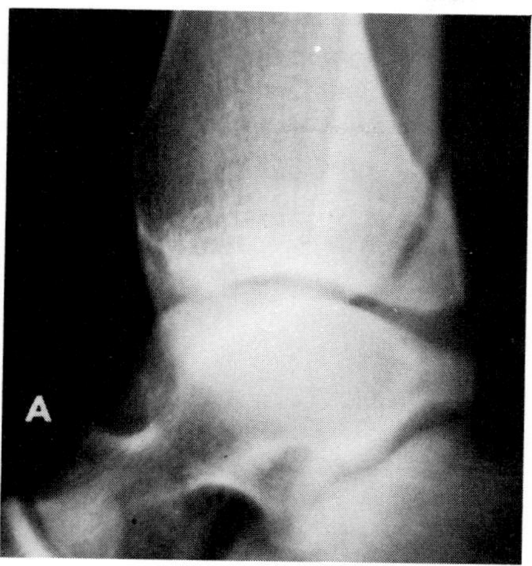

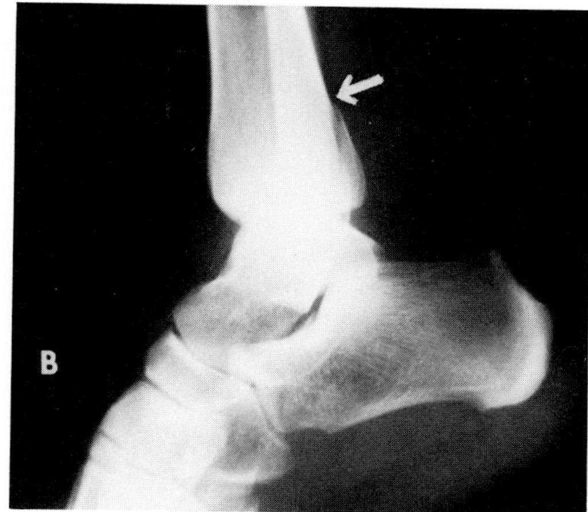

Figure 6-79. *A*, The minimal type of posterior marginal fracture; *B*, Undisplaceα fracture of posterior lip of distal tibia.

wedge up the medial border of the heel when applying the permanent cast.

Fractures of Posterior and Anterior Margins of the Tibia with Displacement of the Foot

The fractures of the posterior surface of the tibia are divided into the *classical* fracture, where more than ⅓ of the articular surface of the tibia is broken off, and the *minimal* fracture, where there is less than ⅓ of the articular surface broken free. The classical fracture (Fig. 6-78) must often be reduced and maintained by open surgery because the displacement tends to recur. If experienced, try reduction and check position by x-ray. If the displacement recurs call for a specialist.

Reduction is not difficult if the fracture falls into the minimal fracture classification (Fig. 6-79). Have the patient flex the knee by allowing the leg to hang over the edge of the operating table. Apply backward pressure on the leg above the ankle and pull the foot forward, accompanied by dorsiflexion. Casting is similar to other fractures but should remain immobilized 8 weeks.

When the fracture involves the anterior margin of the articular surface of the tibia with forward displacement of the foot, pull the leg above the ankle forward and push the foot backward while plantar-flexing. This fracture recurs easily and specialty help may be needed for open reduction. Check stability by x-rays.

Sprains of the Ankle

The most common sprain of the ankle is an injury to the external lateral ligament. Sudden inversion of the foot causes the damage. Unusual violence may cause a sprain fracture wherein the lateral ligament jerks away a spicule of the external malleolus. Similar injuries may occur to the internal and the tibiofibular ligaments.

Suspect a *moderate sprain* on:

–swelling of the ankle
–local tenderness over the ligaments
–pain on normal motion
–only slight joint laxity

The injury is more likely to be a fracture when tenderness exists over the bony malleoli. Tenderness over the dorsum of the foot in front of the ankle indicates a tear of the tibiofibular ligament. With a minor sprain there is no excessive mobility.

Suspect a *severe sprain* with rupture of the ligament on aggravation of the above signs plus:

–great joint laxity and/or abnormal motion beyond the joint's normal limits
–pain on active or passive motion
–excessive rotation of the talus between the malleoli

Under normal circumstances the talus does not move sidewise. Verify excessive mobility with anteroposterior x-rays of the ankle while the foot is forcibly inverted or everted. This can best be done after infiltrating the tender areas with 10 ml of 1 percent Xylocaine.

TREATMENT OF ANKLE SPRAIN. Order ice packs and apply a plastic bag filled with ice chips for 10 min intervals. Protect the skin with a towel. Apply cold also by immersing the foot and ankle in 45° F water for 20 min. Later, when the swelling subsides, use heat. Better still use hot and cold contrast baths after the first 21 to 48 hr. Fill two pails, one with hot water (105 to 110° F) and the other with cold water (45 to 50° F). Immerse the ankle for 5 min in hot water and then 1 min in cold water. Alternate 3 to 4 times.

Infiltrate the tendon and surrounding soft tissue with 10 ml of 1 percent Xylocaine and optionally mix the Xylocaine with 150 turbidity units of hyaluronidase (Alidase).

If the sprain is minor, protect the ankle with adhesive dressing and allow immediate ambulation. If the sprain is moderate but has not produced a ruptured tendon, immobilize with adhesive taping and keep weight off the foot by crutches until the swelling subsides.

Apply adhesive taping in basketweave pattern (see following). This taping allows swelling to occur without interfering with the foot's circulation.

Later, after the swelling subsides, the mortise of the joint may be more effectively protected by the western wrap or the figure-of-eight (see following).

After applying the western wrap and the swelling has subsided, start exercises and ambulation (see later in this section).

Consultation should be sought when the sprain is severe and associated with joint laxity unless the family physician has had experience treating such injuries. The decision to surgically repair or to cast must be made. As time passes the ligaments shorten and the tissues become more difficult to approximate. Consequently, do surgical repair early and have the patient use a walking cast for 2 weeks, following up with appropriate support and exercises.

If examination indicates that surgery is not necessary for a stable and painless ankle, apply a plastic walking boot for 3 to 4 weeks. Apply the cast as though a fracture existed, molding the plaster about the ankle with the pressure of the palms. After removing the cast, continue support with adhesive taping. Start exercises as outlined later in this section.

Basketweave Taping. The Gibney method of applying adhesive in a basketweave pattern is useful as a first support after an injury or for mild or moderate sprains because the open face allows swelling to take place. However, it does not protect the ankle's mortise.

Immediately after injury apply tape and ice. Have the patient hold her ankle at 90° while you tape. Shave the ankle first and paint or spray with an adherent. In an adult start with 1½ in tape applied vertically, parallel with the Achilles tendon. Horizontal adhesive strips 1 in wide are used to crosshatch the vertical ones. Apply the adhesive 8 in above the malleoli. For a few hours cover the adhesive wrap with an elastic bandage. This helps the adhesive to mold and fit the ankle.

In mild sprains with only ligament stretching allow the patient to walk after the initial injury. If the sprain is moderate with only an incomplete ligament tear the use of crutches is advised.

The Western Ankle Wrap. Use the western wrap after initial swelling has subsided. It prevents inversion and eversion but allows extension and flexion.

Walking Figure-of-Eight Bandage. A figure-of-eight adhesive walking strap should be used after the initial swelling has subsided. Keep the ankle at right angles. If not done previously, shave the ankle. Cover the foot and ankle with gauze or Kling to protect the skin. Pull two strips of adhesive around the heel paralleling the Achilles tendon. Apply two horizontal strips of adhesive from the instep, behind the ankle and ending on the opposite side of the instep. Apply the figure-of-eight, starting above the internal malleolus, crossing the instep, continuing under the arch and up over the instep and ending above the external malleolus. Cover the anterior ankle and adhesive ends with short individual strips.

Other Traumatic Causes of Pain About the Heels and Ankles

Differentiate the common sprains, strains and fractures from the following:

–ankle joint effusion from various causes with characteristic bulging near the talotibial junction and in front of the lateral and medial malleolar ligaments
–chronic stenosing tenosynovitis of the peroneal nerve sheath, which causes pain on inversion of the foot and tenderness and swelling behind and below the lateral malleolus
–recurrent slipping of the peroneal tendons as they curve under the lateral malleolus (The patient describes pain or clicking on dorsiflexion.)
–rupture of the Achilles tendon, which occurs about 2 in above the calcaneal insertion
–calcaneal fractures where the hollows beneath the malleoli disappear
–retrocalcaneal bursitis causing pain and swelling on the back of the heel
–infracalcaneal bursitis (policeman's heel) with pain in the ball of the heel
–tarsal-tunnel syndrome, causes numbness, pain and paresthesia to the sole because of compression of nerves in the tunnel under the medial malleolus (Verify the diagnosis by electromyography.)

With recurrent slipping of the peroneal tendons, the patient describes pain or clicking on dorsiflexion. In rupture of the Achilles tendon the patient complains of sudden severe pain and inability to walk. Palpate the tendon to detect the telltale gap by a visible proximal lump. While the patient lies prone on the examining table with his foot hanging over the edge the injured foot is dorsiflexed. Simmond's test results in the absence of plantar flexion when the calf is squeezed.

Casting an Ankle

Clean the skin of the foot and inspect for any infection on skin and between the toes. Position the patient so that his knee is flexed and the ankle at right angles. It is convenient to place the outer border of the patient's foot on your knee. Generally, plaster need not cover the basis of the big and little toes nor come higher than 1 in below the tibial tubercle. Mark the skin with ink, indicating these limits of the cast prior to applying the cast.

Start the soft-roll just below the knee and roll downward avoiding wrinkles. Overlap each strip about 1 in; never double back. Roll down to the midportion of the toes. Roll up and down again, completing three layers of soft-roll. Apply three extra layers over the malleoli, the first metatarsal and the tibial tubercle. Cut the soft-roll back to the marks previously made on the skin. The cut over the tibial tubercle should be to a point 1 in distal to the tubercle and the cut over the first metatarsal to the head of the metatarsal.

If the ankle has considerable swelling apply a molded sugartong splint and cover with an elastic bandage. This may be tightened as needed. In 2 or 3 days, as the swelling subsides, cover the sugartongs with a circular plaster cast. Skip this step if the swelling is not unusual and proceed to a circular plastic cast.

Start the circular wet plaster roll just distal to the tibial tuberosity. Roll down, overlapping each roll about 2/3 the width of the previous roll. While wrapping, keep the plaster roll close to the leg. Roll down to the heads of the toes. Rub the plaster smooth after each roll. Stroke in the opposite direction to which the roll was applied. Continue with the second roll up the leg and the third down. After the third layer is complete, mold the cast to the ankle, giving special care to the heel. Continue to keep the ankle at right angles; take care not to plantar flex the foot. Allow the cast to set.

When the cast is set enough to hold its shape, construct the toe platform. Roll the plaster from the lateral side of the foot around the toes and to the medial side. Make this 4 to 5 layers thick. Leave a generous margin jutting out in front of the toes. After the toe platform has set slightly, mold the excess plaster back under the toes. Now all toes should be free and visible with a substantial platform on which to rest. A short piece of plaster should be rolled around the edge of the cast and the platform, thus incorporating all parts into one cast. Keep the platform from falling into plantar flexion leaving the toes unsupported. Smooth all edges.

Prepare a foot pad 1 to 2 in longer than the foot and 8 to 10 layers thick. The thickness depends on the weight of the patient. Fix the pad to the sole of the cast. Tuck the medial margin of the foot pad under to fill in the arch. The extra length will be used to fold back over the end pieces of the Stryker heel to be applied later. Fix the foot pad with a one-thickness roll of plaster. Bisect the sole with imaginary lines.

Place the Stryker heel on the cast centered over the bisecting lines. Fold the overlaps of the foot pad over each end of the Stryker heel. Proceed to fix the heel to the cast. Use a 4 in roll of plaster to fill in all spaces where dirt might accumulate and to fix the cast and heel together. Smooth all edges.

Instructions for the patient:

- Elevate the foot for 24 hr.
- Call the physician if toes become cold, cyanotic or painful.
- Cast will break if weight bearing is started before the cast is completely dry (24 to 48 hr).
- Wear a high-heeled shoe or cowboy boot on the other foot to even leg height.
- Leave the cast uncovered.
- Use crutches initially because of pain and increase weight bearing as tolerated.
- Keep cast out of water. Tub baths are preferable with the leg hanging out of the tub.

Rehabilitative Ankle Exercises

Patients with any of the preceding fractures and sprains will need rehabilitation. Some individuals will need specialized physical therapy. The average case which the family physician treats will need only the rehabilitative exercises mentioned here.

Some exercises can be done while the patient is still in bed. Have the patient start with the simple ones and proceed with the more strenuous ones as tolerated.

While the patient is in a supine position, instruct him to alternately point the injured foot towards the head of the bed and then towards the foot of the bed with his knee flat against the bed. Repeat ten times.

Instruct the patient to rotate his feet outward and then inward to their full extent without pain. Again repeat ten times. Continue the ankle exercise by having the patient rotate his foot full circle—in, down, out and up ten times. Some physicians then have the patient trace imaginary letters of the alphabet.

Ask the patient to sit on a stool. Spread a towel on the floor with a book on the far end. Have the patient pull the book towards himself by tugging on the towel with his foot. Add more books to the towel as he gains strength.

With the patient still sitting on a stool, have him pick up part of a roll of gauze or small sponge with his foot and place the object somewhere else. Then he should pick up the object again and place it in another site. This can be done with marbles or any small objects.

Test weight bearing as his ankle picks up strength. Have the patient stand on his toes with feet straight ahead. If he can tolerate this exercise without pain or swelling continue with the same exercise while toeing in. Finally, as tolerated, continue the exercises by toeing out. Each of these exercises is to be done ten times.

As toleration grows, the patient exercises to increase strength and flexibility in his ankle. With the patient sitting on a hip-high table or stool, attach a 1½ lb weight to tennis shoe laces with a painter's ladder hook. The patient should flex the ankle as high as possible, hold for 2 sec, rotate outward and return to normal. Repeat ten times. Increase the weight and height daily as tolerated, perhaps up to 15 lb. Repeat the exercise but reverse the action by bringing the foot up and rotating inward.

Fractures of the Metatarsals and Phalanges

The metatarsal is usually fractured by a crushing injury (Fig 6-80) such as in a foot that has been stepped on or run over. Seldom is there displacement. These fractures nearly always require a below-knee walking cast.

Another type of metatarsal fracture is the stress fracture, also called march foot.[4] Prolonged weight bearing (as in prolonged walking or marching) can produce the fracture, usually of the second or third metatarsal. It is a hairline fracture of the shaft of the metatarsal with no displacement. Pain is evoked by flexion or extension of the toes but tapers off with rest and nonweight bearing. It is difficult to visualize the fracture initially on x-ray film but as healing occurs the callus formation can be observed more readily. Rarely is casting necessary; the fracture heals spontaneously. Rest is essential and the foot may be taped. If there is severe pain a walking cast for 4 weeks will help.

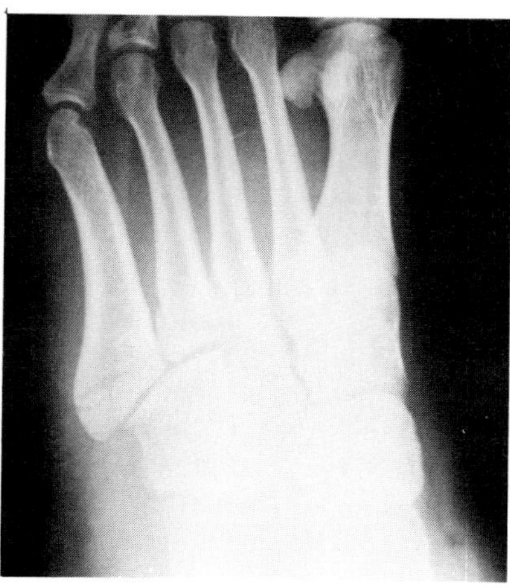

Figure 6-80. Fracture of the fifth metatarsal.

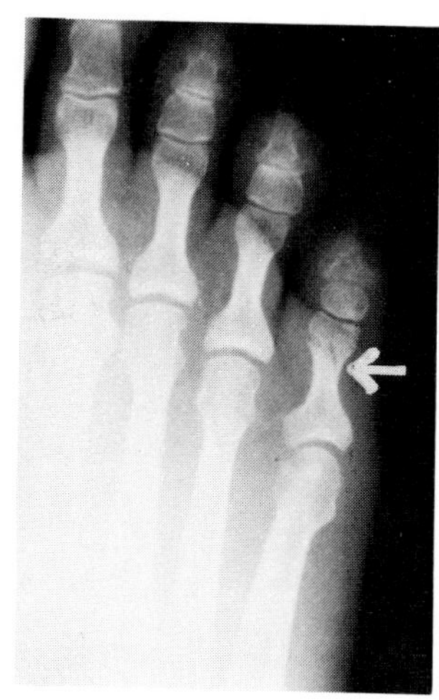

Figure 6-81. Fracture of proximal phalanx, fifth toe.

A fracture of the proximal phalanx is shown in Figure 6-81.

Strapping the Great Toe. Keeping the ankle at a right angle and using ½ in adhesive tape, begin to tape on the under and medial side of the great toe and pull the tape across the toe joint and under the foot. Continue with ½ in tape, starting on the underside of the toe near its lateral side. Bring the tape up and over the toe and onto the foot. Reinforce by repeating the first two strappings with 1 in adhesive. Encircle the front of the foot with individual tape strips, molding the adhesive to the natural contour of the foot.

HEAD AND SPINE INJURIES

Head Injuries

Never underestimate the clinical importance of head injuries no matter how insignificant they appear. The primary concern of the family physician is to diagnose head injuries properly. When a patient has suffered head trauma (Fig. 6-82) observe him for an expanding intracranial lesion. The wisest course is to hospitalize the patient for 24 to 48 hr and record the vital signs every hour or oftener if indicated. Do a general physical examination.

First check the patient's vital signs, noting any evidence of shock. A rising blood

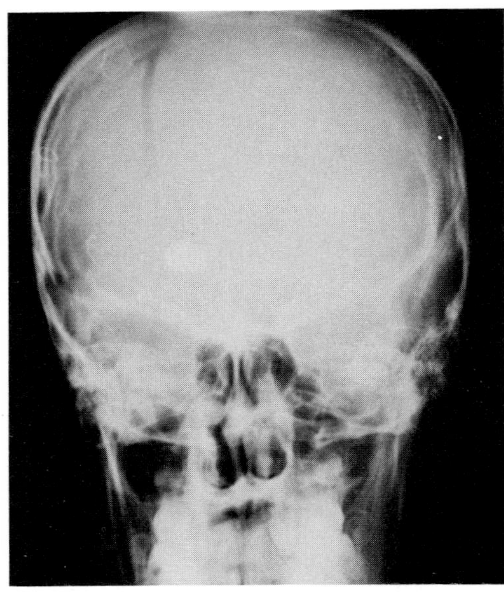

Figure 6-82. Gunshot wound of the right skull with bullet lodged near the third ventricle.

pressure or pulse pressure or slowing respiration and pulse rate may indicate a tonsillar pressure cone. Treat shock (see Chapter 5) and determine extent of other injuries. Do a neurological screening examination.

Check the patient's degree of consciousness. Consciousness may be graded as follows:

1—Alert, oriented
2—Verbally responsive but confused
3—Responsive only to painful stimuli
4—Comatose and unresponsive

A deepening unconsciousness is suggested by a change from one level to another, and represents the clinical manifestations of an expanding intracranial lesion.

Examine the patient's eyes, including the fundi for hemorrhage and venous pulsations and the pupils for size, equality and reaction to light. Remember papilledema takes 48 hr to develop. Retinal hemorrhage indicates increased intracranial pressure; dilatation of a pupil plus a sluggish light reflex follows the development of a tentorial pressure cone; and visible venous pulsations of the retina augur against increased intracranial pressure.

Inspect the bony ridges over and about the eyes and ears. Bruising of these areas may overlay fractures and bruising over the mastoids a basilar skull fracture.

Lift the eyelids and let them close. Lagging of one lid suggests hemiplegia; resistance to opening hysteria.

In a coma the eyes remain fixed or oscillate slowly from side to side. In hysteria there is no oscillation; the eyes may wander but fix momentarily from time to time.

Conjugate deviation of the eyeballs is toward the affected side in destructive lesions of the frontal lobe and away from the affected side in irritative lesions.

Bilateral widely dilated pupils occur in severe post-traumatic shock but also in massive cerebral hemorrhage, encephalitis and in some kinds of poisoning.

Bilateral pinpoint pupils suggest morphine poisoning or a pontine hemorrhage.

A unilateral unreactive pupil indicates a rapidly expanding lesion on the ipsilateral side as in subdural or middle meningeal hemorrhage of brain tumor.

Look and listen for changes in speech, facies weakness, hemiparesis or sensory changes. Such symptoms are related to an expanding intracranial mass.

Perform two tests: skull percussion for tenderness and the rotary jolt test. If either causes lateralized pain suspect a subdural hematoma. Perform the rotary jolt test after excluding injury to the cervical spine by forcefully rotating the head laterally.

Explore any scalp lacerations with a gloved finger to establish the presence and extent of a depressed skull fracture.

If during these first hours the patient shows any signs of deepening unconsciousness, order a skull series and cervical x-rays. AP and PA views reveal fracture lines and establish early the location of the calcified pineal gland. Later this may be of utmost importance when comparison views are necessary. A shift of more than 3 mm on rotated x-ray is significant in determining changes in pressure.

Suggestions on studying skull x-ray films are:

- –study periphery of calvarium and base
- –study lines, channels and sutures
- –study any calcifications within the skull, including the position of the pineal gland
- –note size and shape of sella turcica
- –study all bony ridges such as orbits, sphenoid ridge, temporal bones, paranasal sinuses and mandible (Figs. 6-83 and 6-84)

A baseline for the vital signs should be established. If the x-ray demonstrates a linear skull fracture, especially in the temporal region, with headaches, vomiting and deepening unconsciousness, suspect an epidural hematoma. This may suddenly become serious. Request a neurosurgical consultation and order an echoencephalogram and brain scan.

If the x-ray study reveals a closed depressed skull fracture and the patient is conscious and without focal signs there is no immediate danger. If the patient's vital signs become unstable or focal neurological signs develop, request a neurosurgical consultation.

If the skull fracture is open and depressed, the patient may develop an infection and he requires antibiotics and a neurosurgical consultation.

An echoencephalogram will detect changes in the walls of the third ventricle. Echoencephalograms are especially helpful when x-ray studies do not show a calcified pineal gland.

Lumbar puncture carries certain dangers and, therefore, should not be done routinely on all head injuries. It may precipitate a tentorial or tonsillar pressure cone.

The patient may be discharged from the hospital if the x-rays do not show any fractures and he does not develop any symptoms. Warn the patient that he may still develop an expanding brain lesion and to notify a doctor at the first sign of headache, vomiting or drowsiness.

If the patient did not have a severe head injury and is drowsy following the injury, rule out other causes of unconsciousness, i.e. diabetes coma, uremia, drug overdose or alcoholism.

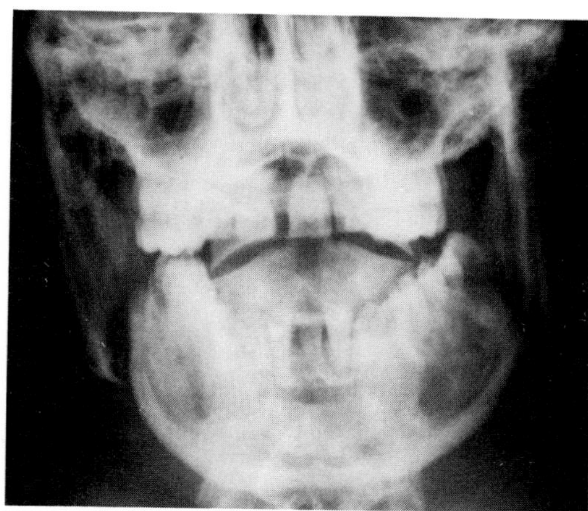

Figure 6-83. Bilateral fracture of the jaw.

But even without an obvious severe head injury, the patient should be observed for persistent headache and vomiting. If symptoms occur watch for an expanding brain lesion. Consider hospitalization. If no symptoms occur and the patient stays fully alert, send the patient home. Have relatives wake the patient every 2 hr to check his responses. If he develops symptoms have him return to the emergency room.

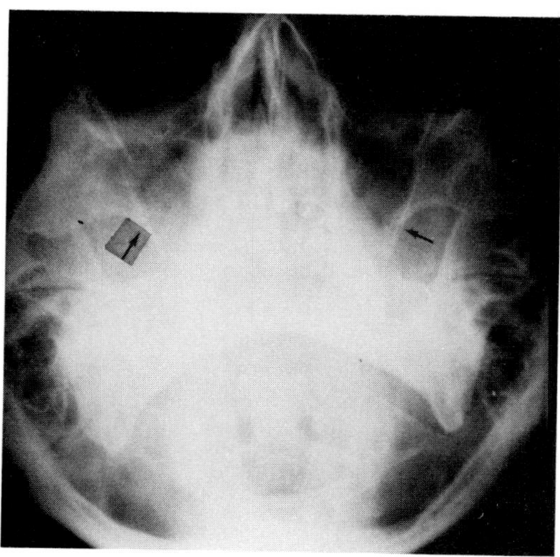

Figure 6-84. Bilateral fractures of the maxilla.

Subdural Hematoma

With a linear fracture and the development of any focal neurological signs following the injury suspect an acute subdural hematoma and request a neurosurgical consultation. A lumbar puncture is most helpful in diagnosing a subdural hematoma, a condition most frequently missed. In this injury look for red cells in the spinal fluid, xanthochromic fluid or elevated protein. Occasionally an electroencephalogram is helpful, but arteriography is usually needed to confirm the diagnosis. Differentiate a traumatic lumbar puncture from intracerebral hemorrhage by the criteria in Table 6-1.

A subdural hematoma is one of the most frequently missed serious head injuries. It exhibits the signs and symptoms of an expanding intracranial mass with a time lapse after the head injury. There is not much difficulty in diagnosing the immediate accumulation of blood in the subdural space. But minor head injuries may be followed by a latent period of days, weeks or months before the onset of headaches and then it may simulate a brain tumor. Search for localizing signs of an expanding lesion. In some instances the patient suffers attacks of drowsiness, mental confusion or coma. For reasons which are not completely understood, intermittent drowsiness tends to be progressive even after the hemorrhage has ceased. Gradually coma develops. Aphasia and hemiparesis may appear as a result of compression of the brain.

Arteriography is done to detect whether the cerebral vessels fail to reach the inner skull because of an intervening clot. Often a craniotomy is needed to confirm the diagnosis. Treatment is surgical evacuation of the clot.

Family physicians must be alert to a delayed cerebral hemorrhage following head trauma. An intracerebral hematoma is the most common pathologic finding. Half the patients will give the history of having been unconscious for a short period of time following the trauma. Cerebral vascular accidents then occurred after an asymptomatic period of up to 30 days after the trauma.[4]

Extradural Hemorrhage

The source of an extradural hemorrhage is usually a ruptured middle meningeal artery. The most characteristic history is of head injury with loss of senses followed by a rapid recovery of consciousness. After a so-called lucid interval a gradually increasing coma supervenes with progressive hemiplegia, fixed dilated pupils and death unless treatment is prompt.

Remember there may be no lucid interval. When the head is severely injured consciousness may not be regained.

Thus in any case of head injury it is more important to keep track of the level of consciousness than it is to be monitoring the pulse and blood pressure. This means a constant grading of the level of consciousness by observing the nature and strength of the

Table 6-1. Criteria in Differentiation

	CSF pressure	*Blood in tubes*	*CSF clotting*	*Xanthochromia*	*Repeat puncture at higher level*
Intracerebral hemorrhage	Often increased	Blood in all tubes	No clotting	Positive after 8–12 hr	Same as initial puncture
Traumatic lumbar puncture	Low	Blood in first tube	Clots	None unless patient is icteric	Clear

Table 6-2. Subarachnoid Cerebral Hemorrhage

Symptoms	*Signs*	*Laboratory findings*
Sudden, severe head pain Dizziness or drowsiness Nausea and/or vomiting Stiff neck Confusion, irritability Photophobia	Semiconscious or unconscious Nuchal rigidity Kernig's sign Bilateral pyramidal tract signs Semiparesis or hemiplegia	Bloody or xanthochromic cerebrospinal fluid Angiography for an expanding subdural or extradural hematoma. aneurysm or an anomaly

Treatment	*Follow-up*
Turn patient on affected side; do not move more than necessary Elevate head slightly Loosen clothing about throat Keep from chilling Hospitalization and observation	Advise patient against further participation in strenuous exercise or contact sports

stimulus required to rouse the patient. If coma is deepening, even though the patient has never been fully conscious, suspect extradural hemorrhage.

Extradural hemorrhage should be suspected when a skull fracture is discovered before the deepening coma. Again carotid arteriography may demonstrate the lesion. The treatment is trephining of the skull and evacuating the clot.

Subarachnoid Cerebral Hemorrhage

A blow to the head as may occur in football may cause a laceration to the cerebral substance, a cerebral aneurysm or an arteriovenous anomaly. The danger is continued or recurrent hemorrhage and death. Symptoms and signs are indicated in Table 6-2.

Neck Injuries

Neck injuries, including fractures and fracture-dislocation, occur as a result of diving into shallow water, parachute jumping, contact sports and automobile accidents. Check for restricted neck motion, deformities, neurologic signs or symptoms and tenderness over the cervical musculature or upper thoracic spinous processes. Inspect the patient for other injuries, especially about the head.

Unlike cases of thoracic or lumbar injuries of the spine, where it is important that the patient be placed supine on a rigid support, a patient with a suspected neck injury may be either supine or prone. The important thing is to apply some form of traction. Every ambulance should have a halter, pulley and weights. Adjust the incline of the stretcher so that the patient's weight serves as countertraction. In an emergency one individual should be assigned to hold the patient under the occiput and chin and apply such traction as he is able.

Order roentgenography in suspicious cases. Inspect films for atlas fractures, odontoid process fractures, neural arch fractures in C_3 with dislocation of C_2, compres-

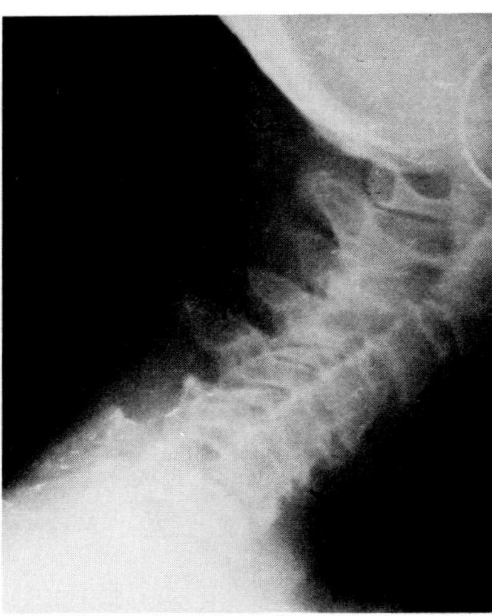

Figure 6-85. Old compression fractures of C_6 and C_7 with fracture of the posterior arch and spinous process of C_7.

sion fracture of C_4, C_5 and C_6 (Fig. 6-85), rotatory fractures of articular facets and fractures of lower cervical spinous processes.

Examine the cervical spine with the patient seated. Inspect the neck from front, sides and back for deformities and pathological posture. Ask the patient to point to the site of his pain. Test active motion of the neck by asking the patient to turn chin to right, to left, up and down and then point each ear to its respective shoulder joint. Palpate the paracervical muscles for spasm and the spinous processes for tenderness. With the finger or rubber hammer percuss the spinous processes for tenderness. Auscult the moving joints for crepitus.

Common Cervical Injuries

Fracture of a spinous process (Fig. 6-86) causes sudden severe pain from neck to the shoulder aggravated by movement with exquisite tenderness over the injured process.

Flexion fractures of C_5 occur on violent hyperflexion of the neck. This injury can cause sudden death or quadriplegia.

Partial dislocation from hyperextension follows a blow on the forehead hyperextending the neck and rupturing the anterior longitudinal ligament. The injury results in intense pain, and one spinous process may appear more prominent. Paraplegia is common. X-ray diagnosis is essential.

A patient with a fracture of the atlas supports his head with his hands and is unable to nod. He will also have a severe occipital headache. Depend on clinical examination rather than on x-ray pictures entirely. The injury can cause sudden death.

Fracture of the odontoid process frequently causes sudden death following injury to the brain stem. Peculiarly enough the patient can walk without supporting his head. The diagnostic sign: inability to rotate the head. The diagnosis should be made clinically and immediately. Completely immobilize the neck to prevent sudden death.

Cervical spine strain follows a forcing of an abnormal range of cervical motion as happens in "spearing" in football. Signs and symptoms include tenderness over involved area, muscle spasm, limited motion and some loss of strength. Rule out fracture and dislocation. If seen early inject long-acting local anesthetic; if seen later use a steroid with or without a local anesthetic. Some patients recover faster with a temporary cervical collar or with light cervical traction at night. Physical therapy is important. Reassure the patient, for recovery may take 8 weeks. A well fitted cotton collar may permit the athlete to participate earlier.

Cervical disc rupture follows a blow to the head along its longitudinal axis as in spearing, lifting or straining.

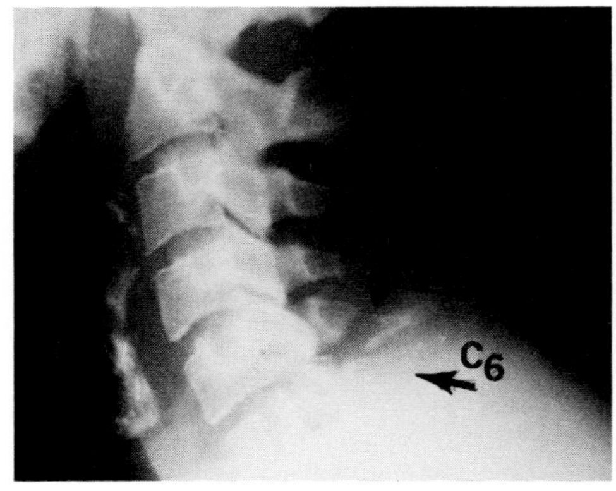

Figure 6-86. Fractures of the spinous processes of C_5 and C_6.

Signs and symptoms include:

–weakness in upper extremities
–possible bladder and bowel impairment
–pain radiating to neck, shoulders, arm, forearm or hand (Provoke the radicular pain by thumping the top of the head or by thrusting the head downward.)
–possible loss of deep reflexes of biceps or triceps
–possible tetraparesis or tetraplegia with some sensory losses
–possible paralysis of specific muscles of upper extremities
–increased cerebrospinal protein

The two MG changes may show nerve root damage after 3 wk of compression. X-ray may show only a narrowed disc. A myelogram usually shows a defect in the involved interspace.

Treatment is cervical traction, physical therapy and analgesics. Surgery if there is no relief from conservative treatment.

Whiplash Injuries

"Whiplash" is only a legal term. A far better term is cervicoligamentous muscle strain or simply extension strain of the neck. This injury to the cervical area occurs when an automobile in which a person is riding is struck suddenly and unexpectedly from the rear. As a result of inertia, the head tends to stay in the same position while the body is rammed forward. This tends to whip the neck. When this happens the spinous processes tend to kiss each other posteriorly; anteriorly the anterior longitudinal ligament may be sprained or strained. Fractures rarely occur. Nerve roots involved are C_5, C_6, C_7 or C_8.

Obtain a careful history and document. Describe any preexisting symptoms or injuries. Record the exact mechanism of injury, the immediate symptoms or signs and the delayed symptoms or signs.

Do a careful physical examination including a description of any abnormal posture of the neck, degree of limitation of motion and in which direction, site of localized tenderness, degree of involuntary muscle spasm, any neurologic findings and low back injuries.

A key to estimating the extent of the injury is how far the patient can extend his neck. Have the patient put his head back, and then gently pull the head a little farther. If pains radiate down the arm, be more guarded in outlook and treatment. This type of pain is much more likely to be radicular and/or discogenic in origin.

Check for low back injuries although the patient may be able to touch his toes. Search for low back injury by having him extend his back for 10 sec. This is another extension injury and he will not be able to maintain the required posture for 10 sec.

Evaluate the following differential features of the injury: emotional shock, musculoligamentous strain, injury to disc, fractures or dislocations of spine, injury to nerve roots and injury to spinal cord.

Roentgenoscopy should include the skull and cervical spine, a view of the odontoid process, oblique views of each side to study the intervertebral foramen and, if not shown clearly with the preceding, a special view of the C_7 to T_1 junction.

Base treatment on proper diagnosis. Initial immobilization by bed rest for 5 to 7 days is preferable to a cervical collar. Physical therapy with heat (preferably warm packs) and gentle massage. Give analgesia with aspirin or other favorite analgesia. Antispasmodics and muscle relaxants may be used but do little good. Give steroid injections when 1 to 2 ml will cover the tenderness. Expect no relief if injection is given in the center or on the edge of a large painful area. Avoid repeated injections of trigger points.

The patient should do light exercise to diminish edema and prevent muscle atrophy. While in bed have the patient roll his head back and forth. Consider the use of a cervical collar for 2 to 3 weeks when the patient ambulates.

Begin traction only if it helps. Try traction for radiation pains. A double pillow may help relieve aches that radiate into the shoulders or arms. Obtain the most effective traction by raising the head of the bed about 45° and breaking the bed under the knees.

Apply traction from overhead bars with the neck slightly flexed.

Finish all the above treatment by 6 weeks. Many patients suffer ailments of iatrogenic origin because doctors insist on prolonged and useless rest.

Returning Athletes to Sports after Injuries

Family physicians serving certain sports events must decide on the spot which injured players may return to the game after neck injuries. The AMA sports committee lists its criteria in Table 6-3.

Withhold any athlete with possible fracture, internal hemorrhage or ligamentous sprain severe enough to limit good function from playing, pending accurate diagnosis and evaluation.

Head injuries are difficult to assess. If a boy is unconscious for a period of more than a few moments, remove him from competition and do not permit him to return that day. Do not allow contact for 1 wk.

If a boy shows signs of concussion, i.e. dizziness, nausea, weakness, confusion and loss of memory, withhold him from competition until all signs disappear. If the symptoms have been present more than a few minutes, withhold him for at least the rest of the day. The symptoms may occur without a period of unconsciousness and may actually occur without any known injury.

If a boy is momentarily dazed but clears promptly and has no symptoms or any clinical signs, permit him to return to competition on that day. Withhold from competition for 7 days after the disappearance of all signs and symptoms any boy who sustains a significant concussion. If signs or symptoms persist beyond a few minutes of the injury order a complete neurologic work-up including skull films and electroencephalograms.

Vertebral Fractures

These fractures (Figs. 6-87 and 6-88) occur as a result of auto accidents, tobogganing accidents, epilepsy or tetanus.

Examine with the patient lying supine, working your fingers along the spine, pressing each spinous process as though lifting the patient. If the pressure causes pain, treat as though the patient had sustained a compression fracture. Evaluate distal sensation and motor and sphincter control. Elicit the reflex by lightly pricking the skin near the anus and watching for a "wink" reflex.

Order bed rest for a few days until the patient is comfortable if there is no neurologic deficit. Call a neurosurgeon immediately if a neurologic deficit does exist. Expect a very little improvement if immediate paraplegia occurs. If neurologic deficiency extends, the patient should be decompressed. No surgery is indicated if progressive improvement occurs.

Table 6-3. When to Return Athletes to the Game

	Return to game	*No return*
Obvious deformity of neck	–	+
Tenderness		
over cervical spinous process	–	+
over upper thoracic spinous process	?	?
over the trapezius	?	?
over the sternocleidomastoid	?	?
Restricted neck motion	–	+
Weakness of extremities	–	+
Numbness in extremities	–	+
Pain radiating down arm	?	?

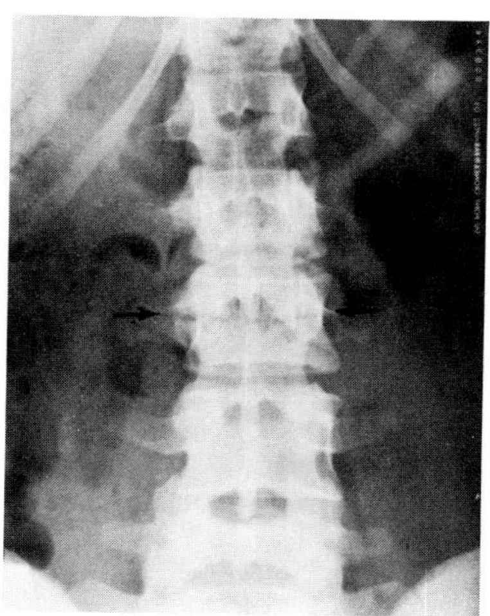

Figure 6-87. Seatbelt fracture of posterior elements of L_3 (transverse fracture).

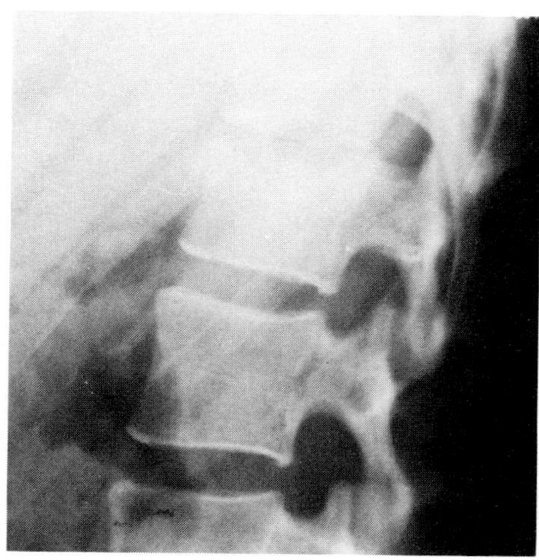

Figure 6-88. Compression fracture of the first lumbar vertebra.

Pelvic Fractures

Pelvic fractures (Fig. 6-89) occur as a result of auto accidents or a child being run over by a vehicle. Check immediately for hematuria, catheterizing if necessary. Check the patient's abdomen for rigidity and bowel sounds to rule out internal injuries and check the lower extremities for neurovascular competence.

If hematuria is present or you are unable to pass a catheter seek urologic consultation. Seek a general surgical consultation if there are evidences of internal injuries. Treat by bed rest. A sling is more uncomfortable and can produce more harm than benefit.

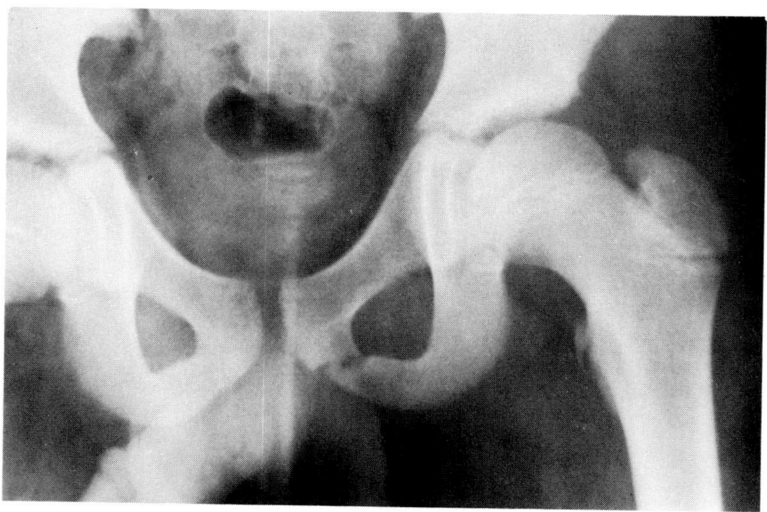

Figure 6-89. Fracture of the descending ramus of the left pelvis.

BURNS

The treatment of burns is the same whether they be by fire, boiling water, electrical currents or chemicals.

General Evaluation

Evaluate the depth and extent of the burn. Treatment will depend on these two factors. Estimate the depth of the wound by the following observation: *First Degree*—superficial erythema partial thickness burn; *Second Degree*—blistering (skin hypersensitive), partial thickness burn; *Third Degree*—charring, dead white (insensitive), full thickness burn.

Base the differential diagnosis on history, appearance and reaction to pin prick or hair pulling.

Estimate the extent using the *Rule of 9's:*

- –burn of head—9%
- –burn of left upper extremity—9%
- –burn of right upper extremity—9%
- –burn of front of trunk—18%
- –burn of back of trunk—18%
- –burn of left lower extremity—18%
- –burn of right lower extremity—18%

For children under one year of age use *Rule of 19's:*

- –burn of head—19%
- –burn of each lower extremity—18%

For each year over 1, subtract 1 percent from head and add ½ percent to each lower extremity.

Classification of burns: A minor burn is a second degree or partial thickness injury affecting less than 15 percent of the body surface or a third degree or full thickness injury affecting less than 2 percent. *Prognosis:* 40 percent burn in 40-yr old has a 50 percent mortality; 65 percent burn in a 65-yr old has a 100 percent mortality.

Prevention and Treatment of Infections

Soon after a burn, the area is invaded by staphylococci and streptococci organisms. These organisms come from the skin and hair follicles. By the end of a week look for the invasion of gram-negative organisms, i.e. Pseudomonas and Proteus. In deep burns, the danger of C. tetani is always present in the nonimmunized. Most third degree burns develop infections. First and second degree burns need not if properly cared for.

Classify infections as local or invasive. In local infections pus may cover the burn but there is no redness in the surrounding area. The local infection can destroy any remaining viable tissue if not treated. With an invasive infection not only is the wound covered with pus but also the surrounding tissues are red and swollen. This type of wound may lead to lymphangitis, lymphadenopathy and septicemia.

Serious burns should be cultured whenever the bandage is changed or every 2 or 3 days until the time of danger is over. Clinical observation of the wound is important. Pseudomonas is accompanied by the production of blue-green, foul-smelling, water-soluble pigments known as pyocyanin and pyoverdin. These are bacterial pigments and are fluorescent. Early invasive infections by Pseudomonas can be recognized by daily inspection under a Wood's light.

Whenever the burned area is less than 15 percent of the body surface consideration should be given to early debridement and skin grafting as a means of combating subsequent infections.

Treatment of Early Noninfected Minor Burns

If not infected or otherwise complicated a partial thickness burn will heal within 2 to 3 wk without much scarring. Cleanse the wound with warm water and bland soap, removing all dirt and loose dead skin. Break all blisters except those in the palm of the hand and remove all dead epithelium. Apply a bactericidal ointment such as polymyxin B-Bacitrocin-neomycin ointment under a bulky dressing covering the entire wound. Furacin-impregnated gauze strips have worked well for me. Change the dressing every 3 to 5 days. If the burn is moderate in size order a systemic antibiotic such as penicillin to protect against hemolytic streptococcus infections. Immunize against tetanus in even small third degree burns if the patient's tetanus immunization is not up-to-date.

Treatment of Locally Infected Minor Burns

Rest with burned area elevated, especially the lower extremities. Wet saline soaks are helpful. Apply fresh every 4 hr. Keep them moist and warm. Gauze pads are best next to the skin. To maintain warmth, place the aqua-K pad over the dressing. Two or three days of soaks will do wonders in clearing up local infections.

Use an antibiotic cream. Sulfamylon (mafenide acetate) is popular and helpful but is more practical for large third degree burns. Gentamycin, furacin, silver sulfadiazine and ½ percent silver nitrate all have their advocates. Sulfamylon acts against Pseudomonas. An ideal program is to have the wound soaked in warm saline for 20 min and follow with a thick coating of Sulfamylon cream. Wounds heal faster if allowed to remain exposed.

Treatment of Burns with Invasive Infections

Treat the wound locally as outlined above and give systemic antibiotics. While awaiting culture and sensitivity testing give penicillin. Colistin, synthetic penicillins, and gentamycin have all been used for invasive infections or prior to major debridement or grafting.

Treatment of Burns after Infection Is Controlled

If protection only is needed consider either a homograft from a dead body or from an amputated leg or a heterograft of pigskin. Homografts of skin actively kill bacteria in granulation tissue and prepare the wound bed for autografts. Patients are never out of danger until debridement is completed either by daily tubbing or surgery and the wound is covered by living tissue. Consider sheet grafts, postage stamp grafts and mesh grafts.

For small wounds pinch grafts may be applied as an office procedure when the infection is controlled. With the patient on an antibiotic, debride the wound edges and base. Use 2 percent Xylocaine as a local anesthetic. Excise 1 cm pinch grafts from another area of the body and implant on the wound site. Cover the wound with an ointment of 1 percent neomycin, a 0.5 percent hydrocortisone ointment and a Telfa dressing. Place guage sponges over all for bulk and wrap with Curlex dressing. Dress weekly after cleaning with saline. The patient should avoid excessive movement of the part.

Complications

Major burns associated with shock are complicated medical problems. Shock is treated in the usual fashion but major attention must be focused on fluid loss, decreasing blood volume and diminishing urinary output. Proper treatment requires the physician to differentiate between renal shutdown caused by inadequate perfusion of renal vessels that respond to mannitol or necrosis of renal tubules.

Other complications of major burns are:

- –respiratory injuries following smoke inhalations and explosions (tracheal "cast" may suffocate the patient unless a tracheostomy is done)
- –concomitant injuries
- –vascular shut-down in extremities and even the chest with circumferential escharing that may need decompression incisions
- –gastrointestinal complications (ileus or acute gastric dilatation with distension and hematemesis necessitating a nasogastric tube—one or more Curling's ulcers occur after extensive burns)
- –malnutrition (Careful watch must be kept on replacing nitrogen, carbohydrate, vitamin, iron and salt.)

–deformities from burn scars including claw deformities of the hand, neck contractures, ectropion of eyelids and mouth, axillary and wrist contractures (These should all be prevented by the proper use of splints and active/passive exercises.)

–Marjolin's ulcer, a squamous carcinoma in unstable burn scars

REFERENCES

1. Edwards EA: Acute peripheral arterial occlusion. *JAMA* 223:909, 1973.
2. Aufranc OE, et al: Epiphyseal fracture of the proximal humerus. *JAMA* 213:1476–1479, 1970.
3. Lissner B, Griffin JM: A sticky fix for a finger. *Emerg Med* 5:260, 1973.
4. Cailliet R: Foot and Ankle Pain. Philadelphia: F.A. Davis Co., 1968, p. 95–96.
5. Morin MA, Pitts FW: Delayed apoplexy following head injury. *J Neurosurg* 33:542, 1970.

GENERAL STUDY AIDS

Moseley HF: Traumatic disorders of the ankle and foot. *Clinical Symposia* Vol 17, 1965.

Symposium on knee injuries in athletics (unpublished articles for extension course on knee injuries). UCLA, 1967.

Special exhibit committee on fractures, AMA. *Exhibit on fractures* (Scientific exhibit) AMA booklet (3300–256:467–10M).

CHAPTER 7

Musculoskeletal Pain

Several studies of family practice indicate that about 18 percent of all consultations are referable to the musculoskeletal system. Peculiarly enough the complaints are not solely from the elderly. Although there is a steady increase in the number of patients in each decade from 25 years up, the largest number (24 percent of the total) is in the 15- to 24-year-old age group. The complaints in the young are associated with trauma in the men and soft-tissue rheumatism in the women (Table 7-1). In the elderly, osteoarthritis is responsible for 40 percent of the complaints.

FUNCTIONAL MUSCULOSKELETAL PAIN

Family physicians should be able to recognize functional musculoskeletal tension. Its recognition is important in order to save the patient the hazards of anti-inflammatory and steroid medications. The patient appears taut and grim, hunched with contracted posture, anxious with excessive sweating and somewhat disabled with contracted hard muscles. His extremities are cold and there is a fine tremor. Pain is burning or stabbing. Frequent locations of pain are the occiput, paracervical, lumbar, intervertebral or interscapular muscle groups. The spasm frequently relaxes when stretched or massaged. There is no evidence of organic disease. The tension recurs with emotional turmoil or conflict. Patients often explain they are restless, uptight or holding themselves in.

When treating a patient of this type, consider his physical and psychological problems. Attempt to get the patient to talk about himself rather than his ailment. Explain to him the nature of his pain. Use physical measures of treatment such as hot baths and swimming. Spray the area with ethyl chloride or have the patient use other counterirritants. In severe cases, try local injections of Xylocaine into trigger areas. This gives enough relief to allow the patient to focus his attention on something else. About the only drug of value is Valium (diazepam).

HAND DISORDERS

Heberden's Nodes

Probably Heberden's nodes are the most common cause of pain and deformity at the DIP joint. The nodes are a hereditary condition that cause swelling and tenderness. They occur on one or more fingers except the thumb. The nodes are hard nodules, 2 to 3 mm in diameter and on either side of the finger's dorsal midline. The process is a localized osteoarthritis, but their development does not necessarily indicate that generalized osteoarthritis will follow.

Do not treat except when painful. Nothing will change the arthritic process. For relief, inject equal parts of Decadron and Hydeltra-TBA around the nodes.

Table 7-1. The American Rheumatism Association's Classification of Arthritis and Rheumatism

I. Polyarthritis of unknown etiology
   A. Rheumatoid arthritis
   B. Juvenile rheumatoid arthritis (Still's disease)
   C. Ankylosing spondylitis
   D. Psoriatic arthritis
   E. Reiter's syndrome
   F. Others

II. Connective tissue disorders
   A. Systemic lupus erythematosus
   B. Polyarteritis nodosa
   C. Scleroderma (progressive systemic sclerosis)
   D. Polymyositis and dermatomyositis
   E. Others

III. Rheumatic Fever

IV. Degenerative joint disease (osteoarthritis, osteoarthrosis)
   A. Primary
   B. Secondary

V. Nonarticular rheumatism
   A. Fibrositis
   B. Intervertebral disc and low back syndromes
   C. Myositis and myalgia
   D. Tendinitis and peritendinitis (bursitis)
   E. Tenosynovitis
   F. Fasciitis
   G. Carpal tunnel syndrome
   H. Others

VI. Diseases with which arthritis is frequently associated
   A. Sarcoidosis
   B. Relapsing polychondritis
   C. Henoch-Schonlein syndrome
   D. Ulcerative colitis
   E. Regional ileitis
   F. Whipple's disease
   G. Sjogren's syndrome
   H. Familial Mediterranean fever
   I. Others

VII. Diseases associated with known infectious agents
   A. Bacterial
      1. Brucella
      2. Gonococcus
      3. Mycobacterium tuberculosis
      4. Pneumococcus
      5. Salmonella
      6. Staphylococcus
      7. Streptobacillus moniliformis (Haverhill fever)
      8. Treponema pallidum (syphilis)
      9. Treponema pertenue (yaws)
      10. Others
   B. Rickettsial
   C. Viral
   D. Fungal
   E. Parasitic

VIII. Traumatic and/or neurogenic disorders
   A. Traumatic arthritis (result of direct trauma)
   B. Lues (tertiary syphilis)
   C. Diabetes
   D. Syringomyelia
   E. Shoulder-hand syndrome
   F. Mechanical derangement of joints
   G. Others

IX. Diseases associated with known biochemical or endocrine abnormalities
   A. Gout
   B. Ochronosis
   C. Hemophilia
   D. Hemoglobinopathies (sickle cell disease)
   E. Agammaglobulinemia
   F. Gaucher's disease
   G. Hyperparathyroidism
   H. Acromegaly
   I. Hypothyroidism
   J. Scurvy (hypovitaminosis C)
   K. Xanthoma tuberosum
   L. Others

X. Tumor and tumorlike conditions
   A. Synovioma
   B. Pigmented villonodular synovitis
   C. Giant cell tumor of tendon sheath
   D. Primary juxta-articular bone tumors
   E. Metastatic
   F. Leukemia
   G. Multiple myeloma
   H. Benign tumors of articular tissue (Fig. 7-1)
   I. Others

XI. Allergy and drug reaction
   A. Arthritis due to specific allergens (serum sickness)
   B. Arthritis due to drugs (hydralazine syndrome)
   C. Others

XII. Inherited and congenital disorders
   A. Marfan's syndrome
   B. Ehlers-Danlos syndrome
   C. Hurler's syndrome
   D. Congenital hip dysplasia
   E. Morquio's disease
   F. Others

XIII. Miscellaneous disorders
   A. Amyloidosis
   B. Aseptic necrosis of bone
   C. Behcet's syndrome
   D. Chondrocalcinosis (pseudogout)
   E. Erythema multiforme (Stevens-Johnson syndrome)
   F. Erythema nodosum
   G. Hypertrophic osteoarthropathy
   H. Juvenile osteochondritis
   I. Osteochondritis dissecans
   J. Reticulohistiocytosis of joints (lipoid dermatoarthritis)
   K. Tietze's disease
   L. Others

Reprinted with permission from Primer on the Rheumatic Diseases, Amer. Rheumatism Assoc., The Arthritis Foundation, New York, with permission.

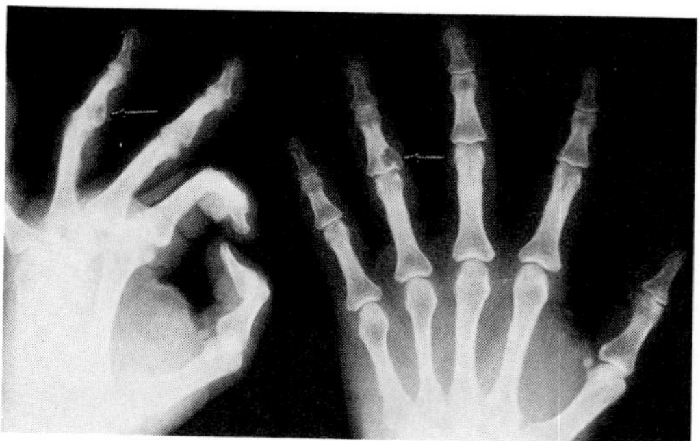

Figure 7-1. Enchondroma of the fourth finger.

Mucous Cysts

Heberden's nodes are often confused with mucous cysts. Both occur about the DIP joint. Mucous cysts, however, are unilateral. The remainder of the joint appears normal. If doubt exists, x-ray the finger and osteoarthritic degenerative changes will be present with Heberden's nodes. More confusion exists when both Heberden's nodes and a mucous cyst are present on one finger.

Treatment of a mucous cyst is the same as for Heberden's nodes—Decadron and Hydeltra-TBA. Do not be misled by the apparent simplicity with which the cyst may be removed. Surgery is radical. Excise the cyst and skin. Replace the skin by a split thickness graft.

Ganglion

Ganglia are small growths of connective tissue arising from tendon or capsule sheaths. They occur about the hands, wrist, and fingers. They usually feel like solid tumors but are distended with a gelatinous fluid.

Aspirate the sticky fluid with a #18 needle after infiltrating the area with Xylocaine, 2 percent through a #25 needle. Scarify the internal capsule with the needle point after aspiration. Last of all inject ¼ ml each of Hydeltra-TBA and Decadron into the ganglion. If the above is unsuccessful, excision under general anesthesia in a hospital is required. Be prepared to trace and excise all the lining of the ganglion, even if tendons and nerves need be displaced. In some instances the tract will lead to the bony periosteum.

Mallet Finger

Mallet finger is a finger which is permanently flexed at the DIP joint. The deformity is caused when the extensor tendor is torn from its insertion on the distal phalanx. Suspect the injury whenever patients complain of an injury to the finger. Splint the DIP joint (not the IP joint) hyperextended with a padded narrow aluminum split for 3 to 8 weeks.

First Carpometacarpal Joint Strain

Think first of this strain when a woman complains of pain and tenderness in the first carpometacarpal joint. X-ray pictures are negative unless the strain is long-standing, in which case the joint irregularities of degenerative arthritis can be seen. Immobilize loosely with an elastic bandage about the wrist and base of the thumb. Three weekly injections of Hydeltra-TBA and Decadron are usually effective in relieving discomfort.

De Quervain's Disease
(Chronic Stenosing Tenosynovitis)

This is a common disorder occasionally confused with carpometacarpal joint strain. De Quervain's disease is a condition in which the extensor pollicis brevis tendon is inflamed. Occasionally small swellings the size of raisins can be felt on the tendon by palpating the snuffbox (Fig. 7-2) at the base of the thumb.

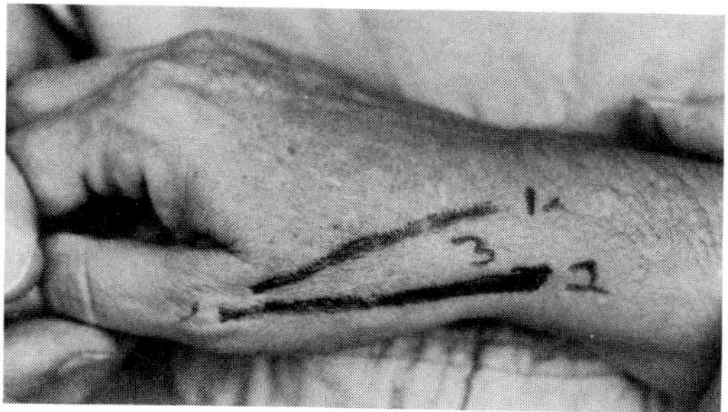

Figure 7-2. *1,* Extensor pollicis longus; *2,* Extensor pollicus brevis; *3,* Anatomic snuffbox.

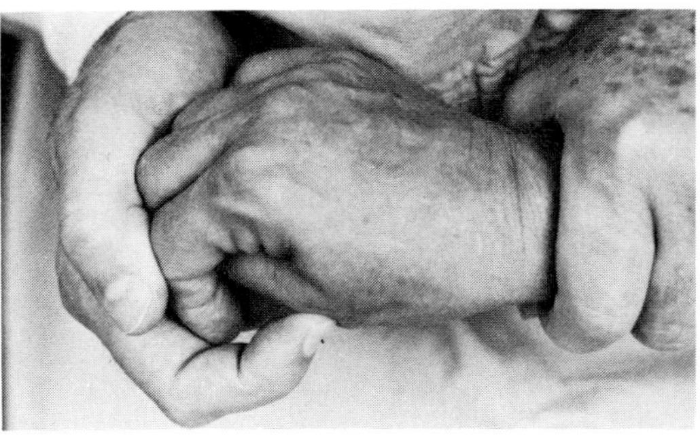

Figure 7-3. Finkelstein's test for DeQuervain's disease. Ask the patient to clench his fist over his thumb. Now push the flexed thumb ulnarward. The test is considered positive for chronic stenosing tenosynovitis if the patient complains of pain at the radial styloid process.

Search for three signs:

–tenderness of the radial styloid process extending for 1 to 2 cm proximally
–positive Finkelstein's test (Fig. 7-3)
–painless passive extension of the thumb

To treat, inject the tendon sheaths of the radial styloid process with ¼ ml each of Decadron and Hydeltra-TBA 3 or 4 times at weekly intervals.

Trigger Finger (Stenosing Tenosynovitis)

Diagnose trigger finger (Fig. 7-4) by finding an area of point tenderness over the flexor aspect of the metacarpophalangeal joint. Palpate for a thickened sheath or nodule. In some cases, on extending the finger, the motion is impeded, locking the finger in flexion. With more pull, the finger finally snaps into extension, sometimes painfully. There may be all degrees of snapping and pain, or no pain at all.

Treatment is simple. Inject the tendon sheath on the flexor side of the metacarpal head. Use Decadron and Hydeltra-TBA, ¼ ml of each, once weekly for 3 weeks.

PAINFUL FEET

Examining the Feet

Give special attention to the patient's feet whenever performing a general examina-

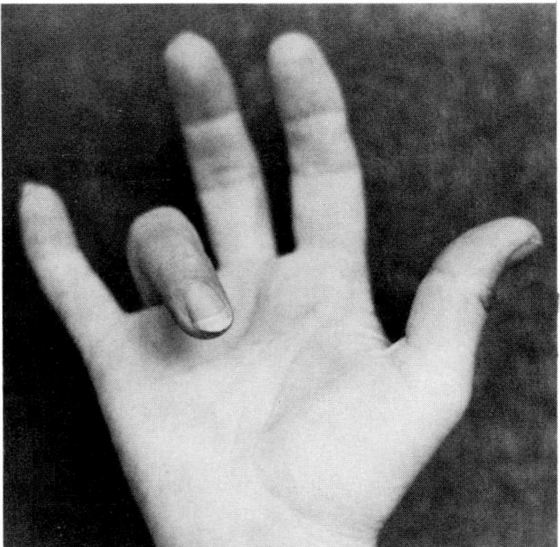

Figure 7-4. Trigger finger, a disease of the flexor tendon of the middle or ring finger.

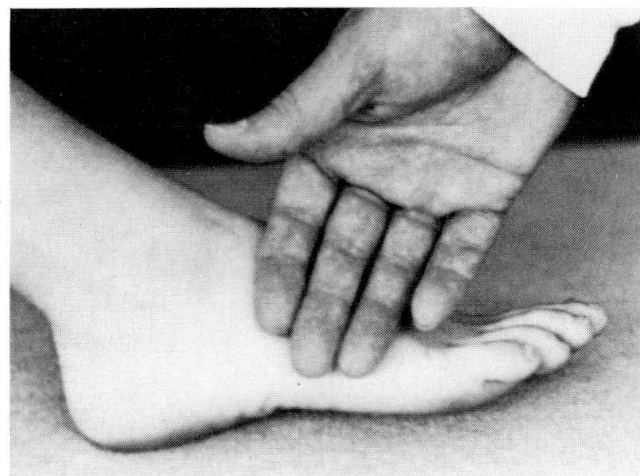

Figure 7-5. Test skin temperature with the back of your hand but first apply your hand to the back of your neck for comparison.

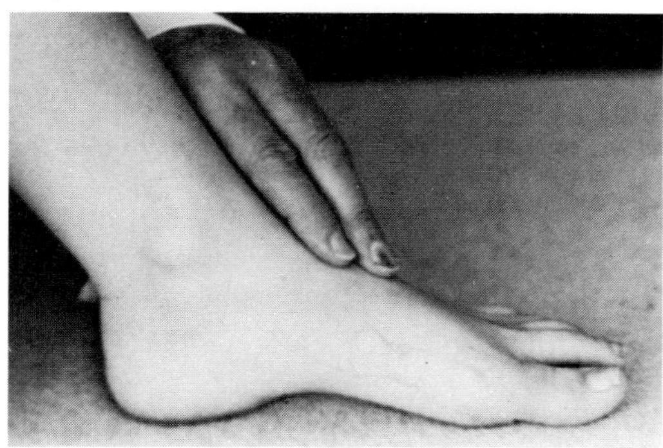

Figure 7-6. Check circulation in the extremity by palpating the patient's pulse.

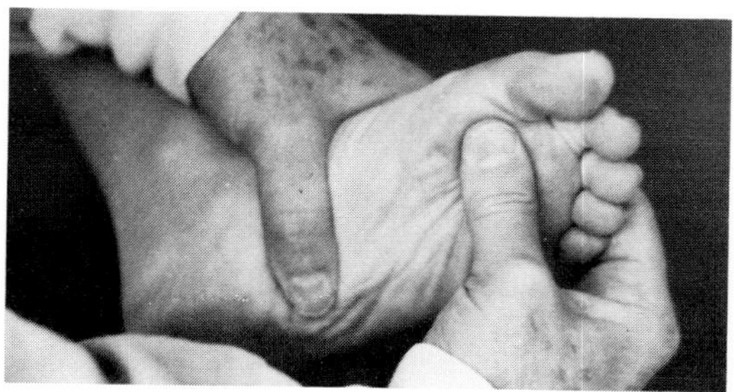

Figure 7-7. Test for general foot motion. Hold the patient's foot around the instep. With your opposite hand grasp the ball of her foot and inscribe a circle with the great toe. This will give you some idea of the efficiency of the joints between the tarsal and cuneiform bones. Practice to palpate for frozen tarsal joints and their metatarsal segments.

tion. Inspect the patient's feet with his shoes and stockings removed and while they are weight bearing and at rest. Drop a plumb line from midpatellar. It should fall between the first and second metatarsal bones. Note and compare the color the skin, the temperature (Fig. 7-5) and turgor. An excessively pale skin indicates restricted circulation, a bluish skin a slow circulation, and redness plenty of blood because of inflammation. Check the circulation by palpating the posterior tibial and dorsalis pedis arteries (Fig. 7-6). Check motor, sensory and vibratory response in both feet. Search for atophy and swelling. Test the motion in all joints (Fig. 7-7)—plantar and dorsal flexion, eversion and inversion. Steady the foot with your left hand while checking the motion of the metatarsal bones (Fig. 7-8) and especially the tarsometatarsal joints.

Pay close attention to the big toe. Test for motion (Fig. 7-9). Learn how much flexion and extension exists in the first metatarsophalangeal articulation. Begin the examination by placing your index finger and thumb at 90° angle. To determine total motion, force the great toe downward to full flexion. With the left hand still forming a right angle push the big toe into full extension. Normally, this arc should range from 90° to 130°. To determine extension only of the big toe, measure the extension arc from a neutral position (Fig. 7-10). Normally this should be at least 45°. If the extension is limited (locked) consider osteochondritis

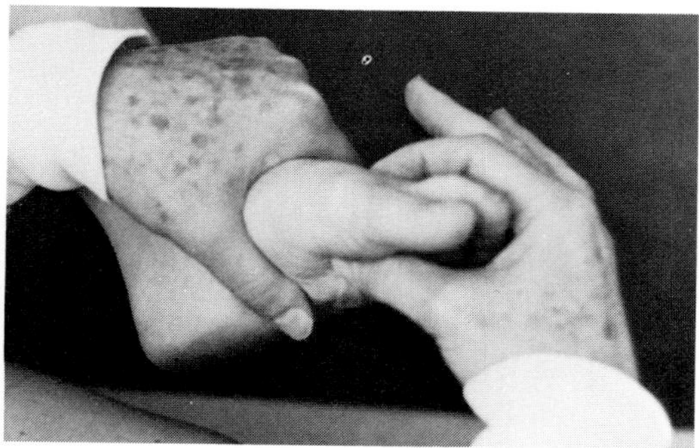

Figure 7-8. Tightly hold the patient's foot with your left hand and with your right grasp the head of each metatarsal and move it up and down. Determine the range of motion of each metatarsal by this movement. Greatest motion occurs in the bases of the fourth and fifth metatarsals as they articulate with the cuboid.

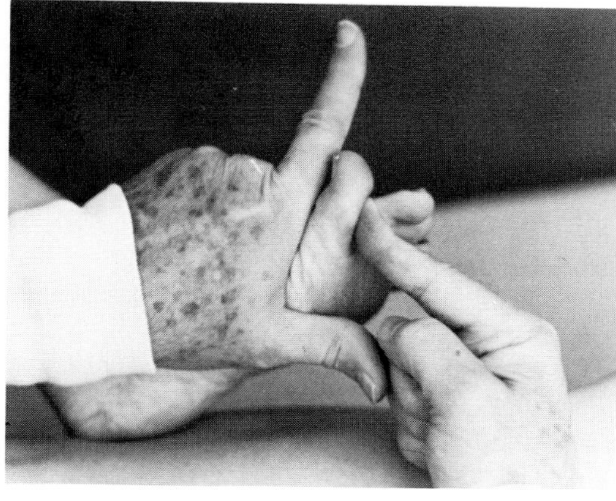

Figure 7-9. With your left index finger and thumb at a 90° angle, push the big toe with your other hand into full extension.

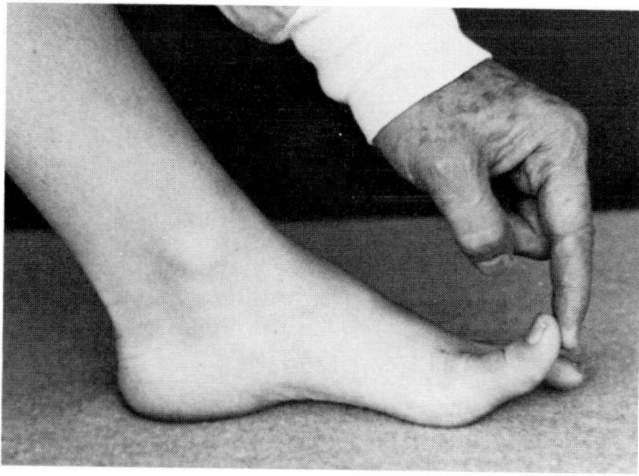

Figure 7-10. Normally extension should be at least 45°.

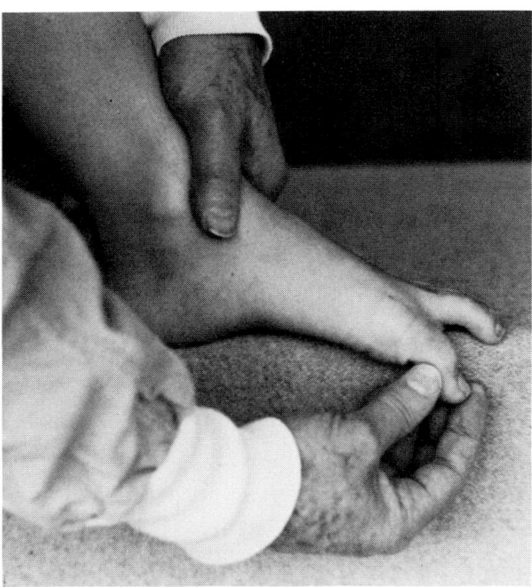

Figure 7-11. Check plantar flexion.

(hallux rigidus or hallux limitus), a bony lipping on the dorsal brim of the joint surface of the head of the first metatarsal bone. Dorsal extension is important in walking and 30° is sufficient for ordinary activity but not enough for good running. Plantar flexion of 45° is superfluous (Fig. 7-11). It is necessary, however, to have strong muscular power to perform the act of plantar flexion because this motion is used against the ground in the third stage of walking when the body weight is thrust forward.

Next determine alignment of the great toe in relationship to its metatarsal bone. Normally this should be a straight line on the mesial side of the foot. Determine the outward flare of the big toe from the midline by placing your finger as shown in Figure 7-12. Place the index finger of your left hand in a position so that its edge is parallel to the long axis of the first metatarsal bone. Next place the tip of your right index finger on your left index finger, forming a right angle. Now observe the inner edge of the great toe and its relationship to the right angle. From this you can determine whether the big toe is 30°, 45° or 60° out of line. Thrust the great toe toward the midline as far as possible with your right thumb (Fig. 7-13) to determine the lateral motion of the joint. A bunion joint is at least 45° out of line.

Motion of the smaller toes as a group is important. Determine flexion of the smaller toes using the position of the big toe in neutral position as 0° (Fig. 7-14). The foot has a tendency to contract in foot disturbances and the smaller toes draw up and cannot be brought down beyond the neutral base position. If there is limited flexion, examine each toe for hammer toe, ankylosis and dislocation of the proximal phalanx.

Test for subluxation or displacement of the tarsal bones. The most important displacement is a spreading of the bony elements of the transverse tarsal arch with a

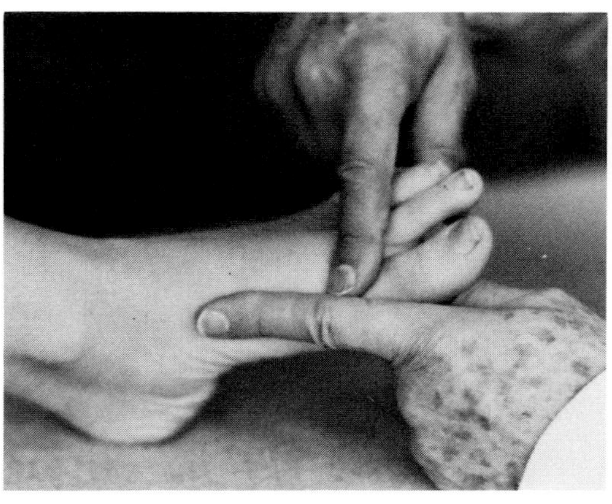

Figure 7-12. Determine the outward flare of the big toe from the midline.

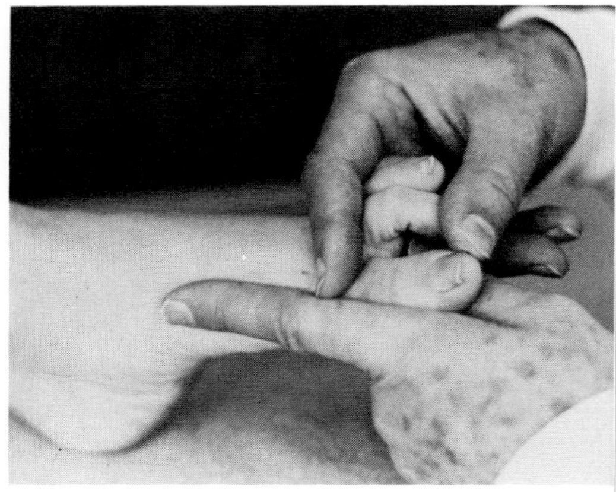

Figure 7-13. Thrust the great toe toward the midline to determine the lateral motion of the joint.

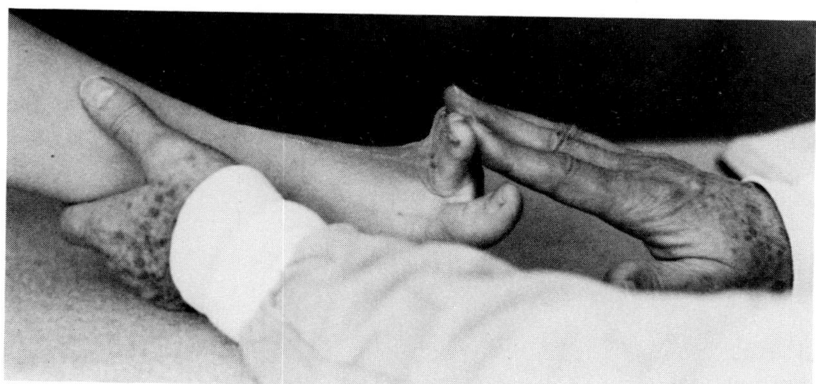

Figure 7-14. Determine flexion of the small toes.

downward dropping of either the first cuneiform or the cuboid. If you are not experienced in detecting displacement, palpate for soreness under the tuberosity of the cuboid (Fig. 7-15). Soreness indicates subluxation. The same holds true for the first cuneiform. The most common bony lesions are an inward and downward rotation of the cuboid and a downward slipping of the first cuneiform bone (Fig. 7-16).

Have the patient stand so you can examine him for flatfeet. Position his feet about 4 in apart and parallel. Check the height of the medial longitudinal arch. Is it high or flat? If flat, does it resume normal shape when weight is removed? Have your patient stand on one foot without support for a minute (Fig. 7-17). Observe the action of

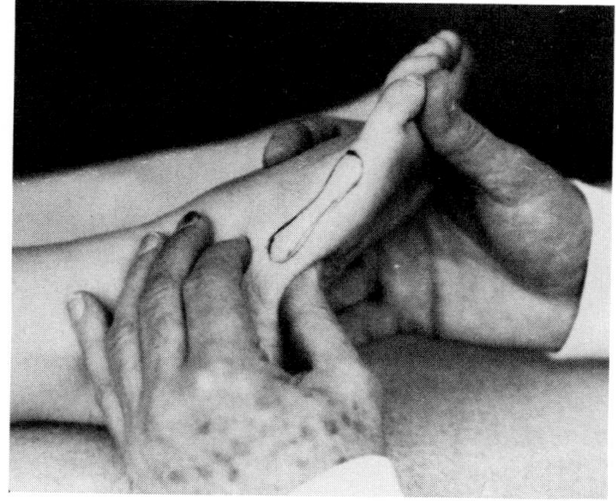

Figure 7-16. Examine the cuneiform bone.

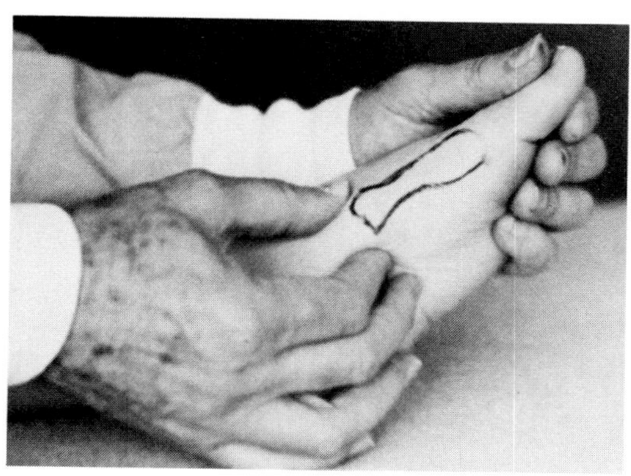

Figure 7-15. Palpate for soreness under the tuberosity of the cuboid.

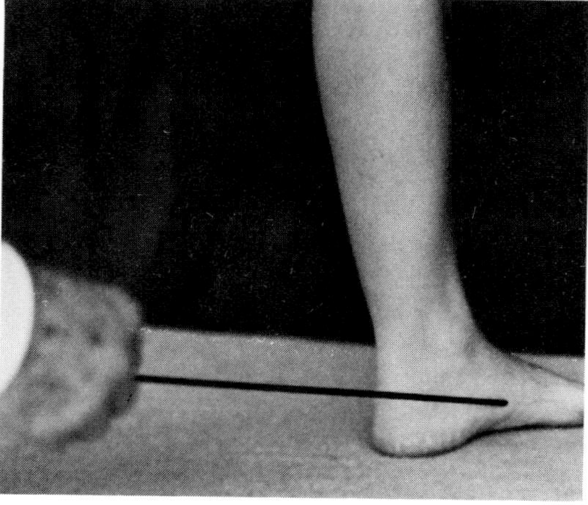

Figure 7-17. Have your patient stand on one foot so you can observe the action of the inner spring arch.

the innerspring arch as it adjusts, keeping the weight balanced on the pivoting joint in the outer weight-bearing arch. Unbalanced posture is common in foot trouble, often creating low back symptoms.

Look at the feet from behind. Is there bowing of the Achilles tendon? This is a dependable sign of pes planus. Have the patient stand on his heels to test the anterior leg muscle and shortening of the Achilles tendon. Eversion is limited in rigid flatfeet, inversion by spasm of the peronei. Observe how the patient walks (Fig. 7-18). Correlate the walk with the result of your foot tests. For instance, the patient in hallux rigidus may turn his ankle outward to prevent weight bearing on the great toe joint.

Determine if the patient is wearing proper fitting shoes. If the foot has good function, the shoe will show wear on the lateral edge of the heel and sole. Fair function of the foot wears the heel and sole evenly. And poor function will wear down the medial side and tilt the heel into a valgus position.

Thrombophlebitis is a definite cause of foot trouble. Figure 7-19 indicates the sites of communicating branches of the veins.

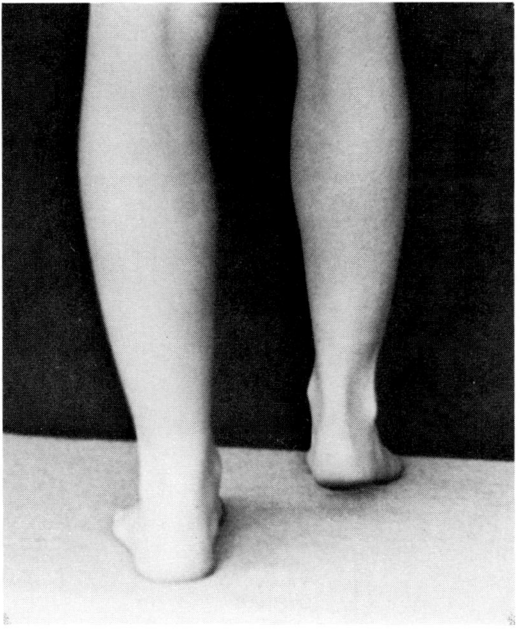

Figure 7-18. Observe how the patient walks.

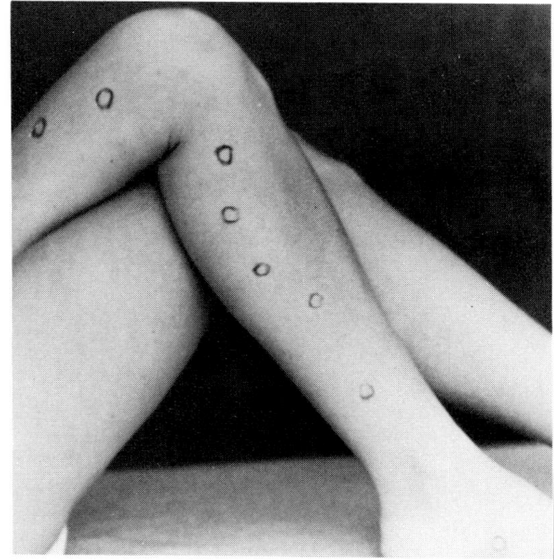

Figure 7-19. Circles focus on the course of the veins with probable sites of communicating branches.

When these points are painful, the finding is most suggestive of chronic phlebitis.

Remember foot problems may reflect systemic disease such as gout, diabetes mellitus, arteriosclerosis, rheumatoid arthritis, osteoarthritis and infections.

Corns

Hard and soft corns are caused by friction. Soft (interdigital clavus) are the result of two bony prominences rubbing together, plus moisture. Soft corns will disappear when the offending exostoses are removed. Hard corns are conical shaped keratin fingers pointing into the dermis. They are caused by chronic friction, usually from improper fitting shoes.

Plantar Callosities

These patches of thickened epidermis occur under metatarsal heads. Usually they cause little or no pain and are difficult to treat. The cause is unequal distribution of weight over the metatarsal head. Before suggesting surgery; try metatarsal bars (Fig. 7-20) or metatarsal pads in an attempt to equalize weight bearing between the meta-

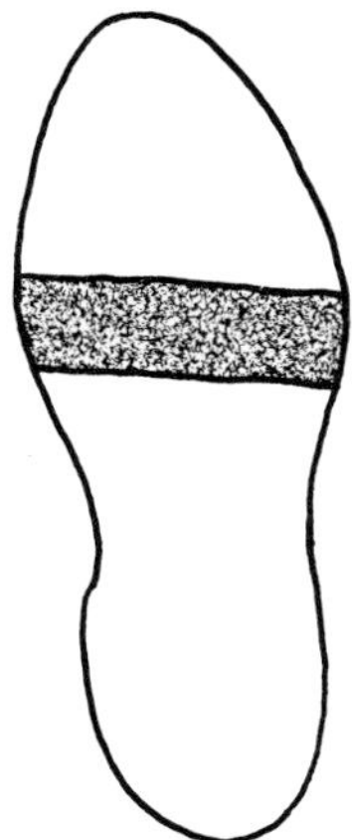

Figure 7-20. For relief of metatarsalgia or metatarsal callosities, prescribe a 3/16 in thick bar placed on the sole of the shoe behind the metatarsal heads.

tarsal heads. Soaking the callus each evening with lanolin or baby oil helps. Don't allow the patient to pare the callus down with a knife or razor blade. Suggest sandpaper or an aluminum type nutmeg grater for this purpose. If these simple measures do not help, refer the patient to an orthopedist.

Plantar Warts

Differentiate warts from plantar callosities and corns. Warts are caused by virus infection and their treatment differs from that of corns. A tip in differentiating: pinching warts from the sides cause pain but digital pressure is not particularly painful although weight bearing is; Plantar corns have an opposite response in that pressure causes pain and squeezing does not. There is no ideal method of removal of plantar warts. I prefer electrocoagulation. I have found b.i.d. applications of trichloroacetic acid by toothpicks too prolonged and generally ineffective. Other physicians seem to obtain better results from this method. I have never had a true wart drop off after injecting with Xylocaine; others claim they do. Surgical excision is effective if the wart is small enough. Occasionally in cases of recurrence, I have a competent radiologist radiate the lesion. This is helpful, especially if combined with paring down the surrounding keratin before each treatment.

Perforating Neurotropic Ulcers

Ulcers may occur almost anywhere on the soles but most frequently under a metatarsal head. Do not be misled by its painlessness and do not treat locally without a searching general examination for systemic causes such as diabetes mellitus, peripheral neuritis, pernicious anemia and spinal cord tumor.

Ingrown Toenails

Paronychias are common and are the result of improper trimming of the nail of the great toe. The lateral edge of the nail plate grows into the nail fold and produces irritation. Finally infection is set up at the corners as the nail grows out. Teach your patients to trim their toenails straight across and not down at the edges.

Minor degrees of irritation and infection may be relieved by soaks and placing cotton under the edge of the nail until it grows out. But generally, once the nail fold is severely infected, surgical excision of 3/16 of an inch of the nail's edge plus the accompanying fold is needed to cure the disease (Fig. 7-21).

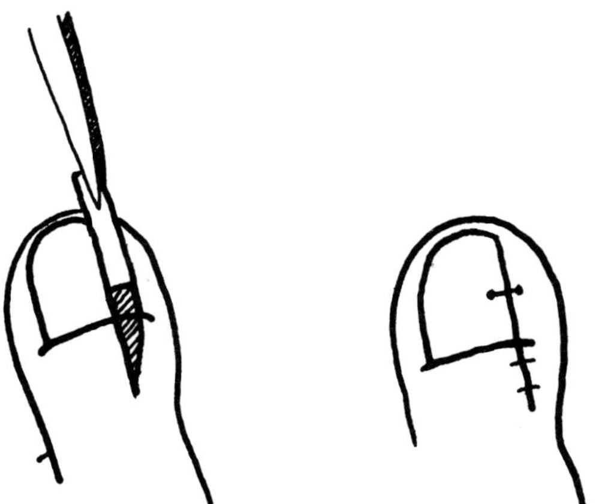

Figure 7-21. Excision of an ingrown toenail usually can be done under local anesthesia. A Penrose drain around the base of the toe clamped by a hemostat will provide hemostasis. With a pair of straight scissors incise the lateral quarter of the nail up to and including its base and matrix. A second incision is made up the skin at a 45° angle, including all diseased tissue. Curet granulation tissue from the wound, including all the matrix. One or two sutures will be sufficient.

Merely removing the nail is not enough. Surgical excision can be done under local anesthesia using a rubber band for a tourniquet. Excise the outer portion of the nail with scissors; then open the nail bed with a scalpel and thoroughly currette. One or two sutures are needed to close the wound and perhaps one suture through a hole in the remaining nail edge.

Fungus Toenails

Fungus infections are found in older patients who are unable to care for their nails properly. Removing the nail is insufficient. Remove the entire nail bed.

Heel Pain

Pain in and about the heel is often caused by an inflamed bursa. Pain, swelling and tenderness near the insertion of the Achilles tendon may result from a *retrocalcaneal bursitis*. Look at the shoes the patient is wearing. Usually the heels are too high or, with men, their boots are stiffbacked. *Policeman's heel* (infracalcaneal bursitis) is the result of excessive walking, usually in an obese patient. Pain is present in the ball of the foot. On palpation, you will find tenderness over the tuberosity of the calcaneus. A *heel spur* is a forward growth of bone at the attachment of the plantar aponeurosis and short foot muscles (Fig. 7-22). Some physicians remove this so-called spur to relieve pain in the heel. This is a faulty practice because heel spurs have nothing to do with pain.

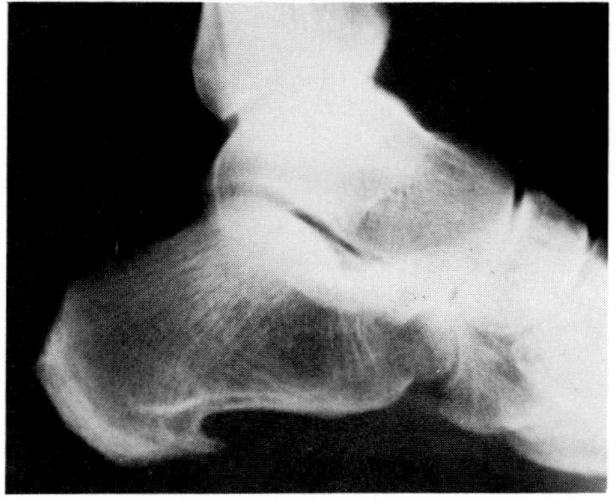

Figure 7-22. Heel spur, a forward growth of the bone at the attachment of the plantar aponeurosis and short foot muscles. Heel spurs are not painful.

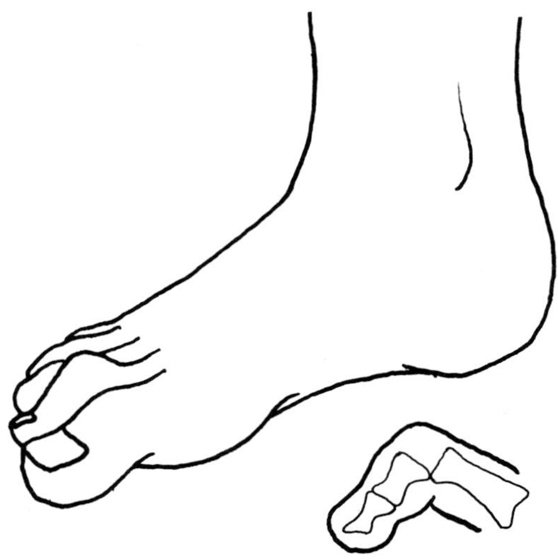

Figure 7-23. Hammer toe.

Another cause of heel pain is *tarsal-tunnel syndrome*. It often occurs after fractures or dislocations of the foot or ankle, sprains with subsequent edema, tenosynovitis, foot strain or chronic stasis of the posterior tibial vein. Compression of the nerve in the tunnel behind and inferior to the medial malleolus causes numbness, burning pain, paresthesias and occasionally paresis of some small muscles of the feet. Prove the diagnosis by measuring nerve velocities.

Hammer Toes

This deformity is so named because it resembles a hammer (Fig. 7-23). Only the second toe is usually involved. It is bilateral and often accompanies hallux valgus. Except for a poor cosmetic result, the best treatment is excision of the proximal phalanx. Probably the best course for a family physician is to refer the patient to an orthopedist to resect the proximal I-P joint and thread a Steinmann pin through the bones to maintain correct position. The pin must be left in for 8 weeks and removed after fusion has taken place.

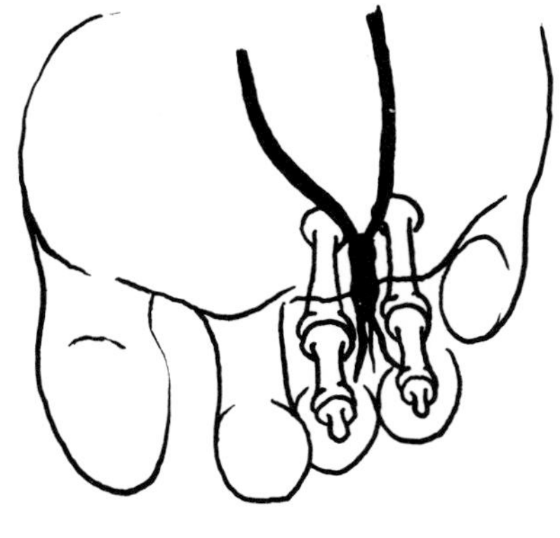

Figure 7-24. Plantar neuroma.

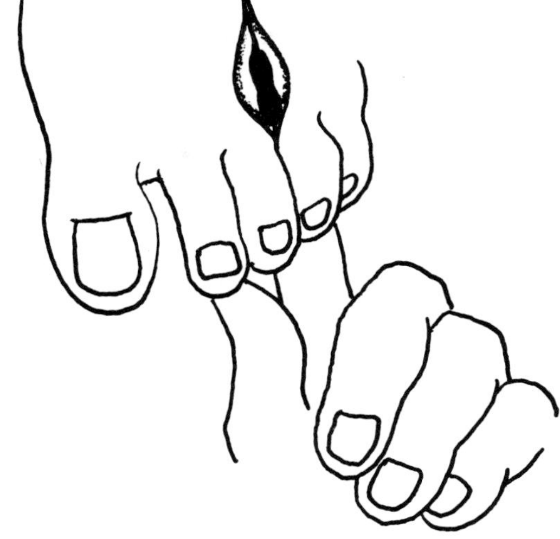

Morton's Neuroma (plantar's Neuroma)

This neuroma (Fig. 7-24) usually causes the patient great pain, numbness, tingling and a burning sensation. The patient often attempts relief by taking off his shoe and rubbing the foot. The burning sensation may become so intense the patient will put his foot in a bucket of cold water. X-rays are normal. Try to palpate a small tumor between the third and fourth toe. Usually there is tenderness between the same toes near the metatarsal heads. The treatment is simple and effective surgery. Make a 1 in incision on the dorsum of the foot between the third and fourth toe just proximal to the web. Using your left hand, make pressure from below and pop the neuroma out. Tell the patient to expect some numbness between the toes because of excision of the nerve. Allow the patient to walk on the foot as soon as tolerated. A metatarsal bar may be tried and injection of ¼ ml each of Hydeltra-TBA and Decadron into the site, but surgery is needed in 50 percent of the cases.

Bunions

Bunions are more common in the female than in the male. The patient most likely to develop a bunion is the one who has some degree of metatarsus varus. When this type of foot is squeezed into a pointed shoe, the stress necessary to produce a bunion begins. The bursa over the medial aspect of the MP joint is irritated and becomes painful. As the stress continues, the great toe is forced laterally. As the medial side of the joint capsule stretches, the joint actually becomes dislocated. The long extensor to the great toe is pulled laterally and shortened and acts as a bowstring fixing the toe in a lateral position. The awkward position of the great toe crowds the second toe (Fig. 7-25) and trouble develops in both toes.

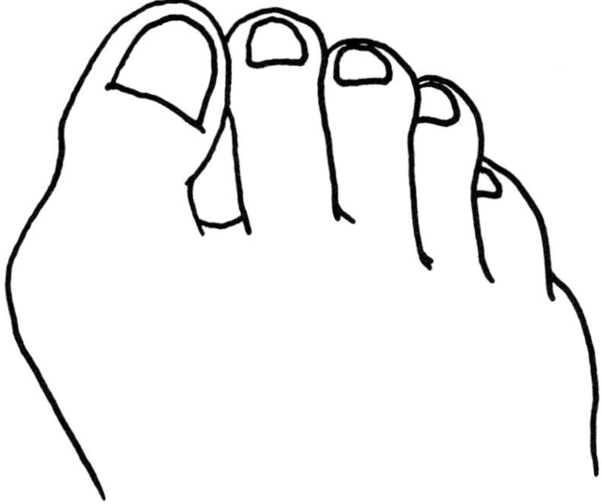

Figure 7-25. Bunions are caused by congenital adduction of the metatarsals and incorrect shoes.

If no infection is present inject a painful bunion with small doses (¼ ml) of corticosteroid. Surgery generally is necessary, although there are numerous splints and exercises prescribed. Do nothing until the blood supply is checked.

There are several operative procedures for bunions. The three that give the most consistent results are the techniques devised by McBride, Mitchell and Keller. The most popular is the Keller operation. Possibly all three should be used as circumstances differ. Results are not uniformly good. It is wise to refer these patients to a good orthopedist.

Other Uncommon Conditions

You should be aware of the following conditions that cause pain in the feet:

- –Calcaneal fractures from landing on the heel during a fall
- –Arthritis in its various manifestations
- –Metatarsal stress fracture (march fracture caused by excessive walking or standing)
- –Infections, including those of the deep fascial spaces
- –Ganglia
- –Dupuytren's contracture of the foot
- –Absense of middle phalanx
- –Overlapping of the fifth toe and bunionette
- –Fractured phalanx
- –Gout
- –Subungual exostosis of great toenail and subungual globus tumor
- –Ram's horn nail—an overgrowth of the toenail

SINGLE JOINT PAIN

Finger Joint

The commonest cause of single finger joint pain is trauma. Traumatic arthritis produced by a small fracture into a joint is an example. This is often called baseball finger because the injury occurs by a baseball or other object striking the end of the finger.

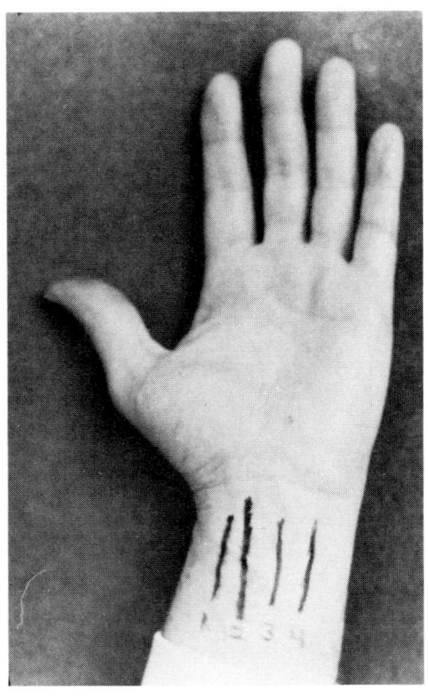

Figure 7-26. Tendons of the left volar wrist: *1*, Flexor carpi radialis; *2*, Palmaris longus; *3*, Flexor digitorum sublimis; *4*, Flexor carpi ulnaris.

Wrist

Most commonly the wrist is affected by trauma, such as sprains, strains, traumatic synovitis, fracture, tears of ligaments, tendons (Fig. 7-26) and capsules and joint dislocations. Such trauma originates from sports or occupational injuries.

Osteomyelitis

Osteomyelitis of the wrist usually occurs in childhood (Fig. 7-27). Staphylococci are

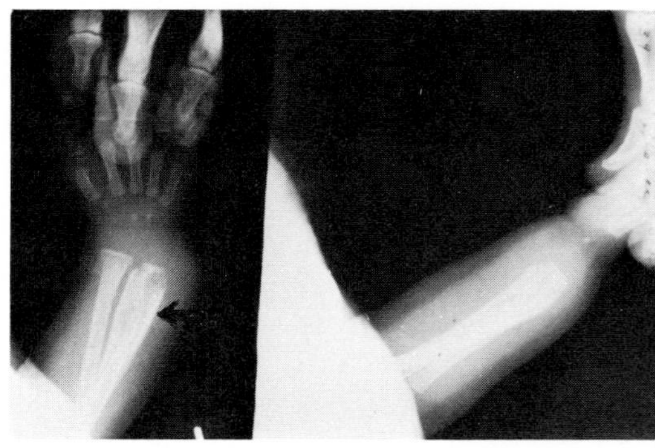

Figure 7-27. Osteomyelitis of the wrist.

the chief offenders. Onset is sudden with fever and pain. You may be able to locate an area of increased warmth by passing your fingers over the skin.

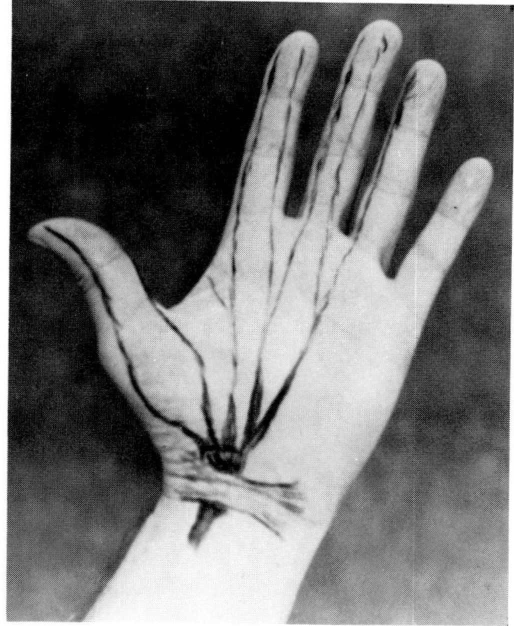

Figure 7-28. Distribution of the median nerve.

Carpal Tunnel Syndrome

Look for carpal tunnel syndrome whenever the patient complains of awakening from sleep with a severe paresthesia in the distribution of the median nerve (Fig. 7-28). In other cases a deep aching occurs in the forearm. Early in the disease, when the patient attempts to use his hand, wrist or forearm, he experiences paroxysms of pain and paresthesias. As the disease progresses the patient loses some motor function such as finger and thumb opposition, pinching, grasping and release. In time, thenar eminence atrophy occurs.

Verify the diagnosis by (1) holding the patient's wrist in extreme palmar flexion for 60 sec, thus reproducing the patient's symptoms (Fig. 7-29); (2) percussion over the median nerve (Tinel's sign) (Fig. 7-30); and (3) electromyographic testing. The latter measures the motor conduction velocity. The usual conduction delay from the proximal wrist to the thenar eminence is less than 5 m sec. In carpal tunnel syndrome, the delay may average around 8 or 9 m sec. Alterations in sensory conduction also occurs.

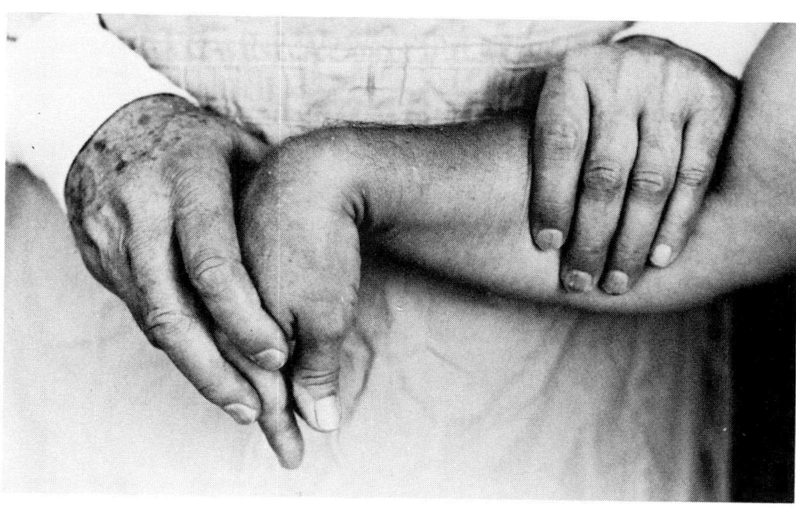

Figure 7-29. Testing for carpal tunnel syndrome. Hyperflex the wrist for 60 sec. Consider carpal tunnel syndrome if the patient's symptoms are reproduced or made worse. If her symptoms are relieved by extension, the diagnosis is practically verified.

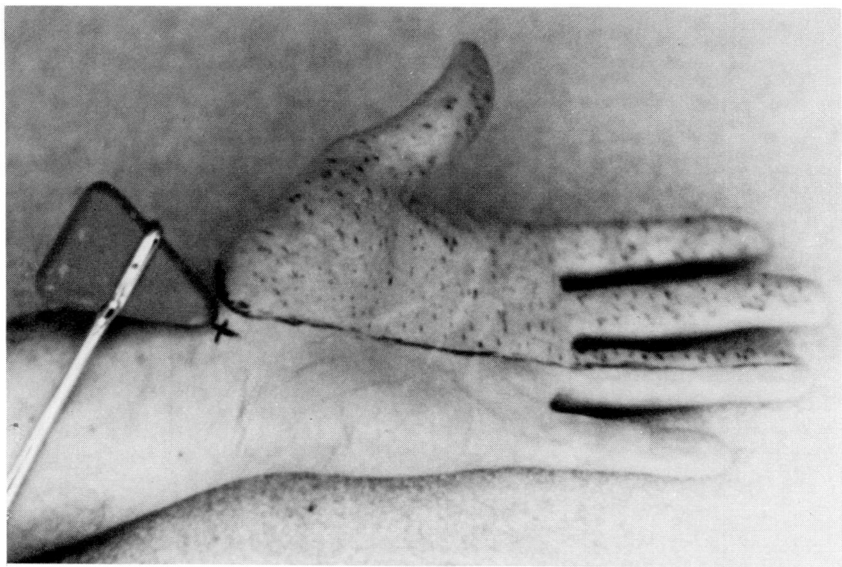

Figure 7-30. Tinel's sign of carpal tunnel syndrome. Percuss the radial side of the palmaris longus tendon. Tinel's is considered positive if a tingling sensation is produced by the tap.

Whenever you find a carpal tunnel syndrome, check out the possibility of systemic lupus erythematosus, rheumatoid arthritis, amyloid infiltrations, multiple myeloma, acromegaly, diabetes, and hypothyroidism as well as local causes of trauma, cysts, ganglions and neuromas.

Try conservative treatment, immobilizing the wrist in dorsiflexion while giving diathermy, microtherm and ultrasound. If this approach doesn't work, suggest surgery. It consists of sectioning the transverse carpal ligament and exploring the carpal tunnel carefully for neoplasms, cysts, ganglia or granulomatous inflammation.

Elbow

This joint is readily injured because of its unprotected and vulnerable location. The olecranon bursa is a frequent site of trauma. Inspection and palpation secure the diagnosis. The bursa is tender, warm to palpation, distended and crepitant. Chronic ole-

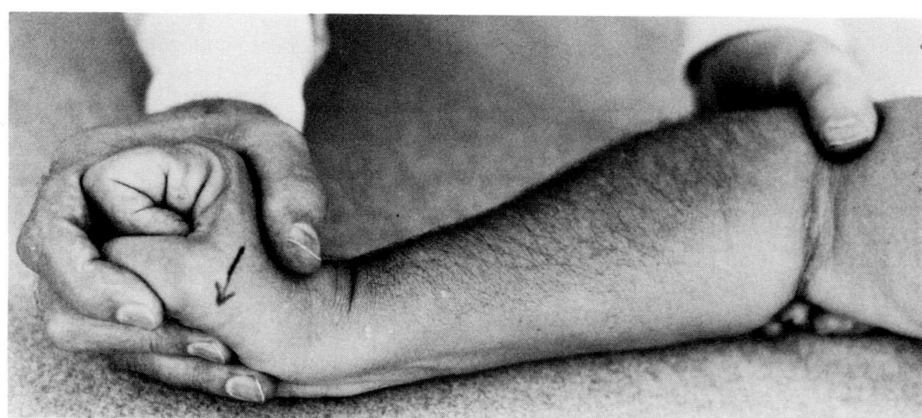

Figure 7-31. Cozen's test for tennis elbow.

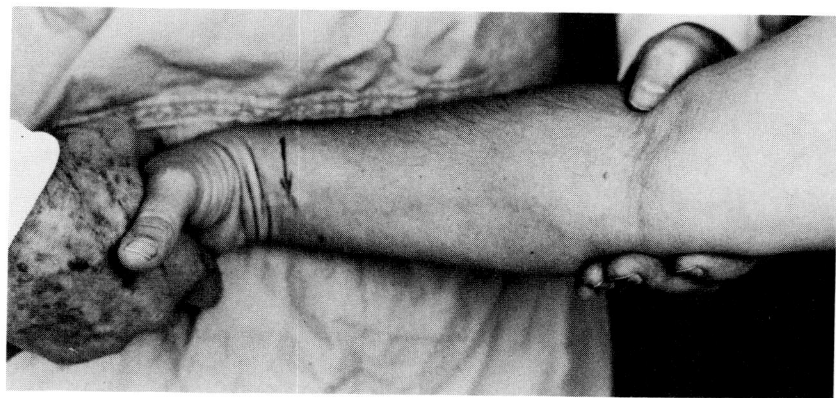

Figure 7-32. Mill's maneuver for tennis elbow.

cranon bursitis is common with rheumatoid arthritis and gout. Synonyms are miner's or student's elbow.

Epicondylitis

Another common cause of elbow pain is epicondylitis, tennis elbow, which results from severe and repeated pulling of the forearm muscle tendons at their insertion into the humeral epicondyle. Tenderness is sharply localized to the epicondyle and found by the tip of an unopened pen. Pain is also accentuated by forceful contraction of the muscles of the forearm. Extending the wrist as in picking up small objects will cause pain, but lifting heavy objects when the wrist is flexed causes little or no pain.

In Cozen's test for tennis elbow (Fig. 7-31) ask the patient to clench and extend his wrist. With your right hand attempt to flex the patient's wrist against his resistance. Pain in the lateral epicondyle during the maneuver is considered a positive test. In Mill's maneuver (Fig. 7-32) the patient is asked to extend his elbow with the wrist flexed. Attempt to pronate the wrist against the patient's resistance. A positive test is indicated if the patient complains of pain in the lateral epicondyle.

Tennis elbow is caused by inflammation in any of the structures in and around the radiohumeral joint: chronic radiohumeral bursitis, tendonitis of the cojoined extensor tendon attached to the lateral epicondyle, synovitis, partial rupture of the origin of the extensor muscles with secondary periostitis of the lateral epicondyle or gout.

In milder forms of the disease, immobilize or ask the patient to abstain from activities that require prolonged grasping and traction movements with the forearm. Some physicians give ultrasound or microtherm treatment. I prefer cold applications and some active exercise to keep the joint and tendons from freezing.

Most times you will need to resort to more active treatment. If done skillfully, local injections (Fig. 7-33) of Xylocaine with or without a steroid will shorten the disease. Occasionally 2 weeks of oral steroids will be necessary. Surgical treatment consists of re-

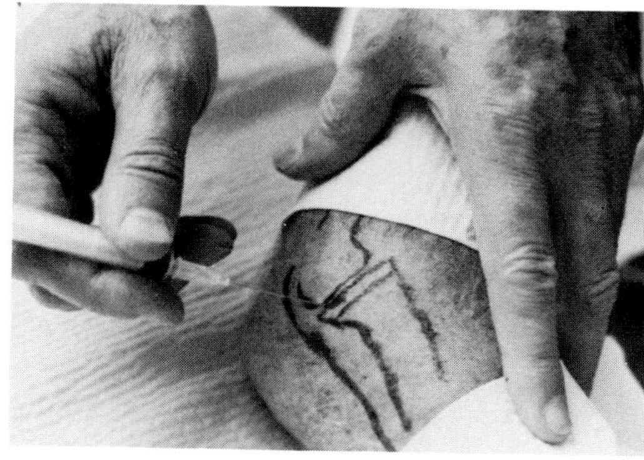

Figure 7-33. Injection treatment of tennis elbow. Injection should not be made into the lateral epicondyle. For a radiohumeral bursa injection, attempt to find the pictured site.

lease of the common extensor origin from the epicondyle and excision of any inflammatory tissue between the tendon and joint capsule. Surgery is usually delayed until after the patient has had a trial of immobilization with a cast or sling.

To put these treatment modalities in their proper perspective, consider the following. Injection of an anesthetic and steroid will relieve pain greatly or completely in about 95 percent of the cases if done properly. About 32 percent will require additional injections and about 6 percent of these will need surgery.

Find the region of greatest tenderness by using the point of an unopened pen. When the point is located, press the pen into the skin, marking the area with the small circular indentation of the pen. Through the center of this mark inject 2 percent Xylocaine in and around the area until tenderness disappears and gripping becomes painless. Through the same needle, inject 10 to 15 mg of hydrocortisone. Finish by manipulating the joint carefully. When the Xylocaine wears off, the joint may be painful for 10 to 15 hr. Analgesics and ice bags are used to alleviate this discomfort. When the pain and tenderness is rather diffuse and the disease is chronic, prescribe an oral anti-inflammatory drug such as phenylbutazone. When the disease is extremely painful, consider the application of an extension splint on the wrist for 1 to 2 weeks.

Shoulder

Not all shoulder pain is arthritis or bursitis or painful stiff shoulder. Learn to make a precise diagnosis. In family practice you will encounter painful shoulders frequently and can treat most of them after learning a few principles.

Calcific Tendonitis

The most common cause of the painful shoulder syndrome is calcific tendonitis of one of the tendons inserting into the greater trochanter of the humerus. Most commonly this is the tendon of the supraspinatous muscle.

Start your examination by asking the patient to put his hand behind the small of his back or behind his neck. This movement abducts and rotates the arm, movements particularly restricted in supraspinatus tendonitis. Next, with your fingers palpate the entire shoulder for tenderness. The patient has poor pain localization in the shoulder and will be surprised when you find tenderness beneath the acromial tip or in the notch between the greater and lesser tubercles of the humeral head.

One useful finding is elicited by asking the patient to stand with his arms hanging loosely at his side. Ask him to slowly elevate his extended arm through an arc from 0° to 180° in the coronal plane of the trunk. Obviously, if the patient can do this painlessly, it is good evidence there is no serious injury or disease of the shoulder. If he is unable to raise the arm even 10°, look for a fracture, a dislocation or a complete rupture of the supraspinatus tendon. If he is able to lift the arm painlessly the first 60°, but is stopped with pain between 60° and 120°; or can't get by 90°, suspect chronic supraspinatus tendonitis or a partial rupture of the same tendon.

Pain throughout the range of elevation indicates arthritis.

Finally, in calcific tendonitis, x-ray films will show calcium deposits in the tendon.

If the calcium deposit ruptures through the peritendinous tissues, it may localize in the subacromial bursa that lies over the supraspinatus tendon. Then the condition is complicated by calcific bursitis. Frequently, calcific tendonitis and subacromial bursitis coexist (Fig. 7-34). Infrequently, bursitis ex-

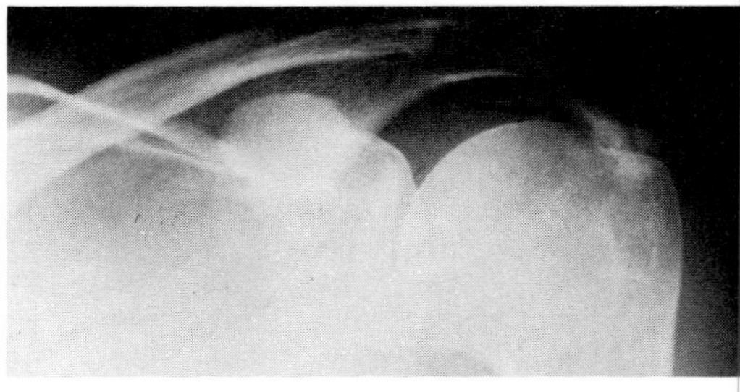

Figure 7-34. Chronic supraspinatus tendonitis and subacromial bursitis with calcifications.

ists alone, producing similar shoulder pain. You will find it impossible to know whether the lesion is in the tendon, the bursa or both from the character of the pain and its localization.

Persistence of tendonitis and/or bursitis of the shoulder may cause irritation of other fibrous structures around the shoulder joint capsule and a chronic adhesive capsulitis may develop. The shoulder then becomes motionless, painful and stiff—the so-called *frozen shoulder*.

Trauma

Trauma may cause tears in the tendons attached to the humeral trochanter or in the musculotendinous cuff of the shoulder joint. When this follows trauma the patient is unable to abduct the shoulder. Tears of the glenohumeral joint capsule account for a large percentage of cases of shoulder pain. Pain in this case is localized to the subacromial region.

Bicipital Tenosynovitis

Another tendon frequently involved in shoulder joint pain is that of the biceps muscle. Bicipital tenosynovitis is characterized by pain and tenderness over the bicipital groove and around the long head of the biceps tendon. The pain is initiated by movement of the arm, requiring contraction of the biceps muscle, and there is persistent tenderness over the lesser tuberosity of the humerus.

Thoracic Outlet Syndrome

The thoracic outlet syndrome (scalenus anticus syndrome) is basically a brachial plexus neuralgia caused by contracture or hypertrophy of the scalenus anticus muscle, cervical rib (Fig. 7-35), congenital elongation of the C_7 transverse process, costoclavicular syndrome caused by pinching of the brachial plexus and other structures, congenital fibrous bands, poor posture in the obese patient or those with kyphoscoliosis or Wright's hyperabduction syndrome.

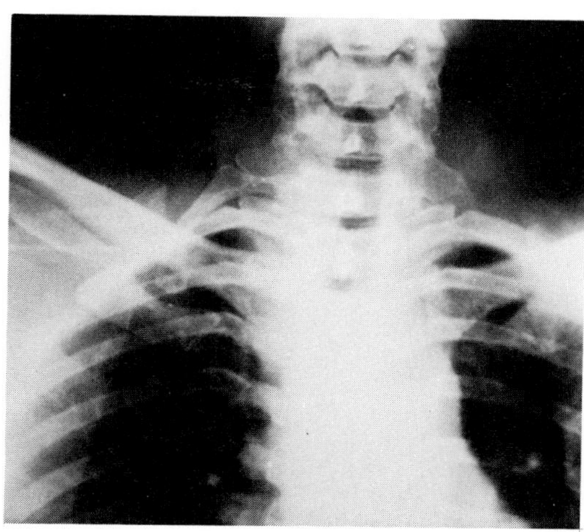

Figure 7-35. Cervical ribs (on right) in addition to producing spasm of the scalenus muscle may directly compress the subclavian artery, thus diminishing the radial pulse.

Symptoms consist of weakness and atrophy of the intrinsic muscles of the hand. Ask the patient about annoying paresthesias of the arm and forearm along the distribution of the ulnar and median nerve dermatomes. Tingling and numbness may be the first complaint, but eventually hypesthesia and even motor weakness develop. In advanced cases, the fingers become cyanotic, pale and cold as the radial pulse diminishes, suggestive of a true Raynaud's syndrome.

The scalenus anticus syndrome can be detected with the Adson's vascular compression test (Fig. 7-36). Turn the patient's head toward the affected side and elevate the chin. This position will squeeze the subclavian artery between the scalenus anticus muscle and the cervical rib. Monitor the patient's radial pulse while the head is held in this position. A positive test is indicated by an obliteration or diminution of the pulse.

Conservative treatment consists of physical therapy but these cases do better after sectioning the scalenus anticus muscle and removing cervical ribs, fibrous bands, adhesions and lipomas. Occasionally, a resection of the first rib through a posterior thoracoplasty is necessary.

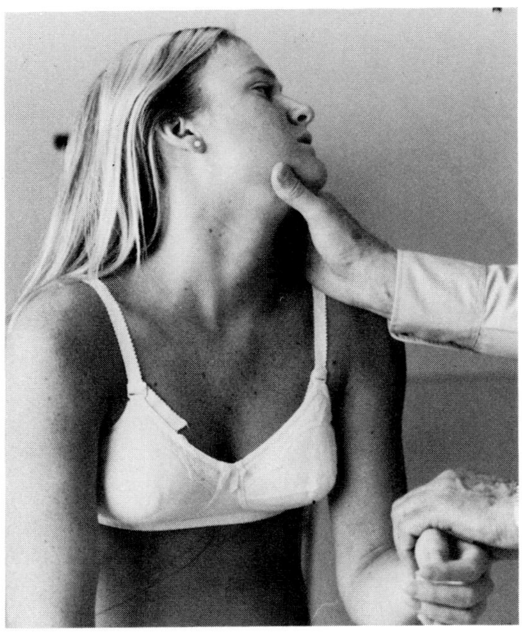

Figure 7-36. Adson's vascular compression test for scalenus anticus syndrome.

Shoulder-Hand Syndrome

Although rare, keep in mind the possibility of a shoulder-hand syndrome (sympathetic reflex dystrophy, Sudeck's atrophy). The single most important factor in the management of this disagreeable disease is early recognition. Watch for it following myocardial infarction or during the course of chronic pulmonary disorders, including malignancy. It is also associated with cerebrovascular disease and subsequent to trauma. Its exact cause is debated.

The disease occurs in three stages: (1) A painful shoulder plus swelling and pain in the fingers and hand. The edema is not of the pitting variety but more of an induration. The hand may be cyanotic but warm. (2) The shoulder improves and swelling of the hand decreases but flexion and stiffness progress. Superficial vasoconstriction causes a fall in temperature; x-ray examination shows a patchy osteoporosis of the long bones of the upper extremity. (3) Atrophy of the skin and subcutaneous tissues with increasing contractures of the palmar and digital fascia. Finally, the upper extremity becomes almost useless. Differentiate the disease from carpal tunnel syndrome and dorsal outlet syndrome.

Treatment can be long and complicated. It consists of: Xylocaine block of the stellate ganglion and/or local injections of Xylocaine into trigger points; extensive physical therapy administered by a competent physical therapist and right-sided epidural anesthesia, which interrupts the sympathetic innervation to the extremity.

Other Causes of Shoulder Pain

- brachial neuritis (Fig. 7-37)
- osteoarthritis of the 4th, 5th or 6th cervical vertebra produced by osteophytic lesions pressing on spinal nerves that innervate the shoulder
- diseases of the gallbladder, liver or pleura
- cardiac or coronary artery disease
- fractures and dislocations of the shoulder structures (See Chapter 6)

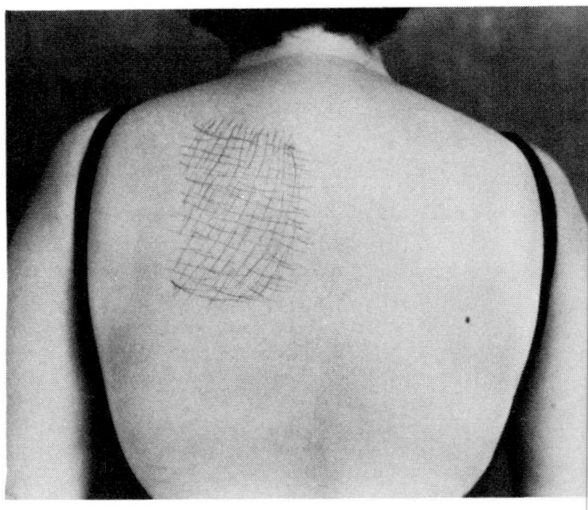

Figure 7-37. The most common site of referred pain following a ruptured cervical disc.

Ankle

The ankle joint is subject to sprain of either the lateral or medical aspect of the joint depending on whether the foot was forced into eversion or inversion. Pain or clicking during dorsiflexion of the ankle with

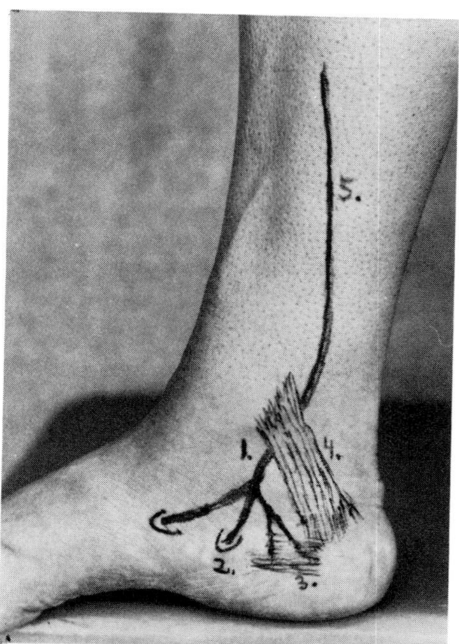

Figure 7-38. Anatomy of the tarsal tunnel syndrome: *1,* Medial plantar nerve; *2,* Lateral plantar nerve; *3,* Origin of the abductor hallucis muscle and the calcaneal branches of the posterior tibial nerve; *4,* Flexor retinaculum; *5,* Posterior tibial nerve.

eversion is produced by recurrent slipping of the peroneal tendons. In addition to these causes and fractures of the bones, chronic stenosing tenosynovitis of the peroneal tendon sheath is a possibility whenever inversion of the foot causes pain.

Tarsal Tunnel Syndrome

The tarsal tunnel syndrome is the lower extremity's counterpart of the carpal tunnel syndrome and is produced by compression of the posterior tibial nerve as it passes through the tarsal tunnel (Fig. 7-38). In this condition, the patient complains of pain in the sole of the foot and numbness and tingling in the foot. Sensory loss and weakness of the intrinsic muscles of the foot develop as the disease advances. Don't confuse the diagnosis with arthritis in the ankle, but consider the possibility when evaluating patients with painful feet or ankles.

Secondary tarsal tunnel syndrome may be associated with callus following a fracture, hypertrophy of the abductor hallucis muscle or tenosynovitis. Surgery is the preferred treatment.

Hip

This is a difficult joint to examine directly because of its deep location. The patient may point to an area seemingly unrelated to the hip (Fig. 7-39). Distinguish hip from low back pain. Low back pain is more often associated with pain in the sciatic or obturator nerve distribution whereas patients with disease of the hip may complain of pain along the anterior aspect of the thigh or in the knee. This pain radiates along the

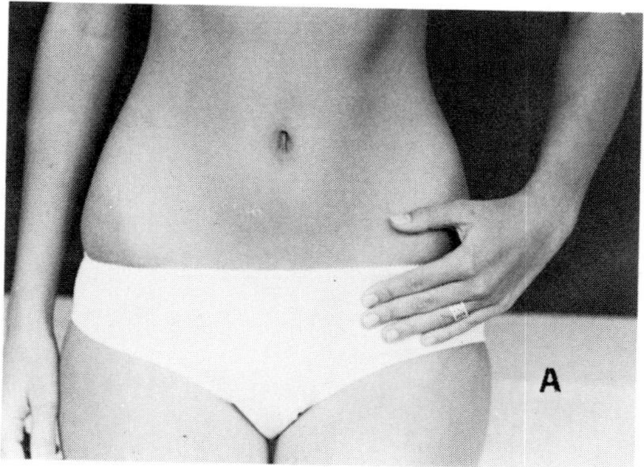

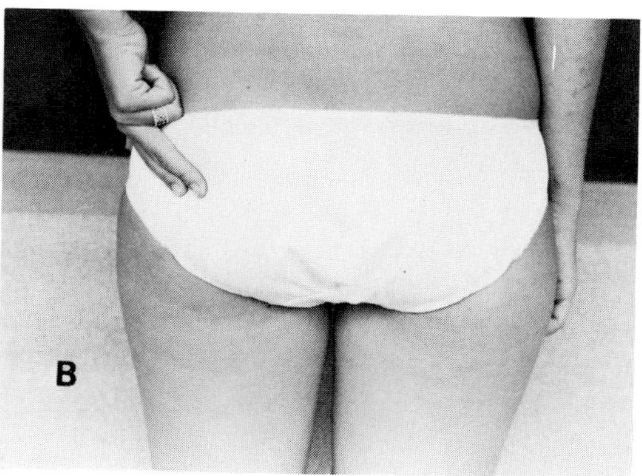

Figure 7-39. Sites of hip pain. Ask the patient to point to the painful area and she will usually point to the, *A*, inguinal area or, *B*, the buttocks or both.

femoral nerve. Pain in the knee should always prompt examination of the hip.

Examination of the Hip

With the patient standing, locate the greater trochanters of the femur (Fig. 7-40). Place your thumbs on the anterior superior iliac spines and allow your fingers to wrap naturally around the body curve. Your finger tips will encircle the greater trochanters of the femur and the distances can be compared accurately. Ascertain the distance between the anterior superior iliac spine and the greater trochanter (Fig. 7-41). This is best done by placing one finger on the greater trochanter and the thumb on the spine. You will be able to detect small differences in heights of the trochanters. The degree of shortening can be measured by placing objects under the short leg until the pelvis is horizontal.

With the patient supine, grasp the lower end of the supine patient's thigh and rock it back and forth (Fig. 7-42). This maneuver helps to locate the pain. Other more strenuous tests may be omitted if the initial examination proves positive.

To test for rotation with flexion, flex the patient's hip and knee into right angles

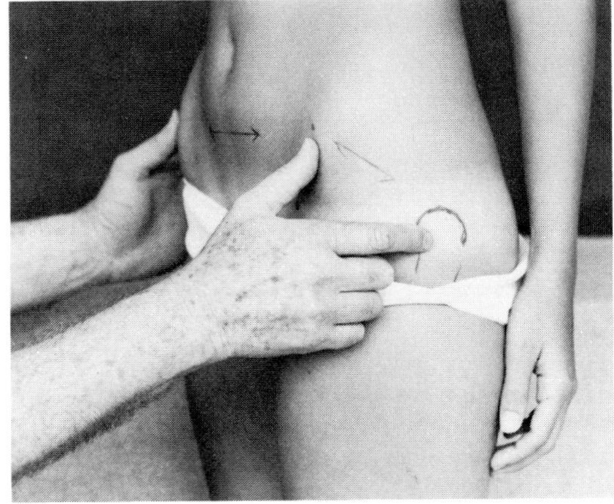

Figure 7-41. Ascertain the distance between the anterior superior iliac spine and the greater trochanter by placing one finger on the greater trochanter and the thumb on the spine.

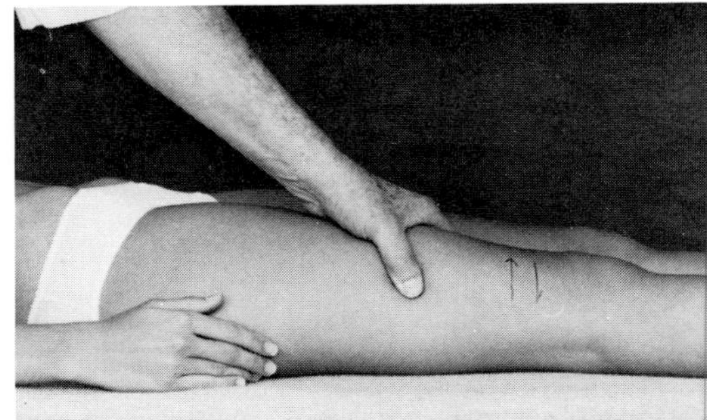

Figure 7-42. This maneuver helps to locate hip pain.

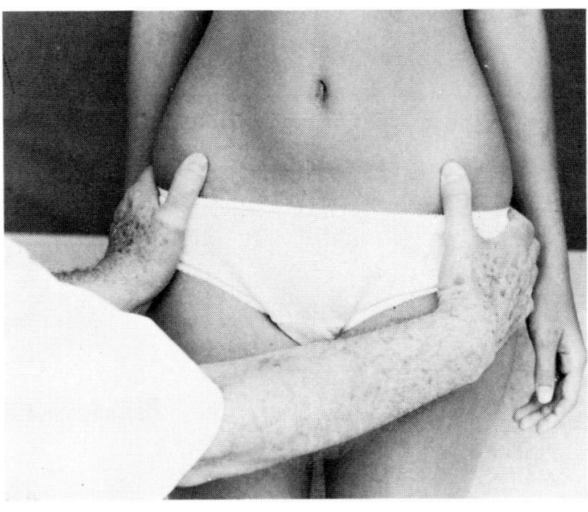

Figure 7-40. In locating the greater trochanters of the femur, allow your fingers to wrap naturally around the body curve.

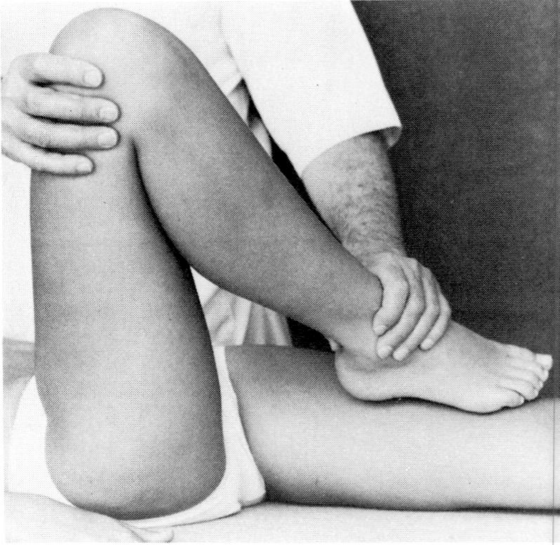

Figure 7-43. Test for rotation with flexion.

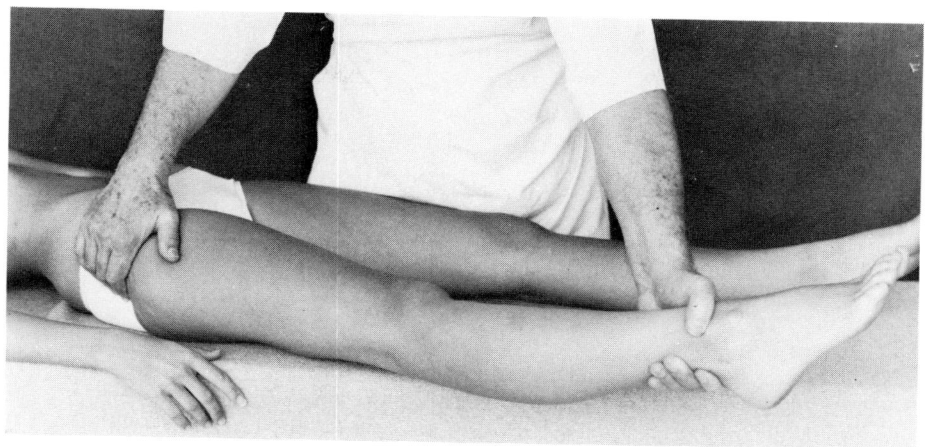

Figure 7-44. Test the angle of abduction. Compare the movement with the opposite leg.

while she is supine and move her knee from side to side (Fig. 7-43).

To test the angle of abduction (Fig. 7-44), place one hand on the iliac crest to palpate for pelvic movement. Grasp the patient's ankle with your other hand. Move her leg outward in abduction until her pelvis moves. Compare the movement with her opposite leg.

To test the degree of adduction (Fig. 7-45), with the patient's leg still in extension, grasp the ankle of one leg and move it across the other in adduction. A normal hip will allow the thigh to cross the midthigh of the opposite leg.

To test for extension of the hip, turn the patient into the prone position. Place one hand on the back of her pelvis and lift her limb into extension with the other hand (Fig. 7-46). A normal hip will extend about 15°.

In the anvil test (Fig. 7-47), the patient is in the supine position. Raise her leg and strike the calcaneous with your fist in the direction of the hip. A painful response may help locate early disease of the joint.

Measure the length of the lower extremity by stretching a tape measure from the anterior superior iliac spine to the medial malleoli of the tibia (Fig. 7-48). Compare with her opposite leg. To measure the circumference of her leg, mark off similar levels on both legs using the

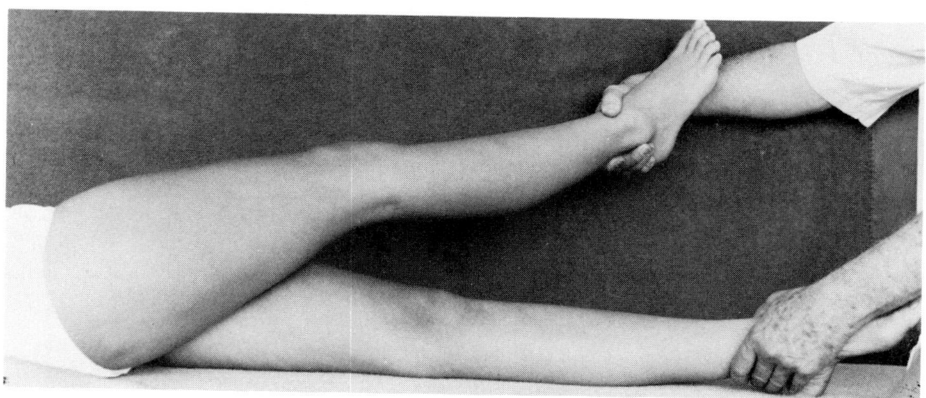

Figure 7-45. Test the degree of adduction. A normal hip will allow the thigh to cross the midthigh of the opposite leg.

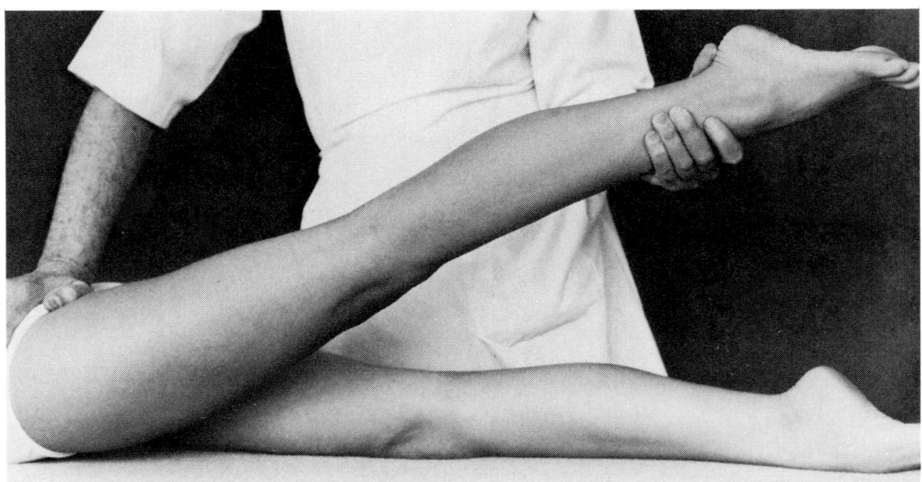

Figure 7-46. Test for extension of the hip. A normal hip will extend about 15°.

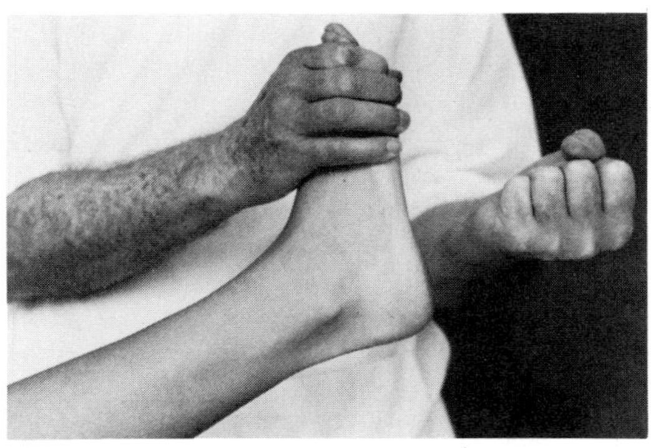

Figure 7-47. The anvil test. A painful response may help locate early disease of the joint.

anterior iliac spine as a common base (Fig. 7-49). Check the girth at these levels and compare with the opposite leg.

To determine tilting of the pelvis, sit in front of the standing patient with your thumbs on the anterior superior iliac spines (Fig. 7-50) and observe whether an imaginary line between the spines is horizontal.

The greater trochanter of the femur can be located by drawing a line, Nelaton's

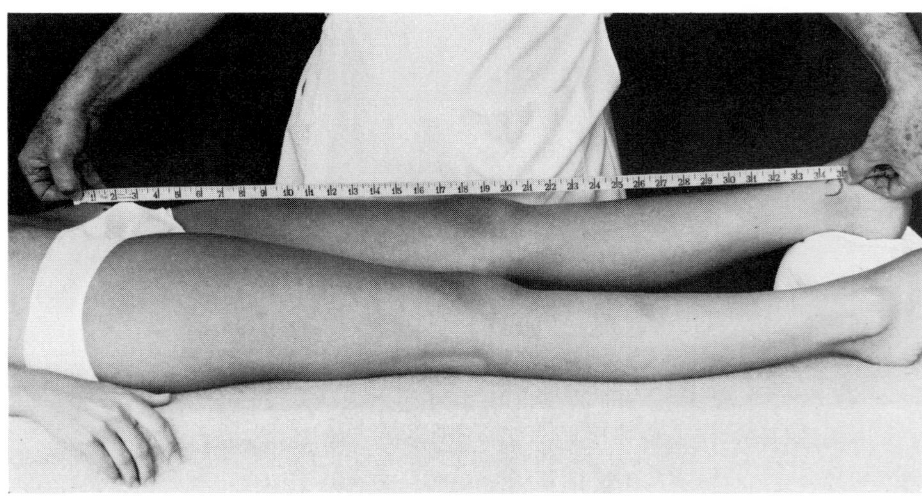

Figure 7-48. Measure the length of her lower extremity with a tape measure.

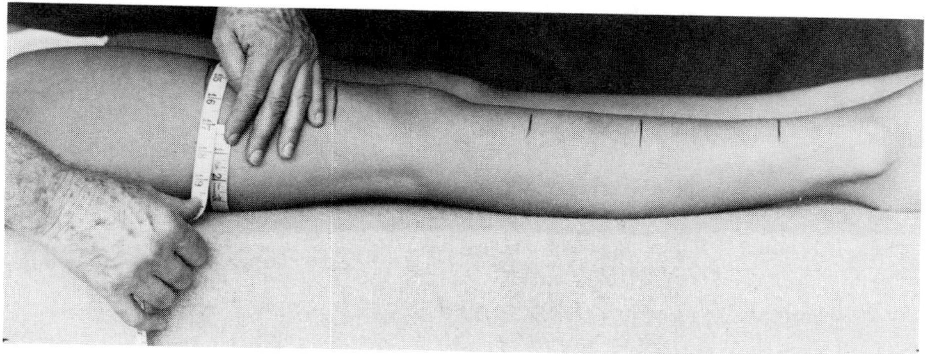

Figure 7-49. Measure the circumference of her leg and compare with her opposite leg.

line, from the anterior superior spine to the ischial tuberosity (Fig. 7-51). When the thighs are flexed the line passes through the tip of the greater trochanter. Allow an upward deviation of 1 cm as normal.

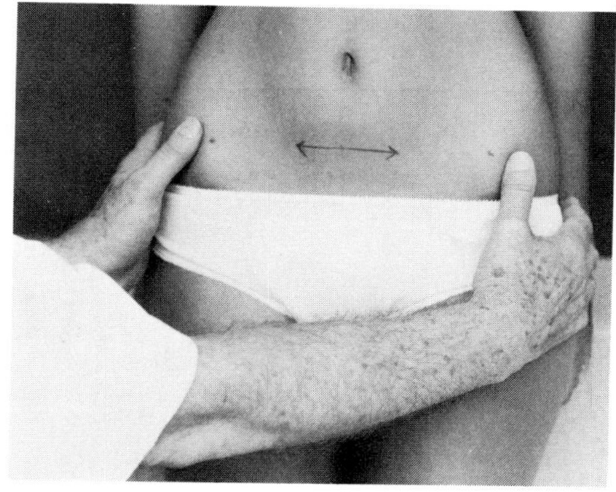

Figure 7-50. Observe whether an imaginary line between the spines is horizontal or not in determining tilting of the pelvis.

Causes of Hip Pain

There are a variety of causes of hip pain. Some conditions are idiopathic, but the majority can be designated to a specific disease or condition of the hip (Table 7-2). Steroid therapy subsequent to disease elsewhere in the body may cause a painful situation in the hip. Alcoholism is another factor.

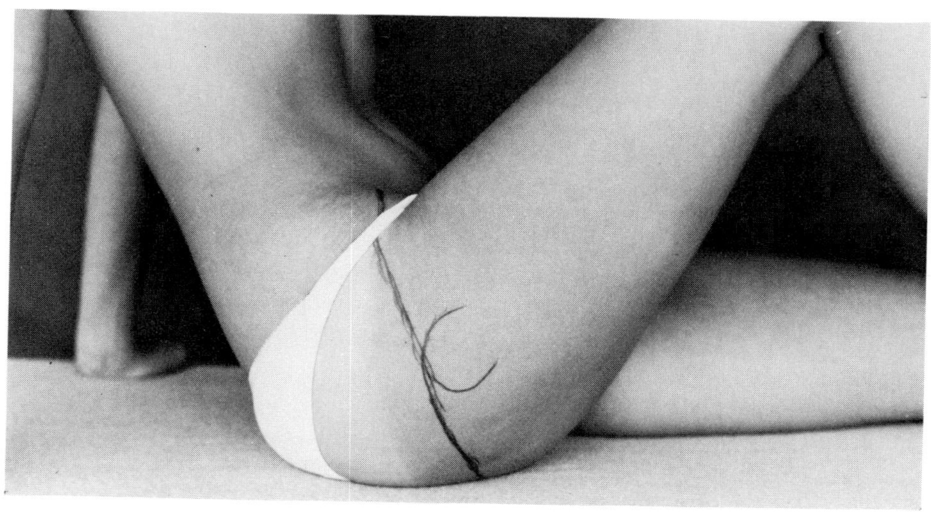

Figure 7-51. Nelaton's line.

Table 7-2. Painful Hip Conditions by Ages

0–4 yr
- Congenital dislocations
- Idiopathic synovitis
- Septic arthritis

4–11 yr
- Avascular necrosis (Legg-Calve-Perthes disease)
- Septic arthritis
- Juvenile rheumatoid arthritis (6 mo to adolescence)

Adolescence
- Slipped femoral capital epiphysis
- Septic arthritis

Adults
- Arthritis
  - Osteoarthritis
  - Septic arthritis
  - Rheumatoid arthritis
  - Tuberculous arthritis
- Fractures and dislocations
- Strain or tension in the hip joint capsule from previous trauma
- Trochanteric tendonitis or bursitis
- Psoas abscess and bursitis
- Avascular necrosis
  - Hemoglobinopathy (sickle cell disease)
  - Gout
  - Caisson's disease
  - Gaucher's disease
  - Hyperlipoidemia
  - Diabetes

Osteoarthritis (Malum Coxae Senilis)

The chief symptom of this condition is boring pain in the groin, buttocks or around the greater trochanter. The pain may radiate to the posterior thigh, the inner thigh or the leg. It must be differentiated from lumbar disc disease and knee problems.

After the patient rests the hip may become stiff but this disappears with exercise. Gradually the patient may develop a limp of which he is unaware. Attempts to separate the patient's thighs cause pain. Passive motion is restricted in all directions.

There is controversy at the present time between the surgery-minded and the medical-oriented therapist regarding the best therapeutic modality. Neither extreme is appropriate: patients do not need "to live with it" nor should all patients require surgery.

Some simple protective measures may prevent the loss of early functional capacity. They are:

- –weight reduction (the hips may bear as much as 2 to 4 times the body weight under normal activity).
- –use of a cane in the opposite hand
- –use of one or two crutches
- –forgo the use of intra-articular cortisone (hip joint appears to be particularly vulnerable to infection)
- –simple exercises such as with a stationary bicycle
- –proper rest periods

Marked decrease in pain often results from a regimen of total rest in bed for a few days, then the use of crutches for a few weeks followed by the use of a cane. Aspirin or Indocin are valuable agents in hip pain.

Consider surgery if pain cannot be adequately controlled by these methods, if the patient's disability is due to limited motion or if the patient is totally dissatisfied with limitation of activity. The pain, however, must be enough worse than that expected subsequent to surgery to make the risk, time and stress involved in treatment worthwhile.

Operative treatment for arthritis is chosen from mold arthroplasty, osteotomy or total hip replacement in those over 50 years of age. Operative treatment for avascular necrosis may be early bone graft, prosthesis or total hip replacement.

Total Hip Replacement

Criteria for selection of patients: (1) Pain or disability from widespread rheumatoid arthritis or allied diseases in patients of any age in whom the disease state, osteoporosis and general condition preclude partial prosthesis or (2) malum coxae senilis, avascular necrosis of the femoral head or both in patients over 65 years whose general or local condition prohibits the immobilization and rehabilitation required following arthroplasty or fusion.

As a general guide following total hip replacement the patient will have nonrestricted weight bearing after 10 days and will be hospitalized 18 days. He should be able to walk without pain or crutches following the operation.

Knee

Pain occurs in the knee more often than in any other joint because of its anatomic and mechanic vulnerability. Trauma is most frequently the cause of knee pain. Numerous intra-articular structures may be strained, torn or otherwise injured. Considerable diagnostic information may be gained by careful inspection and palpation of the joint. Conditions revealed may be neuromyxofibroma, popliteal aneurysm, anserine bursitis or cyst of the medial or lateral menisci. Search for hip joint disease whenever the patient complains of dull, aching knees without evidence of disease in the knees.

Swellings which occur anteriorly are prepatellar bursitis (housemaid's knee), infrapatellar bursitis (clergyman's knee) and liposynovitis infrapatellaris (Hoffa's disease).

Traumatic diseases of the knee and ankle are discussed in Chapter 6.

Tenderness about the patella indicates injury to the infrapatellar fat pad. Tenderness at a point midway between the patellar and the internal collateral ligament is characteristic of a tear of the anterior semilunar cartilage. Tenderness of the medial aspect of the knee at the joint line suggests an injury to the internal collateral ligament. Locking of the knee usually follows an injury in which a tear creates a loose body in the joint. In a child, pain localized at the site of the patellar tendon is characteristic of a partial separation of the tibial tubercle (Osgood-Schlatter's disease).

Consider hemophilia whenever a hemorrhage occurs into the knee joint following only light trauma. Osteoarthritis causes dull, aching pain aggravated by climbing or descending stairs or hills and walking on uneven ground. Neuropathic joint disease is another possibility.

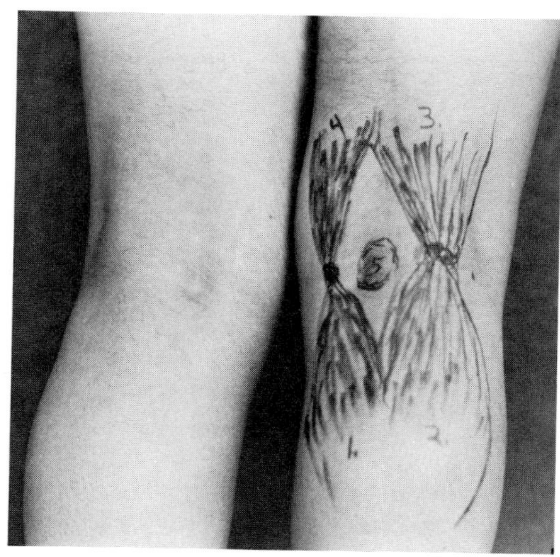

Figure 7-52. The popliteal fossa: *1*, Medial head of the gastrocnemius; *2*, Lateral head of gastrocnemius; *3*, Biceps femoris; *4*, Semimembranosus; *5*, Baker's cyst.

Search for cysts behind the knee joint. Morrant Baker's cyst appears directly posterior to the joint in the popliteal space (Fig. 7-52). It is not visible when the knee is flexed but look for it as the patient stands with the leg extended. The cyst is a diverticulum of the synovial sac protruding through the joint capsule of the knee.

Do not confuse Baker's cyst with popliteal abscess and semimembranosus bursitis.

Osteoarthritis of the Knee

Osteoarthritis is a frequent cause of severe disability in the elderly. The pathology is mainly a degeneration of the articular cartilage. To diagnose the disease, order an x-ray study. It will show a pronounced narrowing and loss of joint space with widening on the opposite side.

The typical clinical picture is a patient who is between 50 and 60 years of age, short and obese, who complains of pain in the medial or posterior portion of the knee. Pain is increased by walking. Examine the knee.

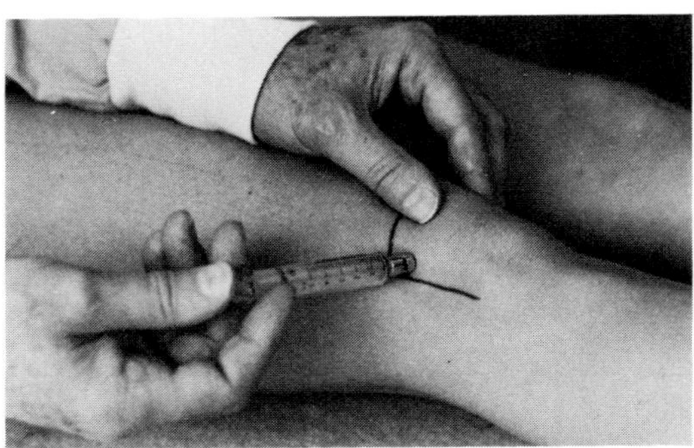

Figure 7-53. Aspirating or injecting the knee joint.

It may be a little swollen and warmer than the opposite knee. Occasionally you will find an effusion because of irritation of the joint with loss of articular cartilage.

Treatment depends on the severity of symptoms and stage of the disease. Salicylates and judicious steroid injections into the knee joint are beneficial (Fig. 7-53). The lateral approach is considered the best for aspiration or injection of the knee joint. Raise a wheal with a 25 gauge needle and 1 percent Xylocaine. To aspirate, use a 20 to 22 gauge needle at least 2 in long. Insert the needle through the wheal inferiorly and medially. Some prefer to nick the skin with a scalpel at the site of injection to keep the needle from carrying a skin plug into the joint.

Surgery consists of osteotomy of the tibia and fibula to shift the weight to the opposite side of the knee joint. Age is not a contraindication. No internal fixation is necessary and by the second week the patient can bear weight in a long-leg cast assisted by a walker.

At this stage, synovectomy and joint debridement are in order. Don't expect surgery to halt the progress of the disease. About all you can promise the patient is a 50-50 chance that the procedure will relieve his pain. Expect further degenerative changes.

Rheumatoid knee

The rheumatoid knee has few features similar to the most benign osteoarthritic knee. Convery and Clawson divide the progressive knee disorders into four phases.[1] The family physician would do well to do the same.

Phase I: X-ray studies are negative except for evidence of soft tissue swelling. Look for the disease in the synovium where there is hypertrophy and joint fluid. Treatment of this phase is medical (salicylates to tolerance), night splints, aspiration of excess joint fluid to prevent distention of ligaments and capsule with an 18 gauge needle and occasional use of intra-articular steroids. In a chronic rheumatoid disease, multiple injections of steroids have been known to cause steroid arthropathy.

Phase II: In this phase, x-ray evidence of the disease is noticeable in the articular cartilage and adjacent bone. Look for the small translucent areas of bony invasion beneath the collateral ligaments where granulation tissue from the proliferating synovia penetrates the joint cavity in tonguelike projections called pannus. This causes fibrosis and ankylosis. It is during this stage of disease that surgical intervention becomes helpful. The procedure of choice is surgical excision of the synovial membrane (synovectomy). This will reduce pain and slow the progression of the disease.

Phase III: For the first time the x-ray pictures will show invasion of subchondral bone along with all the other pathological factors in the soft tissue and articular cartilage.

Phase IV: Expect to find a complete loss of articular cartilage and considerable bone destruction. From here on the patient has little to look forward to except massive damage, angulatory deformities and flexion contractures. The usual attempt at synovectomy and debridement ends in miserable failure. At this point an orthopedist might consider arthroplasty with metallic interpositional prostheses. These might be a tibial plateau prosthesis, a femoral condylar prosthesis or total knee replacement. The last carries a high complication rate. Arthrodesis will provide complete relief and stability but rising and sitting down are extremely difficult. If the patient has general RA and is disabled in upper extremities, arthodesis may completely disable him.

RHEUMATOID ARTHRITIS (RA)

Recognizing Early RA

First establish whether a true arthritis or synovitis is present. This may be difficult during the first 2 or 3 months of the inflammation. Usually there is a prodromal illness lasting a variable time during which the patient complains of fatigue, weight loss, sweating, especially of the palms and soles, and malaise. There may be a low-grade fever and an elevated sedimentation rate during this time.

Morning stiffness is characteristic of RA but does occur in other conditions as well. This complaint is so constant that it can be used as a quantitative guide to the course of the condition. Ascertain the time of day the patient's joints are as ''loose'' as they will become and subtract from that the time she rises. For instance, if her joints become loose at 11 o'clock, subtract from 11 the time she arises—perhaps 7 o'clock. This will indicate 4 hours of stiffness. As the patient's RA improves or worsens, this figure will lessen or increase respectively.

Other signs are pain on motion, tenderness of joints and swelling of at least one joint. Search for accumulations of synovial fluid, for its presence almost always indicates synovitis. RA is a symmetrical polyarthritis. Symmetrical swellings in the MCP and the PIP joints are typical. The hands and ankles become involved as the disease advances. Palpate the subcutaneous tissues over the posterior surface of the radius for nodules. These occur in about one third of those with RA.

Check the blood for the rheumatoid factor. This factor appears during the first 6 months of the disease. Finding the rheumatoid factor gives useful objective evidence of RA but, on the other hand, a negative test does not rule out RA. The test is negative in a third of patients with definite RA. It is positive in up to 3 percent of normal persons, 30 percent of those with SLE and in those with syphilis. X-ray studies are confirmatory if the typical articular erosions are discovered.

Even with the above signs and symptoms, you should not be content with the diagnosis of RA. Attempt to rule out other causes of arthritis. Three diseases—systemic lupus erythematosis, polyarteritis nodosa and scleroderma—may be nearly indistinguishable from RA. Also, RA, in addition to occurring alone, may complicate osteoarthritis and gouty arthritis. Chronic gonorrhea affecting the prostate or salpinx may cause a polyarthritis, and the inexperienced may be trapped by hypertrophic pulmonary osteoarthropathy.

In the differentiation of RA and rheumatic fever, keep two points in mind: (1) rheumatic fever responds to salicylates almost miraculously but RA never responds so completely and (2) the development of a permanently deformed joint nearly always favors the diagnosis of RA.

If your preliminary investigation does not verify a true synovitis, weigh the possibility of other causes of a widespread extra-articular rheumatism, such as multiple myeloma, metastatic carcinoma, polymyositis, polymyalgia, polymyalgia rheumatica, sarcoidosis, psoriasis, purpura, serum sickness and the joint tenderness associated with hepatitis or rubella.

As the joints become permanently involved, the hand of the RA patient becomes characteristic (Fig. 7-54). There is moderate-to-marked swelling of the MCP and PIP joints of both hands. The patient may develop large ridges across the knuckles while much of the soft tissue atrophies. In contradistinction, in osteoarthritis a knobby swelling of the PIP and DIP joints develop, leaving the MCP joints unaffected. Look for other tell-tale abnormalities such as nodules, ulnar drift, swan neck and boutonniere deformities (Fig. 7-55). Be able to identify other afflictions that affect the hand such as the diffuse, painful swelling of the shoulder-hand syndrome, the painless nodular fasciitis of Dupuytren's contracture, the periarticular soft-tissue tophi of gout and the clubbing of pulmonary hypertrophic osteoarthropathy.

Remember RA is a systemic disease. It is important to do a complete physical examination. The diagnosis is made chiefly on

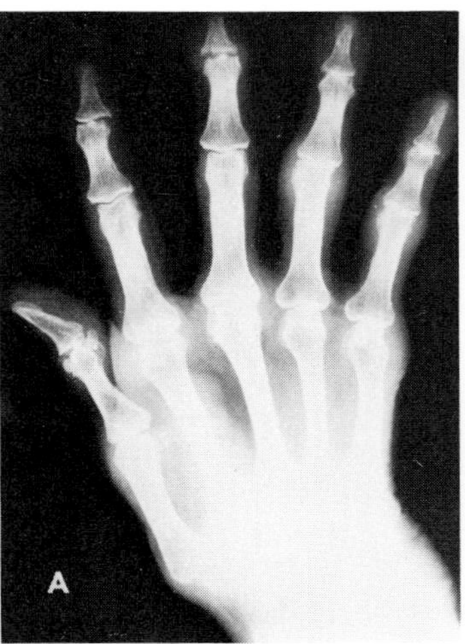

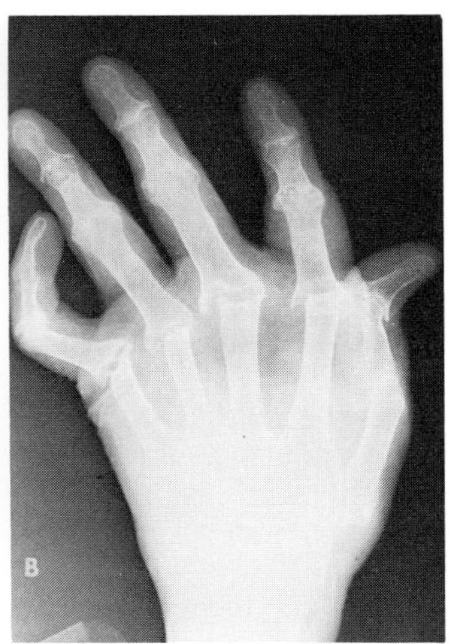

Figure 7-54. *A,* Advanced rheumatoid arthritis. Low-grade tenosynovitis is manifest as fluctuant swelling of the tendon sheaths. In 20 to 30 percent of the patients, subcutaneous rheumatic nodules develop which are found over joint prominences and tendon sheaths. *B,* Marked rheumatoid arthritis of the hand. The disease usually is progressive over a period of several years. Finally complete fixation of the joint, ankylosis, results. Notice the ulnar deviation.

clinical grounds are x-ray and laboratory studies are used to corroborate the clinical impression.

There is no skill involved in palpating joints for RA. The main problem is to assess the joint for heat, tenderness, erythema, and swelling of the joint and/or the surrounding tissues. Follow an orderly routine. Exert a constant amount of pressure on each joint while eliciting tenderness. This can be done by squeezing each joint just enough to blanch the distal third of your fingernails. Be sure to record your findings for future assessments.

Further palpation will tell you whether there is increased heat in the joint. An increase of 1° C can be sensed with the extensor surface of your fingers. The bony enlargement of osteoarthritis can usually be distinguished from the boggy swelling of RA

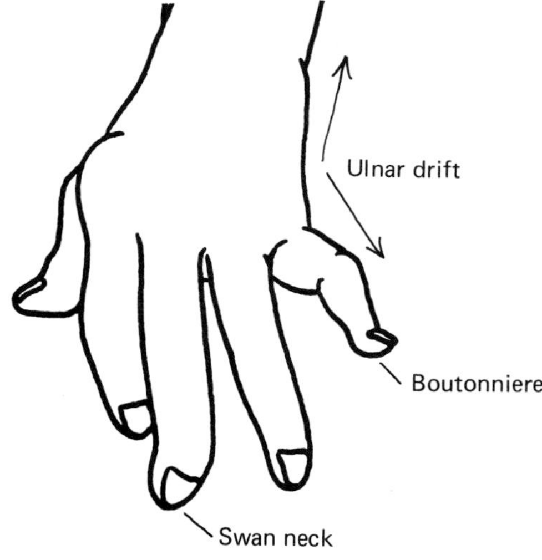

Figure 7-55. Deformities of rheumatoid arthritis. Boutonniere deformity is the result of hyperflexion of the PIP joint and hyperextension of the DIP joint. Swan neck deformity results from hyperextension of the PIP joint and hyperflexion of the DIP. Note ulnar drift.

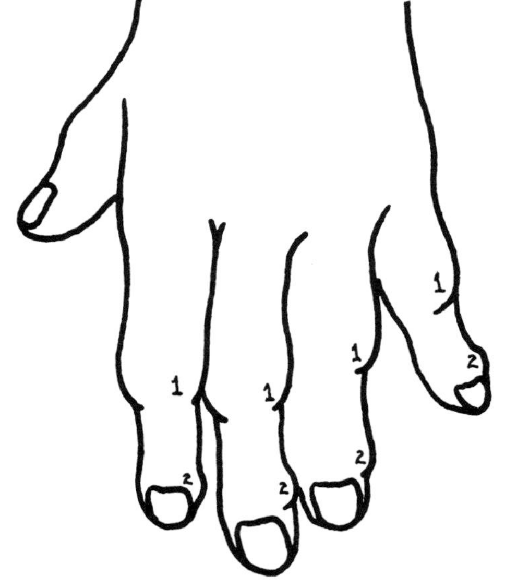

Figure 7-56. *1,* Bouchard's nodes of rheumatoid arthritis; *2,* Heberden's nodes of osteoarthritis.

(Fig. 7-56). After a little practice, you can differentiate between intra-articular effusion, synovial thickening or diseased periarticular disease.

Extra-articular signs of RA are peripheral neuropathy, osteoporosis, rheumatoid vasculitis, amyloidosis, splenomegaly, tunnel syndromes, pericarditis, myocarditis, digital vasculitis, skin ulcerations, coronary arteritis, cardiac valve nodules, lymphadenopathy, Sjogren's syndrome (which must present two of the triad: arthritis, xerostomia and keratoconjunctivitis), scleromalacia, episcleritis, iritis, keratoconjunctivitis, pulmonary rheumatoid nodule, myopathy and pulmonary fibrosis and pleural effusions.

Mortality in rheumatoid arthritis is twice as great in a 5-yr period in patients who have one or more extra-articular complications. These patients also suffered from more persistent joint inflammation, had higher titers of the rheumatoid factor and showed x-ray evidence of more severe joint disease. A search for extra-articular disease will be fruitful in about 76 percent of patients with severe rheumatoid arthritis.[2]

Variants of RA

Reiter's syndrome is the triad of RA, nonspecific urethritis and conjunctivitis. *Psoriatic arthritis* develops in some patients who have chronic psoriasis. It is similar to RA with more destruction of the terminal phalanges. Tests for rheumatoid factor are negative. *Ankylosing spondylitis* (Marie-Strumpell disease) is a localized RA of the spine and pelvis. Rheumatoid factor is not usually present. *Sjogren's syndrome* is diagnosed when the patient presents with two of the three classical symptoms, i.e. RA, xerostomia, and keratoconjunctivitis. The rheumatoid factor is present even when there is no arthritis. *Juvenile RA* (Still's disease) is a childhood condition. Children have more complications of the internal organs, especially the heart. *Felty's syndrome* is a combination of RA, splenomegaly and leukopenia. The rheumatoid factor may be present in high titers.

Laboratory Tests

Rheumatoid Factor (RF)

This factor (autoantibody to IgG) can be demonstrated in the serum of most patients with RA. There is pro and con evidence that the amount of RF found in the serum correlates with the degree of disease activity. There is full agreement, however, that the presence of RF does correlate well with the presence of nodules. Only about 20 percent of patients with juvenile rheumatoid arthritis have the RF in their serum.

Remember the presence of the RF only supports the diagnosis. It is not pathognomonic. Positive findings in diseases other than active RA are often transient and usually of low titer.

Checking for RF in synovial fluid is useful. It is found in the fluid from the affected joints of adults with RA but not in fluid from patients with gouty arthritis, Reiter's syndrome, systemic lupus erythematosis or juvenile RA.

To detect the RF use SCAT (sheep cell agglutination test) also known as the Rose or Rose-Wagler test. Its principle lies in the ability of the RF to agglutinate sensitized sheep erythrocytes. The amount of RF is measured by using serial dilutions of the patient's serum. There are several variations of the test, but SCAT remains the basic one.

The Latex test is probably less accurate but is useful for screening.

Antinuclear Antibody (ANA)

The lupus erythematosus cell (LE) is a manifestation of antinuclear activity. Nuclear material from damaged leukocytes is phagocytized by living leukocytes, thus producing the characteristic inclusion body of the LE cell. The finding of LE cells is not diagnostic of SLE even though such cells may be found in 60 to 80 percent of the patients. Up to 40 percent of the patients with RA may also have positive LE cell preparations. Other diseases with a positive test are scleroderma, rubella arthritis, drug reactions, polyarthritis, etc. If you get a report of a large number of LE cells, it is only suggestive of SLE or one of these overlap syndromes.

The two most widely used laboratory procedures for detecting ANA are the LE prep (to detect LE cells) and the fluorescent antinuclear antibody test (FANA). When levels of ANA are low, LE cells may not be found. If this is the case, order the more sensitive antibody detection test, FANA. The sensitivity of the FANA may reveal antibodies when LE preps are negative; conversely, when LE cells are found ANA can always be detected by FANA.

The typical LE cell is a polymorphonuclear leukocyte containing a large round inclusion body that stains purple red. The finding of large numbers of LE cells is significant and should be reported.

FANA is a highly sensitive technique for demonstrating ANA by immunofluorescence. It involves the use of leukocytes on blood smears as antigens. Visualization of the fluorescing nuclei is done by fluorescent antibody microscopy.

Total Serum Complement (C^1)

In your attempt to sort out the various autoimmune diseases, C^1 may provide data of diagnostic and prognostic importance. The principle: RF or ANA combines with antigen and fixer C^1, producing a large *immune complex* that has toxic, irritating and inflammatory properties.

Its clinical importance is to differentiate gout, rheumatic fever and RA (where C^1 is increased) from SLE, other arthritides, scleroderma and dermatomyositis (where C^1 is either normal or decreased).

Erythrocyte Sedimentation Rate (ESR)

The ESR remains one of the most sensitive indicators of acute inflammation. Normal Westergren for males is 1 to 3 mm and for females 4 to 7 mm per hour. Normal Wintrobe for males is 0 to 10 mm and for females 0 to 20 mm per hour.

A rapidly rising ESR is more indicative of an acute inflammatory process than is an ESR that remains high. But it is a useful screening test for inflammation, which along with C-reactive protein are simple lab tests for the investigation of arthritic problems. Basically ESR helps to differentiate active RF, SLE, RA and gout from the degenerative joint diseases.

C-Reactive Protein (CRP)

This test is nonspecific, somewhat like ESR, but more sensitive. During the stress of inflammation in the body, there appears in the serum an abnormal protein that reacts with the C-polysaccharide of pneumococci from whence it gets its name. It is detectable in the blood 6 to 24 hours after strong inflammatory stimuli such as infection, myocardial infarction, surgical procedures and even typhoid immunization.

In acute rheumatic fever the test can serve as a guide to the infection's activity. In fact, the disappearance of CRP may herald subsiding infection. In any acute inflammatory change or necrosis, CRP precedes the rise of ESR and, with recovery, CRP again precedes the fall of ESR. In acute myocardial infarction, CRP appears within 24 to 48 hours, begins to fall by the third day and disappears in 1 to 2 weeks. In RA it exhibits an inconsistent increase.

Joint Fluid Analysis

Most physicians instinctively culture any abnormal discharges from the body. But many will aspirate joint fluid and discard it without a second glance at the specimen. Examine the joint fluid carefully. It is in this fluid that the disease state can be examined at its primary site. The information will greatly aid in establishing a diagnosis and instituting treatment.

The technique of joint aspiration has been described in another section. Usually the fluid will flow through a #20 gauge needle. But if a joint is infected, the fluid may be too tenacious to flow through a needle with a smaller bore than a #16 or #18. Septic joints are frequently missed because too small a needle was used.

First look at the aspirated fluid. Is it a normal clear yellow? Is it bloody? Blood from a traumatic tap will be unevenly distributed throughout the syringe, may clot during aspiration and will decrease with continued aspiration. Is the fluid turbid? Turbidity increases with the degree of inflammation present. Consequently, fluid from an osteoarthritic joint may be clear, while fluid from a RA joint may not. Is the fluid milky as is found in gout? Is it frankly purulent indicating a septic joint?

Remember a joint contains very little fluid, so that the presence of an effusion indicates some abnormality. Effusions due to trauma or degenerative diseases, unless bloody, are similar to normal fluid in appearance. Turbidity is due to white blood cells and provides a rough approximation of the count.

Now check the viscosity of the fluid (Fig. 7-57). This may be done in two ways. Place a drop of the fluid between your thumb and index finger. Slowly separate the fingers, observing how far the fluid will stretch before it snaps. Normal fluid may stretch an inch before breaking. The second method is to allow the fluid to drip slowly from the syringe. Normal fluid will form a string several inches long. It acts like syrup. Inflammatory fluid is less viscous and runs from the needle more like water.

These observations have taken only a few seconds. Now what laboratory tests should you request? Don't get carried away and order everything you've read about.

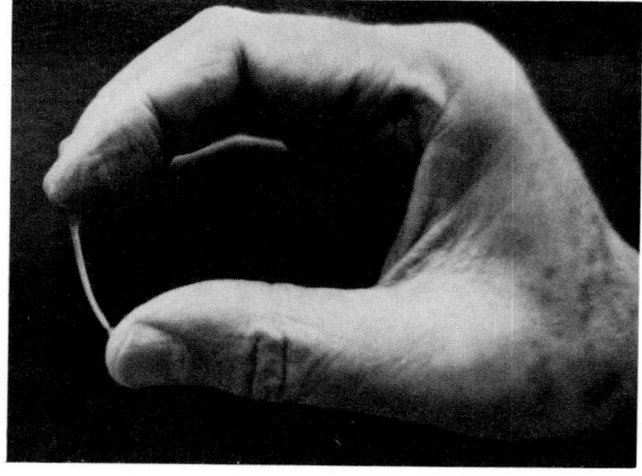

Figure 7-57. Testing viscosity of joint fluid. Viscosity decreases as joint inflammation increases.

Put about 5 ml in a tube with an anticoagulant (10 percent EDTA in normal saline is best) for a white cell count. Perform the count in the same manner as the white cell count on blood except use normal saline rather than 2 percent glacial acetic acid. Normal synovial fluid contains relatively few cells. Effusions caused by trauma or degenerative joint disease have a white count of less than 2,000 per cubic mm. In inflammatory conditions such as RA, Reiter's syndrome and gout, the fluid will contain from 5,000 to 50,000 per cubic mm. Septic joints may exceed 100,000 cells per cubic mm. The differential count is of no importance; most of the cells will be polymorphonuclear leukocytes. If the white cell count is not high, little will be gained by culturing the fluid. In the interest of economy, request the laboratory to culture only those samples with a high white count.

Another simple procedure that gives a fair indication of inflammation is the mucin clot test. The test technique is inexpensive and quick. Drop a little glacial acetic acid into the fluid. In normal fluid a mucin clot forms and drops to the bottom of the tube. If inflammation is present to any significant degree, there is formation of a flocculent precipitate that whirls about like snowflakes when the tube is shaken.

Last of all, put a drop of fluid on a slide and cover with a cover slip. Crystals are usually visible using a light microscope, but polarizing the light will improve your recognition of the crystals. Although I haven't tried it, I've been told that placing one lense from sunglasses on the eye piece of the microscope, and the other lense below the stage a polarizing effect can be produced. An easier way is to purchase a Bausch and Lomb Light Polarizing film #31-52-62-26, which can be inserted into the eye piece and the condenser of a standard microscope.

The most important crystals to be seen and recognized are the needleshaped sodium urate crystals of gout and the rhombus-shaped calcium pyrophosphate crystals of pseudogout (Fig. 7-58).

A glucose determination on the fluid is usually worthless. The total protein content

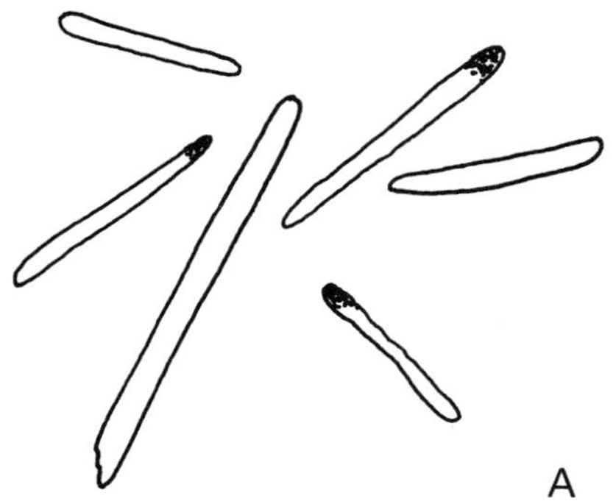

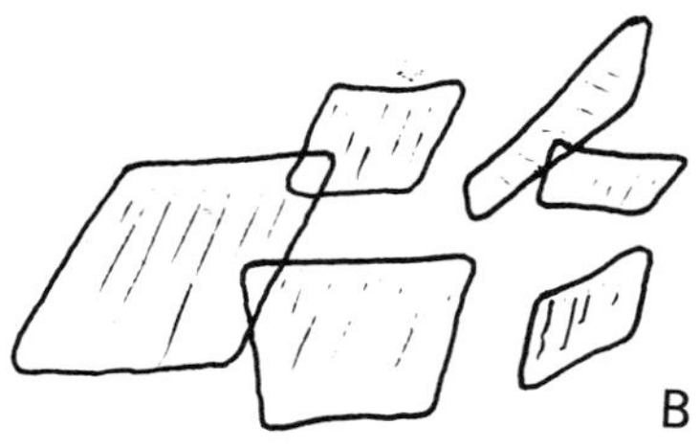

Figure 7-58. Crystals seen in *A*, gout, and *B*, pseudogout.

of the fluid is of no diagnostic help. Unless you have attracted a large arthritic following and have an interest in working out the in-depth details of complex joint problems, skip the immunologic studies. If you need 5 or 6 immunologic tests to make the diagnosis, you are in trouble and should refer the patient to a specialist.

Approaches to Treatment

I am intrigued by the *five levels of therapy* as advocated by Smyth.[3]

Level I is the basic therapeutic program and consists of salicylates to tolerance, therapeutic exercises, heat, patient and family education and appropriate emotional, systemic and joint rest. The objective of this level of treatment is relief of pain, suppression of inflammation, maintenance of function and prevention of deformities. Dr. Smyth considers as essential the education of the patient and his family to the nature and course of the disease.

Level II consists in raising the level of treatment, adding to the basic Level I modalities. There should be more intensive physical and occupational therapy. Employ heavier analgesics such as Librium, relaxants, tranquilizers and Darvon. Have a trial period of anti-inflammatory agents such as Indocin, Butazolidin and antimalarials. Attempt to quiet the most severely inflamed joints with intra-articular steroids. Use orthopedic devices, utilizing splints, bars and canes. The second level of therapy is directed toward patients who have a moderately severe disease that affects multiple joints along with constitutional disturbances and disabilities.

Level III adds oral steroids and gold salts if the preceding levels of treatment have not helped. These patients may be considered candidates for short periods of hospitilization and preventive surgical procedures.

Level IV therapy, Dr. Smythe considers, is outside the realm of chemotherapy. He suggests that 2 to 6 weeks in a rehabilitation center, particularly one devoted to the care of arthritics, is often helpful in slowing the course of the disease. The basic program is an intensification of all modalities with twice-a-day physical therapy given by skilled technicians. This is also the stage wherein reconstructive surgery has an important part in the treatment of RA.

Level V is not within the treatment provcine of the family physician. It is at this time that the patient may be subjected, with his consent, to experimental therapy, including drugs and surgical procedures.

Schumacher,[4] after studying laboratory animals, reports that exercise increases the inflammation in the affected joints of patients with gout. His study should put to rest the rest-exercise controversy. Complete rest rather than exercise is good therapy for acutely inflamed joints.

Sigler and co-workers[5] recommend the institution of gold salt therapy for any patient with sustained active inflammation and evidence of disease progression, and the earlier the better. They report that usually side effects are apparent in the first few months with very few cumulative effects.

The most commonly used preparations are Myochrysine (gold sodium thiomalate) 50 mg per ml, and Solganal (aurothioglucose suspension) 50 mg per ml. Dosage schedule: 25 mg intramuscularly each week for the first 2 weeks. If well tolerated, 50 mg intramuscularly each week.

Monitoring consists of asking the patient before each injection whether he has developed any rash, itching, mouth ulcers or metallic taste in his mouth. Check the patient's urine for protein before each injection and his white blood count before alternate injections.

Discontinue gold therapy if rash, leukopenia or proteinuria appear. If rash is questionable, a trace of protein present or white count falls to 3,000 to 3,500, withhold dose for 1 week and recheck. Gold rash is pruritic.

If no contraindication, continue weekly injections until arthritis is controlled, then gradually increase time intervals and give 50 mg each month as a maintenance dose.

If the arthritis has not responded by the time you have given 1 g of gold discontinue treatment. The majority respond to treatment after receiving 500 to 800 mg.[6]

SYSTEMIC LUPUS ERYTHEMATOSUS (SLE)

In 1971 the American Rheumatism Association identified 14 signs and symptoms related to SLE. Any four of these items can make the diagnosis approximately 90 percent accurate:

- –facial erythema, butterfly rash (a red, scaly rash can appear on other areas open to the sun)
- –Raynaud's phenomenon (severe blanching on exposure to cold)
- –alopecia
- –photosensitivity
- –ulcer of the oral or nasopharyngeal cavities
- –discoid lupus
- –arthritis noticeable more as an morning stiffness of the fingers than as a deformity (most frequent joint complaint in SLE)
- –L.E. cells
- –persistent false positive serological test for syphilis
- –proteinuria
- –hemolytic anemia, leukopenia or thrombocytopenia
- –cellular casts
- –pleuritis or pericarditis
- –psychosis or convulsions

Helpful tests to verify SLE are[7]:

- –antinuclear antibodies check (a negative result rules out SLE)
- –L.E. cell check
- –biopsy of normal appearing skin
- –elevated serum globulin check by electrophoresis
- –complete blood count including a platelet count
- –sedimentation rate
- –immune system tests: Coomb's (direct), cold agglutinins, latex fixation and serological test for syphilis
- –tests usually included in a complete workup: chest x-rays, EKG, blood urea nitrogen and creatinine clearance

For treatment use prednisone or prednisolone.

HYPERURICEMIA AND GOUT

Hyperuricemia is defined as an elevation of the serum uric acid over 6.9 to 7.5 mg/100 ml in men and 5.7 to 6.6 mg/100 in women. Only about a third of the patients with hyperuricemia (elevated serum uric acid or SUA) ever develop clinical gout.

Primary SUA is an inherited metabolic disorder of purine metabolism transmitted through the female. It produces gouty arthritis. Consequently, when one member of a family has gout, suspect other members. Sex ratio in gout: 95 percent males; 5 percent females. In females, gout occurs after the menopause. Undiagnosed gout is prevalent. If you are not finding approximately 6 cases of gout per 1,000 patients, you are probably not recognizing all the cases of gout in your practice.

Secondary SUA is associated with ailments other than gout, such as polycythemia vera, lymphoma, leukemia, multiple myeloma, psoriasis, hypertension, pernicious anemia, sarcoidosis, primary hyperparathyroidism and myeloid metaplasia. The above disorders occur as a result of overproduction of uric acid following marked cellular proliferation and breakdown of nucleoprotein.

The gouty patient produces too much (overproduces) or excretes too little (underexcretes) uric acid. Normal urinary excretory values for adult males range from 250–600 mg/day. An overproducer will excrete more than 10 mg/kg/day while on a low-purine diet.

Renal urate excretion is decreased in underexcretors by diuretics, aspirin (small doses), ketosis, lactate, nicotinic acid and pyrazinamide.

Renal urate excretion in overproducers is increased by probenecid, sulfinpyrazone, methicillin, aspirin (4 g/day), coumarins, acetohexamide, zoxazolamine, iopanoic acid and tubular disease.[8]

Patients with hyperuricemia are more likely to have arteriosclerosis with hypertension and cardiac hypertrophy than others of the same age. Renal disease from urate deposits in the parenchyma is a complication of hyperuricemia; renal stones occur in 10 to 20 percent of the patients.

When confronted with a patient with hyperuricemia, check serum triglycerides and glucose. Patients with gout are more apt to have faulty metabolism of both fats and carbohydrates.

Today the frequent use of diuretics presents a problem, thiazide-induced gout. From a clinical point of view, the acute attack of gout is the same whether it occurs in a person who has hyperuricemia and takes thiazides or in a person whose level of uric acid has been increased secondary to taking thiazides. The problem results in differentiating patients who develop gout while taking thiazides from patients who develop some other kind of arthritis and, because they are taking thiazides, have an elevated uric acid. These patients are often diagnosed as having gout when actually they may have osteoarthritis, rheumatoid arthritis or one of many other diseases with arthritic manifestations.

Clearly differentiate between hyperuricemia and gout. Patients taking thiazide diuretics have an elevated uric acid level. A few of these people develop clinical gout and this gout is similar to any other clinical gout. Some people believe that the only patients who develop gout while taking thiazide diuretics are those who are predisposed to gout. Others believe that the persistent elevation of uric-acid level may eventually lead to gout in normal individuals.

Initial Symptoms of Gout

The chief complaint usually is a sudden onset of severe pain in *any* single joint. Gout is not limited to the M-P joint of the great toe. The ankles, knees and the olecranon bursae are frequently involved in attacks of gout. The pain may begin abruptly, become intense and in a few days disappear completely.

Presumptive diagnosis can depend on one of the following: inflamed joint with extension of inflammation beyond the actual joint, abrupt attack of acute arthritis lasting 2 to 7 days with no residual joint involvement, relief within 24 hr after taking colchicine and serum uric acid levels above 6 mg %. Remember, however, that gout can exist when the serum uric acid level is normal.

In the colchicine test give the patient two 0.5 mg tablets of colchicine at the start of pain. Continue with a 0.5 mg tablet every 2 hours night and day until relieved or until the onset of nausea, vomiting or diarrhea. This will occur after 10 to 16 tablets.

A positive diagnosis of gout can be made by finding one of the following: positive therapeutic response to the colchicine test, subcutaneous or bony tophi (Fig. 7-59), intracellular urate crystals in either synovial fluid (see Fig. 7-58) or in tophi and x-ray evidence of discrete punched-out lesions of bone. These appear late and in only 30% of the cases.

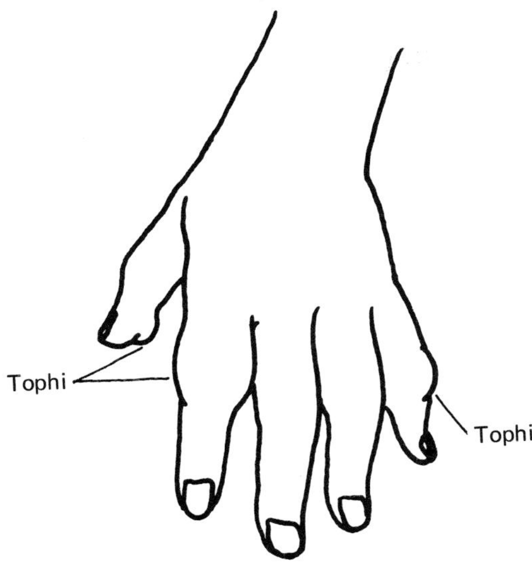

Treatment

Treat acute attacks as outlined for the colchicine test. Start uricosuria therapy 1 week after the initial acute attack.

Give half of a 0.5 g tablet of probenecid (Benemid) b.i.d. for one week and then increase to 0.5 g tablet b.i.d. if the test dose is tolerated. If needed, increase the dose every 4 weeks by 0.5 g until serum uric acid is below 5 mg percent or 24 hour urinary uric acid excretion is above 700 mg percent. Note: Do not give probenecid in conjunction with aspirin and do not start probenecid therapy during the initial attack. For maintenance dosage, consider the following schedule: If serum uric acid is above 6 mg percent increase probenecid to 3 tablets per day; if serum uric acid is below 6 mg percent, continue the drug at 2 tablets per day; and if the serum uric acid is below 5 mg percent and the patient has been free of acute attacks for 6 months, reduce to lowest maintenance dose.

Continue colchicine, 0.5 mg tablets 1 to 3 times daily until the patient has been free of attacks for 1 year. In stable cases, probenecid and colchicine may be given together. Urge the patient to drink at least 6 to 8 glasses of water a day.

Alkalinize the urine by suggesting the patient take 30 to 120 g of soda bicarbonate in divided doses. The patient should determine his dose by checking his urine with nitrazine paper. Hydration and alkalinization will prevent the formation of kidney stones. Put the patient on a restricted purine diet.

In spite of the above, if the patient develops another acute attack, start one of the following four: (1) Give 100 mg capsules of phenylbutazone alka (Butazolidin Alka) stat. Follow up with 2 capsules every 2 hours for 2 doses. Do not repeat for 72 hours. (2) Some prefer oxyphenbutazone (Tandearil). (3) Give indomethacin (Indocin) 50 mg t.i.d. until the attack subsides or inject intra-articular prednisolone TBA 2 to 20 mg plus Xylocaine. (4) Give 100 units of ACTH to start, then 50 units every 6 hours until relieved. ACTH cannot be used alone without precipitating an acute attack. To prevent this complication, administer colchicine for 5 days after ACTH is stopped.

There are several drugs to lower serum uric acid. Do not start them during acute gouty attack or in patients with renal stones. One such drug is allopurinol (Zyloprim) 200 to 600 mg a day in divided doses best for the overproducers. At the start of therapy, the drug may precipitate an acute attack unless colchicine is being given simultaneously. Warn the patient of this possibility. Patients become asymptomatic after several weeks of therapy. Another is probenecid (Benemid) 250 mg (1/2 tablet) b.i.d. If needed after 7 days, increase probenecid to 500 mg b.i.d. Best given in the underexcretor. Sulfinpyrazone (Anturane) can be given 50 mg (½ tablet) b.i.d.

ANKYLOSING SPONDYLITIS (AS)

AS is not difficult to diagnose if you train yourself to think of the possibility. A rheumatologist has no special equipment or knowledge not possessed by the ordinary family physician to aid him in the diagnosis. There are no complex laboratory values to interpret. The diagnosis can be made by performing your regular examination with attention to the back and joints and the proper

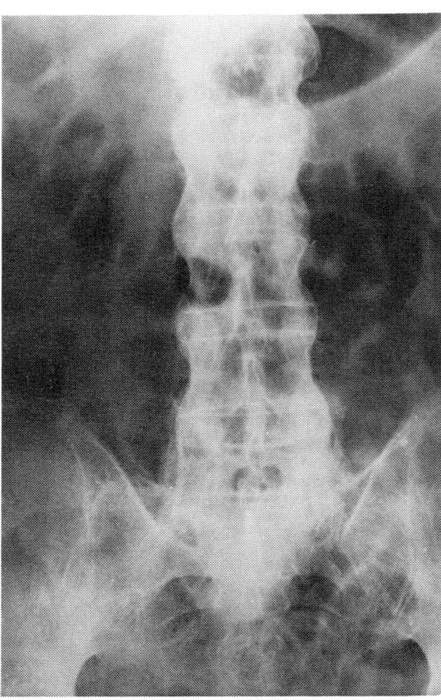

Figure 7-60. Ankylosing spondylitis.

interpretation of an x-ray study of the pelvis and lower back (Fig. 7-60).

The disease is 10 times more common in men than in women. It is frequently thought of as being a disease of old men because the disabling kyphosis may not appear until years after the inception of the disease. However, AS starts its course early, sometimes between 15 and 35 years of age.

The disease starts in one of three ways and this may be the cause of the confusion associated with early diagnosis. Clinically the commonest initial complaint is of low back pain, usually awakening the patient from his sleep in the early morning hours. This is associated with a general morning stiffness of the spine usually relieved by activity. In a less number of cases the early complaints are of peripheral joint pain and stiffness, especially of the hips, knees, ankles and heels. In about 2 to 3 percent of the cases the disease starts as recurrent attacks of iridocyclitis.

In whatever fashion the disease starts, the patient eventually develops an intermittent nocturnal low back pain and stiffness. Systemic symptoms may include fatigue, low grade fever, mild anemia, anorexia and weight loss. Sooner or later the following tests become positive.

Digital pressure over the sacroiliac joints causes pain, one of the first signs of sacroiliac involvement.

The patient becomes unable to lock his knees and touch his toes. Some evidence of the progress of the disease may be elicited by serial measurements of the distance from fingertips to floor.

Ask the patient to place his heels and back against the wall, and then attempt to touch the wall with the back of his head without raising his chin above carrying level. Inability to touch head to wall suggests cervical disease.

In the Schober test, make a mark on the spine at the level of the iliac crests. Make another mark on the spine 10 cm above the first mark while the patient stands. Now have the patient bend forward as far as possible and measure the distance between the two marks. A positive finding is indicated by an increase of less than 5 cm between the marks. This is a sign of lumbar disease.

A decreasing chest expansion is detected by measuring at the nipple line. Chest expansion of less than 4 cm is a clue to early costovertebral disease.

The only laboratory test of possible value may be done on fluid aspirated from a peripheral joint and is done to help differentiate AS from rheumatoid arthritis. Synovial fluid complement values are higher in AS running to 90 or 130 hemolytic units. In RA, the values remain below 50. Of course, ESR is elevated as it is in other collagen diseases.

Final verification of the diagnosis usually depends on x-ray demonstration of the disease process in the sacroiliac joints. Stereoscopic views are helpful for early, adequate visualization. Look for early widening of the sacroiliac joints with blurring of the margins, later sclerosis of the adjacent sacrum and ilium and, finally, complete destruction of the joint space. The spine may also become affected with all the vertebrae eventually becoming joined by bridges of bone, the so-called *bamboo spine* (Fig. 7-61).

Some features which differentiate AS from RA:

–greater prevalance in males (9:1)

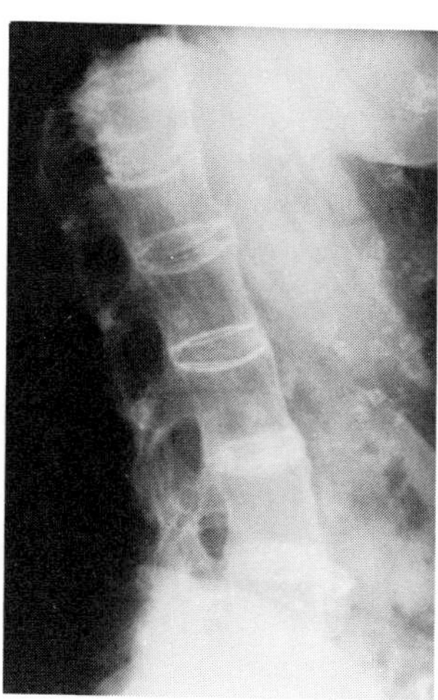

Figure 7-61. Bamboo spine with rheumatoid arthritis and ligamentous calcification in left spine.

- –infrequent involvement of small peripheral joints
- –involvement of spine in every patient
- –early and constant bilateral sacroilitis on x-ray film
- –stiffness more prominent than pain
- –no subcutaneous nodules
- –higher incidence of recurrent iritis
- –negative serum RF
- –lack of response to gold and antimalarials
- –selective response to local irradiation
- –greater frequency of aortitis and conduction defects

Treatment consists of anti-rheumatic drugs and extensive physical therapy. Aspirin is the drug of choice for patients with mild disease. Give 4 to 6 g doses, sufficient to relieve discomfort. For those who cannot take aspirin and for those with more advanced disease, the drugs are Indocin (indomethacin) and Butazolidin (phenylbutazone) or Tandearil (oxyphenylbutazone). Indocin may be given in daily doses of 25 to 200 mg per day. Butazolidin and Tandearil may be effective in doses ranging from 100 to 400 mg daily. The latter two require monitoring by complete blood counts weekly for 2 months and monthly thereafter. Indocin and Butazolidin are so consistently effective that if significant relief is not obtained, question your diagnosis of AS.

Stay away from corticosteroids. The above drugs are much more effective and have less side effects. Topical steroids, however, may be useful when single joints are involved. In the event the patient develops iridocyclitis or vasculitis, oral steroids should be prescribed.

Do not use antimalarial or gold compounds. They are ineffective in AS as well as muscle relaxants. Narcotics are unjustified and so is x-ray therapy.

The prevention of deformities is accomplished by energetic and continuous physical therapy such as postural training; the use of bedboards; removal of all pillows; proper rest and exercise periods.

Choose physical therapy or even a sports activity to prevent future deformities, prevent further loss of range of motion in specific joints, maintain correct posture and mobility of spine and reduce stiffness.

Suggested sports for specific patients are bowling, horseshoes, lawn bowling, croquet, miniature golf, pitch and putt, paddle tennis, table tennis, badminton, fly or surf casting, archery, skeet shooting and swimming. In the latter, help select the proper strokes for the individual.

LOW BACK PAIN

Your approach to the patient with low back pain is important. Low back pain is not always the result of abnormality of an intervertebral disc. Kraus[9] estimates that 84 percent of patients with low back pain have no organic pathology. He contends that most patients suffer from muscular deficiencies as a result of tension. No more than 10 percent of your patients with low back pain should be referred for consultation or surgery.

Take a careful history as you would for any diagnostic problem. However, it can be delayed temporarily if the patient is in acute distress. At a minimum, even on the first visit, ask the following questions: Where is the pain? Exclusively in the back? Does it radiate down the leg or legs? Where? Ask the patient to describe the exact location.

How did the pain start? Sudden or insidious? Did it begin after an injury or some unexpected stress? A sudden onset should cause you to think of possible intrinsic trauma of joints or muscles. If the onset was insidious with stiffness think of disease rather than trauma. Obtain as clear a description as possible for what happened. If there was trauma or an accident, when did it happen, where, and what were the circumstances? Question the patient about other similar attacks. If he has recurrent back pain does it recur after strains or stress? After increasing activity? For no apparent reason?

Now find out about the characteristics of pain: Does sneezing or coughing aggravate it? If so, suspect nerve-root compression. Is the pain constant or intermittent? Does bed rest relieve or increase it? Pain relieved by lying down points toward simple mechanical problems. If the pain is increased or not relieved, think of a more serious disability. Does the pain occur only when the patient walks and go away when he stops or stands? This is the type of discomfort that accompanies a circulatory problem. Ask the patient how he gets out of bed in the morning. Does he roll to his side and come up with his feet on the floor as in myositis? Or does he ease out of bed onto his knees and climb up as in neurological damage?

When taking this short history don't overlook the possibility of systemic disease. Ask about pains in other joints. Prostatitis? Cystitis? Menopause? And before you go too far ask about other treatments he has tried and whether he was relieved by any. Review his past and present illnesses. Record all findings for many of these cases turn out to be legal or insurance problems.

General Examination of the Back

While the patient is standing do an anterior inspection (Fig. 7-62A). Observe

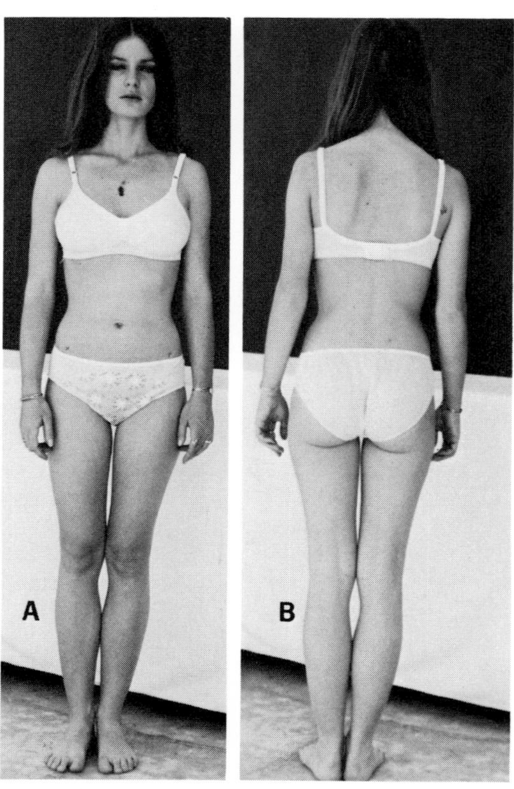

Figure 7-62. *A*, Anterior inspection; *B*, Posterior inspection.

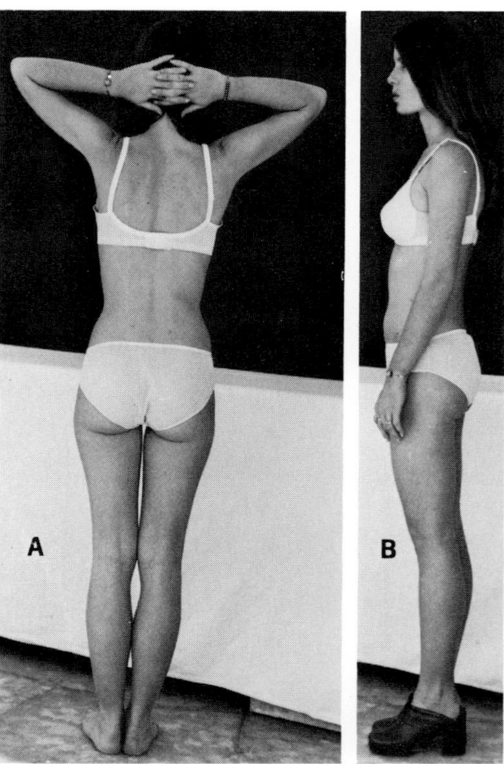

Figure 7-63. *A*, Evaluate lateral spinal motion; *B*, Profile inspection.

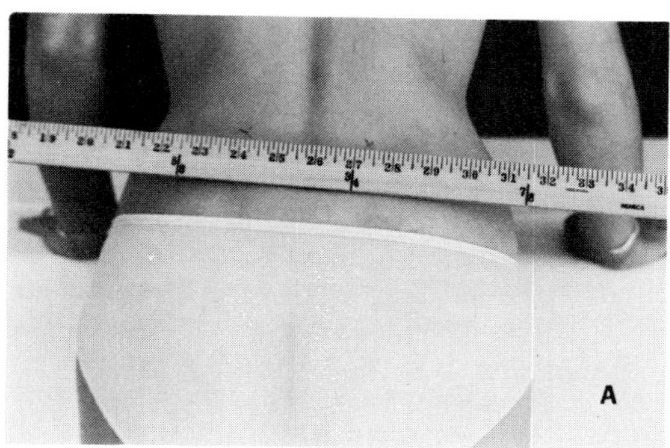

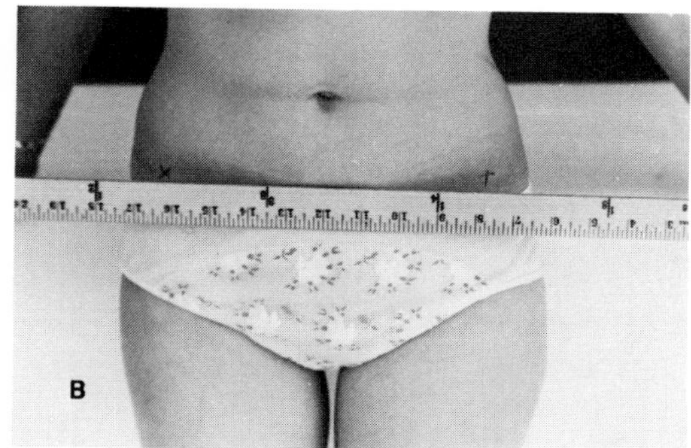

Figure 7-64. Measure the level of the *A*, posterior-superior spine and, *B*, anterior-iliac spine.

whether the abdominal muscles are firm, pendulous and relaxed. Is the pelvis level? Are the feet normal? Have the patient take a few steps and check arches and the presence of pronation. Posteriorly inspect (Fig. 7-62B) for deformities, scoliosis, kyphosis and flattening of lumbar lordosis. Palpate for para vertebral spasm. Is it unilateral or bilateral? Is there a dropping of the gluteal fold on the affected side?

Evaluate lateral spinal motion (Fig. 7-63A). Observe the distances between the elbows and the hips at rest and in lateral flexion. Lateral flexion is restricted in sprains of the muscles on ligaments. The patient is limited in bending away from the bad side. The opposite is the case in lateral disc protrusions. Make a profile inspection with the patient standing (Fig. 7-63B). Inspect for forward tilting of the pelvis both with and without heels. Note also if trunk flexion is limited. If so, is it due to neuropathy, ankylosis, spastic musculature or, as is often the case with wearing of high heels, to shortening of the hamstring, gluteal or calf muscles?

Test for pelvis tilt by measuring the level of the posterior superior and anterior iliac spines (Fig. 7-64). If they are not level by half an inch or more it may be assumed that one leg is shorter.

Have the patient stand on one leg (Fig. 7-65). When the patient with backache stands on his "good" leg the pain of lumbosacral disease will be aggravated. When he stands on his "bad" leg the pain of sacroiliac disease is increased.

Rotation of the trunk upon the pelvis often locates the painful area. Ask the seated patient to lock her hands behind her head (Fig. 7-66), fixing the scapula. This permits rotation of the trunk using the arms as levers. In cases of lumbosacral strain, there is little

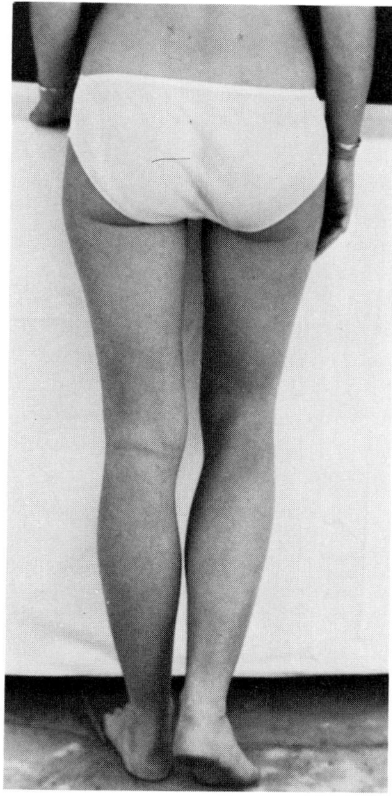

Figure 7-65. Differentiating lumbosacral disease and sacroiliac disease.

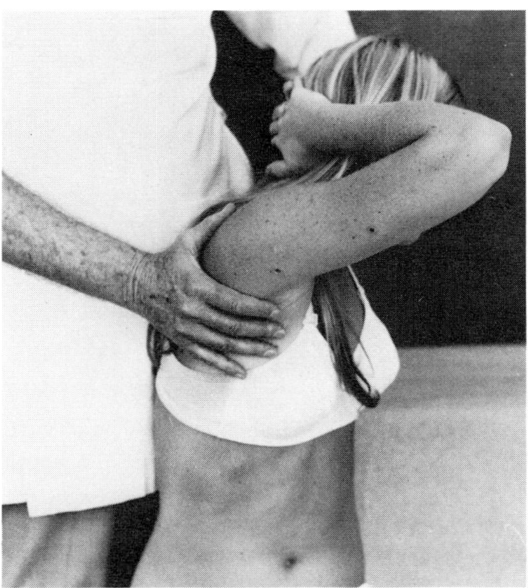

Figure 7-66. Rotation of the trunk upon the pelvis often locates the painful area.

impediment on rotation to the involved side but pain is produced in extreme rotation away from the area of involvement.

In Soto-Hall's sign, with the patient supine, flex the spine by bringing up the head and progressing caudally (Fig. 7-67). The location of pain indicates the level of pathology.

In Goldwaite's sign, place one hand under the lower back of the supine patient. Flex the leg as indicated in Figure 7-68 and then apply leverage to the side of the pelvis. Pain before motion of the lumbar spine indicates sprain of the sacroiliac joint. If motion is detected before pain either the sacroiliac or sacrolumbar joint is involved.

With the patient prone do Ely's test. Flex her knee and press her heel against her buttocks (Fig. 7-69). Check for pathology in either the sacrolumbar or sacroiliac joints, depending on where the pain occurs.

Muscle Function Check

Ober's test for contracture of the fascia lata requires the patient to lie on her side with the lower leg extended. Steady her with your hand on her greater trochanter. Flex the upper leg at the knee with your other hand and abduct and then hyperextend her thigh (Fig. 7-70). Gradually slip the hand back, allowing her leg to fall toward the table. Contracture of the fascia lata is shown by the inability of her knee to touch her opposite leg.

To test trunk mobility the patient is seated with legs extended. She should be able to touch her knees with her head without pain (Fig. 7-71). This movement is restricted if

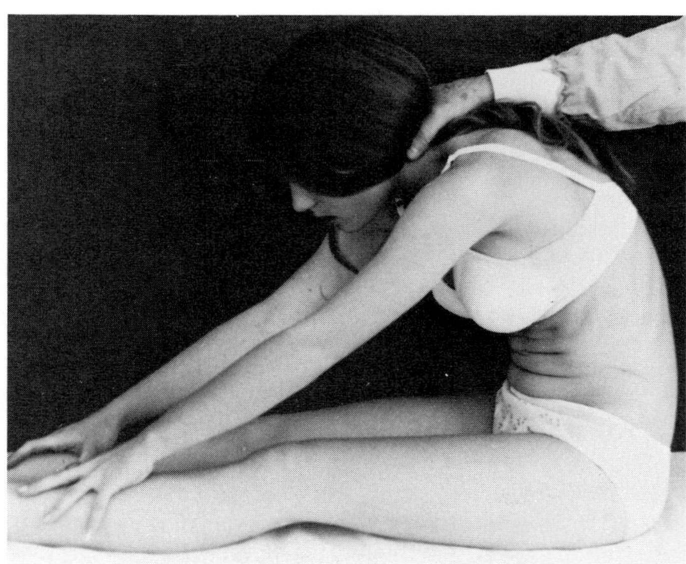

Figure 7-67. Flexing the spine in Soto-Hall's sign.

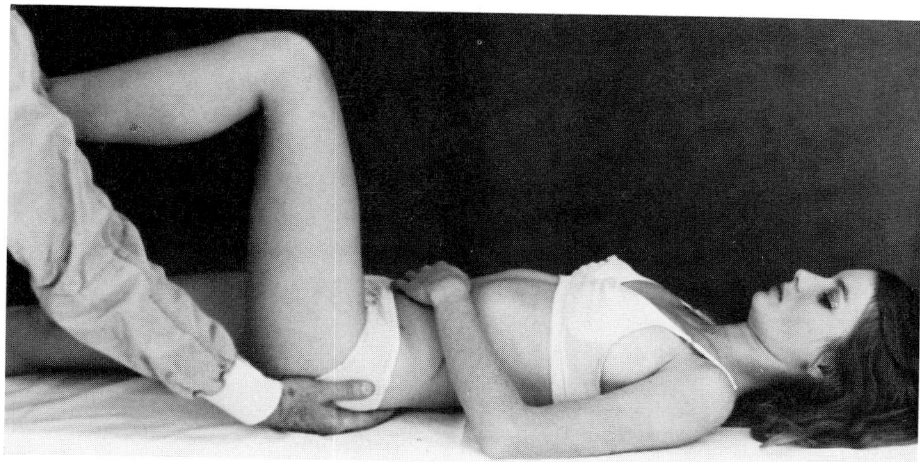

Figure 7-68. The procedure for Goldthwaite's sign.

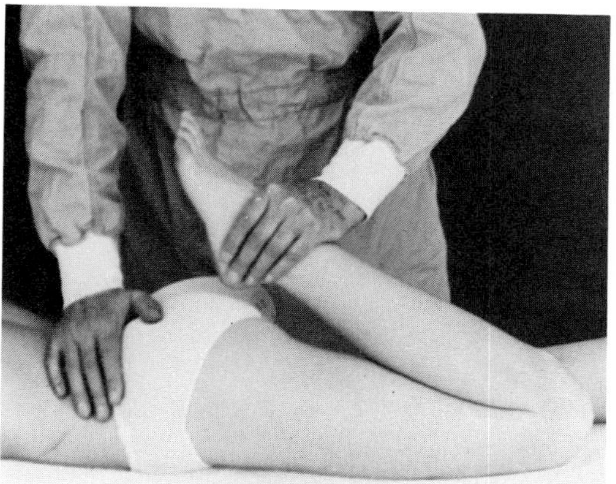

Figure 7-69. Ely's test for pathology in the sacrolumbar or sacroiliac joints.

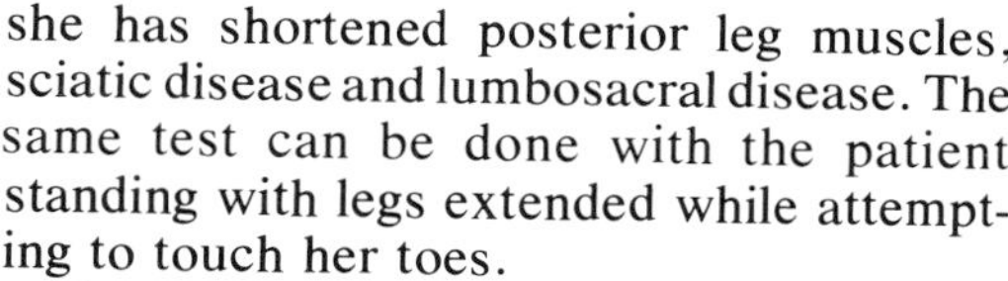

she has shortened posterior leg muscles, sciatic disease and lumbosacral disease. The same test can be done with the patient standing with legs extended while attempting to touch her toes.

Test for short posterior leg muscles with the patient seated with her legs over the side of the table (Fig. 7-72). Flex her trunk to its limit. Grasp one ankle and hold her knee in place with your other hand. Slowly extend the knee joint. If her posterior leg muscles are shortened, the patient cannot maintain a flexed position while the ankle is extended.

The Ely test to determine shortening of the anterior fascial structures of the thigh is

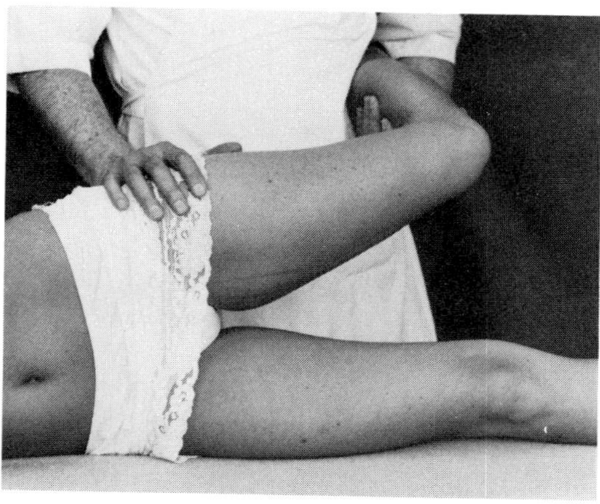

Figure 7-70. Ober's test for contracture of the fascia lata.

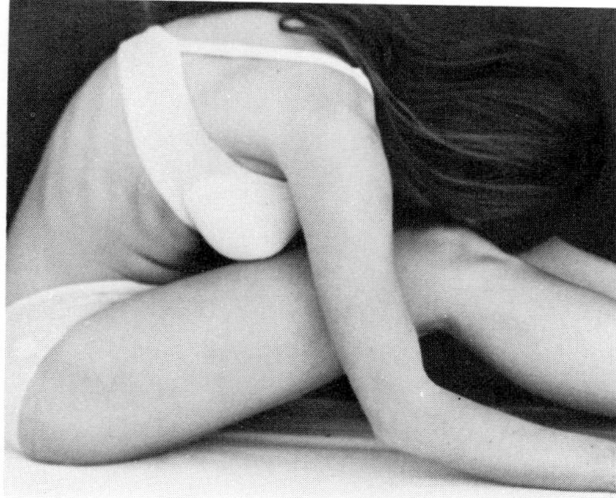

Figure 7-71. The healthy patient can touch her knees with her head without having pain.

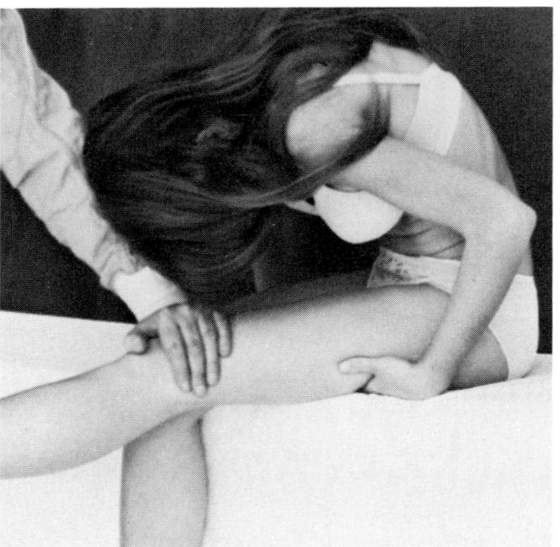

Figure 7-72. Seat the patient to test for short posterior leg muscles.

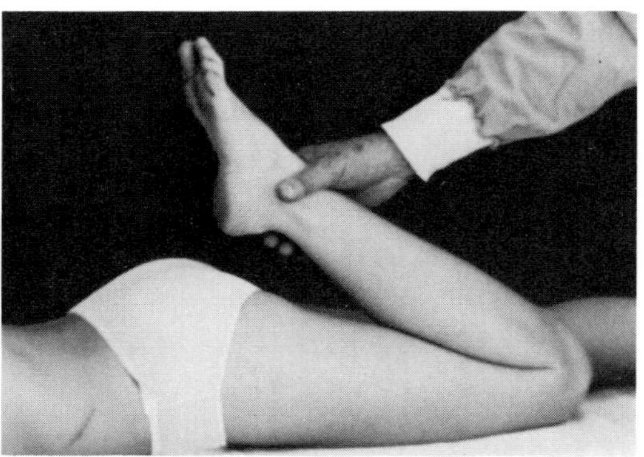

Figure 7-73. In the Ely test the degree of motion is limited by the extent of contraction in the anterior thigh structures.

done with the patient prone. Bend the patient's leg, bringing the heel up to touch the buttocks (Fig. 7-73). The degree of motion is limited by the extent of contraction in the anterior thigh structures. Do not allow the pelvis to tilt or elevate.

Sciatic Nerve Check

These signs are demonstrated with the patient supine. In Lasegue's sign (Fig. 7-74) extension of the knee causes pain along the course of the sciatic nerve. If the sign is positive, examine the patient for causes of sciatic neuropathy. In Linder's sign (Fig. 7-75) passively flex the patient's head. Increased pain in the lumbar or sciatic area indicates sciatic disease. In Bragard's sign flex her stiff leg at the hip. Dorsiflex her foot (Fig. 7-76) when her hip is fully flexed. An increase in pain indicates a neural etiologic factor; if pain is the same a muscular etiologic factor is evident.

Lumbosacral Check

In lumbosacral disease the lower back is rigid and tender to pressure (Fig. 7-77). This is not true in sacroiliac disease. To test for lumbosacral strain place the patient in the position illustrated in Figure 7-78 with pillows under her hips to separate the spinous processes. Palpate her spine for tender areas. In strain the tenderness is usually located above or below L_5. Always consider lumbosacral strain when the patient com-

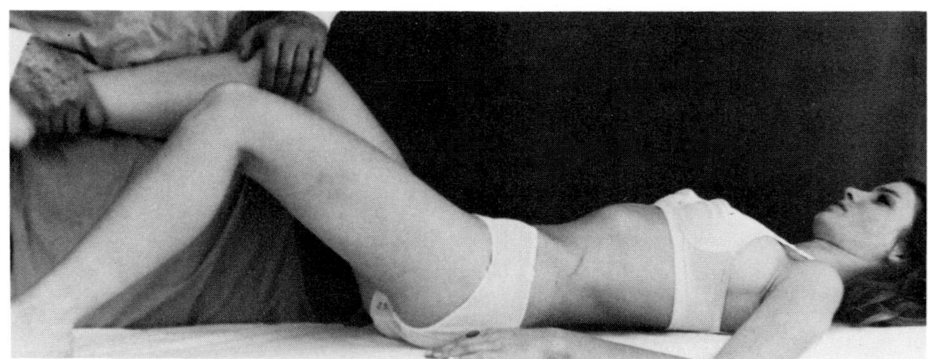

Figure 7-74. If Lasegue's sign is positive, examine the patient for causes of sciatic neuropathy.

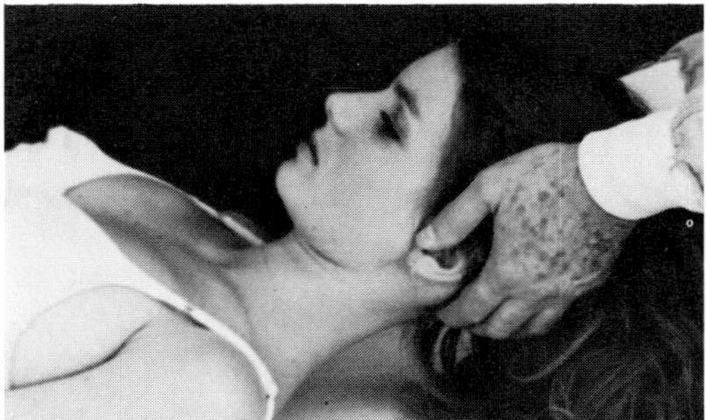

Figure 7-75. Linder's sign to determine sciatic disease.

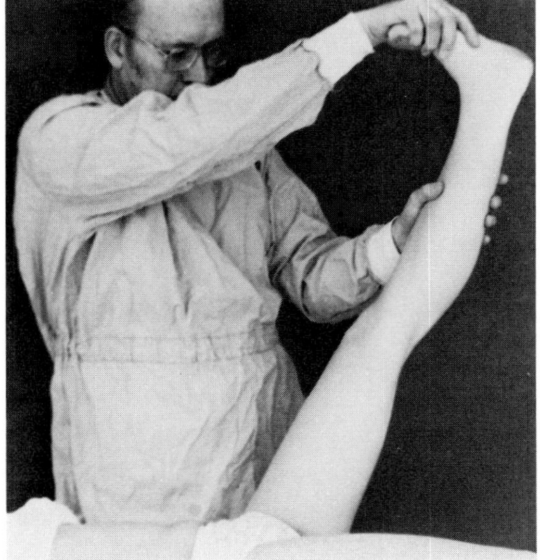

Figure 7-76. Dorsiflexing the foot in Bragard's sign.

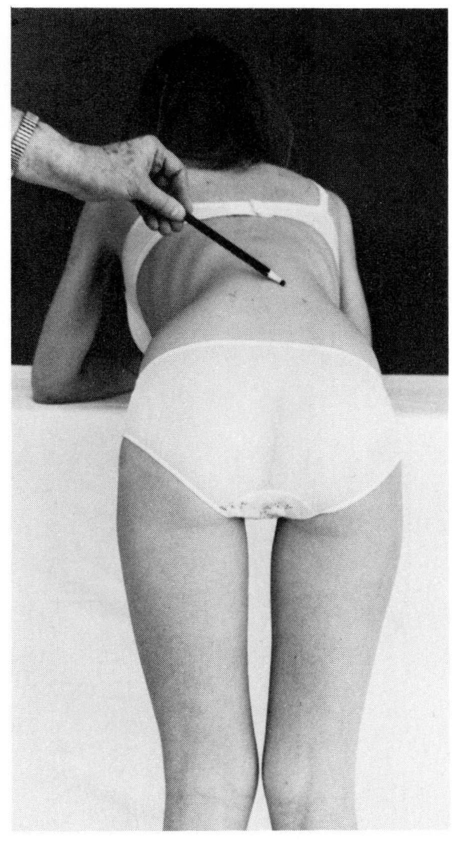

Figure 7-77. Determining rigidity of lower back.

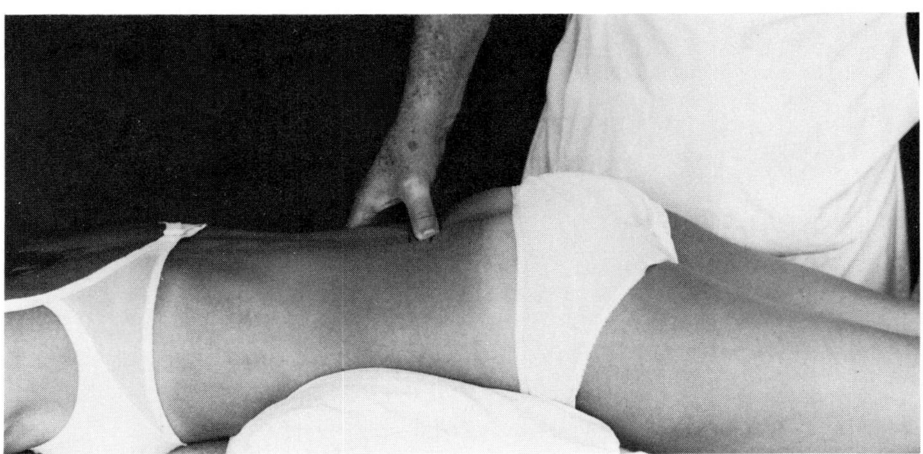

Figure 7-78. Testing for lumbosacral strain.

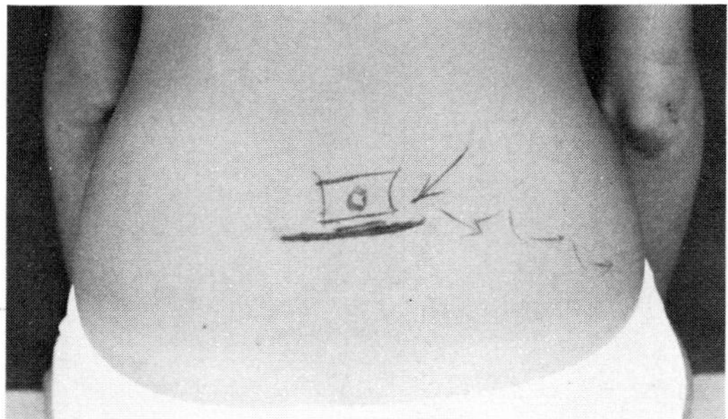

Figure 7-79. Site of lumbosacral strain.

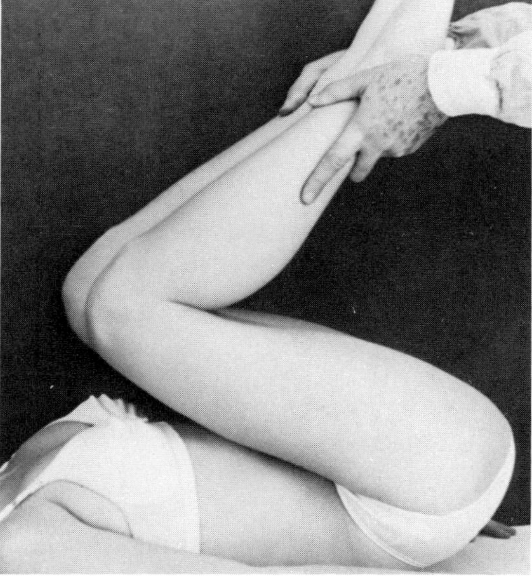

Figure 7-80. This maneuver tests for painful motion in the lumbosacral and lumbar joints.

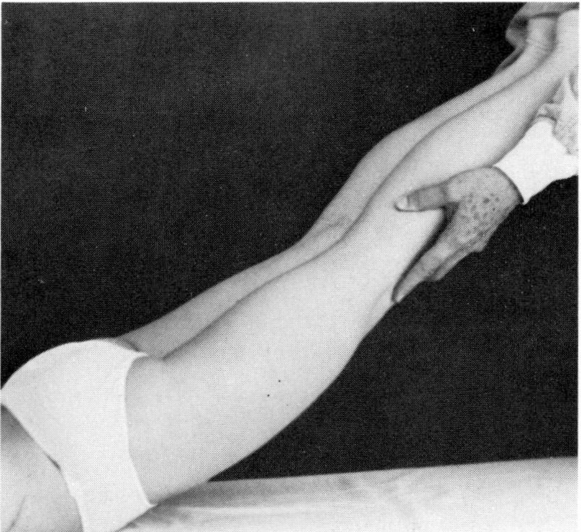

Figure 7-81. Reverse Lasegue's sign.

plains of an aching pain near L_5 or S_1 that radiates laterally (Fig. 7-79).

In the position indicated in Figure 7-80, movement of the lumbosacral joint may be tested without movement of the sacroiliac joints. Consequently, this maneuver tests for painful motion in the lumbosacral and lumbar joints. Pain indicates lumbar spine disease such as arthritis and malignancy.

In a reverse Lasegue's sign (see Fig. 7-74) raise her legs with your hands proximal to her knees (Fig. 7-81). Limitation of hyperextension suggests midlumbar spinal nerve disease or lumbosacral malfunctioning. In Gaenslen's sign have the patient rest on her back with her legs hanging either over the edge of the table or to one side of the table. One leg should be flexed and on the table; the other is then hyperextended (Fig. 7-82). An increase in pain indicates lumbosacral disease.

Sacroiliac Check

To examine the lower back specifically, start the examination with the patient seated and with her back toward you as illustrated in Figure 7-83. Locate her sacroiliac joints either by locating the dimples in the overlying skin or by palpation. With your hands on the iliac crest, trace the posterior extension of the crest toward the posterior iliac spines. If your thumbs then are moved about 1 in toward the spine they will be over the superior notch of the sacroiliac joints.

With the patient prone, fasten her pelvis against the table with your hand. Now flex her knee and hyperextend her hip by lifting up at the ankle (Fig. 7-84). Apply the test to both sides. The test puts a strain on the sacroiliac joints. Raising both legs together produces a strain in the lumbosacral joint. As the pelvis is raised from the table there is a strain in the lumbar joints.

Gaenslen's sign of sacroiliac disease (Fig. 7-85) is useful because, in producing anterior torsion strain, the sciatic nerve is not stretched and, therefore, may be used as a differential sign between sciatica and sacroiliac disease. Have the patient lock her pelvis by holding one knee flexed against her abdomen. Lower the leg of the suspected

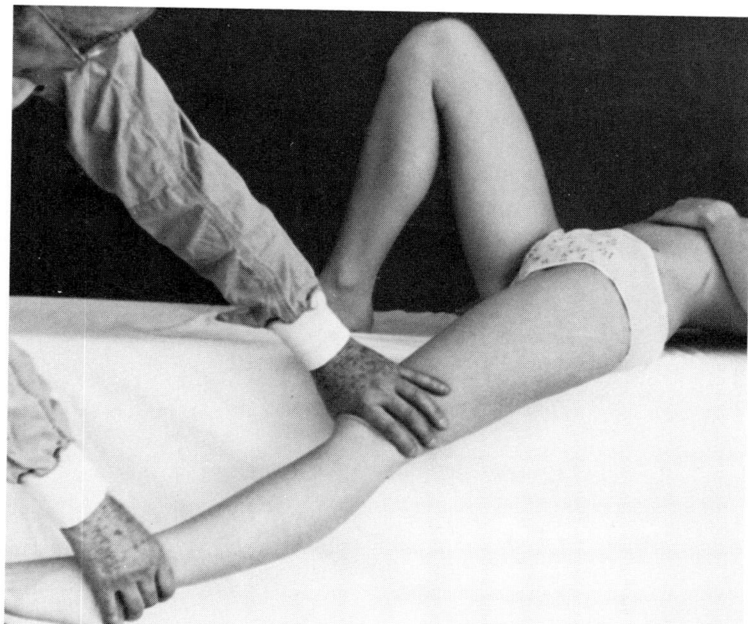

Figure 7-82. In Gaenslen's sign one leg should be flexed and the other hyperextended.

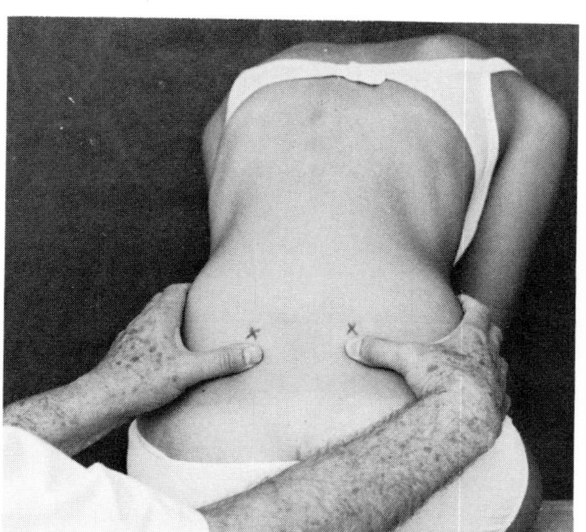

Figure 7-83. Examination of the lower back.

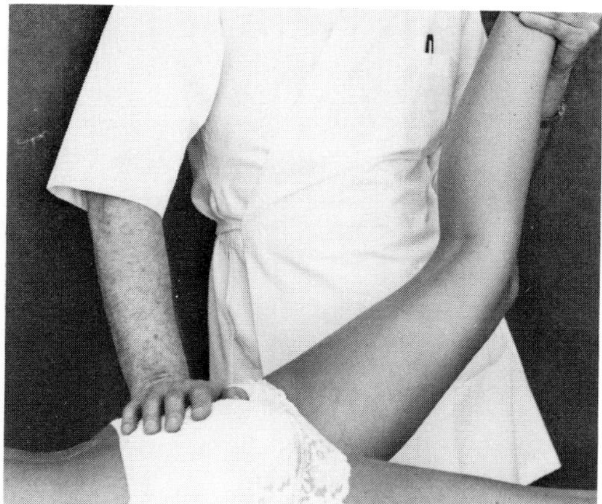

Figure 7–84. Fasten the patient's pelvis against the table with your hand and flex her knee.

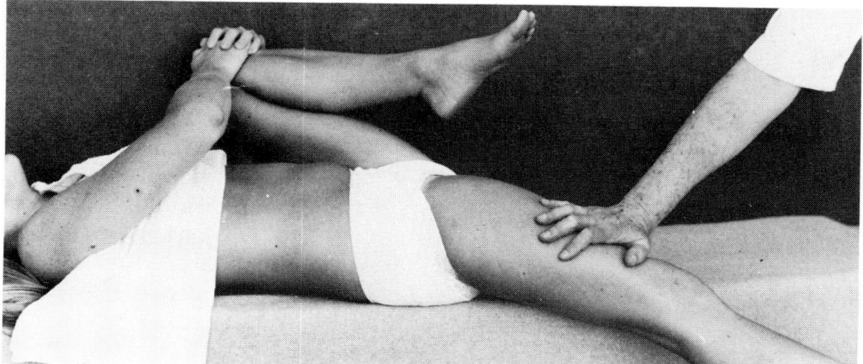

Figure 7-85. Gaenslen's sign may be used as a differential sign between sciatica and sacroiliac disease.

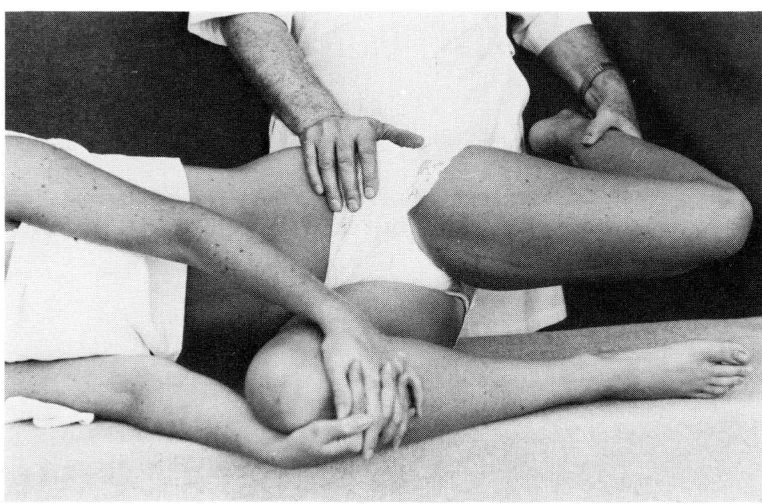

Figure 7-86. Repetition of Gaenslen's test with the patient in the lateral position.

side with one hand on the thigh and the other on the ankle. Pain is produced if the sacroiliac joint is diseased. The side-lying test is a repetition of Gaenslen's test with the patient in a lateral position (Fig. 7-86). Have the patient lie on her painful side with her lower knee pulled up into acute flexion. Flex her upper knee holding the patient's leg with your other hand on her thigh. Continue hyperextending her upper leg. Strain is placed on the lower sacroiliac joint. The time of appearance of pain is important in interpreting the strain. In the compression test put pressure on the iliac crests (Fig. 7-87). Increased pain indicates sacroiliac disease.

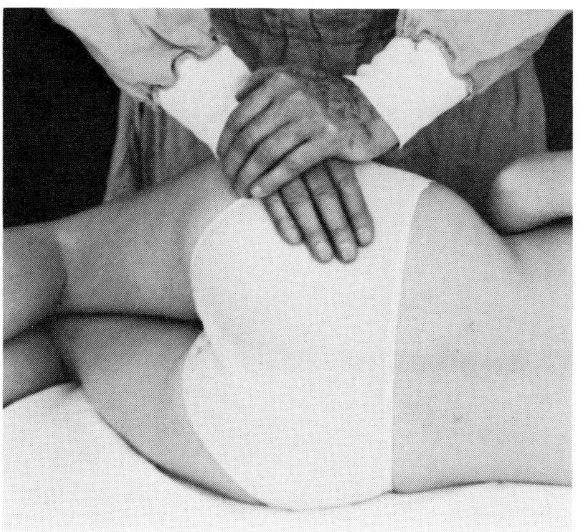

Figure 7-87. Iliac compression test.

Ask your patient to assume a comfortable supine position. Perform the straight-leg raising (SLR) test by flexing her extended leg on the trunk without moving her pelvis (Fig. 7-88). This stretches the hamstring muscles and produces a torsion between the sacrum and ilium. Sacroiliac disease produces pain. In unilateral sacroiliac soreness, pain is produced when the leg is raised to a little beyond 45° from the horizontal. If you raise the leg even further (Fig. 7-89) the sacrum is carried along with the ilium of the tested side so that torsion is made on the opposite sacroiliac joint. Therefore, raising the leg of the good side will produce pain in the opposite sacroiliac when the leg is pushed beyond 45°.

Hip Check

In Patrick's test or Fabere sign, with the patient supine, place her external malleolus over the patella of her opposite leg. Press down on her flexed knee (Fig. 7-90). Increased pain indicates hip disease. La Guerre's test spots hip disease. Abduct her hip with her knee flexed and then externally rotate (Fig. 7-91). If there is no hip disease, sacroiliac disease may be localized.

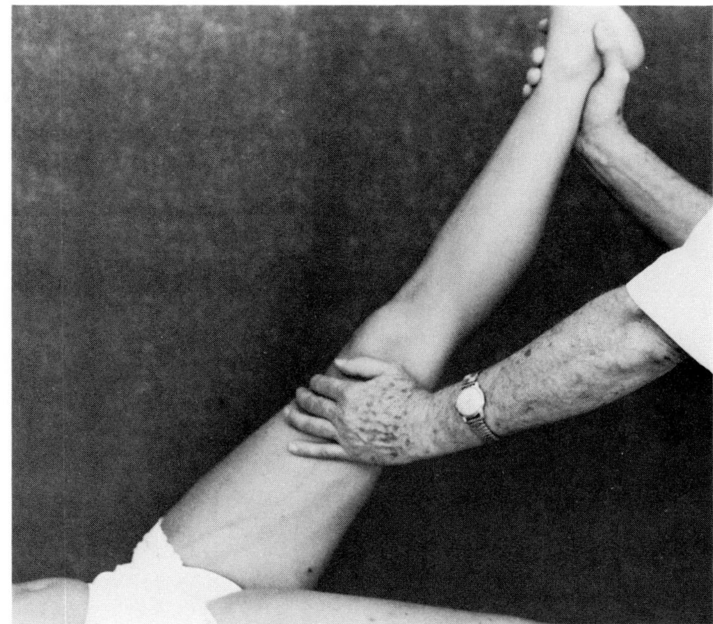

Figure 7-88. Straight-leg raising test.

To test trunk mobility, have the patient seated with legs flexed (Fig. 7-92). Diseases of the lumbar area do not restrict trunk flexion while seated but pain in this position on trunk flexion suggests hip joint pathology or severely restrictive lesions of the lumbar spine.

In another test for trunk mobility the patient is prone. With her knee flexed, pull up on her ankle, hyperextending her hip (Fig. 7-93). Increased pain is evidence of hip joint disease, contraction of the anterior fascia lata or acute disease of the iliopsoas.

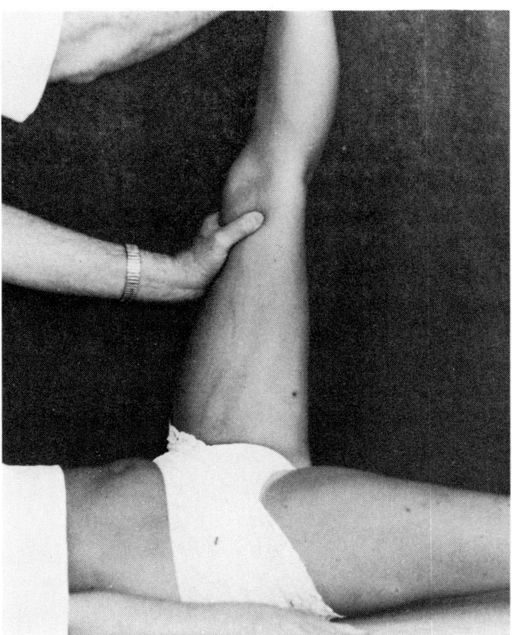

Figure 7-89. Raising the leg on the good side beyond 45° will produce pain in the opposite sacroiliac.

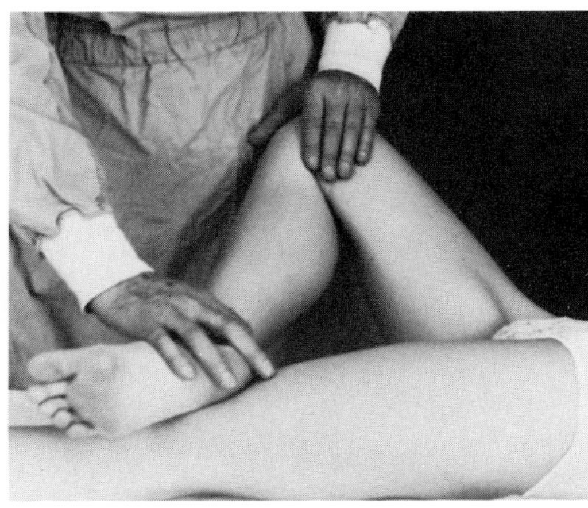

Figure 7-90. Patrick's test (Fabre sign).

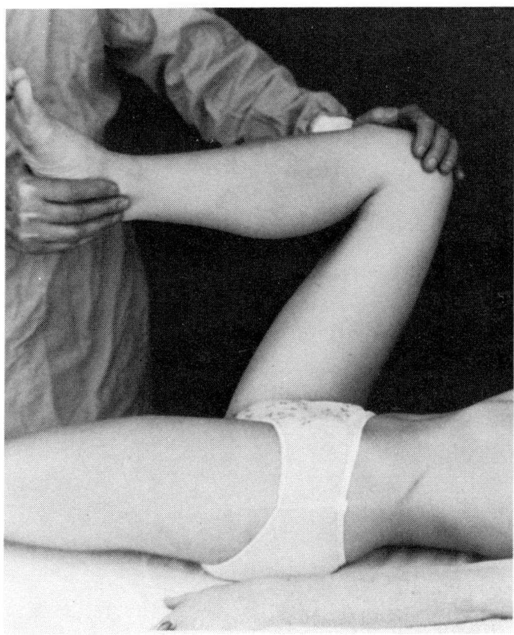

Figure 7-91. La Guerre's test for hip disease.

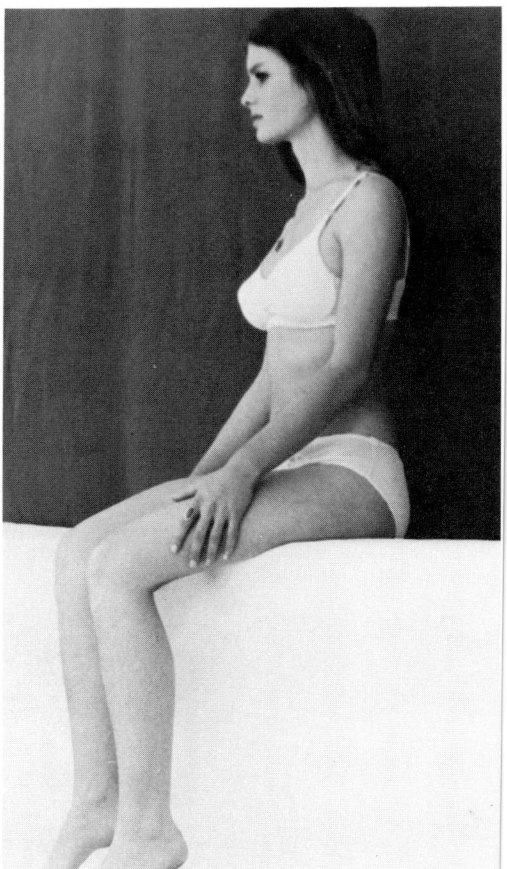

Figure 7-92. Test for trunk mobility.

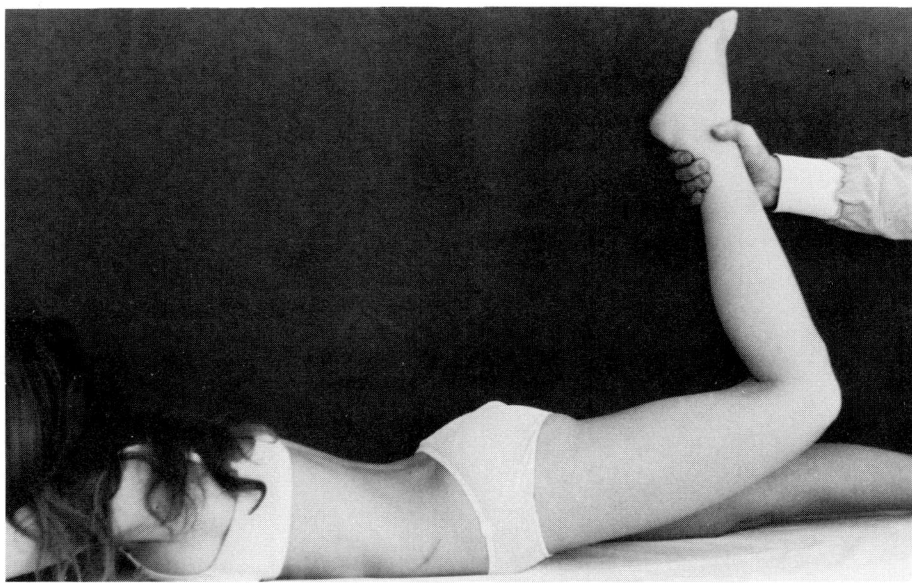

Figure 7-93. Test for trunk mobility with patient in prone position.

Acute Disc Problem

A patient with an acute disc problem will walk into your office with a bent stance and usually listing to one side. Any attempt he makes to straighten up causes severe pain. With his shirt off, one hip appears to be higher than the other.

The pain may have started after coughing, sneezing or straining and is aggravated by the same. He usually doesn't remember any injury to his back. Within a week or two the pain begins to radiate down a leg, causing shock-like pain and numbness along some segmental distribution of the sciatic nerve. Neurologic complications include dragging of a leg or a slapping of the foot against the floor as he walks. Occasionally the patient complains of his foot being too weak to depress the accelerator on the car.

Pain Radiation in Lumbar Disc Disease

In L_4 disease there is pain radiation and hypoalgesia as indicated in Figure 7-94. There is numbness and motor weakness of the great toe and anterior leg with pain in the gluteal region below the iliac crest.

Pain radiation and hypoalgesia occurring in disease of L_5 is indicated in Figure 7-95. Usually there is no change in deep reflexes. There is numbness in the three middle toes. There is pain in the gluteal region between the ischial tuberosity and femoral trochanter and numbness in the lateral leg.

In disease of S_1 there is pain in the medial gluteal region over the ischial tuberosity with radiation of pain and hypoalgesia as shown in Figure 7-96. Numbness occurs in the posterior leg and little toe and motor weakness in the plantar flexors. There is reduced Achilles tendon reflex.

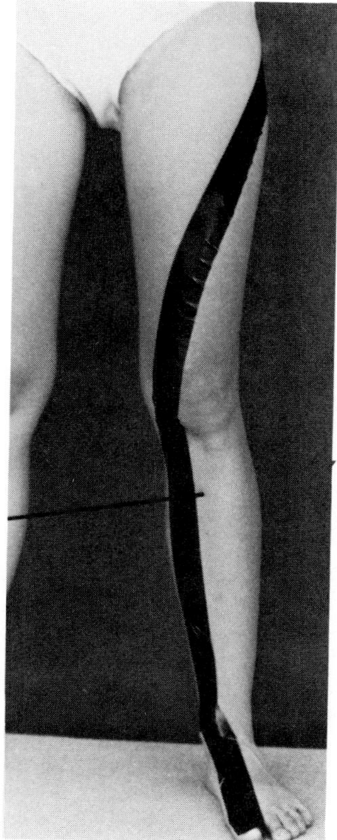

Figure 7-94. Pain radiation and hypoalgesia in diseased L_4.

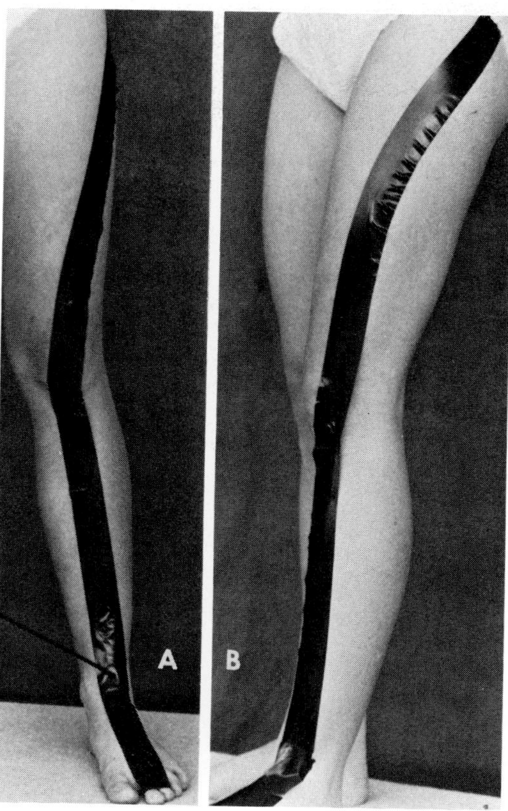

Figure 7-95. Diseased L_5 with *A*, pain radiation and hypoalgesia and, *B*, pain in the gluteal region.

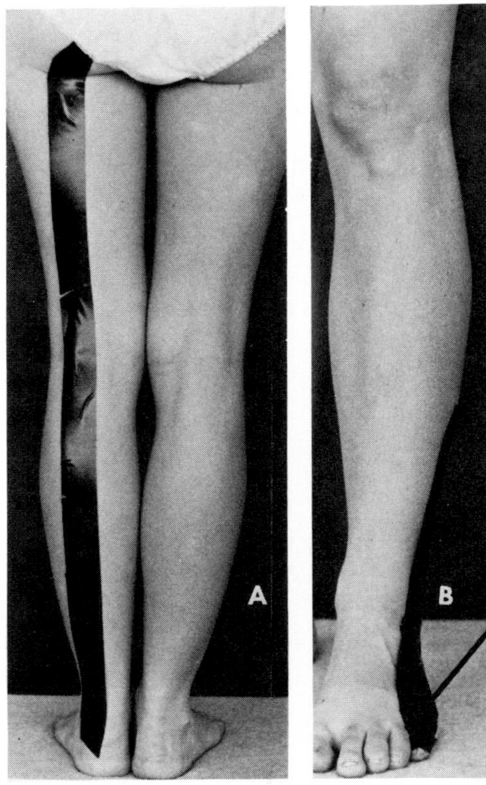

Figure 7-96. Disease S_1 with *A*, pain in medial gluteal region and, *B*, numbness in posterior leg and little toe.

Disease of S_2 causes pain in the medial gluteal fold with radiation and hypoalgesia as outlined in Figure 7-97. There is weakness and the plantar flexion reflex is reduced. Numbness and pain radiation may occur in the posterior thigh and labium majora.

Examination

Do not put the patient through numerous back tests. The diagnosis can be suspected by a detailed history and a few simple tests of the extremities.

Examine the patient first while standing. It is unlikely he has serious back disease if he can touch his toes. Determine the loss of flexion, extension and rotation. Ask him to lie on his back on the examination table and to straighten one leg, then the other and finally both together. All these produce pain when a disc is herniated.

If in doubt or if you suspect the patient may be a malingerer, ask the patient to sit on the side of the examination table. Repeat the SLR test without the patient's knowledge. Ask your patient if her feet bother her and casually pick them up for inspection, thus stretching the sciatic nerve without the patient's knowledge. Magnuson's test is a pointing test for malingering. Ask the patient to point to the painful spot; mark the area with a grease pencil. Later during the examination ask her to point to the painful spot again. Consider malingering if she points to a different spot, but organic disease is a possibility if she points to the same spot. Another check for the exaggerator or

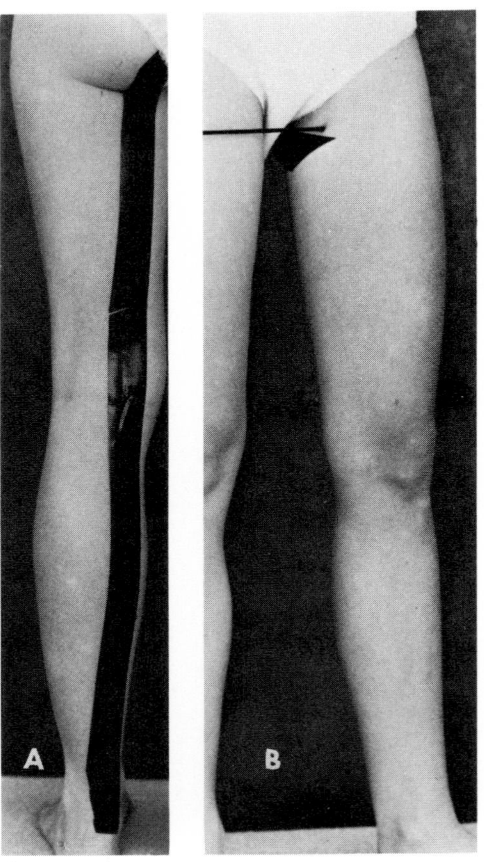

Figure 7-97. S_2 disease results in *A*, pain in the medial gluteal fold and down the leg and, *B*, numbness and pain radiation in the posterior thigh and labium majora.

the malingerer is a toe-and-heel walk. Ask the patient to stand on one leg at a time and do a toe-and-heel walk. A patient with organic disease (even disc herniation) can do these tests fairly well. If she is a malingerer or is exaggerating and is attempting to impress you with the seriousness of her problem, she will be unable to perform these tests.

Remember that SLR depends on other factors, i.e. stoicism, degree of passivity of the iliopsoas muscle and tightness of the hamstrings. SLR may be more useful as a follow-up record during recovery than as a diagnostic test.

Palpate the intervertebral spaces of L_4, L_5 and S_1. More than 90 percent of disc problems occur in these areas. Symptomatic disc herniations are extremely rare in other segments of the spine. Plain film often demonstrates narrowing of the intervertebral space and local spurs (Fig. 7-98).

Tap each space with the reflex hammer. Resulting disc pain occurs in the hips, buttocks or follows the distribution of the sciatic nerve. Lumbar sprains, however, cause local pain in and around the site of injury.

Palpate the entire spine and not just the areas the patient states are painful. This can be done by pushing your hand under the patient's back and, with your fingers, palpating each vertebra for tenderness.

Check the range of motion of the arms, hands, legs, feet and hips. Record your findings.

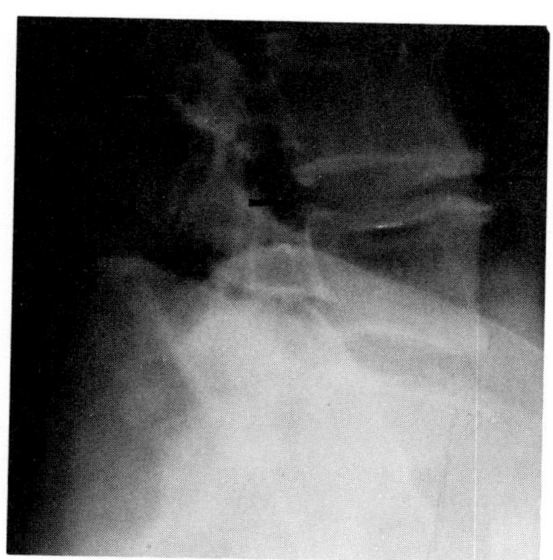

Figure 7-98. Degenerative disc disease and disc herniation.

Do not fail to check chest expansion. If markedly limited, consider the possibility of ankylosing spondylitis.

Check the leg length and circumference of the thighs and calves. Inequality in leg length may indicate a mechanical strain on the lower back. Unilateral muscle atrophy suggests nerve-root involvement.

Check sensory loss. In L_4 and L_5 disc injury, you may find a loss to pin prick sensitivity in the upper foot and the big toe on the affected side (see Figs. 7-94 and 7-95). In L_5 and S_1 disc disease, look for sensory loss along the distribution of the pain, i.e. in the outer lower leg and outer three toes (see Fig. 7-96).

Check for muscle weakness. In L_4 and L_5 herniations, look for weakness in the big and little toe extensors. In addition he may be unable to walk on his heels because of foot drop. In L_5 and S_1 disease, look for a decrease in the ankle and Achilles reflex and even some calf atrophy. In severe neurological involvement, he is unable to walk on tiptoes.

Examine the peripheral pulsations in the legs for arterial insufficiency.

Do a gynecological examination in the female and a prostatic examination in a male.

Do a Naffzinger's test: bilateral compression of the jugular veins aggravates the local pain.

A few cases will be emergencies. Hospitalize these patients promptly. Findings that require hospitalization and consultation are paralysis, loss of bladder or bowel function and dislocations and fractures with evidence of nerve involvement.

Some orthopedists believe the performance of painful back tests such as Patrick's and Lasegue's are unnecessary when the patient has an acute back problem. These orthopedists prefer to observe how he or she undresses, stands, walks, and especially how the patient rises from and sits on a stool. Diagnostic information can be obtained this way to a discerning eye. The same men limit their neurological check to the evaluation of deep leg reflexes and the eliciting of sensory changes. They give attention to the degree of briskness or lack of response to the deep reflex, to the fatiguability of the knee jerk response on five alternate tendon taps, and to any inequality in response between the two sides.

In a younger patient with a backache, there are the following possibilities:

- idiopathic or postpolio scoliosis
- scoliosis from unequal leg length
- congenital lesions of the spine leading to a scoliosis or a kyphoscoliosis
- Scheuermann's adolescent epiphysitis

In older patients check out:

- atrophic, rheumatoid or ankylosing arthritis
- flatfeet or a painful plantar wart
- traumatic disorders of the spine
- spondylolisthesis with strain on adjacent ligaments and articulations
- osteoporosis
- osteomyelitis (staphylococcal)
- osteomyelitis (tubercular, Pott's disease)
- primary sarcoma
- secondary metastic carcinoma from thyroid, breast, kidney or prostate
- multiple myeloma
- intervertebral disc disease
- fibrositis, myofibrositis or muscular rheumatism
- fibritis secondary to osteoarthritis
- faulty body mechanics
- pain secondary to abdominal or pelvic disease i.e. aortic aneurysms, tumors, gallbladder disease and gastrointestinal tract disorders including complications of peptic ulcer disease, pancreatitis and uropathies
- malingering
- psychoneurosis

Any patient who has back pain not relieved in the first day or two of treatment deserves an x-ray study of the lumbar spine and the lumbosacral area. Routinely obtain anteroposterior and lateral views of the lumbar spine. Oblique views are needed to visualize the pars interarticularis on each side. The latter view is not needed on every routine case of low back pain.

In the average case, x-ray studies will be normal, but you will have ruled out congenital abnormalities and diseases of, or injuries to, the bones and joints. If you suspect disease in the pelvis or hips, obtain an AP view of the entire pelvis. I personally don't routinely x-ray every patient who has a backache unless he doesn't respond to treatment within the first two days or has symptoms that are baffling.

Order a spot film of the lumbosacral joint plus stress films of the same area to get all the information available from x-ray films in stubborn cases. Stress films may be obtained by ordering views of the back in flexion, extension and while standing. Standing postural films are helpful in determining if there is a sacral base inclination which may be correctable with a heel lift.

Another x-ray test is the myelogram. If a disc has herniated, myelography will confirm the diagnosis in 70 percent of the cases (Fig. 7-99). It should be done only if surgery is anticipated.

There is a definite trend now toward electromyography that appears to give more specific information regarding nerve root involvement. This, too, is reserved for those patients on whom you anticipate surgery.

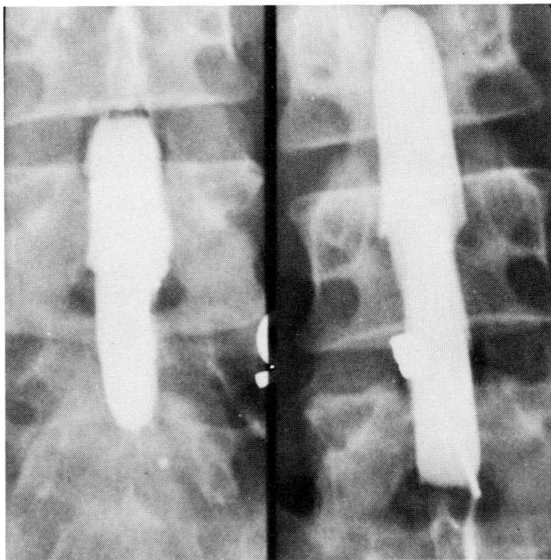

Figure 7-99. Spinal myelogram with slight deformity of L_5.

X-ray as a predictive tool in preemployment examinations is of doubtful value. Redfield[10] reported on the follow-up of 209 employees designated as substandard risks for heavy work by low back x-ray films. Their work records had an injury rate of 32.5 per 1,000 man hours as compared with a 62.3 per 1,000 man hours for a low-risk group. Other studies appear to verify Redfield's conclusions.

Treatment

Ninety percent of patients with low back pain respond to conservative treatment. This means bed rest on bedboards, hot and sometimes cold packs, analgesics, relaxants and injection of trigger points.

Bedboards are ⅝ in thick pieces of plywood. The board should reach the entire length of the bed and from side to side. This generally requires a board 6 x 3 ft for a single bed and 6 x 4½ ft for a double bed. Some patients circumvent this by putting their mattress on the floor during acute episodes of pain.

Kraus[9] warns against putting patients with acute nonorganic low back pain to bed. He believes that some ambulation keeps the back muscle from continuing in spasm with resultant atrophy and shortening. Physiotherapy is his main approach with application of tetanic current first and then 10 min of sinusoidal current second. He finishes his treatment with ethyl chloride spray to all trigger points.

Heat can be applied by hot shower, hot wet towels, heating pad or a hydrocollator steam pack. The latter are inexpensive and can be bought in various sizes. They are heated in hot water and wrapped in a towel before application. Hydrocollators are available from the Chattanooga Pharmacal Co., Chattanooga, Tenn. 37405. Cost ranges from $3 to $11 depending on size and style. A version of the hydrocollator may be used for cold applications.

A patient can also find help by assuming a position wherein her knees and hips are flexed 90° either in bed on bedboards or on the floor with her calves and feet elevated and resting on the seat of a chair. Some obtain fair results from a semi-Fowler position in a special bed with enough pillows under the knees to give relaxed support to their legs.

Analgesics and relaxants commonly used are aspirin, Darvon, Robaxin, Valium, Maolate, Percobarb and Demerol with or without Phenergan.

In many cases the patient can be up and about earlier with a low back support. Women should wear flat-heeled shoes. And it goes without saying that the patient should refrain from lifting or straining the lower back. Teach the patient how to lift. Do not bend over with knees fixed to pick up objects. Always squat. Do not lift loads in front of you above the waist line and lift as much as possible with the legs. Loads above the waist should be carried on the back. Never bend backwards.

After 5 to 7 days of continuous bed rest, all but about 10 percent of patients are on the road to recovery. The 10 percent are the ones who may need further studies to rule out more serious disease. Review in your mind the following possibilities:

- –a ruptured intervertebral disc
- –infection
- –tumor
- –congenital anomaly, i.e. occult spina bifida, spondylolisthesis
- –ankylosing spondylolisthesis
- –arterial insufficiency causing intermittent claudication of the hip
- –a fracture

And finally consider referral for a laminectomy in cases with bowel or bladder weakness, persistent neurological changes or repeated acute episodes.

Patients who have had a "snap" in the back followed by a sharp knifelike pain are often helped by manipulation either with or without local anesthesia. Place the patient on a hard table or on the floor in a side-lying position facing you. Have the patient extend her lower leg while placing her upper foot on the calf of her lower leg. First press and then snap her pelvis forward while pressing downward and forward on her iliac crest with your forearm and making countertraction on her upper shoulder with your other hand. Reverse the pressure by pulling backward and downward on her pelvis while pushing her shoulder forward. Torsion strain of the sacroiliac joints appears to be the condition most often helped by these maneuvers.

Disability evaluation for disorders of the spine are rather stringent: (1) disability following fractures of the vertebra must be accompanied by a description of an appropriate sensory and motor loss; (2) a painful back from osteoporosis must be described in terms of limitation of motion, paravertebral muscle spasm and a compression fracture of a vertebra and (3) ankylosis or fixation of the cervical or dorsolumbar spine must have 30° or more of flexion measured from the neutral position and one of the following: x-ray evidence of calcification of the anterior and lateral ligaments, x-ray evidence of bilateral ankylosis of the sacroiliac joints and abnormal apophyseal articulation.

If a family physician is interested in his approach to diagnosis and treatment by muscle testing and exercises, he may purchase the following: Kraus H, Clinical Treatment of Back and Neck Pain, New York: McGraw-Hill, 1970, and a paperback for patients: Kraus H, Backache, Stress and Tension, New York: Pocket Books Inc., 1969.

Exercises

EXERCISES FOR WEAK BACK MUSCLES (Fig. 7-100). The patient assumes a prone position with her arms at her side palm down. She squeezes her buttocks together and holds for the count of 5 (A). Then she squeezes her shoulder blades together, raises her head and chest as high as possible and holds for the count of 5 (B). She lifts one leg as high as possible (C). She does not hold the position but slowly lowers her leg. After repeating with her other leg she raises both legs as high as possible and slowly lowers them (D).

REHABILITATIVE BACK EXERCISES. A "tail tuck" is done while the patient is in a supine position with arms on chest. She tightens the muscles in back of the hips, tucking her "tail" under. Starting a rolling motion, she flattens her back and lifts her hips a few inches.

To strengthen the abdominal musculature, the patient lifts her shoulders and chest by tightening the abdominal muscles, doing a partial sit-up. Her head should follow the shoulders, not the other way around.

In the low back stretch, the patient grasps her knees and attempts to bring her knees alternately into the adjacent axilla. She then stretches and rotates her lower back.

In straight-leg raising, the patient lifts one leg at a time and attempts to stretch out tightness by lifting her legs higher each time.

The patient stands with her legs crossed one in front of the other but with feet close together. As she relaxes she bends foward, stretching out the tightness in her back. She bounces the tightness out and touches her right toes with her left fingers. She alternates the exercise by changing leg positions.

For low back rotation manipulation, the patient clasps her bent knees and then swings her buttocks from side to side.

Nerve Root Compression Syndrome and Secondary Sciatica

Nerve root compression syndrome from any cause must be accompanied be a description of the pain and limitation of motion that has occurred in the back or neck. Document cervical or lumbar nerve root compression by describing radicular distribution of sensory, motor and reflex abnormalities.

Causes of secondary sciatica are:

- –sacralization of the L_5 vertebrae
- –arthritis of the interarticular joints
- –spondylitis
- –spondylolisthesis
- –tumors of vertebra
- –primary and secondary tumors of the cord
- –herniation of nucleus pulposus
- –arachnoiditis
- –herpes zoster
- –tabes dorsalis
- –pachymeningitis

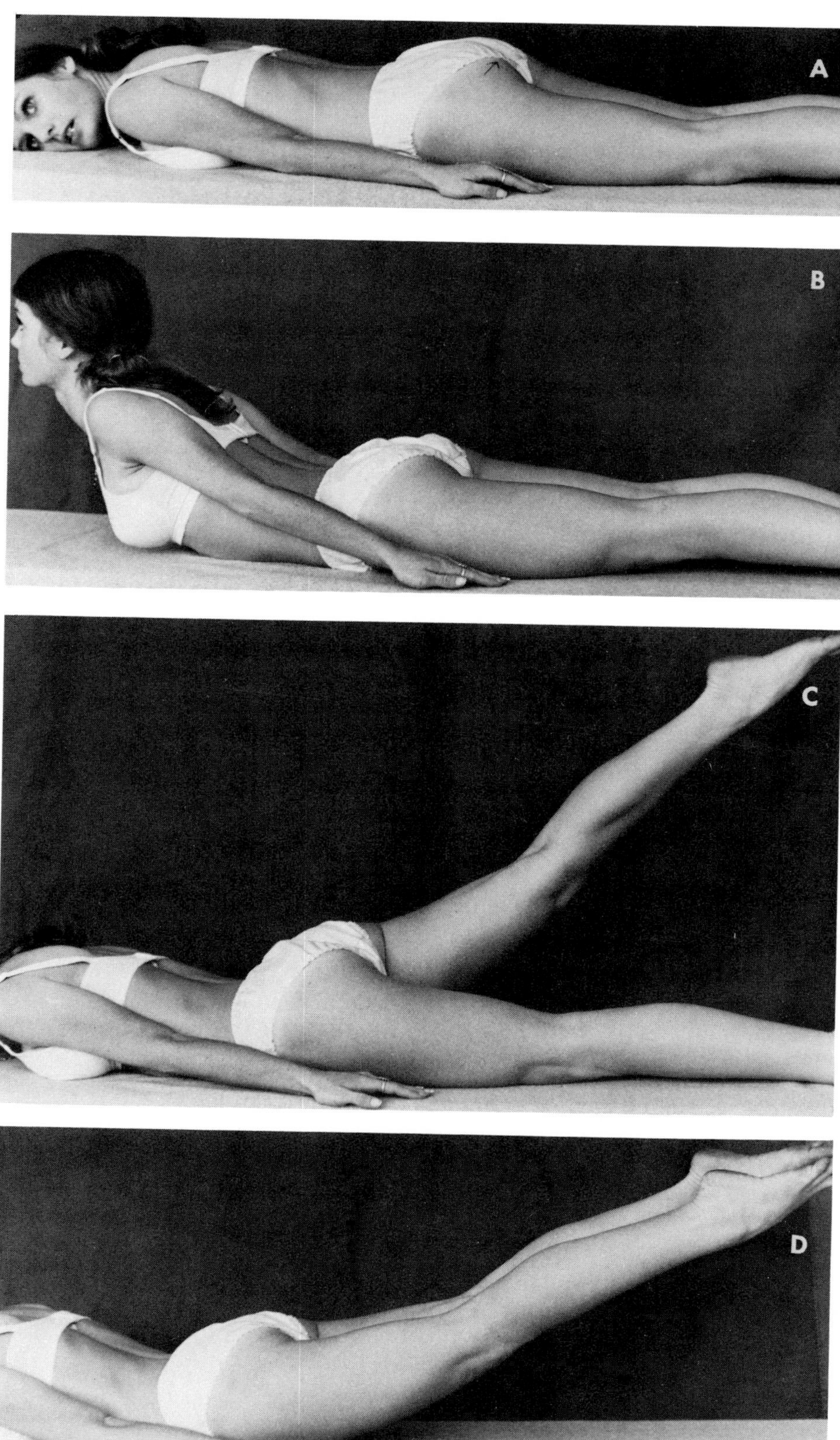

Figure 7-100. Exercises for weak back muscles. (See text for explanation.)

–sacroiliac arthritis or strain
–diseases of the hip
–genitourinary diseases
–rectal impaction

UPPER BACK AND NECK PAIN

When the patient complains of pain in the upper back or in the neck look for:

–ankylosing spondylitis
–herniated or ruptured intervertebral disc
–staphylococcal or tubercular infections of the spine
–Scheuermann's disease of the adolescent
–Sprengel's deformity (winged scapula)
–cervical disc syndrome
–cervical arthritis
–fractures secondary to osteoporosis and tumors
–psychoneurosis
–clay-shoveler's fracture of the spinous processes
–tumors
–scapulothoracic bursitis
–calcified intervertebral disc
–ochronosis (alkaptonuria)

The following is indicative of *cervical arthritis:* (1) Headache in the occipital area due to irritation of the greater occipital nerve, which exits through the third cervical foramen; (2) Involvement of the midcervical spine will produce pain radiating to the entire shoulder-girdle area. (3) Involvement of the lower cervical spine from C_5 to T_2 produces pain which may radiate to the shoulder, arm or forearm. (4) Often there may be diffuse aching in the neck with areas of tenderness over the cervical vertebrae. (5) Irritation of the cervical nerves as they exit through the cervical foramina produce muscle spasm and limitation of neck movement.

Diagnosis of cervical arthritis is usually confirmed by x-ray pictures or cineradiography. Order AP, lateral and oblique views, the latter for study of the foramina. Search for narrowed disc spaces or osteophytes projecting into the foramina. Cineradiography of a degenerated disc shows a subluxating superior vertebrae. A normal disc will rock or roll over the center of the healthy inferior nucleus pulposus.

In *cervical disc syndromes* the most important diagnostic sign you can elicit is the reproduction of the patient's pain by extending the neck and flexing the head laterally toward the painful side. Other symptoms may be so variable as to be almost useless, confusing the examiner with the symptoms of cervical radiculitis, disc rupture, osteoarthritis, shoulder pain due to tendonitis and adhesive capsulitis and even carpal tunnel syndrome.

Cervical arthritis and disc problems may be accompanied by deep reflex changes in the arm or by areas of paresthesia or hypesthesia in the hand. Do a sedimentation rate and check the serum uric acid to rule out gout or inflammatory diseases.

Treat cervical arthritis with salicylates, tranquilizers, sedatives, heat and traction. Traction should start with a 5 lb weight applied for 15 min, b.i.d., and increased to 10 lb for 30 min or even several hours until discomfort is relieved.

Pain Radiation in Cervical Disc Disease

In C_6 disease, pain radiates through the lateral arm with numbness and weakness of the thumb, hypoalgesia as outlined in Figure 7-101 and decreased deep reflexes of biceps and flexor radialis. There is also pain in the upper medial scapula.

In disease of C_7 (Fig. 7-102), pain radiation and hypoalgesia extend from the base of the back neck down the upper part of the arm with numbness and weakness of the second and third digits. The triceps tendon reflex is reduced and there is pain in the upper medial scapula.

With a diseased C_8 disc, there is pain over the medial scapular spine with pain radiation and hypoalgesia as outlined in Figure 7-103. There are no deep reflex changes but there is numbness and motor weakness in the fourth and fifth digits.

Treatment

Treatment of whiplash is described in Chapter 6. Treatment of cervical disc syn-

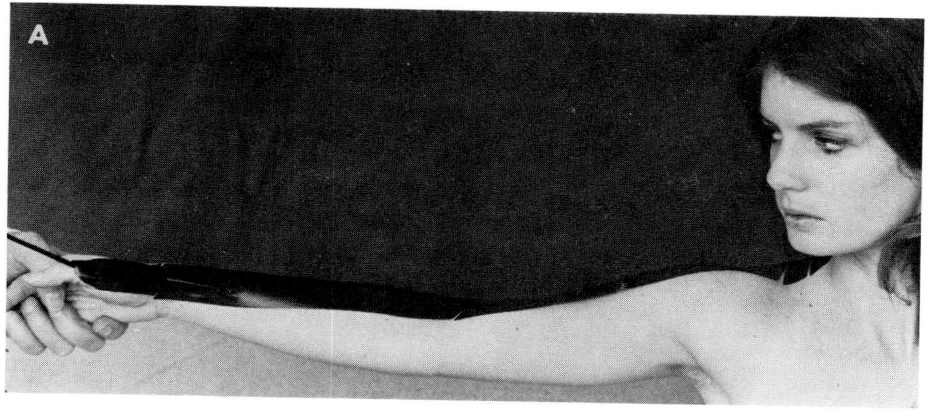

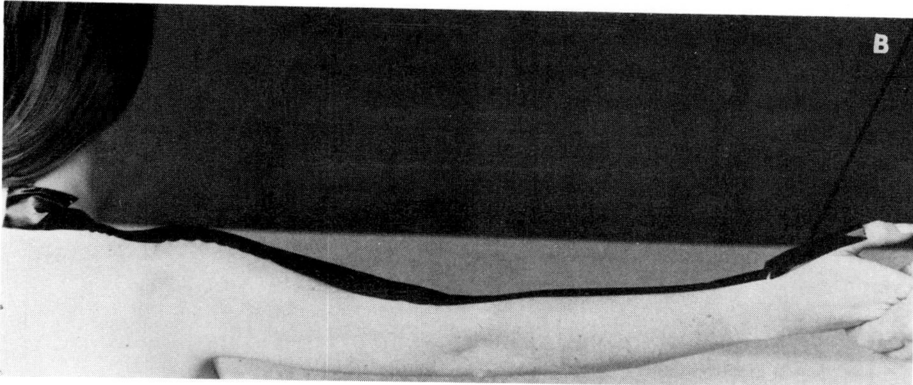

Figure 7-101. Diseased C_6 with *A*, pain radiation in lateral arm and numbness and weakness of the thumb and, *B*, hypoalgesia as outlined and pain in upper medial scapula.

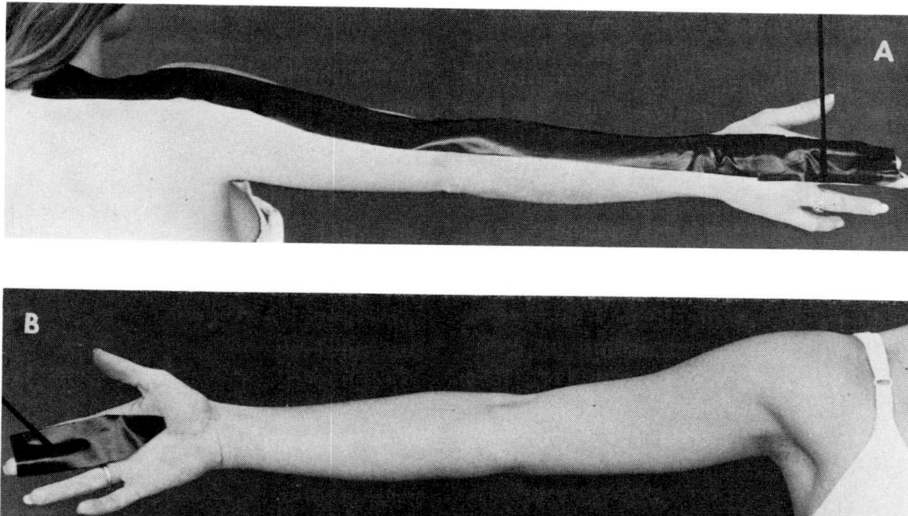

Figure 7-102. Diseased C_7 with *A*, pain radiation and hypoalgesia and, *B*, numbness and weakness of second and third digits.

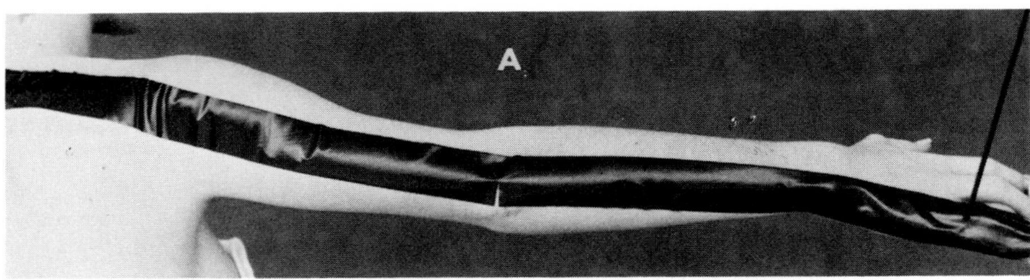

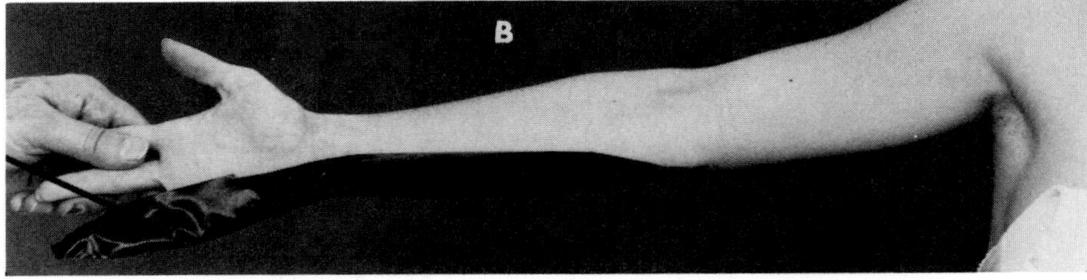

Figure 7-103. Diseased C_8 with pain radiation and hypoalgesia. Numbness and motor weakness in the fourth and fifth digits, *A* and *B*.

drome consists of a variety of the following: analgesics, relaxants, moist heat, massage, ultrasound, injection of trigger points with Xylocaine and Hydeltra-TBA, traction and a collar for neck rest in severe cases. Traction may vary depending on the gravity of the patient's symptoms—at home for 20 min with a 5 lb weight or heavier weights for longer intervals in the hospitalized patient. Bed rest at home with head cradled on a pillow for 4 to 5 days may suffice. Better still, tie an ordinary pillow in the middle with a stocking and place under the patient's head similar to a Japanese pillow.

If you prescribe a collar be sure the patient's neck is flexed slightly and the head placed in a comfortable position. Extending the neck will aggravate the patient's pain.

If other measures fail and if the patient has no counterindication, try prednisone orally for a short period. Some prefer to administer prednisone 30 to 40 mg in one dose every 48 hours which is supposed to diminish the incidence of adverse side effects.

BONE PAIN

Recognize bone pain by the following characteristics: pain increases at night, local tenderness, local swelling and pain intensified by movement.

Differentiate bone pain from articular pain by a careful examination of the painful site and from muscular pain by palpation of muscles between thumb and index finger.

The diagnosis of disseminated disease of bones is usually established by x-ray examination, serum calcium, phosphorus, alkaline and acid phosphatase and the urinary excretion of calcium.

Look for:

- osteoporosis
- multiple myeloma
- hypertrophic osteoarthropathy
- Marfan's syndrome
- Recklinghausen's disease
- Paget's disease of the bone
- osteomalacia
- rickets
- osteogenesis imperfecta (brittle bones)
- osteitis fibrosa cystica disseminata
- dyschondroplasia
- secondary or metastatic carcinoma to bones
- benign osteochondroma (Fig. 7-104)

Osteomyelitis of the Spine

The onset of osteomyelitis is often insidious. The symptoms and signs develop slowly and, even more confusing, x-ray evi-

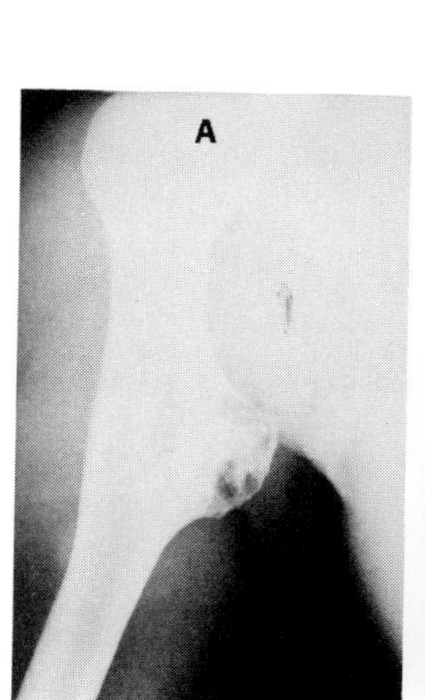

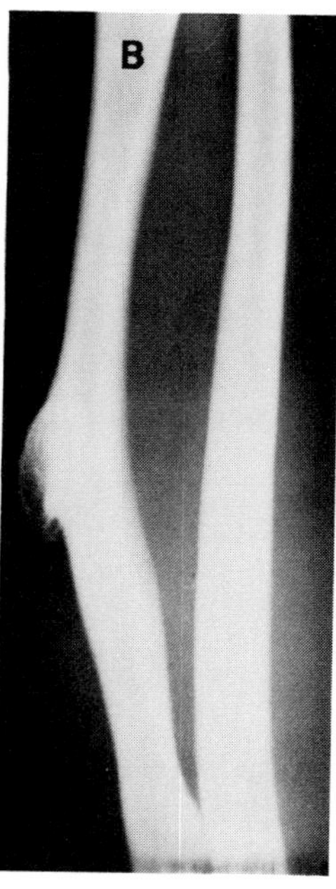

Figure 7-104. Osteochondroma of the *A*, humerus and, *B*, radius.

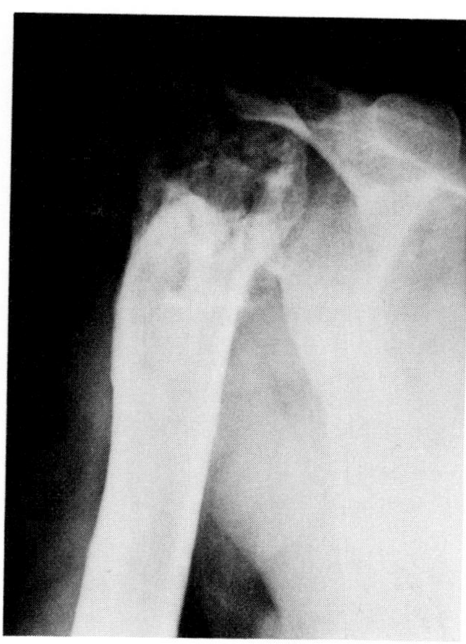

Figure 7-105. Aseptic necrosis of the humerus. Bacteria from superficial infections are carried in the blood and lodge in the terminal capillary loops of the diaphyseal cortex, causing a purulent necrosing process that emerges to the periosteum.

dence of the disease may not develop for 10 days or more after the onset of symptoms. Fever will seldom run higher than 102° and usually a little lower.

The pain is persistent and aggravated by moving or standing and relieved only slightly by analgesics or bed rest.

The earliest x-ray findings are a decrease in the thickness of the intervertebral disc and loss of the normally sharp outlines of the cortical plates of the vertebral bodies. These findings can be easily overlooked without expert interpretation and high quality films.

Strontium-85 scanning is a useful adjunct in detecting bone disease. Strontium becomes incorporated into young reactive bone so that lesions producing new bone give a positive scan. These abnormal scans are found therefore in osteomyelitis, recent fractures, Paget's disease of the bone and metastatic cancer. Abnormal uptakes in metastasis occur before x-ray changes. Fifty percent of osteomyelitis patients will have abnormal scans and normal x-ray findings. Scans, however, can be positive for both metastatic and inflammatory lesions. X-rays can definitely identify the inflammatory disease (Fig. 7-105).

OSTEOPOROSIS

Family physicians seldom refer patients with osteoporosis. But that does not mean these patients receive optimum care. Too often osteoporosis is ignored or misdiagnosed.

The definition of osteoporosis is being revised; so is the concept of the disease. Perhaps the best definition is an atrophy of bone. The volume of the bone remains the same, but its content decreases. The condition afflicts approximately 25 percent of the white female population over age 60 and is responsible for much of the morbidity of aging.

Osteoporosis is usually asymptomatic, but the decreased density of bone predisposes to fracture. It is these fractures and the resulting deformities that are primarily responsible for the symptoms. The common fractures are compression fractures of the

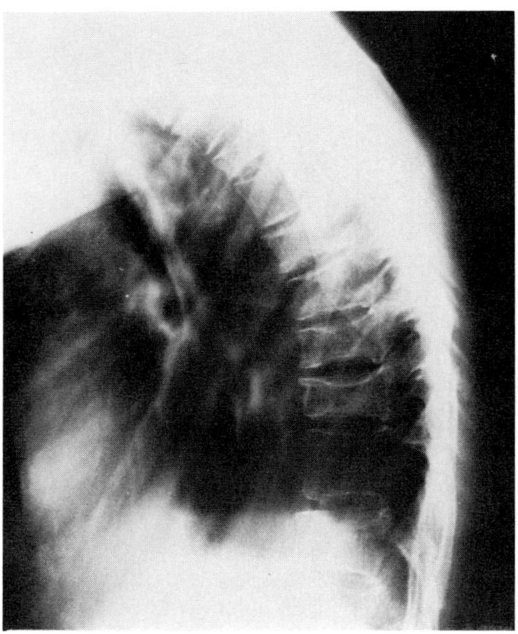

Figure 7-106. Osteoporitic spine with multiple compression fractures resulting from hyperparathyroidism. Excessive parathyroid hormone causes bone resorption.

vertebra (Fig. 7-106) and fractures of the ribs, ischial and pubic rami, upper femur, upper humerus and wrist.

There will be no physical findings prior to fracture. Anterior wedging of the vertebra occurs, causing a loss of height, kyphosis and a loss of normal lumbar lordosis. Fractures of the extremities are more serious. Eighty percent of all hip fractures occur in patients with preexisting osteoporosis.

Some physicians have been able to use the x-ray pattern of the trabeculae in the upper end of the femur as an index of the degree of osteoporosis.[11] The trabeculae in the upper end of the femur are arranged along the lines of tension stresses produced in the bone during weight bearing. As normal bones deteriorate with severe osteoporosis, the trabaculae in the upper end of the femur fade out in definite order. Trabeculae fade earliest where stress is minimal and are retained until the end in areas where stresses are high. Any person whose total bone is physiologic for him will show a normal trabecular pattern, and the pattern changes only as increasing amounts of the original bone are lost.

Another and more practical method is to measure the cortical thickness of bones of the extremities. Measure the cortex with a millimeter ruler. A value less than 45 percent of the total diameter at midshaft usually indicates significant bone loss.

One of the problems in diagnosing osteoporosis is excluding similar clinical and x-ray findings: hyperthyroidism, Cushing's syndrome, acromegaly, multiple myeloma, hyperparathyroidism, osteolytic metastases, immobilization, intestinal malabsorption and rheumatoid arthritis.

One of the newer methods of treating osteoporosis is with the use of sodium fluoride. Symptomatic relief is obtained in about 50 percent of patients who are given this salt. Start with 20 mg per day and work it up to 80 mg over a period of 3 or 4 months. If pain has not decreased in that time, discontinue the drug.

A combination of the following may be tried: Premarin 0.125 mg daily, a high protein diet and calcium 1.0 g daily. Men may be given Durabolin 25 mg intramuscularly weekly or Nilevar 10 mg t.i.d.

Osteoporosis prevention includes an adequate calcium intake described as a minimum of one g/day in the form of pills or a quart of milk, adequate exercise and low-dosage estrogen supplementation starting after the menopause.

MUSCLE PAIN

If your patient complains of muscle pain look for:

–traumatic injury to the muscle
–trichinosis
–influenza
–rheumatic fever
–dengue
–other acute febrile diseases
–hematoma in muscles
–chronic muscle strain
–tonic contractions
–dermatomyositis
–SLE
–polyarteritis nodosa

–polymyalgia rheumatica
–hypoparathyroidism
–muscle contractures from disease, ischemia or inflammation

VARIETIES OF MUSCULAR DYSTROPHY

These diseases are rare and difficult to classify. In fact their classification is still debated. The problem lies in separating the primary muscle diseases from the primary nerve diseases. To make matters more complicated there are some diseases which have characteristics of both. In these diseases, you are dealing with lesions of the final common pathway, i.e. the anterior horn cell, the peripheral nerve, the myoneural junction and the muscle fibers. Muscles weaken and atrophy either if the nerve conduction function has been destroyed or if the muscle fibers themselves have been damaged despite intact nerve conduction.

Both myopathies and neuropathies have certain changes in common, such as muscle weakness, hypotonia, hyperreflexia and wasting. But there are differences. In primary muscle disease look for symmetric muscle weakness and atrophy involving *proximal* muscles of the shoulder and pelvis. In primary nerve disease look for symmetric or asymmetric *distal* muscle involvement, atrophy of the same distal limb muscles, muscle fibrillations or twitchings, sensory changes, cramps and pain.

In order to detect these changes, have the patient completely undress. Inspect the patient carefully for muscle weakness and atrophy. Note the location. Palpate for flabby musculature. Perform the "hand grip" test by asking the patient to grip your hand forcefully and then to let go as promptly as possible. If he hesitates in releasing your hand, you are more likely dealing with a myotonia of neuropathic origin. Also in myotonia (increased muscle tone where the patient is unable to relax after a contraction), when you percuss the thenar eminence the thumb will oppose but relaxation is slow. Percussion of the tongue with a tongue depressor will cause a persistent dimpling of the surface (percussion myotonia). Again, attempt to rule out the myotonias by noting muscle response to electrical stimulation, an exaggerated reaction followed by slow relaxation.

Myotonia occurs in myotonia atrophica or dystrophica, myotonia congenita, paramyotonia-adynamia complex and its varieties and hyperkalemic periodic paralysis, idiopathic. In addition there are nonclinical myotonias which can only be identified electromyographically.[12] Most researchers believe these syndromes are more of a neuropathy and not a myopathy or muscular dystrophy.[13]

Now, with those diseases out of the way, let's go back to the muscular dystrophies. The most familiar variety is *Duchenne's* or *Erb's pseudohypertrophic progressive muscular dystrophy*. These can be identified by the Gower's sign observed when the youngster attempts to get up. When attempting to get up from the floor he uses his hands to climb up his legs. Be sure to rule out the more common cervical spondylosis. When you observe a young adult who has difficulty rising from a chair or who cannot raise his arms above his head, think of *limb-girdle dystrophy* (Erb's).

Not too difficult to identify is the *facioscapulohumeral dystrophy* (Landouzy-Dejerine). Again found in a young adult, its victim develops a lack of facial expression, winged scapulas and atrophic upper arms.

There are the *myotonic dystrophies* discussed above and of a debatable classification. These patients are the ones who have difficulty unclenching their fists repeatedly and have crooked smiles, nasal speech, frontal baldness and testicular atrophy. Their eyelids tend to droop and they have other extraocular pareses.

There is another true muscular dystrophy whose progress depends on the age of the child when stricken. In young children the loss of muscle mass progresses rapidly to death within 2 years and is known as *Werdnig-Hoffman* type of *progressive spinal atrophy*. Muscle denervation leads to a loss of reflexes and hypotonia. In older children and adults, the disease leads only to partial paralysis of a leg. Atrophy proceeds

Table 7-3.

	Myopathy	*Myositis*
Family history	Usually present	None
Age of onset	Before 35	After 35
Course	No remission	Erratic; remissions
Pattern	Symmetrical	Patchy
Nuchal weakness	Spared	Affected
Systemic disturbance	None	Marked
Raynaud's	Rare	Common

slowly and life expectancy is not affected. It is called *Charcot-Marie-Tooth progressive peroneal muscular atrophy*.

Polymyositis (inflammatory myopathy) with its many varieties may not be considered a muscular dystrophy, but it creates problems in differential diagnosis. Polymyositis, whether a myopathy or true myositis (Table 7-3), has features not associated with the myopathies.

Serum enzyme levels may help distinguish the primary muscle dystrophies from the neuropathies, the enzymes tending to be elevated in muscle damage. The *muscle enzymes* are SGOT, SGPT, LDH, CPK and aldolase.

Electromyography helps, but if you suspect a myotonia or lower motor neuron disease, order a nerve conduction study. What is frustrating, however, is that some of these diseases produce changes suggesting both muscle and nerve disease, especially when the myoneural junction is involved. At this point only a muscle biopsy may solve the problem. It is most helpful in diagnosing a slowly progressive muscle disease.

The true myopathies progress inexorably to the patient's death in 5 to 25 years. Sphincters are never affected. Death is usually from intercurrent infections, frequently respiratory infections following inhalation of food or saliva.

FIBROSITIS (NON-ARTICULAR RHEUMATISM)

Synonyms for fibrositis are myofibrositis and muscular rheumatism. Most family physicians diagnose fibrositis when they can find nothing else wrong to account for the patient's symptoms, and perhaps that is the way it should be. Fibrositis is a symptom-complex of acute, subacute or chronic aching, soreness and stiffness.

The cause is not known. It may be related to the psychophysiological disorders. It is often incorrectly diagnosed as spinal arthritis. The disease, if there be such, most often affects the neck, shoulders and low back. The onset may be abrupt so that it causes an acute painful stiff neck or sore stiff lower back. The jar of walking may cause pain of such intensity the patient prefers to remain in bed. Look for a tilt of the head or partial rotation if the disease affects the upper spine and a list or stoop if the lower spine is affected. If the disease comes abruptly, it will usually leave the same way.

When the disease comes on insidiously, however, anticipate a chronic course. Then the symptoms become an ache, increasing after a night's rest when a certain stiffness develops. Question the patient about his activity and you will find that activity causes a decrease in pain and stiffness. However, towards evening, when the patient becomes tired, the symptoms of stiffness and aching recur. Squeeze the involved tissue and the patient registers pain. Press over trigger points and the patient indicates rather widespread discomfort.

Fibrositis is often secondary to osteoarthritis. Remember that osteoarthritis seldom causes pain unless the adjacent fibrous tissue is affected.

Patients with chronic fibrositis seldom get the relief for which they are looking and may drift from doctor to doctor. Most analgesics including the salicylates, Indocin, and even corticosteroids give questionable and certainly variable relief. Injections of trigger areas may be the most beneficial treatment. Reassure the patient concerning arthritis. Calm him with a mild tranquilizer. Regulate his activity to prevent excessive fatigue.

SKELETAL PAIN FREQUENTLY MISDIAGNOSED

Be certain your patient is free of the following diseases.

Peripheral neuritis with or without pernicious anemia.

Early Parkinson's disease with muscle stiffness erroneously diagnosed as degenerative or rheumatoid arthritis. Don't be confused in the latter stages of Parkinson's disease when flexion deformities with ulnar deviation of the fingers occur.

Osteitis fibrosa cystica, Recklinghausen's disease, the bone disease seen in chronic hyperparathyroidism. This disease can be diagnosed early when only vague joint and muscle pains are present. Serum calcium is above 11 in 90 percent of the patients; serum phosphorus is decreased (less than 3 percent) in 90 percent of patients; alkaline phosphatase is normal if no bone disease is present or otherwise increased; urine calcium is increased when the patient is on a low-calcium diet (more than 400 mg on a normal diet); and urine phosphorus is increased unless there is renal insufficiency or phosphorus depletion. Always check serum protein electrophoresis in hyperparathyroidism to rule out multiple myeloma and sarcoidosis. The coincidence of peptic ulcer and renal calculus should prompt a search for hyperparathyroidism. X-ray films show generalized radiolucence of bone, especially of the middle phalanx. Pathognomonic is a jagged, feathery border in the subperiosteal layer of the phalanges.

Hypertrophic osteoarthropathy. Whenever a patient complains of symmetrical arthritis in the peripheral joints think of a possible hypertrophic osteoarthropathy. It often accompanies primary pulmonary malignancy, lung abscess and bronchiectasis. Another tip-off is clubbing of the fingers in addition to the pain in the bones and joints of the extremities. Direct treatment to the primary disease process.

Hypothyroidism can produce a destructive arthritis with joint effusion, lax tendons and ligaments. The disease is completely reversible with thyroid replacement therapy.

Paget's disease of bone (osteitis deformans) is most often asymptomatic. It is often discovered when a routine biochemical panel reveals an increase in the serum alkaline phosphatase. The disease is characterized by increased destruction of bone balanced by a rapid growth of new bone with imperfect architecture. Any bone may become involved with the exception of the hands and feet. Complications include spontaneous and pathologic fractures; single or multiple osteogenic sarcomas in the site of the osteitis; and increased blood flow through the spongy bone, which leads to the same pathophysiologic process as an arteriovenous fistula with cardiac failure. There is no effective treatment unless the recently introduced mithramycin proves useful. It is still experimental, however.

Polymyalgia rheumatica, a disease usually discovered in the middle aged or elderly patient. Suspect the diagnosis when the patient complains of severe pain in the neck and shoulder muscles as well as the pelvic girdle. The typical clinical picture is of recurrent episodes of pain without a great deal of deformity but with some fever and a marked increase in the sedimentation rate. If necessary, it is important to make the diagnosis with a temporal artery biopsy because a certain number of these patients will develop blindness. Treatment of the disease and the prevention of blindness depends on its recognition and the administration of a corticosteroid.

SUMMARY OF NONARTHRITIC CONDITIONS CAUSING MUSCULOSKELETAL PAIN

Such conditions are:

- hyperparathyroidism with Recklinghausen's disease
- hyperthyroidism and hypothyroidism
- hypoglycemia
- general bacterial, viral and rickettsial infections, i.e. brucellosis
- tarsal and carpal tunnel syndromes
- shoulder-hand syndrome
- peripheral neuritis with or without pernicious anemia
- polymyalgia rheumatica
- De Quervain's syndrome
- osteitis deformans (Paget's disease)
- scalenus anticus syndrome (thoracic outlet syndrome)

–osteoporosis
–fragilitas ossium (brittle bones)
–rickets
–osteomalacia
–multiple myeloma
–acute and chronic osteomyelitis

INTRA-ARTICULAR INJECTIONS

General Principles

Approach joints from their extensor surfaces. Choose a site for the needle insertion as far from major arteries, nerves and veins as possible. Shave and cleanse the injection site with a germicidal soap or detergent. Paint the skin with iodine antiseptic. Use sterile gloves and either disposable or autoclaved syringes.

Some joints, particularly if effusion is present, may need little or no local anesthesia. Occasionally an ethyl chloride spray will prove sufficient. Otherwise, raise a skin wheal with one percent Xylocaine and inject a little more anesthetic into the subcutaneous tissue.

Select a 20 gauge needle for aspiration and insert it through the synovial membrane. If aspiration of the joint is unnecessary choose a smaller bore needle (#22 to #26) and one of a suitable length (¾ to 3 in). To prevent carrying a plug of unsterile skin into the joint, a few orthopedists are now first incising the skin with the point of a #11 scalpel blade.

Place the joint in the position which causes maximum distension of the joint space. This will facilitate piercing the capsule. When the needle tip enters the joint, a characteristic movable sensation develops. Sometimes a grating of the needle against the cartilage verifies the position of the needle in the joint. If aspiration becomes difficult, clean any debris from the needle tip by reinjecting a small amount of the synovial fluid into the joint and changing the position of the needle. Aspirate all accessible fluid from the joint space.

If the diagnosis is questionable, save a syringeful of fluid for examination. Otherwise, detach the aspirating syringe and leave the needle in place in the joint. Fill another syringe with the desired amount of steroid, attach the syringe to the needle and inject slowly. A suggested standard solution: 10 ml parental triamcinolone acetonide aqueous suspension, 10 mg per ml (Kenalog remains in suspension) diluted with 50 ml of 1 percent lidocaine (Xylocaine) hydrochloride. If more than gentle pressure on the plunger is needed readjust the needle. Moving the plunger in and out several times will mix the steroid with the synovial fluid.

Withdraw the needle, cleanse the puncture site with alcohol and apply a light bandage. Gently and passively move the limb a few times to spread the drug throughout the joint. If the joint is unstable because of the loss of fluid, apply an elastic bandage about the joint. Ordinarily the patient may resume light activity.

Shoulder Joint and Girdle

Examine the shoulder carefully and make an accurate diagnosis. Before injecting, confirm your diagnosis by x-rays. Certain diagnostic clues are elicited when the patient slowly elevates his arm from 0 to 180° while in the coronal plane of the trunk.

Full motion without pain is good evidence of a healthy shoulder. If the arm cannot be lifted more than 10° and is painful, suspect a fracture, dislocation or a complete rupture of the supraspinatus tendon. If the arm can be raised through its normal 180° but is painful throughout, think of arthritis. Finally, if pain is elicited as the arm is moved from 60 to 120°, look for a chronic supraspinatus tendonitis or a partial rupture of the same tendon.

The patient will feel a jerk and a sharp pain at the insertion of the deltoid muscle as he elevates his arm and approaches the 60° point. However, further palpatation of the deltoid area reveals no tenderness there. The point of tenderness will be at or near the insertion of the supraspinatus tendon. This is typical of supraspinatus tendonitis and determines the site of injection.

Bicipital tenosynovitis usually becomes painful a day or two after excessive use of the biceps brachii. Check the arm for Yergason's sign. With the patient's elbow flexed 90° and rotated to the pronated position, grasp his hand and ask him to supinate against your resistance. If pain is produced in the anteromedial aspect of the shoulder, Yergason's sign is positive.

Choose for injection the point of maximal tenderness, whether it be near the insertion of the supraspinatus, the deltoid muscle or the long tendon of the biceps brachii.

Remember, too, bicipital tendonitis is more common than subacromial bursitis. Inject 2.5 to 3 ml of the standard steroid suspension of Kenalog and lidocaine through a #22, 2 in needle after accurate placement of the needle point in and about the tendon. Use the same technique for injection of supraspinatus tendonitis.

Occasionally the shoulder joint may need aspiration and injection. Effusion of the shoulder joint, though rare, almost always bulges anteriorly. Approach the joint from the anterior position. Insert the needle in the palpable space between the head of the humerus and the rim of the glenoid cavity. The needle is inserted and pointed posteriorly from a point just below and lateral to the coracoid process with the arm slightly abducted and externally rotated. The joint cavity is about 4 cm below the skin surface in the average adult.

Elbow Joint

Injections of steroids about the elbow joint is nearly always for "tennis elbow," or, more properly, radiohumeral bursitis. Symptoms include a throbbing pain in the lateral aspect of the elbow aggravated by extension of the wrist as in lifting small objects.

On palpation, tenderness is found over the lateral epicondyle or distally near the radial head. To verify check Mill's maneuver. Have the patient hold his arm in extension with the wrist flexed. Attempt to pronate his forearm against his resistance. The sign is positive if pain is felt in the lateral epicondyle. Cozen's test is done differently. Have the patient extend his wrist and clench his fist. Hold his forearm steady with your left hand while attempting to flex his wrist against his resistance. Again, a positive test is indicated by reproduction of the pain in the lateral epicondyle.

Before injecting the area, carefully localize the point of maximal tenderness. For this purpose, use the tip of a closed pen. When the point is found, press the point into the skin firmly enough to leave a small circle. Use the center of the circle for the insertion site. Use a #26, ¾ in needle and inject about 1½ ml about the site. Remember that tennis elbow is tendonitis plus periostitis. Therefore, attempt to inject 0.5 ml under the periosteum of the epicondyle.

Wrist Joint

Approach the wrist joint from its dorsal surface. The most conspicuous dorsal prominence is the ulnar styloid process. On the radial side of the wrist proximal to the base of the thumb is the anatomic snuffbox. In the hollow, palpate the radial artery and the radial styloid process. On the ulnar side of the extensor pollicis longus tendon is a prominence formed by the articular margin of the radius, called the dorsal radial tubercle (Lister's tubercle).

Have the patient's forearm resting prone on a table so the hand hangs over the edge flexing the wrist. Prepare and drape the dorsal aspect of the wrist by the usual aseptic technique. Palpate Lister's tubercle on the ulnar side of the extensor pollicis longus and infiltrate the skin with local anesthesia.

Enter this complex joint with a #22 to 24 gauge, 1½ in needle at a point just distal to the radius and just ulnar to the anatomic snuffbox. If the needle can be easily inserted to a depth of 1 to 2 cm and feels free, it probably is in correct position. There is another choice entry site. If there is marked synovial bulging on the ulnar surface of the wrist, enter the joint by inserting the needle just distal to the ulnar styloid process and proximal to the pisiform bone.

Other conditions about the wrist joint that may be helped by steroid injections are chronic stenosing tenosynovitis (De Quervain's disease), acute nonsuppurative tenosynovitis, also near the snuffbox, and radial styloiditis.

In De Quervain's disease the tendon sheath of the extensor pollicis brevis is painful. In chronic cases, palpate the snuffbox for one or two swellings, the size of orange seeds. A chronic inflammation involves all layers of the tendon sheath. Examine for three signs: (1) Tenderness extends from the radial styloid process proximately for ½ to 1⅓ cm. (2) Try Finkelstein's test. Have the patient clench his fist over the flexed thumb and then forcefully stretch the wrist into ulnar deviation. If this maneuver causes pain near the radial styloid process, the Finkelstein's test is positive. The pain from the maneuver may be transmitted down the thumb or toward the elbow. (3) Passive extension of the thumb should be painless. Stretch and palpate the tendon and then carefully inject into the tendon sheath rather than into the tendon substance.

In acute nonsuppurative tenosynovitis of the snuffbox a painful 4 cm sausagelike swelling appears. The tendons involved are the extensor pollicis brevis and the more radial abductor pollicis longus, both on the radial side of the snuffbox. Palpate the sheath for crepitus. Again be careful to inject only the sheaths of the tendon.

Inject radial styloiditis with one ml of the standard solution. Use a #26, ¾ in needle and inject about the radial styloid process. After the injection, splint the thumb for 24 hours for maximal relief.

Knee Joint

The knee joint is the easiest joint to aspirate and inject. Have the patient lie down on the examining table and fully extend his knee. After the usual aseptic precautions and local anesthesia, insert a #20, 1½ to 2 in needle into the anteromedial surface of the knee.

Select a point approximately 1 to 2 cm medial to the inner border of the patella and on a line with its midpoint. Direct the needle laterally and slightly posteriorly and distally. Aim for the opening between the posterior surface of the patella and the patellar surface of the femur. The needle point may crepitate on the undersurface of the patella, a distinctive sensation demonstrating successful entrance into the joint.

If the patella is ankylosed or if there is a marked flexion deformity of the knee, attempt to aspirate and inject the knee joint by inserting the needle in an anteroposterior direction on either side of the inferior patellar tendon. Slowly advance the needle through the fat pad into the knee joint space between the condyles of the femur.

Miscellaneous Injection Sites

Inject the occipital ridge for tension headaches or occipital nerve neuritis. Carefully localize the point of maximal tenderness. Inject about 2 ml of the standard solution using a #26, ¾ in needle.

If the scapular attachment of the levator scapulae muscle is painful, inject 4 to 5 ml of the standard solution using a #22, 2 in needle.

For pain in and about the posterior iliac spine and iliac crest, inject 8 to 10 ml of the standard solution through a #22, 3 in needle.

Calcaneal bursitis may be helped by the injection of 2 to 3 ml of the standard solution. Use a #22, 1¼ in needle.

Inject and needle the painful trigger points of the upper or lower back. These painful points are usually caused by varying degrees of fibrositis, myositis and lumbosacral strain. One or two injections in the area of the trapezius or rhomboid muscles of the upper back and the erector spinae muscle of the lower back may save the patient several days of disability and make systemic treatment unnecessary.

Indications for Intra-articular Injections of Steroids

Inject any accessible affected joint except the intervertebral joints. Intra-articular injections are usually done for one form or another of rheumatoid, osteo, gouty or traumatic arthritis.

Intra-articular injections are particularly useful when only one or two peripheral joints are affected.

Occasionally systemic treatment for the arthritides is contraindicated, and intra-articular injections of steroids may be the only safe treatment.

Think of intra-articular injections when maintenance systemic therapy gives satisfactory relief in all but a few of the most severely involved joints.

Soft tissue injections of steroids are useful in painful conditions of muscles, joints, and connective tissues. These include:

- –bursitis, including bunion
- –coccydynia
- –minimal Dupuytren's contracture
- –epicondylitis
- –exostosis such as calcaneal spurs
- –fibrositis including myositis, fibromyositis, lumbago and dorsal lumbar and lumbosacral strains and sprains.
- –hallux rigidus and limitus
- –heloma
- –muscle trauma
- –strains and sprains including the ankle and the collateral ligament of the knee
- –various forms of tendonitis
- –tensor fascia lata syndrome
- –acute torticollis
- –trigger finger
- –painful "trigger points"
- –whiplash injuries occasionally

SOME USEFUL DRUGS FOR MUSCULOSKELETAL PAIN

Probenecid (Benemid) 0.5 g tablets. Dose: 0.25 g b.i.d. for 1 week and 0.5 g b.i.d. thereafter. If necessary, every 4 weeks the daily dosage may be increased by 0.5 g to a total of 2.0 g per day. Do not increase when symptoms are controlled or the excretion of urates are more than 700 mg per day. Keep urine alkaline with potassium citrate 7.5 g daily and increase fluid intake. Start its use at any stage of gout except during an acute attack. Do not give with salicylates. A false-positive Benedict's test for glycosuria may occur. Do not give to patients with uric acid kidney stones or with blood dyscrasias.

Sulfinpyrazone (Anturane) 100 and 200 mg per capsule. Dose: 100 to 200 mg b.i.d. with meals or milk. May increase to 800 mg daily within 1 week or decrease to 200 mg for maintenance after blood urate level is acceptable. Use for reducing blood uric acid level; it has little or no anti-inflammatory action. Do not give to patients with an active peptic ulcer. Encourage adequate fluid intake and alkalinization of urine with sodium bicarbonate 3 to 7.5 g daily. Do not give with salicylates or citrates.

Allopurinol (Zyloprim) 100 mg tablets. Dose: 100 mg b.i.d. in mild gout to 600 mg daily in moderately severe tophaceous gout. May be used with other anti-inflammatory agents, including salicylates. Watch for hepatotoxicity by checking SGPT and serum alkaline phosphatase. Attempt to keep urinary output at 2 L and the urine neutral to slightly alkaline. This is potentially a dangerous drug; learn how to use it properly.

Indomethacin (Indocin) 25 and 50 mg capsules. Dose: 25 to 50 mg t.i.d. May use in small doses (25 mg b.i.d.) with an uricosuric agent for prevention of acute attacks. Use only in rheumatoid arthritis (unpredictable), ankylosing spondylitis, 25 to 200 mg daily; osteoarthritis of the hip, 150 to 200 mg daily; gout, 150 to 200 mg daily; Reiter's syndrome, 75 to 200 mg daily. Indocin is unpredictable in bursitis, tendinitis, synovitis, rheumatoid arthritis and psoriatic arthritis. Indocin is associated with the following side effects:

- –headache in 20 percent of the patients
- –somnolence rarely
- –skin rashes and hypersensitive reactions rarely
- –gastrointestinal symptoms, i.e. bleeding, ulceration (perforation in 15 percent of the patients and diarrhea in 5 percent)
- –confusion (rare)
- –dizziness (rare)
- –hallucinations (rare)

Patients sensitive to aspirin should not receive Indocin because of cross-sensitivity. Indocin may mask infections. Be cautious.

Phenylbutazone (Butazolidin) 100 mg tablets. Dose: 300 to 600 mg daily for 1 week to determine response. Discontinue if there is no response. If there is satisfactory response, decrease to a maintenance dose of 100 to 200 mg daily. In no event give more than 400 mg daily. Use for rheumatoid arthritis, spondylitis, osteoarthritis, psoriatic arthritis and painful shoulder. Do not use in patients with cardiac, hepatic, renal or blood problems or those on anticoagulants or sulfonylureas. Monitor the blood count and discontinue when either the hemoglobin or white blood cells decrease.

Oxyphenbutazone (Tandearil) 100 mg tablets. Closely related to Butazolidin. Observe all the precautions as with Butazolidin.

Some phenylbutazone combinations. Butazolidin Alka Capsules minimize gastric irritation. Use with the same care as in Butazolidin. The formulation: 100 mg each of phenylbutazone and aluminum hydroxide, 150 mg magnesium trisilicate and 1.25 mg homatropine methylbromide. Sterazolidin capsules give the anti-inflammatory and analgesic effect of phenylbutazone and prednisone. Formulation is the same as above but with only 50 mg phenylbutazone and 1.25 mg prednisone. Use with the same care as when using any steroid or phenylbutazone.

Colchicine in 0.5 and 0.65 mg tablets is considered a specific for acute gout. The main adverse effect of colchicine is on the gastrointestinal tract but adjustment of dosage usually gives sufficient relief that it can be used intermittently to terminate acute attacks. Dose: 1.0 mg every 2 to 3 hours for 4 to 5 doses.

Colchicine combinations: Colbenemid tablets is a combination of 0.5 mg colchicine and 500 mg probenecid. Dose: 1 tablet daily for 1 week and then b.i.d. if needed.

Muscle Relaxants

The following are frequently used drugs as muscle relaxants in joint and skeletal problems. Their pharmacologic effects vary in effectiveness. I prefer to use something more reliable as aspirin, codeine or Percodan.

Chlorphenesin carbamate (Maolate) 400 mg tablets. Dose: 2 tablets t.i.d.

Methocarbamol (Robaxin) 500 and 750 mg tablets. Dose: up to 3 or 4 tablets q.i.d., average 500 mg t.i.d. Robaxisal-PH is a formulation of methocarbamol, aspirin, phenacetin, phenobarbital and hyoscyamine sulfate.

Mephenesin (Tolserol) 250 and 500 mg tablets. Dose: 1.5 g q.i.d.

Orphenadrine citrate (Norflex) 100 mg tablets. Dose: 100 mg b.i.d. Norgesic tablets are a formulation of 25 mg orphenadrine, 225 mg aspirin, 160 mg phenacetin and 30 mg caffeine.

Chlorzoxazone (Paraflex) 250 mg tablets. Dose: 2 tablets q.i.d.

Carisoprodol (Soma) 350 mg tablets. Dose: 1 tablet q.i.d.

Metaxalone (Skelaxin) 400 mg tablets. Dose: 2 tablets q.i.d.

REFERENCES

1. Convery FR, Clawson DK: The rheumatoid knee. *AFP* 4:52, 1900.
2. Gordon DA, et al: Extra-articular features of rheumatoid arthritis. *Am J Med* 54:445–452, 1973.
3. Smyth CJ: Arthritis: five levels of therapy. *Ch Dis Management* Feb. 1, 1972.
4. Schumacher, Jr., HR: et al: New studies back up old arthritis treatments. *JAMA* 219:1409–1410, 1972.
5. Sigler JW et al: Gold therapy. *JAMA* 219:1410, 1972.
6. Healey LA: Rheumatoid arthritis: which drug will do what. *Med Times* 99:203, 1971.
7. Deaton JG: Systemic lupus: improved tests sharpen diagnosis. *Res/Int Consult* 1:43, 1972.
8. Healey LA: Hyperuricemia: what it means . . . what to do about it. *Consult* 11:21–23, 1971.
9. Kraus H: Clinical Treatment of Back and Neck. Pain. New York: McGraw-Hill, 1970.
10. Redfield JT: Low back x-ray doubtful as useful employment screen. *Med Tribune,* 1971.
11. Singh M, et al: X-ray evidence of osteoporosis. *J Bone Joint* Surg 51 [Am]:457–467, 1970.
12. Bhatt GP: Myotonia—a review of its clinical implications. *Calif Med* 114:16–22, 1971.
13. Engel WK: Myotoma—a different point of view. *Calif Med* 114:32–36, 1971.

GENERAL STUDY AIDS

Karten I: Pitfalls in the diagnosis and treatment of rheumatoid arthritis. *Med Times* 98:137–146, 1970.

Cozen L: Office treatment of hand disorders. *Med Times* 98:195–199, 1970.

Calabro JJ, et al: Ankylosing spondylitis. *AFP* 2:88, 1970.

Montgomery RM: Morton's toe. *Cutis* 8:463, 1971.

Owen DS, et al: Management of gouty arthritis and hyperuricemia. *GP* 38:132–138, 1968.

CHAPTER 8

Neurologic Signs and Symptoms

CRANIAL NERVES

Olfactory Nerve (I Cranial)

The olfactory nerve is not a rewarding nerve to test because it is not often primarily involved in the disease process.

To test the function of the nerve, ask the patient to identify familiar odors—cloves, peppermint, tobacco and coffee—with his eyes closed. Test one nostril at a time. I often use a bar of scented soap, which is usually close at hand. However, the patient's ability to separate odors is more important than identifying odors.

Be sure the nostrils are patent. The ability to smell is often temporarily upset with acute and chronic rhinitis or derangements that may persist for weeks after other symptoms have subsided. Anosmia may occur with head injuries, viral infections of the respiratory tract, meningioma in the olfactory groove and tabes dorsalis.

Repugnant smells are part of the uncinate fits in epilepsy and indicate a lesion involving the uncus in the temporal lobe. These fits are also associated with repugnant tastes and smacking movements of the lips.

Optic Nerve (II Cranial)

Too many family physicians neglect to test the function of the optic nerve. The tests for this nerve are time consuming but rewarding. To save your time, teach your nurse to check visual acuity and to screen visual fields. Ophthalmoscopic examinations of the retina and fundus you must do yourself.

Check the function of the optic nerve by testing the patient's visual acuity, evaluating his visual fields (Fig. 8-1) and inspecting his fundus and retina.

Visual acuity is best tested in the office using the standard Snellen charts, providing the illumination is adequate and sufficient distance from the chart is arranged. Snellen testing is described in more detail in Chapter 3.

Screen the visual fields by the direct confrontation test. Seat your patient one meter in front of you at eye level. Ask him to cover his left eye with his hand or with a piece of paper. Ask him to fix his right eye on the bridge of your nose. Close your left eye. Flick a cotton applicator at arms distance out his visual field and then bring it slowly toward the midline, asking him to signal when he first sees the applicator from the corner of his eye. Compare his response with yours. Repeat, bringing the applicator in toward the midfield from all directions. Then test the second eye similarly. The confrontation test results are easily interpreted if you remember the principles in Figure 8-2.

Visual field defects are found in almost all optic nerve afflictions and are called

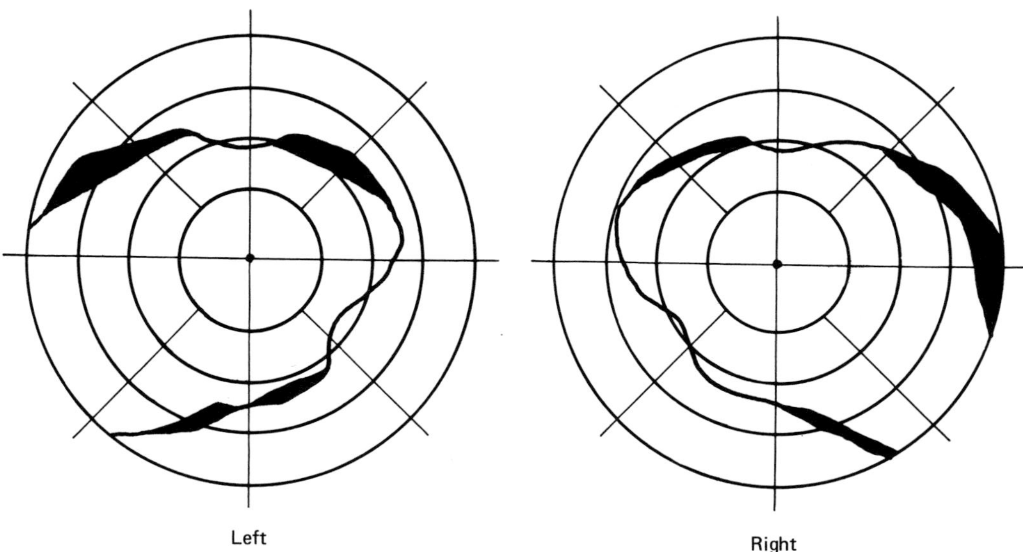

Figure 8-1. Normal visual fields showing the characteristic flattening above and on the nasal sides.

scotomas in optic and retrobulbar neuritis or hemianopsias, which are mainly bitemporal or homonymous. Look for a loss of both temporal fields of vision in bitemporal hemianopsia (Fig. 8-3). This defect is caused by compression or disease of the optic chiasm in or above the sella turcica. In most instances the lesion is a primary pituitary tumor growing in the sella turcica (Fig. 8-4). Rule out other space-occupying lesions: meningioma, adenoma, arachnoiditis, aneurysm, hypophyseal stalk tumor, trauma with laceration of the optic chiasm, pressure of a dilated third ventricle or pressure of a posterior fossa tumor.

The patient has a homonymous hemianopsia if you find a loss of the temporal field in one eye and the nasal field in the other (Fig. 8-5). This defect represents a lesion in the optic tract somewhere between the optic chiasm and the occipital lobe. Optic tract disease usually arises from tumors, aneurysms or injuries. In the temporal or occipital lobes, homonymous hemianopsia is caused by encapsulated tumor, glioma, abscess, softening of brain tissue, hemorrhage, multiple sclerosis or encephalitis.

Suspect damage to the optic nerve or retina if, on careful examination of the visual fields, you find a defect in a single eye. In concentric symmetric contractions of the visual fields (tunnel vision), suspect glaucoma (Fig. 8-6).

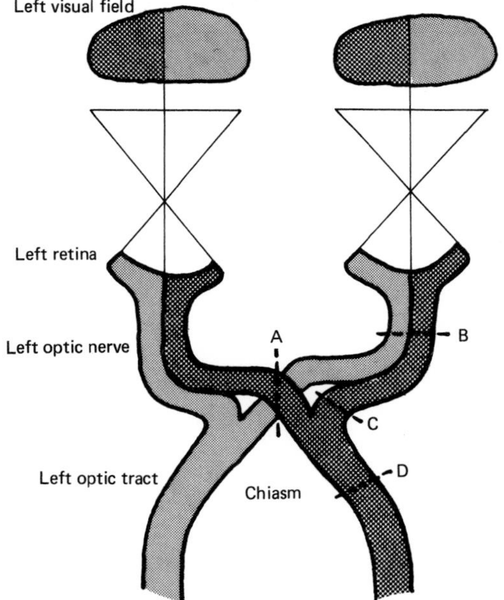

Figure 8-2. Locations of lesions: *A*, Bitemporal hemianopsia; *B*, Total blindness, right eye; *C*, Right nasal hemianopsia; *D*, Left homonymous hemianopsia.

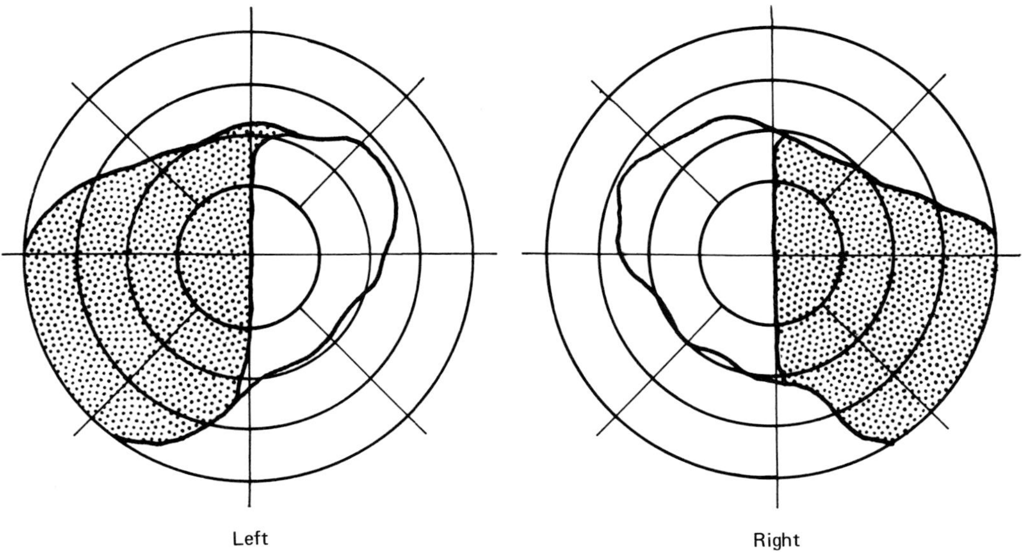

Figure 8-3. Bitemporal hemianopsia. Deficient portions are stippled.

In summary:

–Loss of one field without light perception indicates optic nerve disease.
–Bitemporal hemianopsia is the classical sign of compression at the optic chiasma produced by pituitary tumors.
–Homonymous hemianopsia is produced by lesions between the chiasm and brain.
–Quadrantic hemianopsia is often associated with lesions of the radiation fibers. Upper quadrantic defects suggest temporal lobe involvement; lower quadrantic defects suggest parietal.
–Tunnel vision (loss of peripheral field) occurs when retinal fibers are compressed by glaucoma.
–A homonymous hemianopsia with ipsilateral central scotoma as a result of compression of the optic chiasm and the posterior part of the ipsilateral optic nerve may be caused by chromophobe adenoma, craniopharyngiomas, anterior communicating aneurysm, meningiomas of the medial wing of the sphenoid or localized arachnoiditis.

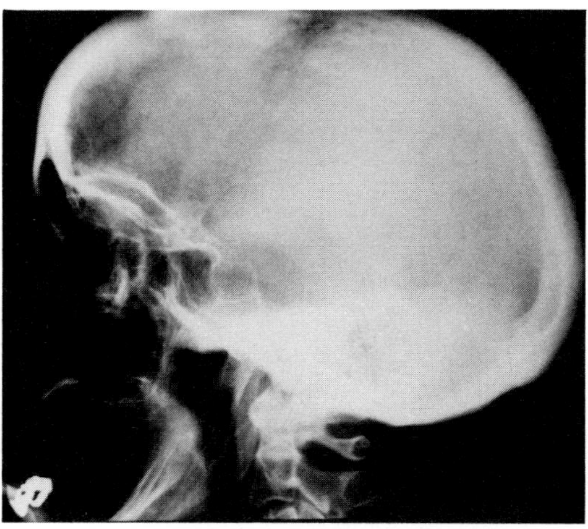

Figure 8-4. Enlarged sella turcica, suggesting tumor.

Using the Ophthalmoscope

Remember that successful ophthalmoscopy depends on the adjustment of three variables: the refractive error and active accommodation of the patient; the refractive error and active accommodation of the examiner; a selection of the proper lens for the structure to be examined, i.e. +10 for cornea, +6 for lens, +2 for vitreous and 0 to −4 for fundus.

With the above in mind adjust the lens to +10 diopters. Keep the sighthole close to your eye or glasses. With the ophthalmo-

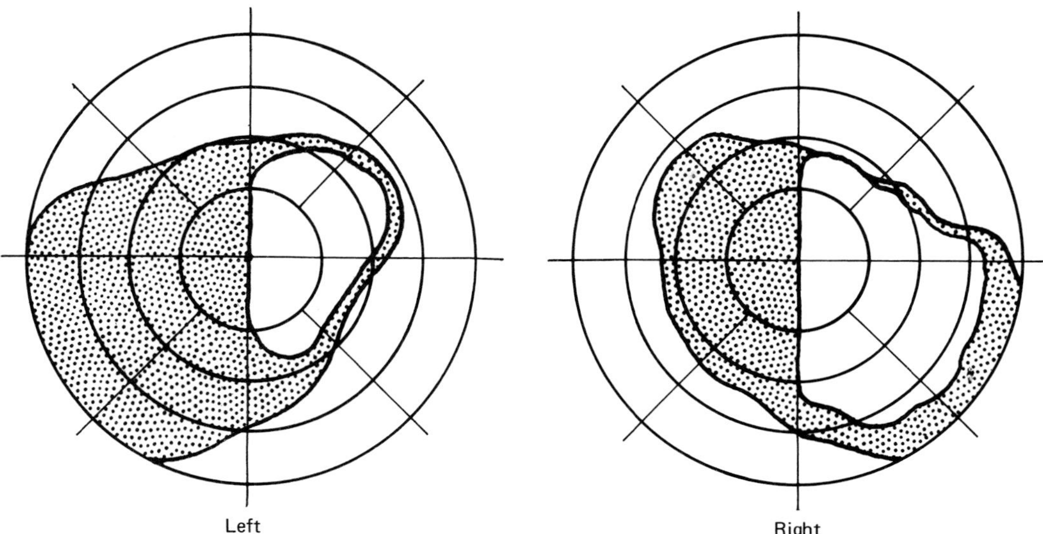

Figure 8-5. Left homonymous hemianopsia. Deficient portions are stippled.

scope light on but the room darkened, move to within 12 in of the patient's eye. Shine the light into the patient's pupil to see the red retinal reflex. Search for dark spots showing against the red background. Change your position, either forward or backward until the black spots are clearly in focus. These spots are opacities in the lens or vitreous.

When you have focused clearly, ask the patient to look up. As he does so, notice whether the spots move up or down. If the spots move up, the opacities are in the cornea or anterior part of the lens; if the spots move downward, they are in the posterior lens or vitreous.

When the media has been sufficiently ex-

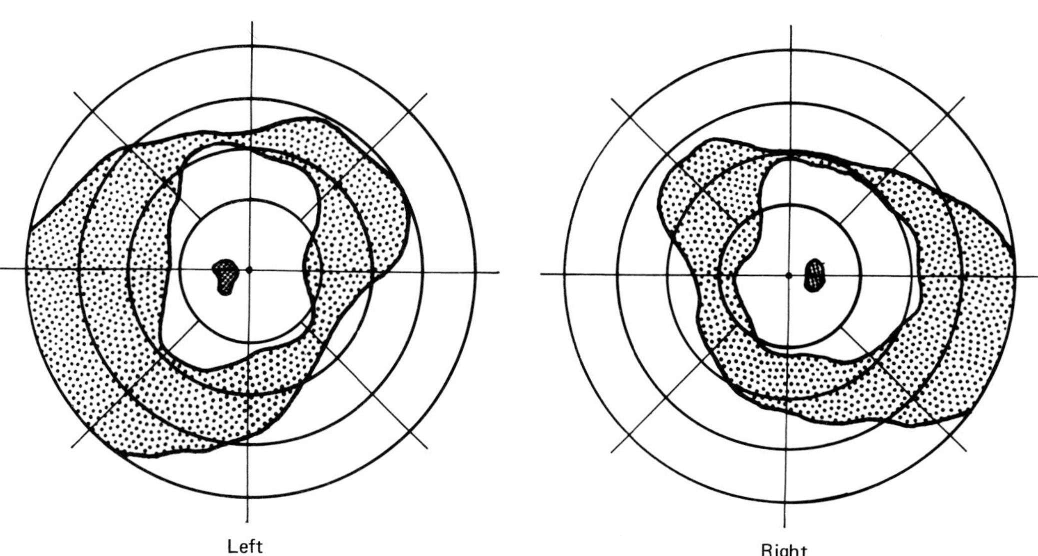

Figure 8-6. Concentric contraction of visual fields in glaucoma. Deficient areas are stippled.

amined, move the ophthalmoscope to within 3 in of the eye. With your index finger on the milled disc of lenses, switch the lenses from +10 to −5 to find the optimal magnification of the retina. This will accomodate for the refractive error of both the examiner and patient.

Find the optic disc. Note its color and outline. Is the edge sharp or blurred? The disc is not always sharply demarcated. The cup is a pale area on the temporal side of the disc. Is the rest of the disc red-orange color? The size and shape of the cup will vary. It is normal to find a crescent of pigment in the retina on the temporal side of the disc.

In the rare instance when the nerve head is elevated (choked disc), measure the elevation by first focusing carefully on the retina some distance away. When that is determined, focus the ophthalmoscope on the edematous nerve head to the point of greatest clarity. The difference between the original and the last reading represents the elevation of the choked disc measured in dropters of swelling (1D, 2D, etc.). About 3D of swelling is equivalent to 1 mm of elevation of the nerve head. Measure other depressions or elevations in the same way, focusing on the arterial reflex in various areas.

Systematically study the arteries and veins. The veins pulsate; the arteries do not. True arteries emerge from the disc; after the second bifurcation, about 1 disc distance from their entrance, the arteries become arterioles. The arteries are bright red, smaller than the veins and have a white reflex stripe. The veins are darker red and about one quarter larger than the arteries. They have no reflex stripe.

Study what occurs when a vein and artery cross. Is there nicking or tapering of the veins?

Now move the light 2 or 3 disc diameters temporally from the disc, and you will be in the region of the macula. Attempt to see this small dark-red area in the retina quickly. Inspection of the macula is uncomfortable and should be done last. In its center is the fovea centralis, a darker spot, which gives off a speck of reflected light. Notice there are no vessels in this area. Retinal pathology is illustrated in Figure 8-7.

From a neurologic standpoint three important observations are made by studying the disc: choking, optic atrophy and retrobulbar neuritis.

Choked Disc

A choked disc (papilledema) is practically always caused by a brain tumor. It is usually, but not always, associated with headache and is accompanied by increased intracranial pressure. A choked disc does not cause a decrease in visual acuity until late in the disease process. This is a helpful point in differentiating a choked disc from optic neuritis.

Other diseases associated with a choked disc are tuberculosis, meningitis, multiple sclerosis, disseminated encephalomyelitis, syphilitic meningitis, hypertension, arteriosclerosis or leukemic retinopathy, subarachnoid hemorrhage and aspirin poisoning. These are rare causes of a choked disc, however. The safe course is to consider a choked disc as being caused by a brain tumor until ruled out.

Optic Neuritis

Optic neuritis produces a papillitis of the disc. Papillitis causes edema of the disc that is indistinguishable from papilledema, but visual loss occurs in papillitis and not with papilledema (Fig. 8-8).

The common cause of papillitis is multiple sclerosis. Rare causes are methyl alcohol poisoning, meningitis and encephalitis.

Inflammation may involve the optic nerve anywhere along its course from nerve head (optic neuritis) as described above to the nerve itself (retrobulbar neuritis). Recognize the retrobulbar form by the following:

- –acute loss of vision in one or both eyes
- –a central scotoma in the visual field
- –a nerve head of normal appearance
- –sudden onset with pain in or over the eye
- –painful eyeball movement

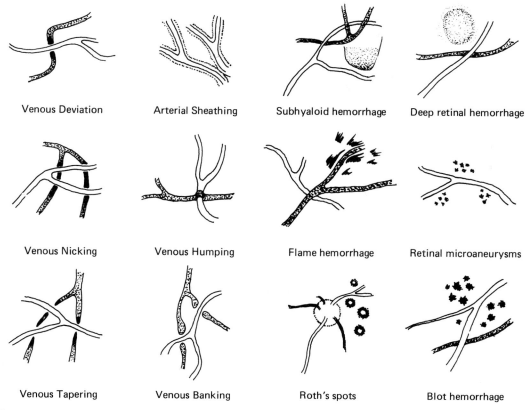

Venous Deviation

Arterial Sheathing

Subhyaloid hemorrhage

Deep retinal hemorrhage

Venous Nicking

Venous Humping

Flame hemorrhage

Retinal microaneurysms

Venous Tapering

Venous Banking

Roth's spots

Blot hemorrhage

Figure 8-7. Retinal pathology.

–headache, unilateral and radiating out over the eye into the forehead and temple

–optic atrophy may follow the acute disease

Causes are variable but in most studies multiple sclerosis tops the list. Search for other causes such as pernicious anemia, diabetes mellitus, alcohol or tobacco poisoning and syphilis.

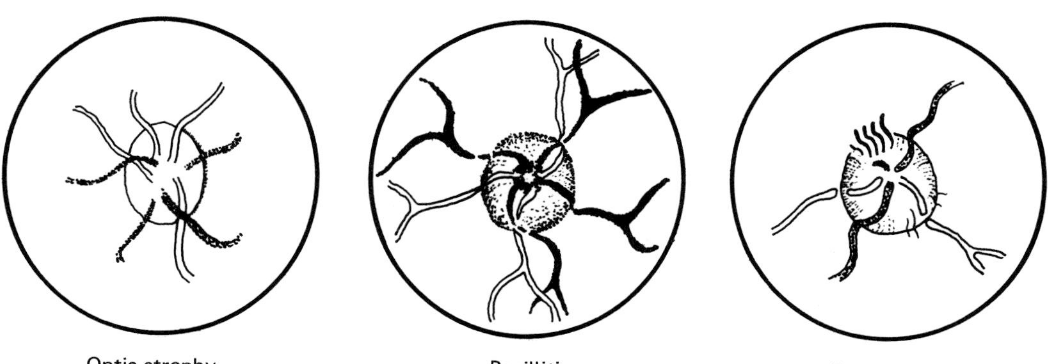

Figure 8-8. Optic disc pathology.

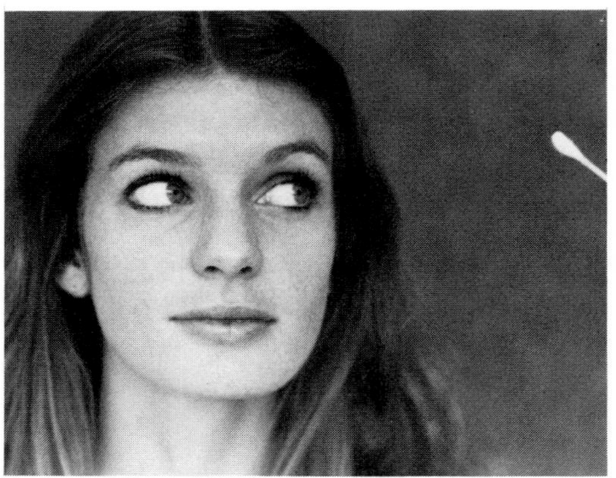

Figure 8-9. Assess ocular nerves III, IV and VI by directing the patient to gaze through all the primary ocular movements.

When the optic nerve head turns pale, think of *optic atrophy*. The disc is white, the borders sharply outlined and the cup and cribrosa visible. Visual acuity is reduced, there may be no perception of light and the direct and consensual reflexes are lost.

Optic atrophy may follow optic neuritis; therefore the causes of neuritis may be considered causes of atrophy. Other causes to be considered are glaucoma, repeated hemorrhage, vitamin B deficiency, pressure from Paget's disease of the skull and tumors and other factors that obstruct the blood supply and thus cause atrophy.

Ocular Nerves (Oculomotor, Trochlear and Abducent Nerves—III, IV and VI Cranial)

Consider these three nerves together. They are intimately associated in supplying the eye and the extraocular muscles (Fig. 8-9). They are frequently affected either singly or in unison in neurologic diseases. Damage may occur in the brainstem, peripherally in their course at the base of the brain and within the orbit.

When evidence of ocular nerve damage is found, search for the following: infiltrating tumors; multiple sclerosis; various encephalopathies; hemorrhagic encephalitis (Wernicke's polioencephalitis); hemorrhage; arteriosclerotic softenings; botulism; meningitis (especially syphilitic); subarachnoid hemorrhage; aneurysms of the internal carotid, posterior communicating or posterior cerebral arteries; meningiomas; trauma; the neuritis of alcohol or lead

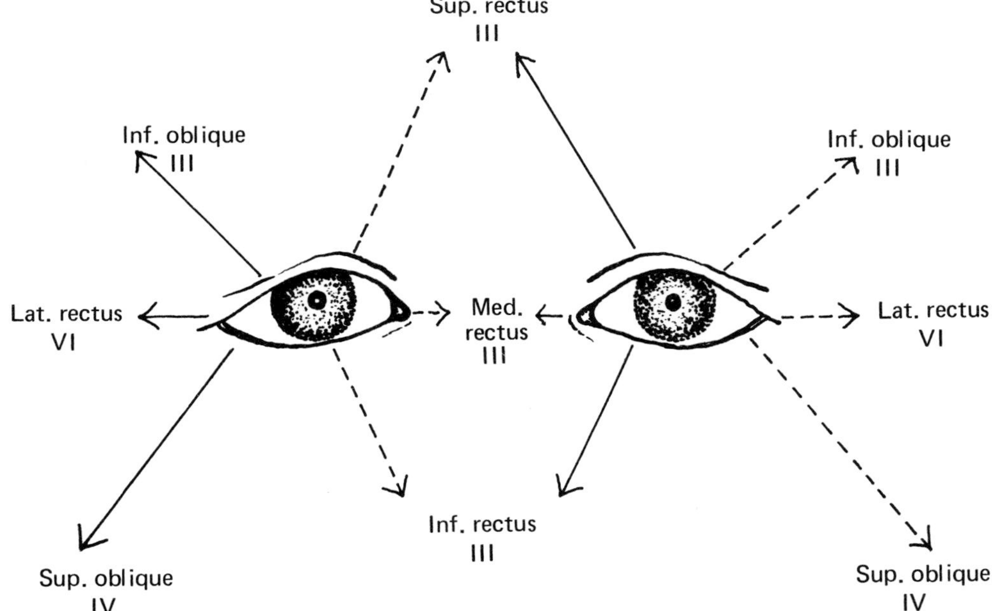

Figure 8-10. The cardinal positions of gaze and their innervation.

poisoning and ethmoid and mastoid sinusitis.

Complete paralysis of all ocular nerves will cause ptosis, immobility of the eyeball, dilated pupils that do not react to light and overreaction of the cervical sympathetic supply. Partial paralysis of the ocular nerves may occur in various combinations, either unilaterally or bilaterally.

Unilateral complete paralysis of the *oculomotor nerve* (III) will cause:

- dilation of the pupil
- ptosis of the eyelid
- inability to open the lid
- inability to move the eyeball upward, inward or downward
- absent pupillary light reflex
- deviation of the right eye downward and outward to the right

The most common cause of oculomotor paralysis is an aneurysm in the circle of Willis.

The *trochlear nerve* (IV) innervates the superior oblique muscle and moves the eyeball downward and outward (Figs. 8-10 and 8-11). This movement is lost in paralysis of the nerve. The patient will tilt his head toward his shoulder in order to prevent dip-

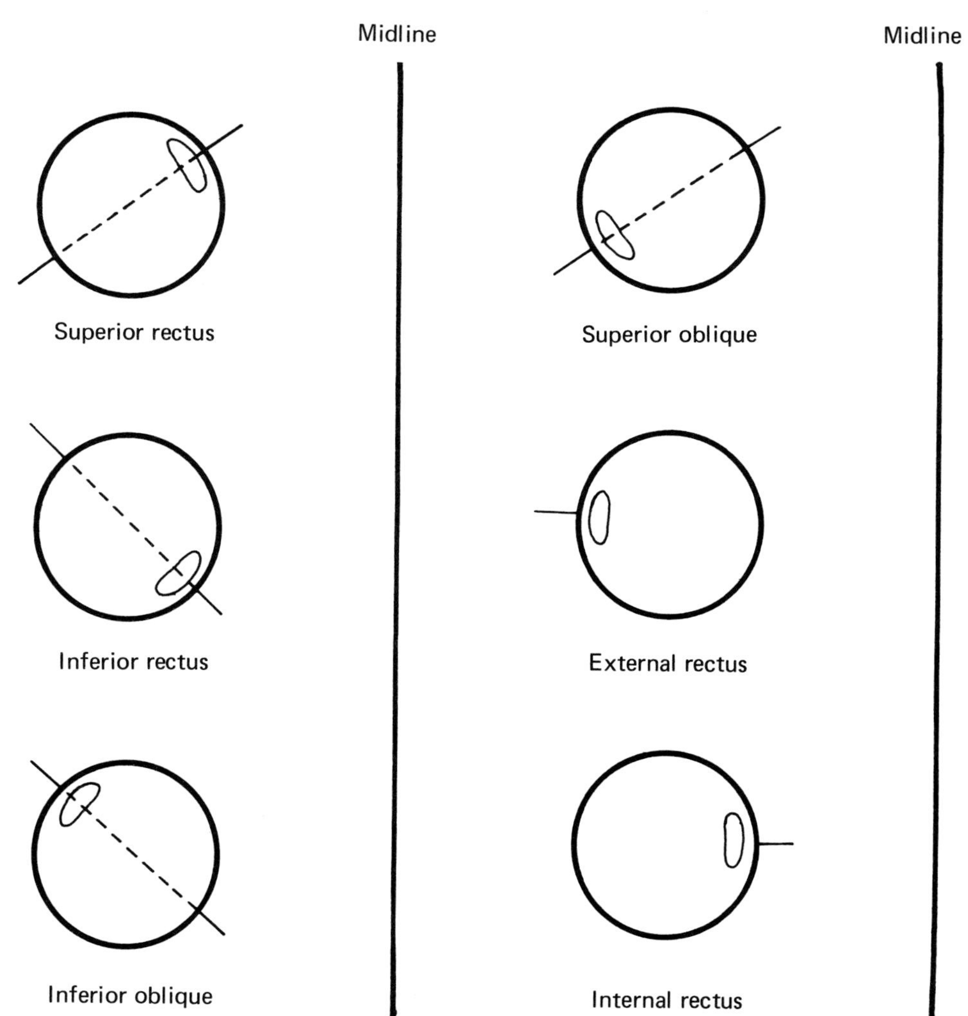

Figure 8-11. Normal ocular movement.

lopia, but do not be misled by this tilt and treat the patient for torticollis. Unfortunately this has happened.

The *abducent nerve* (VI) innervates the external rectus muscle. Paralysis of the nerve results in inability to rotate the eyeball outward. If the paralysis is complete, the gaze cannot be deviated beyond the midline of the affected eye. This is readily recognized by the internal squint, which develops because of the unopposed action of the internal rectus muscle. Diplopia is present and the patient's head is turned in the direction in which the eye muscle has been acting before it was paralyzed.

The *iris and pupil.* The sphincter pupillae is the circular muscle embedded in the iris near the pupillary margin. The sphincter contracts the pupil through parasympathetic (III) stimulation; the dilator (V) widens the pupil by sympathetic stimuli. Mydriasis is dilatation; miosis is pupillary constriction. Miosis occurs when the eye is fixed on a near object, say 20 mm away.

Pupillary reflex is tested preferably in a dark or shaded room by flashing a light obliquely into the pupil. Examine for size, regularity, shape and reaction. Under normal circumstances the pupil reacts quickly to light, the contraction being maintained for a very brief time and then relaxed as the sphincter of the iris fatigues, even with the continued application of light.

A routine examination should include a study of the *consensual reaction.* Under normal circumstances, flashing a light in one pupil results in a prompt contraction of the opposite pupil as well. This is known as a consensual reaction. Test the *accommodation reflex* by watching the size of the pupil as it accommodates to near and far vision.

Malfunction of the pupils occurs in several situations.

Many older people have small, irregular and unequal pupils because of arteriosclerotic changes.

Young women occasionally have benign myotonic pupils that react very slowly to light and convergence. This is known as Adie's syndrome if associated with absent knee and ankle jerks.

Characteristics of Horner's syndrome are a small pupil that does not dilate in the dark, ptosis, possible enophthalmos and decreased sweating on the same side of the face.

An Argyll-Robertson pupil is almost pathognomonic of tabes dorsalis or taboparesis. It is characterized by absent contraction to light, normal or exaggerated contraction to accommodation, miotic pupils, irregular and unequal pupils and absent dilatation with remote pain in other parts of the body.

In ophthalmoplegia interna, the pupil loses the ability to constrict from light or accommodation. It is always dilated. Search for a syphilitic meningitis, vasculitis or virus encephalitis. Lead poisoning and toxins of botulism and diphtheria can cause it.

Oval or unequal pupils occur occasionally in healthy people. In my own practice I have found more physiologic pupillary malfunctions than Argyll-Robertson pupils. Ignore pupils that show minor dilitation or contraction synchronized with the pulse beat. They are of no significance.

Trigeminal Nerve (V Cranial)

The trigeminal nerve is composed of both motor and sensory portions (Fig. 8-12); consequently, look for both motor and sensory symptoms. Fifth cranial nerve function can be assessed by symmetric jaw motion. Check the motor function as the patient bites down on his back teeth.

Motor weakness involving the masseter, temporal and pterygoid muscles may be the result of:

- –peripheral lesions such as trauma, skull fracture or tumor
- –tumor of the cerebellopontine angle
- –infiltrating tumor of the pons
- –encephalitis
- –processes involving the motor nucleus of the trigeminal nerve in the pons

One of the earliest, and sometimes the only, finding in trigeminal sensory loss is the absence of the corneal reflex. Always check

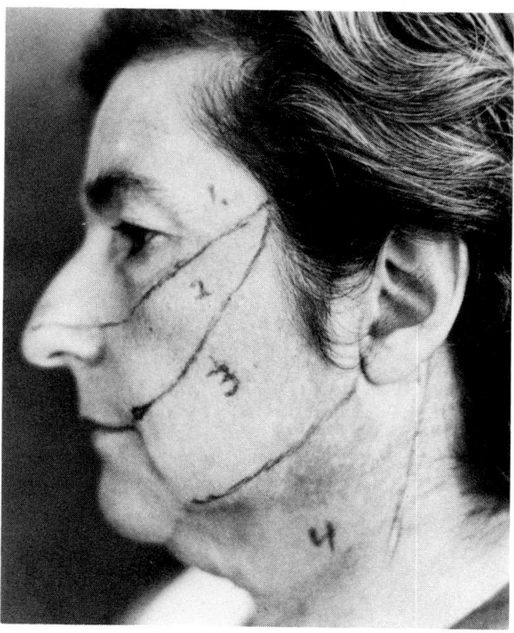

Figure 8-12. Sensory divisions of the fifth cranial nerve: *1*, Ophthalmic branch; *2*, Maxillary branch; *3*, Mandibular branch; and, *4*, Superficial cervical plexus. The occiput and posterior neck is served by cervical nerves. To test tactile sensation have the patient close his eyes and test each area with a shred of gauze. To test pain sensitivity touch with a pin. Compare with other side.

for this reflex. One method to test for the reflex is to ask the patient to look up as you gently touch the cornea with a small piece of gauze. Normally this induces blinking.

Complete interruption of sensory function is rare but may occur with tumors or inflammation of the gasserian ganglion.

Incomplete sensory syndromes involving the face are found with:

- –infiltrating tumors of the pons
- –other conditions that affect the sensory trigeminal nucleus such as multiple sclerosis or encephalitis
- –tumors of the gasserian ganglion
- –herpes zoster ophthalmicus
- –cerebellopontine angle tumors
- –hemiplegia
- –thalamic syndromes
- –syphilitic meningitis
- –acoustic or trigeminal neuromas

Facial Nerve (VII Cranial)

The special anatomy of this nerve must be kept in mind in testing for function. The muscles of the forehead have a bilateral cortical nerve supply. They are, therefore, spared in upper motor neuron lesions affecting the face. In such cases, voluntary facial movements are affected more than involuntary ones such as blinking and smiling. All the facial muscles are affected in lower motor neuron lesions, and both voluntary and involuntary movements are paralyzed. Consequently, the seventh nerve has little localizing value, and associated findings in other nerves must be considered. In brainstem lesions, look for ipsilateral VI nerve palsy. In cerebellopontine angle lesions, look for VIII and V nerve lesions. In lesions of the bony canal, look for VIII nerve lesions as well as loss of taste over the anterior two thirds of the tongue.

Using the actions in Table 8-1, test for function of the upper and lower motor neurons.

Central facial weakness is characterized by weakness of movement of the lower portion of the face on the side opposite the lesion. This is because the upper portion of the face receives innervation from both motor areas, while the lower portion is innervated only from one side of the brain, the opposite motor cortex. Central facial weak-

Table 8-1. Testing for Motor Neuron Lesions

Action	*Motor Neuron Responses* *Upper*	*Lower*
Face resting		
Nasolabial folds	Shallow	Shallow
Palpebral fissure		Widened
Elevation of eyebrow	Present	Absent
Tight closing of eyes	Present	Absent
Frowning	Present	Absent
Showing teeth	Absent	Absent
Whistling and puffing	Absent	Absent
Smiling	Present	Absent
Emotional expression	Present	Absent
Voluntary expression	Weak	Present
Facial paralysis	Central	Peripheral

ness occurs in hemiplegia and focal lesion in the opposite motor cortex.

Peripheral facial paralysis occurs in involvement of the facial nucleus in the pons by polio, encephalitis and infiltrating tumors; involvement of the nerve within the skull as in cerebellopontine angle tumor (acoustic neuroma), meningitis (syphilitic or tubercular) or subarachnoid hemorrhage; involvement of the facial nerve at any point after leaving the skull as in neuritis, skull fractures, tumors of the neck or herpes zoster.

Sensory fibers supply the sensation of taste on the anterior two thirds of the tongue.

Bell's Palsy is an acute lower motor neuron palsy of the facial nerve. To laymen and physicians who have not seen the disease previously the abrupt onset of the disfiguring paralysis of the facial muscles is terrifying. Keep your cool. Reassure the patient. If at the end of a week any movement at all is visible on the affected side assure the patient of eventual complete recovery. Recovery usually takes 4 to 8 weeks but may be as long as a year. Protect the open eye during sleep. Small doses of prednisone may help and electrical stimulation of facial muscles may help prevent atrophy.

Acoustic-Vestibular Nerve (VIII Cranial)

The cochlear division of the eighth cranial nerve has to do with hearing and the vestibular division with equilibrium. Disease of the cochlea is characterized by nerve deafness, loss of air conduction and failure to lateralize sound to the affected ear. Tinnitus may be present for some time before deafness ensues. Nerve deafness is practically always the result of disease of the peripheral portion of the auditory nerve.

Every family physician should purchase and use a simple audiometer. The testing of hearing may be done more accurately by an audiometer than in any other way (Fig. 8-13). Less effective methods are the whispered voice and tuning forks.

For the whispered voice test, position your mouth at the side of the patient's head

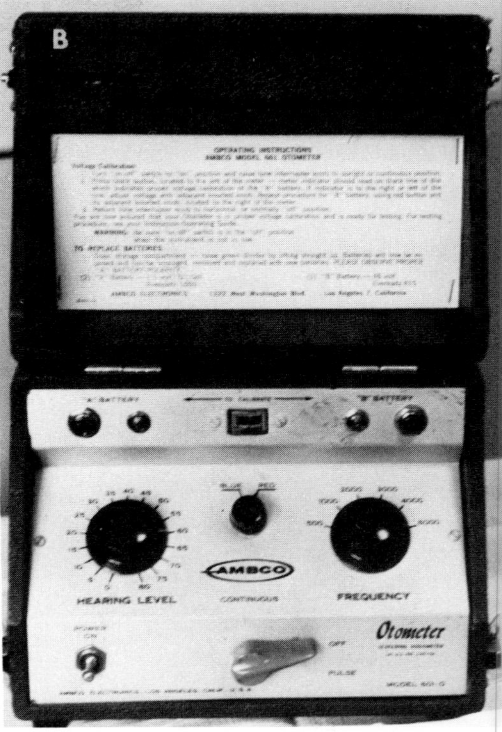

Figure 8-13. *A*, Check hearing with an audiometer, the most effective test to determine the integrity of the cochlear portion of the eighth cranial nerve; *B*, Otometer (Ambco).

about 2 feet from his ear. Ask him to close his opposite ear with his hand. Exhale and then whisper test numbers which he is to repeat. Select loud, medium and soft tones. Using the same intensity for all numbers, find the maximum distance from the ear at which the whispers may be heard.

By using a tuning fork with frequencies between 512 and 1024 cycles per second (Fig. 8-14), you can test for, and distinguish between, perceptive and conductive hearing.

In conduction deafness, bone conduction is louder than air conduction. In nerve deafness, acuity is reduced but air conduction is still the better. Conduction deafness is caused by inflammatory middle ear disease, eustachian obstruction, otosclerosis or Paget's disease of the bone.

Attempt to localize the cause of nerve deafness by checking associated physical signs:

- –Facial palsy and impaired taste would indicate a lesion in the petrous temporal bone.
- –Palsies of the VIII, VII and V cranials would indicate lesions in the cerebellopontine angle.
- –Brain stem palsies plus nerve deafness would indicate nuclear lesions.

Causes of nerve deafness are congenital malformation, fractures of the temporal bone, congenital syphilis, tumors of the cerebellopontine angle (usually vascular or demyelinating problems) or tumors near the corpora quadrigemina.

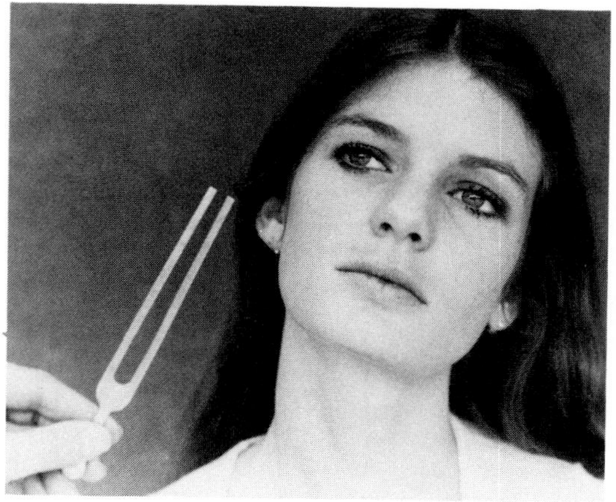

Figure 8-14. Testing hearing with a tuning fork.

The Dizzy Patient

As is the case of most diagnostic problems, a careful history is the most important part of the work-up. For practical purposes, evaluation of the dizzy patient centers around the vestibular system. A disturbance anywhere along the pathway from the end organ to the deep brain may produce dizziness as well as pallor, perspiration, nausea and vomiting. The first problem is to determine whether the lesion is in the peripheral vestibular apparatus, the intermediate vestibular ganglion and acoustic nerve or deep in the brain.

Get the following details: Description of the onset. What was the patient doing? Characteristics of the onset. This would include an exact description of the episode. (Remember, dizziness is a sensation of unsteadiness or light headedness; vertigo is a sensation of whirling within the environment or an environment whirling about the patient.) Be sure of what the patient is complaining. Perhaps he has spots before his eyes, blurred vision, inability to concentrate or blacking out. Does he have a tendency to veer or fall to one side?

Find out about the duration of the attacks. Are they intermittent or continuous? (Intermittent episodes suggest peripheral vestibular disease; continuous dizziness, on the other hand, suggests central disease.)

Is there a pattern? Do symptoms appear when the patient rises from a squatting or sitting position? This is the case in circulatory deficiency, an orthostatic hypotension. Are the attacks related to meals? This suggests hypoglycemia. If nausea and vomiting accompany the attacks of dizziness or vertigo, the problem is more likely to be organic rather than psychogenic.

Is there an associated unilateral hearing loss or tinnitus? These symptoms would suggest a problem in the peripheral organ. A peripheral vestibular disturbance is aggravated by head motion; with central disease, head motion does little to aggravate the symptoms.

Are there associated neurologic complaints? Ask the patient about numbness or weakness on one side of the face or in an extremity. Is there a disturbance of speech? Does the patient stagger between attacks? These symptoms would suggest central nervous system involvement.

In summary, dizziness caused by the peripheral labyrinth is aggravated by change in position and is more intense than is the dizziness of central origin. The pattern of peripheral dizziness is more episodic and recurrent than central dizziness , where it is more or less continual with some variation in intensity. And last of all, central dizziness is associated more frequently with other neurologic complaints than is peripheral disease.

EXAMINATION. Before beginning your examination, consider the possible neuro-otologic disorders for which you are searching (Table 8-2).

Begin your examination with a careful check of the cranial nerves, giving particular attention to the III, IV and VI ocular nerves and to the V, VII, IX, X, XI, and XII cranial nerves.

Do what you can of an audiologic examination. If you do not have an audiometer you will be unable to be accurate. But do perform Rinne's and Weber's tests.

To perform Rinne's test, place the handle of the vibrating fork against the patient's mastoid process while she covers her opposite ear with her hand. Ask her to indicate when she can no longer hear the sound, then hold the vibrating tines near the ear until no sound is heard. Normally, air conduction persists twice as long as bone conduction —called Rinne-positive. When bone conduction persists as long or longer, the test is Rinne-negative.

In Weber's test for hearing perception, place the handle of the tuning fork on the midline of the skull (Fig. 8-15). Ask the patient in which ear she hears the vibration. Right? Left? Both ears? If the sound is heard in only one ear, a conductive loss is indicated in that ear or a perceptive loss in the opposite ear.

Table 8-2. Causes of Dizziness

Peripheral (labyrinthine) causes
Drug toxicity such as with streptomycin
Trauma, concussion and fractures
Chronic otitis media
Labyrinthinitis, including viral infections
Vestibular neuronitis
Positional vertigo
Meniere's disease
Tumors of the cerebellopontine angle, including acoustic neuroma
Allergy
Petrositis
Common central causes
Mild cerebral anoxia
Tumors
Trauma
Demyelinating diseases, i.e. multiple sclerosis
Petit mal
Psychogenic factors
Occlusion of vertebral or basilar arteries or their branches by arteriosclerosis, spasm, thrombosis or external pressure
Hemorrhage of the inner ear or brain
Vascular aneurysm
Hyper- or hypotension
Ophthalmologic causes
Refractive errors
Extraocular muscle imbalance
Simple glaucoma
Endocrine causes
Estrogens
Thyroid diseases
Carbohydrate metabolism
Traumatic causes
Whiplash
Concussion
Skull fractures

Other audiologic tests are pure tone audiometry of air and bone, speech discrimination, small increment sensitivity index (SISI), recruitment, Bekesy audiometry and filtered speech. Further information on these test follows.

Proceed to an evaluation of any nystagmus. The only objective finding in relation to vertigo is nystagmus. True rotary vertigo is almost always accompanied by nystagmus. It is best evaluated by the electronystagmograph, an instrument that records the electric potential of the eyeballs (cornea is postitive; retina is negative). However, gross observation of the nystagmus provides useful information. Search for a spontaneous nystagmus before proceeding with the following checks for it.

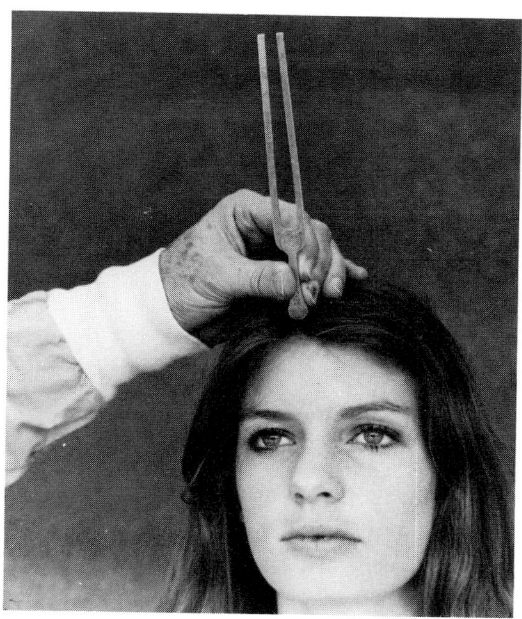

Figure 8-15. Weber's test for hearing perception.

Labyrinthine test for positional nystagmus: Ask the patient to be seated on the examining table. Inspect the eyes for nystagmus. Ask him to lie supine for 30 sec and reinspect for nystagmus. Assist the patient to turn his head and body to one side. Wait 30 sec, and again inspect for nystagmus. Turn the patient to the other side and again wait 30 sec before again checking for nystagmus. Now have the patient drop his head over the top of the table and repeat. Allow him to rest, and finally check him again after sitting up. Remember nystagmus is named for its fast component.

The following is a simple and rapid method for appraising the caloric response of the labyrinth. It is not accurate if spontaneous nystagmus exists. It may be termed the *"minimal" caloric test* and was devised by Fred Lithicum. Instill 0.2 ml of ice water into one ear with the patient's head inclined toward the other shoulder. Twenty sec later ask the patient to straighten his head position and tilt the chin upward 30°. Inspect the eyes while the room is dimly lighted for nystagmus. Wait 5 min and test the opposite side. If there is no response, increase the volume of ice water to 0.4 ml. Continue testing each ear, increasing the volume of ice water by increments of 0.2 ml until a nystagmus is evoked. Compare the volume of ice water needed to stimulate nystagmus in each ear. A significant difference may be 0.2 ml but 0.4 is a definite asymmetric response. Cold water produces nystagmus to the side opposite to the one being stimulated. Use a tuberculin syringe.

Perform the common coordination tests to evalute the cerebellar functions of coordination and balance, i.e. finger-to-finger, finger-to-nose and rapidly alternating movement. Balance is evaluated by the Romberg and tandem Romberg (feet placed toe-to-heel in a straight line). Ask the patient to close his eyes when performing the Rombergs. Remember balance is maintained by three components—visual, proprioceptive and vestibular. A person can manage quite well with any two of the componenets. Closing the eyes will eliminate one of the balancing mechanisms and bring out a deficiency in the other two.

Your ability to do these tests depends on your interest, time and the purchase of equipment. I must emphasize that not all patients with dizziness need as complete an evaluation as outlined. A few puzzling cases will need this thorough evalution. Unless you are interested enough to do the more simple ones frequently, the wisest course is to refer the patient to one who gives attention to these details.

COMMON CAUSES OF VERTIGO. VESTIBULAR NEURONITIS. This causes a few days of intense vertigo. Hearing is not involved. Sometimes it occurs in epidemics or as a result of streptomycin toxicity.

ACUTE TOXIC LABYRINTHITIS. This is the most frequent cause of vertigo. The attack reaches a climax in 24 to 48 hours. Nausea and vomiting occur at its peak. The patient attempts to stay in a horizontal position, which appears to give some relief. Symptoms disappear in 3 to 6 weeks. There is no tinnitus nor reduced hearing. The disease may accompany acute febrile illnesses, pneumonia, influenza, acute cholecystitis, drugs, reactions, alcohol, fatigue and allergy.

VASCULAR SPASM. Transient vertigo may

be caused by vascular spasm. The severity of the attack depends on the extent of the vascular pathology. If an artery or vein ruptures the patient will suffer loud tinnitus, sudden deafness and vertigo with nystagmus. Partial recovery occurs in 3 to 4 weeks.

MENIERE'S DISEASE. This syndrome is characterized by sudden attacks of whirling vertigo, tinnitus and perceptive hearing loss with intervals of complete freedom from vertigo but persistent hearing loss and tinnitus. An attack lasts for hours but not days. Hearing loss is greater on one side, a condition that fluctuates but is slowly progressive. Tinnitus also fluctuates but becomes worse before an attack begins. The disease is self-limited. Labyrinthine tests are normal. No physical signs except deafness and nystagmus are found clinically. Caloric stimulation tests indicate impaired semicircular canals.

The results of treatment are not spectacular. A combination of the following is usually prescribed: vasodilator drugs (Arlidin, nicotinic acid, etc.), diuretics, low salt diet, antivertiginous drugs (Antivert, Tigan, Compazine) and tranquilizers.

ACOUSTIC NEUROMA. Improved surgical techniques, the dissecting microscope and refinements in x-ray diagnosis permit the detection of small acoustic tumors and their removal at an early stage when the operation is reasonably safe.

Suspect a neuroma in patients with a unilateral hearing loss, unilateral tinnitus and some dizziness. The earliest symptom is unilateral tinnitus. Neuromas can usually be differentiated from cochlear lesions, such as Meniere's disease, even while the lesion is small and confined to the internal auditory canal.

Start with a hearing test using a pure tone audiometer. Look for postural dizziness, unsteady gait and attacks of spontaneous vertigo. In most patients you can find a loss of labyrinthine function even in early stages. Do the positional tests for spontaneous nystagmus and the caloric tests mentioned previously. The response to labyrinthine stimulation is decreased or absent on the involved side. Refer the patient, if you are not familiar with the technique and interpretation of the caloric tests.

Check for a loss in speech discrimination by using a standarized word list. In the following list, a tumor patient may recognize only 30 percent of the words but a patient with normal recognition may recognize 90 per cent.

Standard Word List

an	twins	poor	owl
yard	could	him	it
carve	what	skin	the
us	bathe	east	jam
day	ace	thing	high
toe	you	dad	isle
felt	as	up	or
stove	wet	bells	jaw
knees	deaf	hunt	me
not	them	ran	chew
mew	give	there	see
low	true	earn	none

The following are other helpful tests generally done by an otologist. The *Bekesy test* evaluates the patient's response to continuous and interrupted tones. In patients with a neuroma, the appreciation of the continuous tone diminishes sharply as compared with the interrupted tones. *Recruitment* is determined by the alternate Binaural Loudness Balance Test. Recruitment is an abnormal sensitivity to increases in loudness. It is characteristic of cochlear lesions but is uncommon in acoustic neuromas. The *Short Increment Sensitivity Index (SISI)* checks the patient's ability to detect small increments in loudness. The percentage of increments detected is low (0 to 20 percent) in the normal ear or with neuromas and high (40 percent) in cochlear lesions.

Perform the following tests for facial nerve involvement. Carefully check for facial muscle weakness. As a neuroma enlarges, it displaces the facial nerve and impairs its motor function. Do the tear test, which compares the distance of saturation on strips of dry filter paper (Fig. 8-16). Involvement of the facial parasympathetic nerve fibers by a tumor decreases tearing on the affected side. The sensory portion of each facial nerve can be easily and accu-

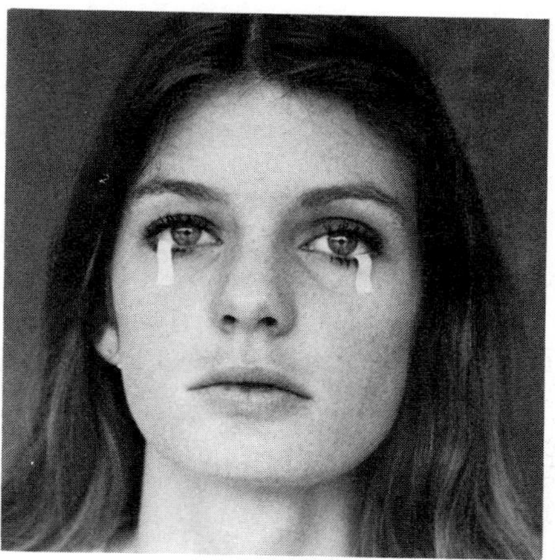

Figure 8-16. Schirmer's test for rate of tear production or lack of tears. A small strip of filter paper is folded over the lower eyelid. If the paper remains unwet for 15 minutes, suspect keratoconjunctivitis sicca.

rately tested by the use of a electric galvanic taste tester.

Look for involvement of other parts of the nervous system as the tumor enlarges.

- –A decrease in corneal sensitivity on the side of the lesion is the first sign of fifth nerve involvement.
- –A diplopia indicates sixth nerve involvement.
- –Dysarthria, dysphagia and hoarseness indicates tenth nerve involvement.
- –Peresis of one or more limbs (pyramidal tract) with hyperreflexia and pathologic Babinski's sign indicates brainstem involvement.
- –Ataxia and incoordination points toward cerebellar involvements.
- –Papilledema indicates interference with the circulation of the cerebrospinal fluid.

X-ray examination of the petrous bone can be especially helpful if done properly and interpreted skillfully; ordinary x-rays of the petrous bone are insufficient. Films should be selected by use of the image intensifier; contrast examinations of the cerebellopontine angle and posterior fossa are needed; and localized tomograms and pneumoencephalography with tomography of the petrous bone should be done.

Cranial Nerves IX, X, XI and XII

The last four cranial nerves, IX, X, XI and XII, are in close proximity. Often, when one is involved, all or others are involved in the same pathology. Individual lesions do occur, however. Consequently, when you examine a patient for disease in and around these areas expect to find a combination of the following signs:

- –loss of special and ordinary sensation to the posterior third of the tongue and soft palate and some degree of anesthesia in the tonsillar fossa (IX cranial nerve)
- –weakness or paralysis of the levator palati or vocal cords (X cranial nerve)
- –weakness of the sternocleidomastoid and weakness and wasting of the upper fibers of the trapezius (XI cranial nerve)
- –deviation of the tongue to the affected side on protrusion (XII cranial nerve)

In lower motor neuron disease the tongue fibrillates and atrophies; upper motor neuron lesions cause stiffness.

Glossopharyngeal Nerve (IX Cranial)

Interference with the ninth cranial nerve decreases the sensation of taste over the posterior third of the tongue, decreases the sensation of pain, touch and temperature over the throat, palate, pharynx and tonsils and causes a small loss of motor function for swallowing.

The glossopharyngeal nerve is seldom diseased alone. Syphilis, tumors, neuritis, fractures and local diseases of the pharynx may affect the nerve.

Be alert to the possibility of a *glossopharyngeal neuralgia*. It can be confused with trigeminal neuralgia, chronic sore throat and otalgia. The chief complaint is paroxysmal pain in the throat radiating to the ear. Eating, talking or yawning seems to set off the pain. Nothing can be found on examination. Other symptoms and other cranial nerves are involved if there is a cerebellopontine angle tumor or aneurysm. The true nature of the disorder is revealed by the regular provocation of pain by a trigger zone in the tonsillar region or pharynx.

Vagus Nerve (X Cranial)

Although the vagus nerve has many functions, swallowing and phonation are the only tangible functions that can be tested during an examination. The symptoms of damage to the vagus nerve depend on the level at which the insult occurs.

The brainstem and cranial parts of the nerve may be attacked by infiltrating tumors, syphilis, tuberculosis, poliomyelitis, multiple sclerosis, syringomyelia, encephalitis, thrombosis of the posterior inferior cerebellar artery, amyotrophic lateral sclerosis, progressive bulbar paralysis, aneurysms of the vertebral or basilar arteries, basal skull fractures, hemorrhage, gunshot wounds and surgery.

If a patient comes to you complaining of hoarseness and difficulty in swallowing, look for a high unilateral lesion of the vagus nerve. The lesion is bilateral if the patient is unable to swallow and has lost his voice. Ask the patient to open his mouth. If you suspect vagus lesions look for a unilateral drooping of the palate on the affected side. Now ask him to say *ah,* and the palate will move over to the sound side. No movement of the palate, of course, would indicate bilateral paralysis. Watch closely to see whether the faucial pillars converge equally. Further information may be gained by touching the back of the tongue with the tongue blade to elicit the absence or presence of the gag reflex. Touch the mucosa of the pharynx with an applicator to determine areas of anesthesia.

Now ask the patient to swallow water. Does the larynx (Adam's apple) elevate properly? Does the patient regurgitate? There will be no rise in the larynx in patients with bilateral paralysis. Continue the examination by looking indirectly at the vocal cords. The cord on the affected side will be abducted. In bilateral paralysis the voice is lost. The patient will be dyspneic and struggling with an inspiratory stridor.

More often the family physician must deal with damage to the recurrent laryngeal nerve. It has been my experience that surgeons prefer to share the care of a patient whose recurrent laryngeal nerve was damaged during a thyroidectomy. There are other causes of damage to this nerve—stab wounds, gunshot injuries, tumors, aneurysms, enlarged glands and other mediastinal diseases.

Recurrent laryngeal nerve damage causes little or no difficulty with swallowing but big trouble with phonation and breathing. These patients usually need a tracheotomy. In bilateral paralysis the vocal cords are immobile and there is aphonia, dyspnea and inspiratory stridor. The cords lie halfway between abduction and adduction. Adductor paralysis occurs in hysteria.

Accessory Nerve (XI Cranial)

The accessory nerve is seldom involved alone but may be associated with other cranial nerve lesions. The most likely problems to involve this nerve are gun and stab wounds to the neck, fractures and dislocations of the cervical vertebrae, surgical operations on the neck, tumors at the base of the brain, aneurysms, poliomyelitis, syringomyelia, amyotrophic lateral sclerosis and neuritis.

To detect damage look for weakness or paralysis of the sternocleidomastoid or trapezius muscles. Paralysis of the sternocleidomastoid causes a flatness on the affected side of the neck, failure of the muscle to stand out on rotation of the neck and loss of muscle strength. You must look for the weakness. Do not expect the posture of the head to be changed.

Paralysis of the trapezius muscle causes drooping and inability to raise the shoulder, weakness in shrugging the shoulders, difficulty in raising the arm above the horizontal, atrophy and flatness of the neck. There may be partial winging of the scapula.

The eleventh cranial nerve is tested by having the patient attempt to move her head toward the midline against resistance (Fig. 8-17). Palpate the tension of the sterno-

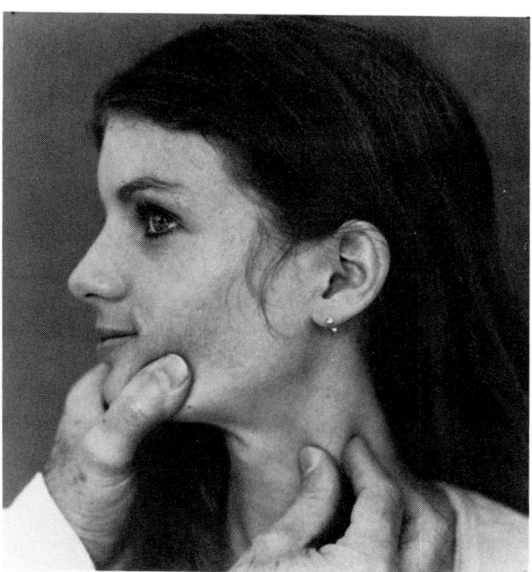

Figure 8-17. The patient attempts to move her head toward the midline against resistance.

cleidomastoid muscle. Ask the patient to elevate (shrug) the shoulders against resistance by your hands (Fig. 8-18).

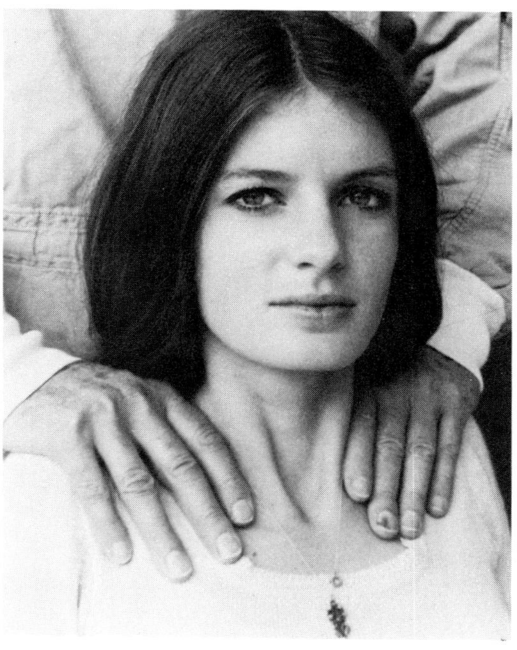

Figure 8-18. The patient elevates her shoulders against resistance.

Hypoglossal Nerve (XII Cranial)

Attempt to distinguish between central and peripheral weakness of the hypoglossal nerve. Central weakness is probably more often associated with a hemiplegia than with other causes. In this instance the tongue deviates to the affected side and there is little atrophy or fasciculations.

Peripheral weakness, on the other hand, is usually associated with many of the same problems as are the IX, X and XI cranial nerves, i.e. syringomyelia, progressive bulbar paralysis, amyotrophic lateral sclerosis, tumors, thrombosis of the anterior spinal artery, poliomyelitis, syphilis, aneurysms, meningitis and neuritis.

In peripheral weakness there is atrophy of the tongue and fasciculations. Look for early atrophy along the edges of the tongue plus fine fasciculation. Later the atrophy is obvious with an actual shrinking of the tongue on the affected side. Detect weakness of the tongue by asking the patient to press her tongue against one cheek and then the other while your hand resists from the outside as you palpate for any weakness. Ask her to stick out her tongue. If the tongue protrudes to one side, the weakness is on that side. Test lingual speech by asking her to repeat "round the ragged rocks the ragged rascal ran."

Because all four nuclei, that is IX, X, XI and XII, are involved in bulbar and pseudobulbar palsies, we will, at this point, discuss the motor neuron diseases—progressive bulbar palsy, progressive muscular atrophy and amyotrophic lateral sclerosis. These three clinical entities usually occur in adulthood or in the aged and are sporadic without any heredity background. The three entities represent subdivisions of one and the same disease. The pathology can best be described as a progressive degeneration of the anterior horn cells, the motor nuclei in the medulla and the upper motor neurons in the spinal cord, brain stem and to a lesser extent the cerebral hemispheres. There are never any sensory symptoms.

In *progressive bulbar palsy* look for weakness and atrophy of the muscles supplied by the bulbar nuclei. The result: atrophy and fibrillation of the tongue and paralysis of phonation, mastication and deglutition. The most important sign is a wasted, fibrillating tongue.

Progressive muscular atrophy is characterized by involvement of the muscles supplied by the anterior horn cells, a result of a degenerative process. Look at the patient's hands. Wasting and weakness usually start in the small muscles of the hand. Fibrillations are a striking and constant feature of the disease. The deep tendon reflexes are preserved until the disease is terminal. The disease runs a progressively downhill course.

Amyotrophic lateral sclerosis represents a combination of one or both of the above diseases. The pathologic change is a degeneration of motor neurons in the spinal cord, medulla and motor cortex. In addition to looking for muscular atrophies and fibrillations, check for exaggerated reflexes, ankle clonus, a pathologic Babinski's sign and spasticity.

Consequently, the fundamental pathology is essentially the same in all types of nuclear amyotrophies, the difference lying in the area of the neuraxis predominantly afflicted by the process—spinal cord, brain stem or both.

These diseases must be differentiated from cervical rib, scalenus syndrome, syringomyelia, cervical cord tumor, syphilitic pachymeningitis, hyperthyroidism, thenar neuritis and superior pulmonary sulcus tremor.

CEREBELLAR TESTS

Asynergia is a lack of coordination between parts that usually work together. To test for it (Fig. 8-19A), ask the patient to extend her arm laterally with index finger pointing. Have her bring her arm through a 45° arc (Fig. 8-19B), touching exactly the tip of her nose with the tip of her finger. Past pointing with eyes open or shut indicates cerebellar disease.

Disdiachokinesia, the inability to make finely coordinated alternating movements can be checked out by having the patient quickly pronate and supinate her hands alternately, similar to rattling a doorknob (Fig. 8-20). A pathologic response is indicated by disorganization of the movements.

To test for dysmetria, ask your patient to close her eyes and then alternately touch some stationary object such as her nose or your finger. Normally this is easily accomplished. Deviations to the left or right or past-pointing indicate either labrythine stimulation or loss of positional sense.

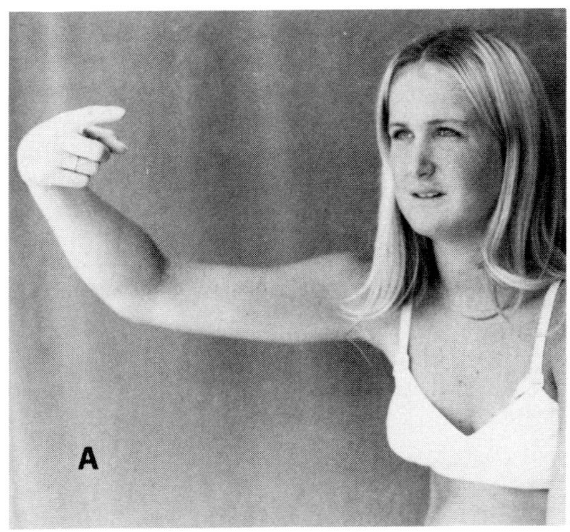

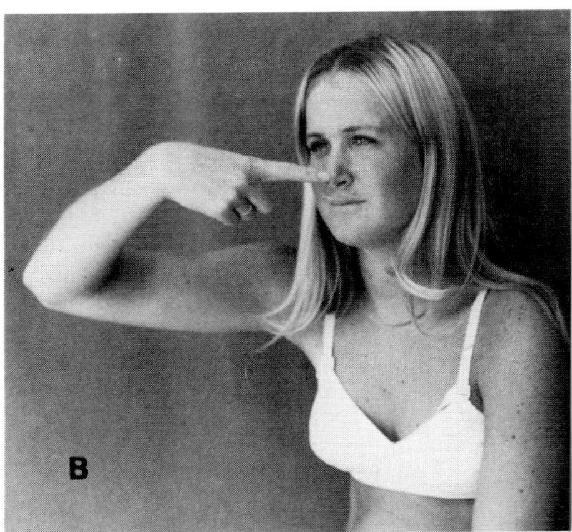

Figure 8-19. *A*, Have the patient extend her arm laterally with index finger pointing. Have the patient bring her arm through a 45° arc, *B*, touching the tip of her nose with the tip of her finger.

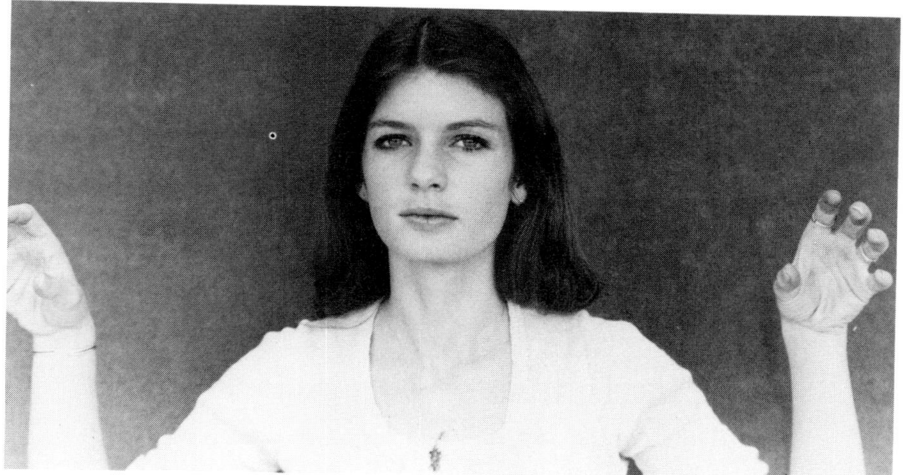

Figure 8-20. Quickly alternating pronation and supination with the hands checks for disdiadochokinesia.

The Stewart-Holmes rebound sign is another test for cerebellar function (Fig. 8-21). Ask the patient to flex her biceps against resistance. Suddenly release her arm. In cerebellar dysfunction, the patient may not be able to control her arm. She may strike herself with her arm or her arm may rebound in several cycles of flexion and extension.

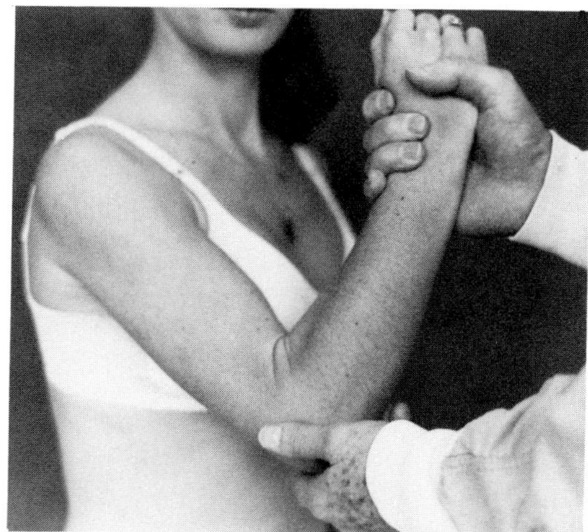

Figure 8-21. Stewart-Holmes rebound sign for cerebellar function.

There are two parts to the heel-to-knee test (Fig. 8-22) for cerebellar and posterior column diseases. First, ask the patient to lift one heel and place it on her opposite knee. This action is jerky and inaccurate in cerebellar disease. Have the patient slide her heel down her leg; watch for tremor. Now have the patient close her eyes to perform the test. In posterior column disease, the

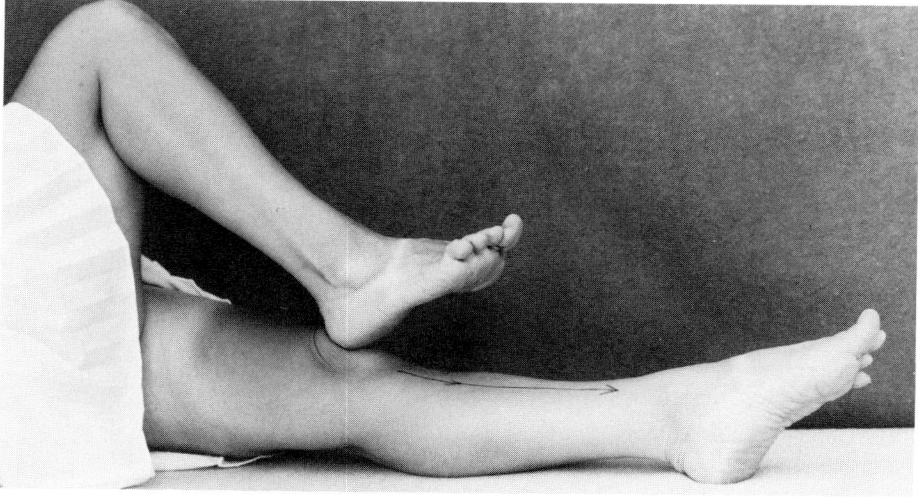

Figure 8-22. Have the patient lift one heel and place it on her opposite knee. As she slides the heel down the skin watch for tremor.

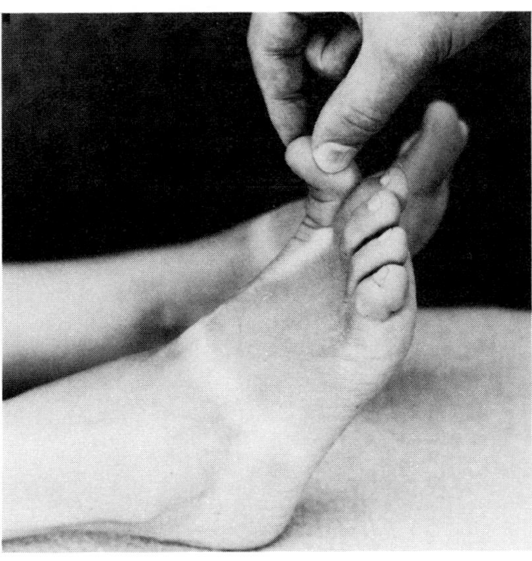

Figure 8-23. Grasp the sides of the patient's toe and alternately flex and extend it.

motions are jerky, the heel slides off the shin and no action tremor is observed.

Test the proprioceptive sense in her toes. Grasp the sides of her toe with your thumb and index finger and alternately flex and extend it (Fig. 8-23). Ask the patient to close her eyes and indicate by word the position of her toe. Refrain from touching the other toes or the dorsal or plantar aspects of the big toe.

EXTRAPYRAMIDAL DISEASE

The pyramidal or corticospinal motor pathway is the main motor pathway for voluntary movement (Fig. 8-24), the other half of the motor system is the extrapyramidal system. There is some fuzziness as to what goes to make up the extrapyramidal system as well as to its function.

It is now generally agreed that the extrapyramidal system is composed of the following: certain parts of the cerebral cortex that have connections with the basal ganglia (a group of large grey masses situated deeply in the brain tissue) and some motor pathways of the brain and spinal cord exclusive of the pyramidal pathways.

The extrapyramidal cortical areas appear to have something to do with the following as determined by stimulation or oblation of certain cortical areas: disturbance of skilled movement, cataleptic type of rigidity, increase in deep reflexes, disability in movements, appearance of pathologic reflexes and some paralysis.

On stimulation of areas, certain stereotyped movements occur such as turning of the head and torsion of the body. Stimulation of other areas causes mouth movements, salivation, chewing and conjugate deviation of the eyes.

Insults to the basal ganglia of the extrapyramidal system cause disorders of muscle tone and movement such as increase in muscle tone, which does not vary during flexion or extension; tremor, which is present at rest, abolished during movement and is rhythmic, occurring six times per sec; slowness of muscular execution; reduced blinking, swallowing and arm swinging; loss of facial expression (in acute chorea the reverse is true); and unwanted movements (chorea). The wrist, ankle and shoulder joints appear to be the earliest and most severely affected.

The *pyramidal system* may be said to deal with the finer adjustments of movement such as performed by the hand and fingers. It is a voluntary system, entirely excitatory. On the other hand, the *extrapyramidal system* is concerned with more stereotyped movements and postural mechanisms in the

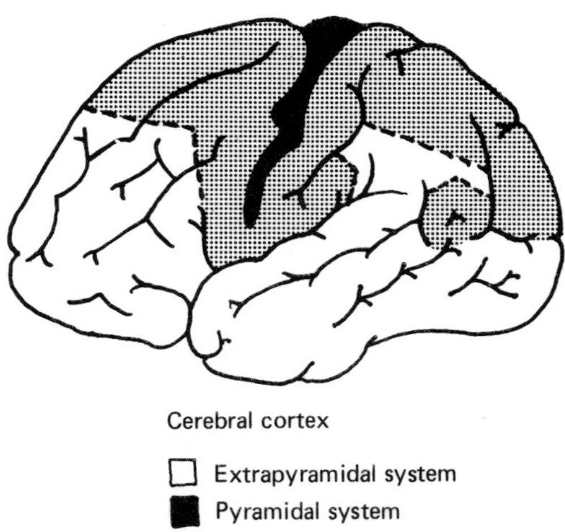

Figure 8-24.

brain stem possibly controlled and modified by the extrapyramidal cortical areas. The functional relationship to the pyramidal system is close; to separate them entirely is nearly impossible.

The diseases of the extrapyramidal system have to do mainly with disorders of movements.

- –paralysis agitans (parkinsonism)
- –Sydenham's chorea (St. Vitus dance)
- –Huntington's chorea
- –hemiballism (hemichorea)
- –symptomatic chorea (unclassified choreas mostly secondary to other diseases)
- –dystonia musculorum deformans (torsion spasm)
- –Wilson's disease (progressive lenticular degeneration)
- –several types of athetosis
- –several indefinite types of extrapyramidal syndromes
- –spasmodic torticollis
- –myoclonias

Huntington's Chorea

This is an adult disease of both sexes. It occurs in the third or fourth decade of life. Suspect the diagnosis when a patient's symptoms are involuntary movements of a fidgety and jerky nature. Grimacing occurs early. Later the arms become clumsy and gait is unsteady and last of all dementia develops. Death occurs approximately 15 years from the start of the disease. It is a hereditary disease. The family physician should be aware of the eugenics of the situation and either counsel the family or refer them for eugenic advice.

Spasmodic Torticollis

You will not as a rule, find this condition to be a diagnostic problem. Rule out eye diseases before treating. Torticollis may be a part of the syndrome of dystonia musculum deformans. It may appear spontaneously or it may follow encephalitis or Parkinson's disease. Watch for a psychoneurotic problem. The application of collars or casts are worthless and should be avoided.

Treatment consists of physiotherapy and a trial of chlorpromazine, meprobamate or reserpine.

Wilson's Disease

This disease, hepatolenticular degeneration, is characterized by degeneration of basal ganglia, cirrhosis of the liver and a brownish ring at the limbus of the cornea.

The disease is a result of increased absorption and/or decreased excretion of copper, which damages the brain, liver and kidney tubules.

Look for this disease in patient's between 15 and 30 years of age. Neurologic symptoms predominant, except in the young where hepatic symptoms appear first. Tremor and rigidity of the limbs are common initial symptoms. The disease is fatal usually within 15 years.

Check serum copper and ceruloplasmin, which is decreased in Wilson's disease. If the urinary excretion of copper is increased, the diagnosis is certain. Kayser-Fleischer rings of the lumbus are also pathognomonic. Suspect the diagnosis in all cases of juvenile cirrhosis and in all cases of disturbances of the basal ganglia.

Penicillamine 1.0 to 2.0 g daily is the treatment of choice. Dietary restriction of copper is important.

Sydenham's Chorea

Sydenham's chorea is an acute disease of the CNS. Suspect the disease by its gradual appearance with irritability, anxiety and occasionally involuntary movements. It is often associated with rheumatic fever; in fact, some consider the disease to be a manifestation of a rheumatic infection. Fortunately the disease is self-limited, running its course in 2 to 3 months. Occasionally purposeless movements will persist for 6 months or longer.

Parkinsonism (Paralysis Agitans)

An attempt should be made to diagnose

parkinsonism in its early stages. Heretofore treatment was unnecessary until the patient needed symptomatic relief. Then little permanent help was given by various anticholinergic drugs. The current trend is to start levodopa therapy as soon as the disease has been diagnosed.

Parkinsonism can be recognized by several extrapyramidal symptoms—rigidity, tremor and slowness of movement.

Rigidity is the most constant feature of the disease and sometimes appears alone. It is first noticable in the face and later in the speech, posture and the patient's movements. Facial expression fades, speech becomes mumbling and monotonous, posture becomes stooped, starting to walk is difficult and when once started a running pace develops. When walking, the patient's arms may hang immobile by his sides. The patient complains of an inability to perform fine finger movements; consequently his writing becomes smaller and illegible. A plastic rigidity is most prominent and is seen early in the neck and shoulders. Detect the rigidity by slow passive flexion and extension of the forearm. A resistance is felt, a sensation as if moving the muscle over a ratchet—the cogwheel sign. The sign is present early and is important to recognize.

Although rigidity of minor degree is nearly always present, tremor is often the first actual complaint. The tremor rate of the disease is about 5 to 6 per sec. Count the tremors per min and divide by 60. It involves the fingers and hands most commonly but finally may involve other parts of the body, especially the arms, head and eyelids. The tremors tend to decrease upon activity and during sleep. Movement abolishes the tremor, but soon after the hand has come to rest the tremor reappears. All tremors are increased by emotional stress, fatigue and anxiety. Watch for the pill-rolling effect in the patient's hands: a rhythmical rubbing between the thumb and fingertips.

Slowness of movement is constant. A long time passes between the desire to act and the initiation of the movement. Watch for this disability as the patient attempts to rise from a chair or attempts to walk or sit down. Extraneous movements such as crossing the legs, gesturing or crossing the arms are lost in parkinsonism.

In the past the syndrome has been classified as to etiology:

- idiopathic (far the most common)
- postencephalitic (has virtually disappeared in recent years)
- arteriosclerotic
- intoxication by manganese and other metals
- carbon monoxide intoxication
- tranquilizers, especially the phenothiazines
- trauma
- intracranial tumors

No longer is there any valid reason for a family physician to wait to use levodopa. It is the most effective agent available today. Don't be too enthusiastic about its effectiveness, however. A third of the patients do not benefit from it or cannot tolerate it. But happily many are benefitted and can continue to work and be useful for years.

Clinicians have advocated several dosage schedules. Most have to do with the rapidity with which the dosage is increased. Possibly a suitable schedule for a family physician would be to start with 250 mg t.i.d. for a total of 750 mg a day. On the eighth day, the dosage is doubled, 500 mg t.i.d. Increase the daily dosage by 750 mg weekly until: the patient receives maximum benefit, develops side effects that prohibit increasing the dosage or the limit of 8 g a day is reached. You may observe changes in the patient's facial expression on 1.5 to 3.5 g per day. But the effective dose is usually around 3 g a day. Most patients can level off at 4 to 5 g a day.

You would be wise to slow up the rate of administration on the first sign of nausea or vomiting with the idea of increasing the rate later. Occasionally, the rate of increase may be as low as 50 mg t.i.d. Some have found that administering the drug seven times a day is more beneficial and results in fewer side effects, but this becomes tedious and unnecessary in most.

Encourage the patient to take the pill or capsule with food or water. Levodopa is tasteless and odorless and may be broken up in the food if necessary. Do not be impatient. Have the patient think in terms of months rather than weeks for improvement. It may require 6 months for the drug to be fully effective. If there is no improvement in 6 months, discontinue the drug. After a year many patients are able to taper off to as much as half or two thirds of the dose and maintain their improvement.

Approximately 25 percent of patients on levodopa therapy experience no side effects at all. All side effects are dose related, are more bothersome at the start of therapy and usually can be controlled by lowering the dosage. None of the side effects are irreversible.

Ask the patient to report gastriontestinal distress, dizziness or lightheadedness on arising, postural hypotension (order elastic stockings), choreiform jerks or restless twitches, insomnia (do not order barbiturates), depression (amitriptyline [Elavil] will help) or harmless brown or reddish urine.

See the patient weekly for the first 6 weeks. Check the blood pressure with the patient standing and while lying down, determine the pulse rate, and do a blood count for leukopenia. After 6 weeks reduce calls to every 2 weeks, and after 6 months see every month. From 6 to 12 months check every 2 months and after one year, every 3 months.

Devise some little test to check the patient's improvement: Have him pick up 10 pennies or open 10 safety pens on each visit and grade his performance. This will help you determine maximum dosage of levodopa.

PYRAMIDAL TRACT DISEASE

The pyramidal tract is synonymous with the corticospinal pathway. It originates in the cells of the cortex and then passes down through the internal capsule, the pons, crosses over in the lower medulla, continues down the cord in the lateral columns, synapsing eventually with the anterior horn cells of the lower motor neuron.

Not all the fibers of the corticospinal or pyramidal tract come from the precentral gyrus. Fibers which originate in the opposite red nucleus, the roof of the midbrain, the brain stem and from the vestibular nucleus have an effect on the anterior horn cell.

Whenever you see a patient who is paralyzed in the face, arm, leg and body, on one side, consider the corticospinal pathway as interrupted on the opposite side of the body *(hemiplegia)*. A *paraplegia* is a paralysis that involves both sides—both arms, or both legs or arms and legs. Paraplegia occurs when both corticospinal pathways are interrupted. If only portions of the corticospinal pathways are diseased or injured, *monoplegia* results. Recognize this by detecting a focal loss of power in the opposite side of the body as you might see in facial weakness, weakness of a hand, an arm or of the face, tongue and arm. A great variety of combinations occurs.

In most instances, monoplegia is a result of disease of the motor cortex. Irritative lesions of the corticospinal pathway produce focal or Jacksonian convulsions.

Interruption of the Pyramidal Pathway

Interruption produces a paralysis involving the opposite face, arm and leg. This paralysis is of the spastic type in contrast to the flaccid paralysis of the lower motor neuron lesion. It involves the arm and leg more than the head, trunk or neck. Occasionally the paralysis is flaccid and, if so, generally transitory. Facial paralysis involves only the lower part of the face. Look for a slowness or weakness in retraction of the mouth and/or a flattening of the normal angulation of the mouth. Ask the patient to say "ah" and the palate will pull to the healthy side. The tongue when paralyzed pushes over to the weak side.

There will be overactive deep tendon reflexes including the biceps, triceps, patellar and Achilles, possibly resulting from a release of the inhibitory effects of the pyramidal influence on the anterior horn cells. Generally speaking the tendon reflexes are increased in proportion to the spasticity of the muscles. Check for ankle clonus.

Cutaneous reflexes are lost, especially the abdominals on the paralyzed side, and pathologic reflexes develop. The most im-

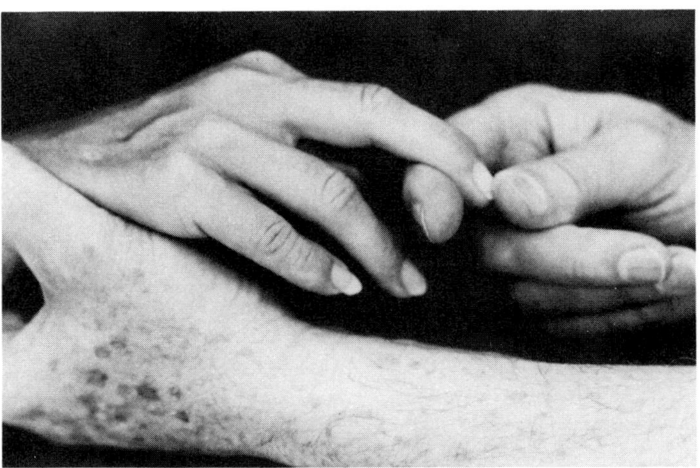

Figure 8-25. Hoffmann's sign for pyramidal tract disease.

portant pathologic reflex is the Babinski sign. A pathologic Babinski always means corticospinal disease no matter what other combinations of weakness, paralysis or deep and superficial reflexes may exist.

Tests for Reflexes

Pathologic Reflexes

To determine Hoffmann's sign for pyramidal tract disease, pronate the patient's hand. Allow her middle finger to rest on your index finger. Flick the terminal phalanx with your thumb while you watch her thumb (Fig. 8-25). If she has pyramidal disease, her thumb will flex and adduct.

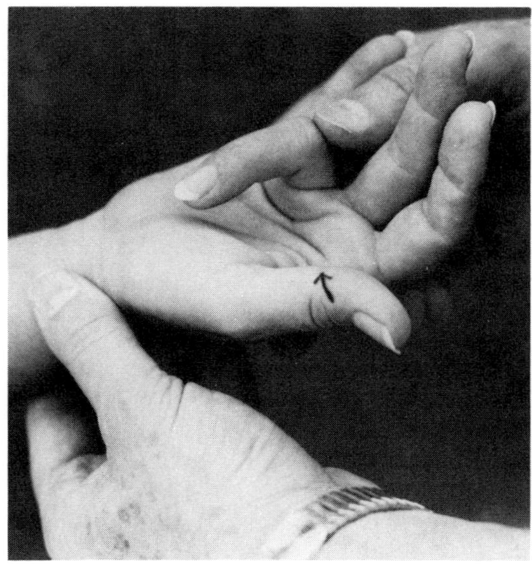

Figure 8-26. Testing Mayer's reflex for pyramidal tract disease.

In Mayer's reflex for pyramidal tract disease, the patient's hand is supinated and her ring finger flexed at the proximal joint. Normally the thumb will flick, adducting and flexing (Fig. 8-26). When the patient has pyramidal tract disease there is no response from the thumb.

Deep reflexes are hyperactive in pyramidal tract disease distal to the lesion. Hyperactive reflex will produce clonus (a hyperactive response to the stretch reflex) because the central inhibition is lost. Lift the patient's knee into slight flexion. Grasp her toes and jerk her foot into dorsiflexion, maintaining the floot inslight tension (Fig. 8-27). Flexion alternating with extension may last as long as tension is held or it may die out.

To establish Babinksi's sign for pyramidal tract disease, stroke the patient's foot with a blunt point along the lateral border curving inward toward the ball of her big toe (Fig. 8-28). A physiologic response is flexion of the big toe followed by flexion of her other toes. A pathologic response is a dorsiflexion of her big toe followed by fanning of all her toes and dorsiflexion of her ankle, knee and thigh.

Grasp reflex is a test for disease of the premotor cortex. Perform the test by placing your index finger into the patient's palm be-

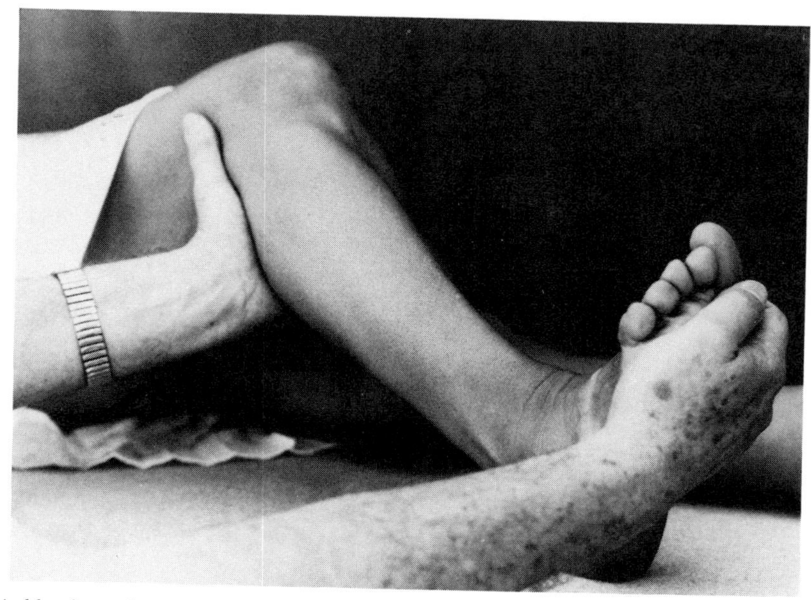

Figure 8-27. Ankle clonus in pyramidal tract disease.

tween her thumb and index finger. Have her grasp your finger as you tickle her palm. If the test is positive, the patient will not be able to let go.

Deep Reflexes of Upper Extremities

The pectoralis reflex checks out the reflex arcs of C_5 to T_1 (Fig. 8-29). The lower cervical arcs, C_7 and C_8, are checked by testing the triceps reflex. Figure 8-30A shows the usual method and Figure 8-30B the alternate method.

The biceps and the brachioradialis reflexes determine the integrity of arcs C_5 and C_6 (Fig. 8-31). Normal response is elbow flexion and supination of the forearm. For the integrity of arcs C_6 and C_7, check the pronator reflex (Fig. 8-32).

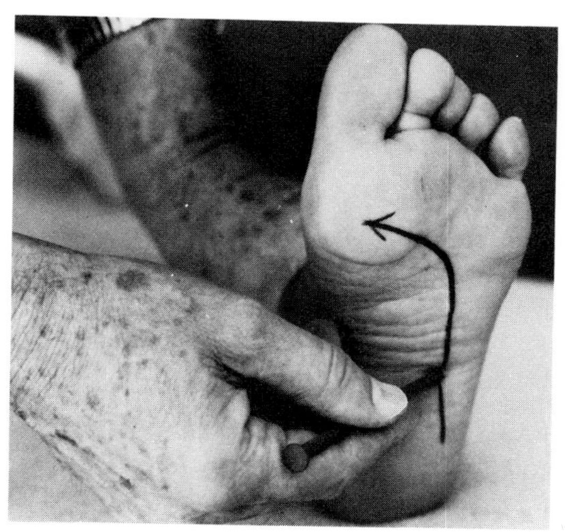

Figure 8-28. Determining Babinski's sign for pyramidal tract disease.

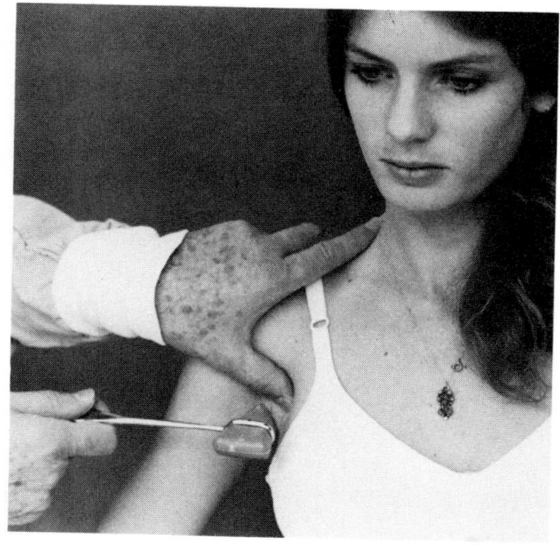

Figure 8-29. Check out the reflex arcs of C_5 to T_1.

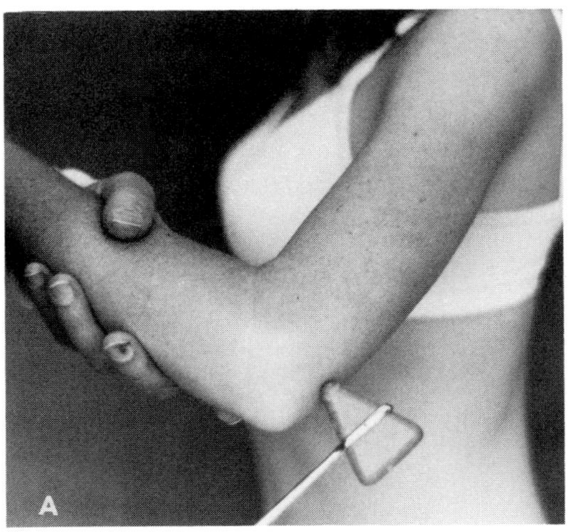

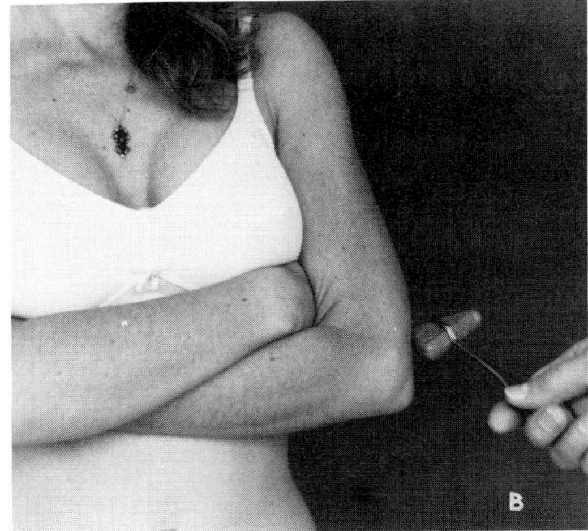

Figure 8-30. *A*, Usual method and, *B*, Alternate method of testing the lower cervival arcs, C_7 and C_8.

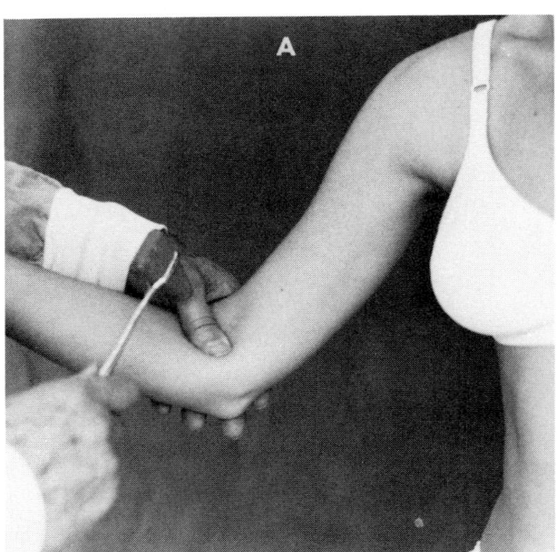

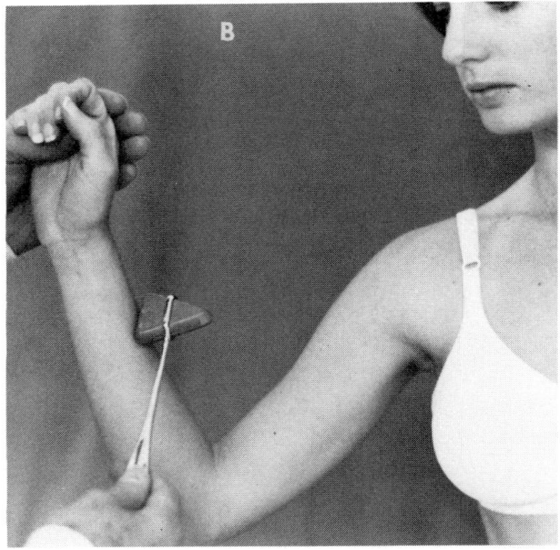

Figure 8-31. *A*, The biceps and *B*, brachioradialis reflexes determine the integrity of arcs C_5 and C_6.

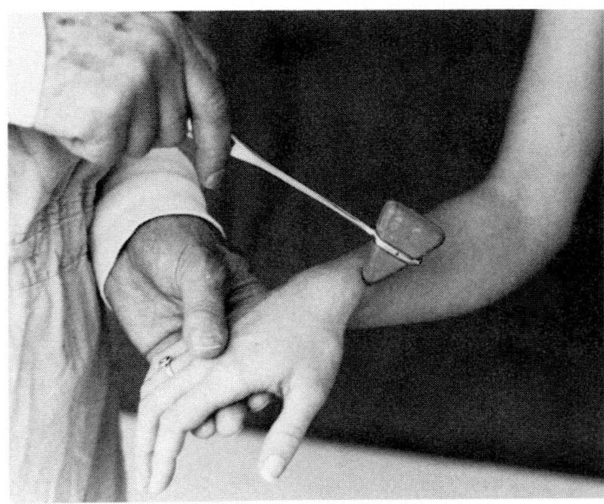

Figure 8-32. Check the pronator reflex for the integrity of arcs C_6 and C_7.

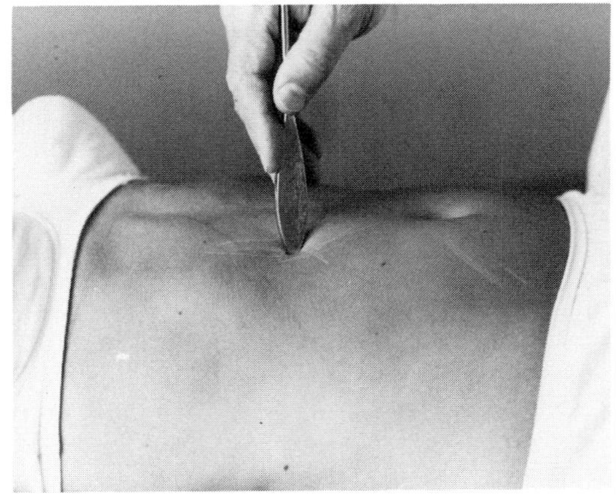

Figure 8-33. Superficial abdominal skin reflexes. Touch the skin lightly.

Superficial and Deep Reflexes of the Abdomen and Lower Extremities

Superficial abdominal skin reflexes are elicited by lightly stroking the skin as indicated in Figure 8-33. Test T_5 to T_8 by testing the upper abdominal skin reflex, T_9 to T_{11}, by midabdominal skin reflex and T_{11} and T_{12} by the lower abdominal skin reflex. Deep abdominal reflexes are tested as shown in Figure 8-34.

Eliciting the knee jerk tests the integrity of the reflex arcs L_2 to L_4. Tapping the petallar tendon causes an extension of the knee. Keep your left hand on the quadriceps femoris and palpate for contraction of the muscle even when the knee does not extend (Fig. 8-35).

Elicit the adductor magnus reflex by tapping the adductor magnus tendon just proximal to its insertion on the medial epicondyle of the femur (Fig. 8-36). Normally the thigh adducts. If response is absent suspect defective reflex arcs L_2 to L_4.

Reflex arcs L_4 to S_2 can be tested by eliciting the hamstring reflex. Check this reflex with the patient supine and her knee flexed about 90°. Tap your fingers, which compress the hamstring tendons (Fig. 8-37). A normal response is flexion of the knee and contrac-

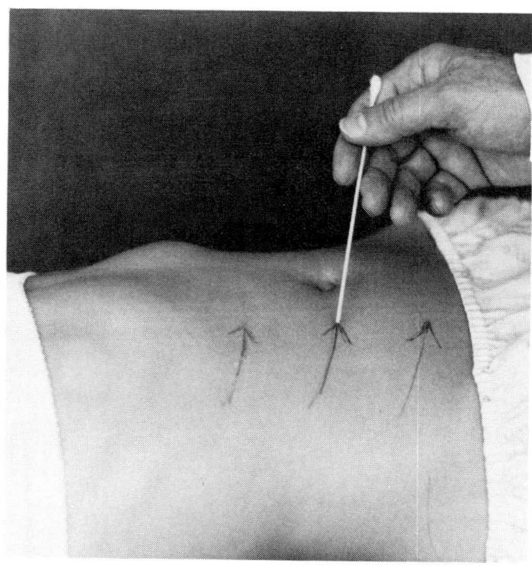

Figure 8-34. Deep abdominal reflexes are elicited by heavy pressure.

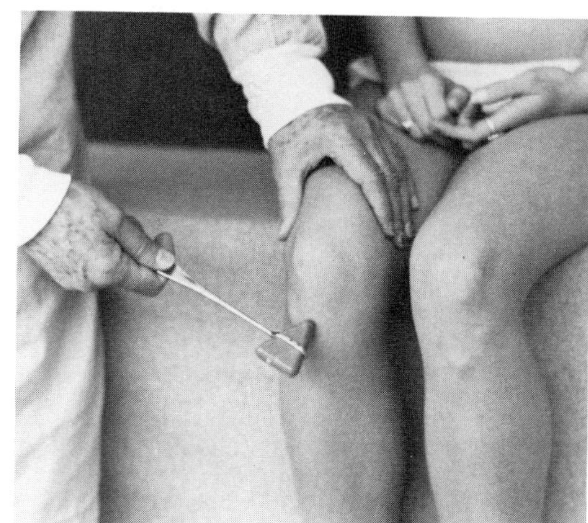

Figure 8-35. Knee jerk test.

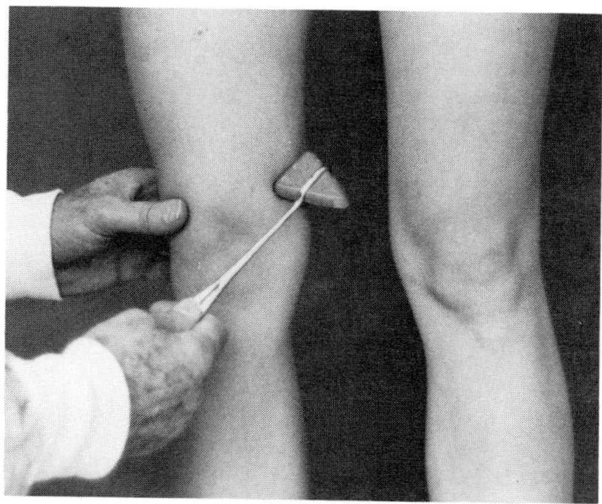

Figures 8-36. Tap the adductor magnus tendon to elicit the adductor magnus reflex.

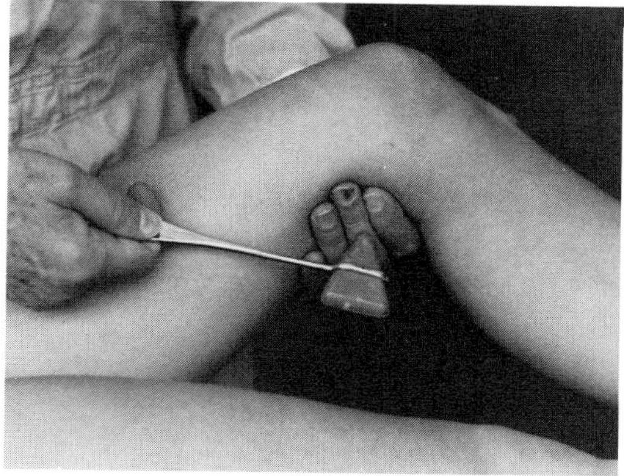

Figure 8-37. Elicit the hamstring reflex to check arcs L_4 to S_2.

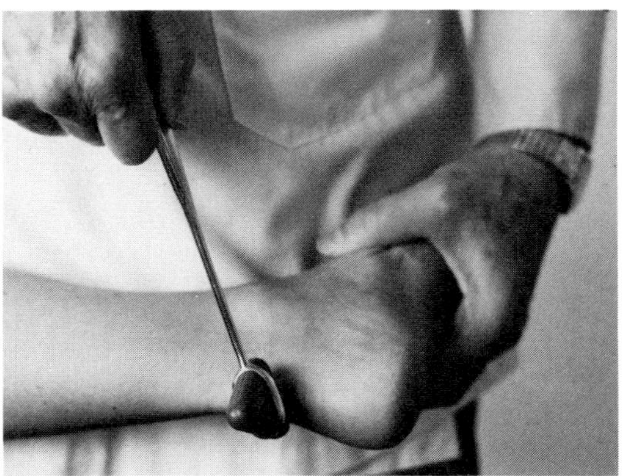

Figure 8-38. Test the Achilles reflex for integrity of the reflex center at L_5 to S_2.

tion of the medial mass of the hamstring muscle.

Test the Achilles reflex for integrity of the reflex center at L_5 to S_2. Testing can be done while the patient is sitting with legs dangling or while she is in a supine position. Grasp and dorsiflex her foot with your left hand. Tap the tendon directly with the broad end of the hammer (Fig. 8-38). Normal response is plantar flexion.

Hoover's sign of hysteria is used to differentiate an hysterical from an organic paralysis. Hold each heel in the palm of your hand with your hands resting on the bed and ask your patient to raise her paralyzed leg (Fig. 8-39). There is no downward pressure of the unaffected foot if the cause is hysteria. However, if the cause is organic, the unaffected foot will press down against your hand.

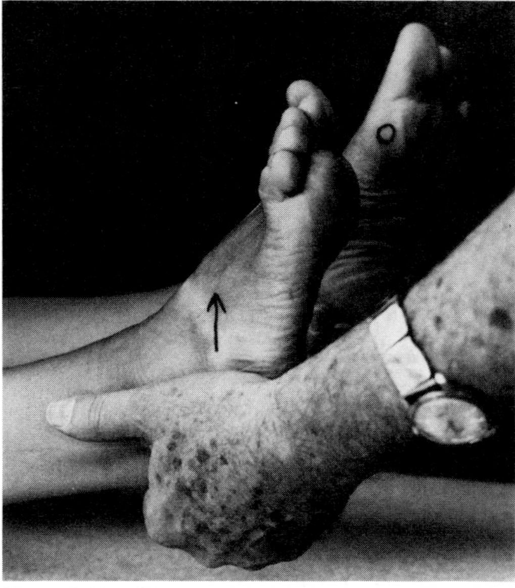

Figure 8-39. Hoover's sign to differentiate an hysteric from an organic paralysis.

Strokes

Strokes (cerebrovascular accidents, CVA). commonly interfere with the proper functioning of the pyramidal pathway. A stroke is defined as a condition in which an acute local abnormality of the blood supply to the brain produces local brain dysfunction or damage.

When confronted with this problem, consider first whether the symptoms were caused by ischemia or by hemorrhage. What you do depends on this decision. There are no physical signs to distinguish between the two. Your opinion must be based on the history, so listen carefully.

Thrombosis of a cerebral artery, occurring on the basis of atherosclerosis, is the single most common cause of a stroke, accounting for more than 50 percent of all cases.

Sites of cerebral artery thromboses in order of occurrence are:

–several small arteries (by far the most common)
–middle cerebral artery (one fifth of the cases)
–basilar artery (one tenth of cases)
–internal carotid artery
–posterior cerebral artery
–anterior cerebral artery

In cases of infarction of the carotid system a third of the patients will have had intermittent episodes lasting 5 to 30 minutes previous to the main attack. The onset is over minutes or hours and is painless. The patient may have hypertension, diabetes or atherosclerosis. Generally there is no loss of consciousness. Focal symptoms may vary from a monoplegia to a hemiplegia, hemianesthesia, homonymous hemianopsia or an aphasia if the dominant hemisphere is involved. Consider the possibility of a dysarthria. If a transitory ischemic attack lasts longer than 12 hours, some permanent disability will result.

One physical sign which should tip you off to involvement of the carotid artery system is the finding of a bruit over one or both carotid arteries. Do not be misled by considering a unilateral bruit as being on the diseased side. The opposite side may be occluded and, consequently, no bruit is heard there while extra blood being forced into the opposing artery may cause a bruit.

Another useful diagnostic technique to detect early carotid artery disease is ophthalmodynamometry. This is usually done by an ophthalmologist or someone accustomed to the procedure. A finding of decreased central retinal artery pressure in one eye indicates a decreased vascular supply to that side.

An infarction involving the vertebral-basilar system may occur with symptoms indistinguishable from carotid artery infarction, but attempt to identify it with the characteristics that follow. There are warning attacks in about two thirds of the patients. The warnings consist of the following characteristics: diplopia, weakness and numbness alternating from side to side with different attacks, dysphagia and dysarthria, vertigo and blurred vision or bilateral homonymous hemianopsia and no physical signs between attacks. The actual infarction may begin over a period of minutes or hours. Focal neurologic signs begin step-wise or in a stuttering manner. Signs are ocular rotational defects, visual field defects, nystagmus, dysarthria, dysphagia, monoparesia or hemiplegia often involving both sides and numbness involving both sides.

When confronted with this type of patient, give consideration to the possibility of an infarction caused by an embolism. The history includes

- –absence of prodromal manifestations in most cases
- –sudden onset of cerebrovascular symptoms without pain (within seconds or a few minutes)
- –severe focal neurologic symptoms
- –source of emboli is usually in the heart
- –embolic phenomena elsewhere in the body (extremities, lungs, kidneys, spleen, etc.)
- –fairly swift improvement in some cases

Cardiac arrhythmias, valvular heart disease and silent myocardial infarctions play important roles in cerebral embolism. For this reason as well as others, order an ECG on every stroke patient.

Physical signs usually associated with the source of the embolus are heart disease with auricular fibrillation, signs of subacute bacterial endocarditis, trauma with fat embolism and pulmonary lesions.

Focal signs are hemiparesis to hemiplegia, hemianesthesia, homonymous hemianopsia and aphasia if the dominant hemisphere is involved.

Attempt to distinguish the above-described attacks of infarction from strokes of hemorrhagic origin. As indicated previously, treatment of the acute attack depends in great measure on this differentiation. The most common cause of intracerebral hemorrhage is hypertension. Subacute bacterial endocarditis occasionally will do the same.

Sites of intracerebral hemorrhage in order of frequency are:

- –basal ganglia (by far most common site)
- –cerebrum
- –cerebellum
- –pons

Not all hemorrhages are intracerebral. Some occur in the subarachnoid space and are most frequently caused by a congenital aneurysm. Eight-five percent of the aneurysms arise from the internal carotid at the origin of the posterior communicating artery, at the first bifurcation of the middle cerebral artery or at the bifurcation of the internal carotid into the middle and anterior cerebral arteries.

The most common cause of all intracranial hemorrhages is trauma. This can occur subdurally or epidurally. And do not forget the possibility of the rare arteriovenous abnormalities.

The history of intracerebral hemorrhage varies somewhat from other kinds of strokes. The onset is generally sudden while the patient is involved in some activity. Generally there is a severe headache but, if not, at least the patient complains of head discomfort. Consciousness is altered. There is a rapid progression of focal symptoms to hemiparesis and hemiplegia. Loss of movement in all extremities may occur or the signs and symptoms of a decerebrate rigidity appear. Hypertension is present and may be severe. Cerebrospinal fluid is bloody in 75 percent of the cases.

In your differential diagnosis consider the following possibilities: brain tumor, subdural hematoma, epidural hematoma, brain abscess, meningitis, encephalitis, postictal states, metabolic defects and coma, convulsive disorders, Meniere's disease, syncope, multiple sclerosis or hysteria.

Treatment

In all kinds of strokes give consideration to the following supportive measures:

- Keep the airway open (an occasional tracheotomy may be needed).
- Consider preventive administration of antibiotics.
- Watch for a fluid inbalance (decide early on the type of nutrition needed).
- Write definite orders for skin care.
- Consider the most appropriate bladder and bowel care.
- Keep the patient in head-up position.
- Early (first day) physiotherapy.
- Correct faulty cardiac output, hypotension, etc.
- For the acute complete stroke, maintain normotensive blood pressure at pre-infarct levels, or 10 mm above if cerebral hemorrhage is excluded.
- Avoid sedation and prolonged sleep.

Use vasodilating agents in treatment of infarction not resulting from embolus. Five percent carbon dioxide may be inhaled at 10 min intervals for 10 min for first 24 hr. Consider the administration of papaverine, nicotinic acid or intravenous histamine. All are safe but not very effective. Stellate ganglion block is not used much anymore. Anticoagulants are definitely of value in slow strokes, transit focal ischemic attacks and recurrent thromboembolisms. Because of the stuttering start of infarctions in the vertebral-basilar system, anticoagulation is especially indicated. In one study, 58 percent of the patients died without anticoagulation while only 8.5 percent of those receiving an anticoagulation drug died. Use heparin intravenously or as a continuous drip for rapid action. For long term treatment, switch to coumadin or dicumarol. Monitor appropriately with either the Lea and White or prothrombin blood checks. Be very careful in selecting cases for anticoagulation. You must be absolutely certain the pathology is not caused by a hemorrhage. If in doubt, don't give an anticoagulant. It is better to miss a few thrombotic cases than to administer anticoagulants while the patient is hemorrhaging. There is no certain way to tell who should receive and who should not receive anticoagulation therapy.

Treatment of intracerebral hemorrhage is surgical, if possible.

Treatment of infarction caused by embolus is basically similar to infarction. Treat the source of the embolus, administer vasodilating drugs and consider anticoagulation.

If you are called to see a patient who is in a coma, possibly from a stroke, do the following:

- establish an adequate airway
- maintain blood pressure
- draw blood for glucose, BUN and electrolyte determination
- administer glucose or lactated Ringers
- check respiration for Cheyne-Strokes or apneustic breathing
- check the pupils
- look for flaccid paralysis on the involved side and a decrease in deep reflexes
- take the blood pressure in the legs to rule out aortic coarctation in the hypertensive patient
- listen for bruits over the carotids, vertebrals, supraclavicular areas and skull

- –order skull x-rays for fracture or a shift in the pineal body
- –do a lumbar puncture for blood, pressure, culture, protein content and a serological test
- –ophthalmodynamometry for pressure determination in the internal carotid artery
- –electroencephalography
- –brain scanning
- –echoencephalography for midline shifts or to demonstrate subdural or intracerebral mass lesions

Apneustic breathing usually accompanies low pontine disease whereas irregular or ataxic breathing results from medullary dysfunction.

Bilaterally fixed dilated pupils are due to severe cerebral hypoxia or midbrain or bilateral third nerve compression. A unilateral dilated pupil indicates a mass in the supratentorial region, such as a tumor, hematoma or large infarct with swelling. Pinpoint pupils indicate pontine lesions in absence of opiate intoxication. A unilateral small pupil associated with Horner's syndrome should cause a search for occlusion of the posterior inferior cerebellar or vertebral arteries. Conjugate deviation of the eyeballs is toward the affected side in destructive lesions of the frontal lobe and away from the affected side in irritative lesions.

In strokes, look for flaccid paralysis and a decrease in deep relfexes on the involved side. Spasticity and hyperreflexia do not develop until hours or days after the acute attack. Early spasticity should lead you to suspect a tumor or subdural hematoma.

Patients who die within the first week following a cerebrovascular accident are more likely to die because of bleeding into the cerebrum, the brain stem or the ventricular or subarachnoid spaces. Patients who die after the first week are more likely to die of infarction or thrombi; their deaths are much more likely to be associated with pneumonia, pulmonary emboli, aspiration pneumonia, peptic ulcers, acute or chronic pyelonephritis, thyroiditis or decubitus ulcers.[1]

PREVENTION. The main goal in stroke care is to prevent a completed stroke by treating the progressive stroke or transient ischemic attacks. Recognizing the early signs and symptoms is the most important step in proper treatment. Consider that arterial insufficiency may be caused by obstruction of the blood flow in the carotid system. In these cases an angiogram can be done to determine whether corrective carotid surgery is indicated.

Transient ischemic attacks last a few seconds, several minutes or, in a few instances, hours. The usual duration, however, is 2 to 10 minutes. Each attack resembles the previous one. The symptoms begin in the same part of the body. The area affected at the onset of the attack usually shows the most neurologic deficiency and is the last part to return to normal. The symptoms of the transient ischemic attack characterize the final deficit that occurs in the completed stroke.

There is evidence that a program of prevention can be built on detecting those patients in your practice who have had transient cerebral ischemia (TCI). In screening patients over 40 years of age search for evidence of the following neurologic deficiencies:

- –transient limb paralysis
- –disorders of speech
- –sensory losses
- –visual deficits or diplopia
- –loss of consciousness
- –dizziness
- –drop attacks

In one study, approximately one fifth of the patients having TCI developed a complete stroke or died of ischemic heart disease during the following 3 to 5-year period.[2]

Symptoms of transient ischemic attacks and strokes vary according to the vessel or system involved (Table 8-3).

Thirty to forty percent of strokes develop in association with arteriosclerotic plaques localized in the internal carotid artery near the common carotid artery bifurcation. Often these lesions can be removed surgically. If these extracranial lesions could be

Table 8-3. Symptoms of Transient Ischemic Attacks by Arteries or Systems Involved

Internal carotid	*Middle cerebral*	*Posterior cerebral*
Weakness†	Weakness†	Homonymous hemianopia
Numbness†	Numbness†	Scintillating scotoma
Dysphasia	Tingling†	
Transient blurring or blindness‡	Dysphasia	
	Homonymous hemianopia	

Anterior cerebral	*Basilar-vertebral**
Weakness in legs†	Vertigo
Numbness in leg†	Mono-, hemi- or quadri-plegia
Reflex incontinence	Numbness§
Confusion	Diplopia (blurring or scotoma)
	Staggring or ataxic gait
	Dysphasia Dysarthria
	Deafness
	Temporary confusion or loss of memory

* Usually bilateral
† Opposite side
‡ Diseased side
§ Either side or alternating

detected and remedied prior to the stroke, 40 percent of the annual 200,000 deaths from stroke could be prevented.

The family physician has an important role in the prevention of acute strokes. He is in the position to be the first to recognize transient cerebral ischemia, minor neurologic stigmata and ischemic amaurosis. When patients exhibit such symptoms plus carotid bruit, consider having the patient studied for a carotid endarterectomy. In one institution the mortality rate over a 12 year period was only 1.4 percent, a safe enough procedure considering its benefits. Patients who have had an acute stroke are less favorable candidates for endarterectomy.[3]

Arteriography is the procedure of choice in selecting candidates for surgical correction. It is the family physician's responsibility to find the patients who might benefit by arteriography. A reliable sign is the identification of a bruit over the bifurcation of the common carotid artery in the neck. A bruit is usually due to a marked stenosis of the artery, especially in the older patient. One cheerful note regarding extracranial artery disease: stenosis is four times as common as complete occlusion and consequently more likely to correction. A third of stenotic lesions occur at the bifurcation of the common carotid, a fifth at the origin of the vertebral and only 4 percent in the middle cerebral artery. Operative treatment does not benefit the completed stroke and is best limited to recurring attacks with mild residuals and evidence of stenotic lesions. For the incomplete stroke, observe paresis for 12 hours: if it increases treat the same as a complete stroke; if it decreases give no further treatment.

Use anticoagulants for the progressive stroke, if hemorrhage has been excluded.

For recurrent stroke, give a mixture of 5 percent carbon dioxide and 95 percent oxygen for 5 min every 15 min, to shorten the attacks and anticoagulants for 6 mo for long term prevention. It is in these cases that you might consider surgery.

For the asymptomatic or incompletely recovered patient, try a low caloric, low cholesterol diet and have the patient avoid prolonged sleep and sedation.

Rehabilitation

Commence rehabilitation immediately after the cerebrovascular accident. Aim your first nursing orders at preventing decubiti and contractures.

Ask the nurses to turn the patient every 2 hours and check the skin for redness. Unless the patient's position is changed every 2 hours, deformities will begin. Help the staff develop a system of communication with the aphasic but alert patient. Request that the patient be fed from the good side and that he attempt to feed himself. For the alert patient, place a calendar and clock on a bedside table positioned on his good side. Open the curtains to allow the patient to orient himself to the time of day.

Proper positioning is extremely important because the result of poor positioning can take years to correct and, in many cases, may never be corrected. Poor positioning begins to take its toll immediately following the stroke. If any joint stays in one position too long, the muscles will atrophy and the joints will stiffen and may never return to normal.

When patients are in the side-lying position (Fig. 8-40), insist on the following: The use of a small, flat pillow to keep the patient's neck straight. Straighten the shoulders into good body alignment. Prevent pull on the shoulder and support the upper arm by placing a folded pillow under the arm. Maintain the patient's wrist in an extended position and place the hand around a folded washcloth with the thumb opposing the fingers. Straighten the lower leg to prevent contracture of the knee. Place the unaffected foot against a footboard to prevent "dropped" foot. Protect the ankle with a sheepskin pad. Place the upper leg on a thick pillow to prevent hip-joint strain.

Check for the following when patients are in the supine position (Fig. 8-41): Position the patient so his feet are against the footboard of the bed to prevent dropped foot (Fig. 8-42). Place the trochanter roll next to the body between hips and knees. Point the knee cap toward the ceiling. Use a flat pillow to straighten the neck and place a pillow under the arm to abduct the arm. Position a flat pillow under the calves to position legs and knees and place a rolled towel in the patient's hand to keep the wrist extended.

Most hospitals will have a hemiplegia kit available from central supply. These kits include cones for hand positioning, heel protectors, trochanter rolls, footboards and posterior molded splints for night.

Start bowel and bladder training as needed.

Order that all joints be put through their gross range of motion each day, preferably during bathing time. Begin teaching the patient early to exercise his own extremities by himself. Don't allow the patient to become increasingly dependent; don't do for him what he can do for himself.

Attempt to get the patient up in a chair within 3 to 4 days. Transferring the patient from bed to chair or wheelchair requires practice. Start by rolling the chair to the patient's unaffected side. When seated in the chair, examine the patient's balance. Support the affected side. If the patient has lost his sense of balance, seat him on the side of the bed. Have him rest his good hand on the bed and lean on it for support. He will tend to fall toward the affected side. Pillows may be used to support him in a wheelchair. If the above is not practical, have a family member stand in front of the patient and push him back into position as needed. Ask

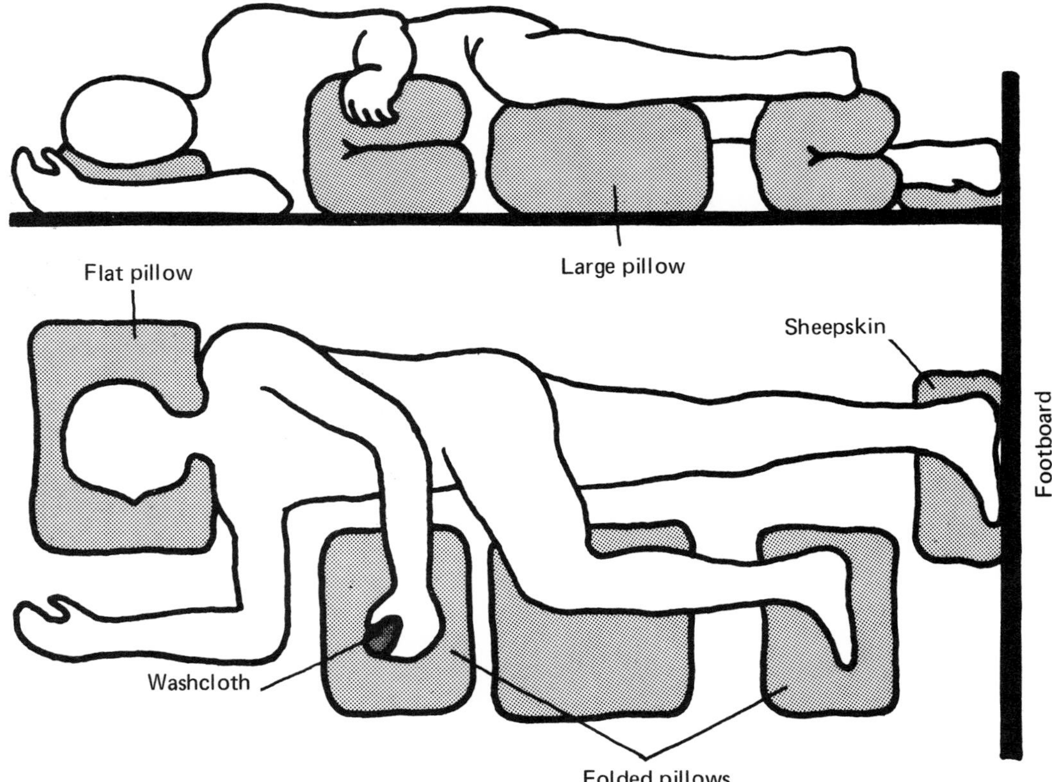

Figure 8-40. Note the important points with the patient in the side-lying position.

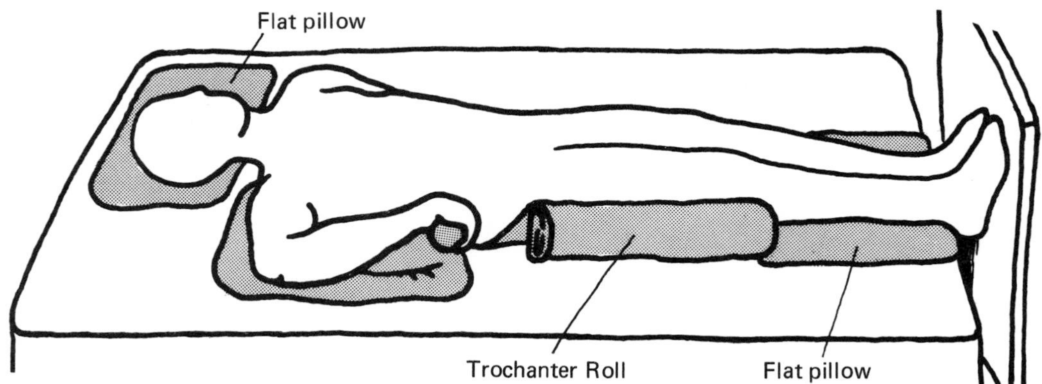

Figure 8-41. Note the important points with the patient in the supine position.

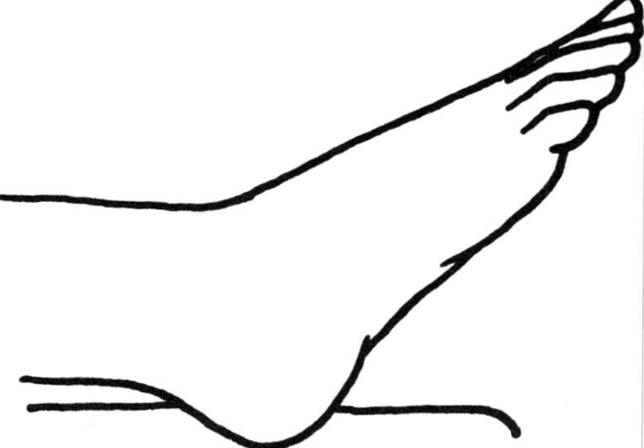

Figure 8-42. Improper positioning of foot. Patients who are allowed to lie in bed with their feet in a "dropped" position may not be able to stand or walk again following recovery from a stroke.

the patient to practice sitting one-half to one hour b.i.d. If the patient continues to fall to one side, have an ophthalmologist examine him for a hemianopia or a disturbance in verticality, wherein the patient does not see objects in their true vertical position.

Order active-assistive exercises. The patient is asked to contract a weakened muscle to the best of his ability. A therapist or family member then moves the extremity passively to complete the unfinished range of motion. Repeat the exercise several times during a 15 to 20 minute exercise period, preferably several times daily. Encourage the patient to assist by using his unaffected arm or leg to carry the weak side through its range of motion. Teach him to move in bed by reaching over the weak side and grasping the side rails for leverage. Have him practice sit-balancing by pulling himself up with the aid of a trapeze bar or a knotted cloth or sheet attached to the end of the bed.

As the acute phase passes, evaluate in more detail the patient's disability. Therapists usually classify the stroke patient as follows:

–*Independent* if the patient performs activities alone in a reasonable time. The patient should feel confident alone and initiate essential activities.
–*Supervised* if he requires verbal assistance.
–*Assisted* if he requires the assistance of one person to perform essential activities.
–*Unable* if he requires the help of more than one person.

Other evaluations which you or the therapist should undertake are an estimation of the patient's cerebration and motivation and, consequently, his ability to cooperate, his ability to stand, walk and transfer to a commode, his equipment needs and his speech.

How to you decide whether a patient has the mental capacity to learn? A patient who has bowel incontinence usually has extensive brain damage and will probably have trouble learning. Global aphasia prevents the patient from understanding what is said to him and, consequently, he will be unable to learn. Loss of memory, lack of judgment, disorientation and lack of motivation are other signs of loss of mental capacity. In the absence of these clinical signs, the patient, even with extensive residual disabilities, may be amenable to limited training. If he can learn to perform some of his self-care activities, it may be possible for him to remain at home rather than be placed in an institution.

The family physician should be able to set realistic rehabilitation goals. First, remember, some patients will continue to improve for 6 months—a few will take 12 months. Evaluate his sense of balance, his muscle power and his ability to coordinate before a patient attempts to walk. He must be able to stand upright, to resist the effect of gravity, to flex and extend the hip and to move one leg at a time in a forward direction.

Evaluate the patient in a standing position. If he requires two people to keep him standing, discontinue further standing exercises. If one person can keep him erect, even though somewhat shaky and unbalanced, continue to have him practice standing. Teach the patient how to stand erect by pushing against a solid object with his good side. Again, someone can stand in front of him and push him back erect as he tends to veer or fall toward his bad side.

Then have the patient stand holding onto a chair or other solid support and practice raising one leg and then the other as in stepping. If you find the patient's knee is unstable and he is unable to support his weight, order a long leg brace or a Handy-Standies knee cage to stabilize the knee. A tibial strap, which can be obtained from major suppliers, will help the patient walk if his foot drops. Gait training consists in teaching the patient to rest his weight on his good leg, then when set to bring his weak leg forward and finally drag his good leg up to it. As the patient improves, other methods may be suggested.

A short leg brace may be needed for the patient with a weak ankle, either with the heel turned out or in and with or without foot drop. Many times a brace can be used to stabilized a weak knee. For long term dorsiflexion, a short leg spring brace is best. If the ankle is spastic or is limited in motion by a shorted heel cord, use a short leg stop-brace. If he has weak quadriceps, brace the leg with a double Klenzak ankle joint.

If the arm hangs down as dead weight, order a Rancho, bucket or cuff webbing sling for support. If the patient has web space contractures, a cock-up or outrigger splint is useful. If he has flexion contractures, use a pancake splint. If the patient has hand and arm disability, have the patient transfer small objects from one pile to another or place them in a cup. Teach him to lift objects with this thumb and index finger, then thumb and middle finger and finally the thumb and little finger.

The patient with moderately severe speech handicaps will recover to a predicted level of communication within 6 months if he has an interested family, is medically stable and has no major physical disability.

A patient will not recover well or will recover slowly or fail to reach his potential if his family is uninterested, he is agitated or depressed over his disability or there is severe involvement in all areas of communication.

Every effort should be made to prevent painful limitation of motion in the shoulder. Daily range of motion exercises should start immediately and continue unabated. Teach patients with good rehabilitation potential to use the reciprocal pulleys so the good arm can help exercise the weak one. If good physical therapy is available and the shoulder continues to freeze up, consider surgery. This consists of resecting about 1 inch of the musculotendinous junction of the subscapularis muscle where it overlies the anterior capsule of the shoulder joint.

The elbow is another joint which often becomes flexed and contracted. A patient, who is otherwise in good condition but has elbow contraction which affects his walking and posture, may have his elbow flexion reduced by transecting the brachialis muscle or elongating the tendon of the biceps and brachialis muscles.

Many patients with upper extremity paralysis also show sensory losses, i.e. position sense or discrete object identification in the hands. If a patient still shows major impairment in sensation 3 months after his stroke, it is likely that the sensory defect will be permanent. No matter how much motor function he has left, this sensory loss will eventually cause a loss of hand function. In this event, attempt to teach the patient how to use the good hand for self-care.

The most common disability which follows a CVA is a calf muscle weakness resulting in an inverted and plantar flexed position of the foot. This is seen especially when the patient walks and may cause tripping and falling. If the muscle spasticity is of moderate degree, order a short leg brace. A double upright brace with a limited range ankle joint will also give stability to the weak ankle.

Focus your attention on exercises and aids designed to help the patient learn to walk, talk, dress, eat, use the toilet and transfer from bed to chair. The best approach is to determine as soon as possible the specific goals the patient can reach. Then call upon the visiting nurse or physical, occupational or speech therapists to work with the patient. If such professionals are not available, instruct a family member to teach and exercise the patient.

Reappraise the patient's progress occasionally and set new goals if indicated.

SUPERFICIAL SENSATION

Disturbances of superficial sensation may be caused by lesions of the spinal roots, peripheral nerves, spinal cord, brain stem, thalamus and cerebral cortex.

Root Lesions

Posterior spinal root lesions cause pain along the distribution of the root. Sneezing, straining or coughing—whatever increases intraspinal pressure—increases the pain. Posterior root lesions also cause disturbances in sensation along the root distribution. Irritative lesions cause hyperesthesia. Such a disease may also cause loss of touch, pain and temperature.

When suspicious of root pain think of three categories of causes: (1) infections such as syphilis, pachymeningitis (tuberculosis or syphilis) and herpes zoster; (2)

bony deformities as in osteoarthritis, vertebral fractures, metastatic carcinoma, bone tumors and tuberculosis of the spine; (3) compressions of extra- and intramedullary tumors, herniated nucleus pulposus, extradural abscess and metastatic cancer.

Spondylosis

In cervical spondylosis, pain is at first confined to the neck but later radiates down the arm. It is intermittent, aggravated by straining and coughing and appears in the muscle predominantly supplied by the root involved. In C_6 lesions, root pain radiates down the outer arm and causes tingling in the thumb and index finger. In C_7 lesions, root pain radiates down the posterior aspect of the arm and forearm and causes tingling in the index and middle fingers. And in C_8 root lesions, pain radiates down the inner arm and forearm and causes tingling in the ring and little fingers.

Examine the patient's neck for restricted movement and the muscles supplied by the root for weakness and fasciculations. C_6 lesions depress the biceps and supinator jerks; C_7 lesions depress the triceps; and C_8 lesions depress the finger jerks, providing they were originally present. Although cervical spondylosis is the commonest cause of nerve root troubles, search for primary spinal tumors and metastatic growths.

Spondylosis, as in the neck, is the most common cause of root pain in the lumbar vertebra. L_4, L_5 and S_1 are the most common sites of the *lumbar spondylosis syndrome*. The symptoms are similar to that described for the cervical vertebra, i.e. intermittent pain aggravated by coughing, straining and jolting with paresthesias at the periphery of the dermatome involved.

In L_4 root lesions, pain radiates down into the anterior thigh and inner leg with weakness of the quadriceps and a depressed knee jerk; in L_5 pain radiates down the outer thigh and leg with weakness in the extensor hallucis longus; and in S_1 pain radiates down back of the thigh into the calf with weakness of plantar flexion and a depressed ankle jerk. Muscle cramps are common.

Peripheral Nerves

If a peripheral nerve is severed, a complete loss of all sensation occurs—touch, pain, heat, cold, position and vibration. Nerves that are only incompletely severed cause incomplete sensory loss in the distribution of the peripheral nerve involved.

Peripheral Neuritis

The chief symptom of this condition is pain along the course of the involved nerve. Paresthesia and hyperesthesia accompany the pain. Palpate for tenderness of the muscles, tendons and nerve trunks, which, in some degree, is always present. In severe cases, there may be a loss of touch, pain, heat, cold, position and vibration. The tendon reflexes are decreased or lost. Inspect for trophic changes, loss of subcutaneous fat, loss of skin corrugations and brittle nails.

Mononeuritis

This is a neuritis involving a single nerve or nerve trunk. The causes are varied and numerous but are usually of local origin. The cervical rib and the scalenus anticus syndromes are examples of mononeuritis produced when the brachial plexus is compressed by a cervical rib or by the scalenus anticus muscle. Other varieties of causes are mechanical (trauma and tumors), infections and toxic.

Sciatica

Sciatica may be divided into two groups: primary and secondary. Determine the difference by palpating for nerve and muscle tenderness along the course of the sciatic nerve in a patient who has had an acute onset of pain and a decrease in the Achilles reflex on the affected side with or without muscle atrophy or sensory changes. This is the picture of primary neuritis. Table 8-4 gives causes of secondary sciatica.

Table 8-4. Causes of Secondary Sciatica

Pelvis	*Vertebrae*	*Spinal cord*	*Muscles and fascia*
Sacroiliac strain or arthritis	Spondylitis	Primary intra- and extra-medullary tumors	Tense fascia lata
Hip diseases	pyogenic	Herniation of nucleus pulposus	Faulty posture
Prostatic and GU infections	tubercular	Pachymeningitis	Myositis of pyriform and gluteal muscles
Rectal diseases	Spondylolisthesis	syphilitic	
Hernias	Secondary or primary tumors	tubercular	
Tumors or cancers of the pelvic organs	Congenital abnormalities	Arachnoiditis	
	Arthritis	Hypertrophy of ligmentum flavum	
	Sacralization of L_5		

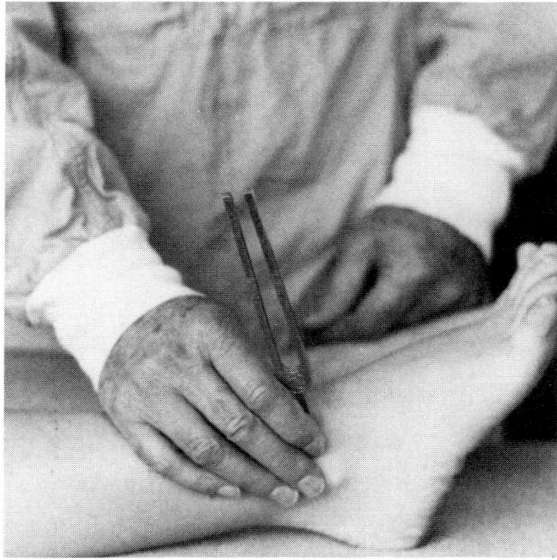

Figure 8-43. Test for vibratory sense.

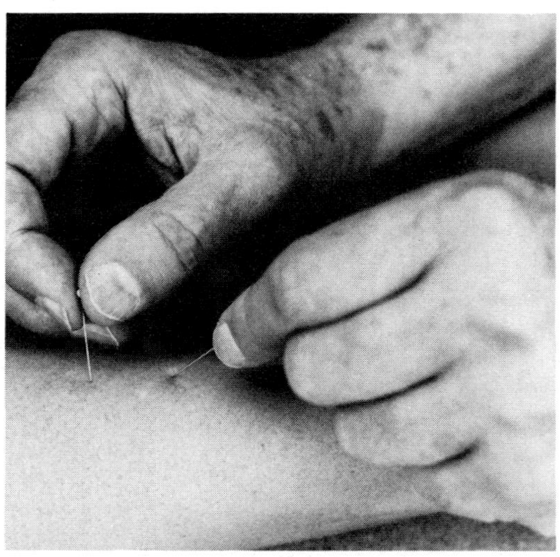

Figure 8-44. Two-point discrimination.

Polyneuritis

Polyneuritis is a multiple neuritis and, as a rule, is the result of a systemic dysfunction caused by a metabolic disorder, a viral or bacteriologic infection, toxic chemicals or a nutritional deficiency. Some common polyneuritic syndromes which you should keep in mind are alcoholic neuritis, neuritis of pernicious anemia, porphyria, diabetic neuritis, chemical neuritis (toxic), uremic neuritis, acute infectious polyneuritis, neuritis of sprue, beriberi and pellagra (nutritional neuropathies) and cancer by invasion or pressure of a nerve.

Diabetes mellitus is the most common cause of peripheral neuropathy. The syndrome is characterized by the fact that it is symmetric, distal and sensory and there is early decreased vibratory sense (Fig. 8-43), two-point discrimination (Fig. 8-44) and loss of ankle jerk. It is often associated with femoral neuropathies and low back pain, pressure neuropathies and oculomotor neuritis and head pain.

Spinal Cord

The clinical symptoms of spinal cord disabilities depend on the extent and level of the lesion. Disease of the gray matter of the cord, the commissural area, causes a loss of pain and temperature sensation. Because the loss follows interruption of the sensory fibers as they cross over from the spinothalamic tract, the loss is bilateral. Only lesions within the spinal cord substance can produce this syndrome, i.e. syringomyelia, syphilitic meningomyelitis, hematomyelia, intramedullary tumor of the spinal cord, and concussion of the spinal cord.

Lesions in the spinothalamic tract cause a loss of pain and temperature sensations on the opposite side of the body. This tract conveys only pain and temperature and, when involved in a destructive lesion, cuts off all segments below the level of the lesion. Look for intramedullary tumors, myelitis, hematomyelia, tubuerculoma and multiple sclerosis. Extramedullary diseases may compress the cord from without.

Hemisection of the spinal cord (Brown-Sequard syndrome) causes a loss of position and vibratory sense on the side of the lesion and a loss of pain and temperature on the opposite side. Trauma as well as intramedullary and extramedullary tumors may cause the syndrome but usually in a less pure form than described above. The loss of pain and temperature on the opposite side is common with little loss of position and vibration sensations on the same side.

Transverse Section of Cord

Complete transverse section of the cord accompanies trauma and many diseases —tumors, syphilis, multiple sclerosis and disseminated myelitis. Motor paralysis and complete sensory loss occur below the level of the lesion. There is sphincter loss or disturbance with retention of urine and feces. Superficial and tendon reflexes are decreased.

Thalamus

The thalamus is the end station of all forms of sensation. A minor vascular lesion of the thalamus may cause sensory disturbances on the opposite half of the body. If the lesion is small and discrete it may affect only the hand, causing tingling, burning or freezing sensations.

Sensory Cortex

A discrete, irritative lesion in the sensory cortex produces epileptic-like symptoms. For example, episodic tingling electric shocks in the hand may be caused by cortical lesions. Because the centers for the hand and mouth are so close together in the cerebral cortex, the corner of the mouth and the hand may be affected at the same time. At other times, the numbness may spread from the fingers up the arm to the mouth. Insufficiency of the carotid or vertebral-basilar arteries may produce such sensations in the hand. Electroencephalograms help to diagnose an epileptic focus. Angiograms of the great neck vessels are mandatory if transient cerebral ischemia is suspected.

HEADACHES

The variety of causes and types of headaches is sampled in Table 8-5.

Intracranial Headaches

Intracranial structures in which headaches can occur are the dura mater at the base of the skull; venous sinuses and tributaries; pain fibers of V, IX and X cranial nerves and cervical nerves; anterior and middle meningeal dural arteries; and about one quarter of the circle of Willis.

If pain is in the anterior two thirds of the head, look for disease above the tentorium. If pain is in the posterior one third of the head, look for disease below the tentorium.

Mechanism of headache production by intracranial disease:

- direct pressure on pain sensitive cranial and cervical nerves
- traction or tension from direct and indirect displacement of pain sensitive structures
- increasing CSF pressure from obstruction to its free flow
- distention or dilitation of intracranial arteries
- inflammation in and about pain-sensitive structures

Table 8-5. Headaches

Causes	*Types*
Cerebral hemorrhage	Space-occupying lesions (traction headaches)
intracerebral	Inflammatory headaches (meningitis encephalitis)
subarachnoid	Muscular contraction headaches (tension headaches)
subdural	Vascular headaches
epidural	migraine and its variants
Cerebral thrombosis	cluster headaches
Cerebral embolus	hypertensive headaches
A-V fistulae	lower-half headaches
Aneurysms	Nonmigraine vascular headaches
ENT and dental disease	febrile or toxic
Neuralgia	hypoglycemic
trigeminal	hangovers
glossopharyngeal	postepileptic headaches
occipital	
bacterial	
Metabolism	
temporal arteritis	
polyarteritis nodosa	
polymyalgia rheumatica	

If a headache is accompanied by any of the following signs and symptoms, search for intracranial pathology:

–fever
–headache aggravated by a cough, straining or a change in position
–stiff neck
–a change of a previous headache pattern for the worse
–seizure or coma
–a neurologic sign, especially if the sign outlasts the headache
–personality change
–headache that always recurs in exactly the same location
–headache that suddenly needs more or stronger medication for relief

Intracranial Tumors

Characteristics of intracranial tumors are headaches that:

–are precipitated by changing positions, bending forward, coughing or straining at stool
–are steady, nonthrobbing, deep, dull and awaken the patient from sleep
–are generally intermittent but occasionally continuous
–start abruptly or change suddenly
–are severe but less violent than migraine, meningitis, tic douloureux and ruptured aneurysm
–occur with or without nausea

Diagnosis is made on the basis of a neurologic work-up plus x-ray or other studies.

GLIOMA/GLIOBLASTOMA. Fifty percent of all intracranial tumors are gliomas. Glioblastomas account for one third of all gliomas and astrocytomas for another third. Glioblastomas are the most malignant and most rapidly growing primary intracranial neoplasms with symptoms occurring within days or within a few weeks. Look for papilledema. Order skull x-rays which may show demineralization of the dorsum sella and for shift of the pineal. Request a brain scan; this is usually positive. An arteriogram is usually diagnostic.

ASTROCYTOMA/CEREBELLAR ASTROCYTOMA. Cerebellar astrocytomas occur in children of any age. Headache aggravated by postural changes or by straining and coughing is an initial sign. Vomiting is a frequent second sign followed by cerebellar signs, their characteristics depending on the tumor's location. Cerebellar signs are papilledema, evidence of chronic increased intracranial pressure on x-ray films and diplopia and deficits in cranial nerve functions. Fortunately astrocytomas can be excised and the patient will survive and enjoy a useful life.

MENINGIOMA. This is an intracranial tumor of the elderly and accounts for 15 percent of the primary intracranial tumors. Meningiomas are classified as benign tumors but they become large before producing symptoms. Consequently, surgery for their removal carries a high morbidity and mortality. Symptoms depend on the location of the tumor plus convulsions and mental changes. Occasionally these symptoms occur before the headache.

CHRONIC SUBDURAL HEMATOMA. This hematoma occurs as a result of trauma sometimes sustained weeks or months previous to the onset of symptoms. Alcoholism and blood dyscrasias are often associated with the lesion. Signs and symptoms include headaches, impairment of intellectual function, hemiparesis and papilledema.

Expect some degree of headache following a cerebral concussion. But if the headache lasts for more than 3 weeks and is accompanied by mental or neurologic changes, thoroughly investigate.

Treatment is surgical evacuation. Consider that most untreated patients die and many are seriously impaired. This is tragic when you consider that subural hematomas are completely curable if recognized in time.

You will need to order the usual tests: x-ray studies of the skull for a shifted pineal or fracture in patients with a unilateral hematoma, a brain scan and, most definitive, arteriography.

OCCIPITAL LOBE TUMORS. These tumors are often confused with migraine and other kinds of headaches. Many patients complain only of visual impairment. A slowly progressive loss in one field of vision may develop unnoticed by the patient. A routine examination may uncover a homonymous hemianopsia with or without papilledema. Flashing lights and auras with the headaches may confuse the diagnosis with migraine headaches. Always hesitate to make the diagnosis of migraine without carefully considering the possibility of an occipital lobe tumor.

METASTATIC TUMORS. This type accounts for 10 to 20 percent of intracranial lesions. Primary sources are lungs, breast, thyroid, liver, stomach, kidney, colon and rectum. Carcinomas of the breast and lung account for 60 percent of the primary sources. The onset is rapid and the symptoms are dependent on the location of the tumor in the brain. In great measure, the diagnosis depends on finding a primary site. Occasionally a secondary lesion overshadows in significance the primary site. In a considerable number of cases you will be unable to find the primary lesion.

INTRASELLAR TUMORS. This type of tumor accounts for 10 percent of intracranial masses and arises most commonly among young and middle-aged adults. The patient often describes the headache as "bursting," and as located in the frontal or temporal area. Search for visual field loss because of the frequent involvement of the optic nerve, chiasm or tract. Inquire carefully into signs suggesting glandular changes. Order a skull x-ray to detect changes in the sella turcica.

Other Intracranial Tumors

BRAIN ABSCESS. An abscess may be ushered in with symptoms of cerebral edema such as headaches, nausea, vomiting and convulsions. Don't expect a multitude of signs and symptoms. When suspicious, search for a recent systemic, pulmonary, sinus or ear infection, a history of drug abuse or even a subacute bacterial endocarditis.

Check a lung x-ray for pulmonary abscess; do an EEG, a brain scan for one or more foci and arteriography for the presence of an avascular mass.

ARTERIOVENOUS MALFORMATIONS. Malformations may vary from a large mass occupying most of a cerebral hemisphere to tiny vascular anomalies. Although present at birth, the first symptoms rarely occur before adolescence or early adult life, or may not occur at all. Prior to rupture, symptoms are caused by vascular dilitation or by the stealing of blood from normal areas. Complications are subarachnoid hemorrhage, seizure disorder and progressive neurologic involvement.

Keep in mind that headaches do not occur before a hemorrhage or a seizure in 75 to 90 percent of the cases. When headaches do occur they are on the same side as the lesion and may simulate migraine even, in a few cases, with an aura. If the work-up suggests an arteriovenous malformation, the most suitable therapy is excision.

ANEURYSMS. These are found in about 2 percent of the cases. Many are found incidentally at autopsy. An unruptured aneurysm does not always require surgery. Aneurysms at the junction of the internal carotid and posterior communicating arteries compress the third cranial nerve, producing oculomotor palsies and irritates the dura, causing a painful headache.

A ruptured aneurysm causes an acute emergency with diffuse headache radiating to the neck, back and even into the legs. The headache is usually preceded by sneezing or straining. Whatever happens as to consciousness and neurologic deficiencies depends on the extent of the hemorrhage. Fifteen percent of patients with a ruptured aneurysm die following the first attack; 40 percent or more die following the second attack.

Most patients show signs of meningeal irritation, confusion, agitation, photophobia and Kernig's sign. Confirm blood or discoloration in the spinal fluid by a lumbar puncture. Localize the lesion by angiography. If you confirm the diagnosis of a ruptured aneurysm, its size, shape and location will suggest the surgical treatment, i.e. clipping, reinforcing or a proximal arterial ligation.

RULING OUT INTRACRANIAL TUMORS. To rule out intracranial tumors do the following practical examinations:

- –physical examination
- –neurologic examination, including a study of the fundi and the optic discs
- –skull x-rays for bone demineralization, erosion, sclerosis, displacement of the pineal or abnormal calcium deposits
- –echoencephalogram
- –brain scan
- –EEG

Echoencephalography, because of the ease of its performance, is being used more frequently for the screening of space-occupying intracranial lesions. The screening of approximately 1800 mental patients identified 12 patients with a shifted cerebral midline structure. Echoencephalographic screening is much more likely to identify patients with unilateral or asymmetrical cerebral atrophy from various causes than it is space-occupying lesions.[4]

If you still suspect an intracranial tumor and the above are normal, request in addition a right carotid or brachial arteriogram, a determination of ventricular size and a lumbar puncture (only when you suspect bleeding or a brain tumor).

Functional Headaches

While some headaches have an organic cause the great majority are functional and, for practical purposes, are of two varieties: tension and vascular headaches. These two types account for 95 to 98 percent of all headaches with the great majority being of the tension type.

Tension headaches

Characteristics of tension headaches are:

- –insidious onset without predictability
- –may be related to conscious emotional stress
- –patient first aware of a vague aching but pain gradually becomes pressing and viselike
- –patient localizes pain with difficulty
- –bilateral-symmetrical and simultaneous
- –pressure and soreness behind the eyes
- –may wax and wane
- –no relief from ergot preparations
- –nausea or vomiting and photophobia often confuses the diagnosis with migraine
- –headache associated with muscle contractions in the neck and scalp

Drug therapy for tension headache is usually less than satisfactory. There are no specific drugs for the relief of pain due to sustained muscular contraction. Combinations of analgesics plus a barbiturate with or without dextroamphetamine are useful if used with caution.

Aspirin, 300 to 600 mg every 4 hr p.r.n.
Darvon, 65 mg every 4 hr p.r.n.
Zactirin, 100 to 200 mg every 4 hr p.r.n.
Valium, 2 to 5 mg q.i.d., p.r.n.

Display interest, patience and concern. Explain the mechanism of pain. After a careful physical examination, dispel any lingering doubts as to etiology—allergy, constipation, vitamin deficiency, etc.

Migraine or Vascular Headaches

In one family practice, 15,000 patients were screened for migraine and 1,200 patients with migraines were found, an average of 8 percent. There are all gradients of migraine complaints from the most severe and disabling illness to trifling symptoms. It is safe to assume that less than half the migraine victims ever consult a physician.

Background of the patient:

- headaches start early in life
- family history of migraine
- past history of motion sickness
- headaches precipitated by ingestion of alcohol, certain foods, vasodilator drugs and oral contraceptive pills
- history of periodicity of headaches

Headaches are more common in females but somewhat relieved by pregnancy and the menopause. Some pregnant women do have excessive and prolonged vomiting. Others suffer at least one toxemia of pregnancy. In any event, these women become nauseated and vomit more easily than nonmigrainous women.

Characteristics of the attack are:

- headache preceded for 15 to 30 min by auras, scotomas or numbness
- headache pain is unilateral, builds up over a period of 2 to 3 hr and may last 2 to 3 days, or occasionally the headache stops during the first good night's sleep
- headache is throbbing or pulsating, or pounding in rhythm with the heartbeat
- associated with photophobia, nausea and vomiting

TREATMENT OF MIGRAINES. TO ABORT AN ATTACK. Oral ergotamine preparations: *Cafergot* (ergotamine tartrate 1.0 mg plus caffeine 100 mg) 2 tablets at onset and 1 to 2 every 30 min for maximum of 6 to 8 tablets. Nausea and vomiting common. *Ergotrate* (ergonovine maleate 0.2 mg tablets) 2 tablets every 1 to 2 hr to a maximum of 8 tablets each attack; less nausea.

Sublingual ergotamine preparation: *Ergomar* (ergotamine tartrate 2 mg) 1–3 tablets in 1 to 2 hr at onset of symptoms; very effective.

Aerosol ergotamine preparation: *Medihaler-Ergotamine* (ergotamine tartrate) 1 to 2 puffs at onset and repeat in 10 to 15 min p.r.n. Expensive but effective.

Suppository ergotamine preparation: *Cafergot suppositories* (ergotamine tartrate 2 mg) Rapid absorption; no nausea. Useful when patient is vomiting.

Injectable ergotamine preparation: *Gynergen* (ergotamine tartrate 0.5 mg/ml) Dose: 0.25 to 0.5 mg IM or SC. When instituting treatment, find dose needed to control attack and then administer total dose at onset in subsequent attacks. 2 ml maximum per week. Nausea occurs frequently. *DHE*-45 (Dihydroergotamine mesylate) Dose: 0.5 to 1.0 mg IM or IV. Less likely to cause nausea than Gynergen. May repeat in 1 hr p.r.n. Maximum dose 3 mg. Patient may be trained to self-administer.

PROPHYLACTIC TREATMENT. *Sansert* (methysergide) 2 mg tablets. Dose: 2 mg daily may control and avoid nausea. May need 2 mg t.i.d. and, if so, patient will need monitoring—BUN, creatinine and IVP checks to prevent retroperitoneal fibrosis. Intermittent use may prevent complications.

Diet control by eliminating foods with significant tyramine content—red wine, chocolate, lima and Italian beans, cheddar cheese, chicken liver, raisins, avocadoes, plums, fish and nuts.

In the elderly try Hydergine sublingual tablets, 0.5 mg, maximum 3.0 mg daily.

Dilantin (diphenylhydantoin) 300 to 500 mg daily, May be useful if EEG pattern is dysrhythmic, otherwise of questionable value. Antihistamines, i.e. *Benadryl* 150 to 200 mg daily or *Periactin* (4 mg tablets) 20 to 24 mg daily. Both may cause drowsiness. Increase dose slowly over a period of weeks. Tolerance may develop.

CLUSTER HEADACHES. These headaches are called cluster because of their tendency to occur several times a day for 6 to 8 weeks and then not to recur for as long as 6 to 12 months. Cluster headaches come on suddenly, reach their maximum intensity in 5 to 10 minutes and disappear in 1 to 2 hours (Table 8-6). The pain is sudden and violent and accompanied by coryza and a vasomotor flush of the face.

Treatment of cluster headache has not been standardized. Try one of the following. Use some of the drugs suggested for migraine to abort cluster headache. *Aristocort* (triamcinolone) 16 mg daily stops the headache in 18 hr if used in conjunction with ergotamine. *Medrol* (methylprednisolone) 16 mg daily every other day in a slow-release preparation. Use Sansert 2 mg t.i.d. along with the Medrol. Try *Delalutin* (hydroxyprogesterone caproate) 500 mg IM each week for several weeks during the period of attacks; also heavy doses of chlorpromazine 400 to 500 mg per day during the attacks.

Histamine desensitization is done over a period of 21 days by giving intravenous histamine. Add histamine diphosphate, 3 mg to 250 ml of saline and administer fast enough for the patient to get a flush but not fast enough to produce a headache.

MENINGITIS

Prompt recognition of meningitis is crucial. If you establish the diagnosis early, successful treatment usually follows. Delay increases the mortality and morbidity rates. Diagnosis is not difficult, except in infants and the young when the classic symptoms are absent. The triad of an intense headache, a stiff neck and vomiting is almost always present.

The type of bacterium and even the signs and symptoms vary somewhat with the age of the patient. Definite clinical signs of meningeal irritation are absent in infants under 2 months of age. Suspect the disease in any baby who suddenly becomes fretful or irritable and vomits or takes his feedings poorly. A high-pitched cry, usually recognized by the mother, should create further suspicion. Signs of the disease in these young patients are often limited to a full or bulging fontanelle. Don't be misled by the afebrile infant. The temperature may be subnormal in shock. Escherichia coli is the most frequently identified organism in infants under two months. Others are streptococci and bacteria of the klebsiella-aerobacter group.

In patients between 2 and 12 months of age, symptoms are more classic—fever, headache, vomiting and perhaps convulsion. If you delay treatment, confusion and coma result. You can generally find a stiff neck and elicit Kernig's sign (Fig. 8-45) and Brudzinski's sign (Fig. 8-46) on physical examination. In severe cases, the patient may

Table 8-6. Differentiation of Cluster and Migraine Headaches

Migraine	*Cluster*
Pain builds up over a period of time	Comes on suddenly
Occasionally awakens the patient during the night	Does not occur during sleep
Woman's disease	Man's disease
Associated with nausea and vomiting	Seldom upsets the stomach
Patient finds relief when lying down	Patient walks the floor
May last several hours or days	Disappears in 1–2 hr

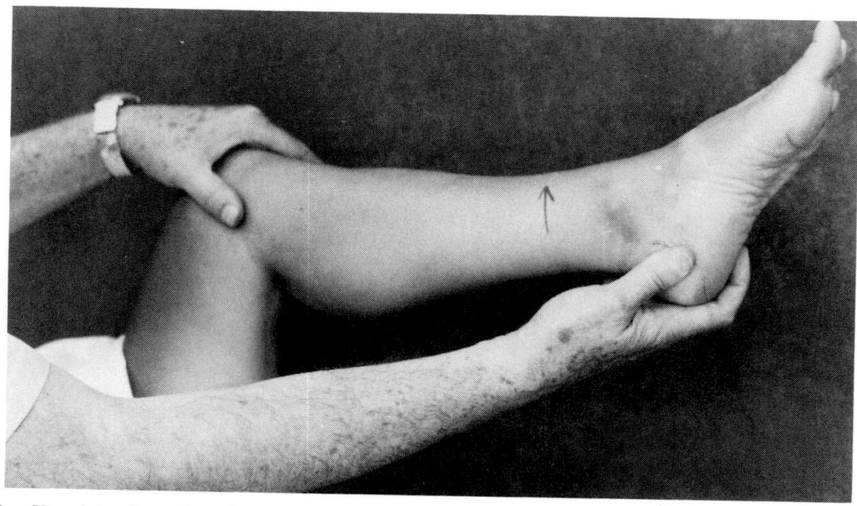

Figure 8-45. Kernig's sign of meningeal irritation. Flex the patient's knee and thigh to 90°. Hold the hip steady while attempting to extend the knee. If the patient has meningeal irritation, she will resist extension because of pain in the hamstrings.

develop purpuric lesions, ranging in size from a few millimeters to many centimeters. Occasionally the rash appears even before signs of definite invasion of the meninges occur.

Hemophilus influenzae is the most common cause among older infants and young children. H_1 influenzae, Neisseria meningitidis and Diplococcus pneumoniae are responsible for over 95 percent of bacterial meningitis in patients over 2 months of age. In diagnosis consider the following: skull fractures, sinusitis, mastoiditis, acute endocarditis or dermal sinuses and injuries of dura from neurosurgical or orthopedic procedures.

When you suspect meningitis, promptly order cultures of both blood and cerebrospinal fluid (CSF). Do this before giving antibiotics. To establish the etiologic diagnosis and direct the appropriate treatment, you must know the number and types of cells present and the glucose and protein content of the CSF. If antibiotics have been given for one or more days before you suspect meningitis, you can be misled. There will be minimal changes in the CSF glucose and protein content. In fact, organisms in the CSF will

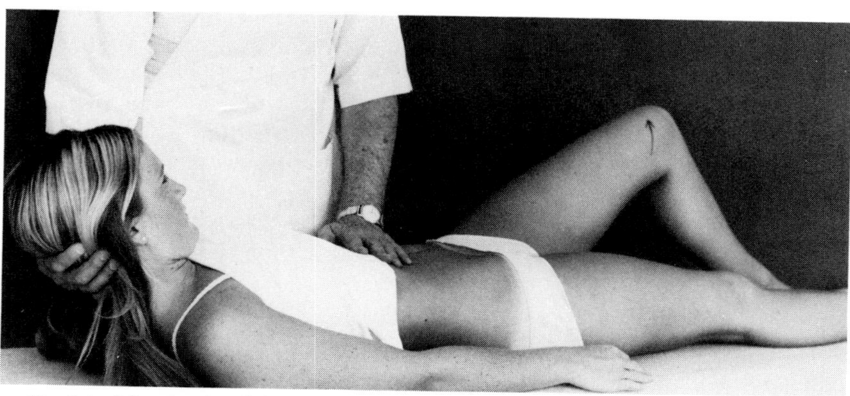

Figure 8-46. Brudzinski's sign is elicited by placing the patient on her back and raising her head passively. Brudzinski is positive when the patient involuntarily flexes her thigh. A positive test indicates meningeal irritation.

go undetected or the predominant cell will have changed to the mononuclear.

To get the needed information, do a spinal tap. Order the following: gram stain on smear of the CSF, a differential cell count, an assay of the CSF's sugar and protein content, culture of the fluid and test of isolated organisms for sensitivity to drugs. If the CSF is clear or slightly hazy, order a wet preparation for yeast forms, india ink study for fungi, and cultures for fungi and tuberculosis. If the CSF is cloudy or milky, order a culture for anaerobic and microaerophilic organisms. Differential diagnosis is simple with the above information. Without this data, you will never be certain of diagnosis or be able to properly treat a patient with meningitis.

In meningismus, the fluid is essentially normal, although CSF pressure may be somewhat up. An important differential point: meningismus disappears after a lumbar tap.

You can begin treatment early if care is taken in interpreting the gram stain. Differentiate gram-positive pneumococcus, gram-negative meningococcus and pleomorphic gram-negative coccobacillary. A study of the CSF should help you differentiate between the following: Aseptic meningeal reactions, acute purulent meningitis, tuberculous meningitis, mumps meningitis, choriomeningitis of viral origin and polyneuritis.

Remember that a positive blood culture is common in H. influenzae meningitis and up to 50 percent of cultures are positive in other bacterial infections. A slide agglutination test is usually positive on the CSF of patients with H. influenzae infections.

Unless you are familiar with the different antibiotics selected for treatment of meningitis and their best route of administration, seek consultation but do so promptly.

Viral meningitis requires only symptomatic treatment; fungal meningitis requires amphotericin B; and tuberculous meningitis requires strenuous treatment with a combination of streptomycin, isoniazid, pyridoxine and para-aminosalicylic acid. Since most cases of bacterial meningitis are pneumococcal or meningococcal in origin, penicillin G is the best all-round choice, 1 to 2 million units, IV every 2 hours. But this is an oversimplification: seek advice. Treatment should be started with at least two drugs. New information suggests that ampicillin alone may be as effective as combination therapy; in fact, ampicillin appears to be the drug of choice in the treatment of a purulent meningitis not acquired in the hospital. Treatment should continue 7 to 14 days in the case of bacterial infection to months or even permanently in other varieties.

In infants less than 2 months of age start treatment with gentamicin and ampicillin. Continue until the organism has been identified.

Treatment tips on hospital acquired bacterial meningitis: without organism identification, start with gentamicin and oxacillin; if gram-negative bacilli are identified on a slide, start with gentamicin and chloramphenicol; and, if pseudomones is suspected, begin with gentamicin and carbenicillin.

In all forms of meningitis give close attention to supportive treatment: adequate airway; electrolyte control; prevention of cerebral edema by urea or mannitol therapy; monitoring of vital signs and their correction, possibly by means of a central venous catheter and the administration of saline, albumin, dextran or blood; and consideration of heparin for intravascular clotting defects plus steroids, both of which are controversial as routine measures.

A positive response to treatment is indicated when the CSF examined 24 hours after instituting treatment is sterile. Don't worry if the white cell count and protein level is still up or even higher than on the diagnostic tap. The glucose level will definitely be higher if treatment is effective.

The prognosis in newborns is poor. There is an 85 percent mortality, even with antibiotics. Streptococcal and staphylococcal infections carry a high mortality. In pneumococcal meningitis, mortality is around 30 percent and higher in the elderly or in those who have greatly abnormal CSF protein and sugar.

Meningococcal meningitis is generally the most benign form with the lowest mortality rate. Pneumococcal meningitis carries a higher mortality than the meningococcal variety and is associated with complications secondary to bacteremia.

Prophylaxis must be given those who came in patient contact. Sulfonamide prophylaxis has been used for years but is no longer reliable for universal use. Prescribe sulfa now only when the organism is sulfa-susceptible. Penicillin G or V, ampicillin or erythromycin all appear to prevent secondary cases among household contacts. Secondary cases of H. influenzae meningitis occur but no proven method of prevention has been established.

Recognize any neurologic deficiencies in patients before dismissal. In children, test for visual and hearing impairments as well as motor disabilities. One test is not enough. Repeat the check every 3 months for a year. Watch for intellectual loss. If the problems are recognized early and proper rehabilitation started, the losses are minimized.

COMA

Think of unconsciousness as a void of consciousness and the range of consciousness as extending from alert wakefulness through clouding (obtundity) and stupor to precoma and coma. The deepest state of unconsciousness is coma in which the patient lies motionless and unresponsive to stimuli with deep and superficial reflexes lost and with urinary incontinence.

Think of the following as possible causes of coma: alcohol; trauma; cerebrovascular lesions; poisoning, carbon monoxide, drugs; diabetes; epilepsy; meningitis and other infections; pneumonia; cardiac decompensation; exsanguination; neurosyphilis; uremia; eclampsia; neoplasms; hypoglycemia; hepatic failure; brain abscess; subdural hematoma; sunstroke; functional, hysteria and psychotic states and endogenous or exogenous toxins.

An approach to diagnosis. Interview anyone you can find who knew or was with the patient. Ask the ambulance driver to bring any knowledgeable person along for questioning. All facts are important. Where was the patient found? When? Were there any empty drug bottles nearby? Was there evidence of trauma? Where did he last eat? Who prepared the food? What were his symptoms before coma developed? What past diseases did he have? Epilepsy? Diabetes? Alcoholism? Addiction? Cancer? Psychosis? Suicidal tendencies?

Perform a careful general examination, especially noticing the respiratory excursions and the skin color. Jaundiced? Cyanotic? Cherry-red? Inspect and palpate for lacerations, gunshot wounds, bruises and skull fractures. Smell the patient's breath for alcohol, paraldehyde, the bitter almond odor of hydrocyanic acid, acetone, ammonia and fetor oris.

Examine the tongue for lacerations sustained during an epileptic convulsion. Inspect the ears for a bloody or purulent discharge; the mouth and throat membranes for infections or the discoloration of poisoning.

Do a screening neurologic check. Test for meningeal irritation by checking for nuchal rigidity and for the Kernig's and Brudzinski's signs. Check each limb for muscle tone as you search for signs of hemiplegia.

Check the deep reflexes but remember that in deep coma all reflexes are lost and the Babinski's signs are pathologically bilateral. Deep reflex evaluation is not particularly helpful unless some reflexes are retained.

Check the patient's response to painful stimuli. This is most helpful in estimating the depth of coma. Elicit this response by making pressure with your index finger just below the mastoid process. Test other deep pressure sense losses by squeezing the patient's testicles or his Achilles tendon. On forceful flexion of the terminal phalanx of the finger or toe on the paralyzed side, the patient will not be able to withdraw the limb while, on the normal side, forceful retraction of the limbs occurs.

Give special attention to inspecting the patient's eyes. Check for lid lag. Attempt to open the lids. This is resisted in hysteric patients. Do the eyes fix from time to time as in hysteria or do they oscillate slowly? How about the size of the pupils? If pinpoint, think of morphine poisoning or a pontine hemorrhage. If one pupil is unreactive, think of an expanding lesion on the same side such as a subdural hemorrhage, brain tumor or middle meningeal artery hemorrhage. Pupils that fail to react to light are a bad omen. Inequality of the pupils is common; its significance is difficulty to evaluate. If both pupils are widely dilated, think of trauma, massive cerebral hemorrhage, encephalitis, atropine poisoning and far advanced brain tumor. Conjugate deviation of the eyeballs is toward the lesion in destructive disease in the frontal lobe but away from the lesion in irritative ones.

Watch for signs of facial muscle paralysis. Does the mouth droop on one side? Does the cheek on one side puff out on expiration? Press on the supraorbital notch to elicit muscle action while watching for assymetry of contraction.

Check the fundi for evidence of choked disc or neuroretinitis.

While completing the above ask for the following:

- catheterization and urinalysis (Install a Foley for output monitoring)
- blood count and blood chemistries (a minimum blood check: blood glucose, BUN and carbon dioxide content)
- assays for barbiturates, bromides, salicylates and tranquilizers if poisoning is suspected
- x-ray of skull and chest if indicated
- gastric lavage for all poisonings
- lumbar puncture for bleeding, infection and for diseases that may have altered the body chemistry

If you find the patient has increased intracranial pressure by fundoscopic examination or if you suspect an intracranial mass, delay a lumbar tap. Otherwise you risk causing decerebrate rigidity or even a failure of respiration. If a mass is definitely suspected, an arteriogram is more in order.

Some signs and what they suggest:

Soft eyeballs—diabetes
Bulging fontanels—meningitis
Muscular twitchings—uremia
Kussmaul breathing—diabetes
Increased respiration—pneumonia
Wounds on tongue—epilepsy
Decreased blood pressure—trauma
Increased blood pressure—CVA, uremia
Positive Kernig's sign—CVA, meningitis
Stiff neck—CVA, meningitis
Vomiting—CVA, poisoning
Convulsion—epilepsy, CVA, syphilis, alcoholism
Hemiplegia—CVA
Irregular pulse—cardiac decompensation
Slow pulse—Stokes-Adams syndrome

THE ELECTROENCEPHALOGRAM (EEG)

An EEG has its best known value in seizure disorders. An interseizure record is valuable to confirm the seizure diagnosis and to help locate the area in the brain where the seizures originate. An interseizure recording is also helpful in petit mal attacks, particularly if the recording happens to be made during an attack. You can expect 20 percent of interseizure records to be normal. Antiepileptic drugs may inhibit the brain wave recordings but are not likely to blot out the underlying disorder.

If the patient has a brain abscess, there is between 90 to 95 percent chance it will show on an EEG.

If the patient has a malignant tumor, there is a 75 to 80 percent chance it will show on an EEG tracing. EEGs are more likely to be abnormal when the tumor is supratentorial than infratentorial and with gliomas than with meningiomas. EEGs will localize tumors in 5 percent of the cases when other methods fail and will verify the location suggested by other tests in 80 percent of the cases.

The EEG may help when you suspect increased intracranial pressure and are delaying a spinal tap. The tracing reflects increased intracranial pressure fairly accurately. Pressure may then be decreased by hypertonic agents and the EEG repeated. The best time to perform a tap can thus be chosen.

Check EEGs following head injuries for diffuse or focal abnormalities. Serial EEGs are excellent for determining prognosis in severe head trauma and are helpful in distinguishing between concussion, contusion and intracerebral bleeding.

In CVAs, the EEG is not often directly helpful. When the diagnosis is in doubt, however, a persisting or progressive EEG abnormality should alert you to the possibility of a tumor. EEG changes after an infarction resolve rapidly and generally indicate a good prognosis.

In a subdural hematoma it is rare to find a normal EEG; it is abnormal in 85 to 95 percent of the cases. But the tracing in no way indicates the type of pathology present. The best that can be said is that a normal EEG makes a subdural hematoma unlikely.

When subarachnoid bleeding is massive enough to cause symptoms, the EEG is nearly always abnormal. In the comatose patient, then, the EEG may help distinguish between subarachnoid hemorrhage, focal lesions and some systemic diseases.

Occasionally an EEG will give warning of an impending encephalopathy in hepatic and renal failure. EEG changes parallel the severity of the metabolic encephalopathy.

Remember many epileptics have normal EEGs and many normal patients have abnormal EEGs. The patient's slightest activity may affect the tracing, even the opening or closing of the eyes. In general, abnormalities revealed by EEGs indicate total cerebral malfunctioning rather than any specific pathologic process. A frontal tumor may cause electrical activity in the temporal lobe and an epileptic scar on one side of the brain may produce a response from its mirror region. Occasionally perfectly normal brain waves are recorded from parts of the brain that have been removed.

Generally the EEG is one of the least precise of the various diagnostic procedures in neurology. Do not depend on any single neurologic test if there are others that may help substantiate the diagnosis. Brain scans and cerebral angiograms are of much greater value than an EEG in locating lesions. Think of CSF examinations, x-rays of the skull and spine, pneumoencephalograms and electromyograms as well as careful history and physical examination in arriving at a diagnosis.

MULTIPLE SCLEROSIS (MS)

There is an important and large group of diseases of the CNS classified as the demyelinating diseases. The pathology of this group is a focal or diffuse disturbance of the myelin sheaths (white matter) of the nerve fibers in various regions of the nervous system and to a lesser degree affecting the neurons or their processes.

Multiple sclerosis appears in four clinical types, listed here in order of frequency: (1) Attacks and remissions wherein the disease waxes and wanes over a long period. Remissions may or may not be complete. The history must be sought for. Look for signs in multiple systems of the CNS. (2) The chronic progressive type wherein there are no remissions. (3) The stationary type. (4) The acute forms wherein the onset is sudden, often resembling a febrile disorder and usually with symptoms of loss of vision, hemiplegia and paraplegia. Retrobulbar neuritis accounts for the loss of vision and this may be associated with loss of abdominal reflexes, loss of vibratory sense in the legs, hyperreflexia and perhaps a pathologic Babinski's sign.

In 1965, Schumacher and his committee published six criteria needed to make the diagnosis. These have since become controversial but they help point up the nature of the disease. They are:

- Objective signs and symptoms caused by abnormalities of the CNS.
- Involvement of two or more parts of the CNS, usually the pyramidal, cerebellar and sensory pathways.
- Signs and symptoms as a result of disease of the white matter.
- The disease must have started while the patient was between 10 to 50 years of age.
- Two or more attacks lasting 24 hours and more than a month apart or slow stepwise progression of symptoms and signs over a 6 month period.
- A neurologist or someone familiar with neurologic diseases must decide the symptoms could not be better explained by another disease.

Some Signs and Symptoms

Major dysfunction is a result of damage to the pyramidal tracts. Look for spastic paresis in the legs plus a pathologic Babinski sign. Cerebellar involvement causes ataxia, intention tremor, dysmetria and poor alternating movements. The typical patient has a spastic-ataxic gait and poorly coordinated hand movements. Signs are bilateral, symmetric and more often in the legs. Brain stem involvement produces nystagmus, usually horizontal in type, dysarthria and diplopia.

Sensory pathway involvement is common. Check for a loss of vibratory or positional senses. Again the signs are mainly in the legs and are symmetric. The patient often describes a numbness ("feels different"). Usually you can't find a sensory loss in these numb areas. If you can't, don't call the patient hysterical.

Don't delay considering MS while you await the development of the Charcot triad (nystagmus, scanning speech and intention tremor). You cannot employ these findings in making a diagnosis for they do not always appear. Obviously, when they do all occur, the diagnosis is certain.

Optic atrophy is a common finding and occurs early in the disease. Don't waste time looking for a pallor of the temporal halves of the optic nerve head. Do inquire into a history of retrobulbar neuritis. The patient may present with this disease. This is of great importance in recognition of early MS.

Some signs and symptoms listed in order of their usual frequency.

- –increased deep reflexes in legs
- –diminished or absent abdominal wall reflexes
- –chief complaint of weakness and stiffness in one or both legs
- –nystagmus
- –bilateral Babinski's
- –tremor of an extremity
- –bladder symptoms
- –hesitant or disturbed speech
- –spastic gait
- –pain, numbness or tingling

Differential diagnosis:

- –spinal cord tumors
- –encephalomyelitis
- –CNS syphilis
- –Devic's disease or neuromyelitis optica
- –primary anemia
- –amyotrophic lateral sclerosis
- –hysteria
- –cerebral arteriosclerosis
- –encephalitis
- –brain tumor
- –cerebellar disease

It is difficult to give a prognosis. The average duration of the disease is 5 to 20 years. Individuals with acute cases may die within 18 months. Single symptoms such as diplopia, retrobulbar neuritis and vertigo carry a more favorable prognosis than do combinations of symptoms. Death often occurs from complications of decubitus ulcers or urinary tract infections.

A family physician has a grave responsibility in helping the patient avoid factors that cause fresh attacks. These are respiratory infections, contacts with allergens, pregnancy, chilling, trauma, surgery, emotional disturbances, mental, emotional and physical fatigue and nutritional deficiencies.

Because MS patients are in a delicate state of equilibrium many ordinarily harmless occurrences may precipitate an attack.

EPILEPSY

Some researchers refer to epilepsy as a paroxysmal cerebral dysrhythmia. The term, in some ways, explains what happens, but seizures also occur in patients without recorded EEG changes. However, the electroencephalogram is the most important adjunct we have in clinically appraising the convulsive state.

Grand mal epilepsy is characterized by an aura, a convulsion and the postconvulsive state. The aura is a sensory experience and occurs in about half of the cases. In many the aura serves as a warning of an impending convulsion. Auras are somatic, visceral, visual, olfactory or auditory.

As a rule the seizure develops immediately. Unconsciousness also follows the aura at once. The epileptic fit begins with unconsciousness and occasionally with a shrill cry. The patient falls to the ground. The body is thrown into a tonic state—the individual becomes rigid with arms and legs extended. The patient clenches his jaw, retracts his head and rolls up his eyeballs. Respirations cease and the face becomes flushed or cyanotic. The bladder or bowels may empty during this tonic phase of the attack.

Within half a minute the clonic phase begins: the head jerks forcibly, the arms and legs contract and relax, the jaw jerks, saliva pours from the mouth, the tongue may be bitten and breathing is noisy and stertorous. The seizure may last from 1 to 10 minutes. The fit eventually plays out and the entire episode ends in complete relaxation followed by a deep sleep or confusion lasting for minutes or hours. If these major seizures continue without cessation the attack becomes known as *status epilepticus*. Death may occur in status epilepticus. Grand mal attacks have no localizing significance. They merely indicate an increased irritability of the cortex.

For a prolonged grand mal attack, give Valium (diazepam) IV slowly over a 2 min period not exceeding 10 mg. Wait 5 min and, if needed, give paraldehyde IM, 1 ml per year of age but never to exceed 5 ml. Wait 20 to 30 min. If the convulsions continue, repeat the Valium IV. Again wait 5 min and, if needed, repeat the IM paraldehyde. If the convulsions still continue after a reasonable time, give an IV barbiturate, amobarbital, 30 min after the last paraldehyde. Last of all, if needed, consider giving sodium thiopental or have an anesthesiologist give an ether anesthetic. The quick acting barbiturates stop the convulsions, but give them only when oxygen and other resuscitation equipment is available because of the danger of respiratory depression.

For status epilepticus the attack may go on from 1 to 4 days. The general care of the patient is essential. If the patient is comatose, treat him symptomatically. Do not give anticonvulsant therapy. If he has received unknown doses of therapy get stat blood levels of the barbiturates and of Dilantin. The patient may be comatose from an overdose. Maintain fluid intake by clysis or IV glucose and saline. Catheterize or insert a Foley catheter. Order cool sponge baths, ice bags and cool enemas for fever. Move from side to side to prevent pneumonia.

Motor jacksonian seizures are focal clonic convulsions of a limb, part of a limb, both limbs of one side of the body or of the muscles of the face. Jacksonian convulsions begin as a rule in one of three places: the thumb and index finger, the angle of the mouth or the great toe. An attack beginning in the hand passes up the arm and down the leg. Attacks beginning in the great toe, extend up the leg and, if it continues, down the arm. Attacks involving the face usually begin at the angle of the mouth. You may encounter all degrees of seizures from a twitching of the toe to a generalized convulsion. Consciousness is not impaired unless a general convulsion occurs. Intravenous Valium may help terminate these attacks if prolonged.

Sensory jacksonian seizures are not as common as their motor counterparts. They are characterized by sensations in the parts of the body similar to the motor attacks and proceed along the same tracts as do the motor seizures. The sensory and motor seizures may be mixed. The sensations are numbness, tingling, prickling and vague painful sensations.

These focal motor and sensory jacksonian seizures are of great importance. They usually indicate a lesion in the opposite cortex. In the case of motor seizures the lesion is in the motor cortex and in sensory seizures the lesion is in the opposite parietal lobe.

Petit mal consists of a momentary stare or blank look—indicative of a suspension of consciousness. The attacks may be called spells, blackouts, trances, daydreaming, even thinking by distracted parents. Often they are discovered by a teacher or parent. The attacks come and go abruptly, sometimes frequently, and are of brief duration. The patient is usually able to walk about and take medication and food by mouth. Petit mal status is generally self-limited. Have the patient watched to keep him from harming himself.

In *psychomotor seizures* the patient may be irritable for hours or days before a seizure. The seizure commences with a wild look, an inappropriate phase or a peculiar gesture. The movements during an attack may appear purposeful but are poorly coordinated. They may consist of simple acts such as lip smacking, hand wringing, clutching or plucking at objects.

The attack may last from a few minutes to a few hours. The patient loses his higher level of consciousness and is unaware of what transpires, but he retains motor function and an ability to react in automatic fashion. He may respond to questions but lack understanding. This may be the only objective clue. During the attack the patient may walk for miles or may commit senseless acts of violence. Psychomotor seizures should prompt a search for a brain tumor. The attacks are generally self-limited.

Uncinate fits are rarely encountered and are characterized by disagreeable odors or tastes. There may be movements of the lips and tongue with some impairment of consciousness.

The Family Physician and Epilepsy

The family physician is in the best position to recognize and prevent or treat the emotional problems associated with epilepsy.

Convince the parents of an epileptic child to raise him as a normal child within limits of his disability. Encourage the parents to create an atmosphere wherein the child feels wanted. Remember the emotional problems of epileptics begin at home: parents are fearful of future attacks and brothers and sisters reject the epileptic. Watch for signs of withdrawal and dependency or aggressiveness and hostility. Relieving some of the tensions around an epileptic child will lessen the number of attacks, improve his ability to learn and decrease his hyperactivity and restlessness.

Do not allow the parents to develop secrecy about their child's ailment. Help them meet the problem without shame and embarrassment.

Do not allow the epileptic child to be shut off from activities and social contacts. Otherwise you risk the development of belligerency and inferiority with antisocial tendencies.

Do not allow parents to overprotect an epileptic child. The child does not need constant, strict surveillance nor does he need to be protected from all disappointments.

Do not allow parents to treat the child as something special. The child should be made to live as other children with reasonable restrictions. Do not grant unreasonable demands because of pity.

Do not allow parents to treat this child as they would a child with tuberculosis or acute rheumatic fever. He does not need to rest daily. Instruct the parents to allow the epileptic child to play and conduct himself as his normal associates do. Contrary to general belief, physical activity favorably affects an epileptic disorder. Epileptic patients have fewer seizures when they are participating in normal physical activities such as football and baseball. EEGs of epileptic patients frequently are accentuated during the resting state.

Explain to the parents that there is a small calculated risk when they allow their child to participate freely in all normal childhood activities. They must weigh this, however, against the greater risk of emotional and personality maladjustments.

Remember many epileptics live in a constant state of anxiety for fear of injury during a seizure. Reassure the patient and his family.

Epileptics are also fearful of the state of unconsciousness—of losing contact with their environment—creating embarrassment and apprehension.

Epileptics are also concerned and worried about the effect a seizure may have on their family and friends who see the attack.

Some epileptics who have repeated seizures are afraid of being put in an institution. Again the only treatment is for the parents to express their love and affection and to make the afflicted one feel wanted.

Many epileptics who are fearful of having a seizure in public restrict their activities to the confines of their homes and consequently develop marked antisocial tendencies. In some cases, accidental exposure of the disease has had a beneficial effect upon the epileptic patient.

Epileptics are reluctant to disclose their condition to prospective employers. In fact, many lose their jobs when their condition becomes known. A doctor can do his community duty by helping the general public understand the problems of the epileptic patient.

Remember that some emotional problems are related to the patient's antiepileptic medications. Some patients are kept constantly drowsy and dull. The proper dosage of medication for each patient is that amount which controls his seizures but does not produce untoward reactions. Most patients are better off leading a normal life between occasional seizures than being seizure-free in a perpetual state of drug-induced drowsiness or confusion. In addition, some patients resent the continuous, daily doses of medication.

REFERENCES

1. Brown M, Glassenberg M: Mortality factors in patients with acute stroke. *JAMA* 224:1493–1496, 1973.
2. Karp HR: Transient cerebral ischemia: prevalence and prognosis in a biracial rural community. *JAMA* 225:125–128, 1973.
3. Smith RR, et al: Endarterectomy in cerebrovascular diseases; 100 consecutive cases. *S Med J* 64:1000–1003, 1971.
4. White DN, Clark JM: Amplitude-averaged A-scan echoencephalography of a mental hospital population. *Canad Psychiat Assoc J* 15:453–460, 1970.

GENERAL STUDY AIDS

Rhoton AL, et al: Acoustic neuroma. Adapted from an exhibit presented at AMA's 118th annual convention and reported in *Mod Med* 39:96–109, 1971.

Blonsky ER: Differential diagnosis of Parkinsonism. *Hosp Med* 8:43, 1972.

Livingston S: Insight into the personality of the epileptic youth. *Med Insight* 3:22–39, 1971.

Bunn PA: Meningitis. *Emerg Med* 2:13–19, 1970.

Friedman AP, et al: Chronic recurring headaches in intracranial disorders. A pamphlet sponsored by the Headache Unit of the Montefiore Hospital and Medical Center in the Bronx, NY.

Patel AN: Transient ischemic attacks. *AFP* 4: 97–102, 1971.

Klassen AC: The stroke syndrome: diagnostic procedures. *Med Times* 97: 212–222, 1969.

Thomas G: Dizziness—it may be serious. *AFP* 3: 70–76, 1971.

Braun R, et al: Orthopedic rehabilitation of the stroke patient. *Calif Med* 115: 11–15, 1971.

Rosenthal AM: Home management of the hemiplegic patient. *AFP* 3: 115–119, 1971.

Ford JR, Duckworth B: Physical Management for the Quadriplegic Patient. Philadelphia: F. A. Davis Co., 1974.

CHAPTER 9

Urologic Symptoms and Findings

EXAMINATION

Physical Examination

Anything less than a complete abdominal, pelvic and rectal examination is insufficient to diagnose urologic diseases. Give special attention to the costovertebral angles, the right and left lower abdominal quadrants and to the suprapubic area. While doing a pelvic bimanual examination, do not fail to inspect the urethral opening.

Elicit costovertebral angle tenderness by palpation in the angle formed by the spine and the twelfth rib (Fig. 9-1). Tenderness in this area points toward kidney or paranephritic inflammation. Do not confuse acute myositis or fibrositis with renal disease.

A common problem is distinguishing between an enlarged left kidney and the spleen. Occasionally this will be difficult because both organs have the same general shape. Remember the spleen has a sharp edge but the kidney never has. Neither can you depend on the splenic fissure because the palpable notch may simulate the lobulation of a kidney tumor. Generally, a normal size left kidney cannot be felt through the abdominal wall.

The posteriorly placed kidney can only enlarge forward and downward; the anteriorly placed spleen may be considerably enlarged before it appears below the thoracic cage. On the right, the kidney is lower and, without any enlargement, its lower pole can usually be ballotted. Fist percussion over the costovertebral angles often elicits deep pain when the kidney is inflamed.

Listen for a bruit or murmur over the large arteries of the abdomen. A stenosis of the renal artery often is first detected by a bruit. Move down to the lower abdomen. Palpate and percuss the suprapubic area for a dis-

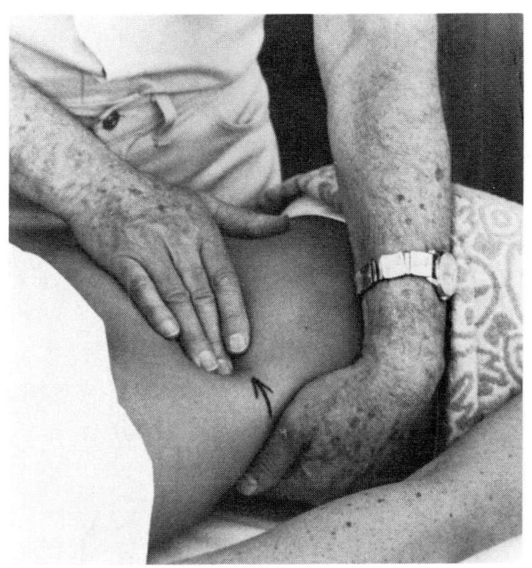

Figure 9-1. Palpation and ballottement of the kidneys. Place one hand around the patient's flank with your fingers in the costovertebral angle. Place your opposite hand on her anterior abdomen and palpate for any unusual masses. The hand on the abdomen should be moved gradually upward toward the costal margin seeking the lower pole of the kidney or tumor. The normal kidney moves with respiration and may be palpable during inspiration. Tap the kidney with the finger in the costovertebral angle and frequently you can feel the kidney ballot against the other hand.

tended bladder or other tumors. Retract the penile foreskin and inspect the urethral meatus, glans and sulcus. Palpate the penis for indurations and nodules. Continue your examination by palpating the spermatic cord, testis and epididymis. If a mass is present in the scrotum, attempt to define it by transillumination.

By this type of examination you should discover the presence of varicocele, spermatocele, beaded vas deferens or nodules, hydrocele, testicular tumors, torsion of testis or hernia. Aspirate all hydroceles and spermatoceles in order to better palpate the testis for cancer.

Last of all do a rectal digital examination to determine the status of the prostate, seminal vesicles and rectum. The normal prostate is slightly tender and somewhat firm but elastic on pitting. Palpate for the three longitudinal grooves, two laterally and one centrally. The seminal vesicles can be felt as bands running at 45° angles from the base of the prostate.

Look for:

- –stony hard prostate of cancer, tuberculosis or calculi (If the grooves have disappeared you have additional evidence of an infiltrating neoplasm)
- –small isolated nodule of early carcinoma
- –exquisitely tender prostate of acute prostatitis
- –tender, bulging prostate of an abscess
- –painful seminal vesicle of seminal vesiculitis

Laboratory and X-Ray Aids

Urinalysis

Any physician who has worked on a medical audit committee knows that attending physicians often overlook or ignore significant urinalysis findings. Cole[1] reports that in 1,000 patients admitted to the University of Alabama Hospital, 163 had urinalysis showing bacteria in the presence of protein, increased leukocytes, erythrocytes or casts. Of those 163 patients, cultures were ordered only on 73 even though 17 had clinical and laboratory evidence of urologic disease. At the same time, the staff ordered cultures on 135 other patients, 30 of whom had neither clinic nor laboratory evidence of disease.

Regard the urinalysis as an important clinical aid. A perfectly normal urine is very significant if the analysis is done properly. For dependable results, urine must be properly collected and stored.

PHYSICAL DATA. COLLECTION. Specimens collected in the office after eating will commonly contain reducing substances and sometimes protein. Urine voided about 3 hours after a meal is most likely to contain pathologic substances and is preferred for general examination. Early morning specimens are more likely to contain mucous and pus not seen later in the day. Midafternoon specimens may be more accurate for urine urobilinogen, an early sign of hepatitis. A word about the preservation of urine for urobilinogen determination. To be certain of its presence, place half a teaspoonful of sodium carbonate in a specimen bottle before collecting the specimen. This will maintain alkalinity. In addition, avoid unnecessary exposure to light. Containers must be chemical clean. Sterilization is not needed unless cultures are to be done.

Examine fresh urine for accurate results. All factors change rapidly if the urine is allowed to sit. Refrigeration at 4° C is the most practical and effective preservative. Special preservatives: Toluene, 2 ml per 100 ml of urine, covers the urine and prevents air contact but does not prevent the growth of organisms; formalin, 1 drop of 40 percent formaldehyde per 30 ml of urine, preserves urinary sediment; concentrated hydrochloric acid preserves the urine for VMA and 17-ketosteroid analysis; the preservative tablet is excellent and does not interfere with most tests.

Have all specimens labeled with the patient's name, date and time of collection. Include on the notation whether the specimen was voided or collected by catheterization.

To collect an uncontaminated urine specimen by the clean-catch method, have the patient cleanse the urethral orifice with an antiseptic solution (Fig. 9-2A). Instruct her to discard the first of the stream as the

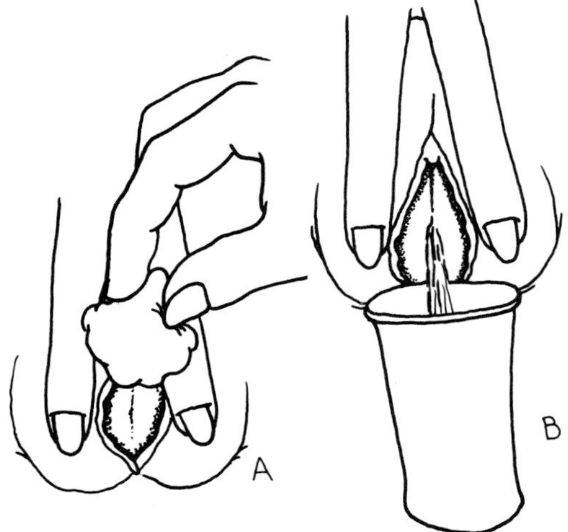

Figure 9-2. The clean-catch method to collect urine. *A*, The anterior urethra harbors bacteria; therefore, cleanse the area to avoid these contaminants. *B*, Instruct the patient to spread her vulva. The urine first passed should not be collected.

distal urethra is usually colonized with bacteria and the first few ml are highly contaminated. Ask the patient to spread the vulva and void into a sterile container (Fig. 9-2B). Finally, ask her to discard the end of the stream since it is expelled with less force and may dribble over the surrounding skin and mucosa causing contamination.

Catheterization may be done on women who are unable to do a careful clean-catch collection (Fig. 9-3) but infection is introduced in certain cases. However, done carefully with proper cleansing, catheterization results in a low degree of contamination. Bladder aspiration (Fig. 9-4) is becoming more popular. This technique cannot be used in patients who are unable to retain their urine until the bladder is distended. The technique is valuable because all cultural growth is significant since no contamination can occur.

Remember you are responsible for the proper collection of all laboratory tests. See that orders are written to obtain exactly what you need.

VOLUME. A 24-hour volume is helpful in determining certain functions. Normally about 170 L of fluid are filtered out by the glomerulus in 24 hours. The tubules reabsorb about 168 L, leaving an adult urine production of 800 to 1,600 ml per 24 hours. The night volume is about half or a third of the day volume. Children under 6 years of age pass about one fourth that of the adult; while those 6 to 12 eliminate about one half the adult output. Consider the patient oliguric if the 24-hour urinary output is between 100 to 600 ml (4 to 25 ml per hour). Anuria is 0 to 100 ml in the same time. Even with dehydration, normal kidneys continue to excrete more than 600 ml daily. Consequently, oliguria and anuria indicate dangerous degrees of renal failure.

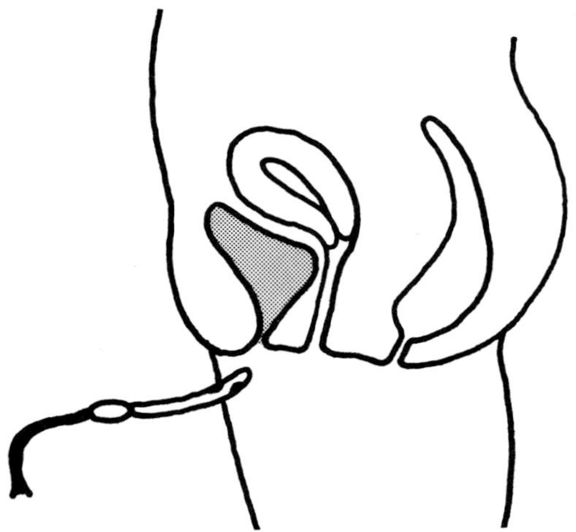

Figure 9-3. Catheterization may be done on women who are unable to do a careful clean-catch collection.

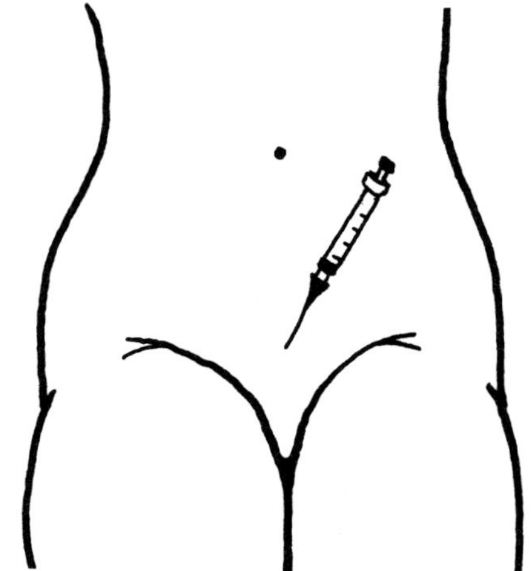

Figure 9-4. Bladder aspiration is significant since no contamination can occur.

Causes of oliguria are dehydration following diarrhea, vomiting and fever; chronic nephritis; acute nephritis; cardiac decompensation; acute renal failure following transfusion reaction; surgical shock; massive hemorrhage; and hypotension following injuries.

If doubt exists as to the renal output, pass a catheter and measure the output. This should always be more than 30 ml per hour (400 ml per day). On the other hand, volumes of 2,500 ml per 24 hours are not unusual in diabetes insipidus.

Causes of polyuria are excessive fluid intake, diabetes insipidus, diabetes mellitus, reflex irritation of urinary tract on passage of stones or with infections, chronic nephritis with hypertension and nervousness.

When fluid intake is restricted (no fluid for 14 hours) an excretion of more than 55 ml per hour would indicate the patient has polyuria.

Nocturia is the excretion of more than 500 ml of night urine with a specific gravity of less than 1.018. Measure day urine from 8 A.M. Roughly measured the day volume should be 3 to 4 times that of the night. Regard a disturbance of this ratio as an early sign of renal decompensation, a physiologic effort to excrete a greater volume in order to clear the blood of metabolic wastes.

COLOR. Normal urine is yellow to amber, darkening with increasing concentration. Yellowish urine appears after ingestion of tetracyclines, pyridine and riboflavin. Orange urine suggests ingestion of the antihelminthic santonin, the anticoagulant phenindione and urbilinogen excretion. Olive-green to yellow-brown urine follows the excretion of bilirubin. Red urine suggests the ingestion of beets, blackberries, aniline dyes from candy, pyridine, aminopyrine (Pyramidon), phenolphthalein (red in alkaline urine, colorless in acid), sulfonal, picric acid, cascara, and inborn errors of chronic cutaneous porphyria and erythropoietic porphyria. Freshly voided hemoglobin or myoglobin also colors the urine red.

Dark-brown or even black urine is seen when the urine contains old blood and hemosiderin. Myoglobin, melanin, porphyrins, homogenistic acid and hydroquinones only turn the urine dark after it is made alkaline. Blue-green urine follows the ingestion of methylene blue, thymol and many other dyes. If a yellow froth is present, think of bilirubin. Orange in acid urine and red in alkaline follows rhubarb taken as a food or a purgative and senna, aloes or Argyrol.

CLOUDINESS OR TURBIDITY. Usually freshly voided urine is clear. Do not make any assumptions from the clarity or cloudiness of the urine; most cloudiness has no pathologic significance. Alkaline urine produced from the ingestion of orange juice will have a murky white sediment that disappears on the addition of acid. The urine will become even more cloudy as it stands and the alkalinity increases.

The white or pink turbidity of amorphous urates disappears on heating; urine cloudy with pus will become more turbid on beating. If enough bacteria are present to produce cloudiness, they have multiplied since the specimen was voided. Blood will cause a reddish-brown or smoky urine.

ODOR. Although certain disease entities produce representative odors, the observation cannot be relied upon for diagnostic purposes. The most useful observation gleaned from the odor is whether the urine is too old to test.

SPECIFIC GRAVITY. The glomeruli excrete 50 gallons of urine per day but the tubules reabsorb all but a L or so. Consequently, estimates of the concentrating and diluting ability of the kidney are a measurement of tubular function. Specific gravity determination is an important part of the urinalysis. A normal kidney can produce urine with a specific gravity ranging from 1.001 to 1.040 depending on what it must do to maintain proper disposition of wastes. A random specific gravity of 1.025 or higher indicates adequate renal concentrating power. If looked for, this measurement can often be found on the patient's chart. This may relieve the attending physician of further checks into renal function.

Watch for the following sources of a misleading determination:

Cold urine. Hydrometers are calculated to record at certain temperatures. For every

3° C above or below the calibration temperature, decrease or increase, respectively, the specific gravity reading by 0.001.

Previous medications and test materials. Diodrast and other dyes used as x-ray contrast substances will cause urine output of high specific gravity as well as PSP. A dose of Epsom salts in preparation for other tests will give a misleading value of kidney function if not known and considered.

Low specific gravity. The commonest cause of a specific gravity below 1.010 is water overloading. The production of urine consistently below 1.008 is known as hyposthenuria. Diabetes insipidus and compulsive water consumption may cause this and even after ordering water deprivation the patient may, for some time, continue to poorly concentrate urine. Hyposthenuria may persist in presence of hypokalemia, hypercalcemia and in cases of chronic pyelonephritis, hydronephrosis and polycystic disease, wherein the tubules have been damaged.

High specific gravity. High solute loads cause specific gravity readings of more than 1.030. The solutes are usually glucose as in diabetic acidosis. A relatively high solute load can be caused by dehydration.

A rough estimate of the total urinary solids may be calculated by multiplying the last two digits of the specific gravity by 2.6. The specific gravity should be determined on a mix of a 24 hour specimen. The product is the number of grams of solid in 1,000 ml of urine. The figure doesn't mean much and is seldom used. The average solids in the urine are about 60 g per 24 hours per 150 pound man.

Use the specific gravity to interpret other urinary findings. The amount of protein in the urine may change from a 3+ reaction in concentrated urine to a trace in diluted urine. All hyaline, granular and cell casts tend to dissolve in diluted urine, and red cells will hemolyze.

Reaction. On random specimens, the urinary reaction means nothing. It could well be dropped. The normal 24 hour urine has an acid reaction of approximately pH 5 or 6. The extremes, in health, are 4.7 to 8.0.

Repeated determinations of the pH are useful in determining if urea-splitting organisms are at work in the urinary tract producing persistently alkaline urine; detecting aldosteronism or primary tubular acidosis; and in therapeutic situations, i.e. the prevention of uric acid calculi by checking on the efficacy of base-producing drugs. Uric acid precipitates in acid urine; or eliminating proteus infection by keeping the urine persistently acid.

For emphasis, more should be said regarding the usefulness of adjusting the pH to aid therapeutic management. The procedure is a grossly neglected aid. Urinary pH has a profound effect on the action of drugs, particularly those administered for urinary tract infections and those administered to dissolve, or at least prevent, the formation of urinary calculi.

The susceptibility of infectious organisms to antibiotics or chemotherapeutic agents varies with urinary pH. Consequently, you must select the drug with the greatest therapeutic effect but also maintain a urinary pH on the level at which the antibacterial effectiveness is greatest. The effectiveness of a drug against a specific organism may be more effective, less effective or not effective at all, depending on the urinary pH.

Consider the following; streptomycin, neomycin, kanamycin and benzylpenicillin are more effective against all organisms in an alkaline pH. Tetracycline, mandelic and hippuric acids are more active in acid reactions. In fact, the effectiveness of the two last mentioned will decrease 3 to 5 times as the pH rises from 5.0 to 5.5. This is important when you consider these acids are potent and are effective against virtually all pathogens in the urinary tract with resistance to their action virtually unknown.

Furthermore, reports now indicate that the commonly used sulfonamides as well as the less commonly used chloramphenicol varies in bacteriostatic effectiveness depending on the pH and the organisms. For instance, these drugs may be effective against A organism when the reaction is acid but against B organism only in a less acid or alkaline reaction.

The effective treatment of urinary calculi by adjusting the pH with diet and drugs has been reviewed in Chapter 12. Only oxalate stones are unaffected by urinary pH.

Drugs other than antibiotics are also affected by urinary pH. Chloroquine, quinine and procaine are more readily excreted in acid urine, while salicylic acid and phenobarbital are excreted to a greater degree in alkaline urine. In salicylism, for example, excretion of free salicylate is increased 10 times with a change of urinary pH from 6 to 7.7. In both salicylism and phenobarbital intoxication, alkalinization of the urine should be employed therapeutically.

On the other hand the antihypertensive agent mecamylamine (Inversine) excretion is depressed in an alkaline urine and, consequently, the retention results in a more profound and prolonged hypotensive effect.

PROTEINURIA. Drop the old term albuminuria because new methods of assay have found that many plasma proteins, except those of high molecular weight, are found in normal urine. Perhaps only 5 to 20 percent of the excreted protein is albumin. Just how excess protein gets into the urine is still not clear. It may be by increased glomeruli filtration or decreased tubular reabsorption or both.

The older generation of doctors were taught that normal urine contains no protein. Popular tests for proteins were insensitive to the small amounts in normal urine. Researchers are still debating what is normal. Even though the literature states that protein is excreted at the rate of 50 to 150 mg per day, recent evidence makes it wise to accept a 200 mg rate as the upper limits of normal.

Now we know that dipstick tests are not "too sensitive." They need to be interpreted properly. Dipsticks give a 1+ reaction with 30 mg protein per 100 ml urine and trace reactions with 10 mg/100 ml. In the case of a healthy subject who excretes 150 mg protein in 1,500 ml of urine (a normal rate) the concentration in the urine will be 10 mg/100 ml and will be picked up as a trace reaction. Therefore, by all means, use the dipsticks (Combistix, Albustix, Uristix). They give you additional information if interpreted properly. The heat-acetic acid test detects concentrations as low as 2 to 3 mg per 100 ml and give more false-positive results. Dipsticks are reliable in yet another way. They do not give false-positives if the patient has been taking sulfa drugs (Gantrisin) or tolbutamide or has had certain x-ray contrast media.

FUNCTIONAL OR ASYMPTOMATIC PROTEINURIA. Proteins appear in the urine when there is no demonstrable renal or systemic disease. This type of proteinuria is often called functional or asymptomatic. The most common of these is the *orthostatic* or *postural proteinuria*. Orthostatic proteinuria is present when the upright urine specimens contain protein and the recumbent specimens do not. Measure the amount while the patient is recumbent in bed at night and compare the finding with the specimen obtained after the patient has been standing or walking for 2 hours. Before diagnosing the condition, repeat the test on two or three occasions to ensure its reproducibility. General opinion favors the view that orthostatic proteinuria is seldom the forerunner of renal disease.

Exercise proteinuria is another functional variety. Severe exercise such as occurs in track, handball, football and basketball produces not only proteinuria but also profound but transient abnormalities in the urinary sediment.

Occasional proteinuria persists in both the upright and recumbent positions and in both rest and exercise. If no disease is found, call it *asymptomatic persistent proteinuria*. These cases call for a full investigation. Renal biopsies generally indicate minor but definite abnormalities in the renal tissue. If these changes are minor and renal function is normal, there is little evidence to suggest that massive proteinuria or renal deterioration is likely.

Other proteinurias classified as asymptomatic are those following prolonged exposure to cold and those occurring during pregnancy. From 30 to 50 percent of women have protein in their urine intermittently during an apparent uncomplicated pregnancy. It disappears shortly after delivery; its significance is not known.

PRERENAL ORGANIC PROTEINURIA. This

is a proteinuria associated with other than primary kidney disease. There is cardiac decompensation with passive congestion of the kidneys. Plasma proteins may be normal and the circulation through the glomerulas is slowed, resulting in a more prolonged contact of the plasma with the glomerular capillaries.

Disease states which increase plasma proteins cause a proteinuria even though the glomeruli and tubules are functioning normally. Muscle injury releases myoglobin. Multiple myeloma creates an excess of immunoglobulins producing *Bence Jones proteinuria*. Hemoglobin in excess of serum haptoglobin causes *hemoglobinuria*.

Other causes of prerenal organic proteinuria are chemical poisoning drugs and fever and severe toxemia. The latter causes cloudy swelling of the renal epithelium. Ascitis and intra-abdominal tumors produce congestion by pressure on the abdominal veins.

Renal Proteinuria. The conditions of renal proteinuria are called primary kidney diseases. In nephritis proteinuria is constant in all forms but the amount does not parallel the severity of the disease. In nephrosis large losses of protein occur in the nephrotic syndrome. Destructive kidney lesions occur in tuberculosis, cancer, etc.

Definitions for massive proteinuria vary, but a sensible interpretation of "massive" in current literature would be in excess of 4 g per day. Massive proteinuria is usually associated with abnormalities of the glomeruli.

Since the advent of measuring serum and urine proteins by quantitative immunochemical techniques, kidney function and its relationship to proteinuria has changed. The type of protein—whether high, intermediate or of low molecular weight—may enable the physician to make a more precise diagnosis.

Small size protein molecules such as myoglobins, beta microglobulin and Bence Jones proteins are filtered out by the normal kidney in large amounts. Those of intermediate size, such as albumin, transferrin and IgG, pass through in small amounts, and those of large size, such as alpha macroglobulin and IgM, do not pass the normal glomerular membrane. Soon kidney diseases may be reclassified on the basis of the size of the molecule that is passing through the membrane.

Postrenal or False Proteinuria. In this classification, protein is added to the urine after being excreted by the kidneys. In this category are pyelonephritis, cystitis, urethritis and vaginal secretions which should be excluded by correct collection techniques.

GLYCOSURIA. Glucose is completely filtered out by the glomeruli because of its small molecular size. Consequently, the concentration of glucose in the glomerulus is the same as that of the arterial blood. During the passage of urine through the renal tubules most of the glucose is reabsorbed. Reabsorption of glucose by the tubules is an active process and under normal conditions occurs at the rate of 160 to 170 mg per 100 ml blood, the so-called "threshold" level. Some glucose does escape reabsorption resulting in a daily excretion of less than 500 mg.

Not all glycosuria is of diabetic origin. Glucose is a reducing substance, a reaction upon which the conventional tests are based. But there are other reducing substances in the urine as well, and these can give a positive test for glucose in the urine. Salicylates and streptomycin in certain concentrations can reduce Benedict's solution and cause confusion. Eliminate this type of confusion by using tests based on the reaction of glucose oxidase. They are available as Clinistix, Testape and Galatest. These tests will detect concentrations as low as 100 mg per 100 ml.

But even with this more specific test, the degree of color change does not always reflect the true concentration of glucose. Other carbohydrate reducing substances still interfere, such as galactose from milk, pentose from fruits, dextrins and proteins. Lactosuria occurs frequently during lactation, and glyucosuria is present normally during the latter months of pregnancy. Transient glycosuria occurs in 10 to 15 percent of normal pregnancies. It is important to differentiate the benign glycosuria of pregnancy from an early or prediabetic state which may become overt during the later months of pregnancy. The absence of hyperglycemia and a normal glucose tolerance curve will rule out diabetes.

If the filtration rate is normal, glycosuria occurs in hyperglycemia as in diabetes mellitus. If the glomerulus is damaged, reducing filtration rate, the urine may be negative for glucose even though hyperglycemia exists. This occurs when renal damage complicates diabetes and in dehydration and shock. If the tubules are defective, glycosuria occurs without hyperglycemia as in the nephrotic syndrome, hereditary renal glycosuria, De Toni-Fanconi syndrome or drug toxemia.

Renal glycosuria is a harmless condition but must be differentiated from *diabetic glycosuria*. It is explained by a lowered renal threshold which allows sugar to spill into the urine even though the blood sugar is within normal limits.

Alimentary glycosuria is only a higher degree of renal glycosuria. The threshold is higher than in renal glycosuria but not high enough to prevent spillage after the ingestion of large amounts of carbohydrates. Remember this when giving intravenous glucose. It is of no consequence unless the glycosuria becomes a misleading finding.

Glycosuria with hyperglycemia occurs in diabetes mellitus, hyperthyroidism, emotional glycosuria, ether and some other inhalation anesthesias and increased intracranial pressure when the patient is in coma. Differentiate the glycosuria of head pathology (injuries, hemorrhages and tumors) from the glycosuria of diabetes mellitus.

KETONURIA. The ketone bodies are acetone, beta-hydroxybutyric acid and acetoacetic or diacetic acid.

In diabetes mellitus and in starvation when carbohydrates are not available for metabolism, fatty acids are not completely combusted and their metabolism stops with the production of ketone bodies. In mild degrees of ketosis, you will only find acetone in the urine. As ketosis increases the other two appear. On the advice of their pathologist many hospital laboratories have dropped the testing of acetone. It is now believed that the nitroprusside test is more sensitive to acetoacetic acid, the most sensitive indication of ketosis. The report is given as follows:

0 = negative
+ = trace
++ = moderate amount
+++ = large amount
++++ = those reactions exceeding standard color charts

Remember the other bit of pathophysiology that is important clinically. Ketone bodies combine with sodium and to a lesser extent with potassium and then are excreted as neutral salts. Consequently, the fixed base of the body is depleted and acidosis results.

Ketonuria occurs in metabolic conditions such as diabetes mellitus, renal glycosuria and glycogen storage disease; dietary problems of starvation and high-fat diets; and conditions of increased metabolic requirements such as hyperthyroidism, fever, pregnancy and lactation.

URINARY SEDIMENT. Sediment analysis is the most important preliminary test in detecting renal disease. Cellular elements collected in the tubules and solidified into a cast suggest chronic renal disease. Red blood cell casts are diagnostic of glomerulonephritis (Fig. 9-5). White blood cells are also found in renal parenchymal disease. Rarely more than 5 white blood cells per highpowered field show up in normal urinary sediment. Consequently when 40 or 50 are found, it is indicative of disease (Fig. 9-6). Oval fat bodies and fatty casts are

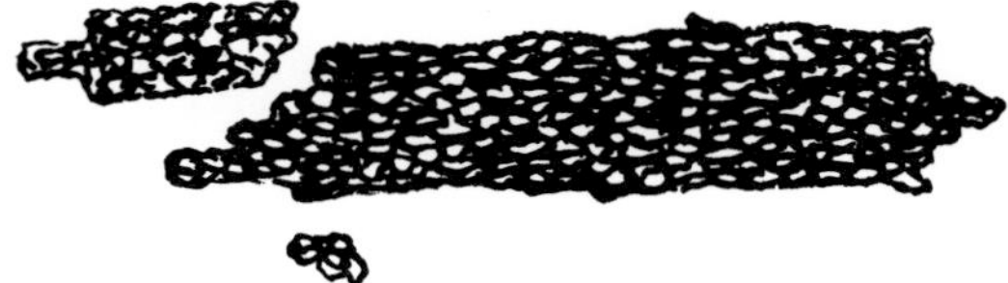

Figure 9-5. Red blood cell casts.

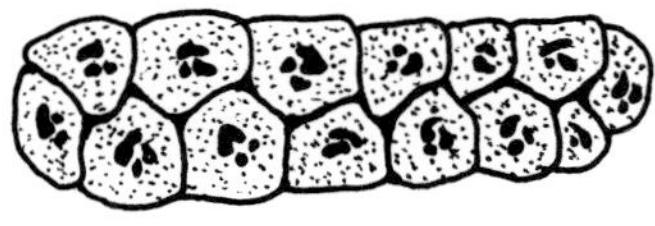

Figure 9-6. White blood cell casts.

indicative of the nephrotic syndrome. Finding hyaline casts should create suspicion of chronic disease. When you find urine pigmented with bile or hemoglobin, the protein of the casts will be stained accordingly.

The common practice of inspecting a drop of urinary sediment without any attempt to quantitate the cellular elements is bad. The specimen loses much of its value as a prognostic test. To roughly quantitate the solids in the sediment adds no expense and little time to the routine microscopic examination.

If you are going to inspect the sediment yourself, a commendable habit, have your technician or nurse prepare the slide as follows: mix the urine thoroughly; centrifuge 15 ml of urine for 3 min at moderate speeds; remove all the supernatant liquid, leaving 1 ml of sediment; mix the sediment with 1 ml of distilled water; transfer a drop of the resuspended sediment to a microscopic slide and cover with a cover slip; and count the number of cellular elements per high-power field.

With this type of report all elements are referred to a 1 to 15 concentration. Now you can compare one report with another with some assurance that the observed element is either increasing or decreasing.

Do this semiquantitative study. If carefully done, you will have no need for the rather cumbersome Addis count. The information you glean from the 1:15 concentration examination is all that you need for every day clinical evaluation.

Staining of the sediment will increase your accuracy and ease of interpretation. Wells and Halsted[2] describe the Sternheimer-Malbin stain and its application. For an excellent study of the morphology of bacterial elements, supplement the wet slide examination with a dry, heat fixed slide stained with one percent methylene blue.

The reporting of unorganized sediment, both amorphous and crystalline, can be misleading and probably should be stopped. Chemical tests are necessary if you need to identify any inorganic sediment in the urine.

Elements of the sediment of no great importance are epithelial cells, mucus threads, spermatozoa in male urine and trichomonas vaginalis. Epithelial cells (Fig. 9-7) are not of much help diagnostically. An excessive number of vaginal epithelial cells in a clean-catch specimen indicates contamination. Determining the site of origin of epithelial cells is mostly guesswork, and if you located the site there is no way for you to know what is a significant number. Mucus threads are often formed as the urine cools. Their origin is generally conceded to occur from the precipitation of mucoprotein. At best, their presence could indicate inflammation in the lower urinary tract. Spermatozoa in male urine means nothing and trichomonas vaginalis in female urine indicates a contaminated urine specimen.

Be chiefly concerned about the number of pus (Fig. 9-8) and red blood (Fig. 9-9) cells, the bacteria and the kind and number of casts. A normal individual excretes about 750,000 leukocytes and 70,000 erythrocytes in 12 hours. This is enough to produce 2 or 3

STERNHEIMER-MALBIN STAIN*

Solution I:	Gentian Violet (85% dye content) Crystal Violet 3.0 g 95% Ethyl alcohol 20.0 ml Ammonium oxalate 0.8 g Triple distilled water 80.0 ml
Solution II:	Safranin 0 (95% dye content) Safranin 0 0.25 g 95% Ethyl alcohol 10.0 ml Triple distilled water 100.0 ml

Note: Mix three parts of Solution I with 97 parts of Solution II. If the mixture is filtered each month it can be kept for three months. Solution I and II unmixed can be stored for years. The stain works best when the urine reaction is between pH 4 to 8.

*Adapted from Wells BB, Halsted SA: Clinical Pathology, ed. 4. Philadelphia: W. B. Saunders, 1967, p. 280.

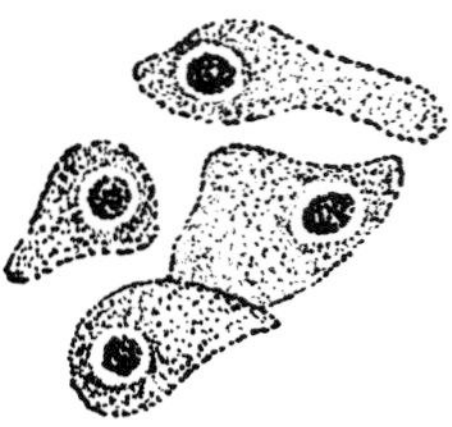

Figure 9-7. Epithelial cells.

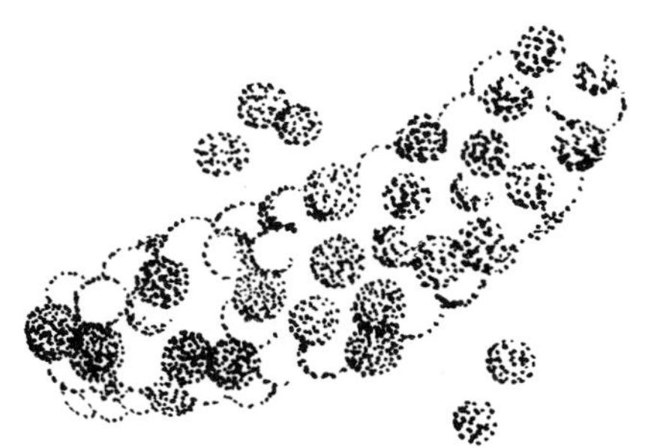

Figure 9-8. Pus cells and pus cast.

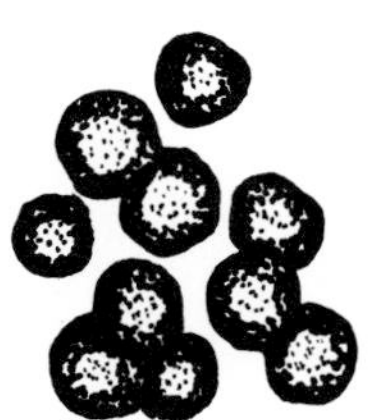

Figure 9-9. Red blood cells.

leukocytes per high-power field and only an occasional red blood cell.

Most laboratories report whether or not the leukocytes "clump." Technicians and doctors impute considerable importance to clumping. Clumping is a function of the reaction of the urine. Generally disregard the finding.

Don't confuse erythrocytes with yeast cells. This is easily done. In an alkaline urine, or even a highly diluted urine, red cells are quickly destroyed. If hematuria is questionable, check for it by using a chemical test. This, too, is not always sensitive enough to detect every case of hematuria.

IDENTIFICATION OF CASTS. Casts are formed in the distal and collecting tubules and represent the shape of the tubular lumen in which they are formed (Fig. 9-10). If protein concentration in the tubule is high and the filtrate is acid, the protein precipitates and forms *hyaline casts*. When searching for hyaline casts, decrease the light and the microscopic condenser; otherwise the light may burn out their outline. A true hyaline cast has no cells. A few hyaline casts are often found in the urine of normal people. As hyaline casts are being formed, however, debris including red, white and epithelial cells may become caught in the protein matrix producing hyaline casts with these various cellular elements within. Classify these as *cellular casts*.

An excessive exfoliation of the tubules, the tubular epithelium, piles up in the lumen and forms casts which, as they proceed down the urinary tract, degenerate and lose their outlines, thus becoming *granular casts*. Cellular and granular casts in excess are found only in renal disease. If the tubular epithelial cells are heavy with fat droplets, as in the nephrotic syndrome, they produce on desquamation oval fat bodies or *fatty casts*.

Normally red cells appear in the glomerular filtrate in such scant numbers that their presence is barely discernible. When the glomeruli are diseased or inflamed both red cells and fibrinogen escape into the filtrate. In any appreciable number they will form clots in the tubules. As the clots loosen and pass, the cells lose their outlines and finally appear in the urine as a homogenous, yellow to orange cast.

What is a significant bacteriuria? This is important. Considerable evidence establishes a correlation between significant bacteriuria and pyelonephritis. An associated pyuria does not always help. Significant bacteriuria is not always found with a significant pyuria. Nor do clinical symptoms always appear helpful. A significant and clinically important bacteriuria often shows up in the asymptomatic patient. Confusion

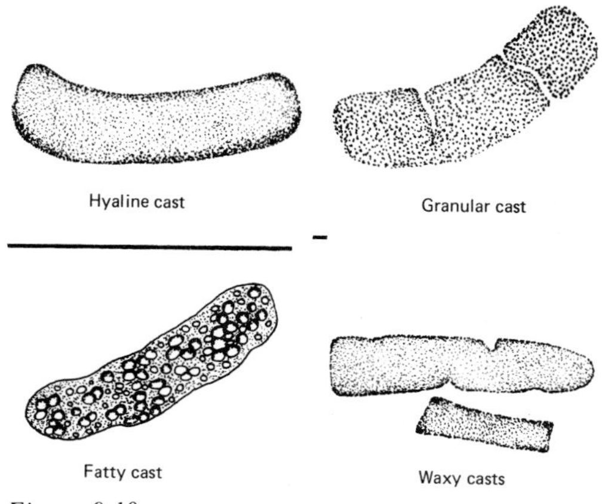

Figure 9-10.

is compounded when a significant bacteriuria appears on the report of a patient with no known urinary tract infection.

What to do? More on this later, but, if suspicion is high and has been increased by the finding of pyuria and/or bacteriuria, request a gram stain on the centrifuged urine. If organisms are detected the bacteriuria is significant. Order a complete bacteriologic work-up.

Renal Function Tests

Remember the two parameters in renal function: glomerular filtration and tubular reabsorption. A quick review of filtration and reabsorption will put the renal function tests in proper perspective.

In 24 hours the glomeruli excrete 600 g of sodium. The tubules reabsorb all but $^1/_{100}$ of that leaving the urine with only 6 g. In the same time, the glomeruli excrete 50 gal of water and the tubules reabsorb all but a L or two. The glomeruli excrete 35 g of potassium; the tubules reabsorb all but $^1/_{18}$, leaving 2 g in urine. The glomeruli excrete 200 g of glucose; healthy tubules reabsorb nearly all, leaving no practical amount in the urine. Even with urea the tubules reabsorb about ½, leaving 35 g per 24 hr in the urine.

Renal function tests usually assess either filtration or reabsorption. They indicate only the degree of impairment. Rarely do they indicate the cause of renal disease. In addition they are relatively insensitive; there may be considerable damage before the tests so indicate.

Don't overlook the routine urinalysis for help in estimating renal function. Albumin and casts indicate damage to the glomerulus. High specific gravity in absence of diabetes mellitus signifies good tubular function.

BLOOD UREA AND BLOOD CREATININE TESTS. Determine the blood urea and blood creatinine. Elevation indicates interference with glomerular function either primarily or secondarily. In interpreting the result, keep in mind that a low-protein diet may cause a low reading. The test is not very sensitive; glomerular filtration must be reduced approximately 30 percent before the blood urea rises. Perform the tests. These are simple to perform and often give as much information as other more elaborate ones. (Normal range blood urea, 15 to 40 mg/100 ml; normal creatinine, 0.7 to 1.5 mg/100 ml.)

The creatinine clearance test is probably the most practical method of measuring the glomerular filtration rate (GFR). The rate of clearance of creatinine from the blood almost exactly parallels the GFR. But creatinine clearance can be correlated with the serum creatinine concentration. There is a linear relationship between these two quantities. Consequently, in most cases the strictly accurate urine collection and the additional time and expense of the clearance studies make the simple serum creatinine determination more valuable.

Remember these conversion factors: Correlate 1.0 mg percent creatinine level with 100 percent creatinine clearance. If the clearance falls to 25 percent of normal, the serum creatinine will rise to 2.0 mg percent. As this relationship is linear, every 7.5 percent decrease in clearance represents a rise of 0.1 mg percent in serum creatinine, an increase of 1 mg/100 ml in 1 year indicates a loss of one half of the patient's kidney function.

Serum creatinine varies from patient to patient, depending on muscle mass. A 100 pound patient may be normal with a creatinine of 0.8; a healthy hard working man, all muscle, may be normal at 1.6; a little fat girl without much muscle tissue may have a creatinine of 0.6. But if the 100 pound girl shows up with a creatinine of 1.3, the finding is an abnormal one.

Family physicians are occasionally deterred from ordering 24 hour creatinine clearance studies because of the inconvenience of the 24 hour control period. Richardson and Philbin[3] reported a favorable correlation between 1 hour and 24 hour clearance rates. They contend that 1 hour creatinine clearance studies are more easily supervised than 24 hour studies. After an extensive study they concluded that carefully controlled 1 hour clearance studies can be used instead of 24 hour studies to determine glomerular filtration rate.

THE PHENOLSULFONPHTHALEIN TEST. The phenolsulfonphthalein (PSP) test is the best routine clinical quantitative estimate of renal function. A mistake that is often made is to have the patient empty his bladder when the intravenous dye is injected. The amount of urine in the bladder makes no difference. A quantitative collection of dye is greatly improved by having urine in the bladder at the time excretion begins. The test can be extended to 1 or 2 hours, but it adds nothing to the information obtained by the 15 minute excretion. Use only the 15 minute check. Less than 25 percent excretion of dye in 15 minutes is definite evidence of renal impairment. A 25 to 50 percent excretion is borderline.

PSP testing also allows a urologist to check each kidney separately. He does this by inserting separate catheters into the ureters and doing a PSP or creatinine clearance in each kidney. This could well prevent the catastrophe of removing a kidney when the contralateral one is poorly functioning.

How to interpret NPN, BUN, serum creatinine, creatinine clearance, serum uric acid and PSP in relationship to renal disease. The NPN of blood[4] includes all nitrogen that is present in a filtrate after removal of protein. The NPN includes urea, uric acid, creatinine, creatine, amino acids, glutathione, nucleotides, etc. The major component is urea (45 to 50 percent). Only a small fraction is accounted for by creatinine (1 percent) and uric acid (3 percent).

Then why has practice shifted away from NPN determinations in renal disease? Because urea is the element in which we are interested and the relationship between urea and NPN is too variable to be helpful. Because of the variation, NPN now has been discarded in favor of BUN and serum creatinine determinations.

The two tests' results must be properly interpreted. BUN and serum creatinine may at first remain normal, even while the creatinine clearance is decreasing. Then suddenly, without warning, great further renal damage may rise steeply.

Comparing serum uric acid to BUN and serum creatinine is frequently helpful. Disproportionately high uric acid levels are seen in gouty nephropathy, uric acid calculi with obstruction, myeloproliferative disorders and in renal disease associated with lead intoxication. A high uric acid in uremia plays a role in the pericarditis associated with renal failure. In addition, hyperuricemia is an early sign of toxemia in pregnancy. What hyperuricemia indicates in hypertension has not been finally explained.

The best single overall measure of function, particularly in chronic renal disease, is the creatinine clearance test. In addition to reflecting function changes the test throws light on the glomerular filtration rate—considered the most clinically significant aspect of renal excretory function.

The popular BUN test is an "unexcelled measure of excessive excretory demands upon renal function." BUN does not reflect renal function changes, but it does afford the best single measure of uremia. A significant use in BUN, however, does not occur until 75 percent of renal function has been lost. Remember that fluctuations in load levels result from diet or changes in body protein balance: in growing children the excretable load is depressed; in severe stress the load may be enhanced. These fluctuations do not mean kidney damage.

Most clinicians prefer the phenolsulfonphthalein (PSP) dye excretion test when a general screening test is indicated. This test yields information on the presence of even the slightest damage to the renal system, beginning with the kidney and ending at the bladder. It is of little value in following progressive renal function changes.

A practical point: PSP is depressed if performed after an IVP. The effect lasts 8 hours or longer. Drugs such as nitrofurantoin (Furadantin), Pyridium and BSP interfere with the determination of PSP.

CONCENTRATION TESTS. The ability of the kidney to concentrate urine is one of the more sensitive tests for early loss of function. The test can be done easily; in fact it is often made and recorded on the chart without the attending physician being aware of its determination. If the patient is given no water after 5 P.M. and urine samples collected at 7, 8 or 10 A.M. the following morning, one of the determinations will show the maximum concentration of which the kidneys are capable. One specimen should concentrate to 1,025. Interference with the test should be expected in pregnancy, severe water or electrolyte imbalance, adrenal cortical insufficiency, chronic liver disease, formation of edema, cardiac decompensation, shock or poor patient cooperation.

Contraindications to its use are the ill patient or elderly in whom water deprivation might further endanger their health. A 14 hour water deprivation can be an uncomfortable experience for the very ill or those with fever.

Another method of conducting the concentration test, which is helpful under certain circumstances, is the Pituitrin method. Some discomfort of forced dehydration can be overcome by the Pituitrin injection method of concentrating the urine.

Dilution tests are never so helpful as the concentration tests. Dilute urine is always a late sign of kidney malfunction and occurs after other symptoms and signs have been positive for some time.

Often neither test need be done. Watch the hospital record. If the specific gravity varies as much as 10 points in its last two figures or concentrates to 1,025 in any one specimen, you are justified in assuming renal function is normal.

Intravenous Pyelogram

X-ray studies using an intravenous contrast media delineates:

- –changes in kidney position
- –abnormalities in architecture of the renal collecting system
- –variations in kidney size or number
- –variations in density
- –variations in contour
- –abnormalities of function
- –difference in excretory function of one kidney as compared with the other
- –other pathologic conditions in the pelvis (Fig. 9-11)

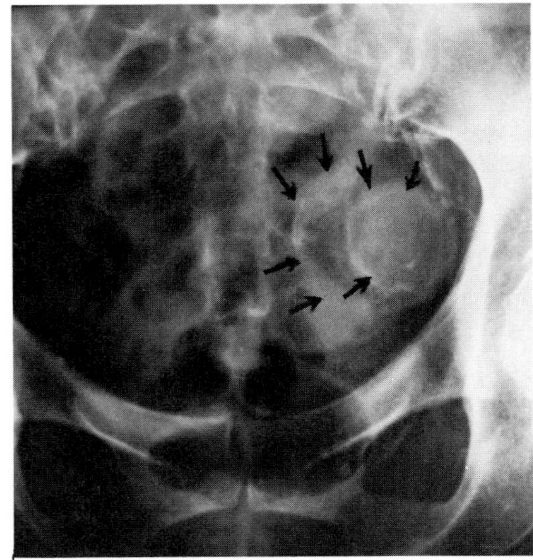

Figure 9-11. Two eggshell aneurysms discovered in the left pelvis.

The value of excretory pyelography in early or moderate azotemia is that it can:

- –detect morphologic variations in the urinary tract
- –establish the existence of obstructive urinary tract disease as a cause of azotemia (Fig. 9-12)
- –determine the adequacy of the contralateral kidney
- –confirm the intrinsic renal process as a cause by ruling out obstructive disease
- –alert to the possibility of greater renal damage than may have been indicated by the BUN

The latter is especially true with patients on a low-protein diet whose BUN's may show only slight to moderate elevation even in severe disease.

Renal Biopsy

If significant doubt exists after the renal study as to the nature of the disease, consider renal biopsy by the precutaneous route. Many now feel the study is safe, convenient and reliable. Its main interest is to distinguish between glomerulonephritis and periarteritis, disseminated lupus erythematosus, pyelonephritis, capillary glomerulosclerosis, diabetes, sarcoidosis or amyloidosis.

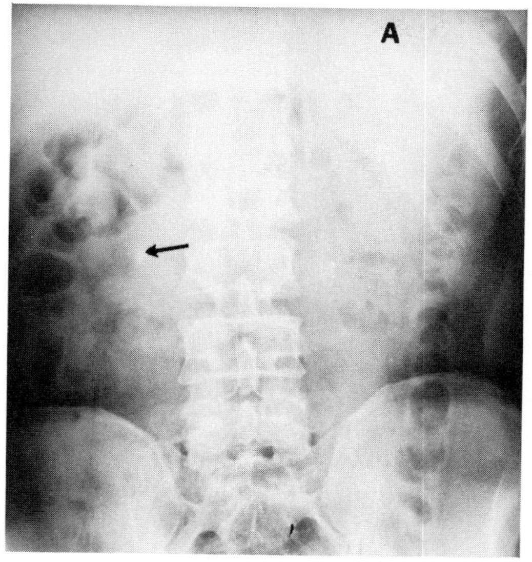

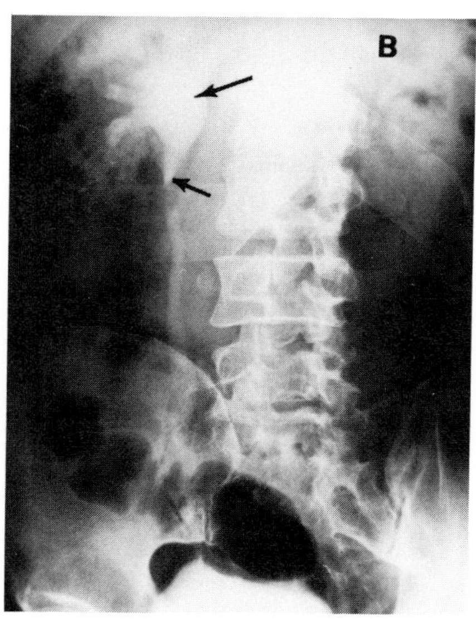

Figure 9-12. A ureteral calculus was suspected in a patient because of pain and hematuria. *A*, Plain film of abdomen shows what appears to be an opaque stone in upper ureter. *B*, Intravenous pyelogram verifies a stone in the right ureter with a hydronephrosis. Note, however, the apparent dilated ureter below obstruction suggesting an obstruction in the lower ureter also.

CHRONIC RENAL FAILURE

Diagnosis

In this day of renal dialysis and kidney transplant, the family physician can only go so far in the management of chronic renal insufficiency. He should be able to make the diagnosis and at least institute treatment with the assurance of some temporary improvement.

For evaluation, start with a creatinine clearance and serum creatinine for determination of the glomerular filtration rate (GFR). Other assays should be made but let this determination be your guide. If the GFR rate is greater than 25 ml/min, little difficulty is experienced by the patient. He may be asymptomatic and the disease is recognized during a check-up or incidentally when help is sought for another disease. If the GFR is between 5 to 25 ml/min the outlook is fair. Ordinarily, good conservative management will keep the patient asymptomatic. If the GFR is less than 3 to 5 ml per min, the patient will develop renal failure. The treatment of this group should be directed by a specialist.

Symptoms are far reaching and can be easily overlooked because they may appear in other organ systems. Instances are:

- –pericarditis, the most frequent cardiovascular disability
- –pleuritis and pleural adhesions and effusions
- –anemias and clotting defects
- –gastrointestinal signs and symptoms, including nausea and vomiting
- –osteosclerosis, osteomalacia and poor callus formation
- –neurologic and psychiatric signs and symptoms
- –a persistent pruritus
- –drug accumulation in body tissues
- –retinal signs such as papilledema, retinal hemorrhage, thickening of the arteries, variations in calibre, tortuosity, increased light reflex, notching of arterovenous crossings and soft exudates near macula

Treatment

Treatment should be guided by the following laboratory assays and the patient's clinical condition. In order to stabilize the patient do these tests daily and then taper off as the patient's condition improves.

First there is need to establish whether systemic acidosis is present and, if it is, whether it is of the uremic or hyperchloremic variety. This can be complicated because of the vast number of bodily variables. In general uremic acidosis is associated with glomerular disease and hyperchloremic acidosis with tubular disease.

Classify the acidosis and plan treatment by observing daily weight fluctuations, intake and output, concentration and dilution of urine and ability of kidney to maintain sodium balance.

The patient's ability to concentrate and dilute the urine is determined by observation of the specific gravity of the urine under test conditions. In glomerular disease the concentrating ability of the kidney is maintained longer than with tubular disease.

In glomerular disease there is a tendency to retain sodium, which increases the possibility of edema formation and attendant strain on the cardiovascular system. On the other hand, tubular disease decreases sodium output. All this can be determined by serum sodium assay and occasionally urine sodium determination.

In primarily glomerular disease, watch weight and water balance to determine the need for sodium and/or water restriction. If acidosis exists, some sodium may be given as the bicarbonate. If the disease is predominantly tubular, the same parameters should be used to determine the need for supplementary salt.

Somewhat the same conditions prevail in maintaining potassium balance. Again, in glomerular disease the serum potassium increases because of the kidney's decreasing ability to excrete the electrolyte. In contrast the tubular problem is of opposite action. The tubules waste potassium and cause a hypokalemia. Electrocardiographic tracings pick up the toxic limits of potassium variation. Use EKG tracings to decide on whether potassium supplementation is necessary.

Fortunately, the kidneys are usually able to maintain potassium balance even in moderately advanced disease but for hyperkalemia, when it does develop, treat with (1) intravenous glucose with insulin to cover the glucose; (2) Kayexalate retention enema (mix 30 g in 200 ml 10 percent glucose and retain for at least 2 hr; and (3) intravenous sodium bicarbonate (150 mEq/L given by a specialist). Potassium restriction is not usually necessary with a GFR greater than 10 ml/min.

The treatment of acidosis in renal failure is tricky. Here again you must distinguish between the tubular, hyperchloremic acidosis and the glomerular, uremic acidosis (Table 9-1). The acidosis should be corrected in either case. Take your time in doing so. To attempt a quick correction may be hazardous. Twelve to 24 hours is physiologically acceptable. Administer sodium bicarbonate by mouth or intravenously. (Ampoules 44.6 mEq may be given directly or with other fluids—except those with calcium.)

Be on the alert for correctable causes of the renal failure. The hyperchloremic, tubular type often is caused by some obstructive urinary lesion. Rule out:

–benign prostatic hypertrophy
–carcinoma of the prostate
–pelvic carcinoma
–bladder tumors

Table 9-1. Characteristics of Acidoses

Hyperchloremic acidosis	*Uremic acidosis*
Decreased plasma bicarbonate Normal or moderately increased urinary ammonia Increased urinary sodium and potassium Decreased acidic urine although severe systemic acidosis exists Increased chloremia	Decreased plasma bicarbonate Decreased urinary ammonia Decreased urinary sodium and potassium Continued acidic urine, reaching limits of 4.5 to 5 pH Increased serum ammonia

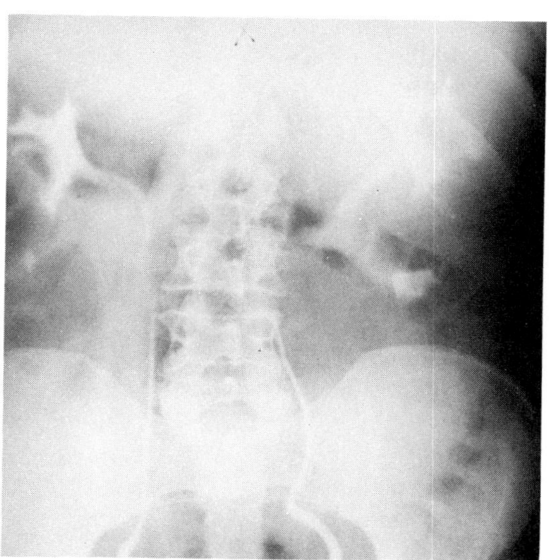

Figure 9-13. Polycystic disease of the kidneys. Pyelogram reveals blunted calyces with oval and crescentic compression of kidney tissue. There is hypertension and bilateral enlargement of the kidneys. The disease is inherited as a mendelian dominant. Hematuria may be the first symptom.

- –strictures and stones
- –toxic drug reactions
- –gout
- –myeloma
- –polycystic disease (Fig. 9-13)
- –pyelonephritis

The uremic, glomerular type is more frequently associated with the acute and chronic nephritides, diabetes, SLE and amyloidosis.

There is a significant correlation between pregnancy and chronic glomerulonephritis The disease worsens rapidly as soon as the patient becomes pregnant and it can be expected that the mother will lose considerable kidney function. Birth control pills will do the same. On termination of the pregnancy or on stopping the pills, kidney failure usually stops.

Do not restrict the diet of those patients who have a GFR of 25 ml or more per min. Moderately restrict protein in those whose GFR is 5 to 25 ml/min. Forty to 60 g/day of protein will be about right. Give high caloric foods with extra vitamins and the essential amino acids. The latter can best be accomplished by using eggs and an electrolyzed whey formula. Mehbod and coworkers[5] suggest a diet which allows 28 g of protein of which 90 percent is of high biologic value and supplies 112 calories. Carbohydrate and fats make up the rest of the 2,200 calories. Free fluid in the diet does not exceed 600 ml. Sodium is limited to 500 mg and potassium to 2,000 mg daily. (See Appendix for 7-day menu.)

Further restrict protein intake to less than 20 g in those with a GFR of less than 5 ml/min.

Kidney Transplantation

Surgical teams are now getting over 70 percent graft survivals and 90 percent patient survivals in kidney transplantation. A San Francisco team claims its last 175 transplants have been successful.

The key to saving more lives of patients with chronic renal failure lies in obtaining live kidney donations from the public. Donors usually come from volunteers in the patient's family. The family physician has a responsibility in educating his patients to the importance of kidney donation and to signing a pledge card. Dialysis in a patient can't be carried on forever; death occurs among its users also. A great number of patients go on dialysis in hopes of eventually getting a kidney.

The best donors are healthy young people, but they are the least likely to carry a donor's pledge card. They believe it's unnecessary to sign a donor's card because death does not seem imminent. In this circumstance, the family physician can urge the parents to carry a card. The card might remind them of the possibility of kidney transplant if one of their children should die.

ACUTE RENAL FAILURE

Classify the causes of acute renal failure as prerenal, renal and postrenal. Acute renal failure is not always due to primary renal disease which has caused sudden renal deterioration. A large number of bodily insults may cause sudden impairment of renal function with oliguria.

Some causes without reference to their being pre-, post- or renal are the following: surgery; trauma; burns; concealed accidental hemorrhage; anesthesia; septicemia, particularly with E. coli and staphylococci; severe dehydration; renal obstruction; pyelonephritis; sulfonamide overdosage; hypotension from any reason; nephrotoxins; acute glomerular nephritis; renal artery thrombosis; severe vomiting and diarrhea; transfusion reactions that cause free circulating hemoglobin; and neoplasms (Fig. 9-14).

The important concept: Recognize that acute renal shut-down may suddenly follow or be part of the pathophysiology of any of the above mentioned states. Recognize it by beginning oliguria, a urine volume of less than 400 ml/24 hours. Recognition is all important because acute renal failure is immediately reversible if detected early. Blood volume, blood pressure, central venous pressure and urinary output are all useful and practical guides.

This emergent renal disease has two phases: the oliguric phase, which may last 1 to 21 days, and the diuretic phase, which may develop quickly. Treatment of each phase is different.

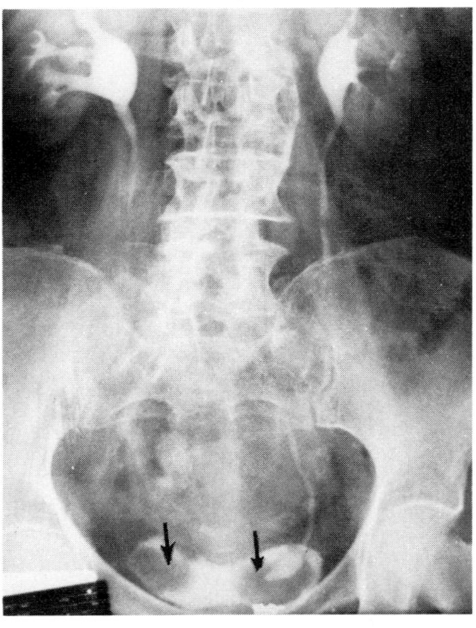

Figure 9-14. A bilateral papillary transitional cell carcinoma which was mistaken for possible urethroceles. Tip off should have been the irregular outline.

Oliguric Phase

The clinical picture is:

- –oliguria (less than 400 ml/24 hr)
- –urine specific gravity between 1.010 and 1.015
- –a pH of around 7.0
- –albumin 1 to 2+
- –red cells and their casts and leukocytes in the urinary sediment

During this stage, restoration of volume deficit may be all that is necessary for treatment. At this point, distinguish between renal failure and simple dehydration. In renal failure, the specific gravity is around 1.010 and the urea content less than 600 mg/100 ml. In dehydration, the specific gravity is above 1.015 and the urea content above 2.0 g/100 ml.

Occasionally one can tell whether acute damage is being superimposed on chronic renal failure by an x-ray or tomography study. In the event there is chronic damage, the x-ray will show the outline of contracted kidneys.

In a few days, systemic changes occur. They are:

- –hypertension
- –dulling of the sensorium
- –increased pulse and respiration
- –vomiting
- –decreased serum bicarbonate
- –increased serum creatinine, BUN and potassium
- –increased anemia

Ideally, the best way to manage these patients is by peritoneal dialysis or hemodialysis. With this treatment given 3 to 4 times a week, a patient will not become uremic and complicated electrolyte imbalances will not occur.

Pending such treatment or where dialysis is not available, attempt the following nondialytic management. Recognize first that great danger lies in overhydrating these patients. A mere replacement of fluid and electrolytes is sufficient. This can be accomplished by giving a 25 percent glucose solution in water. First give enough to replace insensible loss. This is about 500 ml in an adult. It may take 1,000 ml if the patient is feverish and sweating. Add to this the volume of urine passed in the previous 24 hours. If the solution nauseates the patient, replace it with lactose which is less sweetening. If neither can be done, try an intragastric drip. For vomiting, give 50 mg chlorpromazine IM.

Of course the dextrose can be given intravenously, but there are hazards involved. In order to give 100 g of dextrose per day, it will be necessary to utilize 25 to 50 percent solutions because of the need to restrict volume. Consequently, to prevent chemical phlebitis and sclerosis use a polyethylene catheter advanced at least to the brachial vein or to the right atrium. To prevent clotting add 500 units of heparin and 5.0 mg of hydrocortisone to each bottle.

Daily electrolytic determinations and EKG tracings will warn of an impending hyperkalemia. There is some debate but many believe hyperkalemia is what kills these patients. Others believe that many deaths are iatrogenic, that is, caused by fluid overloading. If plasma potassium levels appear to be rising, add 10 units of insulin to each bottle of 50 percent dextrose. Another prophylactic measure is to give sodium polystyrene sulfonate (Kayexalate) by mouth in 15 g doses, 2 to 3 times daily. It is possible to give Kayexalate by enema if the patient can retain the fluid for 2 hours. Kayexalate is a resin which exchanges sodium for potassium in the bowel. Some add sorbitol, an osmotic cathartic, to the resin given, again as an enema. The latter combination will require the mixture to be installed above the rectum by a catheter with a balloon to help the patient retain the solution.

The most common cause of death is infection rather than metabolic failure. Do not give prophylactic antibiotics but promptly treat infection when it occurs. Choose the antibiotic after identification and sensitivity testing. Do give the antibiotics excreted by the kidneys in smaller doses.

Anemia is a common occurrence; however, there is a tendency for the hematocrit to stabilize around 25 to 30 percent. If need arises, give small transfusion of freshly drawn packed red blood cells.

With this regimen, most patients can be maintained until the phase of diuresis occurs. Dialysis is required if neurological signs of drowsiness, twitching, etc. occur; BUN rises above 200 mg; plasma proteins rise above 7.5 mEq/L; or plasma bicarbonate falls below 15 mEq/L.

Don't make the mistake of giving up on those patients who suffer a prolonged oliguria. Treat them aggressively with the expectation that diuresis will occur. There was a recent report of five patients whose output was less than 500 ml/day for 31 to 72 days and who required multiple peritoneal dialysis and hemodialysis but recovered renal function. One patient achieved normal renal function, and the other four recovered to live comfortably independent of hemodialysis.[7]

Diuretic Phase

Change treatment objectives when the diuretic phase begins. Recognize the new phase when diuresis of more than 2 L occurs. Experienced observers believe the diuresis indicates improvement, but the patient may continue ill with increasing concentrations of urea and creatinine.

Treatment during this time can be relaxed a bit; electrolytes and fluids need not be precisely replaced. Perhaps some loss is due to the release of occult edematous fluid accumulated during the oliguric phase. Give the patient only enough to replace insensible loss and to provide a urinary output of about 2,000 ml, a total of about 2,700 ml. Order an occasional check of sodium and chloride in the urine for excessive losses which should be replaced. A good replacement solution contains sodium, chloride and lactate or bicarbonate.

HEMATURIA

Causes of hematuria are listed in Table 9-2.

Family physicians must learn to recognize hematuria as a dangerous symptom. Order a complete investigation whenever a patient has one episode of gross hematuria or 2 or 3 red blood cells in the urine on more than one occasion.

Differential Diagnosis

Before planning a comprehensive urologic study, consider the type of bleeding, how it occurred and with what other common urinary finding it was associated. Consideration of these facts may point you in the right direction.

Did you find the hematuria on a routine microscopic examination in an asymptomatic patient? Consider the possibility of mild trauma, recent vigorous exercise or a recent systemic infection. Look at the patient's penis or the urethral orifice for a simple caruncle.If you cannot find an explanation, repeat the urinalysis several times. If microscopic red blood cells persist, start a complete investigation. Search the sediment for red blood cell casts. If you find one, you can be more certain of the need for the evaluation. Is the hematuria associated with colic? (See Renal Calculi in Chapter 12.) If the patient is a child, search for glomerulonephritis or, if the patient is an adult past 40, a tumor or stone.

Table 9-2. Causes

From the kidney
- Acute glomerulonephritis
- Chronic glomerulonephritis
- Infarction of the kidney
- Subacute bacterial endocarditis
- Nephrotic syndrome
- Pyelonephritis
- Hypernephroma
- Bleeding diseases
- Anticoagulant overdosage
- Trauma
- Renal vein thrombosis
- Calculi (Fig. 9-15)
- Sickle cell disease
- SLE and other collagenoses
- Anaphylactoid purpura
- Hypoprothrombinemia
- Septic and other embolic phenomena
- Renal tuberculosis
- Malignancy
- Idiopathic hematuria
- Cystic disease
- Leukemia and other blood dyscrasias

From the collection system
- Urethritis and prostatitis
- Benign or malignant tumors of the bladder (Fig. 9-16)
- Nephrolithiasis (see Chapter 12)
- Acute bacterial infection
- Foreign bodies
- Prostatism

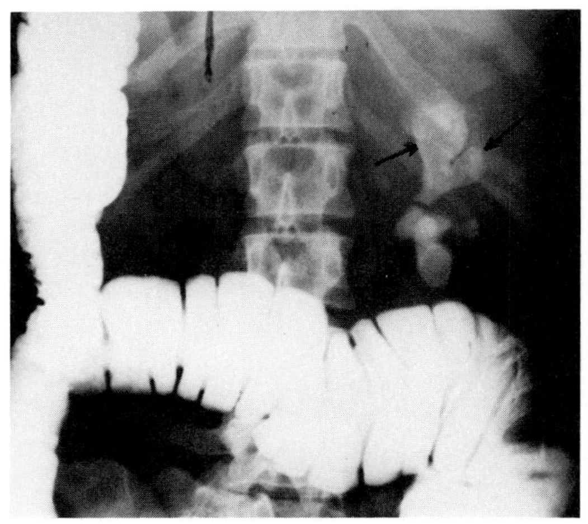

Figure 9-15. A staghorn calculus. Other calculi of the renal pelvis are calyceal and renal pelvis calculi.

The relative amount of hematuria as compared to the amount of proteinuria may be significant. A heavy proteinuria with a relative minor hematuria suggests glomerular disease such as chronic glomerulonephritis or the nephrotic syndrome. A relatively greater amount of blood than proteinuria, on the other hand, suggests tuberculosis (Fig. 9-17), cancer or stones (Fig. 9-18). These relationships are not inviolate because red cells, in considerable number, will produce proteinuria.

The relationship between leukocytes and red cells is not as definite. A high-power microscopic field dominated by leukocytes, however, speaks for infection, but nephritis and nephrosis can produce a considerable number, too.

Order a complete blood count including a platelet count, the latter to rule out certain blood dyscrasias. The presence or absence

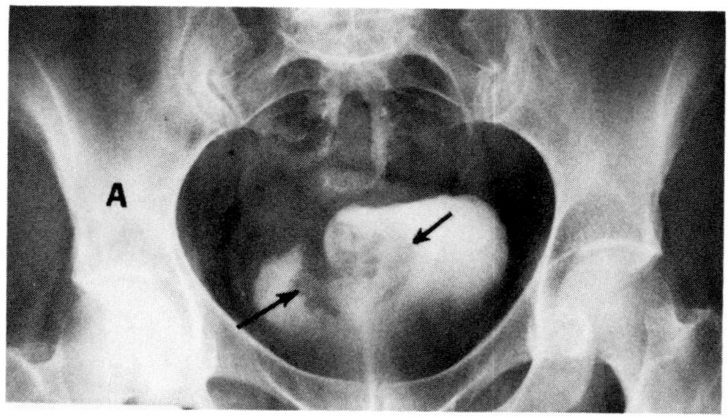

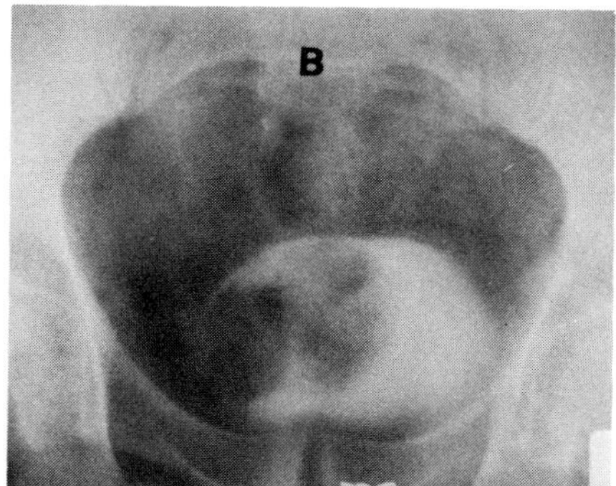

Figure 9-16. *A*, Bladder cancer; *B*, Six months later.

of leukocytosis will be helpful. Is there an anemia? Could it be dilutional as a result of an edema as in acute glomerulonephritis? How about the anemia of azotemia?

No matter the patient's age or size, obtain several blood pressure readings. Remember, hematuria, hypertension and edema equals acute glomerulonephritis. Unilateral kidney disease and chronic insufficiencies cause a hypertension which is reversible if a nephrectomy is done before the healthy kidney is damaged. Proceed with the following tests: culture of throat and other suspicious areas plus acid-fast inoculations and cultures, x-ray of chest, tuberculin skin test, antistreptolysin titer,

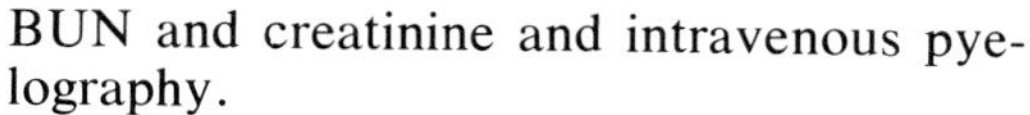

BUN and creatinine and intravenous pyelography.

If the diagnosis is not yet clear continue with consultation and cystoscopy plus retrograde pyelogram, cinecystourethrogram, urine cytology for malignant cells, renal biopsy, aortography to visualize the renal tree, retroperitoneal air insufflation, nephrotomography and renal scan.

In aortography a clear area suggests a cyst, puddling of the dye a neoplasm. A radiologist can deduce several other findings from the study.

Retroperitoneal air insufflation of 1,000 to 1,500 ml of air permits visualization of the retroperitoneal area. Failure of the gas to

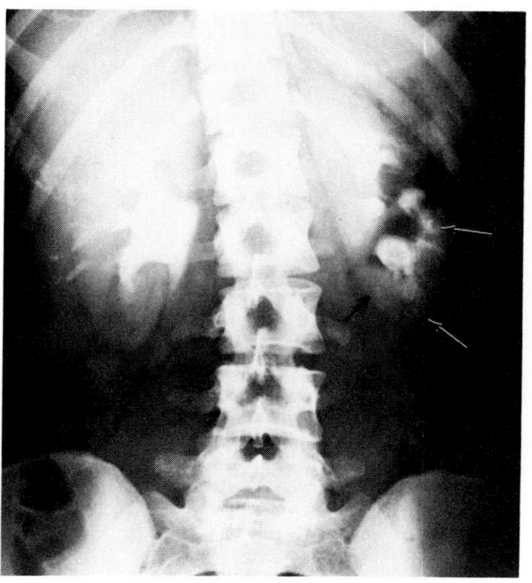

Figure 9-17. Tubercular deformity of the left kidney with an associated papillitis.

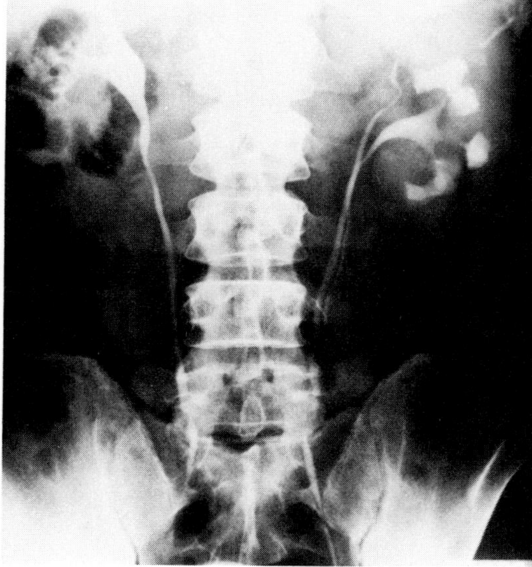

Figure 9-18. Kidney stones in left lower calyx; double collecting system.

diffuse around the kidney suggests local extension of the tumor.

Nephrotomography is a procedure wherein x-ray films are taken at different planes through the kidney while contrast media is given to opacify the mass. It is of limited value.

A renal scan outlines the renal circulation and may be useful to confirm the presence of a small mass. The procedure cannot differentiate between a cyst or tumor.

If you have narrowed your diagnosis to nephritides, tumors or cysts classify them according to Table 9-3.

Remember 95 percent of all renal neoplasms are malignant. Wilm's tumor is practically the only tumor of childhood; most tumors occur after 40 years of age. Renal tumors have few if any symptoms until far advanced. In any event it isn't wise to wait and see when blood is found in the urine. Tumors, stones and infections account for 75 percent of causes for hematuria. Tumors alone account for 20 percent.

Check these clinical findings: Find out if the patient notices more blood at the beginning or at the end of urination. If he states there is more blood at the beginning, think of bleeding distal to the bladder neck and proximal urethra. If bleeding occurs throughout micturation, think of upper urinary tract problems. And if bleeding is mainly at the end of micturation, think of bleeding from the bladder neck or prostatic urethra.

The same findings can be observed by the 3-glass test. Ask the patient to void successively into three specimen glasses. The test result is similar to that described above. Blood in the first glass indicates bleeding below the bladder neck, blood in all glasses indicates bleeding above the bladder neck and blood mainly in the third glass indicates bleeding from bladder neck and trigone.

The Child with Acute Glomerulonephritis

Ninety percent of the children with AGN make a complete and permanent recovery. The first signs to disappear are the fever and edema followed closely by the hematuria and later the hypertension. Proteinuria is the last to go.

Of the 10 percent who do not recover: few become increasingly worse with mounting hypertension and deepening uremia and die within a year, a few develop anuria and die unless treated with dialysis, a few apparently recover but continue to pass albumin and, years later, may develop chronic renal failure or the nephrotic syndrome.

You may see an occasional child who has hematuria 2 to 3 times a year following respiratory infections. In between attacks, the urine will be normal. Patients like this most likely have a focal glomerulonephritis related to respiratory infections. Do not treat. The outlook is good and no restrictions of diet or of activity need be imposed. Be sure the patient does not have lupus erythematosus. If doubt exists, a renal biopsy will make a definite diagnosis.

Table 9-3. Classification in Hematurias

Nephritides	*Tumors*	*Cysts*
Acute post-streptococcal glomerulonephritis	Benign adenoma	Solitary polar, intramedullary, parapelvic simple cyst all appearing uni- or bilaterally
Acute glomerulonephritis associated with other systemic disease, i.e. polyarteritis nodosa, anaphylactoid purpura and radiation to the kidneys	Fibroma	Polycystic disease
Chronic glomerulonephritis	Lipoma	Multicystic disease
Rapidly progressive glomerulonephritis	Leiomyoma	Medullary sponge kidney
Focal glomerulonephritis	Myxoma	Echinococcus disease
Diffuse membranous glomerulonephritis	Hemangioma	
Diffuse membranous glomerulonephritis associated with systemic disease	Hamartoma	
	Malignant Wilm's tumor	
	Hypernephroma	
	Sarcoma	
	Transitional cell carcinoma	
	Squamous cell carcinoma	

Insist that all measures be taken to prevent infections and, when they do occur, treat them strenuously with antibiotics. Many physicians advocate giving phenoxymethyl penicillin, 240 mg, daily orally for several years to prevent further streptococcal infections. Remove grossly diseased tonsils when the patient has recovered.

URINARY RETENTION

When the patient's complaint is urinary retention, look for a prostatic malignancy, benign prostatic hyperplasia (BPH), drugs that may upset the urinary system, central nervous system damage, strictures, diverticula of the bladder, retained calculi or tumors (Fig. 9-19 and 9-20).

Drugs that cause damage to the kidneys are anticholinergic agents, sedatives, antihistamines, antihypertensive drugs, peripheral vasodilators and anti-Parkinsonism drugs. Central nervous system damage may result from diabetes, pernicious anemia, multiple sclerosis, tumors of the brain or spinal cord, tabes dorsalis and senility with arteriosclerotic brain ischemia.

Benign Prostatic Hyperplasia

If you have adjusted yourself to changes in nomenclature, you know that prostatism became benign prostatic hypertrophy and now is benign prostatic hyperplasia with several variations, i.e. benign stomal, benign glandular or nodular hyperplasia. The concept of this disease has not changed. The word *prostatism* now appears to be a catch-all term referring to any obstruction to the urinary flow by the prostate. Benign prostatic hyperplasia, fibrosis of the prostate and carcinoma of the prostate are the three most common prostatic abnormalities causing prostatism.

Patients come to you for one of the following symptoms listed somewhat in the order of their appearance:

–decreased force of urinary stream with increased emptying time
–difficulty in initiating the urinary stream particularly in the mornings

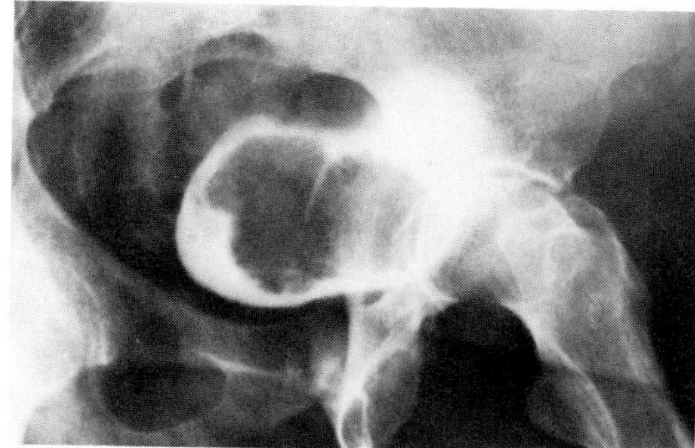

Figure 9-19. Epidermoid carcinoma of the bladder, oblique view.

–awakening at nights to empty the bladder
–increased sensation of incomplete bladder emptying
–sudden acute retention of urine (in about 30 percent of the patients this is the first symptom)
–incontinence of urine (paradoxical dribbling with voiding at intervals caused by impairment of the sphincter mechanism and overflow incontinence resulting from an obstructive threshold that prohibits the complete emptying of the bladder)
–secondary complications of obstruction, i.e. cystitis, pyelonephritis, reflux, hydronephrosis and bladder diverticula
–symptoms of uremia

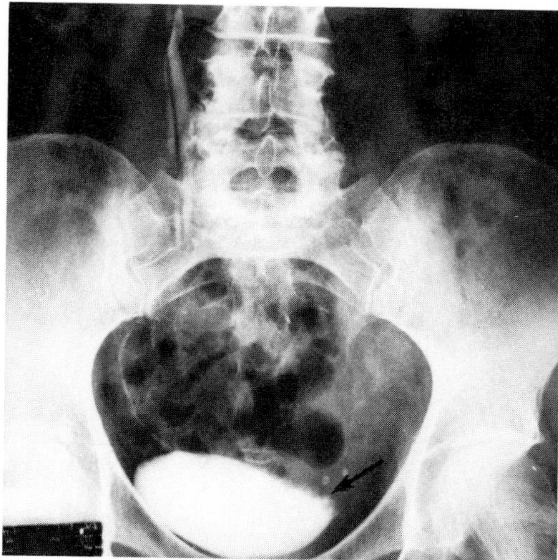

Figure 9-20. Bladder tumor on the left side with nonfunctioning left kidney and duplication on the right.

Digital Rectal Examination

Do the digital rectal examination with the patient in any position that allows you to insert an index finger into his anus. If performed in the office, the ambulatory patient may bend over and place his elbows and forearms on the examining table. This puts him in the proper position for the examination. In the hospital and with debilitated patients, a lateral decubitus will serve equally well. The knee-chest position allows deepest penetration. Place some disposable tissues on the examining table; occasionally excess prostatic fluid will need to be wiped from the meatus. Keep microscopic slides nearby to collect a drop of the fluid for study.

Insert the lubricated finger into the anus examining the orifice and canal. Make a note of any hemorrhoids or fissures. Palpate the rectal mucosa as high as your finger will reach for areas of induration, masses or bleeding.

Begin a detailed examination of the prostate. Remember there is no fixed size. Prostatic size varies from patient to patient. In addition, the size has little to do with the magnitude of the patient's complaints. Large lateral lobes may not cause obstructive symptoms, while the median or subtrigonal lobe may cause complete obstruction with only minimal enlargement.

After estimating the size of the prostate and the laterally placed seminal vesicles, proceed to evaluate the consistency of the gland. It should be compressible. Irregularities, hardness or nodularities are abnormal. In 50 percent of the patients with these findings, cancer is present. In the other 50 percent, a calculus or another benign condition exists.

The normal gland is like a shield 2 in wide. It is surrounded by a sulcus. The lobes are bisected by a midline raphe. Normally the seminal vesicles are not palpable. Whenever you are able to outline the vesicles, be suspicious of inflammation or tumors (Fig. 9-21).

Palpate the membranous urethra and the apical portion of the prostate as you withdraw your finger.

Digital rectal examination is not diagnostic but it is important for two reasons: the determination of the presence or absence of prostatic carcinoma and the determination of an appropriate surgical procedure in treating BPH. BPH affects primarily the median and lateral lobes (Fig. 9-22). Infrequently do the anterior and posterior lobes enlarge except in carcinoma.

Fibrosis of the Prostate

This condition occurs earlier in life than BPH. Apparently the cause is a fibrosis following prostatitis. Often strictures are present because of the close proximity of the urethra and prostate.

Carcinoma of the Prostate

Carcinoma usually begins as a palpable hard nodule in the posterior lobe and infiltrates into other lobes, the seminal vesicles and the bladder. As it grows, the entire gland becomes hard as stone. Carcinoma occurs in 15 to 30 percent of all males past the age of 50. Some family physicians depend on the serum acid phosphatase to aid in the diagnosis of prostatic carcinoma. They should

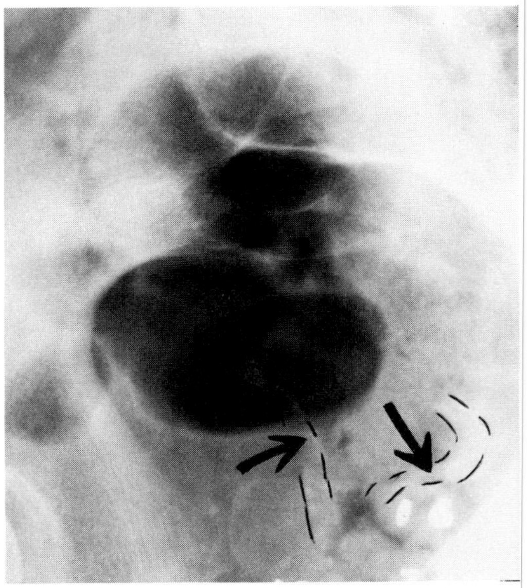

Figure 9-21. Calcified seminal vesicles lightly outlined in oblique view of pelvis.

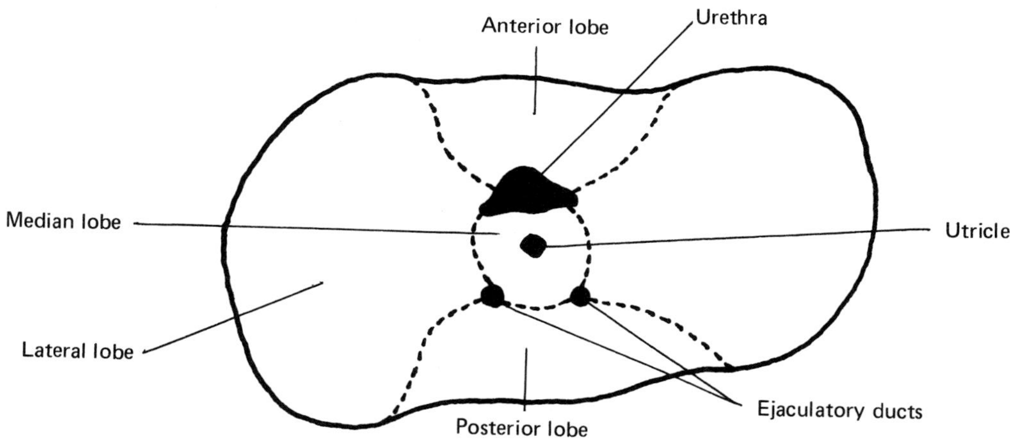

Figure 9-22. Cross section of the prostate.

remember the acid phosphatase does not increase unless the carcinoma has metastasized to the bone (Fig. 9-23). When this occurs, the enzyme rises in 60 percent of the patients only.

In all cases, do an examination of the urinary tract as previously outlined. Give particular care to eliciting signs of obstruction and clues to where the obstruction might be. It takes 240 ml of residual bladder urine in order to detect its presence by percussion. Check the penis and its meatus for evidence of stenosis which may have followed long-forgotten injuries. Tap the costovertebral angles for evidence of pyelonephritis or hydronephrosis.

Laboratory Aids

The family physician should proceed with the basic work-up. Intravenous pyelography is a most helpful examination. A carefully timed postvoiding exposure permits an estimation of residual urine in the bladder without further instrumentation. While doing the intravenous pyelogram order an x-ray study of the pelvic bones for osteoblastic bony metastases. Do an excretory cystourethrogram as the final stage of an intravenous pyelogram. This is helpful in detecting urethral strictures.

Catheterization and sounding occasionally may be needed to determine residual urine and the size of the urethral lumen. Do not do them routinely. In an unhealthy urinary tract these manipulations may be followed by a stubborn infection or complete urinary shut-down. There is some systemic danger in a rapid decompression of a bladder which has carried 400 ml of urine for a protracted period of time.

Occasionally a Papanicolaou smear of the prostatic fluid may show exfoliative cancer

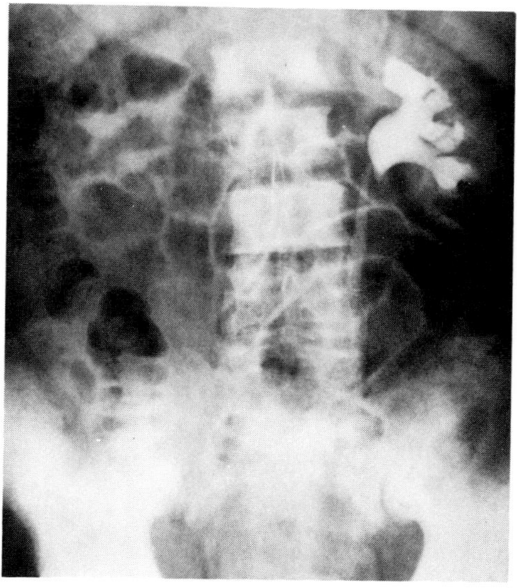

Figure 9-23. Prostatic cancer metastasized to the bone in an AP view. The patient's left kidney (on right side of plate) is hydronephrotic. The patient was injected IV to reveal excretory passages; therefore, the film indicates the patient's right kidney is nonfunctioning.

cells. Be careful because prostatic massage in the presence of cancer may disperse cancer cells into the lymphatics and venules.

By now you have probably arrived at a diagnosis. After all the tests are completed, the diagnosis is usually made by palpating the prostate gland with an index finger.

Leave the following tests to the urologist. Some of them may help him plan on what and how much to do.

Cystoscopy. Usually it doesn't tell much more than you have already learned.

Tissue biopsy using the Vim-Silvermann biopsy needle. This is usually done when the patient is anesthetized for the cystoscopic examination. However, the procedure can be done transrectally in the office, without prior preparation or anesthesia.

Cystometrography to evaluate the neuromuscular integrity of the bladder.

Uroflometry to measure the rate of bladder emptying.

Retrograde urethrography gives about the same information as the voiding cystourethrogram.

Chronic Bacterial Prostatitis

In men, chronic bacterial prostatitis (CBP) is caused primarily by gram-negative bacteria. CBP from whatever bacteriologic etiology is a major source of recurring UT infection. Symptoms and findings include voiding symptoms, dysuria, low back or perineal pain and asymptomatic bacilluria.

Often family physicians do not attempt to localize the site of the infection but begin their treatment on the assumption there is a lower GU tract infection.

An attempt should be made to identify the site of infection, i.e. urethra, prostate, bladder or some combination of these areas. Knowing the location helps the physician to prevent recurrence but also to differentiate it from *prostatosis,* a new term identifying a syndrome with similar symptoms but wherein no pathogen can be identified.

Collect four specimens for culture: (1) the first voided urine for urethral culture; (2) a midstream specimen for bladder culture; (3) a prostatic culture collected by prostatic massage; and (4) the first voided urine following massage again for prostatic culture. Culture the four specimens for gram-negative organism and interpret as indicated on Table 9-4.

If the bladder urine culture is more than 1000 colonies per ml, treat 3 or 4 days with an antibacterial and then check for localization. Prostatic pathogens are not sufficiently affected by antibacterials not to culture out. If no pathogens are found, consider the diagnosis of prostatosis.[8]

Scrotal Enlargements

Enlargements of the scrotum may be caused by varicocele, hydrocele, torsion of spermatic cord, acute epididymitis, acute funiculitis, acute epididymoorchitis, tumors of the testes (seminoma, teratoma or interstitial cell tumors) or tumors of the spermatic cord (lipoma and sarcoma).

Examining the Testicles[9]

Suspect cancer of the testicles when the patient complains of unilateral backache, a tender lymph node in the inguinal area or a

Table 9-4. Bacterial Culture for Gram-Negative Infections

Area of infection	*First voided urine*	*Midstream voided urine*	*Prostatic massage*	*First voided urine after massage*
Urethra or Prostate	↓*	0	↑	↑
Urethra	↑	0	↓	↓
Prostate	0	0	↑	↑

* ↑ = increased culture count; ↓ = decreased culture count.

heavy feeling in the scrotum or when a patient begins to wear a scrotal support to relieve a dull ache. Benign conditions of the scrotum usually cause more pain than cancer.

Inspect the entire genitalia for skin sores, chancre, rashes, enlarged glands or epithelial carcinoma.

Palpate the scrotum for the *bag of worms* characteristic of varicocele. A primary varicocele will empty when a patient lies down; a secondary one empties slowly if at all. The latter will require an exhaustive examination to pinpoint the cause. A fluctuant, pear-shaped, painless cyst that transilluminates could well be a simple hydrocele. Aspiration and testing of the fluid is in order to rule out cancer in the hydrocele. Palpate the vas for granulomas which often follow vasectomies and the area above the testicle for a freely movable cyst, a spermatocele. Again try transillumination. An examiner should be able to palpate a cancer of 1 cm or more. With one hand, lift a testicle and palpate it with the thumb and index finger of the opposite hand. Compare the two testicles in size and consistency. Consider any abnormality cancer until proven otherwise. An undescended testicle is significant because of the increased incidence of cancer in the undescended one. Ask for a surgical consultation in such cases.

ALBUMINURIA AND EDEMA

Causes of albuminuria and edema are in Table 9-5.

Table 9-5. Causes

Nephrotic syndrome
Nephrotic stage of chronic glomerulonephritis
Diabetic nephropathy (Kimmelstiel-Wilson syndrome)
Systemic autoimmune disease lupus erythematosus
Nephrotoxic agents, i.e. mercurials, tolbutamide, versanate and probenecid
Tuberculosis
Syphilis
Amyloidosis
Multiple myeloma
Nephropathy of pregnancy
Thrombosis of renal vein or inferior vena cava
Constrictive pericarditis
Congestive heart failure
Malaria
Poison oak and ivy
Chronic pyelonephritis
Idiopathic
Congenital

Nephrotic Syndrome

Contrary to what many older physicians were taught, the nephrotic syndrome (nephrosis) is not a disease of the tubular epithelium. The primary abnormality is believed to be increased permeability of the glomerular basement membrane to serum proteins. The syndrome is characterized by heavy proteinuria, low serum proteins and edema.

The train of pathophysiologic events in the nephrotic syndrome is an interesting one. It illustrates how a small problem in one part of the body can grow until the health of the entire body is at stake. First, and as yet from some unexplained cause, damage strikes the glomeruli. The glomerular sieve is punctured in such a way that serum protein is allowed to escape. First through the sieve are the smaller albumin molecules. Later as the glomerular damage increases the larger globulin molecules also escape. At this point, measuring the clearance of proteins of different molecular weight presents a picture of the kind and amount of glomerular damage.

The loss of the serum proteins into the urine triggers the onset of other problems. The loss of protein lowers the osmotic pressure of the serum, thus causing a diffusion of fluid into the tissue spaces—edema. With the escape of fluid, blood volume decreases, causing a release of excess aldosterone. This, too, in its turn causes the retention of more salt and water increasing the edema. The loss of gamma globulin which contains antibodies creates in the patient an unusual susceptibility to infection.

In children the onset is insidious. The only early symptom may be a periorbital edema more noticable to the parents than to you. Even this may wax and wane. Certainly, when parents go to the trouble of bringing a child to the office because they think his eyes look tired or funny, do at least a urinalysis.

The diagnosis isn't difficult. The hallmark: massive proteinuria with daily excretion of 5 to 20 g daily. With the large amount of protein passing through the kidney, hyaline and finally granular casts occur in abundance. The absence of hematuria is an important point in excluding glomerulonephritis. A decrease in serum albumin to the critical level of 2.09/100 ml starts the edema.

Another peculiarity of the nephrotic syndrome is the increase in the blood lipoids. When the laboratory reports a milky serum, don't become so enthusiastic about phenotyping and the prevention of heart disease that you forget about checking for the nephrotic syndrome. For practical purposes, the determination of blood cholesterol is a satisfactory index to the total lipemia.

This is one renal disease in which a renal biopsy may be of real help. Frequently only by the histologic pattern can the cause and prognosis be classified. Many patients may have an idiopathic type of disease with little pathologic damage; they will respond well to steroids. Others will be found to have other diseases, most commonly chronic glomerulonephritis. Those with advanced proliferative disease are inevitably steroid resistant.

Because of the meager laboratory findings early in the disease, there is a tendency to classify the albuminuria as functional or the functional albuminuria as organic. Review the causes of albuminuria previously mentioned and eliminate the nonpathologic albuminurias before diagnosing the nephrotic syndrome.

PYURIA

Causes of pyuria are cystitis and pyelonephritis. The urinary tract extends from the urethral meatus to the renal parenchyma. It is filled with a column of urine. The tract is so made that organisms can either pass up or down. Pyelonephritis is a result of organisms passing upward from the bladder to the kidneys (Fig. 9-24). The pathophysiology of pyelonephritis is not known for certain. Patients who have some obstruction, either congenital or acquired, have a higher incidence of pyelonephritis than those who do not.

Under the age of 1 year, the prevalence of bacteriuria is 1 to 2 percent in both males and females. At this age search for a congenital abnormality. After girls reach teenage, bacteriuria increases by 1 percent a decade. At 50 years of age 10 percent of women have bacteriuria.

Family physicians should not be too concerned where cystitis leaves off and pyelonephritis begins. Most urologists spend little time in attempting to differentiate the two. The only sure way is finding histologic evidence of invasion of the renal interstitium by polymorphonuclear leukocytes. In clinical medicine this is not practical. The most inexpensive way, and possibly as certain as any, is the finding of leukocytes in hyaline casts. This simple observation distinguishes upper urinary tract infections from the lower as well as can be done.

Ronald and Boutros[10] recently advocated a therapeutic test which may prove to be of some merit. The test consists of a single intramuscular injection of 0.5 g of kanamycin. They claim this injection generally cures infections confined to the bladder. They consider infections that relapse within 2 weeks with the same causative organism to be of the upper urinary tract.

As a side observation, the doctors found that bladder symptoms, i.e. frequency and burning, had little predictive value as to whether the infection was a lower or upper tract infection. But upper tract symptoms agreed with the final diagnosis in 19 out of 20 patients.

Their final recommendation was to give all urinary tract infections kanamycin. This will cure your patient in a majority of cases. Recheck the patient in 2 weeks. If the patient is infected with the same organism, treat in the conventional way.

Patients with cystitis or pyelonephritis or both come to your attention in one of several ways. They may come to the office ill with typical signs and symptoms of a urinary tract infection, such as dysuria and tenderness in the costovertebral angle. Diagnosis is not difficult.

Others come in ill but with none of the

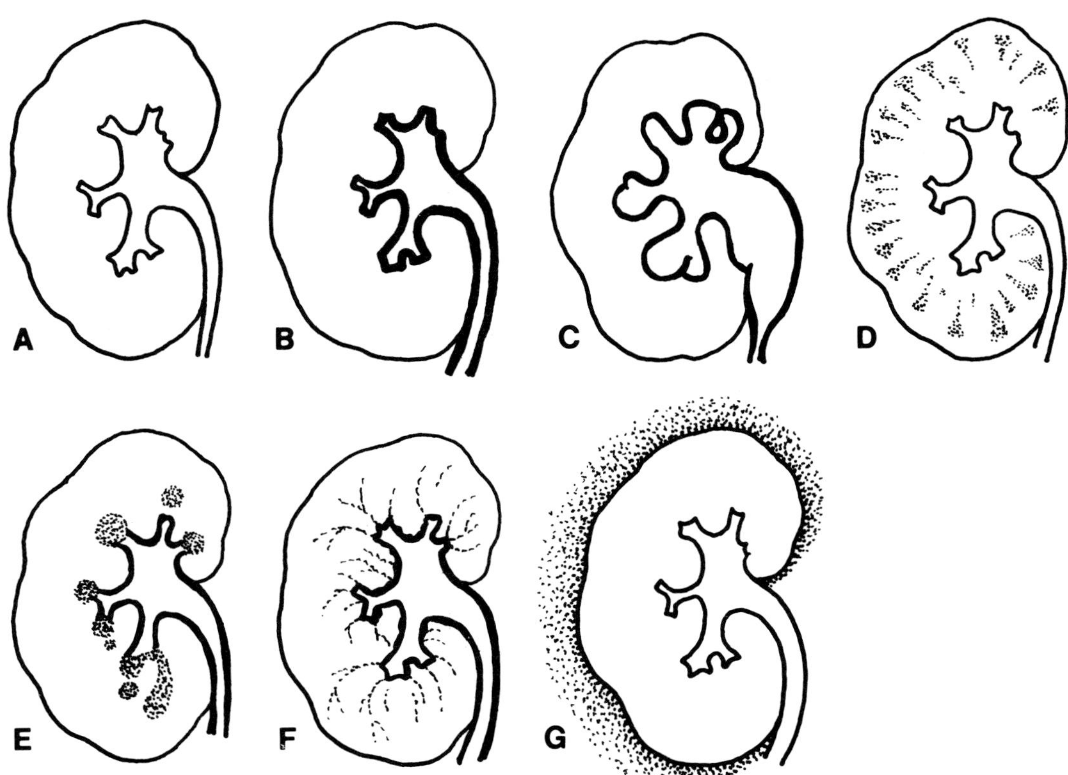

Figure 9-24. A normal kidney, *A*, and various types of renal infection: *B*, Pyelitis; *C*, Infected hydronephrosis; *D*, Cortical abscesses; *E*, Pyonephrosis; *F*, Diffuse pyelonephritis; *G*, Perninephric abscess.

hallmark symptoms of a urinary tract infection. After eliminating diseases in other systems, you finally locate an infection in the urinary tract. Other patients appear, perhaps for some other reason, but have minimal urinary symptoms. The woman who considers herself in good health but must stop frequently to void is a good example. And finally the iatropic patient in whom a urinary infection is found on a routine urinalysis.

There is some debate as to what constitutes a urinary tract infection. For family physicians who are not interested in debating, the wise course is to consider that urine is normally sterile. But because sterile urine is difficult to obtain except by suprapubic puncture certain arbitrary standards of bacteriuria have been set. From a practical everyday treatment standpoint these standards work out suprisingly well.

Bacterial contamination should not exceed 10,000 bacteria per ml. Infected urine usually contains 100,000 or more bacteria per ml. If you want to be a stickler for detail and win no praise from your patients, do as the researchers do and demand that more than 100,000 organisms of the same type be found on 3 consecutive clean voided specimens before making a diagnosis.

In 1970, Finch and Finch[11] studied the midstream urine specimens for UTI in patients suspected of having UTI and routinely in maternity cases. They set the following standards:

- bacterial counts below 10,000 bacteria/ml are almost certainly not infected
- bacterial counts of pure growth of above 20,000/ml are probably infected
- mixed growths above 100,000 bacteria/ml should be repeated after further instruction on collection.

In their study, the incidence of pyuria in infected urines was low. Twenty-eight percent of the females and 29 percent of the males had a significant number of pus cells.

These rather demanding standards do not mean that all urine must be cultured and colonies counted before starting treatment. On a gram stain of uncentrifuged urine, one or more bacteria per high power field correlates with 100,000 or more bacteria per ml. At any rate, and by whichever route, an enumeration of the bacterial count in the urine is the single most important diagnostic procedure in the management of these patients.

Use the following standards (urine clean-voided, first in A.M. or after strenuous exercise). If fewer than 10,000 organisms per ml, disregard the findings as contaminants. If between 10,000 and 100,000 per ml, repeat the test. The test is inconclusive. Organisms could be contaminants or pathogens. If over 100,000 per ml, consider the patient as having urinary tract infection.

Dye tests and the TTC for UTI screening have now fallen into disrepute because of the high rate of false negatives. A new simple incubator test for office use is reported to be about 90 percent accurate. In these tests, a strip of filter paper is dipped into the urine and then touched to an agar surface in a small plastic cup. It is then incubated for 10 to 24 hours at 37° C. A colony count of 3 to 25 is considered suspicious; over 26 is positive. Testuria may be obtained from Ayerst Laboratories, 685 Third Ave., N.Y. 10017; Quantikit from Quantikit, P.O. Box 3932, Portland, Ore. 97408; Uro-Bacti-Lab. from Bacti-Lab., Box 1179, Mountain View, Calif. 94040. I personally would recommend the Quantikit.

If the patient's symptoms are severe, start treatment with either a sulfonamide or a tetracycline. Change to a specific antibiotic after sensitivity studies are completed. After the first course wait 3 to 4 days and reculture. If infection is still present continue appropriate antibiotics. Double the treatment time. Do the same at the end of each course, successively doubling the treatment time until the urine remains uninfected.

No one suggests an old time remedy anymore: hydration. Before the day of antibiotics, water was the mainstay of UTI. No treatment regimen is complete without increasing the patient's water intake.

Do urine cultures or gram stains every 3 months for patients whose attack was their first. Continue with bacteriostatic therapy, i.e. nitrofurantoin, nalidixic acid or methionine (with acidification) for those who have had repeated attacks.

Remember that everything that "burns" isn't a UTI. Take a careful history and rule out:

- –traumatic injuries from truck, motorcycle or auto riding, or traumatic insertion of a tampon
- –a neurogenic bladder which may cause intermittent spasms of pain
- –a stone in the prostate or urethra
- –allergenic foods
- –Trichomonas vaginalis
- –atrophic vaginitis
- –strictures
- –prostatic hyperplasia
- –Hunner's ulcer
- –urethral caruncle

Watch your high risk patients and you will not make many mistakes. High risk patients include pregnant women, preschool girls, diabetics, patients with neurogenic dysfunction, patients with urinary calculi, men with BPH and patients who have been catheterized or who have indwelling catheters. After four days probably all patients with Foleys have UTI. Somewhere between 5 and 10 percent of pregnant women have UTI and even a higher percentage if catheterized before or after delivery. Between 24 to 40 percent of pregnant women with bacteriuria will develop acute pyelonephritis.

Dolan and Meyers[12] recently reported that family physicians were not performing the basic tests before referring patients to urologists. They set the following guidelines: The diagnosis of UTI is not possible without a positive quantitative culture or gram stain of bacteria on unspun urine.

An intravenous pyelogram, a voiding cystourethrogram, BUN, serum creatinine, 2 hour PPBGT and LE cell preparations should be done after the second attack in women and after the first documented attack in men.

Pyuria is a good index of urinary tract infection; however, bacteriuria can occur without pyuria and pyuria can occur without urinary tract infection. Six to ten white cells per high-powered field should be considered suspicious; over ten cells per field is definitely abnormal.

It is usually impossible to differentiate cystitis from pyelonephritis and the work-up should be the same.

The drug of choice would be sulfisoxazole or ampicillin for 2 to 4 weeks for the first urinary tract infection.

Zinner[13] in 1971 reported enhancement of the antibacterial effect of erythromycin when the urine was alkalinzed. Thirty-seven patients with chronic gram-negative infections were treated with erythromycin estolate and alkalinization of the urine. The infecting gram-negative bacteria were eradicated in 73 percent of the patients during therapy. Seventeen patients remained culture negative 3 weeks after treatment and 14 had negative cultures 2 to 6 months after treatment. You might try this as an alternative in some of your stubborn gram-negative urinary tract infections.

BACTERIURIA IN PREGNANCY

Bacteriuria is one of the most common complications of pregnancy (Fig. 9-25). It poses the question of how far a doctor should go in treating an asymptomatic patient with nothing more than bacteria in her urine. Bacteriuria does identify the population at risk and, consequently, should not be ignored.

Several workers have found that if bacteriuria remains untreated during pregnancy, postpartum urine cultures will remain positive in 35 to 50 percent of women 3 to 12 months after delivery. The incidence of bacteriuria varies between 2 and 7 percent depending somewhat on the patient's socioeconomic status. It also rises with increasing age and parity.

It has been fairly well established that when bacteriuria is treated during pregnancy there is virtually no risk that pyelonephritis will develop later in pregnancy. In contrast, about 20 to 30 percent of untreated cases of bacteriuria will develop symptomatic infection.

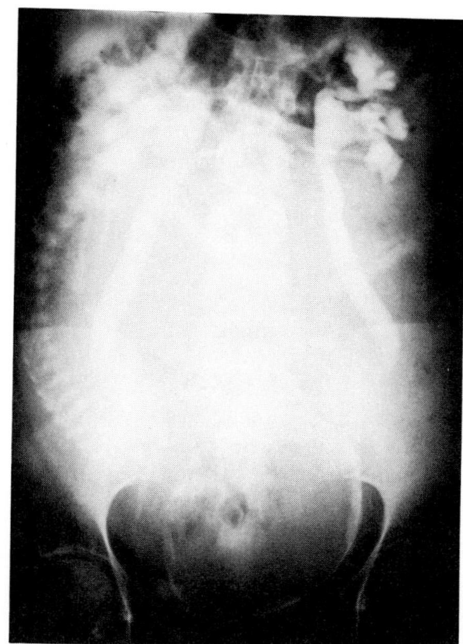

Figure 9-25. Pyeloureterectasis of pregnancy. Most common site is on the right side.

On the same stain a count of more than 5 white blood cells per high-dry field is significant. Therefore, finding bacteria or 5 white blood cells or both appears to be the best screening technique now available. This will detect 96 to 98 percent of urines with significant bacteriurias.

X-RAY EVALUATION OF THE URINARY TRACT IN CHILDREN

Remember the more thoroughly the urinary tract is examined by radiologic techniques, the less likely will it be necessary to request retrograde pyelography. Depend on intravenous pyelography for the upper urinary tract, providing a large-volume dose of the contrast media, fluoroscopy and multiple films during peak excretion are employed. For the lower urinary tract, order cystourethrography, again with fluoroscopy and sequential spot films.

With these techniques such abnormalities as meatal, urethral and bladder neck obstruction can be identified. With these extended radiologic techniques, request retrograde studies only when the urinary tract or a portion of it cannot be visualized by intravenous pyelograms or cystourethrography.[14]

VESICOURETERAL REFLUX

Vesicoureteral reflux occurs in association with GU infections, lower urinary tract obstructions, neurogenic disease and occasionally following surgery. The ureteral orifices are usually displaced to a lateral and superior position. It is estimated that 1 percent of white girls are affected. As suggested reflux is not a single disease entity. The edema following an infection may be a factor in reflux and, if so, will improve on antibacterial therapy.

The diagnosis is made or suggested by a cystogram. Surgery is indicated whenever a dilated ureter, a hydronephrosis, a persistent infection or a defective ureteral orifice is found.[15]

THE PROBLEM OF URINARY CATHETERS

The use of a urinary catheter carries a significant risk of introducing an infection into the genitourinary tract. A single catheterization carries a risk of approximately 1 to 2 percent. An indwelling catheter will cause a similar infection in 90 percent of cases within 4 days. A sterile, closed drainage system will delay the infection 7 to 14 days.

Prophylaxis by either antimicrobial drugs or by irrigation is of questionable value. Monitoring the urine by frequent culturing and treating those who become infected is possibly the best course to pursue. Infection is inevitable and the antimicrobials only help to determine the pathogen involved.

SOME USEFUL DRUGS

Most antibiotics can be used for specific urinary tract infections. Manufacturers have prepared many combinations of anti-infectives plus analgesics, antispasmodics and/or urinary acidifiers. Some are listed below:

Urobiotic capsules contain 125 mg oxytetracycline, 250 mg sulfamethizole and 50 mg phenazopyridine HCl. Dose: 1 to 2 capsules q.i.d.

Azotrex capsules, practically the same as Urobiotic, but usually a little less expensive.

Pyridium Tri-Sulfa-A tablets contains 167 mg sulfamerazine, 167 mg sulfadiazine and 167 mg sulfamethazine with 150 mg phenazopyridine. Dose: One tablet q.i.d.

Azo Gantanol tablets contains 500 mg sulfamethoxazole and 100 mg phenazopyridine HCl. Dose: 2 tablets every 12 hr.

Azo Gantrisin contains 500 mg sulfisoxazole and 50 mg phenazopyridine. Dose: 2 tablets q.i.d.

Neg Gram capsules, nalidixic acid for gram-negative infections. Capsules 250 and 500 mg. Dose: 500 to 1000 mg q.i.d. (Study side effects before prescribing.)

Furadantin contains nitrofurantoin. Tablets 50 or 100 mg. Dose: 100 mg q.i.d. For prophylactic use, may use smaller doses, i.e. 50 mg b.i.d. (Study side effects before prescribing).

Mandelamine tablets contain methenamine mandelate 500 or 1000 mg. Dose: 0.5 to 1.5 gm q.i.d.

Pyridium tablets contain only phenazopyridine HCl 100 mg. Dose: 2 tablets t.i.d., a.c.

REFERENCES

1. Cole W: *Fam Pract News* Feb:30, 1973.
2. Wells BB, Halsted JA: Clinical Pathology, ed. 4. Philadelphia: W. B. Saunders, 1967, p. 280.
3. Richardson JA, Philbin PE: The one hour creatinine clearance rate in healthy men. *JAMA* 216: 987, 1971.
4. Dunea G, Freedman P: The NPN level of the blood in renal disease. *JAMA* 203:123, 1968.
5. Mehbod H, Baskin M, Moss J: Diet in uremia. *Am Fam Pract* 4:76, 1971.
6. Belzer FO, Kountz SL: Kidney transplant center thrives on advertising. *JAMA* 219:1404, 1972.

7. Sieglar RL, Bloomer HA: Acute renal failure with prolonged oliguria—an account of five cases. *JAMA* 225:133, 1973.
8. Meares, Jr., EM: Bacterial prostatitis vs "prostatosis": a clinical and bacteriological study. *JAMA* 224:1372–1375, 1973.
9. Rowen RL: Adequate examination of the testicles. *Res/Int Consult,* May:15–16, 1973.
10. Ronald AR, Boutros P: Diagnostic test shows site of urinary tract infection. *JAMA* 219:17, 1972.
11. Finch RM, Finch J: Bacteriological counts of urine in general practice. *J Roy Coll Gen Pract.* 19:201–210, 1970.
12. Dolan, Jr. TF, Meyers A: PG education held failure in GU infection. *Med Tribune/Med News* 12:1, 1971.
13. Zinner SH: Erythromycin and alkalinization of urine in treatment of urinary tract infections due to gram negative bacilli. *Lancet* 1:1267–1268, 1971.
14. Shopfner CE: Pyelo-cystourethrography: methodology. *Pediatr* 46:553–565, 1970.
15. King LR: Vesicoureteral reflux: a radiographic sign common to multiple diseases. *JAMA* 220: 854, 1972.

GENERAL STUDY AIDS

Cimino JA, et al: Diagnosis and treatment of common urinary tract infections (five installment programmed instruction course that begins in AFP 5:169, 1972).

CHAPTER 10

Cardiovascular Problems

HEART SOUNDS

Palpating the Heart

Recent observations confirm that palpation of the heart's impulse is more accurate in determining left ventricular volume and mass (hypertrophy) than the electrocardiogram, chest x-ray, fiberoptic apexcardiogram or by biplane angiographic determinations.

In 1858, Dr. Thomas Watson in his *Principles and Practice of Physics* wrote: "There is no sign of hypertrophy so sure as that afforded by the heart's impulse. You feel, not a smart, quick and sudden knock, but a steady, heaving, irrepressible swell, which is perfectly characteristic. You may always infer increased thickness of the walls of the organ when you meet with this regular heaving motion, and the extent to which the whole heart is enlarged in such cases may be conjectured by the extent of space over which the heaving impulse is perceptible."

What is the *point of maximal impulse* (PMI)? The PMI is produced by the intraventricular septum striking the anterior chest wall as the heart tenses and rounds up during contraction. The septum is composed mainly of left ventricular fibers and, therefore, the impulse represents left ventricular events. The left parasternal impulse (LPI) is uniformly created by the anterior wall of the right ventricle. You cannot rely on palpation, however, to distinguish between right, left or biventricular hypertrophy because either or all may modify the spatial relationships as rotation around the vertical axis occurs.

Practice and learn to identify the following characteristics of the PMI or LPI: location, size, duration of outward thrust, ectopic beats and parasternal lift near the left lower sternal border (right ventricular impulse).

You will find the PMI in the fifth interspace within the midclavicular line in patients with a heart of normal size and configuration (Fig. 10-1). Learn to evaluate the size of the impulse when palpating. The PMI of a normal heart should cover less than a 3 cm area. The amplitude of the impulse should be a brief tap only, less than one third to one half of systole.

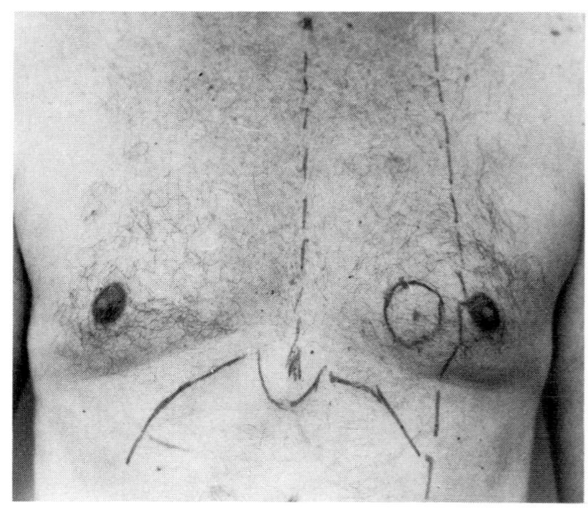

Figure 10-1. PMI in a normal size heart, located inside the midclavicular line in the fifth intercostal space.

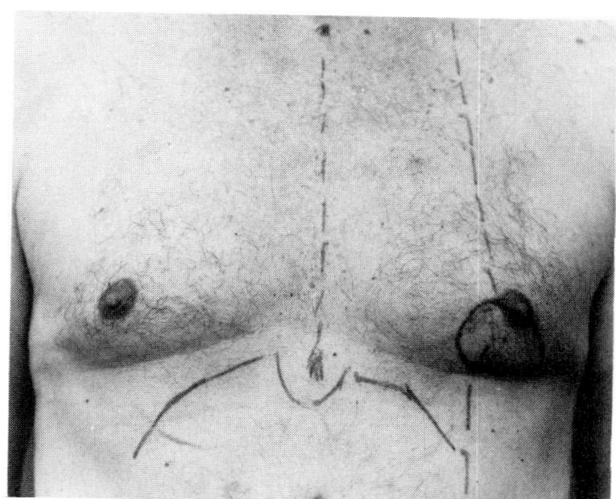

Figure 10-2. The PMI in hypertrophy from pressure overload. The important clue is the duration of the outward thrust.

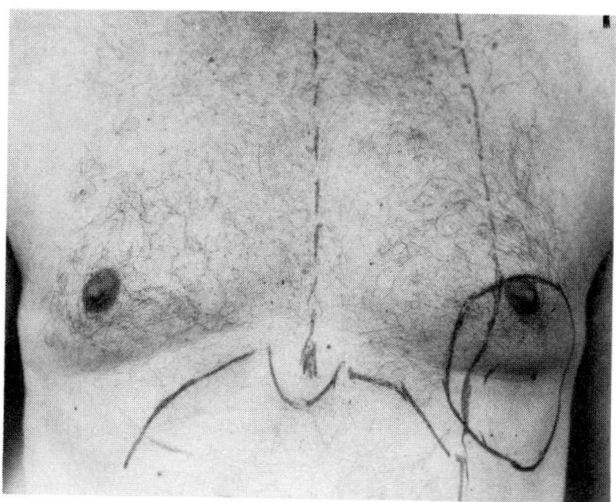

Figure 10-3. The PMI in volume overload.

When cardiac enlargement occurs, the PMI moves downward and outward, often into the sixth intercostal space and outside the midclavicular line (Fig. 10-2). The amplitude is a sustained forceful thrust covering an area up to 3.5 cm. The duration of the impulse is over one half of systole. Pressure overload occurs with systemic hypertension and aortic stenosis. These conditions often do not produce a general overall cardiac enlargement but a specific left ventricular enlargement. Remember *the important clue is the duration of the impulse*. Associate left ventricular overload with mitral insufficiency, aortic insufficiency, ventricular septal defects and A-V fistula.

Palpate for the PMI outside the midclavicular line in a lower interspace in volume overload (Fig. 10-3). The size of the impulse may increase to 6 cm. Volume overloads can usually be separated from pure pressure overloads by the greater amplitude of the former, best described as a dynamic outward movement. Pure pressure overloads, as described, are noted for their duration, volume overloads for their amplitude. Of course mixed types occur as cardiac disease progresses. Of course, mixed types do occur and at times other conditions may cloud the findings (Fig. 10-4).

Now palpate for right ventricular overload. Evaluating the lift caused by right ventricular hypertrophy appears to be more re-

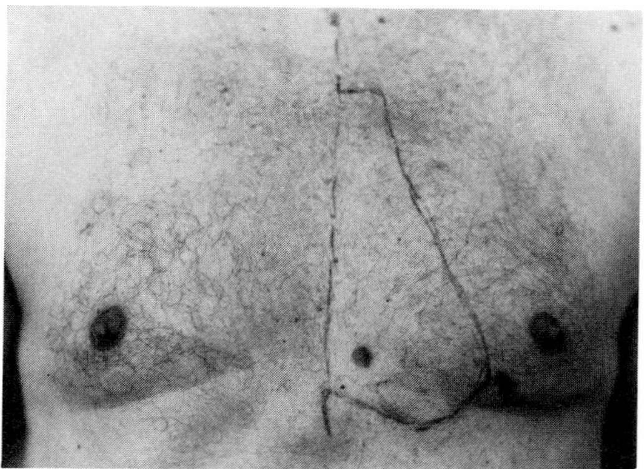

Figure 10-4. The ectopic impulse of a ventricular aneurysm close to the left border of the sternum. These infarctions produce paradoxic pulsations medial to the normal PMI at the apex.

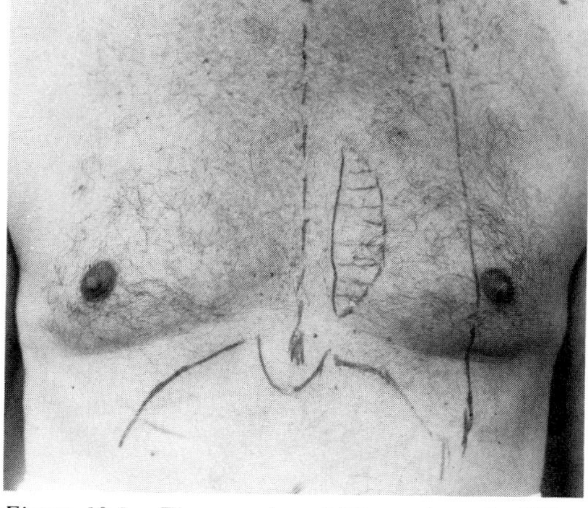

Figure 10-5. The parasternal lift consists of a lifting motion adjacent to the left sternal edge. The sustained thrust felt best in the palm of the hand suggests a pressure problem.

liable in diagnosing this condition than using the electrocardiogram. Place your hand over the lower parasternal border and palpate for the characteristic sustained systolic lift against the entire hand (Fig. 10-5). The degree of pulmonary hypertension varies with the duration of the lift. In fact, the findings are similar to those described for left ventricular problems. Recognize right pressure overloads by the duration of the impulse, right volume overloads by the amplitude of the impulse.

Last of all, locate the PMI before auscultating for mitral valve disease. You will often miss mitral murmurs if the bell of your stethoscope is not placed directly over the PMI.

Listening for Extra Heart Sounds

Cardiac events, which do not produce audible sounds normally, may, under abnormal circumstances, produce audible sounds. For instance, the fourth heart sound may be the only positive finding in patients with symptomatic coronary artery disease; a midsystolic click may be the only clinical evidence of mild mitral regurgitation; and the third heart sound may be the earliest clinical manifestation of left or right heart failure.

The fourth heart sound (atrial sound of presystolic gallop) is produced in the ventricle by the force of the atrial contraction, possibly resulting from distention of the ventricular muscle, stretching of the chordae tendeneae and/or falling together of the valve cusps. An effective atrial contraction can produce the sound. You will never hear the sound in patients with atrial fibrillation. The atrial sound is heard 0.08 to 0.10 seconds after the beginning of the P wave of the ECG. Listen for the sound just preceding the first heart sound. The sound is accentuated by: (1) increased resistance of the ventricle to distention as in hypertrophy; (2) forceful atrial contraction; and (3) prolongation of the P-R interval.

The left-sided fourth heart sound is best heard with the patient in the left lateral position with a bell stethoscope applied lightly to the cardiac apex. The sound is increased on expiration or exercise. Consequently the fourth heart sound is increased by mild bed exercise, during which there is an increase in the interval between the sound and the first heart sound. This is in contrast to the splitting of the first sound which diminishes as the heart rate increases. Left-sided fourth heart sounds are associated with hypertension, aortic stenosis, myocardiopathies, mitral regurgitation and myocardial infarction with sinus rhythm. Listen for the right-sided heart sounds in the third and fourth left intercostal spaces. They are often increased during inspiration. Increase the pressure of the bell of the chest to help distinguish the sound from splitting. This will decrease the intensity of the sound and may cause it to completely disappear. High frequency sounds such as occur in splitting persist unchanged. Right-sided atrial sounds are present in patients with right ventricular hypertrophy secondary to pulmonary stenosis or pulmonary hypertension.

The third heart sound (ventricular gallop, protodiastolic gallop) is produced by both the left and right ventricle. The sound is produced during diastole shortly after the second heart sound. The sudden filling of the ventricle and partial closure of the atrioventricular valves create the ventricular vibration.

The left-sided third sound, like the fourth heart sound, is best heard with the patient in the left lateral position with a bell stethoscope on the cardiac apex (Fig. 10-6). Expi-

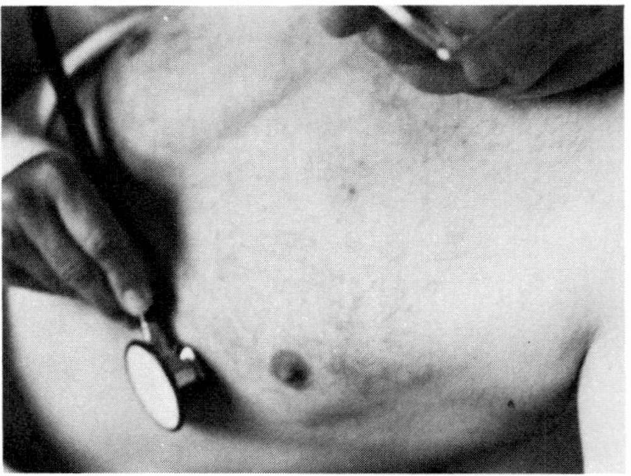

Figure 10-6. Protodiastolic gallop sound (ventricular gallop, third heart sound): the rhythm sounds like the gallop of a horse.

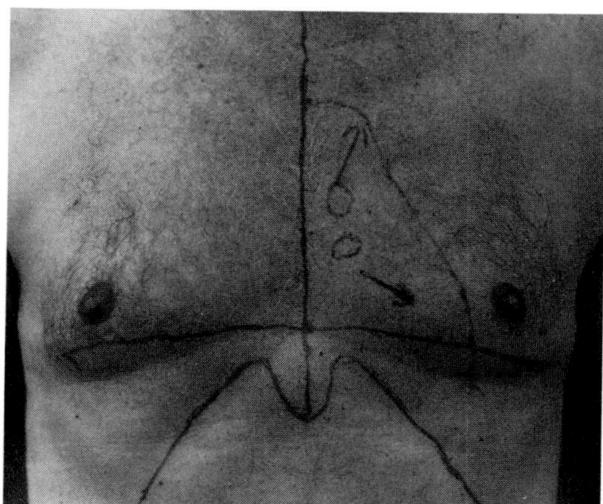

Figure 10-7. The opening snap is a brief diastolic sound which is usually due to stenosis of an A-V valve, most commonly the mitral valve. The snap is usually best heard at the lower left sternal border. It radiates to the base of the heart and is audible at the ventricular apex.

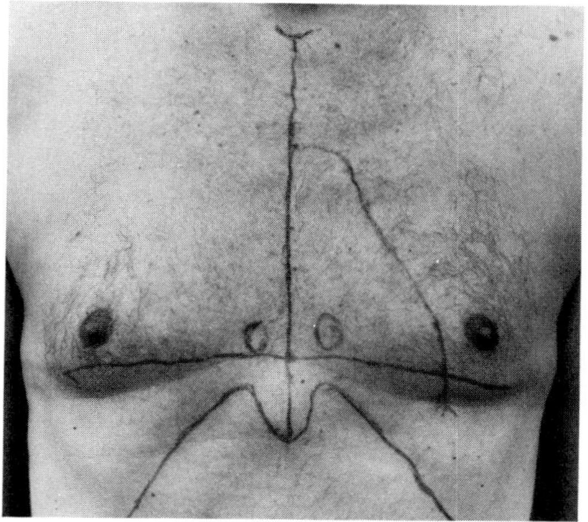

Figure 10-8. The opening snap of the tricuspid valve is best heard near the midline along the lower left or lower right sternal border.

ration increases the intensity of the sound. In some young people, the sound may be a normal finding. In patients past 40 years of age the finding usually indicates ventricular decompensation or A-V valve imcompetence. Mitral regurgitation is a common cause.

Listen for the right-sided third sound at the lower left sternal border or just beneath the xiphoid. It increases with inspiration. Its significance is the same as described above for the left-sided third heart sound.

Think of the fourth heart sound as occurring just before the first heart sound, and the third heart sound just after the second sound. The opening snaps of the mitral and tricuspid valves (Fig. 10-7 and 10-8) occur when the ventricular pressure falls below that in the atrium. The rapid filling phase of the ventricle starts with the opening snap.

It is a brief early diastolic sound which is usually due to stenosis of an A-V valve, commonly the mitral valve.

The opening snap of the stenotic mitral valve is usually best heard at the lower left sternal border although it is frequently heard at the apex.

Do not confuse the snap with the third heart sound which occurs near the same time, nor with the delayed pulmonic component of the second heart sound. Differentiate the opening snap by its radiation to the base of the heart, its intensity along the lower left sternal border and its persistence when the patient stands while the third heart sound disappears.

The aortic ejection sound is usually best heard at the left ventricular apex and at the second right intercostal space during expiration (Fig. 10-9). It occurs at the end of left ventricular contraction when the ventricular pressure exceeds the aortic pressure and the aortic valves open. Listen for it immediately after the first heart sound. A stenotic semilunar valve which is flexible will open with a snap. Excessive distention of the aorta by ejection of a greater amount

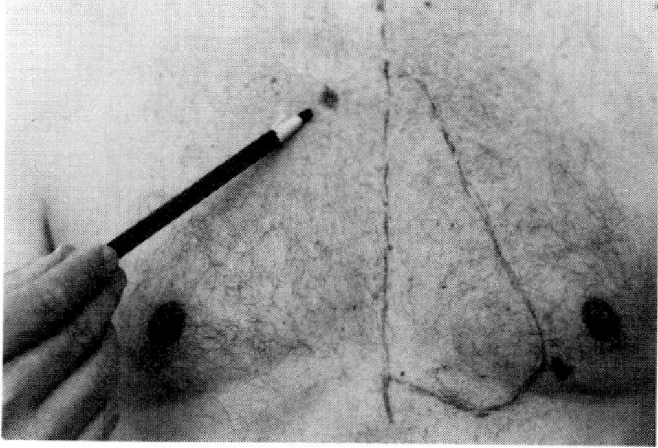

Figure 10-9. The aortic ejection click is a sound produced at the time of the opening of the semilunar valves and ejection of blood into the great vessels.

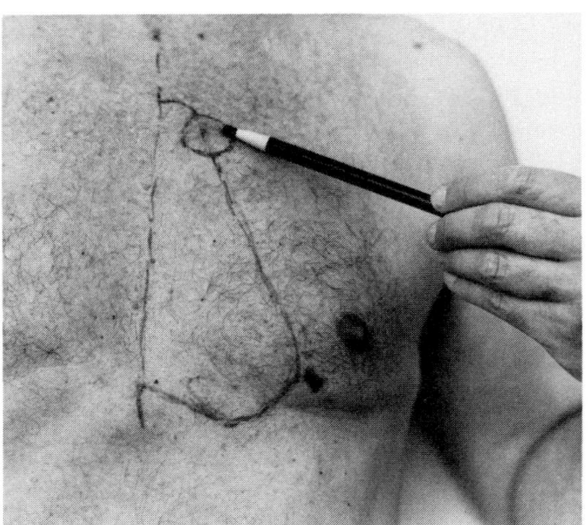

Figure 10-10. The pulmonic ejection click is usually heard best during expiration. Its location is in the pulmonic area near the sternal border.

of blood than usual will produce vibration and sound.

Ejection sound may also arise from the pulmonary circulation (Fig. 10-10). In this event the sound occurs immediately after the first sound but over the pulmonic area left of the sternum during expiration. Both aortic and pulmonic ejection sounds occur in the presence of semilunar valve stenosis and in conditions associated with dilitation of the aortic or pulmonary artery.

Midsystolic clicks appear to be of importance. Recent evidence indicates that the sound may result from unequal lengths of the chordae tendenae of the mitral valve. They are best heard along the lower left sternal border and at the apex at the middle of systole.

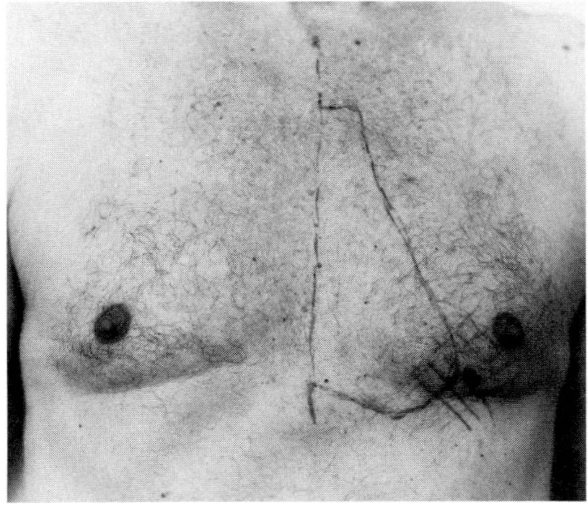

Figure 10-11. Mitral regurgitation.

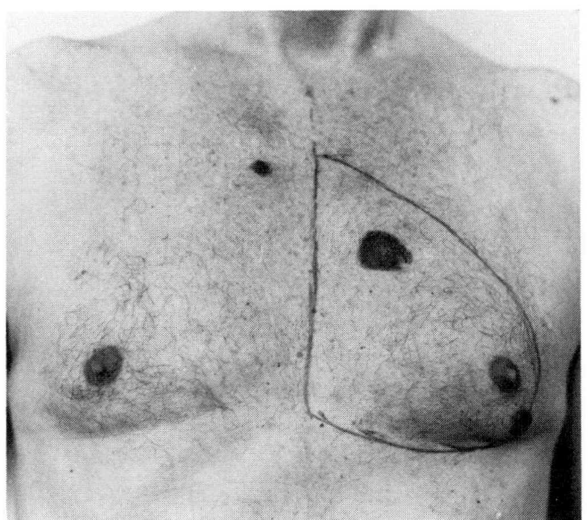

Figure 10-12. Severe aortic regurgitation.

Differentiate midsystolic clicks from the second heart sound by identifying the first and second heart sounds elsewhere on the chest. After the proper timing has been established, move the stethoscope to where the click is heard and the second sound will be clear. The click is definitely midsystolic.

When once identified, consider the finding as evidence of mild mitral valve regurgitation (Fig. 10-11). In mitral valve regurgitation the PMI always is at the apex. The murmur is holosystolic in time, high pitched and flowing and heard best with the bell stethoscope. Administer antibiotic prophylaxis before and after dental procedures, surgery and deliveries.

Severe aortic regurgitation (Fig. 10-12) is identified by a high-pitched diastolic murmur heard best in the third left interspace. In addition a rough systolic murmur is usually heard in the second right intercostal space. There is some controversy regarding the origin of a rumbling mid-diastolic and presystolic murmur at the apex and lateral from the apex. These murmurs may represent a mild degree of mitral stenosis or an Austin Flint murmur.

Splitting of the Second Heart Sound

The second heart sound is referred to as

the "key to cardiac auscultation." If you haven't already done so, learn to recognize the splitting of the sound and the effect respiration has on it.

Auscult in the second left intercostal space. Remember you are listening to two sounds: aortic and pulmonic valve closures (Fig. 10-13). They are nearly synchronous in time during expiration and split during inspiration. During the split is the time to compare the intensity of the two sounds. Unless you can hear and identify the two sounds, it will be impossible for you to compare and state your result in the commonly used formula $A_2 > P_2$. Therefore A_2 refers to aortic valve closure and P_2 to pulmonic valve closure. Get it straight: A_2 and P_2 do not refer to the second sound in the aortic or the pulmonic areas. Another mistake: once you understand the meaning of the two terms, i.e., that A_2 and P_2 are single sounds caused by single valve closures, the term split P_2 means nothing. A single sound cannot be split. Splitting refers only to the splitting of A_2 from P_2 usually determined while listening to the second sound during quiet inspiration.

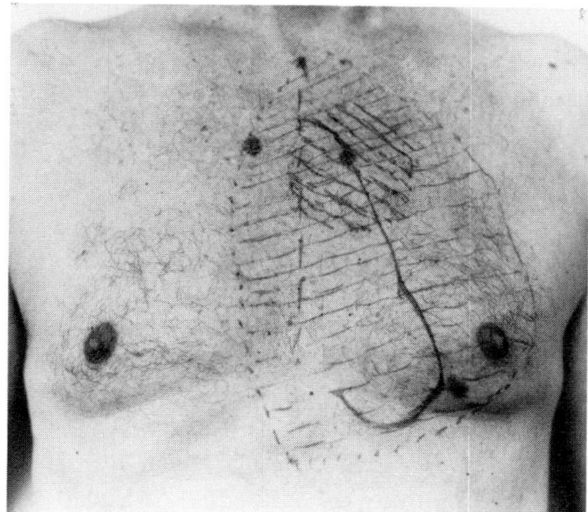

Figure 10-13. Composition of the second heart sound. The area shaded by the single lines indicates where the aortic second sound is heard. The crosshatched area indicates the area where the pulmonic second sound is heard. Consequently, in the left second interspace, the second heart sound is composed of both aortic and pulmonary sounds. In this area, on inspiration, the pulmonic second sound is delayed, causing a split from the aortic sound.

From Figure 10-13 you can see that the comparative intensities of the two sounds may vary from place to place over the precordium. In the shaded area P_2 may be greater than A_2 but not necessarily so. Over the aortic and apical area, A_2 is greater than P_2.

Splitting of the second sound on inspiration is caused by a change in the intrathoracic pressure on respiration. Inspiration decreases intrathoracic pressure, which in turn increases the filling of the great veins, the right atrium and the right ventricle. To handle the increased volume, the right ventricle must increase the stroke volume and, in doing so, ventricular contraction takes longer, delaying the pulmonic second sound.

While this sequence of events is going on, action of the lungs accommodates for the increased volume resulting in little or no change in left ventricular timing. The net results are a separation of A_2 and P_2, the A_2 occurring first and P_2 following.

Expiration with increased intrathoracic pressure reverses the above changes and again a melding of the two sounds occurs. It is nearly needless to say that splitting can only be heard in the dark area wherein P_2 and A_2 are superimposed (represented by the shaded area of Fig. 10-13).

Conditions which alter the physiologic splitting of the second sound follow:

1. Right bundle branch block causes splitting even during expiration; however, further splitting occurs on inspiration. In this case the splitting is due to a delayed activation of the right ventricle.
2. Left bundle branch block causes splitting during expiration, which disappears on inspiration, paradoxic splitting, the reverse of normal splitting. The delay in activation of the left ventricle cancels the physiologic delay of the right ventricle and A_2 and P_2 become synchronous.
3. Atrial septal defects cause a "fixed" splitting—splitting of equal degree during both expiration and inspiration. Respiration causes no change in right atrial dynamics which is not transmitted to the right atrium.
4. Pulmonic valvular stenosis also causes a fixed splitting during expiration and inspiration.

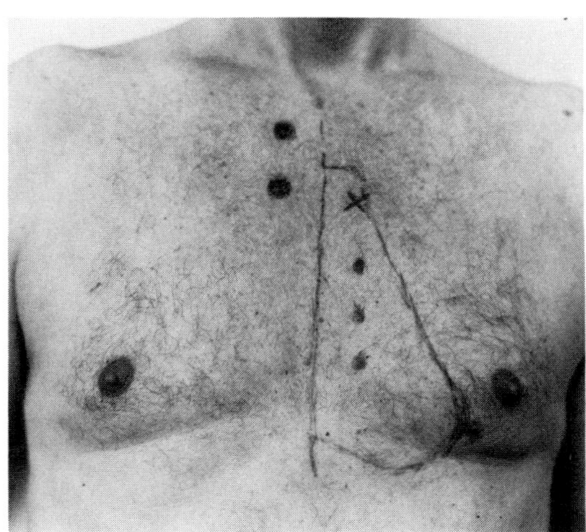

Figure 10-14. The systolic murmur of aortic stenosis is a harsh systolic murmur heard best in the first and second right interspaces, but it can be heard at the apex. Along the left border of the sternum the murmur is often less intense than at the apex. A third heart sound may be heard at the apex.

5. Aortic stenosis (Fig. 10-14), if severe, splits the second sound during expiration but the sounds are unified on inspiration. Again a type of paradoxic splitting. The left ventricular contraction becomes greater, slowing its timing and meeting the delayed physiologic timing of the right ventricle.

6. In the tetralogy of Fallot only a single sound is produced and that of aortic origin.

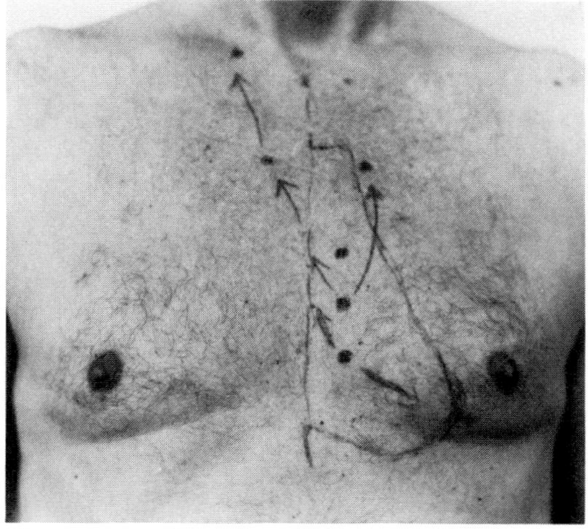

Figure 10-15. Innocent systolic murmur is best heard along the left sternal border and at the apex. It is early and midsystolic only, medium pitched, rough or vibratory and radiates to the apex, aortic ar^a, pulmonic area and often the neck.

There is no splitting either with expiration or inspiration. This is explained by the decreased intensity of P_2.

A family physician must practice to distinguish all these sounds and murmurs from innocent systolic murmurs (Fig. 10-15).

ATHEROSCLEROTIC HEART DISEASE

Occurrence and Prevention of AHD

In North America 1 out of every 5 men will have a major coronary episode, such as myocardial ischemia (MI) or sudden death, before age 60. The probability multiplies with increased risk factors; the more of the following factors present, the greater the patient's chances of developing coronary disease. About 25 percent will die within 3 hours of the onset. Another 10 percent will die within the first week. Among these who are fortunate enough to get well and go back to work, 20 percent will die in the first 5 years.

AHD in men between 35 to 55 years of age is 6 times more common than in females. After the menopause women become as susceptible to CHD as men. Since 1900 there has been only a small percentage gain in the life expectancy of 40 year old males. Higher susceptability to AHD is the single most important factor preventing the male from keeping pace with the life expectancy gains made by women. Menstruating women do not have CHD unless they have hypertension, hypothyroidism or diabetes mellitus.

In attempting to prevent disease, you will be foiled constantly by the psychologic frailties of your patients. The prevention of heart disease is a prime example. Patients insist on serial checks of their cholesterol while continuing to smoke, refusing to exercise and scoffing at losing weight.

Hyperlipemia

Researchers now agree that the elevation of serum lipids leading to premature atherosclerosis is a result of habitual and excessive intake of cholesterol and saturated fats. This conclusion stemmed from

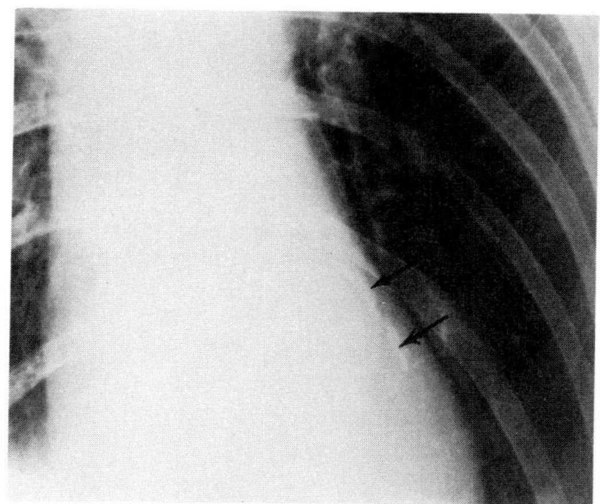

Figure 10-16. X-ray film of the heart showing calcification of the left coronary artery.

the simple observation that atherosclerosis and AHD (Fig. 10-16) were common among people of the world whose diet was rich in meat, dairy products and eggs—all foods high in cholesterol and saturated fats. The converse of this observation also proved true. Populations whose diets consisted mainly of high starched grains and tubers proved to have a low incidence of AHD.

Hypercholesterolemia alone is associated with a high incidence of AHD. Mass screening to determine the serum cholesterol is sufficient in attempting to identify high risk patients in a community. This determination can be made without fasting the patient. It is less expensive to perform and subject to less errors than other measurements of serum lipids.

In your office, however, when evaluating an individual, collect blood for both a cholesterol and triglyceride determination after preparing the patient by the following means. Test results are more dependable if the patient has not been taking a contraceptive pill, thyroid or barbiturates. Instruct the patient to eat a dinner low in fat and without alcohol the night before. If possible select patients for testing who have been on a normal diet for 1 to 2 weeks and have maintained their weight for the same time. Have them fast for 15 hours and report for venipuncture.

Remember that the result of cholesterol testing is erratic. Before subjecting the patient to long and expensive therapy, check cholesterol three times, requesting the patient to report for venipuncture on the same day of the week, the same time of day and with the same time relationship to meals.

Both measurements will assist you in guiding the patients. The findings in the population at risk is a moderate hypercholesterolemia with or without a hypertriglyceridemia, but without chylomicronemia.

At this point, rule out the conditions which produce hyperlipemia:

–contraceptive pills
–alcoholism
–uncontrolled diabetes mellitus
–hypothyroidism
–nephrosis
–biliary obstruction
–pancreatic disease
–myeloma

There is a genetic factor involved in hypercholesterolemia and hypertriglyceridemia. Its importance as compared to diet has not been completely evaluated. But even patients with familial hyperlipemia respond to dietary restrictions. Consequently, for practical purposes, both for diagnosis and treatment, check the blood relatives of a patient found to have hyperlipemia.

Remember at age 45 to 50 the ideal cholesterol level is 220 mg/100 even though your laboratory suggests a normal range of 120 to 300. Birth cholesterol level is 80 to 90; at age 25 it should be around 160. No research has shown there is a critical level below which no risk exists. Therefore, strive to get your patients' cholesterol level as low as possible without making them sick. Below 200, the risk of AHD is greatly diminished.

If both the serum cholesterol and serum triglyceride are normal, do no further testing. The patient is not at risk at least from hyperlipidemia. If either the serum cholesterol or serum triglyceride is elevated, order lipoprotein electrophoresis. In this event the serum should be stored in a refrigerator overnight.

Although lipoproteins can be measured

Table 10-1. Hyperlipoproteinemia

	Types				
	I	*II*	*III*	*IV*	*V*
Triglyceride	Elevated	Normal	Elevated	Elevated	Elevated
Cholesterol	Normal	Elevated	Elevated	Normal*	Elevated
Physical findings	Eruptive xanthoma	Corneal arcus in lower 180°; xanthelasma; tendon xanthomas	Palmar xanthomas; subcutaneous xanthomas	None	Eruptive xanthomas; xanthelasma; subcutaneous xanthomas; tendon xanthomas
Predominant	Chylomicrons	Beta-lipoproteins	Abnormal beta-lipoproteins	Pre-beta-lipoproteins elevated	Both pre-beta-lipoproteins and chylomicrons elevated
Sensitivity	Fat	Fat	Both fat and carbohydrate	Carbohydrate	Both fat and carbohydrate

*Latent type occasionally can be diagnosed until patient is fed a high carbohydrate diet.

and classified by either ultracentrifugation or paper electrophoresis, the latter is simpler and less expensive and is the test usually done except in large medical centers. A drop of plasma to be tested is placed on filter paper and put into an electric field. The field causes the lipoprotein to migrate on the paper strip at rates determined by factors such as their electrical charges, particle size, paper absorption, etc. Differences in the migrating rates of the lipoproteins result in their accumulation into distinct bands. The laboratory technician then classifies the hyperlipemia as one of the five types suggested by Fredrickson (Table 10-1). Normal findings are:

Beta, ~85 percent
Alpha, ~15 percent
Pre-beta, small amounts
Chylomicra, absent

Type I is a rare familial disorder appearing in early childhood. A low fat diet clears the hyperglyceridemia. Type II is a common disorder, accounting for 40 percent of all hyperlipoproteinemias. The disease has a genetic component but also occurs secondarily in myxedema, nephrosis, cirrhosis and multiple myeloma. Patients with type II hyperlipoproteinemia may develop atherosclerosis early in life, which causes an increased incidence of coronary heart disease. Dietary cholesterol must be reduced to less than 300 mg per day. Do not restrict carbohydrates nor protein intake. So include a high ratio of polyunsaturated fat. This type of diet means cutting eggs, most dairy products, shellfish and fatty meats from the diet.

In type III hyperlipoproteinemia, select a diet that will reduce the patient to normal weight. Once this is accomplished, maintain the patient on a diet in which 40 percent of the calories are from carbohydrate and 40 percent from fat. Restrict cholesterol to less than 300 mg per day. Eliminate candy and concentrated sweets. Reduce ingestion of saturated fat and increase unsaturated fats.

Patients with type IV should also be reduced to normal weight. Subsequently maintain the patient on a diet of 300 to 500 mg of cholesterol per day, a preponderance of unsaturated fat. Reduce the calories from carbohydrates to about 40 percent. Eliminate alcohol. No matter what you read, the causative agents of type IV are not clear. One place or another, you may hear that sensitivity to carbohydrate, obesity, glucose intolerance and hyperinsulinism are etiologic conditions. Don't be surprised if the patient does not respond to treatment. Although the above causes may be present in one or more patients, none of these conditions is common to all cases of type IV disease.[1]

Patients with type V hyperlipoproteinemia often have a primary disease such as diabetes mellitus or alcoholism with a secondary elevation of cholesterol and triglyceride. Help the patient reduce to his ideal weight. Fifty percent of the maintenance calories should come from carbohydrates and not more than 25 to 30 percent from fats. Allow no more than 300 to 500 mg of cholesterol per day and eliminate alcohol entirely.

In all types except type I prescribe clofibrate with or without nicotinic acid as a trial. It is least helpful in type II hyperlipoproteinemia but some response in cholesterol reduction may occur. In type II consider other drugs, particularly in the more serious cases, i.e. dextrothyroxine, sitosterols, nicotinic acid and cholestyramine. All the latter mentioned drugs are difficult to give because of the large doses required or the unpleasant side effects. For instance even nicotinic acid should be given in doses to 3 to 6 g/day to be effective; dextrothyroxine 4 to 8 mg/day; and the sitosteroids 18 to 25 g/day.

Type III responds fairly well to clofibrate, type IV and V less well but should be given a trial along with nicotinic acid. The dosage is 2 g/day in divided doses. Remember that clofibrate may cause nausea or other gastrointestinal symptoms, skin rashes, alopecia, leukopenia, elevated transaminase, elevated creatinine phosphokenase (CPK), muscle soreness and occasionally ventricular irritability resulting in an arrhythmia. Reduce the dosage of anticoagulants when giving clofibrate because of its potentiating effect. Reduce anticoagulants to one third or one half the usual dosage.

Before leaving the subject of cholesterol and its causative relationship to CHD, consider the following statistics. The average incidence of the first major coronary event (first fatal or nonfatal myocardial infarction) in a population whose cholesterol level is below 250 is around 50 per thousand. In those whose serum cholesterol ranges from 250 to 299 the incidence increases to about 115 per thousand. And those whose serum cholesterol is above 300, the incidence rises to 160 per thousand.

Some proprietaries frequently prescribed are the following:

Atromid-S (clofibrate). Dose: 500 mg q.i.d. When giving, monitor serum lipid levels. If no significant response in 3 months, discontinue treatment. If gradual increasing levels of transaminase occur, discontinue. Be careful in giving the drug to diabetic patients. Atromid-S will reduce xanthomas even though not reducing plasma lipid levels and the continuation of the drug is warranted if the lesions are slowly disappearing.

Choloxin tablets (sodium dextrothyroxine). Dosage: start with 1.0 to 2.0 mg daily and increase monthly by 1.0 to 2.0 mg increments to a maximum of 6 to 8 mg daily if necessary for control of cholesterol. Do not give to the patient with organic heart disease. Give only to euthyroid patients. Liver or kidney disease is a contraindication. Be careful in diabetics; oral antidiabetic drug dosage is required. Probably not wise to give when patients are on anticoagulants except under strictest control. You might give it a trial with type IV or V when diet and clofibrate do not work.

Cumid and *Questran* (cholestyramine resins) reduce cholesterol and tend to relieve the pruritus of biliary obstruction.

Other controversial proprietaries are:

Cytellin. Each tablespoonful contains 3 g Cytellin (sitosterols). Dose: 15 ml before meals.

Nicalex tablets. Each tablet contains 500 mg nicotinic acid in form of aluminum nicotinate. Dose: 2 to 4 tablets t.i.d.

For you and your patients, the National

Heart and Living Institute provides six booklets on the dietary management of the five types of hyperlipemia. One is especially prepared for physicians, the others for patients and includes sample menus. Write: Office of Heart Information, National Heart and Living Institute, Building 31, Room 6A03, National Institutes of Health, Bethesda, Maryland 20014.

The local branch of the American Heart Association has the following four publications: "The Way to a Man's Heart," "Recipes for Fat-Controlled, Low Cholesterol Meals," "Planning Fat-Controlled Meals for 1200 and 1800 Calories" and "Planning Fat-Controlled Meals for Approximately 2,000–2,600 Calories."

Cigarette Smoking

Both men and women in their fifties who have a heavy smoking history and who are still smoking have three times as many heart attacks and five times more sudden deaths than nonsmokers. Stopping smoking for 1 year returns these people to the nonsmoker's risk curve. Pipe and cigar smokers do not have a greater risk than nonsmokers. Adjustment for hypertension and hyperlipemia does not account for these findings, although smokers have more atherosclerosis than nonsmokers at autopsy.

The incidence of a fatal or nonfatal myocardial infarction in nonsmokers, those who have quit smoking or in those who smoke only a pipe or cigar is under 50 per thousand. In those who smoke no more than half a pack a day, the incidence rises to about 60 per thousand. The incidence rises to about 80 per thousand in those who smoke 1 pack a day, and to 130 per thousand in those who smoke more than one pack of cigarettes per day.

The standard cigarette weighs 1 g and contains 20 mg nicotine. Research suggests that 35 percent of the nicotine is destroyed at the burning tip, 35 percent is lost in the side stream, 22 percent enters the mouth, and 8 percent remains in the unsmoked portion of the cigarette. Others suggest that only 10 percent is absorbed by the noninhaler and 90 percent by the person who inhales.

The main physiologic effects of smoking are an elevation of blood pressure and pulse rate, a decrease in skin temperature and a flattening of the T waves of the electrocardiogram. Peculiarly enough, even though ordinarily alcohol causes vasodilitation of the peripheral blood vessels, the vasoconstriction from smoking could not be prevented by alcoholic vasodilitation.

The American Medical Association from work done in its clinical laboratory reports that filtered cigarettes remove only about 5 percent of the nicotine in the main stream of the smoke.

It is only fair to report that in spite of these facts, some researchers suggest that *stress* which results in compulsive smoking is the causative factor and not the cigarettes per se. These researchers back their hunch by observing that there has been no decrease in the average age or death among physicians since many have stopped smoking.

For patient education, suggest they contact the local heart association to obtain two pamphlets: "How To Stop Smoking" and "What Everyone Should Know About Smoking and Heart Disease."

Hypertension

Hypertension after the age of 45 years is a greater risk factor than hypercholesterolemia. An elevated diastolic pressure is more significant than an elevated systolic pressure. The incidence of a major fatal or nonfatal myocardial infarction in patients whose diastolic pressure is below 85 is around 50 per thousand. In patients whose diastolic pressure is between 85 and 95 the incidence rises to 80 per thousand; in those whose diastolic pressure is 94 to 104 the incidence is 100 per thousand; and in those with a diastolic pressure about 105, the incidence leaps to about 180 per thousand, nearly doubling in incidence.

In the Framingham study, men aged 45 to 62 with blood pressures more than 160/95 had five times more ischemic heart disease than men whose blood pressures were under 140/90.

The question of how far to go in working-up a hypertensive patient depends a great deal on the patient's age. In patients aged 15 to 30, do every test necessary to rule out remediable hypertension. After 40, remediable hypertension is less frequent; consequently tests are less fruitful. For openers do a history and physical and routine laboratory checks plus serum potassium, palpate femoral pulses for coarctation of aorta, listen for bruits, order an intravenous pyelogram and obtain an ECG.

Because of the ease of treatment, hypertension should be the first line of treatment. A sustained diastolic blood pressure of 95 mm of Hg requires medical treatment—diet first and then, if needed, mild drugs to quiet down a labile systolic hypertension. Start with a thiazide diuretic and a low sodium diet. Vary the sodium intake according to the severity of the disease. A labile systolic hypertension generally responds to weight reduction, sedatives, tranquilizers and/or mild hypertensive drugs.

For patient education, have your patient contact his local heart association and obtain "High Blood Pressure."

Obesity

Someone recently said that a mesomorph who gets heavy has only three choices: reduce, get castrated or die of arteriosclerotic heart disease. There is a definite relationship between ischemic heart disease and obesity. The relationship, however, is somewhat obscure because hyperlipemia, diabetes mellitus, obesity and hypertension are so physiologically interwoven as to make distinction difficult.

The question that remains unanswered is whether an obese person who is nonhyperlipemic, nonhyperglycemic, nonhypertensive and nonhyperuricemic is still at risk. The findings to date are equivocal. A *little* obesity probably adds little risk. In any case, obesity is associated with other risk factors and weight reduction is an important adjunct in controlling obesity-related risk factors.

Determine obesity by skin fold measurements taken in at least six places. From this you can determine percentage body fat.

Abnormal Glucose Tolerance

Patients with diabetes mellitus have twice as much hypertension and twice as many heart attacks as nondiabetics. This is of considerable importance when you realize that one in 80 Americans has diabetes mellitus.

Diabetes as well as hyperlipemia can be genetic risk factors. Consequently, all young people, particularly males, whose parents have had early coronary disease, should have their blood sugar tested along with serum cholesterol and triglyceride.

There are some questions that remain unanswered about the role of asymptomatic hyperglycemia as a coronary risk factor. The relationship between diabetes and coronary, cerebrovascular and peripheral vascular disease has been studied and verified.

Age

Sooner or later age catches up and produces coronary or cerebral antherosclerotic symptoms. Levine studied 20 fathers and 21 sons and recorded their ages at the onset of angina pectoris. The statistics are rather discouraging. He found that the sons developed angina 13 years earlier, on the average, than had their fathers. In addition the sons died 14 years earlier. The genetics that account for this are not clearly understood.

Physical Activity

There is no proven relationship between increased exercise and a decreased risk factor. About the best that can be said is that sedentary people are more susceptible to sudden death than active people.

For patient education regarding exercise and to keep exercising within proper limits refer your patients to the following sources: "Creative Walking" from your local heart association and "Exercise Equivalents," by Loring Brock, M.D., from the Colorado Heart Association, 1375 Delaware, Denver, Colorado. For one dollar you can get the

"Physician's Handbook for Evaluation of Cardiovascular and Physical Fitness" from the Tennessee Heart Association, 205 22nd Avenue, Nashville, Tennessee, 37203. This booklet will give you the facts necessary to promote physical activity by your patients either before or after a heart attack.

Hyperuricemia

There is evidence to suggest that coronary artery disease is related to a uric acid level of more than 6.9 mg percent. No one has discovered whether the increased uric acid level caused by diuretics and drugs will cause an increase in ischemic heart disease. Hyperuricemia, like other factors, is usually associated with other risk factors, i.e., obesity, hypertension and hyperglycemia. There is research tentatively indicating that hyperuricemia operates as an independent risk factor.

Pulse Rate

A study in Chicago attempts to link a resting pulse rate of more than 80 beats per minute with an increased incidence of coronary heart disease. As the heart rate in selected persons varied above 80 beats so did the incidence of coronary heart disease.

Positive Family History

Many factors are involved, but most major studies reveal a tendency for ischemic heart disease to attack blood relatives.

Electrocardiographic Changes

From a Chicago study there is evidence that 10 percent of healthy males between 40 and 59 years of age have abnormal resting ECG's. The abnormal patterns were bundle branch blocks, arrhythmias, left ventricular hypertrophy and nonspecific T wave changes, i.e., low voltage, diphasic or flat T waves. The ECG response to exercise and the resting ECG provide helpful information relative to coronary risk. A significant number of middle-aged adults with normal resting ECG patterns exhibit an ischemic response (depression of the ST segment) to moderate exercise. These people are at increased risk of developing overt clinical coronary disease.

A word of warning to those family physicians who still depend on resting ECG's to detect coronary artery disease. A recent study from the Good Samaritan Hospital in Phoenix, Arizona, discloses that of 106 patients with triple coronary vessel disease, 17 had perfectly normal ECG's and three patients who had 100% obstruction to one or more coronary arteries also recorded normal ECG's. Therefore a substantial number of patients who have coronary artery disease will have normal resting ECG's. Further their study points out that resting ECG's do not predict the extent of the disease.[2]

Stages of AHD

There are five or six synonyms for AHD: coronary atherosclerotic heart disease, coronary heart disease, atherosclerotic artery disease and ischemic heart disease. Select one which rolls off your tongue easily and reflects that the disease is an atherosclerotic process of the big arteries.

Stage I. During this stage you can find no detectible disease but the coronary arteries are slowly becoming involved in the atherosclerotic process. Most researchers now believe the disease process begins shortly after birth. Some advocate phenotyping at birth either routinely or in infants of high genetic risk.

Stage II. The effect of gradual and progressive coronary atherosclerosis becomes electrocardiographically noticeable when the patient exercises strenuously. Look for ST depression and/or nonspecific T wave abnormalities during exertion. From a preventive standpoint, this is the ideal stage in which to begin treatment.

Stage III. Further coronary artery deterioraton leading to angina pectoris with or without ECG abnormalities. Clincial symptoms of angina, fatigue or depression may prevail with secondary ECG changes or with changes only during pain; or ECG changes may dominate the clinical picture with a variety of specific and nonspecific ECG abnormalities.

Stage IV. Actual myocardial infarction characterizes stage IV. Coronary arteries no longer supply sufficient blood to the heart muscle and the stage is ushered in by an attack of pain accompanied by all the symptoms, findings and complications following myocardial necrosis.

Stage V. Coronary arteries no longer adequate to support a viable myocardium and death results from an arrhythmia or massive infarction. Death occasionally occurs without prior symptoms.

Practical Office Screening for Occult AHD

First, look to the patient's medical history. Have other relatives had heart disease, diabetes, gout, peripheral vascular disease, stroke or AHD? Is the patient a heavy smoker? Is the patient more than 30 percent overweight? Is the patient active? Is he under stress in his work or domestic affairs?

Second, on physical examination does the patient have hypertension of more than 160/95 or an enlarged heart? Is the patient more than 30 percent overweight by skin fold check?

Third, do a screening laboratory work-up:

- –serum cholesterol (nonfasting) of no more than 250mg/100ml
- –12 to 14 hr fasting triglyceride of no more than 175mg/100ml
- –2 hour postprandial blood sugar of no more than 120mg/100ml
- –nonfasting serum uric acid levels of no more than 7mg/100ml
- –x-ray film for an enlarged heart
- –ECG tracing before and after exercise

Remind your patient: the more risk factors present, the greater his chances of developing AHD.

Treadmill Testing

Consider first whether the patient has had a resting ECG. A wise physician will order a resting ECG at least every 2 years on all patients over 40 years of age, men and women alike. On the resting ECG's, look for any type of S-T and T wave changes, any arrhythmia, left ventricular hypertrophy or intraventricular conduction abnormalities.

If the patient has a normal ECG but has one or more of the risk factors previously outlined, order a submaximal exercise test. An abnormal ECG with exercise has the greatest predictive value for coronary disease, and gives you some idea of the efficiency of the coronary circulation.

Submaximal refers to exercising the patient to a pulse rate 15 percent less than his maximal rate as determined by his age. There are charts that indicate maximal and submaximal rates for each age, but the charts are not necessary. If the patient is between 20 to 60 years of age, subtract the patient's age from 220. The resulting figure represents the patient's maximal heart rate. Eighty or eighty-five percent of that figure is the submaximal heart rate and to which rate the exercising should proceed before considering the exercise testing as negative or physiologic.

Do not do treadmill testing in your office unless you are prepared to resuscitate or defibrillate the patient. Treadmill testing has become sophisticated in gadgetry and technique; for best and safest results, refer the patient to a hospital treadmill center.

The old Master's two-step testing is obsolete because the work-load was standardized. This standardized work-load proved, in many cases, to be too little exercise to bring out abnormalities and in others too much and dangerous.

Treadmill testing starts with evaluating a standard 12 lead ECG. If this is normal, electrodes are affixed to the chest wall in lead I, AVF, V5 and V6 positions. An electrocardiogram is then recorded at rest in the supine and standing positions. The patient is often asked to step onto a treadmill with a 10 percent slope set at a speed of 1.7 MPH. The patient walks for 3 minutes at the following speeds in MPH: 1.7, 3.2, 4 and 5.

Blood pressure is taken in both standing and sitting positions and is recorded at 1 minute intervals during exercise and for a period of 8 minutes after exercise.

The study is terminated whenever

–chest pain develops
–the patient becomes exhausted or dyspneic
–tachycardia suddenly develops
–multiple PVC's occur
–progressive S-T segment depression develops
–undue increase in blood pressure develops.

If none of these symptoms or findings occur, the patient is urged to continue until his pulse rate reaches 95 percent of the predicted maximal pulse rate.

The test results are indicated as being physiologically normal (negative treadmill) and positive but there is also some correlation with the anatomic location of the disease in the coronary artery. The incidence of a positive ECG response with two or three vessel disease is 94 percent. Ninety percent of patients with isolated disease of the left anterior descending artery have a positive response, but only 50 percent of patients with right coronary artery disease have a positive test. Consequently, patients with angina are more likely to have a negative treadmill test if the disease is localized to one vessel, especially if the stenosis is in the right coronary artery.

A less sophisticated method of testing is the multilevel testing. The equipment necessary is less expensive and can be done in the office providing you can defibrillate and resuscitate.

Take and evaluate a resting ECG. It should be normal. Using lead I, fix the left arm electrode at the left C_5 and the right arm electrode at the right C_5 position. This will pick up 95 percent of the abnormalities. Using 9 inch steps have the patient step for 3 minutes at the rate of 10 steps/minute. Evaluate his heart rate, blood pressure and ECG. The patient may rest or continue depending on his fitness. Continue the exercise by stepping at the rate of 20 per minute, then 30 and perhaps 40. Continue for 3 minutes at each level, evaluating before continuing to the next. When the patient's pulse rate reaches 85 percent of the predicted maximal rate, discontinue the test. Be sure to continue ECG monitoring up to 10 minutes after the exercise has been completed. Some abnormalities may be discovered only during this interval.

ECG changes or an unusual increase in blood pressure may occur at any exercise level. Use the same criteria for discontinuing the test as outlined for treadmill testing.

The question arises as to the effect of digitalis on exercise testing: both digitalis and exercise-induced subendocardial ischemia will produce depression of the J junction as well as an ST segment sagging. Differentiation is almost impossible from a single tracing.

If the patient has received a long-acting digitalis preparation prior to exercise tolerance testing but has no evidence of a digitalis effect on the resting ECG, proceed with the testing. If the digitalis effect is definite, cancel the testing. Wait 2 weeks after all ECG evidence of digitalis has cleared and then proceed with testing. The main reason for the cancellation: ischemia sufficient to produce ECG changes plus digitalis might produce a life-threatening arrhythmia under testing conditions.

Coronary Arteriography

As a prelude to surgery, coronary arteriography is now being done to evaluate the prospect of successful revascularization. It is generally agreed that arteriography best be done on all symptomatic patients whose angina is becoming progressively worse. The working criteria varies with different heart teams, however.

When asking your patient to undergo coronary arteriography, assure him that the danger of dying is less than 1:1,000; the danger of myocardial infarction is about 1:800; and in incidence of ventricular fibrillation varies from 2 to 5 per 100. I would consider it wise to reserve coronary arteriography and the subsequent surgery for the angina patient who is becoming incapacitated by the disease.

Angina Syndrome

Treating Angina Syndrome

Angina pectoris results from an unfavorable balance between coronary blood flow and myocardial oxygen requirement. The most common cause of angina pectoris is obliterative coronary atherosclerosis.

NITROGLYCERIN. Plain nitroglycerin is an excellent drug except for its short action. The duration of action of sublingual nitroglycerin is about 20 minutes; consequently, its main use in this form is in aborting attacks of angina.

SHORT-ACTING PROPRIETARIES. Nitroglycerin (glyceryl trinitrate) sublingual tablets in strengths of 1/100 gr (600 mcg), 1/150 gr (400 mcg), and 1/200 or (300 mcg). Onset of action 1 to 2 min. Duration of action 20 to 30 min. Nitroglycerin (Nitroglyn Sublingual).

LONG-ACTING PROPRIETARIES. Isordil (isosorbide dinitrate, ISD). 5 mg sublingual tablets best given t.i.d., p.c. and before proposed exertion or excitement. Duration of action, 1½ to 2 hr. Isordil is prepared as a 10 mg oral tablet. The oral tablet best be taken before meals. There is a 30 to 60 min delay in action and the tablet's effect is attenuated. Sorbitrate (same as Isordil). No nitrates are more useful in preventing angina than Isordil and Sorbitrate.

Cardilate Sublingual (erythritol tetranitrate) in tablets of 5, 10, or 15 mg. Sublingual dose may be increased to 15 mg. Cardilate is similar in nearly all respects to ISD except for more frequent headaches.

P.E.T.N. (pentaerythritol tetranitrate). Dosage: 20 mg tablets q.i.d. on an empty stomach. For prevention of attacks only; not to abort attacks. Onset: 1 hr. Duration 4 to 5 hr. Peritrate (same as P.E.T.N.). These last two preparations are relatively weak in action, but are useful for patients who are hypersensitive to the more potent nitrates.

All sustained-action oral preparations of the above mentioned drugs have proved disappointing (ineffective or unsatisfactory). Do not prescribe these inferior but expensive formulations.

THE BEST MEDICAL TREATMENT. Nothing appears to be a more effective prevention of angina than a combination of propranolol (Inderal-Ayerst) and isosorbide dinitrate (ISD). The drugs are additive, complementary and synergistic. If you prescribe the combination properly tailored for individual patients, the therapeutic effects will far exceed anything you have used before. Dosage: propranolol 20 to 100 mg orally before meals and ISD 5 mg sublingually after meals.

Some Clinical Findings During an Attack

Ausculate the heart, identifying the second heart sound near the sternum in the second or third interspace. At this point, with the use of the diaphragm of the stethoscope, you can best hear any splitting of the second sound. During angina, listen for a paradoxic (reversed) splinting, i.e. widening on expiration and narrowing on inspiration. Listen while the patient breathes normally and then have him breathe a little heavier.

Move the diaphragm of the stethoscope to the point of maximum intensity. Locate the PMI accurately by palpation. Any murmur that appears or becomes worse during angina is significant. Usually, however, the murmur is systolic in time, either holosytolic or late systolic and becoming holosystolic.

Now have the patient turn onto his left side in the left lateral recumbent position or resting on his left elbow. Listen for two abnormal sounds—a presystolic and/or a midsystolic gallop. You will hear the presystolic gallop best just medial to the apex beat with the bell stethoscope. If inexperienced, a presystolic gallop may be difficult to distinguish from a split first sound. Some differences: the split of the first sound is narrower than the sounds of a presystolic gallop. The sound of splitting radiates to other areas while presystolic gallop is confined to the medial area of the PMI. Positional changes do not effect first sound splitting, but elevating the legs, thereby increasing filling, increases while standing decreases the gallop.

To hear the midsystolic gallop continue the examination with the bell stethoscope and with the patient in the left lateral recumbent position. Listen directly over the PMI for a low frequency nearly rumbling sound. As with the presystolic gallop, the middiastolic sound becomes louder during ventricular filling and less distinct during ventricular emptying.

Then either palpate the femoral and/or the radial pulses for pulsus alternans or listen for it while taking the patient's blood pressure. I happen to think it easier to check for it while determining the systolic blood pressure. It's easy. When the systolic tones come through, do you hear each beat or every other one? Allow the air to escape from the cuff very slowly in order to detect the condition. In palpating the radial or femoral pulses, exert pressure until the impulses disappear. Then very slowly release the pressure over the artery until you can feel the every-other-beat of pulsus alternans.

Another controversial maneuver done for diagnostic purposes is massaging of the carotid sinus during angina. It is reported the carotid sinus massage during angina will ease the pain and slow the pulse. If it occurs the findings are diagnostic. Some tips to avoid complications are:

- do not massage the sinus more than 5 sec or after the pulse slows
- massage only one side at a time
- monitor the heart rate by auscultation while massaging
- if the pulse slows but pain continues the diagnosis is not verified
- if the pulse slows and the patient indicates the pain is less the diagnosis is verified

To do the test, lightly palpate the carotid pulse, following it upward to the upper border of the thyroid cartilage. Generally at this point a bulge can be detected over the carotid artery. Have the patient extend and turn his head to the opposite side. Press and massage the artery against the spinous processes of the vertebrae. Use your second, third and fourth fingers for massaging.

MYOCARDIAL INFARCTION (MI)

Treating the Suspected MI Patient as an Emergency at His Home

Relieve the patient's pain with morphine sulfate. Give small doses ($^{1}/_{6}$ gr) intravenously and repeat as needed. Check for arrhythmias. Remember infarction fatalities are most often due to ventricular fibrillation during the first hour. If the patient is having PVC's, he is probably headed for ventricular fibrillation. Give 50 to 100 mg lidocaine (Xylocaine, Astra) intravenously. If the patient has a bradycardia, give him 0.4 to 0.5 mg of atropine intravenously.

If fibrillation occurs in spite of these measures, strike the patient on the lower half of the sternum with one or two sharp blows.

If normal rhythm is not restored, open the patient's airway by tilting the patient's chin up and begin mouth-to-mouth ventilation. If alone, alternate between 15 heart compressions at a rate of once every second and ventilation of lungs twice—a ratio of 15:2.

While waiting for the ambulance, which has cardioversion machinery, give epinephrine, 0.5 ml of a 1:1,000 solution intravenously or by intracardiac injection. If possible, also give 50 ml of 7.5 percent sodium bicarbonate intravenously every 10 minutes.

When the ambulance arrives, start the oxygen and sodium bicarbonate in preparation for cardioversion. If still unsuccessful, give more lidocaine, 50 to 100 mg and, if possible, a slow infusion of 500 mg in 500 ml of glucose in water. If a rate has been restored, 0.4 to 1 mg of atropine will help speed up a slow pulse.

A good resource booklet is the American Heart Association's "Definitive Therapy in Cardiovascular Resuscitation."

Recognizing the Impending Infarction

In one study[3] 84 percent of patients who were later diagnosed as having myocardial infarction had prodromal pain for several weeks prior to the attack; and those who later had cardiac arrest had pain for more than a month. The most common prodrome to infarction was atypical angina of recent onset. Other symptoms were dyspnea, fatigue, palpitation and sweats. Even 93 percent of the patients who later proved to have a lesser brand of coronary insufficiency had the prodromal pain suggesting a steadily increasing angina.

Consider and beware of the following complexities in diagnosing coronary arteriosclerosis. At the University of Virginia,[4] 89 patients were found and studied who had anginal patterns of pain plus several risk factors, i.e., smoking habit, elevated serum cholesterol and/or elevated postprandial blood sugar levels.

The 89 patients underwent selective arteriography. Forty six or nearly half proved to have significant coronary stenosis. Of these 46, 14 had normal resting ECG's. Twenty one of the 46 took the standard double Master's test, and 9 still had negative electrocardiographic findings. And even with maximal exercise, a few never produced positive ECG's. Of the 21, 12 did have a positive ECG result.

Out of the original 89, 43 did not prove to have coronary stenosis by selective arteriography (nearly 50 percent). Thirty one of these 43 took the double Master's test. Twenty five confirmed the results of the arteriographic findings. Six had false positives. Happily enough none of this group were known to have had a myocardial infarction during the subsequent 6 years.

Verifying the Suspicion of Acute MI

Serial enzyme studies plus serial ECG's can reduce the diagnostic error of MI to less than 5 percent. The most widely used enzyme tests are:

SGOT (serum glutamic oxalacetic transaminase), normal range 10 to 40 units per ml. This normal may fluctuate 12 units per ml in 24 hr but is not affected by meals. The SGOT following an infarction may start rising within 6 hr, peaking in 24 to 36 hr. It may increase four to six times normal; when shock is present, to 200 units per ml in 36 hr; and in rather grave conditions to 300 units. The serum level returns to normal in 4 to 6 days. The SGOT enzyme is also elevated after biliary surgery, drug administration, emboli, and during hepatic, pericardial, pancreatic and gallbladder disease.

LDH (serum lactic dehydrogenase), normal range 150 to 400 units per ml. Although serum concentration begins within 6 to 12 hours and peaks in 12 to 48 hr, LDH may persist as long as 6 to 12 days, following an MI. It may reach a maximum of 500 to 3,000 units per ml. LDH, too, may increase in other conditions related to the liver and lungs plus leukemia, lymphomas, carcinoma and pancreatitis.

CPK (serum creatine phosphokinase), normal range 0.33 to 4.49. Serum enzyme rise begins even earlier than SGOT, within 3 to 6 hr, and will peak at 4 to 5 times its normal value. This test is affected by activity, hypothyroidism, renal, brain and muscle disease.

SHBD (serum hydroxybutyrate dehydrogenase) will remain elevated 2 to 3 weeks. An elevated SHRD is fairly specific and gives no false negatives. Confusion can occur when the patient has certain blood dyscrasias or liver disease.

Symptoms in MI

Symptoms to expect in MI are:

- –substernal pain in 90 to 95 percent
- –symptoms of pulmonary congestion in 70 to 90 percent
- –symptoms of heart failure, most likely left heart failure, in 50 to 70 percent
- –symptoms of pulmonary edema in 10 to 20 percent

When a severe pain lasts more than an hour, look for a transmural infarction. When a severe pain lasts for 30 minutes but less than 60 minutes, look for a subendocardial infarction. A pain which lasts only minutes suggests angina pectoris.

Arrhythmias to look for are:

- –ventricular premature beats in 40 to 70 percent
- –sinus tachycardia in 30 to 43 percent

- –atrial tachycardia in 4 to 8 percent
- –total A-V block in 4 to 8 percent
- –bundle branch block in 10 to 18 percent
- –ventricular tachycardia in 6 to 27 percent
- –ventricular fibrillation in 8 to 10 percent

Heart sounds in acute myocardial infarction are:

- –paradoxical pulsation in 80 percent between the left sternal border and apex or along the left heart border as a bulging during ventricular systole
- –atrial gallop or fourth heart sound in 75 percent
- –ventricular gallop or a third heart sound in 70 percent
- –murmur of mitral incompetence in about 55 percent
- –pericardial friction rub in 10 to 20 percent
- –occasional murmurs of papillary or interventricular septum rupture in 1 or 2 percent

To hear atrial gallop, lightly apply a bell stethoscope to the patient's chest. Listen for a low-pitched, low-intensity gallop. Auscult with the patient supine and in the left lateral position. Listen over the apex during diastole for ventricular gallop.

Standing Orders for Suspected MI in Coronary Care Unit (CCU)

Standing orders include the following:

- –bed rest
- –liquid diet 24 hr (specify whether patient can feed self), but no coffee, tea, carbonated beverages or ice water
- –vital signs every 2 hr
- –chart intake and output
- –indwelling venous catheter with continuous intravenous of 5 percent glucose in water
- –ECG on admission if not done in ER
- –ECG monitoring daily for 3 days (record ECG strip hourly and upon appearance of any ectopic rhythm)
- –portable chest x-ray
- –laboratory studies
  Sedimentation rate, CBC, SGOT, LDH, CPK daily 3 days.
  First day only: FBS, BUN, serum potassium, prothrombin time, urinalysis and cholesterol
- –oral temperature.

The attending physician should stipulate the following:

- –morphine sulfate gr $^1/_6$ p.r.n. pain every 3 to 4 hr
- –valium or other sedative for night sedation
- –patient's ability to feed himself
- –may the patient stand to void
- –use of commode with assistance?
- –other activities permitted (read, shave, etc.)
- –oxygen? mask or catheter?
- –laxative? (Pericolace 2 tablets daily)
- –anticoagulants? (Heparin or coumadin or both with proper monitoring)
- –times the patient may sit in chair

The attending physician should grant authority for the following treatments in emergencies:

- –premature ventricular contractions (PVC)—in event of multifocal PVC's or if 6 or more PVC's/minute, give a 50 mg bolus of lidocaine and start lidocaine drip (2,000 mg/1,000 ml).
- –ventricular tachycardia without loss of consciousness—follow above lidocaine orders.
- –ventricular tachycardia with circulatory collapse—resuscitation, defibrillation, follow above lidocaine orders and add sodium bicarbonate 50 ml intravenously.
- –ventricular fibrillation—same as for ventricular tachycardia with circulatory collapse.

Arrhythmias Following MI

The main objective of the coronary care unit is no longer the prompt resuscitation of patients after cardiac arrest. Presently, the number one priority is the early recognition and treatment of arrhythmias likely to precipitate cardiac arrest.

Factors which predispose to cardiac arrhythmia are an enlarged heart (when it does develop the consequences are more severe), any preexisting impairment of the conduction system and myocardial ischemia.

Arrhythmias most often appear within the first few hours following admission. The risk of a fatal arrhythmia is highest shortly after infarction and then gradually decreases. The patient who reaches the coronary unit has, therefore, survived the time of greatest hazard.

Some arrhythmias can be treated on an elective basis unless associated with an inadequate cardiac output with hypotension or failure. Atrial fibrillation or flutter will usually spontaneously revert to a normal rhythm. The best treatment is Cedilanid 0.8 mg IV followed by increments of 0.4 mg every 2 to 4 hours as needed to a total of 1.6 mg. Use all digitalis preparations cautiously in acute myocardial infarction because of reduced toxic threshold. Some suggest giving no more than 70 percent of the calculated digitalizing dose for the first 48 hours. If the patient is not tolerating the arrhythmia, i.e. stroke volume is low, rapid heart rate, hypotension or failure, consider immediate synchronized precordial shock.

Atrial premature complexes (APC's) and paroxysmal atrial tachycardia are not particularly dangerous in themselves but are frequent forerunners of atrial fibrillation or flutter. Usually no treatment is needed if the patient is being monitored. If not, look for changes in heart rate and neck vein distention. Treat as outlined above. Be even more cautious with digitalis preparations. One difference in treatment: precordial DC shock is unnecessary for controlling APC's. If digitalis does not control the rhythm, try quinidine. Give either orally or IM, but for APC's give 0.2 to 0.4 g every 6 hours p.o.

Sinus bradycardia occurs in up to 15 percent of patients with myocardial infarction. Sinus bradycardia is the most hazardous arrhythmia next to ventricular arrhythmia. It can be far from trivial. When the heart rate drops to about 60, trouble can be anticipated. In the patient with vasovagal syncope or AV dissociation, give atropine, 0.5 to 1.0 mg IV, and lower the patient's head. Repeat the atropine two or three times, p.r.n.

If the patient isn't being monitored and the rate is near 30, administer Isuprel 0.2 mg IM, repeated as needed. Do not give Isuprel IV unless the patient is being monitored.

Other methods of administering Isuprel: attempt to maintain blood pressure at 100 to 110 systolic and pulse at a minimum of 40 to 50 beats per minute. Remember, 10 ml equals 2 mg. Therefore, dilute 10 ml in 500 ml of 5 percent dextrose in water. Start administration with 15 to 30 drops per minute and titrate to the patient's needs. For IV push, mix in a 10 ml syringe, 1 ml (0.2 mg) of Isuprel with 9 ml saline and inject IV through a 20 to 22 gauge needle. Sublingual tablets, 10 to 15 mg may be given every 1 to 6 hr. Rectal suppositories, 5 to 15 mg may be inserted every 1 to 6 hr. Injection of 0.2 mg may be administered subcutaneously every 1 to 6 hr through a 25 gauge needle.

If more help is needed, try steroids, prednisone 60 to 80 mg, in first 24 hours tapering to 40 mg thereafter.

(Note other ways to give atropine: Remember 1 ml = gr. 1/150 = 0.4 mg. To give 1 to 2 mg, select a 5 ml syringe and draw up 2.5 to 5 ml solution. Inject by a slow IV push through a 20 to 22 gauge needle. Give also by IV drip in 100 ml of 5 percent glucose and water. To give 0.4 to 2.0 mg, draw up 1 to 5 ml in same syringe and give IM using 21 to 23 gauge needle. To give 0.6 to 0.8, draw up 1.5 to 2.0 ml in a 2 ml syringe and give subcutaneously through a 25 gauge needle.)

Some adjustment in treating bradycardia is needed if the slow rate is the result of AV blocking. First degree block requires atropine as suggested above. Second degree block requires Isuprel 0.2 mg IV diluted in 500 ml of 5 percent glucose in distilled water. Insert a pacing catheter prophylactically. Third degree block or on threatened asystole, start pacing the heart.

Arrhythmias Requiring Emergency Treatment

Ventricular premature complexes (PVC's) that may need treatment may best be anticipated following isolated premature contractions or bigeminy. The decision to treat depends on what is happening. If more than 5 PVC's occur in 1 minute or in salvos, or if coupling occurs, treat immediately with 50 to 75 mg (1 mg/kg) of a 2 percent solution lidocaine by IV push. This is usually effective in 3 to 5 minutes. If needed, repeat 3 times. This may be effective in 20 to 40 minutes. (Note: Use 10 ml syringe for 50 mg and give through a 20 to 22 gauge needle.) In the meantime, start a steady infusion at rate of 2 to 4 mg per minute to maintain effect. The usual maintenance dose of lidocaine is 1 to 2 mg per minute. Peak flow is 4 to 5 mg per minute for 1 to 3 hours. The usual combination is 500 to 1,000 mg lidocaine in 250 to 500 ml 5 percent glucose in water. Titrate the drip rate to the needs of the patient.

Once the PVC's are suppressed, plan for long term therapy with quinidine (0.2 to 0.4 g every 6 hours p.o.), Pronestyl (2.0 to 4.0 g daily divided into 4 to 8 doses and given every 3 to 6 hours) and Inderal (10 to 30 mg p.o. 4 times daily). Reserve Inderal for special situations and consult a specialist. Do not give in cases of bradycardia, asthma or congestive heart failure.

Ventricular tachycardia calls for immediate precordial DC shock followed by the use of one or more of the following: lidocaine, quinidine, Pronestyl or Dilantin. Ask for consultation to plan long-term therapy. Ventricular tachycardia is the forerunner of ventricular fibrillation.

Ventricular fibrillation again calls for immediate precordial DC shock. If unsuccessful, proceed to closed chest cardiac massage and ventilation support with or without intubation. To give external cardiac massage (Fig. 10-17), locate the lower half of the patient's sternum (but not the xiphoid). Place the heel of one of your hands on the area and place the heel of the other hand on the back of your first hand. Lean forward so that your shoulders are over the patient's sternum. Keep your elbows straight. Using the weight of your upper body, press straight downward on her sternum. On an adult, depress the sternum one-half to 2 inches. Establish a regular rhythm of about one compression every 2 seconds.

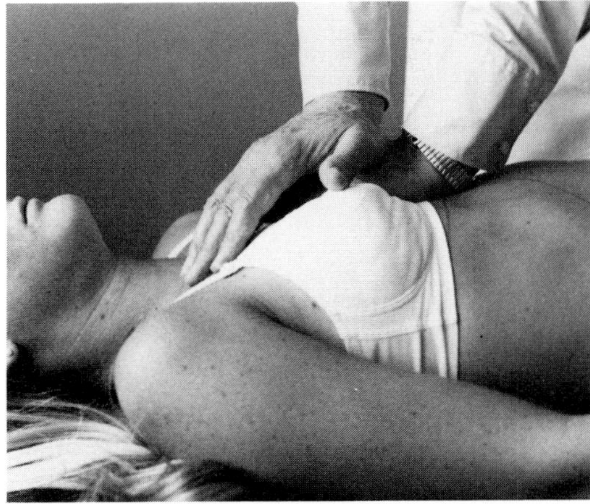

Figure 10-17. Procedure for external cardiac massage.

Premature ventricular contractions do not appear to affect survival in the absence of heart disease. They do, however, increase mortality when they are associated with ischemia of the coronary muscle. Their occurrence during an acute coronary attack may herald ventricular fibrillation with cardiac arrest.

Chest Thump

A sharp blow to the chest (Fig. 10-18) can terminate a ventricular tachycardia. It will do no harm in cases of asystole and may save a life when the arrhythmia is a prefibrillatory ventricular tachycardia.

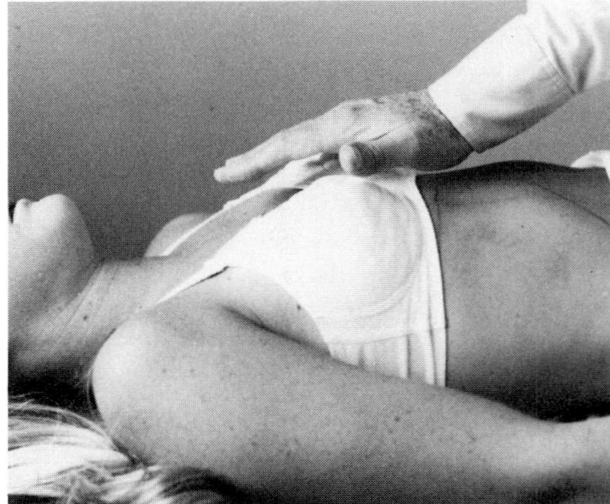

Figure 10-18. A sharp blow to the chest while awaiting a defibrillator occasionally establishes normal rhythm.

If the patient has tolerated the tachyarrhythmia satisfactorily and a cardioverter is available, cardioversion with low energy is more predictable, less traumatic and preferred.

Cardioversion

Cardiovert immediately in ventricular flutter or fibrillation. If the patient is conscious, prepare him by administering 2 to 5 mg Valium IV. Titrate the Valium to the patient's needs. Some patients need 5 mg IV every 5 minutes to a total of 20 mg. Remember these patients usually need assisted respiration and closed chest massage.

Cardiovert for ventricular tachycardia whenever pulmonary edema and/or shock is present, especially when the patient is unable to tolerate the usual drugs.

Cardiovert in supraventricular arrhythmias—if the patient has an extremely rapid rate and falling blood pressure and if he does not respond to digitalis.

In summary, cardiovert for all tachycardias except sinus whenever pulmonary edema and/or shock is present. Some contraindications are digitalis toxicity and AV blocks.

Administer the shock on the downstroke of the R wave or on the upstroke of the S wave. Some cardiologists start with low dosage shock, 100 watt-seconds and build up to 400 watt-seconds while others start out with 400 watt-seconds.

If patient response is not prompt, administer 50 ml undiluted sodium bicarbonate (44.6 mEq/50 ml) every 5 minutes. If still no response, give 5 ml of a mixture of 1 ml of 1:1,000 aqueous epinephrine in 9 ml of saline IV or intracardiac. Continue external massage and assisted ventilation.

Liability can usually be avoided by performing a proper and adequate examination. A misdiagnosis of heart trouble is not actionable unless your care is below the usual standards of skill, care and knowledge. Treatment and diagnosis must conform to your community's standard of care. You do not need to adhere to any particular school of thought as long as the therapeutic program you follow is one accepted by at least a respectable minority of the profession.

Even if the outcome proves disastrous, there is no negligence unless it can be shown that proper diagnosis and prompt treatment would have lessened the impact of the disease.[6]

Lidocaine (Xylocaine, Astra)

Although much has been written regarding the prophylactic value of lidocaine, you should know that those benefits have never been proven. Chopra and coworkers[7] found that on a double-blind study of 82 patients with myocardial infarction the incidence of ventricular tachycardia, fibrillation and mortality were similar in the two groups, even though the initial PVC's were suppressed with lidocaine. Their study provided no evidence to support the routine use of intravenous lidocaine in the management of ventricular ectopic activity after acute myocardial infarction.

Again, just to keep you from developing a smugness regarding the use of lidocaine consider Adgey and coworkers' report[8] which not only points out the ineffectiveness of lidocaine in controlling and preventing ventricular dysrhythmias but the unusually high incidence of bradyarrhythmias that occur during the first hour after an M.I. They believe the resources for coronary care should be directed towards the prehospital phase.

Last of all, there is some evidence to show that lidocaine may be as effective in combatting ventricular dysrhythmias when given intramuscularly as when given intravenously. Bernstein and fellow workers[9] in a carefully controlled study correlating serum lidocaine levels and clinical results proved that effective drug concentrations were reached between 15 to 30 minutes after the IM injection of 200 mg of lidocaine and that therapeutic levels were maintained for at least 60 minutes.

Their point was that lidocaine should be given IM to all patients suffering an acute MI before they are moved to a hospital, again emphasizing the importance of prehospital monitoring and treatment. If one prefers attempting this method, consider 4 mg/kg as a low dosage and 6 mg/kg high. One experimenter has shown that giving the lidocaine intradeltoid produced higher blood levels more rapidly than did intragluteal injection. Therapeutic blood levels persisted for over 2 hours. The high dose levels will produce minor neurologic signs but none of a permanent or major nature.[10]

When to Anticoagulate

For the past decade the family physician has been caught in the cross fire of the coagulators and the anticoagulators. The average clinician gets little help from consulting a cardiologist regarding a wise course to pursue. The cardiologists themselves appear to be divided on the question. Few medical questions have fired as much controversy over so long a time. The issue is still being debated.

In part, some of the confusion regarding the effectiveness stems from the 1950's when at least 20 percent of patients with myocardial infarction developed thromboembolic complications. During those years anticoagulation was useful. In recent years, however, because of coronary care units and more effective treatment of heart failure, earlier ambulation and arrhythmia control, thromboembolic complications have dropped to 5 percent. Consequently, anticoagulation does not appear to have as salient an effect on the mortality and morbidity as it once did.

Although the use of heparin and coumarin compounds have proven their effectiveness in controlling venous thrombosis and pulmonary embolism, their success in reducing mortality in myocardial infarction has been far less.

The Pacemaker

The pacemaker may be used in the following.

- –Adams-Stokes syndrome
- –bradycardia from sinoatrial arrest and in block or bradycardia if the rate is slow enough to cause symptoms and if it is resistant to drug treatment
- –first degree AV block with bundle branch block or bilateral branch block
- –complete heart block with prolonged QRS and slow ventricular rates
- –second degree block of the Mobitz type II.

Only small numbers of patients with myocardial infarction will need pacemakers, something on the order of two or three out of every 200 patients. Remember the risks: ventricular arrhythmias, perforation, sepsis and knotting and breaking of catheter.

Try every reasonable method of arrhythmia control before resorting to pacemaker implants. This implies the skillful use of drugs and a wise choice of patients. Consultation is more useful in selecting patients than is needed for the actual implantation.

Patient Education and Care During the Post-Hospital Period

Moss[11] emphasizes the clinician's responsibility in two areas: (1) long-term anti-arrhythmic prophylaxis, and (2) patient education.

He points out that PVC's are the tip-off to possible dangerous ventricular arrhythmias. A frequency of more than 10 PVC's per thousand normal beats is associated with a ten-fold increase in sudden death. If you find even one PVC during hospital rounds, you can be certain that many could be documented by the use of an electrocardiographic tape recorder.

Long-term antiarrhythmic therapy includes:

- –Pronestyl 500 mg p.o. every 4 hr.
- –quinidine sulfate 400 mg p.o. every 6 hr
- –Dilantin
- –Inderal (The physiological effect of Inderal is somewhat unpredictable; watch carefully.)
- –monitoring for hypokalemia, especially patients on digitalis and diuretics
- –elixir of potassium chloride 15 mEq two to three times daily helps to replace

potassium loss (Many believe that potassium ingestion is as important in arrhythmia control as is Pronestyl or quinidine.)

Patient education can best be carried out during a series of short consultations during the patient's last 4 to 5 days of hospitalization. Moss urges that the patient be educated along the following lines:

- –general information regarding the nature of heart attacks
- –hazards of smoking
- –diet for weight control
- –physical activity
- –need to minimize all emotional stress
- –use, type and dose of all medications, best by writing
- –explanation of prodromal signs and symptoms of complications and what to do about them

Weight control is important. The patient needs to reduce calories, avoid saturated fats and have an adequate unsaturated fat intake, reduce sodium ingestion and limit coffee to no more than two to three cups daily.

Physical activity consistent with the patient's age and extent of his disease should be outlined in detail. In general, instruct the patient to refrain from physical effort that causes chest discomfort or breathlessness. Explain that his day's activities should not leave him exhausted. Have the patient begin activity by walking about the house a minute or two hourly gradually increasing to 5 minutes. Ask him to rest 2 hours after his noon meal and to sit up as much as possible. Request the patient to refrain from stair climbing for the first 7 to 14 days at home and then begin by counting five after making a step before proceeding to the next. Gradually reduce the count to three counts as tolerated.

Your responsibility does not end here. You are to be congratulated on protecting your patient during the first dangerous hour of his infarction and guiding him through the coronary unit and regular floor care to home. But now some of your less spectacular work begins: establishing for your patient the proper long-term health habits. The restoration of preinfarction function is not sufficient for secondary prevention. When the patient goes home the rather unappreciative job begins of helping the patient change risk-taking behavior in the areas of weight control, blood lipids, dietary habits, cigarette smoking and personal stresses.

Few family physicians will be able to organize as detailed a program as it put on by the Coronary Heart Disease Rehabilitation Center at San Diego State College. For the ordinary patient such a program is not necessary providing his doctor takes as active an interest in his rehabilitation as he does in his hospital care.

By the third postinfarction month, the patient should have been evaluated and certain rehabilitation objectives outlined. This evaluation should include:

- –determination of blood chemistries including the lipid phenotyping
- –skin fold measurements at six sites for estimation of body fat
- –pulmonary function studies
- –psychologic evaluation, or at least your appraisal, of the patient's emotional problems including degree of depression, anxiety and somatization

After this evaluation instruct the patient on how best to meet his needs employing the dietitian and other specialists as needed. Whatever long-term plans you formulate should be explained in detail to both the patient and his wife. The cooperation and understanding of the patient's family is essential to successful rehabilitation. Remember the goal is to achieve and maintain a higher level of physical fitness than was present at the time of the infarct.

The next order of business is to determine the exercise prescription. This can best be done by controlled treadmill testing, bicycle ergometer testing, postexercise blood studies including lactate determination.

The bicycle ergometer test is done to estimate the maximal oxygen uptake, a good index of cardiac performance, the idea being to train the ventricles to put out an increased stroke volume. The maximal oxygen uptake is used to chart the patient's progress at 3, 6 and 12 month intervals during the first year and twice yearly thereafter.

The follow-up testing is necessary to assess not only improvement but also to detect those patients who do not respond to routine rehabilitation or who are actually deteriorating. In this case the exercise program will be stopped and a complete reevaluation be done, including coronary cinearteriography. From these exercise-failure patients, select candidates for surgical bypass.

In any event, from the data obtained from these preexercise tests a practical approach to the intensity of exertion is worked out. When exercising is begun, whether it be light conditioning, walking, jogging or swimming, the *exercise heart rate* should not be exceeded. The patient may need 3 months of exercise at one level before moving up to another level of exercise.

According to reports, the San Diego group[12] uses the Karvonen formula to determine the exercise heart rate. Exercise heart rate: (maximum heart rate − resting heart rate) × 60 to 70 percent + resting heart rate = exercise heart rate in beats per minute.

Exercising consists of a 20 minute warm-up period of stretching and conditioning of the joints and periarticular tissues for the endurance phase. At first heart rate monitoring is done frequently. Patients may group themselves for jogging and swimming depending on heart rate response. After the exercise period, the patient is encouraged to take a 5 minute cooling down period. Between workout days, the patient is encouraged to play golf or walk 1 hour at 4 miles per hour.

When to Consider Arteriosclerotic Heart Disease Disabling

The following are disabling heart problems (based on Social Security regulations):

Myocardial infarction associated with consistent ECG abnormalities (or consistent abnormalities of serum enzymes) and one of the following: chest discomfort on effort, relieved by rest or nitroglycerin or another documented myocardial infarction within 6 months following previous infarction.

Persistent heart block or recurrent arrhythmia as evidenced by ECG (in absence of digitalis) with cardiac syncope.

Angina pectoris, associated with resting ECG abnormalities, in the absence of digitalis (in the presence of digitalis, the predigitalis ECG should be evaluated), and showing one of the following: (1) depression of the ST segment to more than 0.5 mm in any leads, I, II, a VF, V^1 to V^6; or (2) elevation of ST segment to 2 mm or more in any leads I, II, III, V^1, V^5, or V^6; (3) inversion of the T wave to 5.0 mm or more in any two leads except leads III, a VR, V^1 and V^2; (4) inversion of T wave to 1.0 mm or more in any of leads I, II, aVL, V^2 to V^6 *and* R wave of 5.0 mm or more in lead aVL *and* R wave greater than S wave in lead aVF; (5) second or third degree heart block; or (6) left bundle branch block as evidenced by QRS duration of 0.12 seconds or more in leads I, II, or III *and* R peak duration 0.06 seconds or more (in absence of myocardial infarction) in leads I, aVL, V^1 or V^6.

Angina pectoris associated with standardized ECG exercise test abnormalities in the absence of digitalis (in the presence of digitalis, the predigitalis ECG should be evaluated) showing one of the following: development of depression ST segment to more than 0.5 mm which lasts for at least 0.12 seconds and appears in at least two consecutive complexes in any lead or development of bundle branch block.

Chest discomfort on effort relieved by rest or nitroglycerin with obstruction or narrowing of coronary vessels observed on angiography or heart enlargement demonstrated by x-ray or ECG.

The Patient's Hospital Chart in Myocardial Infarction

Patients with myocardial infarction are considered major hospital admissions. His chart will most likely be reviewed whether the patient lives or dies. Many patients will need consultation for unexpected complications. It is likely the family physician will lose his privileges in coronary care unless he demonstrates sound judgment, perceptive diagnostic ability and competent therapeutic skill. Document your skill by writing a hospital chart that can't be criticized. Your chart should include:

- –indications for admission and whether the diagnosis is established or not
- –history including specific reference to the patient's pain
- –physical examination observations
- –laboratory work
- –special procedures, including in nearly all cases cardiac monitoring, to be consistent with the diagnosis, cardioversion and pacing
- –estimated length of stay
- –indications for discharge

Spell out details of the pain, i.e. onset, radiation and duration. Was the pain in the left chest? Was it crushing or sharp? To where did it radiate? To the jaw? The arm or hand? Does the patient complain of heaviness or a sensation of weight on the chest? Is the pain accompanied by dyspnea, vomiting, sweating, weakness, syncope, leg pains, hemoptysis or dependent edema? Is there a previous history of angina, myocardial infarction, hypertension or diabetes? How about signs and symptoms of cerebrovascular insufficiency or intermittent claudication?

In your physical examination, record any of the following signs: evidence of shock as displayed by pallor, apprehension, restlessness, pulse rate, sweating, cyanosis, tachypnea, blood pressure and temperature. Describe the heart as to size, rhythm, sounds, murmurs or friction rubs. Give particular attention to any arrhythmia. Describe the type and distribution of pulmonary rales and breath sounds. Are friction rubs heard? Record the size of the liver and spleen. The chart should indicate whether the abdominal aorta or femoral pulses were examined and what the results were. Do not forget to examine and record the nature of the carotid artery pulsation. Can you hear a bruit? Is the jugular vein distended? Is there calf tenderness and/or edema?

Under laboratory work the chart should include the result of any and all preadmission ECG's. Minimal postadmission laboratory studies are CBC, urinalysis, ECG and serum enzymes daily for 3 days if the ECG is not diagnostic.

Other laboratory studies as indicated are blood sugar 2 hr postprandial, serum enzymes, prothrombin or clotting time, serum lipids, serum electrolytes, BUN, x-ray of chest as a minimum and other radiographic studies as indicates such as UGI and gallbladder series, angiocardiography and aortography if dissecting aneurysm is suspected. Radiographic studies are counterindicated in established MI.

In young individuals, free of other diseases, with small infarcts as judged by the ECG and/or enzymes and changes in the white blood count, temperature and sedimentation rate, the probable length of hospital stay should be 14 to 21 days. In other than small transmural infarction, 21 to 28 days.

Verify and record early complications that may extend the patient's hospitalization. These are shock, coronary pain of unusually long duration, cardiac failure, serious arrhythmias, other types of heart disease, unusually large infarction, systemic or pulmonary embolism, perforated interventricular septum, ruptured chorda tendinea, ruptured papillary muscle.

Verify and record late complications (beyond the first week of illness), including cardiac failure, serious arrhythmias, embolism, recurrence of coronary pain suggesting impending infarction, persistent tachycardia, difficulty in regulating anticoagulant therapy, pericarditis and/or effusion, aneurysmal dilatation and persistent RS-T elevation.

Plan on hospitalization for 21 days after control of any or all early complications. Late complications will prolong stay by the length of time required to control them. An extension of the original infarction or a second infarction will require the minimum 21 day period of hospitalization as of their occurrence.

Indications for discharge should be determined and stated: normal pulse and temperature, freedom from pain except for occasional mild angina and ambulant.

HYPERTENSION

Ninety to 95 percent of hypertensive patients have no known cause for their high blood pressure. These are the essential *primary hypertension* cases.

Secondary hypertension implies that the hypertension is secondary to some known inciting cause. Five to 10 percent of these cases are secondary to such problems as vascular rigidity, renal arteriosclerotic abnormalities, endocrine imbalances causing overactivity of pituitary, adrenal or thyroid glands, neurologic and psychogenic conditions and miscellaneous and rare diseases associated with hypertension.

Renal arteriosclerotic abnormalities include acute and chronic glomerulonephritis, acute renal ischemia or infarction, polycystic renal disease, acute tubular necrosis, vascular anomalies and aneurysms, tumors, hyperparathyroidism and vitamin D intoxication, collagen diseases, renal tuberculosis, urinary tract obstruction, renin producing tumor and amyloidosis.

Endocrine imbalances are pheochromocytoma, systolic thyrotoxicosis, Cushing's syndrome, primary aldosteronism, acromegaly and adrenal cortical hyperfunction.

Neurologic and psychogenic causes of secondary hypertension are brain tumors, some antibiotics, acute intermittent porphyria, familial autonomic dysfunction, cerebrovascular accidents and systolic psychogenic hypertension.

Miscellaneous and rare diseases associated with hypertension are toxemia of pregnancy, aortic coarctation, metabolic and hereditary disorders, nephrectomy hypertension and oral contraceptives.

Taking a Patient's Blood Pressure

Have the patient seated and relaxed with arms slightly flexed and the forearms supported on a solid surface at heart level. Apply the cuff snugly to the arm with its lower border about 2½ cm above the antecubital space. Palpate the radial or brachial artery while inflating the cuff. Inflate the cuff 30 mm of Hg above the point of disappearance. Begin deflating the cuff at a rate of 2 to 4 mm of Hg per heart beat.

Listen for the Korotkoff's sounds and monitor the decline in the manometer readings. Observe the manometer reading when the first pulsing blood flow is heard in the brachial artery. The reading at the point when two consecutive tappings are heard is the systolic pressure. Continue to monitor Korotkoff's sounds until they suddenly become muffled and blowing in character. This is recorded as the diastolic pressure. Record as RAS (right arm setting) and LAS or, when taken lying down, RAL or LAL or, standing, RAST or LAST.

In instances where it is wise to take the blood pressure in the leg, a special cuff should be used and applied above the knee while the patient is lying down. Listen for Korotkoff's sounds over the popliteal artery in the popliteal fossa. The systolic pressure is usually 15 to 20 mm Hg higher than the arm pressure.

If the systolic pressure in the leg is equal to or lower than the systolic pressure in the arm, determine if the findings are uni- or bilateral. If it is unilateral, look for a partial occlusion of the iliac or femoral artery on that side of the body. If it occurs bilaterally, look for aortic coarctation or an arteriosclerotic plaque at the bifurcation of the abdominal aorta into the common iliac arteries.

A classification is given in Table 10-2. Notice the systolic blood pressure is ignored in this clinical classification. This concept may be changing. A Massachusetts group[13] after a 14 year study, reports that systolic hypertension is a better indicator of coronary artery disease risk than diastolic hypertension. They unequivocally state that systolic hypertension is not normal in older people, women do not tolerate hypertension well and labile hypertension is dangerous. These findings are all contrary to previous beliefs.

Their conclusion: "Asymptomatic 'hypertension' is both a very common and a very potent contributor to morbidity and mortality in coronary heart disease." Their

Table 10-2. Clinical Classification of Hypertension

	Groups			
	I	*II*	*III*	*IV*
Hypertension	Mild labile	Moderate	Severe (accelerated)	Crisis
Diastolic pressure	90–105 mg Hg	105–120 mm Hg	120–140 mm Hg	140 mm Hg or over
Symptoms	Asymptomatic	Generally asymptomatic but may have certain degrees of retinopathy and tissue damage	Tissue damage in fundi, brain heart and kidney	Acute medical emergency, grade IV tissue damage

definition of systolic hypertension was defined as a pressure of over 160 mm Hg and diastolic hypertension as over 95 mm Hg. Normotension was 140/90. They urged that hypertensives be sought out and their pressure treated as soon as possible.

The Patient's Hospital Chart in Hypertension

The chart should include the history:

–statement on duration of hypertension
–family history of hypertension
–review of CNS symptoms, i.e. dizziness, syncope, sensory or motor deficit
–review of cardiovascular symptoms
–history of exertional pain
–exertional dyspnea
–edema
–genitourinary symptoms
–dysuria
–hematuria
–nocturia

In your report on the physical examination describe the optic fundi (Keith Wagener classification, see following pages), neck veins, lung findings, thyroid size and cervical bruits. In addition give estimate of cardiac size, presence of extra heart sounds, comment on second heart sound, notes on cardiac rate and cardiac rhythm, murmur description, intensity of heart sounds, cardiac classification according to AHA classification (see end of this chapter), ankle edema, femoral pulse and abdominal bruit.

List laboratory studies. The minimum are urinalysis, CBC, blood glucose, serum sodium, serum potassium, x-ray of chest, electrocardiogram, any test for pheochromocytoma, intravenous pyelogram, urine culture, serum creatinine, serum cholesterol, serum calcium and 24 hr proteinuria.

Hypertensive Work-up

Do a complete urinalysis and culture. Take a timed 24 hour collection for catecholamines or VMA (vanillylmandelic acid). If possible collect sample while patient is hypertensive. These assays are done to rule out pheochromocytomas. About half of the patients with pheochromocytomas have intermittent secretion of catecholamines and experience paroxysmal symptoms such as headache, palpitations, perspiration, tremor, nausea and epigastric or chest pain. For this intermittent hypertension collect a random specimen soon after an attack. These are reported in mg/100 ml. But checking mg/24 hours is more dependable.

The 24 hour collection of catecholamines or VMA has a fairly high degree of specificity except in patients who have been taking alphamethyldopa, tetracycline, adrenaline or large doses of vitamin B or who have been ingesting vanilla or fruits. It is wise to have the patient stop all the above for 2 days preceding the test and the alphamethyldopa for at least a week. It is also difficult to get a high degree of specificity in patients who have been exercising vigorously prior to the test and who have progressive muscular dystrophy or myasthenia gravis. VMA determination is probably the best all-round test for this purpose.

Take a complete blood count and sedimentation rate and a serum sodium and potassium. If the serum potassium is normal, give the patient sodium chloride, 2 g q.i.d. orally for 4 days and repeat the serum potassium determination on the fifth day. If the serum potassium remains within normal range, an aldosteronoma is probably excluded. If the potassium is low the patient should be admitted for a complete endocrine evaluation.

Include a 24 hour creatinine clearance or at least a serum creatinine. Serum calcium and 2 hour post 100 g glucose blood sugar are important also. Take x-ray films of the chest and a timed intravenous pyelogram. This should include a 30 second and 2, 5, 15 and 30 minute films plus an erect postvoiding film. The dye must be rapidly injected to obtain a nephrogram phase. And finally take an electrocardiogram.

Depending on the results of the above, proceed with the following as indicated:

- –cystoscopy and voiding cystogram if obstruction is suspected
- –split function kidney tests if indicated
- –rarely kidney biopsy
- –thyroid function tests
- –collagen vascular work-up
- –urinary porphyrins
- –urinary 5-HIAA
- –collection of 24 hour urine for 17-hydroxycorticosteroids and/or aldosterone for primary or secondary hyperaldosteronism.

Primary aldosteronism (Conn's syndrome) is a hypertensive syndrome caused by hyperfunction of the glomerulosa zone of the adrenal cortex. This is most frequently caused by an adenoma, although carcinoma and a diffuse cortical hyperplasia can be the basic disease.

Diagnostic hallmarks of primary aldosteronism are:

- –elevation of urinary aldosterone
- –suppression of plasma serum activity before and after a period of salt restriction
- –normal levels of 17-hydroxycorticosteroid excretion

Diagnostic hallmarks of secondary aldosteronism are:

- –elevation of urinary aldosterone
- –elevation of plasma renin activity

The important point is that primary aldosteronism requires resection of an adrenal tumor for cure whereas, in secondary aldosteronism, the renal circulation or disease of the renal parenchyma must be investigated.

Renovascular Hypertension

Disturbances in the renovascular mechanism account for 5 to 10 percent of the hypertensive population. Suspect the problem in patients who develop hypertension under 30 or over 50 years, suddenly develop more serious symptoms and findings, have an accelerated hypertension or develop symptoms of a vascular accident such as flank pain, renal trauma, peripheral arterial emboli or in patients with an abdominal or flank bruit.

There are numerous laboratory tests for diagnosis, but the most helpful are an intravenous pyelogram, angiotensin test and measurement of the pressor substance. In the pyelogram look for disparity in kidney size, delayed opacification in rapid sequence films or a delayed washout during diuretic pyelograms. These criteria will identify 70 to 90 percent of cases. The angiotensin infusion is a helpful screening test. The concept is that a diminished responsiveness to exogenous angiotensin in the presence of increased endogenous angiotensin (angiotensin II is the powerful peripheral vasoconstrictor whose action is responsible for the hypertension of renal origin). The most definitive test is the measurement of the pressor substance. The elevation of renin activity in peripheral plasma and a two-fold gradient between the afflicted and normal side is indicative of a lesion correctable by surgery.

Keith-Wagener Classification of Hypertensive Retinopathy

Class 0: Normal.

Class I: Mild generalized narrowing of the arterioles with no narrowing less than half the diameter of the vein. Branching of arterioles at angles—less than 75°.

Class II: Generalized narrowing of arterioles to less than a third of the vein size. Frequent segmental constrictions of the arterioles to less than half the caliber of proximal arterioles. There may be nicking of the veins where the arterioles cross.

Class III: Same as class II except with hemorrhages and/or exudates. There are often circular or flame-shaped hemorrhages. The exudates are actually microinfarcts. Findings of class III indicate accelerated hypertension.

Class IV: Same as classes II and III with papilledema. Although papilledema is the hallmark of malignant hypertension, it may also be present in a rise of intracranial pressure and occasionally its cause is undetermined.

Electrocardiographic Changes in Hypertension

Labile hypertensives usually have normal ECG's. *Mild primary* (essential) hypertensives may have left atrial (P wave) abnormalities. This is consistent with an atrial diastolic gallop a forerunner of hypertensive heart disease. *Moderately severe* hypertension will show electrocardiographic evidence of left atrial abnormality and/or left ventricular hypertrophy.

These changes merge into more severe changes including left axis deviation, tall R in aVL, depressed ST segment in V5-V6, inverted T in I and aVL and inverted T in V5-V6.

These changes may occur in patients with angina as well as those digitalized. As the severity of the disease progresses the pattern becomes one of left ventricular hypertrophy with prominent ST-T changes in I, II, aVL, aVF and V4 through V6 and the depressed ST segment in V5 and V6 extends to I, aVL and V4 through V6. Even when left ventricular hypertrophy cannot be seen, severe hypertension can be recognized by finding changes in the P wave. They may resemble the mitral P, i.e. a wide wave which becomes notched with peaks exceeding 0.04 seconds.

Treatment

Treatment of Borderline Hypertension

Whether there is value in treating borderline hypertension has not been fully decided. Possibly 15 percent of young people with a blood pressure around 145/90 will develop hypertension in 10 to 15 years. The best approach is to insist that potential hypertensives receive medical attention but not necessarily drug treatment.

First of all, attempt to establish a reliable baseline by repeated measurements. Whenever possible have the patient determine his blood pressure either by himself or by other members of the family while at home. If once decided that the patient has hypertension, observation and treatment become a life-time proposition.

Preventive measures may be all that are necessary. Should the patient reduce? Is the patient's cholesterol elevated? Blood sugar? Uric acid? Does the patient's resting heart rate run consistently above 80? Does he ingest too much salt? All these factors should be determined and corrected.

If the blood pressure continues to rise over a period of months or years consider drug therapy. Primary drugs are diuretics or reserpine. If the patient also has an increased resting heart rate of over 90, propranolol 40 mg b.i.d. may inhibit both the pressure and heart rate.

If the patient can take a diuretic, there is no need to require a low sodium diet. Less diuretic will be needed, however, if the patient will abandon table and cooking salt.

Treatment of Hypertension

First prescribe a thiazide or chlorthalidone. Remember chlorothiazide and hydrochlorothiazide are short acting diuretics and need be taken twice daily. Chlorthalidone, methyclothiazide and polythiazide are long acting and need be taken once daily.

Chlorothiazide (Diuril). Dose: 500 to 1,000 mg b.i.d. Dispensed in 250 or 500 mg tablets.

Hydrochlorothiazide (Hydrodiuril and Esidrix). Dose: 50 to 100 mg b.i.d. Dispensed in 25 and 50 mg tablets.

Bendroflumethiazide (Naturetin). Dose: 5 mg daily for 1 week and continue with 2.5 or 5.0 mg daily. Dispensed in 2.5 and 5.0 mg tablets.

Hydroflumethiazide (Saluron). Dose: 50 to 100 mg daily. Dispensed to 50 mg tablets.

Methyclothiazide (Enduron). Dose: 2.5 to 5 mg daily. Dispensed in 2.5 to 5.0 mg tablets.

Polythiazide (Renese). Dose: 1.0 to 4.0 mg daily. Dispensed in 1.0, 2.0 and 4.0 mg tablets.

Chlorthalidone (Hygroton). Dose: 50 to 100 mg daily. Dispensed in 50 to 100 mg tablets.

Diuretics will cause a loss of 3 to 4 pounds of weight, body regulatory mechanisms will adjust and further depletion of salt and water do not occur. Monitor the patient's weight for the first week to confirm the loss. Blood pressure decline occurs as early as the third day or may be delayed 6 weeks after initiating treatment.

Start elderly patients on half the maximum dose and increase as tolerated.

The response to diuretic therapy is variable. Expect, however, a reduction of 15 to 20 mm of Hg systolic and 10 to 15 mm of Hg diastolic in nearly all patients. Many, of course, will respond more.

Generally thiazide diuretics have little harmful effects. Many patients will develop an altered glucose tolerance curve which reverts to normal when the drug is discontinued. There is no evidence that true diabetes can result from thiazide diuretics.

Be aware of serum potassium depletion in every patient taking diuretics and complaining of fatigue. Monitor the potassium level in all patients with arrhythmic tendency. Maintain normal serum potassium levels. The first step is to substitute half the daily dose of the thiazide for a potassium-sparing diuretic such as Dyrenium (50 mg) or Aldactone (25 mg). Aldactazide and Hyazide contain the above added to hydrochlorothiazide (25 mg), given two per day.

Also monitor the serum uric acid while the patient is taking diuretics. Gout will occur when the uric acid level reaches 10 mg percent. If serum uric acid increases, add probenecid 500 mg b.i.d.

If blood pressure drop is insufficient on diuretics alone, probably the safest and most effective drug addition is alphamethyldopa (Aldomet). Reserpine 0.25 mg daily may be tried, but because of its unpredictable benefits and the side effects of depression, nasal stuffiness and tendency to promote weight gain its use is being replaced by Aldomet. Do not use Aldomet and reserpine together.

Aldomet has a short action span, never more than 6 hours and occasionally as low as 3 hours; consequently, it should be given three times daily always added to a basic diuretic background. Start with 250 mg t.i.d. After 3 to 4 days its full effect can be seen; if necessary increase to 500 mg t.i.d.

Undesirable side effects are orthostatic hypotension, drowsiness which is generally temporary, nausea and vomiting. All these effects occur rarely. The drug does alter the serum proteins and produces a positive Coomb's test in about 10 to 15 percent of patients but rarely does an anemia occur.

Methyldopa (Aldomet). Dose: 250 mg t.i.d. adjusted at 3 to 7 day intervals. Dispensed only in 250 mg tablets.

Some reserpine preparations in common use:

Reserpine (Serpasil). Dose: 0.25 to 0.5 mg daily. Dispensed in 0.1, 0.25, 1.0 and 2.0 mg tablets. Doses as high as 1.0 mg should only be used initially.

Reserpine (Eskaserp). Dose: Usually one 0.25 mg spansule b.i.d. to start and 1 daily for maintenance. Dispensed in 0.25 and 0.5 mg spansules.

Syrosingopine (Singoserp) (an altered reserpine which is claimed to be as antihypertensive as reserpine but with less of its undesirable properties). Dose: 1 to 3 tablets daily; maintenance, ½ to 3 tablets daily. Dispensed only in 1.0 mg tablets.

If combinations of the above drugs do not result in effective regulation of the blood pressure, try guanethidine as the next level of treatment. Guanethidine is a sympathetic blocking agent and causes long and irreversible blockage of sympathetic discharges at the nerve endings. Consequently accept postural hypotension with orthostasis as part of the treatment.

Guanethidine sulfate (Ismelin). Dose: 10 mg for 5 to 7 days, 20 mg for 5 to 7 days, 30 to 37.5 mg for 5 to 7 days, 50 mg for 5 to 7 days, and then 62.5 to 75 mg daily as necessary for ambulatory patients. Hospitalized patients may receive more rapid treatment. Adjust the dose upward as needed until the standing morning blood pressure is as low as can be tolerated by the patient because of dizziness and syncope on arising. The average maintenance dose is between 37.5 and 50 mg daily. The tablets are dispensed in 10 and 25 mg tablets. (Study the drug pharmacology before prescribing.) As the drug becomes active, reduce the Aldomet; continue the basic diuretic therapy.

Other drugs occasionally used but which have no advantages over the ones suggested and may be less effective or more dangerous are: Apresoline (hydralazine), Eutonyl (pargyline) Protalba or Veralba (protoveratrine), Unitensen (cryptenamine), Ansolysen (pentolinium) and Priscoline (tolazoline).

What about the elderly with a systolic hypertension and a high pulse pressure? Consider this patient as having an arteriosclerotic hypertension. Do not treat unless the patient is symptomatic, i.e. having dizziness, occipital headaches, epistaxis. Often only a diuretic is necessary. Remember antihypertensive drugs may have a heavy impact on the elderly.

In patients with a dissecting aneurysm of the aorta, treat energetically. Statistics show that medical treatment that lowers the blood pressure is more effective than the surgical approach. Parenteral reserpine, guanethidine and large doses of diuretics are often necessary to lower the blood pressure.

A word of caution regarding the patient with hypertension and renal failure (azotemia): lowering the blood pressure always reduces the glomerular filtration rate and raises the blood urea. Proceed with lowering the pressure but slowly and with caution. Monitor the blood urea and serum creatinine. Allow some rise in these products as long as you do not precipitate a uremia and as long as urinary excretion remains more than 750 ml per day. Consider using one of the slower acting antihypertensive drugs.

Arfonad (trimethaphan camphorsulfonate). A ganglionic blocker and peripheral vasodilator. Try a controlled infusion accompanied by constant monitoring of the urinary output. Arfonad is dispensed in 10 ml vials of 50 mg per ml. Administer in 0.1 percent concentration in 5 percent dextrose. Start the infusion at a rate of 60 drops (3 to 4 mg) per minute and then adjust to desired level.

Management of the Hypertensive Crisis

If there is need to reduce the blood pressure within an hour a hypertensive emergency is said to exist; if reduction can be delayed 24 hours treatment is spoken of as being urgent.

Hypertensive crises that require parenteral administration of antihypertensive drugs are:

- hypertensive encephalopathy
- acute pulmonary edema
- dissecting aneurysm
- hemorrhagic cerebrovascular accident
- head injury
- some cases of pheochromocytoma
- eclampsia
- when hypertensive drugs cannot be given orally as in the unconscious or postoperative patient
- when hypertension is accompanied by acute left ventricular failure, aneurysm, intracranial hemorrhage or severe epistaxis

Consider the following as *urgent* reasons for reducing the blood pressure:

- the resting diastolic blood pressure is 130 mg Hg or more

–heart failure without pulmonary edema
–grade III or IV retinopathy
–preeclampsia

Useful drugs

Reserpine is the agent most commonly used because it is convenient for intramuscular injection, rarely causes hypotension, it is not orthostatic and its reaction in emergency lowering of blood pressure is slow enough not to be dangerous. A delay of 2 to 3 hours between injection and maximal effect may be considered a disadvantage. Reserpine may cause a profound sleep bordering on coma. Because of its delayed action and the doctor's anxiety to reduce the blood pressure in an emergency, the frequent doses may cause hypotension.

Serpasil can be given in a dose of 1.0 to 2.5 mg IM. Dispensed in 2.0 and 10 ml with 2.5 mg per ml. Give every 4 hours as needed.

Hydralazine is especially effective in managing a hypertensive encephalopathy. Reduction in pressure usually occurs within 30 minutes when given intramuscularly and within two minutes when given intravenously. Do not give when the hypertension is associated with acute coronary insufficiency or left ventricular failure.

Ansolysen (pentolinium tartrate). Dispensed in 10 ml with 10 mg per ml. Dose: 2.5 to 3.5 mg IM. It is a ganglion blocking agent. Marked hypotensive effect within 30 to 60 minutes. May also be given IV by titration from a syringe for prompt hypotensive effect. Continuous IV infusion may be used for a smooth and precise control of blood pressure. In heart failure, Ansolysen may reduce blood pressure. When administering, monitor the blood pressure frequently.

Arfonad, (trimethapan camphorsulfonate) (see previous explanation of its use).

All antihypertensive drugs listed are enhanced by the simultaneous administration of a diuretic. The diuretic of choice is Lasix (fursemide) because it can be given IV. It is rapidly effective and does not cause an acute decrease in glomerular filtration rate. The usual dose for this purpose is 40 to 120 mg.

Two drugs, diazoxide and sodium nitroprusside, will probably replace the presently recommended drugs when released for commercial use.

Diazoxide acts as a direct vasodilator without depressing cardiac output or renal blood flow—one 300 mg vial given in a single IV dose takes effect within 5 minutes and lasts for 2 hours.

Diazoxide is a rapid-acting vasodilator drug that is effective in the management of hypertensive emergencies. Before treatment, hospitalize the patient and continue hospitalization until the hypertension is controlled by orally effective drugs.

Preparation: Hyperstat IV in 20 ml containers supplying 15 mg/ml. In adults, inject 300 mg (5 mg/kg of body weight) within 30 seconds for maximal response. Repeat at intervals of 30 minutes to 24 hours as needed.

The major adverse reactions are sodium and water retention plus hyperglycemia. To prevent fluid overload, administer IV fursemide 30 to 60 minutes before each injection of Hyperstat. Begin more permanent oral antihypertensive agents at any time.[14]

Sodium nitroprusside (a vasodilator) made by dissolving 60 mg sodium nitroprusside in 25 ml of 0.9 percent sterile sodium chloride solution and refrigerated in sealed and dated brown bottles is stable for 1 month. Immediately before use, add two bottles to 500 ml of 5 percent dextrose in distilled water. Give IV continuously. It takes effect within 2 minutes and lasts for the duration of the infusion.

Don't use

–reserpine or methyldopa in hypertensive encephalopathy
–Ansolysen or Arfonad in eclampsia or preeclampsia (Apresoline is the drug of choice.)
–reserpine or Aldomet in head injuries (Ansolysen and Arfonad are the drugs of choice.)
–Apresoline in myocardial infarction or acute left ventricular failure (Use Ansolysen and Arfonad.)
–reserpine or Aldomet during intracranial hemorrhage (Others may be used without danger.)

Do

- –determine blood urea nitrogen and creatinine (If BUN is more than 50 mg per 100 ml repeat daily.)
- –monitor blood pressure at minute intervals until pressure stabilizes.
- –prepare one L of 5 percent dextrose in distilled water containing 1 ampule of levarterenol. (Keep at patient's bedside in event of excessive drop in pressure.)
- –stop antihypertensive treatment when the blood pressure drops halfway from starting blood pressure to 150/90 (This should relieve complications.)
- –discontinue parenteral therapy and start oral therapy as soon as possible

THE CARDIOMYOPATHIES

Thirty years ago young physicians were warned to avoid the diagnosis of myocarditis. At the time there were those who questioned whether the condition existed even when it appeared most logical. Now primary myocardial disease is known to exist, both in an inflammatory and a noninflammatory nature. Consequently whenever a disease process attacks the heart muscle and spares the surrounding structures (valves, pericardium and coronary vessels) it is now appropriate to speak of the process as a *primary myocardial disease* or a *cardiomyopathy*.

In 1970 Mattingly[15] proposed a classification of the cardiomyopathies. His classification was based on etiology and included inflammatory causes as well as metabolic, infiltrative, neuromuscular and idiopathic causes (Table 10-3). Study his classification and be on the alert for cardiomyopathies in your practice. Perhaps some of the patients who you are now treating as arteriosclerotic heart disease cases can be reclassified as a cardiomyopathy. Look for them among your patients who present as AHD except for the expected angina.

About 360 L of blood per day are diverted through the coronary arteries of an average sedentary man. This allows for large contact with the heart of any infections, bacteria, toxins, drugs and other products of metabolism. Several pathologic types are known to exist.

The *hypertrophic* variety is one in which a left or biventricular hypertrophy occurs causing little or no symptoms for years. The *obstructive* variety is basically an extension of the hypertrophic. Classification for the obstructive type depends on the above findings plus a hypertrophic septum that obstructs left and also right ventricular outflow. The *congestive* variety is recognized by large biventricular dilatation. A

Table 10-3. Classification of Causes of Cardiomyopathies

Inflammatory	*Metabolic*	*Infiltrative*
Bacterial Viral Parastic Nonspecific Hypersensitivity Brucellosis	Thyrotoxicosis Nutritional Hormonal Electrolytic Thiamine deficiency	Amyloidosis Glycogen storage disease Hemochromatosis Neoplastic disease

Neuromuscular	*Idiopathic*
Muscular dystrophies Friedreich's ataxia	Idiopathic hypertrophy Idiopathic hypertrophic subaortic stenosis Familial cardiomyopathy Alcoholic cardiomyopathy Endomyocardial fibrosis Postpartum cardiomyopathy

good example is the thinning and stretching of the cardiac walls following amyloid deposits.

Findings and symptoms are not diagnostic but are generally recognizable: Cardiomyopathies are more common in men. They occur with occasional palpitation, dizziness or syncope and there is evidence of heart failure as the disease progresses. Look for ECG changes such as QRS, ST segments and T wave changes. Arrhythmias are common.

Treatment should be the standard care of all failing hearts—diuretics, digitalis and dietary salt and sodium restrictions. One word of caution: digitalis toxicity is more likely to occur. Consequently prescribe the shorter-acting glycosides. While digitalizing, monitor the heart by ECG tracings.

If you study the list of causes, some are seen to be remedial. Be prompt with specific treatment for any systemic disease; the damaged heart may recover entirely. Order bed rest. It appears to be more helpful than in other forms of heart disease.

HEART FAILURE

Symptoms of Heart Failure

The symptoms of heart failure are itemized by standard textbooks as follows:

- –acute shortness of breath
- –orthopnea
- –persistent hacking cough
- –frothy sputum
- –blood-stained sputum
- –cyanosis
- –possible chest pain even without myocardial infarction
- –skin cool, moist and blanched even without shock

A layman can diagnose a heart attack from those symptoms. Where you should be of help is in preventing such a disaster by recognizing subtle signs of failure in the patient who walks into your office. It's true, many attacks appear to come on suddenly without prodromal symptoms, but more often than not there will have been signs and symptoms that a sharp-eyed family physician could have recognized.

Respiratory Signs

The respiratory tract often presents the first signs of failure. After all, many clinicians look upon pulmonary edema as a complication of pulmonary hypertension plus a lymphatic inadequacy. The cause of the pulmonary hypertension is a weak or failing left ventricle. The pulmonary hypertension is probably the fundamental cause of death when one excludes a dangerous arrhythmia.

Coughing may be the predominant first feature of left-sided heart failure. Be suspicious if the cough is nocturnal or if it is induced by exertion. Examinations in the office are often conducted with the patient sitting up. Have the patient lie down in order not to miss an important clue. The cough of pulmonary edema may suddenly start when the patient lies back. In the hospital when the patient is in bed have him turn over to the opposite side. Or if the head of the bed is elevated flatten out the bed. These changes in position may be all that is needed to start a hacking cough —an early symptom that you could well miss if not on the alert. Consider the elderly patient who tells you he has bronchitis or a cigarette cough as potentially early failure cases.

And while you are changing the patient's position, listen for moving rales. Rales in the right base may be made to appear in the left base by simply turning the patient. These moving rales are characteristic of heart failure.

Another neglected respiratory symptom often spoken of by the patient but disregarded by the physician is trepopnea. Investigate the patient who tells you he can sleep in one position but not another because of shortness of breath. Trepopnea is probably a result of greater pulmonary engorgement on one side than on the other. In this regard, the left side appears to cause more trouble than the right. The respiratory distress usually starts within 10 seconds to 2 minutes after rolling into the position. Be alert for an increase in respiratory symptoms when you roll the patient over to check his right lung base or to palpate for sacral edema.

And, finally, when was the last time you paid much attention to a wife who told you her husband was holding his breath at night? This classic type of breathing, Cheyne-Stokes, occurs frequently in the elderly with mild failure. It is described as a period of apnea lasting from 10 to 30 seconds followed by a period of hyperpnea lasting 1 to 3 minutes.

Venous Signs

Turning now from the respiratory system to the venous signs, the family physician encounters an entirely different constellation of findings. First examine the patient while sitting up in a chair. Inspect the veins on the undersurface of the tongue. In this position the sublingual veins are normally collapsed. If they are bulging, the venous pressure is 20 cm or more.

With the patient still sitting perform the Gärtner maneuver. Ask the patient to allow his arms and hands to dangle until the veins are distended with blood. When this is done ask him to slowly raise one hand until the veins flatten and disappear. Now measure the difference in cm between the level of the hand and the right atrium. This is a pretty fair estimate of the venous pressure providing there is no venous constriction in the axilla.

Now have the patient recline on the examining table with his head and thorax elevated 45° from horizontal. The Lewis procedure (Fig. 10-19) consists of measuring the vertical height of the cervical venous pulses above the manubrium sterni. Normally they should ascend no more than 1 or 2 cm above this point. In high venous pressures the veins may be distended to the angle of the jaw representing a venous pressure of 25 cm or more. Some clinicians measure the vertical distance above the manubrium in mm to the top of the column of blood in the external jugular vein as the elevation of the venous pressure above normal.

If the left jugular vein only is distended (more likely in the elderly) Sabathie sign is positive. The finding is produced by kinking of the left innominate vein as it passes in front of a dilated aortic arch associated with hypertension or atherosclerosis.

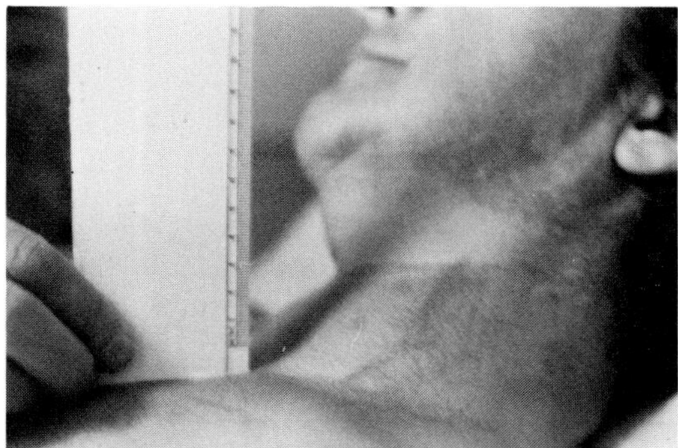

Figure 10-19. Lewis procedure. The venous pulses should not ascend more than 1 to 2 cm above the level of the manubrium sterni. If the veins are distended to the angle of the jaw the venous pressure is usually 25 cm of water or higher.

While the patient is in the 45° degree position, check his hepatojugular reflux (Fig. 10-20). The mechanism of this reflux is not fully understood but an overload on the right ventricle is produced by applying pressure over the abdomen. This overload exceeds the capacity of the already malfunctioning ventricle to handle the increased load without causing an increase in the venous pressure. Before beginning the test ask the patient to continue breathing normally. Breath holding produces a Valsalva effect, the most frequent cause of false

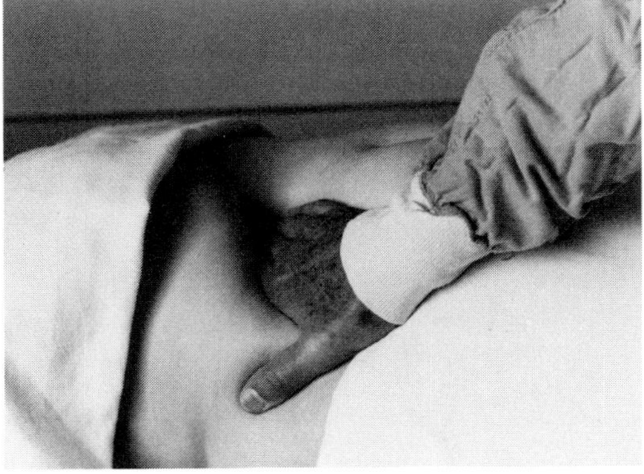

Figure 10-20. Hepatojugular reflex. Place the palm of your hand over the RUQ and apply firm nonpainful pressure for 30 to 60 sec. A positive response for right ventricular failure is indicated by increased distention or pulsation of the neck veins.

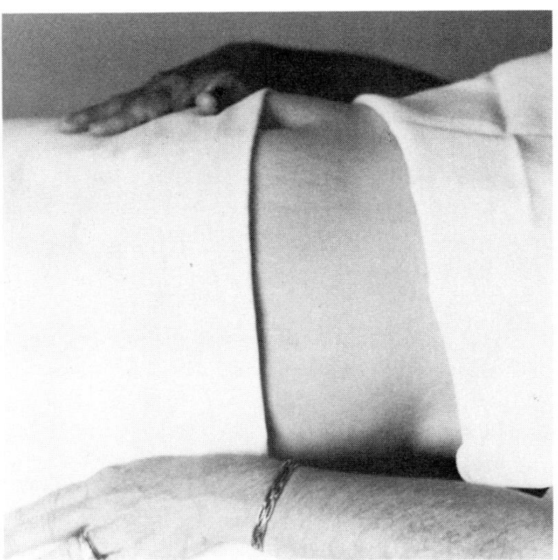

Figure 10-21. Von Recklinghausen maneuver for estimation of venous pressure.

positive findings. Now place the palm of your hand over the patient's right upper quadrant. Exert pressure, preferably up under the ribs toward the liver for 30 to 60 seconds. The test is positive and indicates right ventricle failure if the cervical veins distend or pulsate.

Now put the patient's head down into position on a flat firm surface for the von Recklinghausen check of venous pressure (Fig. 10-21). Ask the patient to place one hand on his thigh and the other on the examination table. Normal venous pressure is indicated when veins on the thigh hand are collapsed and the veins on the table are distended. If the dorsal veins of both hands are distended the venous pressure is elevated; if the veins are all collapsed the pressure is abnormally low.

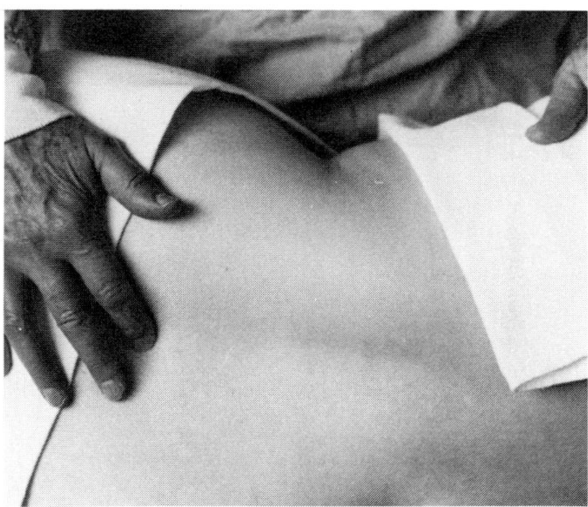

Figure 10-22. Check for sacral and posterior thigh edema in heart patients who are in bed. These areas are often edematous when the legs and feet are nonedematous.

Before leaving the subject of veins, and to be complete, the presence or absence of edema should be determined. Most physicians inspect the patient's ankles for edema but many forget to palpate the sacrum and the posterior thighs for edema in the bed patient (Fig. 10-22). Do so. You may find edema at those points when the feet and ankles are edema free.

Arterial Signs

Of the arterial signs of cardiac decompensation most frequently overlooked is pulsus alternans. The easiest way to identify pulsus alternans is by a careful systolic blood pressure determination. You will miss it if you take the blood pressure hurriedly. What is required is a very slow deflation of the cuff. If, as you take the systolic pressure, only alternate beats are heard for a distance of 2 to 10 mm of Hg or more, the patient has pulsus alternans. (Do not confuse this mechanical pulsus alternans with ECG alternans.) Pulsus alternans can be determined by palpating the radial pulse, but it is not easy. Stick by the blood pressure method. The conditions with which it is most frequently associated are hypertensive heart disease, aortic stenosis and ischemic heart disease. When pulsus alternans is present listen carefully at the cardiac apex for a third heart sound gallop. Both help to establish left ventricular failure.

In my experience the Valsalva maneuver has limited usefulness. First of all you must be careful which patients you select to perform the test. Elderly patients with coronary or cerebral disease should not be asked to exert enough to do the test properly. In addition, it cannot be performed on the dyspneic or unalert patient. It does not pick up early cases of failure. When it once becomes positive, other signs and symptoms are more significant.

Valsalva maneuver is done in different ways, some rather complicated. Forget all the details and do it like most clinicians do. Ask the patient to take a deep breath and push down as if moving his bowels. Have him strain in this fashion for 10 seconds. Then monitor his pulse for a few seconds for bradycardia. If no bradycardia occurs the patient is suspected of having failure.

Cardiac Signs

Three cardiac signs are most important in diagnosing early failure: tachycardia at rest or an undue increase in rate on exercise; a loud pulmonic closure sound; and the identification of the third heart sound (ventricular gallop; protodiastolic gallop).

A failing left ventricle causes pulmonary hypertension which, in turn, causes a violent closure of the pulmonary valve. The sound may become louder than its aortic component even when systemic hypertension is present. It is an easy sign to identify and dependable in predicting left-sided heart failure.

Probably the hallmark of failure is the identification of the third heart sound gallop. At times it is easily palpated and heard. On other occasions, try as you may, it will elude you. The pathologic third sound may diminish or disappear when the patient stands or is propped up in bed. Have the patient lie flat or even raise his legs. Occasionally the triple rhythm can be felt as well as heard. Auscult with a bell stethoscope placed lightly on the cardiac apex. Have the patient hold his breath while lying in the left lateral position. It is diastolic in time, low in pitch and galloping in rhythm.

Unfortunately, watchful observation for all these signs, even by the sophisticated physician, may not be enough. Pulmonary edema may appear without the slightest warning. All the equipment we now use including that for central venous pressure monitoring may warn you too late to start preventive measures.

Pomerantz[16] reports a discovery that may alter this dangerous situation. The technique is based on the hypothesis that changes in lung fluid volume, however slight, should change the electric impedence of the lungs, thereby providing an accurate indicator of developing pulmonary edema.

Pomerantz suggests that high risk patients be monitored during times of critical illness. According to the reports, when a patient is being continually monitored, changes will be observed 45 minutes before ordinary methods detect the same. For needed equipment and suggested technique study Dr. Marvin Pomerantz's original article in *Annals of Surgery* 171:5 1971.

X-Ray Evidence of Congestive Failure

Findings on an ordinary x-ray film of the chest may vary depending on the cause of the heart failure. X-ray signs of heart failure are indirect signs only but can be helpful if interpreted properly. The following signs are not too much for a family physician to learn to recognize:

–cardiomegaly (Figs. 10-23 and 10-24)
–prominence of the pulmonary veins for pulmonary hypertension (Remember this sign becomes observable whenever the pulmonary pressure exceeds 16 mm of Hg.)

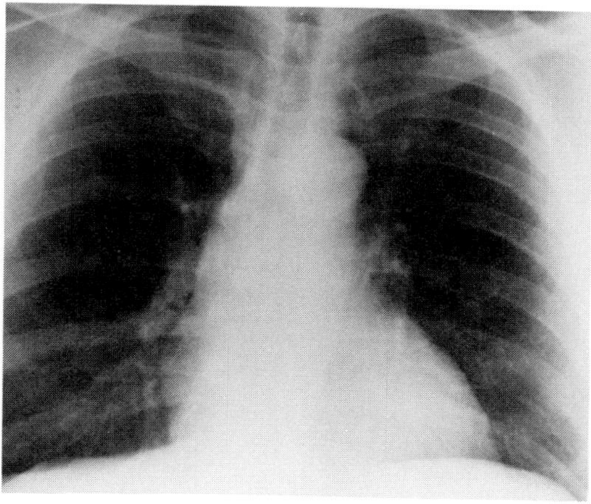

Figure 10-23. Slightly enlarged heart.

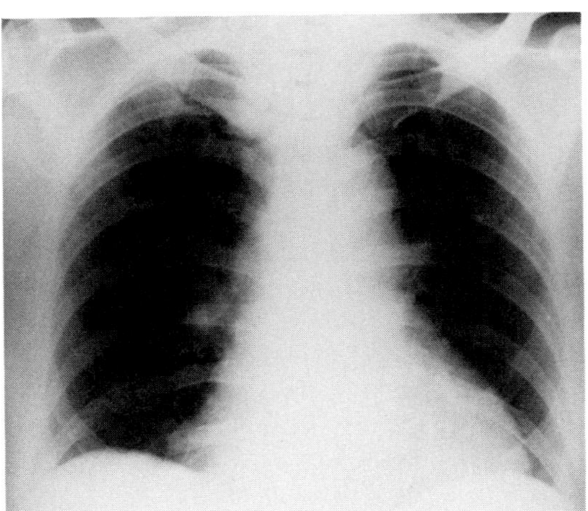

Figure 10-24. Cardiomegaly associated with cardiac decompensation.

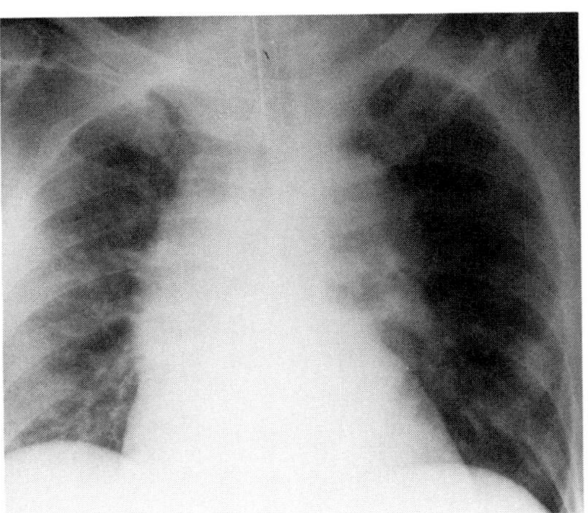

Figure 10-25. Aortic aneurysm with cardiomegaly.

–prominence of the aorta and pulmonary artery (Fig. 10-25)
–prominence of the superior vena cava and azygos vein
–mitral disease (Fig 10-26)
–accumulation of pulmonary fluid either as effusions (Fig. 10-27) or interstitial and alveolar edema (Fig. 10-28)

Pulmonary edema may be unilateral, bilateral or appear as the spectacular "bat wing" variety. If your eyes are sharp, Kerley A and B lines can be seen.

Emergency Treatment of Acute Heart Failure (Pulmonary Edema)

General Measures

Sit the patient up to reduce right ventricular filling. This is simple and effective. If you don't advise it, the patient will usually assume the position on his own accord.

Administer morphine sulfate intravenously or subcutaneously in small doses, grain

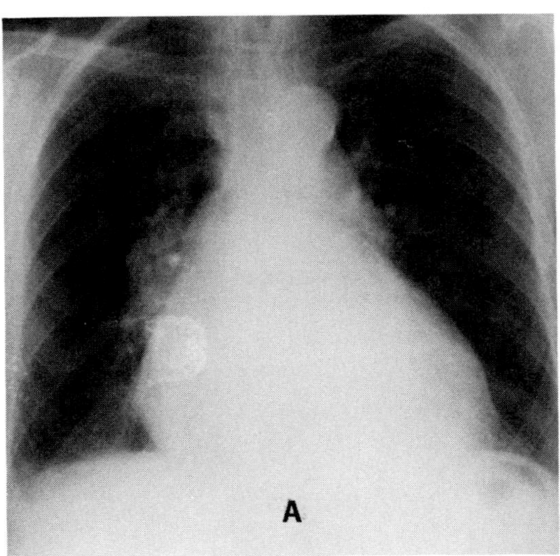

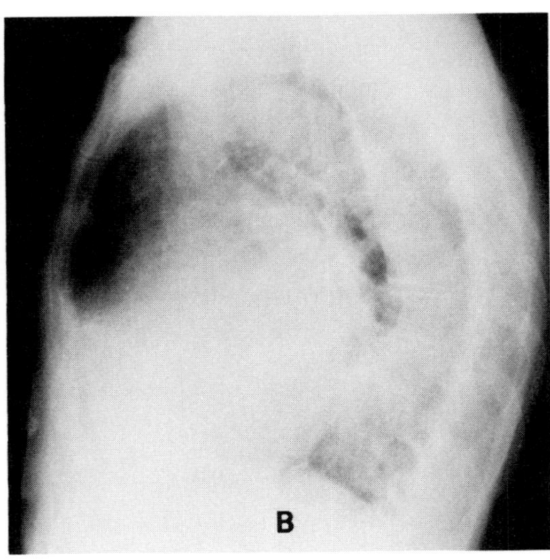

Figure 10-26. *A*, Anteroposterior and, *B*, lateral view of enlarged right atrium with mitral disease probably combining stenosis and insufficiency.

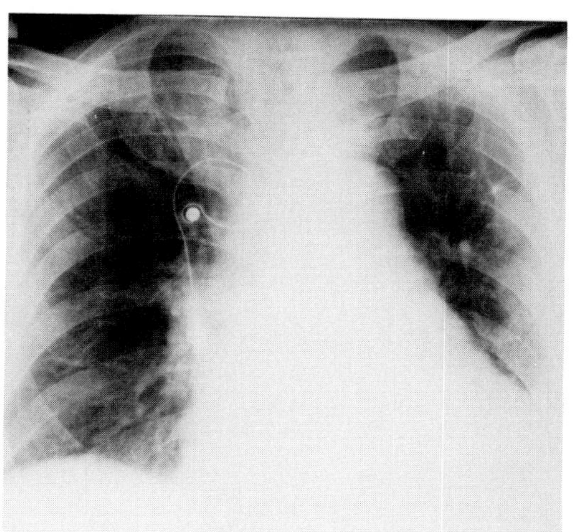

Figure 10-27. Congestive heart failure with effusion and venous hypertension.

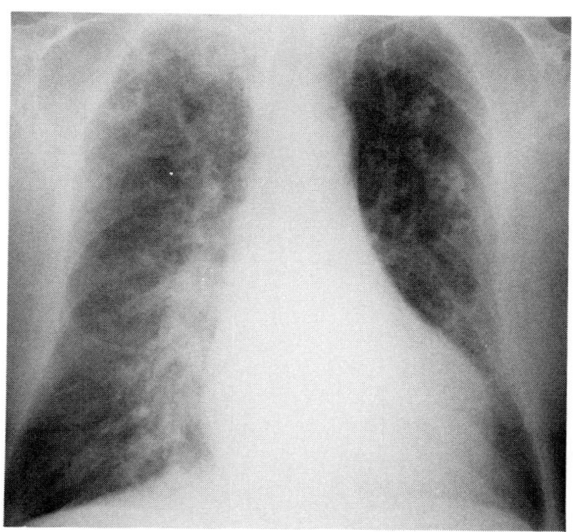

Figure 10-28. Congestive heart failure with enlarged heart and pulmonary edema.

1/6 or less, just enough to allay restlessness.

Give oxygen, 2 to 4 L is sufficient.

Specific Measures

Foremost among the specific measures is the administration of a digitalis preparation as an inotropic agent and, when necessary, to control an arrhythmia. Be careful when the pulmonary edema is a result of myocardial infarction. Give smaller doses than usual. In addition, digitalis is more likely to precipitate a serious arrhythmia when serum potassium is low.

Give a diuretic parenterally-ethacrynic acid, furosemide or even a mercurial. If given at the same time as digitalis, watch for a low serum potassium level and the resultant ectopic rhythms.

Consider venesection of at least 250 to 500 ml of whole blood. For a quick relief of volume load on the left ventricle, place tourniquets on the extremities and rotate every 15 to 20 minutes.

If the pulmonary edema is the result of an arrhythmia, give the appropriate antiarrhythmic drug or use the electroconverter to restore normal sinus rhythm.

If the congestive failure is the result of an acute hypertensive crisis, give antihypertensive drugs.

If pulmonary edema is precipitated by pleural effusion, removing large quantities of blood or other fluids from the pleural cavity may give dramatic relief.

Digitalis

HOW TO PRESCRIBE DIGITALIS. Do not depend on orally administered digitalis when the patient has pulmonary edema. Something quicker acting is necessary. Give deslanoside (Cedilanid-D). Adjust the dose to no more than 0.4 mg every 1 or 2 hours for a total dose of 1.2 mg in the undigitalized patient. A precaution: the full effect of any one dose may not become apparent for up to 4 hours.

In critical cases such as is the case in patients with a rapid ventricular rate with atrial fibrillation or flutter, give 0.4 mg Cedilanid-D every 30 minutes intravenously to a total dose of 1.2 mg. Any decision to give larger doses or additional doses must rest on an inadequate response coupled with negative ECG evidence of intoxication. Remember intoxication sometimes comes from the rate of administration rather than total dosage.

Maintenance dose, once you've obtained maximum benefit, is usually $^1/_{10}$ the digitalizing dose. There is no exact formula to use in switching from Cedilanid-D to a longer-acting digitalis such as digoxin (Lanoxin). Generally you can begin substituting Lanoxin 0.25 or 0.5 mg daily.

The old idea that effective therapy requires a *full* digitalization no longer holds. In fact this idea can cause unnecessary intoxication and even death.

In less critical patients and in those with acute myocardial infarction a slower method of administration is appropriate: give 0.25 mg of oral Lanoxin every 4 to 6 hours to a total of 1.5 mg. Then give a maintenance dose of 0.25 mg daily.

In patients with ventricular premature systoles, give smaller doses plus potassium. If rhythm cannot be controlled with short-acting Lanoxin, switch to long-acting digitoxin 0.1 mg t.i.d. for 4 days. Rapid digitalization with digitoxin requires the administration of 0.6 mg orally. Wait 5 to 6 hours. If no evidence of toxicity appears, give 0.3 mg every 6 hours to a total of 1.2 mg.

Try the following schedule for the patient who is taking Lanoxin but in inadequate amounts: give 0.25 to 0.5 mg of oral Lanoxin 2 to 3 times daily for 1 to 2 days, followed by a maintenance dose of 0.25 mg. Remember the addition of a diuretic may preclude the administration of digitalis or the giving of additional digitalis.

Some don'ts.

- –Don't give digitalis if you plan to eventually use precordial shock.
- –Don't use digitalis for pure mitral stenosis unless it is given for an arrhythmia.
- –Don't give when patient appears to be developing a ventricular arrhythmia.
- –Don't give digitalis when the patient has paired ventricular premature beats, ventricular tachycardia, or in second degree, SA or high grade AV blocks.
- –Be careful about giving digitalis when blocks are present.

Use low dosage digitalis in patients with hypothyroidism, liver disease, acute inflammatory cardiac disease, primary myocardial disease or in alcoholic cardiomyopathy. As a rough rule in renal disease reduce Lanoxin dosage to 25 or 40 percent of the usual amounts. Digoxin preparations are eliminated by the kidneys. On the other hand, digitoxin is metabolized in the liver and, therefore, only needs to be reduced about seven percent in renal disease.

The oral administration of digoxin probably is adequate for most patients who require rapid digitalization since the drug rapidly appears in the blood. Furthermore, the timing of maintenance dosage in relation to meals is not important as the presence of food in the stomach does not influence the degree of absorption of the drug.

The elderly may reach maximum effectiveness by giving 0.25 mg of Lanoxin t.i.d., a total of 0.75 mg, on the first day and then going on with a maintenance dose of 0.25 mg the following day.

Considering the renal excretion rate in a patient with normal functioning kidneys, a patient may take 0.25 mg Lanoxin daily for 10 days and have remaining in his body on the tenth day 0.50 mg.

Remember the prime determinant of the rate of renal excretion of digoxin is the glomerular filtration rate (GFR). The GFR is measured clinically by the creatinine clearance. Neither the serum creatinine nor the BUN clearly reflect the GFR in the elderly. Therefore there is a sound basis for substantially reducing the daily maintenance dose in the elderly, even if the BUN and the serum creatinine levels are normal.

The other factor affecting digitalis dosage is body weight. Studies show that the same intravenous dose of digoxin produced blood concentrations that were twice as high in the elderly as in the younger patients.

LONG-TERM DIGOXIN THERAPY. Review from time to time every elderly patient on long-term digoxin therapy to determine the patient's need to continue such therapy. The principle that if once prescribed the need persists indefinitely is no longer valid.

If the need for digitalis was not definitely mandatory when first prescribed and if the patient continues without evidence of failure or an arrhythmia give the patient a trial period without the drug. One study found that of 22 elderly patients, 17 remained free of congestive heart failure. Digoxin therapy was reinstituted in two patients when borderline signs of failure recurred. Consequently you may find that long-term digoxin therapy is common but often unnecessary.

MANAGEMENT OF DIGITALIS INTOXICATION. Don't get excited if your patient shows digitalis intoxication. Most patients can recover from the effects of mild digitalis toxicity if the drug is withheld for several days. Signs of toxicity might include first degree atrioventricular block, sinus bradycardia and PVC's.

More serious cardiac arrhythmias may require some additional medication. Potassium will help if the patient has developed atrialtachyarrhythmia or ventricular arrhythmia. Monitor continuously by ECG if giving the potassium IV. Do not use in renal failure or in second degree or complete AV block. Propranolol is drug of choice if serum potassium level is normal. Lidocaine is usually effective in quieting digitalis induced arrhythmias. Most patients respond to IV administration of Dilantin within 3 seconds to 5 minutes. Effects last 5 minutes to 4 to 6 hours. Dilantin is probably the most effective and safest of drugs for this purpose. Pronestyl or quinidine may be used when above agents are contraindicated.

Prevention of Acute Pulmonary Edema

Successful prevention of pulmonary edema depends in good measure on the cause. Some causes are remediable, and an observant family doctor can spot and correct them before failure is obvious. Other causes are not remediable; in these cases, good supportive treatment will postpone the unhappy day.

First search for the remediable extracardiac factors:

–hypertension and conditions that cause it
–digitalis toxicity
–hypokalemia from too heavy diuretic therapy
–hyponatremia
–overlooked chronic pulmonary disease with cor pulmonale
–arteriovenous fistula
–beri-beri heart disease in alcoholic patients who may respond to thiamine
–hyperthyroidism, anemia and obesity.

If there is hypokalemia from too heavy diuretic therapy attempt to get along on about half the maximum effective dosages, i.e. hydrochlorothiazide 50 mg b.i.d.; furosemide 40 mg t.i.d.; ethacrynic acid 50 mg b.i.d.; quinethazone 100 mg daily; and chlorthalidone 100 mg daily. Larger doses of diuretics should be given with potassium chloride supplements, up to 200 mEq daily.

Hyponatremia responds to fluid restriction. Limit the patient to 600 to 800 ml per day.

Next search for the remediable cardiac factors:

–atrial septal defects and patent ductus arteriosus
–acquired valvular lesions that can be corrected surgically
–cardiac tumors, ventricular aneurysms and constrictive pericarditis
–cardiac infections

Atrial septal defects and patent ductus arteriosus are two of the most common congenital heart lesions found in adults. Acquired valvular lesions that can be corrected surgically should also receive penicillin prophylactically. Both aortic and mitral valve damage can be corrected. Cardiac tumors, ventricular aneurysms and constrictive pericarditis are surgically correctable. Cardiac infections include tuberculosis of the pericardium, acute myocarditis from childhood diseases and acute and subacute bacterial endocarditis.

Watch for and avoid precipitating factors in patients with known cardiac problems:

–silent myocardial infarctions
–fever
–hyperthyroidism
–acute pulmonary disease
–loss of diuretic responsiveness
–administration of steroids and phenylbutazone with their salt and water retention properties

–administration of beta adrenergic blockers, most commonly propanolol
–development of arrhythmias correctable with proper remedies

Arteriosclerotic coronary artery disease is the most common cause of cardiac failure. If a patient in failure has no hypertension or murmurs, the most likely diagnosis is arteriosclerotic heart disease.

Managing Potassium Imbalance

In a man weighing 60 kg, the total extracellular potassium content is about 48 mEq/l; the intracellular potassium content is about 3,600 mEq. In terms of total body potassium, more than 98 percent occurs intracellularly averaging about 150 to 160 mEq/l while 1.5 to 2.0 percent occurs extracellularly or 4 mEq/l. Thus the ratio of intracellular to extracellular potassium is about 40 to 1.

And yet when we sample the body's potassium, we do so on the plasma and believe we have a true picture of the patient's potassium balance. But a low, normal or high plasma potassium does not always reflect the total body potassium. A small percentage of the intracellular potassium could leave the cells undetected but cause a tremendous extracellular build-up if the potassium remained there. Normally, dangerous extracellular build-up is prevented by renal excretion.

Fortunately, however, it is the changes in the extracellular or plasma potassium that we are most interested in and which cause most abnormalities.

Most potassium leaves the plasma via the kidneys, specifically the glomerulus. The glomerulus freely filters out potassium at the rate of 720 mEq/24 hours. The proximal renal tubules reabsorb most of this. Consequently, the amount of potassium that appears in the urine is dependent on distal tubule secretion. In acidosis, when an excess of hydrogen ion exists, potassium ion secretion is inhibited, while, in alkalosis, when hydrogen ion is diminished, potassium is secreted into the urine.

Normally the concentration of potassium in the extracellular fluid is kept constant, a condition essential to normal neuromuscular activity.

When the concentration of potassium outside the cell wall decreases (or the concentration within the cell wall increases), a muscular paralysis occurs proportionate to the change.

When the concentration of potassium outside the cell wall increases, initiation and propagation of stimuli are deranged. The result is cardiac muscle atony and arrhythmias plus skeletal muscle weakness.

Hypokalemia is said to exist when the plasma concentration falls to 3.8 mEq/l, althrough symptoms resulting from hypokalemia do not occur until the concentration falls to 2.7 mEq/l or below. Symptoms are muscular fatigue and hypotonicity. When potassium plasma concentrations fall below 2.0 mEq/l paralysis may develop. Weakness or paralysis of the respiratory muscles may cause death.

Arrhythmias include premature atrial contractions, premature nodal contractions, premature ventricular contractions, supraventricular tachycardias and ventricular tachycardia.

When potassium levels fall below 2.7 mEq/l, diagnostic electrocardiographic changes occur. These include widening, flattening or inversion of the T wave; pro-longed Q-T interval; and prominent U waves occur.

Treatment

Hypokalemia most commonly results from vomiting or the therapeutic administration of diuretics. In this event replacement calls for potassium chloride. Usually a nasty 10 percent elixir of potassium chloride is prescribed sufficient to prevent losses as determined by periodic evaluation of plasma potassium levels. Each 15 ml dose should contain 20 mEq of potassium chloride. Do not use the enteric coated.

In a patient who tends to develop hypokalemia, foodstuffs cannot be depended upon for prevention because of their low potassium content (orange juice 10 mEq/200 ml; bananas 10 mEq/100 g).

The use of potassium-sparing diuretics may be helpful when indicated otherwise.

Dyrenium (triamterene) 100 mg. Dose: 1 capsule b.i.d. after meals to start, then adjust to needs. Maintenance dose is usually 1 capsule daily or even 1 every other day. May be used with other diuretics. Do not use potassium supplements or potassium rich diets with triamterene. Periodic checks are needed on plasma potassium, BUN, CBC and liver function. Often used with a thiazide diuretic as in Diazide, 25 mg hydrochlorothizide and 50 mg triamterene. Dose: one tablet b.i.d., then adjust.

Aldactone (spironolactone) 25 mg. Dose: 50 to 100 mg daily. For edema, start with 100 mg daily in divided doses. Basically, observe the same precautions as when using Dyrenium. Often recommended for use in conjunction with a mercurial or thiazide diuretic as in Aldactazide tablets. 25 mg hydrochlorothiazide and 25 mg spironolactone. Dose: 1 to 8 tablets per day.

In a hypokalemic emergency when intravenous therapy is called for calculate the total 24 hour dose by the following formula:

Patient's weight in kilograms $\times$ 3 mEq = maximum safe dose in 24 hr.

In any event, the administration of 50 mEq per hour is dangerous and requires constant electrocardiographic monitoring.

If renal tubular acidosis exists, the potassium should be given in the form of potassium gluconate or citrate.

Some proprietary potassium supplements are:

K-Lyte (elemental potassium) supplies 25 mg. When an effervescent tablet is mixed with water, it becomes potassium citrate, bicarbonate and cyclamate. Dose: 1 tablet in 3 to 4 ounces of water. Expensive.

Potassium Triflex Liquid (elemental potassium) 15 mg. supplied by 500 mg each of potassium acetate, bicarbonate and citrate. Dose: 5 ml diluted, 3 to 4 times daily.

Kaon tablets and Elixir. 5 mEq and Elixir 6.6 mEq elemental potassium supplied by potassium gluconate. Dose: 2 tablets or 15 ml in 30 ml of water b.i.d.

K-Ciel Syrup. 6.6 mEq elemental potassium supplied by potassium chloride per 5 ml. Dose: 5 ml in half a glass water.

Foods high in potassium are: *Vegetables:* spinach, squash, potatoes and beans with skin; *Cereals:* all-bran, wheat germ and Boston brown bread; *Meats:* hamburger, beef sirloin and ham; *Fruits:* apricots, peaches, orange juice and bananas; *Fish:* salmon and halibut; *Miscellaneous:* molasses, sunflower seeds, peanuts, watermelon and cantaloupe.

Hyperkalemia

Hyperkalemia is said to exist when the potassium level exceeds 5mEq/l. Significant abnormalities begin appearing when the level exceeds 6.0 to 6.5 mEq/l. Hyperkalemia is often associated with acute renal failure, trauma to large areas of tissue, massive hemolytic attacks, postoperative states, prolonged febrile states, prolonged nutritional deficiences, sodium depletion states, Addison's disease and iatrogenic causes when potassium supplements have been prescribed and not monitored or in switching from one diuretic to a potassium sparing one.

Symptoms are vague: muscular weakness, cramping, occasional paralysis or convulsions. The most common danger is associated with cardiac arrhythmias.

Early electrocardiographic changes are prolonged P-R interval and narrow-based, tall, peaked or "tented" T waves. As the hyperkalemia increases the ECG changes become more complex. Changes noted are absence of P waves; widened, slurred biphasic QRS complexes; tall T waves; and serious ventricular tachyarrhythmias. Electrocardiograms are diagnostic. Start treatment on the basis of positive findings on the ECG. This finding may be more dependable than serum potassium levels.

Treatment

In an emergency do the following within the first few minutes: insert an intravenous, indwelling catheter, give a standard vial of calcium gluconate, give one standard ampule sodium bicarbonate (44 mEq) IV.

A standard vial of calcium gluconate (10 ml vial with 10 percent) has 1 g of calcium gluconate. Give up to one vial per minute for 3 to 4 minutes. This helps neutralize the effect of potassium but does not reduce the hyperkalemia. Discontinue the calcium gluconate if the rhythm reverts.

Now give one standard ampule sodium bicarbonate (44 mEq) IV. When that is finished give 1 ampule of 50 ml of 50 percent glucose. Continue alternating sodium bicarbonate and glucose for at least 2 ampules of each. It will further help to give 10 units of regular insulin either in the glucose or subcutaneously.

All this should take no more than 20 to 30 minutes. The serum potassium probably will have dropped 1.5 to 2.5 mEq.

The intensity of treatment can now be slowed. Give 10 percent glucose in saline during the next hour to hold the benefits of the emergency treatment. Start Kayexalate 15 g orally q.i.d. in small amounts of water. This is a potassium removing cation exchange resin. It may also be given as an enema through an inflated Foley catheter. Give at body temperature 30 g in 150 to 200 ml water every 12 hours. Retain 4 to 10 hours if possible.

Reduce dietary sodium. If more help is needed, obtain consultation regarding possible peritoneal dialysis, especially if hyponatremia or acidosis is present. If acidosis and uremia are present, consider hemodialysis.

CLASSIFICATION (TABLE 10-4)

Table 10-4. Classification of Patients with Cardiac Conditions

*Functional Capacity**

Class I
- No limitations on physical activity.
- No symptoms with ordinary physical activity.

Class II
- Slight limitation of physical activity.
- Symptoms occur with ordinary physical activity.

Class III
- Marked limitation of physical activity.
- Symptoms occur with less than ordinary physical activity.

Class IV
- Symptoms with any physical activity and may occur at rest.
- Symptoms increased in severity with any physical activity.

*Therapeutic**

Class A
- Physical activity not restricted.

Class B
- Ordinary physical activity not restricted.
- Severe or competitive physical activity not advised.

Class C
- Ordinary physical activity moderately restricted.
- Strenuous activity discontinued.

Class D
- Ordinary physical activity markedly restricted.

Class E
- Complete bed rest.
- Confined to bed or chair.

After the American Heart Association.

*Functional capacity is estimated on the cardiac patient's response to physical activity. Therapeutic classification indicates the restriction of activity which is advised based on the severity of the cardiac disorder.

REFERENCES

1. Schoenfield G, Kudzma DJ: Type IV hyperlipoproteinemia. *Arch Intern Med* 132:55–63, 1973.
2. Benchimol A, et al: Resting electrocardiogram in major coronary artery disease. *JAMA* 224:1489, 1973.
3. Hochberg HM: Characteristics and significance of prodomes of coronary care unit patients. *Chest* 59:10–14, 1971.
4. Newton RM, et al: Clinical correlations with coronary arteriography. *Va Med Mon* 97:688–692, 1970.
5. Cardiac arrest: AMA Office of the General Counsel. *JAMA* 216:2217, 1971.
6. Heart Attacks: AMA Office of the General Counsel. *JAMA* 223:365, 1973.
7. Chopra MP, et al: Lidocaine therapy for ventricular ectopic activity after acute MI: double-blind trial. *Br Med J* 3:668–670, 1971.
8. Adgey AAJ: Acute phase of MI. *Lancet* 2:501–503, 1971.
9. Bernstein V, et al: Lidocaine intramuscularly in acute MI. *JAMA* 219:1027, 1972.
10. Zener JC, et al: Blood lidocaine levels and kinetics following high-dose intramuscular administration. *Circulation* 47:984 –988, 1973.
11. Moss AJ: Acute myocardial infarction — pre-

hospital and post-hospital consideration. *Med Times* 98:81, 1970.
12. Boyer JL: Physical activity programs following MI. *Hosp Med* 8:95–112, 1972.
13. Kannel WB, et al: Systolic versus diastolic blood pressure and risk of coronary heart disease. *Am J Cardiol* 27:335, 1971.
14. Kosman ME: Evaluation of diazoxide: (hyperstat I.M.). *JAMA* 224:1422, 1973.
15. Mattingly TW: Diseases of the myocardium. *Am J Cardiol* 25:79–80, 1970.
16. Pomerantz M: Taking the measure of pulmonary edema. *Emerg Med* 3:113, 1971.

GENERAL STUDY AIDS

Maha GE: Diet and drug therapy for hyperlipoproteinemia. *Med Times* 99:49, 1971.

Mendlowitz M: The problem of screening in hypertension. *Mt. Sinai J Med* 38:474–477, 1971.

Chung EK: Guide to managing digitalis intoxication. *Postgrad Med* 49:99–101, 1971.

Pennington JE, et al: Chest thump for reverting ventricular tachycardia. *New Eng J Med* 283:1192–1195, 1970.

Bonanno JA, et al: Principles of antiarrhythmic therapy. *Drug Therapy* 1:15–24, 1971.

Schwartz AB: Management of potassium imbalance. *Drug Therapy* 2:15–24, 1972.

CHAPTER 11

Pulmonary Diseases

UPPER RESPIRATORY INFECTIONS (URI)

Classification

Mogabgab[1] suggests the following classification for URI:

A. Afebrile URI (T↓101° F)
B. Febrile URI (T↑101° F)
C. Pharyngitis (severe sore throat with dysphagia with or without exudate)
D. Laryngitis, tracheitis and bronchitis
E. Atypical pneumonia

Category A is the most common infection in adults and children. In adults the etiologic agent is most often a rhinovirus; in children nearly any virus may be implicated plus beta-hemolytic streptococci.

Category B is more common among children. Again, nearly any virus can be involved. In adults, Influenza A and B are common agents. Arthralgia, myalgia and fever help to distinguish this category from category A.

Beta-hemolytic streptococcus pharyngitis and infectious mononucleosis are frequent infections in category C.

The tracheitis, bronchiolitis or croup of infants and children and many viral infections of adults belong in category D.

Category E could well be classified as a lower respiratory infection because the lungs are frequently involved, commonly with a mycoplasma pneumonia (Eaton agent). In young adults an x-ray film is needed to diagnose this nonbacterial, atypical pneumonia.

Keep in mind in treating adult pharyngitis that about one third of the cases are of unknown etiology, one third are beta-hemolytic streptococcus and the rest viral. The most common viral infection is rhinovirus which accounts for more pharyngitis than adeno- or other viruses.

The etiologic factors are different in children. If the child is under 18 months you can practically forget streptococcus as a cause for pharyngotonsillitis. This infection at this age is certain evidence of a viral infection. From this age on, however, streptococcal infections increase in frequency but never account for the majority of cases.

Although upper respiratory infection is one of the most common of diseases, it is one of the most misdiagnosed too. Many conditions, both grave and insignificant, including cancer, have been erroneously diagnosed as "colds." On the other hand, the most misdiagnosed condition is beta-hemolytic streptococcal pharyngitis (Fig. 11-1).

In a child, suspect streptococcal infection when the disease has begun suddenly with high fever and abdominal complaints. It is not very helpful in differential diagnosis to know whether exudate is present in the throat. Look for petechiae on the soft palate. Neither is the degree of fever a very specific indication of the etiologic agent.

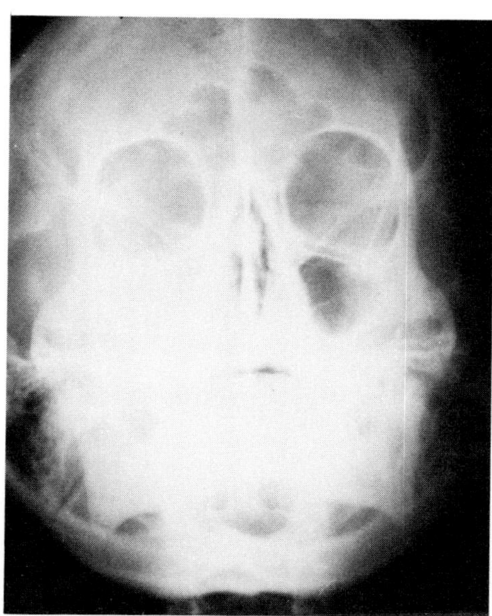

Figure 11-1. Right maxillary sinusitis with air-fluid level and right maxillary cloudiness.

In infants under 18 months, common colds can cause temperatures of over 102°.

There is no certain way to differentiate streptococcal and viral infections except by throat culture. Culture all sore throats if you are going to practice top grade medicine. Considering all the uncontrolled factors of family practice, however, it is not always feasible to culture every throat.

When a throat culture is not possible consider therapeutic tests of aspirin and penicillin. Doctors frequently do this when they tell patients to take aspirin and call back. Although the idea has merit, physicians are often criticized for being lazy in suggesting aspirin. Such is not the case. A child who improves an hour after taking aspirin is not likely to have a streptococcal infection. Conversely, if he remains systemically as ill with only a moderate reduction in fever, suspect a streptococcal invasion.

The therapeutic test with penicillin can be helpful, too. Prescribe penicillin and if the child is not greatly improved and afebrile in 24 hours, stop the penicillin. This is good evidence of a viral infection.

Do not depend on therapeutic tests although they are fairly reliable. Employ them as exceptions in your practice. The wise course is to establish a routine of throat culturing. One good reason not to depend on the therapeutic test of penicillin is that many carriers will be missed. The streptococcal carrier may have an acute viral pharyngitis and consequently not respond to penicillin. These cases, however, should have the ten day penicillin prophylaxis treatment.

Streptococcal infection also occurs in a chronic or subacute form. Suspect the disease in a whining young child with a chronic cold and low-grade fever even though he does not have an exudative pharyngotonsillitis.

Probably not as many acute streptococcal sore throats are missed as mild ones. You can obtain diagnostic help by inquiring as to whether other members of the family have also had a sore throat. A patient who has a coryza and sore throat and has been exposed to another household member with similar symptoms demands a search for a streptococcal infection.

Classic symptoms of a streptococcal infection in an adult are a red throat, tender cervical glands and difficulty in swallowing. Do not confuse streptococcal sore throats with infectious mononucleosis. A debated point is whether leukocytosis can be a dependable sign in differentiating a bacterial and a viral infection. The consensus of opinion is that in children it means little or nothing as there is no established pattern of leukocytosis in either disease. In adults, however, the white count may be helpful. Most researchers claim that 25 percent of bacterial sore throats have no rise in the leukocytes. In adults, suspect a bacterial infection, however, if there is a significant leukocytosis.

Some physicians lapse into the habit of giving antibiotics on a prophylactic basis believing the therapy will prevent secondary bacterial invasion in a patient with lowered resistance. Most authorities claim this is not so. There is no evidence that any viral infections either precede or lower the patient's resistance to streptococcal infection perhaps with one exception: viral pneumonia may become secondarily infected. But don't assume you can prevent or treat any viral upper respiratory infection with antibiotics.

Everything considered, inaugurate a throat culturing routine. Give the patient two prescriptions, one for 24 hours and one for 10 days. Have them fill the first prescription and call back for the culture report when it is finished. If the culture is positive, have him fill the second for a 10 day supply. If the culture is negative, discontinue antibiotics and treat symptomatically.

Treating URI

Prescribe aspirin as a routine for adults and as needed for children. Prescribe a full aspirin dose in children. Force fluids to prevent aspirin poisoning.

Prescribe Actifid (antihistamine-vasoconstrictor combination) for adults to keep air passages open; in children, nose drops such as ½ to ¼ percent Neosynephrine, 2 to 3 drops 4 times daily. Use aqueous nasal drops. Don't use long-acting adult drops nor oral decongestants under 2 years of age. Benedryl is helpful as a sedative for those who cannot sleep because of the nasal congestion. Do not promote the use of nose drops longer than 7 days.

Order warm saline gargles for sore throat. Suggest bed rest only if the patient feels like resting.

If you must give an antibiotic because of patient pressure, give something least likely to cause trouble, perhaps a few doses of penicillin orally. There is seldom a need for injections and if used they should be justified medically and recorded.

Therapeutic Problems Associated With Antibiotic Therapy

A proven case of streptococcal sore throat may not respond when the organism has become antibiotic resistant. Select a different antibiotic or reculture and start over. Some strains of staphylococci produce penicillinase. In these cases, the penicillins will not help. Mixed microbial infection will also cause treatment problems. Do not fail to interpret the culture results in the light of clinic findings. Again the culture may be positive in streptococcal carriers with treatment failure when the patient's acute disease is viral. Do not forget to order sensitivity testing when indicated.

When giving antibiotics, watch for antibiotic allergy or hypersensitivity. Keep in mind:

- the fever of penicillin
- the rash of penicillin, especially that of ampicillin
- the photosensitization of the tetracyclines
- the diarrhea of lincomycin
- the nausea, vomiting and flatulence of any orally administered antibiotic
- the vitamin K and riboflavin deficiencies with long-term ampicillin or tetracycline therapy
- the superinfections caused by all antibiotics

Do not use the following antibiotics in the treatment of upper respiratory infections unless unusual circumstances exist (then their use should be documented):

- chloramphenicol (Chloromycentin) because of the danger of aplastic anemia
- demethylchlortetracyline (Declomycin) because of high incidence of photosensitization
- erythromycin estolate (Ilosone) or triacetyloleandomycin (Cyclamycin or TAO) because of liver toxicity
- sulfonamides because of low tissue levels

Treatment failure also occurs because the patient and/or the doctor does not fulfill his obligations, especially in cases of beta-hemolytic streptococcal infections. The patient fails to take the antibiotic daily for the full 10 days. In this case, you would be justified in giving Bicillin, 1.2 million units by intramuscular injection, despite the pain of the injection. Bicillin C-R is less painful.

Another area of cooperation between you and your patient is in having other family contacts cultured for streptococcal infections. Do not neglect having patients return after treatment for a follow-up nose and throat culture, particularly those who have been treated orally.

Treatment of Beta-Hemolytic Streptococcus Infection

PENICILLIN. Penicillin-V orally 125 to 250 mg 3 to 4 times daily is preferred. It can be given anytime during the day without consideration to meals. It is better absorbed. The price is about the same as other oral penicillins. If penicillin-V is not available use as a second choice penicillin-G.

Trade names for penicillin-V (phenoxymethyl penicillin follow: In capsules and tablets: Penicillin V tablets, Pen-Vee, V-Cillin and Compocillin. In liquid: Penicillin-V Oral (125 and 250 mg/5 ml), Pen-Vee for suspension (90 and 180 mg/5 ml), V-Cillin Pediatric (125 and 250 mg/5 ml) and Compocillin-V oral suspension (180 mg/5 ml). In addition, Wyeth and Lilly manufacture drops.

If you choose the intramuscular route of penicillin treatment, the popular Bicillin is recommended. Bicillin Long Acting Suspension is offered in 300,000 to 600,000 units of penicillin-G benzathine per ml. It is painful. Bicillin C-R 600 and 300 is less painful. The 600 has 300,000 units of penicillin-G benzathine plus 300,000 units penicillin-G procaine per ml. The 300 has 150,000 units of each of the forgoing penicillins in each ml. Penicillin-G, benzathine like procaine penicillin-G has a prolonged effect because of its slight solubility. Because of this property, it has prolonged action at the expense of high blood concentration.

ERYTHROMYCIN. If the patient is sensitive to penicillin, use erythromycin (Erythrocin). It is less expensive than lincomycin (Lincocin) and causes less gastrointestinal symptoms. Popular erythromycin preparations on the market are: In capsules and tablets: Erythrocin stearate filmtabs (100 to 250 mg tabs) and Pediamycin chewable tabs and Erythrocin chewable (both with 200 mg of erythromycin or succinate). In liquid: Erythrocin Granules (200 mg per 5 ml) and Pediamycin Suspension Granules (200 mg per 5 ml).

Estolate preparations are popular, but their use in children is debated because of some evidence that the estolate salt is hepatotoxic. Consequently the succinate is preferred in children.

In case a documented streptococcal sore throat does not respond, think of the possibility of staphylococcal penicillinase-resistant complication. There is plenty of evidence that penicillinase production can be increased by exposing staphylococcus to penicillin. In this case, consider substituting sodium oxacillin (Prostaphlin) or lincomycin (Lincocin) for penicillin.

Do not use sulfonamides. They are not effective against beta-hemolytic streptococcal infections as a treatment agent. Use them only prophylactically. Do not use the tetracyclines because 25 percent of group A streptococci are resistant to them. Never use steroids for upper respiratory infections.

Do not give antibiotics in mild uncomplicated acute bronchitis. Do give when the risk of bronchopneumonia is great: in patient's with chronic bronchitis or bronchiectasis, in children and the elderly or infirm, when another disease complicates the disease as in heart disease and in patients with severe bronchitis.

Infectious Mononucleosis

Mononucleosis is an acute systemic disease characterized by fever, generalized hyperplasia of lymphoid tissue and abnormal mononuclear cells in the blood. Think of the disease as having two stages. The first stage will be 7 to 10 days of fever and pharyngitis; the second is a two week period of drowsiness and weakness (a condition lasting approximately a month).

Do not attempt to diagnose mononucleosis by clinical evidence alone. Seek laboratory confirmation of your opinion. The total white count has little diagnostic significance. In fact, the total count may be normal. Look at the differential. If the lymphocytes are more than 50 percent of the total, suspect mononucleosis. Order a heterophile agglutination test (Paul-Bunnell) for if the antibody titer is above 1:56 the disease is active. A positive test without other laboratory clinical findings indicates a previous infection. For months following an attack of mononucleosis the heterophile titer may jump up whenever the patient has any acute respiratory disease. Do not confuse this with a second or third attack of mononucleosis. Most patients recover within a month with lasting immunity.

Watch the patient's throat during the first stage. He may have a simple lymphoid hyperplasia or a severe exudative pharyngitis, the latter caused by bacterial invasion. This patient will have a severe sore throat, dysphagia, swollen anterior cervical lymph nodes and about a third of the throats will culture out beta-hemolytic streptococci. A few patients will become jaundiced as a result of transient biliary stasis. Other lymph glands over the body may be swollen. One danger: a sudden, tender spleen may rupture easily if traumatized.

Mononucleosis is frequently misdiagnosed as hepatitis when the patient becomes jaundiced. Every case of suspected hepatitis should have a heterophile agglutination test. The jaundice of mononucleosis is not a hepatitis but solely a mononuclear infiltration that depresses hepatic function. Even though the bilirubin goes to 8 mg percent, by the end of the week it begins to subside.

Serious complications are rare, they are a ruptured spleen, hemolytic anemia and thrombocytopenia.

Prolonged bed rest is of no great value. Children should be kept in an environment where they can rest if they feel fatigued. Prohibit strenuous activity to protect the spleen from being damaged.

Do not give ampicillin for bacterial throat infection. This drug, for some unexplained reason, causes the rash so often attributed to the disease. The rash of rubella is often confused with mononucleosis because of the lymphadenopathy. Do give a 10 day course of antibiotics if beta-hemolytic streptococcus is present.

For high fever and severe sore throat give 80 mg prednisone per day, tapering off quickly as the patient improves. Otherwise treat the patient symptomatically, i.e. aspirin, fluids, ice collar, soft diet and hot gargles.

LOWER RESPIRATORY INFECTIONS

Unfortunately the efficacy of antibiotics has diminished the need for family physicians to make a precise diagnosis when treating patients complaining of respiratory infections. This is unscientific medicine. We owe each patient that best diagnosis we can make and treatment tailored to that diagnosis. The injudicious prescribing of antibiotics on the basis of upper and lower respiratory infections is no better than back-fence medicine.

I am listing what is generally conceded to be the eleven most common respiratory infections. Most of your cases of cold or coughs may be classified as:

- –upper respiratory infection
- –tracheobronchitis
- –atypical pneumonia (Fig. 11-2)
- –acute lobar pneumonia
- –bronchopneumonia
- –systemic gram-negative pneumonia
- –purulent bronchitis and respiratory failure
- –slowly resolving pneumonia

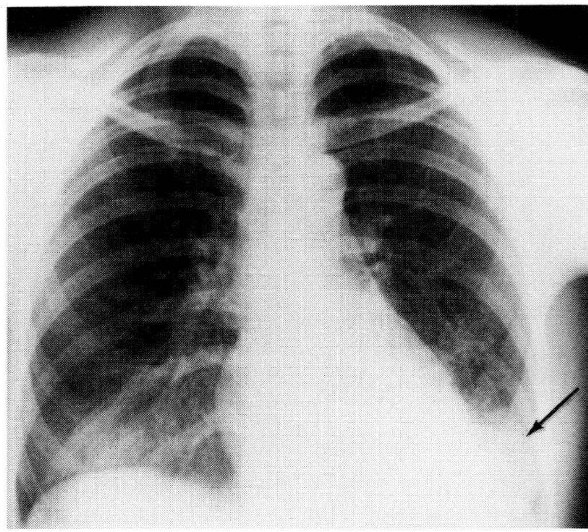

Figure 11-2. Viral pneumonia of the left lower lobe. Interstitial and alveolar infiltrates disappeared completely within one week.

–pulmonary abscess
–emphysema
–chronic pneumonia

The etiologic agents producing these diseases are rhinoviruses, influenza viruses types A, B and C; parainfluenza viruses 1, 2 and 3; adenoviruses types 3, 4, 7 and 21; Mycoplasma pneumonia; bacterial organisms; Mycobacterium tuberculosis; mycobacterial infections; and fungal infections.

Eighty-five antigenic types of rhinoviruses produce 25 percent of the common colds. They are of little danger to the lungs.

Influenza viruses types A, B and C (Fig. 11-3) with many antigenic variants cause 80 percent of acute respiratory diseases in epidemics and about 12 percent in nonepidemic periods. There is no specific therapy. Vaccines are available for prevention but must be antigenically related. Consequently, health departments attempt to identify the strain of organism in the early stages of an epidemic.

Parainfluenza viruses 1, 2 and 3 are responsible for 10 percent of acute upper respiratory diseases. Very seldom do they cause viral pneumonia.

Adenoviruses types 3, 4, 7 and 21 cause 3 to 5 percent of severe respiratory infections (Fig. 11-4) such as viral pneumonia, acute URI and pharyngoconjunctival fever.

Mycoplasma penumonia is responsible for 25 to 50 percent of primary atypical pneumonias. In contrast to atypic pneumonia this disease is responsive to erythromycin or tetracycline. The disease is cold agglutination positive. The laboratory can culture this organism and your diagnosis can be precise.

Bacterial organisms include Streptococcus pneumoniae, Staphylococcus aureus, Klebsiella pneumoniae, Hemophilus influenzae, Escherichia coli, Proteus species, Pseudomonas, Bacteroides and microaerophilic or anerobic Streptococci. These organisms may be involved primarily or secondarily in pneumonias, bronchopneumonia or bronchitis. In order to select the right antibiotic, identify species by gram stain and/or culture of respiratory tract secretions. The course of bacterial disease is often interrupted by stubborn superinfections. Change antibiotics as indicated by repeated cultures.

Myobacterium tuberculoses cause pulmonary infiltrates that are difficult to distin-

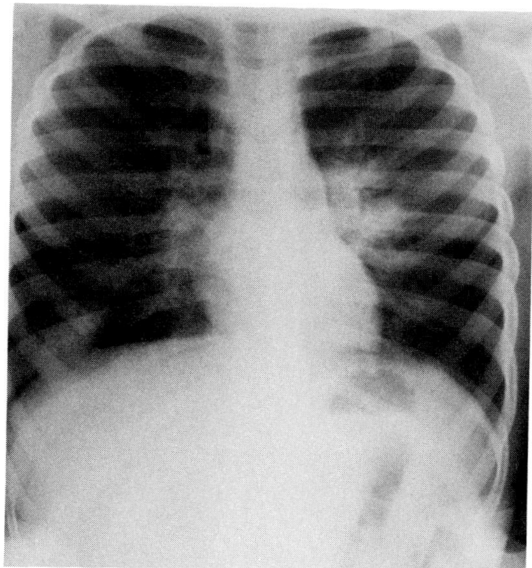

Figure 11-3. Primary influenzal pneumonia, central pseudolobar consolidation, bilateral. Areas of consolidation extend outward from the hilar-areas. The homogenous densities resemble lobar pneumonia, but the irregular borders of the lesions can be seen, suggesting the lesion is not bound by lobar margins.

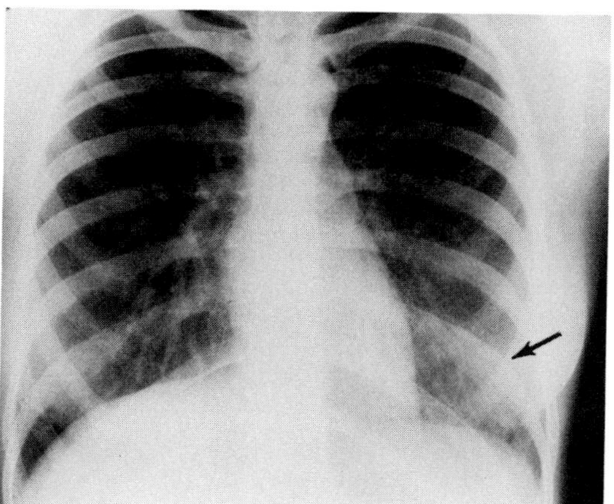

Figure 11-4. Pneumonic infiltrates are the principal x-ray findings in viral diseases affecting the respiratory tract. Roentgenology shows a light consolidation in the posterior basilar segment, LLL pneumonia.

guish from other less virulent mycobacterial species and even viral, bacterial and neoplastic diseases of the lungs. Work out the differential diagnosis of mycobacterial types by comparing the skin reactivity to different mycobacterial antigens and by comparing cross-reactivity at different dilutions of test antigens. Mycobacterial infections must also be distinguished from infections with the weakly acid-fast actinomycete, H. asteroides.

Fungal infections include histoplasmosis in the central and northeastern United States, coccidiodomycosis in the West and Southwest; and blastomycosis in the South and Southeast. The latter include cryptococcosis, candidiasis, mycomycosis and aspergillosis. In fungal infections culturing is often insufficient for definitive diagnosis. If you plan to use amphotericin B, which is toxic to the kidney, the wise course is to verify the diagnosis by biopsy.

Differentiating Atypical and Bacterial Pneumonia

Atypical

Base your diagnosis of atypical pneumonia on the history, physical examination, simple laboratory tests and x-ray studies. Perhaps etiologic agents can be recovered in research centers, but attempting to recover etiologic agents isn't going to help your patient now. More likely, but still not too practical, are serologic studies. These studies are insignificant unless an increasing titer is found. Even if you order a titer at the beginning of the ailment, there is little use in checking in 2 weeks. That is too late in helping plan therapy.

Atypical or viral pneumonia (Fig. 11-5) in untreated patients lasts for about a week and then gradually resolves although x-ray changes often persist for 2 to 3 weeks. However, the elderly and debilitated are prone to develop serious complications.

In atypical pneumonia the white blood count is normal, the sputum smear has few leukocytes or bacteria and the culture is reported as "normal flora." X-ray findings are out of proportion to the physical examination findings if the atypical pneumonia is caused by mycoplasma pneumoniae. A check on the cold agglutinins will show elevation.

Not all types of atypical pneumonia organisms respond to antibiotics, but enough will that all patients should be treated with antibiotics, preferably tetracycline 0.5 mg every 6 hours for 10 days or with erythromycin in the same dosage.

Bacterial

Lobar pneumonia (bacterial) with its explosive onset and bloody sputum is easier to diagnose. The incidence of the disease is

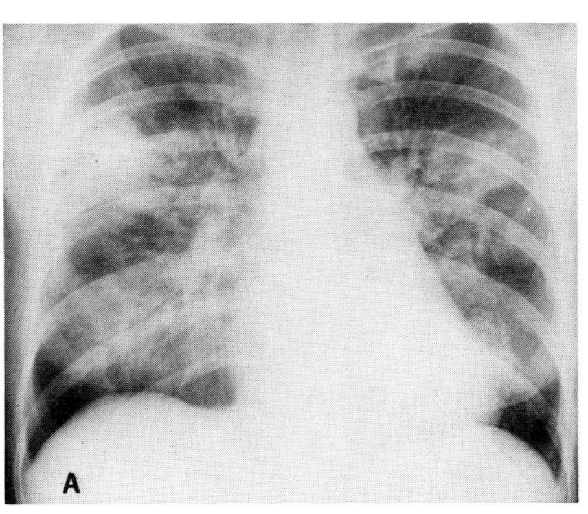

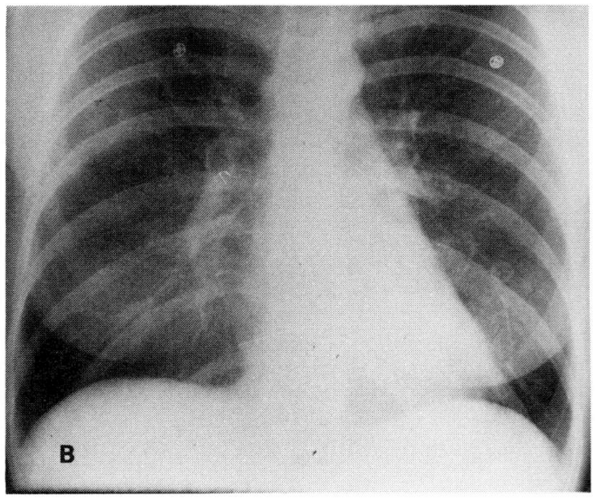

Figure 11-5. *A*, Atypical pneumonia. *B*, Six days later the chest shows no sign of the disease—a remarkably fast clearing for such an extensive atypical pneumonia.

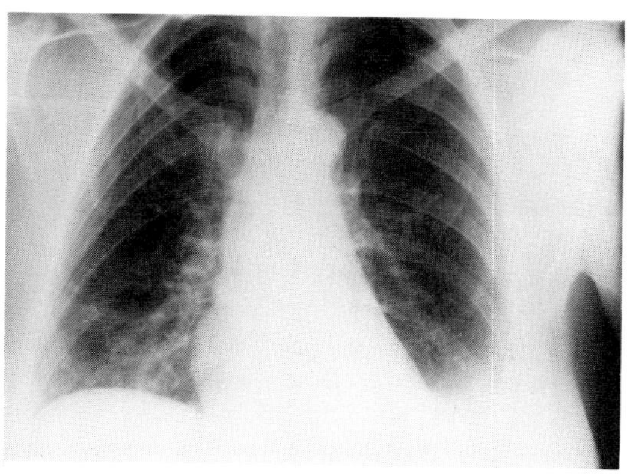

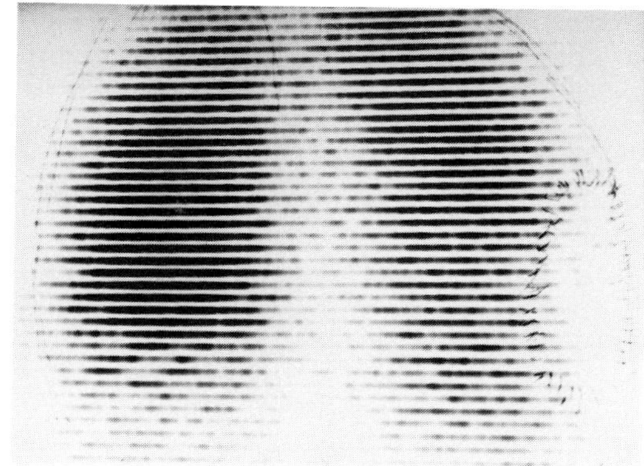

Figure 11-6. *Left*, Infarction in LLL; *Right*, A positive scan verifies the diagnosis.

much lower now, but older physicians could spot the patient with lobar pneumonia from across the room. Look for an elevated white blood count, a sputum smear loaded with leukocytes and bacteria and a heavy growth of the pathogens on sputum culture. An x-ray picture usually verifies your suspicions (Fig. 11-6). Usually you will find one of four organisms: Pneumococcus, Staphylococcus, Klebsiella pneumoniae (Friedlander's bacillus) or Mycobacterium tuberculosis.

Treat this disease as an emergency. It is a serious one with a fairly high mortality. The patient will appear gravely ill and give a history of an acute onset with chills, fever, chest pain, productive cough and some respiratory distress.

Obtain a culture of the sputum as soon as possible. In the meantime, begin antibiotic therapy on the basis of a gram or acid-fast stain.

TRANSTRACHEAL ASPIRATION. Often uncontaminated sputum is difficult to obtain. If so, you will be wise to do a transtracheal aspiration. It is not difficult to do.

Place the patient in the supine position with his neck hyperextended over a pillow placed between his shoulders. Prepare the skin area over the trachea. Raise a wheal in the skin with 1 percent Xylocaine and infiltrate to the trachea.

Using equipment from a Bardic Intracath set, insert a 14 gauge needle through the cricothyroid membrane below the thyroid but above the cricoid cartilage. Thread a catheter through the needle down into the trachea and then remove the needle.

Attempt to aspirate any pulmonary secretions. If no material is obtained, inject 5 ml of saline. You can aspirate an uncontaminated sample of sputum when the patient begins coughing. Remove the catheter and apply pressure over the puncture site for 3 to 5 minutes. This will prevent bleeding and the infiltration of air.

Do an immediate gram stain but also send the specimen for culture. At this point, determine which antibiotic to use by the class of organism seen on the gram stain.

PNEUMOCOCCAL PNEUMONIA. A gram-positive, lancet-shaped diplococci indicates pneumococcal pneumonia. Start the patient on the relatively low dosage of aqueous penicillin G, 600,000 units IM every 6 hours. The low dosage is to prevent superinfection. If the patient is sensitive to penicillin, try cephalothin IV, 1 g every 6 hours or erythromycin IV, 250 mg at the same intervals. Stay away from tetracycline in pneumococcal pneumonia.

STAPHYLOCOCCAL PNEUMONIA. Suspect staphyloccal pneumonia when the stain shows gram-positive cocci. Penicillin-G will not be effective if the staphylococci is a penicillinase producer. This you do not know from the gram stain; therefore, to be effective from the start, prescribe oxacillin or nafcillin, 1 g IV every 4 hours. If the patient is penicillin sensitive, begin with cephalothin IV, 1 g every 3 to 4 hours. Switch the antibiotic to penicillin if the culture shows the staphylococcus is sensitive to penicillin.

GRAM-NEGATIVE PNEUMONIA. If gram-negative rods with large capsules (Klebsiella pneumoniae) are found on the gram staining, think of Friedlander's pneumonia. The disease is rare but the mortality rate is high. Often the disease progresses to chronic suppuration with abscess formation and fibrosis.

X-ray examination of the lungs reveals little information of bacteriologic value. There are no x-ray patterns suggesting the gram-negative organisms of Enterobacter, E. coli or Proteus. The most diagnostic findings occur in the fulminating lobar consolidation, cavitation and empyema of a Klebsiella infection. Pseudomonas pneumonia is characterized by a diffuse alveolar involvement with macrocavitation. A Bacteroides infection is often associated with a massive empyema.[2]

The patient who shows up with a Klebsiella gram-negative organism is frequently either an alcoholic or is debilitated from other causes. Klebsiella pneumoniae is sensitive to several drugs, but the least toxic of the antibiotics to which it responds is gentamicin. Add to this cephalothin, a relatively nontoxic antibiotic. Continue treatment for 2 weeks. Allow the culture to determine antibiotic selection. Abscess formation, emphysema or destruction of a lobe may occur, necessitating surgery.

Pneumonias caused by other gram-negative organisms (E. coli, Klebsiella-Aerobacter group, Proteus and Pseudomonas) are often due to superinfections following antibiotics, steroids or immunosuppressive agents. Tracheotomies are occasionally complicated by these infections. Another hazard is the spread of gram-negative infections following the use of contaminated inhalation equipment.

Start with gentamicin, 1.5 mg/kg IM every 8 hours plus ampicillin, 12 g parenterally daily. In penicillin-sensitive patients substitute cephalothin for ampicillin. If you find the infection is Pseudomonas, continue the gentamicin and replace the ampicillin with carbenicillin, 24 to 30 g IV daily. Many physicians believe that probenecid enhances the effect of the antibiotic. If you choose to do so, give it orally, 0.5 g every 6 hours. Continue treatment for at least 2 weeks.

Now what if you find the gram stain is without any specificity, i.e. loaded with gram-positive cocci, gram-positive diplococci, gram-negative rods? This could well be a necrotizing or aspiration pneumonia. This type of pneumonia often follows aspiration of food, water or vomitus from the patient's mouth into the tracheobronchial tree. Suspect necrotizing pneumonia in patients with infected gums and loose teeth or those who have been unconscious from epilepsy, alcoholism, anesthesia or trauma to the head. Most commonly, look for it a few days after a cold or bronchitis when the patient's symptoms worsen. On examination you will find a patch of rales over the affected area and typical x-ray findings.

Many instances of postoperative pneumonia, pleurisy and atelectasis are in reality manifestations of pulmonary infarction (Fig. 11-6). At first the area of infarction appears as a diffuse shadow but later it becomes organized and casts a sharply defined density on the film. A positive scar verifies the diagnosis. Infarction of a lung segment is caused by a localized obstruction in the pulmonary circulation.

Begin treatment for necrotizing pneumonia promptly with (1) 20 million units of penicillin-G IV or 12 g of ampicillin parenterally daily or (2), if patient is penicillin-sensitive, give 0.75 g of chloramphenicol orally or IV every 6 hours. Continue for 2 to 3 weeks.

H. influenza pneumonia is best treated with ampicillin, 12 g a day in adults and 150 mg/kg a day in children. In this instance administer it either intravenously or intramuscularly.

Pneumonia that complicates influenza is rare because influenza is sporadic. During epidemics of flu, however, pneumonia accounts for most of the deaths. Often pneumonia occurs following aspiration of infected material from the trachea into the deeper bronchial field. Check then for a staphylococcal pneumonia. When this occurs, the patient falls into an overwhelming toxemia called *fulminating influenza pneumonia*.

The patient gives a history of the usual influenza infection; however, rather than improving, he becomes suddenly and acutely ill. Consider the complication an emergency. The patient will need oxygen and other measures to prevent circulatory collapse. Give antibiotics without the aid of culture efforts: benzylpenicillin (1.0 million units), cloxacillin (500 mg) or ampicillin (500 mg). Give these intramuscularly every 6 hours. Further treatment will depend on the patient's response and the result of sensitivity testing. Consider the use of steroids in fulminating cases. In milder cases, the patient may respond to penicillin or tetracycline, 250 mg every 6 hours.

General treatment. The mainstay of treatment is the use of antibiotics as outlined. Other measures are:

- –bed rest
- –forced fluids (2,000 to 3,000 ml daily)
- –codeine sulfate (33 to 65 mg every 4 hr p.r.n.) for aching, fever and headache
- –oxygen by nasal catheter or tent for cyanosis
- –keep temperature under 104° with cool baths, aspirin or refrigerated blanket
- –steam inhalations
- –saturated solution of potassium iodide, 10 drops every 4 hr to loosen secretions

Complications

Watch for delayed resolution with fibrosis and chronic suppuration (Fig. 11-7). If delayed more than 2 to 3 weeks, search for an unusual problem, such as carcinoma, bronchiectasis, tuberculosis, antibiotic resistant disease or system disease (diabetes, cirrhosis, alcoholism or nephritis).

Effusions occur 7 to 14 days after the onset of pneumonia. If needed, treat with daily aspiration and infusion of 500,000 units of benzyl penicillin into pleural cavity.

Empyema is not frequent since the advent of antibiotics. Heart failure is a serious complication.

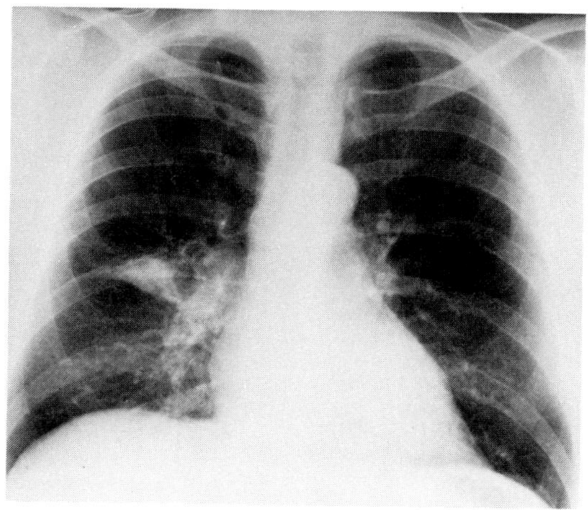

Figure 11-7. Pneumonia unresolved in the anterior segment of the RUL. Pathology: engorgement followed by red and gray hepatization and, finally, resolution and clearing of infiltrate.

Often a lung abscess (Figs. 11-8 and 11-9) starts following inhalation of organisms from pyorrhea, gingivitis or diseased tonsils. Occasionally putrid lung abscesses are caused by infected emboli in the course of sepsis and following abdominal operations. A small particle of clotted blood or pus may become impacted in a small bronchus while the patient is unconscious or is under anesthesia. Before the cavity forms, the x-ray appearance of the abscess is that of pneumonia.

There may be miscellaneous complica-

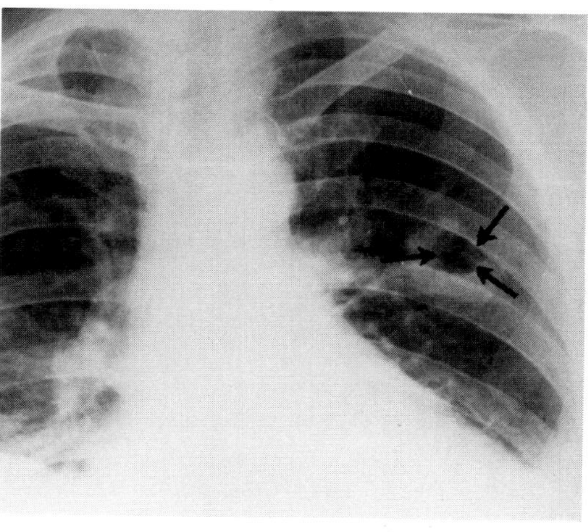

Figure 11-8. Left lung abscess.

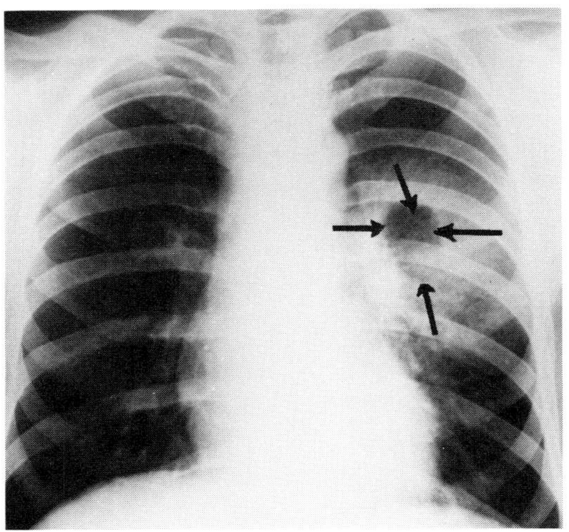

Figure 11-9. Lung abscess.

tions of pneumonia, including pericarditis, endocarditis and meningitis.

INFLUENZA

In 1957 the A_2 subtype influenza appeared. A_2 influenza is the etiologic agent of Asian flu. Harris[3] describes the symptoms of influenza and their incidence as follows:

–cough, 90 percent
–coryza or nasal obstruction, 82 percent
–headache, 72 percent
–malaise, 66 percent
–shivering, 64 percent
–muscular pains, 62 percent
–sore throat, 62 percent
–sudden onset, 46 percent
–expectoration, 40 percent
–anorexia, 37 percent
–hoarse voice, 37 percent
–irritability, 22 percent
–nausea or vomiting, 11 percent

The same researcher lists the following signs in the order of their frequency:

–fever (100° to 102°, duration 2 to 5 days), 100 percent
–injected pharynx, 68 percent
–nasal obstruction, 64 percent
–red, injected conjunctivae, 56 percent
–sputum, 40 percent
–flushed face, 24 percent
–nasal discharge, 20 percent

The incubation period for influenza is generally from 18 to 36 hours following infection.

Vaccination

Influenza vaccination has not proven as effective as with the viruses of smallpox, yellow fever and poliomyelitis. One reason is that the vaccine loses its effectiveness as antigenic properties change. Another cause of ineffectiveness as a prophylactic agent is the time required for the vaccine to produce antibodies, a minimum of 2 weeks and usually longer. In contrast, influenza epidemics spread rapidly. Considering the vaccines must be made after the invading organism has been identified and the public's hesitancy to being vaccinated early, not much help is obtained in controlling epidemics.

Keep high risk segments of the population immunized. They are persons over 65 years of age; persons of any age with chronic diseases such as asthma, diabetes mellitus, tuberculosis and cirrhosis of the liver; and personnel responsible for maintaining critical services in the community: medical and health services, public utilities, transportation, education and police and fire departments.

Contraindications to vaccination include:

–history of hypersensitivity to egg, chicken or chicken feathers
–presence of poliomyelitis in the community
–history of epilepsy or convulsion provoked by fever
–routine use during pregnancy

Influenza vaccination does not lend itself to routine use as is done with other immunization procedures. Vaccinate healthy groups routinely only when influenza epidemics are predicted.

Lederle, National, Parke-Davis, Lilly and Wyeth prepare a bivalent influenza vaccine containing 700 CCA units, 400 CCA units A_2/Aichi/2/68 (Hong Kong variant) and 300 CCA units B (Mass) 3/66 in each ml. It is claimed that Parke-Davis' Fluogen and Lilly's Zonomune Bivalent have less allergenic properties and consequently, less reactions. It is advisable to give Fluogen intramuscularly. All the rest may be given subcutaneously.

For adults not previously immunized, give two injections of 1 ml 2 months apart; for children 6 to 10 years, 0.5 ml; and from 3 months to 5 years, 0.1 to 0.2 ml. For booster give same dose but do not repeat. Vaccination in children is not very effective unless first given 2 weeks apart and then two doses repeated again in 2 months with a total of four injections.

There is still no practical way to differentiate the causative organism of lower respiratory infections. As is the case with most viral diseases, all that is possible is a clinical educated guess. Even a high leukocyte count in peripheral blood does not always indicate bacterial infection. A pleural effusion accompanying pneumonia is more frequent with bacterial disease, but effusions can occur with nonbacterial pneumonia as well. In adults a smear and a culture of the sputum are of value, but children swallow such material and, consequently, it is not often available for study.

Watch for complications in the paranasal sinuses, middle ear, bronchi and lungs either singly or in some combination. The most serious complication is the development of primary viral pneumonia or secondary bacterial pneumonia. Patients with preexisting cardiac or pulmonary disease, the aged and the pregnant woman in the last trimester contribute to the high mortality rate.

The incidence of influenza has been studied in the United Kingdom.[4] Virulence of the organism and host resistance are only two factors determining the frequency and mortality of influenza. The other factor appears to be cold weather. The study does not explain why but does verify the relationship. Perhaps staying indoors, which increases crowding, accounts for a higher incidence. Another suggestion was that lowering of the humidity by artificial heat could be the main factor. No definite suggestions for prevention came from the study.

COCCIDIOIDOMYCOSIS

Contary to popular opinion, coccidioidomycosis is nearly always a mild self-limited disease. The most prominent symptom is a sharp localized but transient pleuritic pain. In one series, half the patients had a cough and a third a low-grade fever. Most patients believe they have the flu, a conclusion which is not always reliable.

Coccidioides immitis lives in the sand and soil of the desert region of the Southwest and in other countries of Central and South America. The fungus produces a pulmonary granuloma. It is usually inhaled with dust, but it may also pass through broken skin or mucosa.

Laboratory aids include a Coccidioidin skin test 1:1000 and the precipitin test. The latter becomes positive in 91 percent of the patients in 3 weeks. During the first week only 50 percent are positive. Complement-fixation titers appear in 80 percent of cases within 1 month. Dissemination is suspected if the titer is positive in 1:16 dilution. Positive dilution of 1:32 indicates dissemination. A titer which keeps rising is diagnostic.

Chest x-ray studies usually confirm the diagnosis but must be taken serially. X-rays taken at 2 to 4 day intervals disclose the following evolution and resolution: circular infiltrate (a smudge) enlarging to a snowball (4 cm), then resolving to a cancer-appearing lesion and finally to a coin-sized lesion that generally disappears in 20 days.

TUBERCULOSIS

The adult type or chronic tuberculosis usually affects the apices and upper lobes of the lungs (Fig. 11-10). This is an area of little ventilation but of high oxygen tension because of an even greater reduction in pulmonary blood flow there. If not treated, many of these soft lesions go on to necrosis, cavitation and fibrosis.

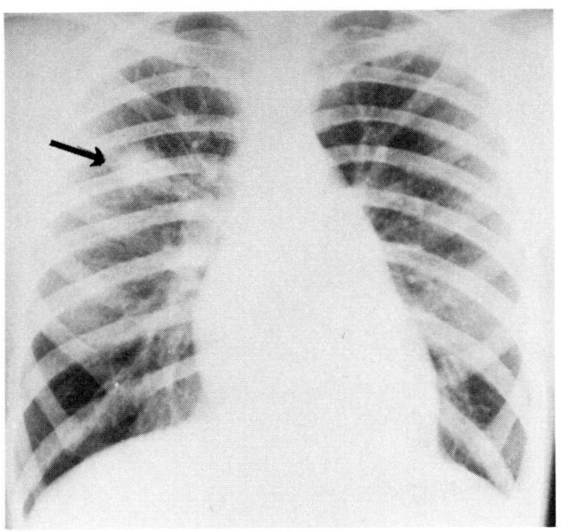

Figure 11-10. Adult type of chronic tuberculosis usually affects the apices and upper lobes.

Pulmonary tuberculosis occurs with chronic fibrosis, cavitation, scarring and calcification and partial collapse of the lung. The disease is encountered most often in persons between 20 and 40 and constitutes one of the most frequent single forms of adult tuberculosis.

Pneumonic tuberculosis affects most often the right upper lobe of young adults but occasionally it is seen in elderly diabetics. The rupture of a caseous lymph node into a bronchus may often start such a spread.

Both lungs are usually involved in infiltrating tuberculosis. Tubercular laryngitis is present in about half of the patients and tubercular enteritis in about two thirds of the patients. If the tubercle bacilli is swallowed in the sputum it can ulcerate the mucosa of the ileum and cecum.

CHRONIC OBSTRUCTIVE LUNG DISEASE (COLD)

The patient with acute bronchitis may get well, may begin recurrent bronchitis or may begin attacks of asthma. Both recurrent bronchitis or asthma can cause damage that results in chronic bronchitis. At this point the disease becomes, for practical clinical consideration, partially, if not wholly, irreversible. Chronic bronchitis can merge directly into pulmonary emphysema or it can proceed indirectly through the bronchiectactic route. The complications of emphysema are bronchopneumonia, pulmonary insufficiency with anoxemia or hypercapnia and cardiac failure.

Think of these entities as being different phases of one long progressively deteriorating disease. Consequently consider COLD as a syndrome that embraces chronic bronchitis, asthma and pulmonary emphysema. These diseases have one symptom in common—undue breathlessness on exertion. Varying degrees of cough and sputum production precede or accompany the dyspnea.

Chronic Bronchitis

Cigarette smoking is a precipitating agent of chronic bronchitis. Seldom will you find chronic bronchitis in nonsmokers. As the disease chiefly occurs after 35 and as patients almost imperceptibly lose their wind the inclination is to blame the aging process rather than increasing respiratory disability. But alveolar hypoventilation and hypoxemia become evident in time and lead to cor pulmonale and eventually heart failure.

JAMA recently estimated that over 34,000,000 Americans are sensitive to cigarette smoke. Of these 16,099,000 are affected with asthma, 16,818,000 with chronic sinusitis, 726,000 with emphysema and 400,000 with chronic bronchitis.[5]

Bronchial Asthma

Bronchial asthma (bronchospasm) is a diagnosis made frequently by the family physician. But bronchospasm has many causes, some of which are disastrous if overlooked. The wise approach is to think of the wheezing patient, especially the young, as having bronchospasm. Then start searching for the cause of the spasm. Suspect a foreign body; pulmonary cysts; tracheoesophageal fistula; congenital lobar emphysema; bronchial stenosis; sequestration of the lung; diaphragmatic abnormalities; cystic fibrosis; mediastinal tumors such as thymoma, neurofibromas, teratoma and lymphoma; achalasia; enlarged mediastinal lymph nodes; hiatal hernia; tuberculosis; adenovirus infections; defects in the immune mechanism; asthmatic bronchitis; recurrent bronchiolitis; and allergies to dust, pollens, dermals and infections.

Laboratory Studies And Tests

Consider any or all of the following in making a diagnosis:

- –chest x-ray studies with high kilovolt (films of the airway, possible with a barium swallow; in children, check thymic shadow).
- –complete blood count with attention to lymphocyte count
- –sweat test
- –Tuberculin and monilia skin tests
- –cultures of the nasopharynx, throat or bronchial secretions
- –x-ray film possibly of nasopharynx for a lymphoid mass in children
- –nitro blue tetazolium dye test for phagocytic dysfunction
- –Schick test and check isohemagglutinins
- –quantitative gammaglobulinemia
- –search for sputum eosinophils with the combined eosin methylene blue stain of Hausel (This test is not absolutely diagnostic although extremely suggestive when obtained from a patient who shows the physical findings of asthma.)

The most important clinical confirmations of the diagnosis of asthma are elicited from two simple therapeutic procedures:

1. Inject 0.3 ml of 1:1,000 dilution of epinephrine subcutaneously. If this injection is followed within minutes by reduction in wheezing, it is evidence of bronchial reversibility and virtually diagnostic of asthma.
2. The other test is the patient's response to steroid therapy. Administer 15 mg prednisone every 6 hours for 2 days. With rare exceptions this will completely reverse the bronchospasm associated with asthma.
3. The best nonclinical objective test for asthma involves the use of the spirometer or peak flow meter. One reading should be made before and one after using a bronchodilator. At least 15 percent improvement indicates a reversible bronchospasm (asthma).

If an apparent asthma does not respond to the usual symptomatic treatment, think of infectious asthma. Although the pathophysiologic process is the same as an asthma caused by other irritants, treatment will differ. Relief will come only with the administration of antibiotics.

To cause the disease, infection does not need to occur in the lungs or bronchi. Sinusitis, tonsillitis and adenoiditis may be the offending agent. Suspect infectious asthma on finding pus, bacteria and eosinophils in the sputum; leukocytosis; fever; asthma occuring subsequent to acute infections; red mucous membranes; a preceding cough in patients with no known allergies; or any negative allergic skin tests.

Give these patients broad spectrum antibiotics for 10 to 14 days. Tetracyclines are recommended.

Pathogenic organisms, generally responsible for bronchial infections are frequently mixed, S. pneumoniae; H. influenza, H. hemolyticus, Streptococci, Staphylocci and E. coli.

Predisposing Factors

Be more suspicious of pulmonary symptoms in men age 45 and over.

A heavy cigarette smoker has 60 to 70 times greater risk of developing an epidermoid cancer than a nonsmoker. A heavy smoker is a person who smokes 40 or more cigarettes per day. One out of 8 of these smokers will develop lung cancer, as compared with 1 in 300 nonsmokers. The incidence of cancer is directly proportionate to the number of cigarettes smoked.

The incidence of cancer is higher in persons exposed to occupational fumes, dust and chemicals such as chromates, nickel and asbestos. Petroleum products are thought to be carcinogenic. Documented evidence now supports the observation that lung cancer has a higher incidence in cities than in rural areas. Even nonsmokers in the city have a higher incidence than nonsmokers who live in a rural area. This statistic implicates urban pollution.

Pulmonary Emphysema

Chronic bronchitis generally precedes emphysema. Cigarette smoking invariably accompanies the coughing and postnasal drainage. The patient maintains his general health, however, until about the age 50. Then gradually exertional dyspnea occurs. Often symptoms become worse after a cold or bout of influenza.

Occasionally, COLD is confused with heart disease and, indeed, as COLD advances, right heart strain may progress to right heart failure with even more dyspnea, hepatomegaly, ascitis or dependent edema. A tip-off in differentiating the two is the type and severity of orthopnea. Uncomplicated COLD patients are not orthopneic. They may, however, sit up during the night to cough up accumulated secretions. The symptom is well worth inquiring into.

Family physicians occasionally spend their time and the patient's money attempting to find an extrapulmonary cause for an emphysematous patient's sudden loss of weight. This frequently happens in deteriorating emphysema. Possibly the patient finds it tiring to eat and the changing circulatory problems create an early satiety. Peculiarly enough about a quarter of the patients develop a peptic ulcer.

The findings on physical examination depend, in good measure, on the stage to which the disease has progressed. Early in the course of the disease the only ausculatory findings are diminution of breath sounds and prolongation of expiration. Later the intermittent expiratory wheezes, rhonchi and musical rales become continuous and annoying.

In percussion of the chest the sound is hyperresonant and the chest is enlarged.

Early in the condition, many patients find some relief by breathing with pursed lips on expiration. Many sit on a chair leaning forward, perhaps with their arms on the chair rests.

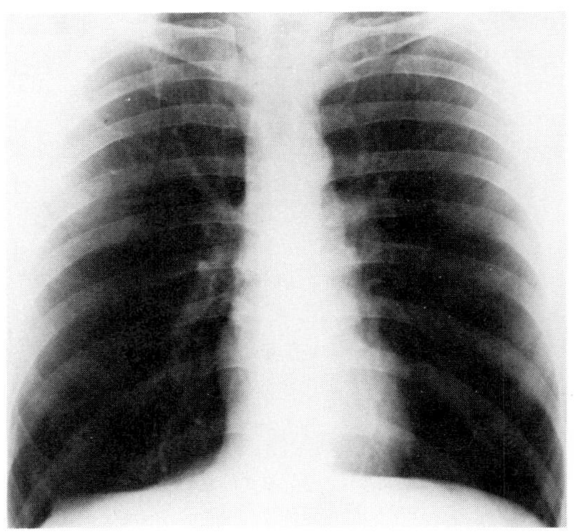

Figure 11-11. A PA film demonstrating typical findings of pulmonary emphysema: flattening of diaphragm, increased radiolucency, widened rib spaces and small heart.

Some patients develop a barrel chest rather early; others do not. The increasing anteroposterior diameter of the chest does not correlate very well with the severity of the disease.

X-ray films do not always tell the true early story. Typical radiologic findings (Figs. 11-11 and 11-12) are:

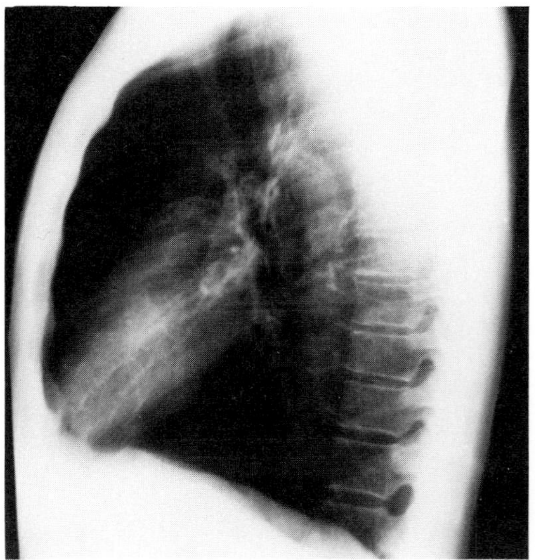

Figure 11-12. Typical findings of pulmonary emphysema. Note the flattening of the diaphragm and increased radiolucency in this lateral radiograph. The heart and aorta are displaced.

–flattening of the diaphragm seen in the A–P view and, even more noticeably, in the lateral view
–increased anteroposterior diameter of the thorax
–increased radiolucency in the retrosternal and retrocardiac spaces
–radiolucency of the lung fields and decreased vascular markings in the periphery of the lungs

Interpret the films by evaluating all these parameters. None of the findings may appear spectacular. The radiologist's interpretation is made after studying all factors.

The EKG is a valuable aid in evalutation. All patients with emphysema do not develop cor pulmonale. If the EKG findings are not typical of cor pulmonale with right ventricular hypertrophy, suspect other forms of heart disease.

Generally these patients can be cared for as outpatients. See them in your office at frequent enough intervals to keep them on a planned program aimed at preventing infections and keeping the sputum liquid and bronchospasm at a minimum. On each visit evaluate the patient's symptoms and attitude. Hospitalize any patient with evidence of confusion, delirium or persistent somnolence. The chief manifestations of the disease are dyspnea, cough and sputum. Evaluate all these factors and adjust medications to meet unfavorable developments. As previously suggested, check a 12 or 24 hour sputum specimen for volume, purulence, cytology and microbiology.

Indications for hospitalization include the aforementioned mental symptoms plus sudden increase in dyspnea and sputum volume or loss of body weight. When dyspnea increases, patients often overuse their Medihaler or even their ephedrine tablets until tolerance develops. In addition, a complicating illness such as diabetes can create hazards of electrolytes and acid-base imbalance which can only be treated effectively in a hospital.

Profile of the Patient with Emphysema

The average age of the patient when first diagnosed as emphysema is 52 years. Prior to the initial diagnosis the patient has suffered a cough for 9 years and had abnormal sputum production for 7 years.

The average patient will discontinue productive work at 53 years, 1 year after the onset of dyspnea. The first acute attack of respiratory failure occurs at 57 years, 5 years after the diagnosis of COLD.

About two thirds of the patients who develop COLD will have smoked cigarettes 31 years before the first attack of respiratory failure.

About 10 percent of the patients will die of bronchopneumonia after the first episode of respiratory failure. Ten percent more will die following the second attack of failure, which usually occurs 8 months after the first attack. Two more will die following the third episode after a 4 month interval between the third and fourth attacks.

Sixty-six percent of the patients will die within 7 years of the onset of COLD and within 2 years of the first acute episode of respiratory failure.

Office Pulmonary Function Tests[6]

Study a Vitalor spirogram for a moment (Fig. 11-13). Notice that the horizontal lines represent liters (L) and, from the bottom to the top of the spirogram, increase in value to approximately 5 L. The vertical lines represent time increasing to 6 seconds

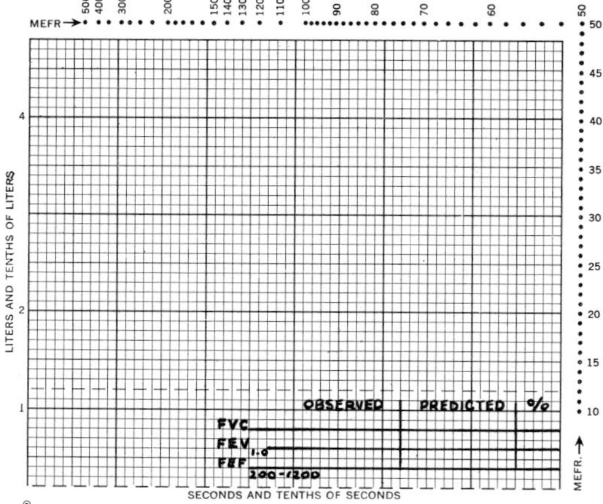

Figure 11-13. Vitalor spirogram.

from the left to the right. There is a dotted horizontal line at the 1.2 L or 1,200 ml level. At the top and the right hand edges of the spirogram there are a series of small numbers running from 10 to 500 and marked either MEFR (maximum expiratory flow rate) or forced expiratory flow rate between 200 and 1200 ml ($FEF_{200\text{-}1,200}$) in the newer terminology. The terms mean the same. And last of all, notice the incomplete form near the center of the spirogram in which observed and predicted percentages of normal are to be recorded for FVC, $FEV_{1.0}$ and MEFR (or $FEF_{200\text{-}1,200}$).

The spirogram is a recording of a patient's forced expiration. The Vitalor is a simple and inexpensive apparatus. Other convenient devices for recording the forced vital capacity are the Wright Peak Flow Meter and the Puffmeter.

The forced vital capacity (FVC) is the volume of a maximal expiration performed as quickly as possible following a maximal inspiration. This one forced expiration, if measured and timed, yields considerable information regarding the functional capacity of the lungs.

To determine the FVC, ask the patient to stand. Adjust the mouth piece to the level of the patient's mouth or allow her to hold it at her natural level (Fig 11-14). She should not bend over or strain upward toward the mouth piece. Do not allow her to proceed until she has assumed a comfortable stance.

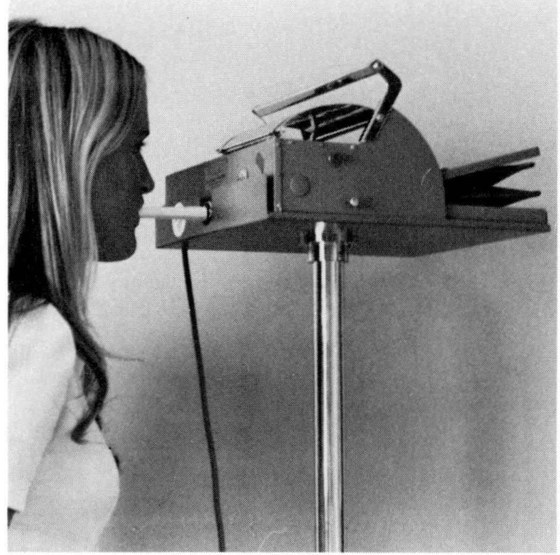

Figure 11-14. Determining forced vital capacity (FVC).

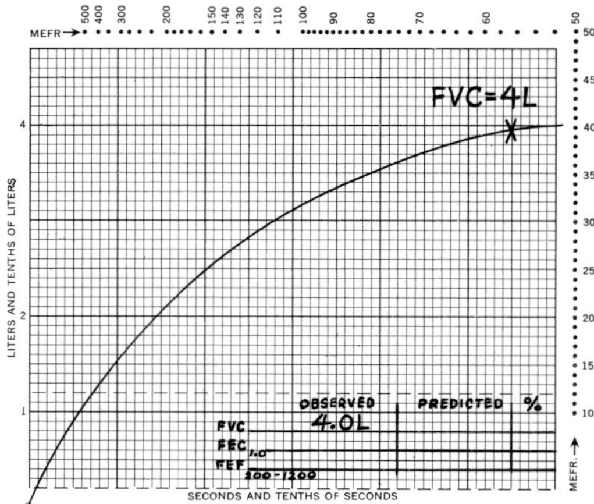

Figure 11-15. Record of FVC on spirogram.

When all is ready, ask her to *completely* fill her lungs with air (forced inspiration) and then to blow *all* her air into the mouth piece as forcefully and rapidly as possible. When she does this, a line is recorded on the spirogram starting at the lower left hand corner and curving upward and across the spirogram to the right side of the graph (Fig 11-15). The line represents 6 seconds of time and measures in L the volume of the patient's expired air.

Near the right margin of the spirogram, the recorded line reaches its peak. The highest point reached is the expiratory volume recorded in liters. This volume is significantly reduced in chronic obstructive lung disease (COLD) caused by the trapping of air in the terminal air sacs. The result is an important standard measurement in evaluating the patient's pulmonary function. Record the finding in the space provided on the spirogram for FVC under *observed* performance. Later it will be compared with a *predicted* performance and the percentage of normal calculated.

Now calculate the Forced Expiratory Volume for 1 sec ($FEV_{1.0}$). For this determination, select and mark off the middle half of the curve. For instance, if the patient has a FVC of 4L, the middle half of this volume would be between 1L and 3L.

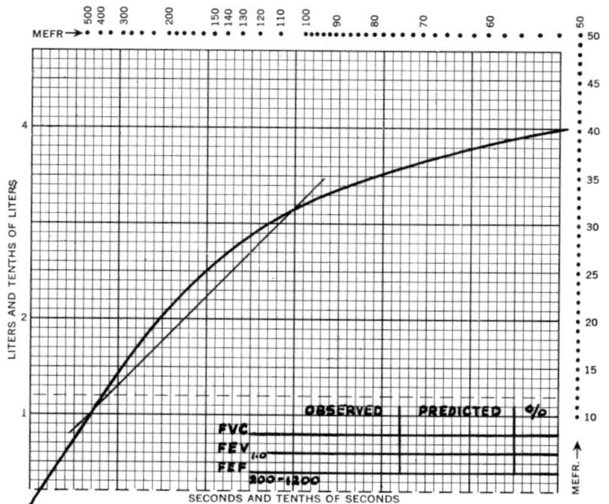

Figure 11-16. Forced expiratory volume for 1 sec ($FEV_{1.0}$)

With a ruler draw a line between the points where the recorded line crosses the 1L and 3L mark (Fig. 11-16).

On this new line, place dots at the 1 and 2 sec vertical lines, thus marking off 1 sec in time. The dots will appear on the 1.3 and 2.3 horizontal L lines (Fig. 11-17).

Now calculate: 2.3 − 1.3 = 1.0L. This figure is the $FEV_{1.0}$—the volume of air exhaled per second during the middle half of expiration. Record this figure on the spirogram as done for FVC.

This is possibly the most valuable clue to the severity of the expiratory airway obstruction. Obtain more information by repeating the test 5 to 10 minutes after

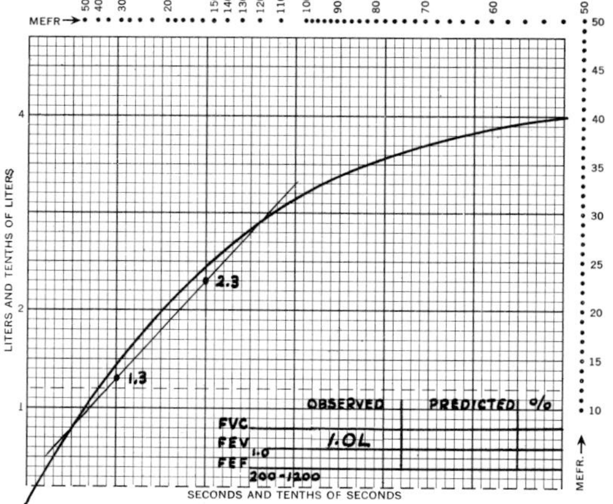

Figure 11-17. $FEV_{1.0}$ = volume of air exhaled/sec during the middle half of expiration.

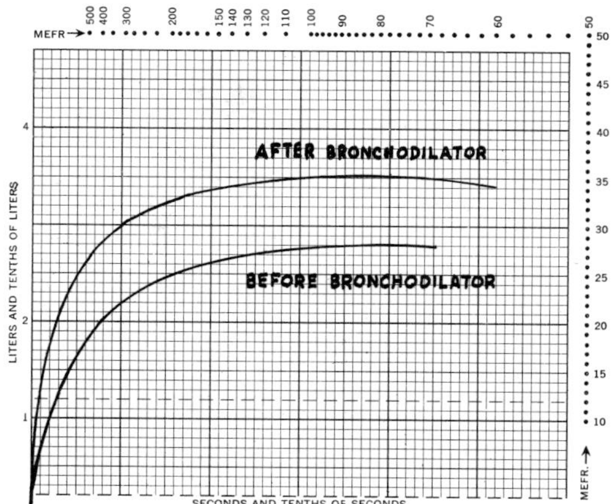

Figure 11-18. FVC before and after the use of a nebulized bronchodilator.

allowing the patient to inhale a nebulized bronchodilator. An increase in either the FVC of $FEV_{1.0}$ of 15 percent is helpful in determining the partial reversibility of expiratory obstruction and whether bronchodilators will be of help (Fig. 11-18). This type of improvement occurs most often in bronchial asthma. COLD shows no such improvement.

Proceed now to calculate the MEFR (maximum expiratory flow rate) now called the $FEF_{200-1,200}$. For this you will use the small numbers about the top and right edge of the spirogram. Again use a ruler and pencil. Make note of the dotted line running horizontally across the spirogram at the 1.2L (1,200 ml) level. With this reference point in mind, establish two points on the spirogram: the first is the dot in the lower left-hand corner and the second is where the tracing bisects the dotted horizontal line. Connect the two points with a ruler but allowing the ruler to extend to the small MEFR numbers printed about the two margins of the spirogram (Fig. 11-19).

The number then found is the $FEF_{200-1,200}$ in L/min. This number is placed in the space on the spirogram marked $FEF_{200-1,200}$ or MEFR. A slowed rate is an early manifestation of COLD. A $FEF_{200-1,200}$ determined by this method is less accurate than if determined by a spirometer. Most physicians, however, do not maintain spirometers in their offices.

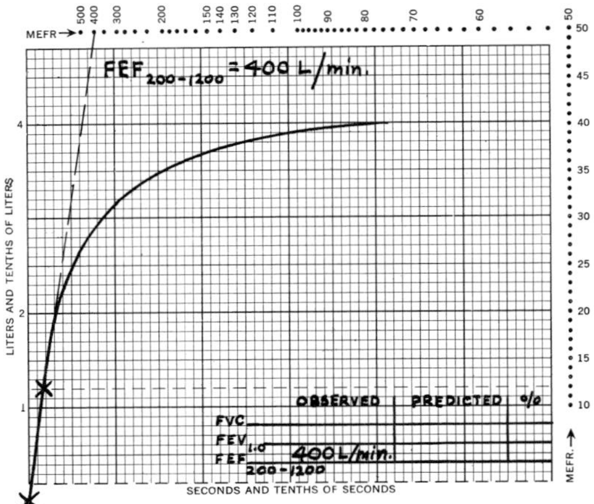

Figure 11-19. Calculations for $FEF_{200-1,200}$, formerly MEFR (maximum expiratory flow rate).

With observed performance now determined and recorded, go about finding what the normal or predicted performance should be for each observed measurement. Obviously, the observed performance without comparison to a norm means little.

Determine the predicted MEFR, $FEV_{1.0}$ and the FVC by reference to the Kory nomograms (as adapted by the National Tuberculosis and Respiratory Disease Association and supplied in the jacket of instructions that accompany the purchase of spirometry equipment). Record of these figures in their appropriate space on the spirogram.

After the observed and predicted performance figures are recorded, calculate the percentage of normal for each. Begin the calculation with the $FEV_{1.0}$.

$$\frac{\text{Observed } FEV_{1.0}}{\text{Predicted } FEV_{1.0}} \times 100\% \text{ of normal } FEV_{1.0}$$

Calculate the FEV and MEFR in the same way using the observed performance as the denominator. Record the results in the appropriate spaces on the spirogram.

These determinations, of course, are not very accurate—the range of normal for people of the same sex, age and height varies as much as 15 percent. Consequently, a person whose predicted FVC performance was 4.4 L may be considered within normal range if she dropped to 4 or even 3.9 L/min. The important point to remember, however, is the significance of a drop, say of a reading of 4.4L 1 year ago to 3.9 now.

A normal person expires at least 83 percent of his FVC in 1 second and 97 percent in 3 seconds. Express the results of ventilatory function tests in volume units such as L, L/min and in percentages. An example: "The patient's $FEV_{1.0}$ is 3.5 L, 106% of the normal $FEV_{1.0}$ predicted by the Kory nomograms" (Fig. 11-20).

Other determinations can be made from the spirogram produced by the simple Vitalor, i.e. vital capacity (VC), forced expiratory volume in T sec ($FEV_{T\%}$), forced expiratory flow in percent ($FEF_{25-75\%}$). These figures add little or nothing to what can be deducted from the FVC, $FEV_{1.0}$ or the $FEF_{200-1,200}$. If you care to purchase a spirometer, a determination of the maximum voluntary ventilation (MVV) may add significant information. But if you need more information than can be found on the above tests, the wise course would be to refer the patient to a pulmonary function laboratory. The tests described here, however, are adequate for the evaluation of lung function in the great majority of patients. More important than any one test would be finding progressively greater impairment on annual examination as done in the family physician's office.

In their manual for physicians, the

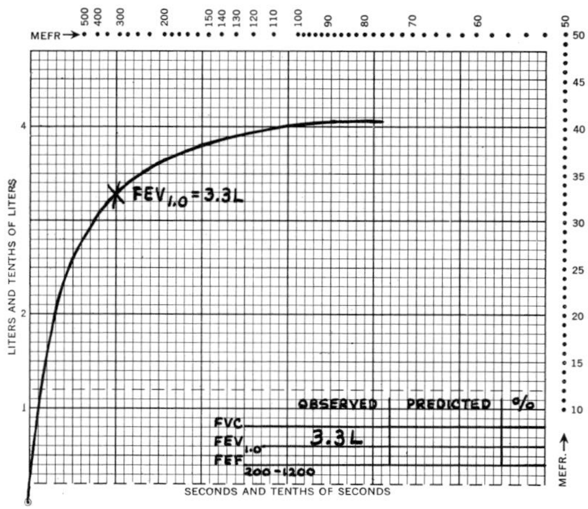

Figure 11-20. Forced expiratory volume ($FEV_{1.0}$).

National Tuberculosis and Respiratory Disease Association advises more extensive testing for the following types of patients:

–those hospitalized because of complications of COLD
–those with diagnostic problems
–those proposed for thoracotomy and/or pulmonary resection
–those presenting medicolegal problems
–those whose history and testing appear unreliable
–those suspected of having an alveolar-capillary block as in diffuse fibrosing pulmonary disease.

Primary Diffusing Capacity

Without careful diagnostic tests, emphysema patients are often hastily diagnosed as having congestive heart failure. For detection of obstructive disorders of the pulmonary circulation, order a pulmonary diffusion capacity test. Decrease in pulmonary diffusion may be the earliest finding in collagen disease, sarcoidosis and in such industrial diseases as asbestosis. Use the test to determine whether the pulmonary capillaries are blocked by emboli.

The test is easily done and is safe for the patient, but its performance requires a trained technician and expensive equipment. All the patient need do is take a breath of carbon monoxide, hold his breath 10 seconds and exhale. The test plus the calculations can all be done in 10 minutes.

The determination of pulmonary diffusion capacity is useful in patients who are dyspneic but have a normal vital capacity and a normal maximal expiratory flow rate. The test is harmless. Use it repeatedly to evaluate treatment or to document the progress of the disease.

Other Pulmonary Function Tests

Single-breath oxygen tests are useful in screening large segments of the population, especially those working in hazardous trades. Abnormal results indicate that not all portions of the lungs are filling and emptying properly.

The single-breath Xenon test can locate pulmonary lesions geographically. Test results may help pinpoint the location of bullae before surgery. The test is done by asking the patient to inhale gas containing Xe^{133}. A detector records the distribution of counts from both lungs. Radiation exposure is similar to that of a chest x-ray.

Purpose of Pulmonary Function Tests

Pulmonary function tests have the following uses:

–early detection of pulmonary or cardiopulmonary diseases such as emphysema, pulmonary fibrosis and pulmonary vascular disease
–to aid in the differential diagnosis on dyspneic patients
–to detect and outline the location and size of regional lung disease
–to evaluate the patient before intra- or extrathoracic surgery
–to detect early respiratory failure
–to monitor patients in acute respiratory care units
–to evaluate, periodically, the worker in a hazardous occupation
–to check on the efficacy of treatment
–to determine the risks of performing other diagnostic procedures

A diagnostic procedure illustrating the latter is Ethiodol, a radiopaque medium, to outline lymphatic vessels. The use of this may temporarily block some capillaries. It is wise to establish the patient's pulmonary diffusion capacity before its administration.

Bedside Match Test for Respiratory Function

Usually the vital capacity is reduced in emphysema. To determine this use a simple match test: Detach and light a match from a standard paper matchbook. When the match is burning steadily, hold it 6 inches from the patient's open mouth. Ask the patient to take a deep breath, hold his mouth wide open and attempt to blow the match out. Do not allow the patient to purse his lips.

Interpretation: Of the patients who have a 1 second vital capacity of less than 1.6 L, 85 percent cannot blow the match out. Of the patients who have a maximum breathing capacity of less than 60 L per minute, 80 percent will be unable to blow the match out.

Bedside Inspection of Sputum

Sputum cannot be examined properly by observing it in a tissue. Collect sputum in a paper sputum cup kept at the patient's bedside. Ask the patient to collect all sputum for 24 hours. No foreign bodies as ashes or cigarette stubs should contaminate the specimen.

Check for color, turbidity, viscosity and odor. Place some sputum in a Petri dish and search for caseous material, Dittrick's plugs, Curschmann's spirals and bronchial casts.

Interpretation: Small amounts of purulent sputum colored green, gray or yellow indicate a resolving pneumonia. Large amounts of fetid sputum accompany lung abscess or bronchiectasis; in the latter the amount of sputum may amount to 200 to 500 ml per day. When it is allowed to stand, it may separate into three layers with mucus on top, clear liquid in the middle and pus on the bottom.

Bloody sputum may appear as blood streaked, bloody or pink. If the sputum is only blood streaked, look elsewhere for the source of the blood, i.e. nose, nasopharynx, etc. If the sputum is pink, suspect mixing of blood and secretions in smaller bronchioles as in pulmonary edema or pneumonia.

Massive bleeding occurs in lung abscess, tubercular cavities, bronchiectasis, pulmonary infarction and embolism, broncheogenic carcinoma and actinomycotic and blastomycotic abscesses.

Currant-jelly sputum is almost pathognomonic for Klebsiella pneumoniae or Type III pneumococcus.

Prune-juice sputum is frequently produced by pneumococcal pneumonias.

Frothy sputum, with or without blood tinge, is typically produced by pulmonary edema.

AEROSOL METHOD. Not everyone with lung disease can produce sputum at will. Recently a satisfactory method of collecting sputum by utilizing an aerosol pump was introduced. The pump is used to nebulize hypertonic saline and prophylene glycol, which the patient inhales. The solution results in the production of bronchial secretions and the urge to cough. This method of collection is more satisfactory than those induced spontaneously. The usual time required to obtain the specimen is 10 to 20 minutes. Three deep-cough sputum specimens can provide 90 percent of lung cancer diagnosis when this technique produces satisfactory specimens.

Treatment

Communicate to the patient your interest and desire to aid him. It is not widely appreciated that COLD commonly manifests itself in mental depression which is hard to recognize. Good communication between you and your patient will be the only way depression can be recognized and treated. A family physician may not be able to cure COLD, but there is no reason to allow the patient to develop hopelessness and despair. Explain to the patient that the aim of treatment is to preserve existing lung function and to help him adapt to the limitations of the disease.

The wise physician will encourage activities within the limits of fatigue and dyspnea. Keep his weight a little below his ideal weight. Generally counsel against changing residences in search of a better climate. However COLD patients are less dyspneic in altitudes under 5,000 feet. In your effort to help the COLD patient, do not waste time or money for allergy testing and desensitization unless there is definite evidence of bronchospasm relieved by bronchodilator therapy. COLD patients who wheeze only on arising, during exertion or during respiratory infections cannot be expected to benefit from stock or autogenous bacterial vaccines.

Help the patient avoid smoking. No medication or therapeutic scheme can do as much to relieve symptoms as putting an end to smoking. Mere reduction of smoking is not enough. Patients must stop just as surely as a patient with alcoholic cirrhosis must stop drinking. Often patients continue smoking because the doctor's attitude toward smoking is too permissive. Avoid other irritants either of the industrial type or of the polluted atmosphere.

Bronchodilator drugs give symptomatic relief. Urge their use if spirometric evaluation confirms their effectiveness. Oral medication is preferred because aerosol inhalers are usually overused. If the patient can be relied upon to control this abuse, nebulized isoproterenol (Isuprel) or epinephrine can be a helpful and handy way to control symptoms. Instruct the patient in the proper use of the equipment. The usual dose is two deep inhalations taken 3 or 4 times daily but in no event more often than every hour. Advise the patient to take the first dose on arising to help loosen the tenacious secretions accumulated during the night. Change to another drug if tolerance develops from overuse.

Intravenous aminophylline is a good remedy for treating bronchospasm. The dose: ½ to 1 g given very slowly intravenously. A more acceptable way is to mix the total dosage with 500 to 1,000 ml glucose and give as an intravenous infusion. Consider giving aminophylline with or without ephedrine as a retention enema or as a suppository. Continued use, however, irritates the rectum and limits its value.

Intermittent positive pressure breathing (IPPB) is ideally suited for the hospital treatment of respiratory failure. Order IPPB to treat pre- and postoperative respiratory complications caused by retained or tenacious bronchial secretions following intervals of hypoventilation. IPPB equipment permits the choice of administering oxygen, air-oxygen mixtures under pressure with or without nebulization of a bronchodilator or a mucolytic or wetting agent. Before ordering permanent home treatment with IPPB equipment, have the patient rent the machine for a month. This therapeutic trial will help you and your patient decide whether the time and expense involved is a worthwhile treatment. Use of the equipment in your office is usually impractical because of the inconvenience, fatigue and expense of several visits daily. Wherever it is used, detailed instructions for its use by yourself or a trained technician is essential.

Whenever a technician is employed to administer the treatment, a physician should write the prescription. Specify:

- –how many times a day the treatment is to be given (average 3 to 4 times daily)
- –how long each treatment is to last (10 to 15 min)
- –what air mixture to use and what percentage (40 percent oxygen is common but can be increased or decreased)
- –how much pressure (Start with 10 to 12 cm of water pressure and gradually adjust to the patient's tolerance. Higher pressures can be used when it would appear beneficial to shorten the time because of fatigue. A respiratory rate of 10 to 12 respirations per minute is most effective.)
- –what bronchodilator to use (isoproternol 1:200 solution is common, 3 to 6 drops (0.2 to 0.4 ml) for each treatment)
- –what wetting agent to use (besides proprietary detergents on the market, 1 or 2 ml of normal saline, 25 percent alcohol or vodka may be used)

Adjust all these variables as needed and as the patient's response is evaluated.

Postural Drainage

If coughing proves insufficient to evacuate sputum, it often helps to have the patient assume postural drainage positions. The goal of this positioning is to make use of gravity to compensate for the impaired mucociliary apparatus that normally propels secretions from more distal airways to the large proximal ones.

Effective drainage of the entire tracheobronchial tree can usually be obtained by utilizing seven basic positions, with appropriate modifications to meet the needs, limitations and response of the individual patient. The basic postural drainage positions are left lateral decubitus Trendelenburg position (Fig. 11-21A), right lateral decubitus Trendelenburg position (Fig. 11-21B), prone Trendelenburg position (Fig. 11-21C), supine Trendelenburg position (Fig. 11-21D), lateral decubitus position (Fig. 11-21E), horizontal prone position (Fig. 11-21F) and horizontal supine position (Fig. 11-21G). A postural drainage position should be maintained for 10 to 15 minutes and should be accompanied and followed by coughing before another position is assumed.

The efficacy of postural drainage techniques is frequently greatly augmented by the use of chest percussion or clapping. The latter consists of rapid forceful repetitive vibration of the chest with cupped hands. If done by an experienced physical therapist, chest percussion is often effective in loosening tenacious secretions. If done properly, chest percussion is not painful. Although considerable practice is required to achieve proficiency with the technique, the patient's

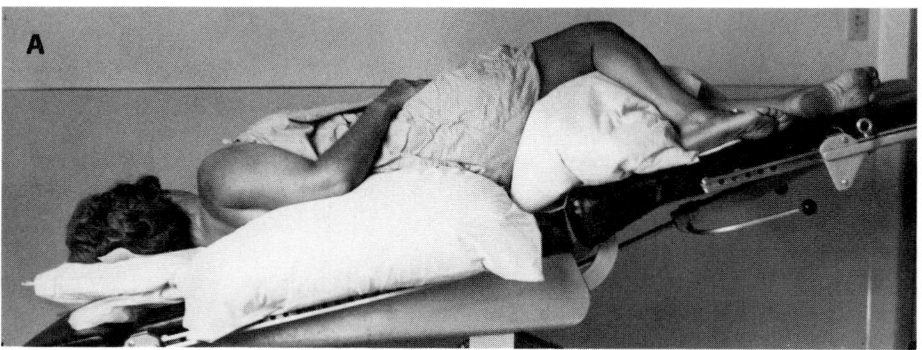

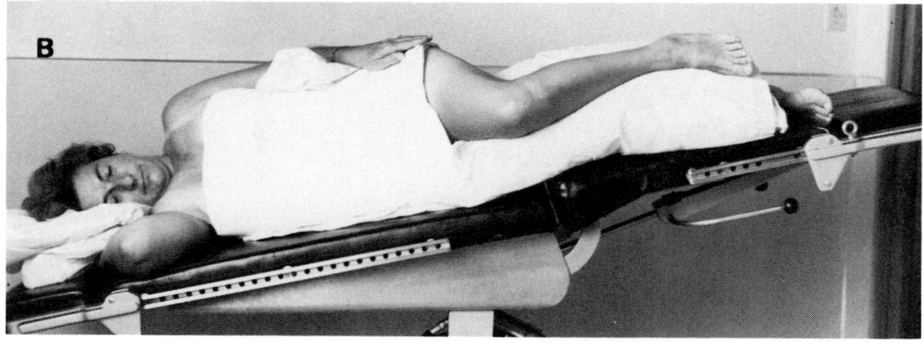

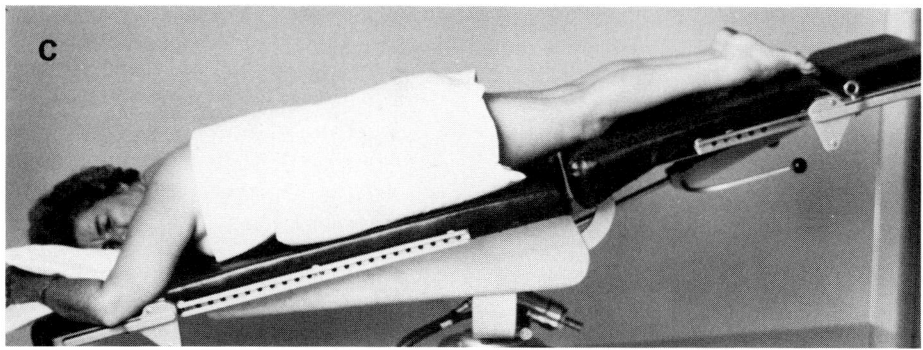

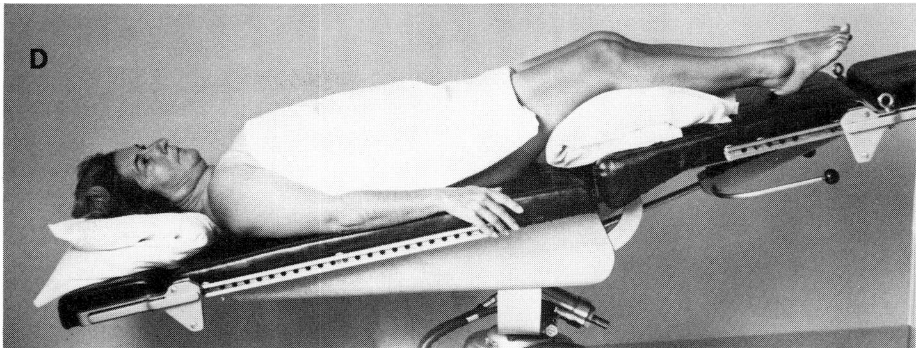

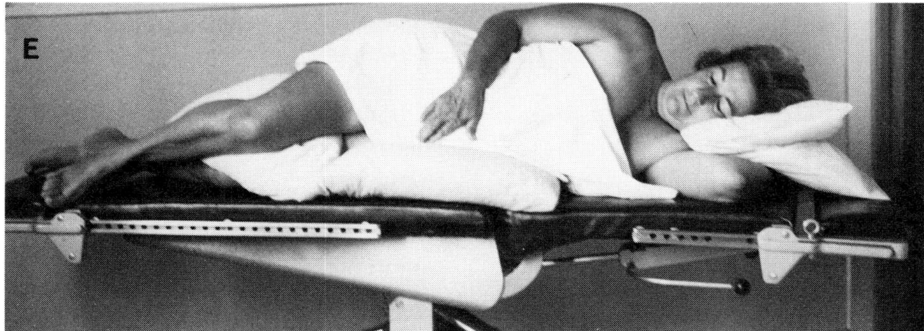

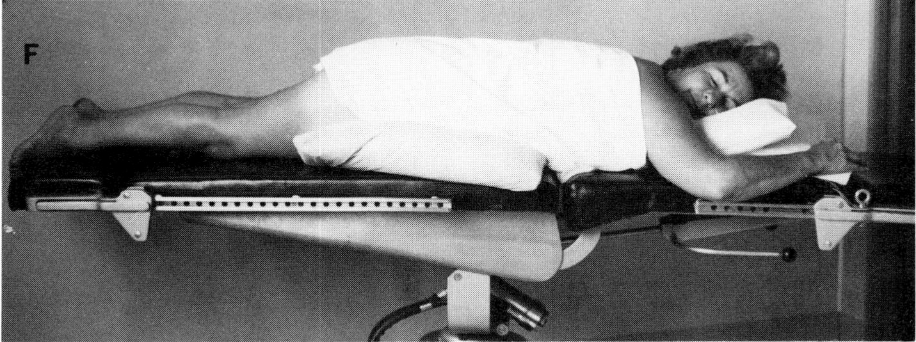

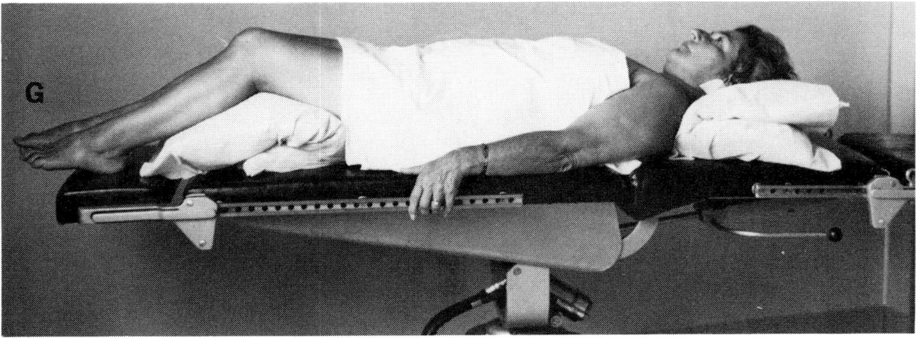

Figure 11-21. Basic postural drainage positions: *A*, Left lateral decubitus (Trendelenburg) position; *B*, Right lateral decubitus (Trendelenburg) position; *C*, Prone Trendelenburg position; *D*, Supine Trendelenburg position; *E*, Lateral decubitus position; *F*, Horizontal prone position; *G*, Horizontal supine position.

spouse is often able to master it or the patient may learn to apply percussion to his own chest.

Prevention of COLD Complications

The patient should be advised to take the following precautions in order to avoid complications:

- –dress warmly and avoid becoming chilled
- –maintain an equitable temperature in the home
- –during cold weather, maintain adequate humidification
- –seek influenza vaccination annually
- –avoid prolonged exposure to high levels of atmospheric pollution
- –stop smoking
- –seek treatment at the onset of any URI
- –make a point to keep all dental and mouth infections to a minimum
- –avoid crowds when respiratory infections are prevalent

Specific Treatment of COLD

The most common cause of tenacious sputum is inadequate hydration. Consequently urge the patient to increase his fluid intake to 3 L per day. Steam and liquid aerosol inhalations are helpful. The heated steam nebulizers available at any drug store are satisfactory. Urge their use, particularly at the onset of any respiratory infection or whenever the sputum volume decreases or suddenly becomes purulent. An old time remedy to liquify sticky sputum is saturated solution of potassium iodide, 10 drops four times daily in a little milk or juice to suit the patient's taste. Watch and discontinue if skin irritation appears.

Recommend courses of antibiotics depending on the patient's need. For home use, give the broad spectrum antibiotics, i.e. tetracycline or ampicillin. For hospital use, administer aqueous crystalline penicillin. At the onset of a cold, order tetracycline 250 mg four times daily for 20 days to prevent Diplococcus pneumoniae or Hemophilus influenzae infection. In severe cases, it is wise to give the patient a prophylactic antibiotic each time other household members get an upper respiratory infection. Many physicians now prescribe the intermittent routine administration of antibiotics the year round or in severe winter climates during the winter months. In this situation tetracycline 250 mg twice daily would be sufficient given the first of each month.

As a rough rule, COLD patients who develop acute bronchitis have a viral infection while those with pneumonia have a bacterial one. Identify any bacterial infection by sputum smear and culture. Do sensitivity testing if staphylococci or gram-negative bacilli are the incriminating organisms. Use penicillin for gram-positive diplococci resembling pneumococci. For straphlococci, use cloxacillin (Tegopen) or methicillin (Straphcillin). For gram-negative infections, start with cephalothin (Keflin) or kanamycin (Kantrex).

For any bacterial infections complicating COLD, begin treatment early and continue for a week. Shorter periods may give a temporary respite from the infection but recurrences are frequent and more resistant to further antibiotic therapy. In patients who do not respond quickly, select another antibiotic or combination of antibiotics after reviewing cultures and antibiotic sensitivity reports.

Antibiotic schedule: (Pen-Vee, V-cillin) Oral penicillin-V, 250 mg every 4 to 6 hours or phenethicillin (Syncillin, Maxipen) 250 mg every eight hours. If patient is penicillin sensitive, use erythromycin (Erythrocin, Ilotycin) 250 mg every 6 hours orally. Intramuscular penicillin: Crysticillin G, 100,000 units stat and procaine G 300,000 units. May give up to 10,000,000 units daily.

Oral oxacillin (Prostaphlin or Resistopen) or cloxacillin (Tegopen) 250 mg plus probenecid, 500 mg every 6 hours.

Intramuscular methicillin (Staphcillin or Dimocillin) 1 g every 4 to 6 hours.

Kanamycin (Kantrex) 15 to 20 mg/kg IM daily or cephalothin (Keflin) 500 mg every 4 to 6 hours IM.

Polymyxin B (Aerosporin) 1.5 to 2.5 mg/kg daily IM.

Steroids are not often helpful to the patient with COLD unless he has a 10 to 15 percent eosinophilia in the sputum and blood. In acute respiratory failure, steroids often prove helpful if given for 2 weeks. Start with 40 mg prednisone daily. Reduce gradually to 10 mg daily; find the smallest therapeutic dose even if tablets must be broken into halves or quarters to do so. If prolonged therapy is anticipated, give a tuberculin test to the patient. Also take care not to reactivate an old peptic ulcer.

Do not deny oxygen therapy to patients with severe respiratory insufficiency. Do supervise its use. Start with a nasal catheter or open mask and a low flow rate—2 L/min. Increase rate by 1 L/min/day if needed. Obviously give oxygen to all patients who are cyanotic or in respiratory distress.

Use digitalis with great caution. Toxic levels can be disastrous. If the patient is fibrillating or has some independent left ventricular disease, order a digitoxin preparation.

Attempt to relieve a nonproductive, paroxysmal cough by expectorant cough mixtures. If tolerated, the saturated solution of potassium iodide given regularly may liquify the secretions and soothe the cough. Enseals of ammonium chloride, 1 to 2 Enseals 3 to 4 times daily can be used similarly. As to ordinary cough mixtures, the guaiacolate derivatives and the elixir of terpin hydrate appear to be beneficial.

Do not prescribe formulations with antihistamines in them. Their drying effect on already tenacious sputum may be enough to put the patient in the hospital.

There is one recent report that when epinephrine, aminophylline, steroids, antibiotics and oxygen fail there may be rather dramatic hope in administering intravenous sodium bicarbonate. In one short series, patients were relieved in 30 to 60 minutes after receiving 90 to 240 mEq of bicarbonate.[7]

Do not overlook the value of humidifying the patient's room, especially when symptoms of infection supervene. Any method to increase the moisture in the air is helpful —a cold vapor apparatus, an ultrasonic nebulizer or a thermostatically controlled water heater. This method of loosening secretions has proven effective. There is controversy over the usefulness of mucolytic agents. If you believe a nebulized mucolytic agent might help try Mucomyst (n-acetylcysteine).

Breathing Exercises for COLD

If the patient learns to breathe properly he or she will find it easier to live with his or her COLD. The following exercises and illustrations are of value to you in teaching the COLD patient how to breathe.

Place the patient in a supine position with her left hand on her chest and her right on her abdomen above the navel. Teach the patient to breathe in and out using the diaphragm only. Ask her to fill her lungs with air without allowing her chest to expand or her left hand to rise. Her hand on her abdomen will rise as she inhales and press up and in when she exhales (Fig. 11-22). Her hand on her chest will remain quiet. She should keep her mouth closed while inhaling

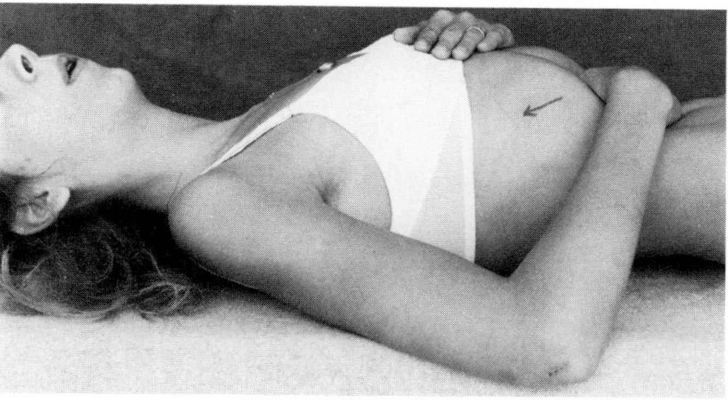

Figure 11-22. While the patient is in proper position she should inhale through her nose and exhale through pursed lips as if whistling.

through her nose but she should exhale through pursed lips as if whistling. Pursing the lips shows the flow of air and allows for more complete emptying of the lungs. Exhaling takes about twice the time as inhaling. While she is exhaling have her push inward and upward with the right hand, assisting the diaphragm in emptying air from the lungs. Have her repeat the exercise four times a day for 10 min at a time. This is the basic breathing pattern. When she has mastered the exercise while lying flat ask her to practice the same exercise while sitting up (Fig. 11-23). If the patient loses control on this basic breathing pattern ask her to stop and recover the breathing pattern. This type of breathing should become automatic.

Another exercise to reinforce the basic breathing pattern is done while the patient is lying on the floor with her knees flexed as far as possible (Fig. 11-24). Repeat the above exercise, again having her use her right hand to assist the diaphragm in expelling air through pursed lips.

Still lying on the floor with knees flexed, the patient locks her arms around her knees as shown. As she exhales through pursed lips have her draw her feet off the floor and pull her knees toward her chest as far as possible (Fig. 11-25). This applies more pressure against her diaphragm and forces air from her lungs. On inhalation she should return her feet to the floor. Repeat the exercise 6 to 8 times.

Have the patient attempt to continue the

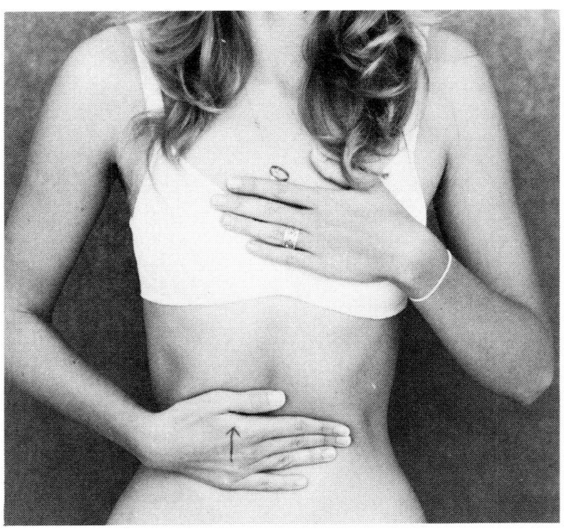

Figure 11-23. Ask her to practice the same exercise while sitting up.

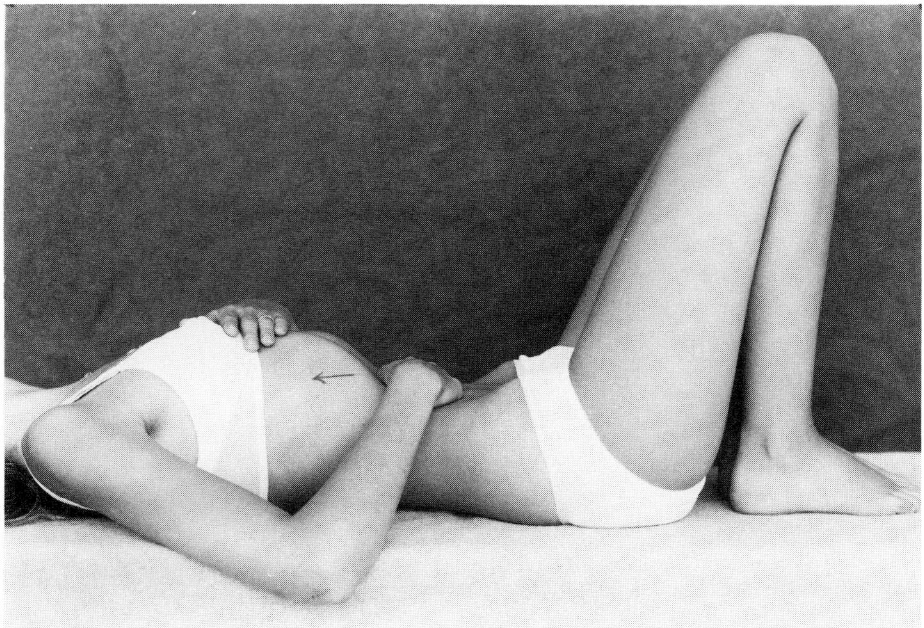

Figure 11-24. While the patient is lying on the floor with her knees flexed have her breathe as in Figure 11-22 with the right hand assisting the diaphragm in expelling air.

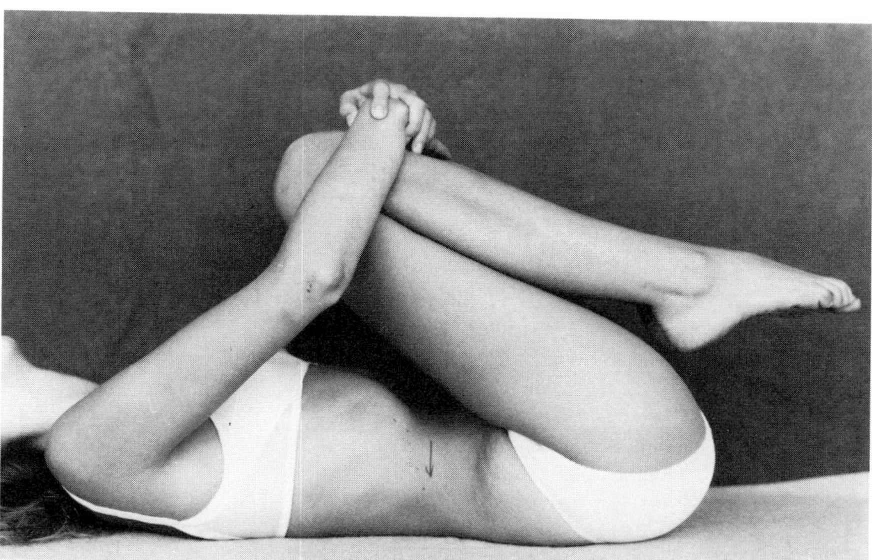

Figure 11-25. Again, while on the floor, the patient locks her arms around her flexed knees. She draws her feet off the floor and pulls her knees toward her chest as she exhales. On inhalation she returns her feet to the floor.

basic breathing pattern while standing and walking (Fig. 11-26). Insist that she inhale through her nose and exhale through pursed lips.

Raise the foot of the bed about 14 in above the head. The easiest way is to put one or two straight chairs under the footboard. Take away all pillows. Place a 5 lb weight on the patient's abdomen and have her practice the basic breathing exercise (Fig. 11-27). Fill a hot water bottle with 5 lb of sand or shot for a weight. As the patient tolerates the weight gradually increase it to 15 lb.

The final exercise is done with a 5 ft long, 3 to 4 in wide, tightly woven band. It should be stiff so it will hold its shape rather than crumple. Have the seated patient put the belt around her waist, crossing it in the back and stretching it out at the sides with her hands (Fig. 11-28). Now have her do the basic breathing exercises, letting the band out as she inhales and tightening it as she exhales. She should do the exercise rhythmically, allowing the band to glide evenly while maintaining a constant pressure. Do the same exercise with the band while standing. Have the patient practice repeatedly until she can do it without concentrating on it. This exercise can also be done without the band. Ask the patient to place her hands on her body with her thumbs to her back and her extended fingers over her lower ribs and abdomen. Compress during exhalation and relax during inspiration.

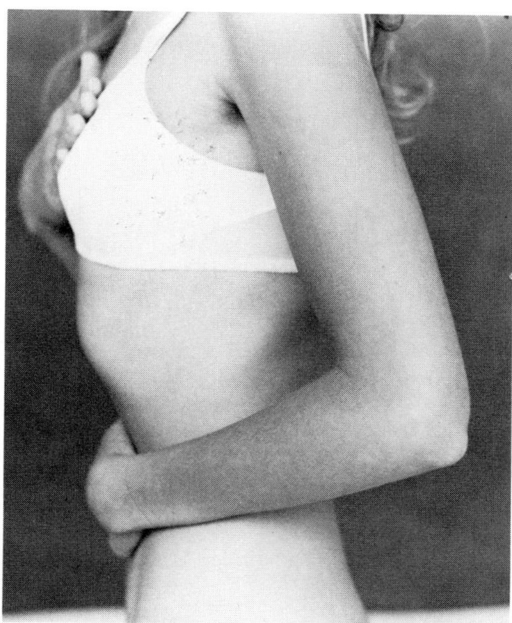

Figure 11-26. The patient continues the basic breathing pattern while standing and walking.

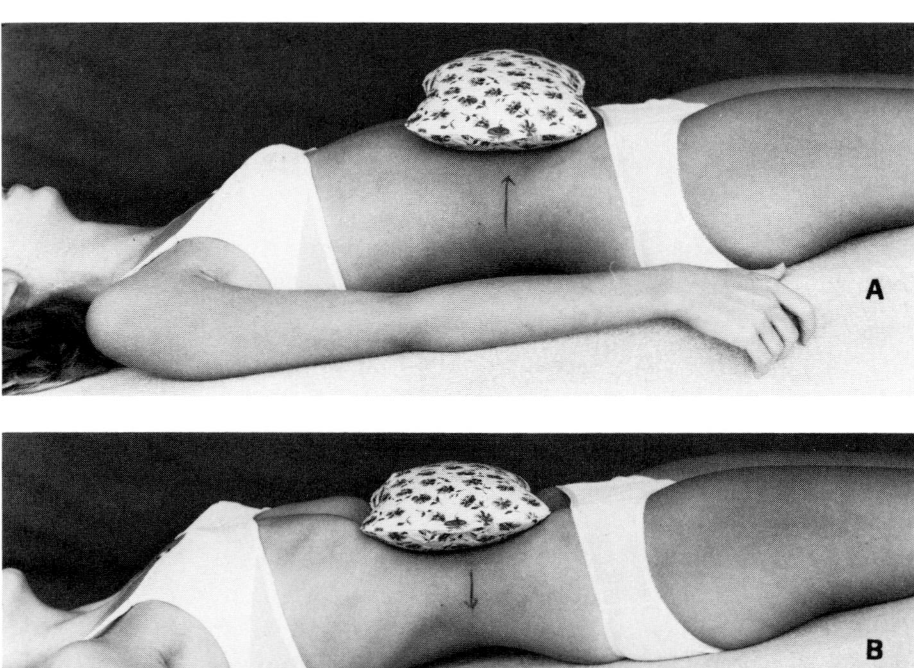

Figure 11-27. *A*, The patient inhales with a 5 lb weight on her abdomen and, *B*, exhales.

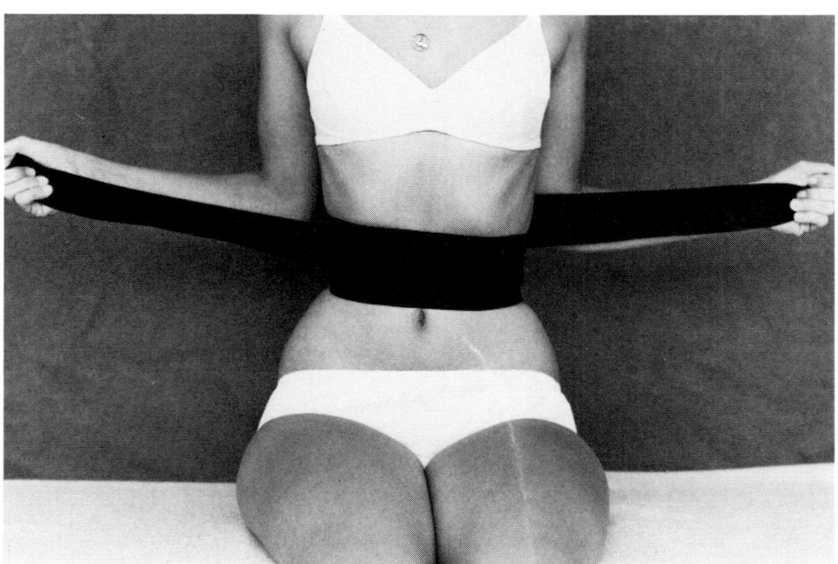

Figure 11-28. Have the patient sit with a 5 ft long, 3 to 4 in wide, band around her waist as illustrated. She lets the band out as she inhales and tightens it as she exhales.

Disability Retirement

The Social Security Administration in its booklet "Disability Evaluation under Social Security" defines disability as the inability to work because of a physical or mental impairment that has lasted or is expected to last at least 12 months or is expected to result in death. The booklet points out that disability need not be permanent. The disability need only be expected to last 1 year.

You will not be able to document your patient's pulmonary insufficiency solely with your office Vitalor. The Social Security criteria includes a report on the patient's maximum voluntary ventilation (MVV) or maximum breathing capacity (MBC) as well as his 1 sec forced expiratory volume ($FEV_{1.0}$). The last can be done on your office Vitalor; the first two require special equipment that family physicians do not usually maintain in their offices.

The equipment consists of a Venturi tube device through which the patient breathes rapidly. This is connected to a rubber balloon filled with a measured amount of air. The amount of air the patient can remove from the balloon in 15 sec is measured and the value for the MVV is obtained from a table accompanying the equipment.

In your report incorporate an appropriately labeled spirometric tracing showing distance per sec on the abscissa and the distance per L on the ordinate. The paper speed to record the $FEV_{1.0}$ should be sufficiently fast for measurement of volume to the nearest 0.1 L. Record the height of the patient. Do not submit test results obtained during or soon after an acute respiratory illness. If wheezing is present on auscultation of the chest, repeat and record the test after giving a nebulized bronchodilator. You must also appraise and report the patient's ability to understand the directions and his cooperation in performing the test. Nothing is left to your judgment.

Verify the patient's impairment of chronic obstructive airway disease (chronic bronchitis, chronic asthmatic bronchitis or pulmonary emphysema with or without abnormal x-ray findings) by submitting MVV and $FEV_{1.0}$ findings equal to or less than the standards in Table 11-1.

Table 11-1.

Height (in)	*MVV equal to or below L/M*	*FEV_1 equal to or < L*
57−	32	1.0
58	33	1.0
59	34	1.0
60	35	1.1
61	36	1.1
62	37	1.1
63	38	1.1
64	39	1.2
65	40	1.2
66	41	1.2
67	42	1.3
68	43	1.3
69	44	1.3
70	45	1.4
71	46	1.4
72	47	1.4
73+	48	1.4

Evaluation of Diffuse Pulmonary Fibrotic Disease

Use a different criteria to report the diffuse pulmonary fibrotic diseases. These include sarcoidosis, Hamman-Rich syndrome and interstitial fibrosis. The report must include vital capacity, arterial pCO_2 and a simultaneous arterial CO_2 saturation, plus diffusing capacity of the lungs for carbon monoxide. The standards which the patient must meet in all three categories are recorded in the previously mentioned "Disability Evaluation under Social Security."

Evaluation in Pulmonary Tuberculosis

Base your evaluation on:

–positive culture on guinea pig innoculation or sputum obtained more than 3 mo after onset of disability
–serial x-rays of lesion of increasing size more than 3 months after onset of disability
–disease far advanced with cavitation and positive culture on guinea pig innocula-

tion obtained at any time following disability
–impairment of pulmonary function as outlined above for chronic obstructive airway and/or fibrotic diseases

ACUTE RESPIRATORY FAILURE (ARF; ACUTE VENTILATORY FAILURE)

ARF occurs whenever the physiologic mechanisms for gas exchange between the atmosphere and body tissues no longer meet metabolic needs. In COLD, ARF may be precipitated by general anesthesia, oversedation, administration of 100 percent oxygen, pulmonary edema, pulmonary thromboembolism, pneumothorax, chest injury, atelectasis or bronchopulmonic infections.

The causes of ARF in patients without COLD may be classified as *primary* as in idiopathic central alveolar hypoventilation and Ondine's curse or *secondary,* hypoventilation from central and peripheral causes. Central depression of the respiratory center occurs from increased intracranial pressure, drugs, trauma and anesthetics. Peripheral diseases that can cause secondary hypoventilation are lung diseases, diseases affecting respiratory muscles and diseases which create a limitation of movement in the thorax.

Ordinarily the body is very sensitive to small changes in pCO_2. A small increase in pCO_2 will double or triple alveolar ventilations. This sensitivity is lost in the above disease states.

When you first see an ARF patient early in the disease he will be dyspneic, cyanotic, alert but apprehensive. Your first inclination will be to treat him as a patient with congestive heart failure with a respiratory infection. If you direct your treatment toward the heart failure and give morphine or a barbiturate, the patient becomes confused, drowsy and may finally lapse into coma. At the bedside in an emergency situation this can easily happen. Even the EKG may be misleading with evidence of myocardial ischemia, right heart strain and various arrhythmias.

ARF is tricky in other ways. The average physician does not perceive cyanosis until the oxygen saturation is below 85 percent. This decrease in pO_2 causes symptoms in the central nervous system and the heart—a tendency toward hypotension, tachycardia and right ventricular hypertrophy and failure. Therefore, blood gas monitoring is essential.

The symptoms from increasing pCO_2 are difficult to distinguish from pO_2 deficiency. But even a 5 to 10 mm Hg increase above the patient's usual level may cause symptoms of drowsiness, confusion, tremors, convulsions and increased cerebrospinal pressure with papilledema.

A study of the blood gases will show the patient is in respiratory acidosis. If detected early, the patient's hypoxemia and hypercapnia can be corrected by voluntary hyperventilation or by 100 percent oxygen administration. Exercise demonstrates very well that these patients have lost their sensitivity and physiologic response to the stimulus of mounting pCO_2. The only mechanism now left to them to simulate gas exchange is the lowering pO_2. But, on the other hand, when pO_2 falls to 26 to 32 mm Hg and arterial oxygen saturation to 60 to 74 percent, lactate begins to accumulate and metabolic acidosis is added to the respiratory acidosis. A pO_2 below 20 mm is not consistent with life.

Now you are caught between maintaining a pO_2 low enough to stimulate breathing yet high enough to prevent severe and complicated acidosis. Clinically this means that oxygen should be given promptly but only enough to maintain pO_2 at 50 to 65 mm Hg. Watch it. Monitoring is essential in this critical state. Changes of 5 percent in inspired oxygen have been found to increase carbon dioxide retention.

The key, therefore, in administering oxygen is to watch the pCO_2. If it is normal or near normal, oxygen can be given without producing hypoventilation. In an acute emergency situation, oxygen administration should proceed carefully, step-by-step, as indicated by 30 to 60 min checks of the pCO_2 As long as the pCO_2 holds steady, oxygen administration may be increased. If the pCO_2 increases, decrease a hold on oxygen consumption. Remember, more than 24 hr of high oxygen (50 to 100 percent) inhalation creates pathologic changes in the bronchial tree including the terminal alveoli. Humidification of inspired gases is essential.

The nasal catheter and cannula administration of oxygen is sufficient to relieve hypoxemia even if given at 3 L/minute. But these methods do not allow for the fine adjustment in oxygen concentration which the Venturi mask does.

To monitor pH, pCO_2 and pO_2 effectively your first decision will be the choosing of the method of arterial monitoring. Does the patient's condition allow for an occasional arterial "stick" perhaps daily, or is the situation critical enough to need gas studies every 30 to 60 minutes? In the latter event, the monitoring should be done by taping an arterial needle in place.

First estimation: If the pCO_2 is 50 mm Hg or lower, ordinary concentrations of oxygen administration can proceed without danger. If the pCO_2 is 50 or above, give oxygen with care. Start with 1 L/min via nasal cannula or catheter. Recheck the pCO_2 and pO_2 in 1 hour. If there is no significant increase in pCO_2 and the pO_2 has risen to 50 to 65 you are doing all right. Continue as you are. If the pO_2 is still low, increase the flow of oxygen to 2 L/min and recheck blood gases in another hour. Continue these checks hourly, increasing the flow rate as indicated until the pCO_2 and pO_2 are right for the patient.

Administer other medications as outlined under COLD treatment.

If the above described oxygen administration does not relieve the patient, start intermittent positive pressure breathing (IPPB). This adds another factor, however, which requires even closer monitoring. If the patient is apneic or uncooperative, IPPB must be controlled by automatically cycling the machinery. Otherwise, simple assistance will be all that is necessary. If more than simple assistance is needed, you need help too. Call for consultation. If no speciality help is available, an anesthesiologist is your best bet. In fact, you may need both.

IPPB can change blood gas concentration rapidly and strikingly. The use of IPPB in patients who are less than critically ill is controversial. The treatments have advantages but also several dangers. Excessive ventilation may result in severe respiratory alkalosis with its train of complicating factors. It is reported to cause a decrease in cardiac output, to rupture alveoli blebs, introduce infection into the pulmonary tract and lead to dependency. It is essential in the critically ill patient. Be conservative in its use otherwise.

Be on the alert for the following at any stage of ARF:

–a clear airway
–cardiac failure
–pulmonary infections
–electrolyte and fluid imbalance

Watch for the need of tracheal suction, endotracheal intubation or tracheostomy. Watch for ECG and treat failure as customary. A venesection will help if the hematocrit is above 60. Get sputum smears, cultures and sensitivity checks for pulmonary infections. Take roentgenograms of the lungs even if only a portable machine is available. Chart fluid intake and output and potassium p.r.n. Give sodium bicarbonate IV for refractory acidosis.

ACID-BASE IMBALANCE*

A family physician should know the theory underlying acid-base balance. The study of two books will accomplish this purpose: Winters RW, Acid-Base Physiology in Medicine, Cleveland: London Co., 1969; Rooth G, Introduction to Acid-Base and Electrolyte Balance, New York: Harper & Row, 1969. Family physicians do not encounter acid-base problems so frequently that the refinements of the Henderson-Hasselbalch equation can be immediately recalled.

For practical purposes, remember the following. Normal values for arterial blood: pH = 7.35 to 7.45. Any figure above 7.4 is

*Some of the ideas for this section were adapted from a programmed computer course on acid-base imbalance designed by Michael A. Bowser, Dept. of Respiratory Therapy, Grassmont Hospital, La Mesa, Calif. Used with the permission of Mr. Bowser.

considered to represent an alkaloses; any figure below represents an acidosis.

pCO_2 = 35 to 45
HCO_3 = 22 to 28
Base excess = −2 to +2

Next recall

–an increase in pCO_2 indicates respiratory acidosis
–a decrease in pCO_2 indicates respiratory alkalosis
–an increase in HCO_3 indicates metabolic acidosis
–a decrease in HCO_3 indicates metabolic acidosis

When one of these major pathophysiologic conditions arises, a compensatory, stabilizing change occurs as follows:

–as pCO_2 increases (respiratory acidosis) there occurs a compensatory HCO_3 increase (metabolic alkalosis)
–as pCO_2 decreases (respiratory alkalosis) there occurs a compensatory HCO_3 decrease (metabolic acidosis)
–as HCO_3 increases (metabolic alkalosis) there occurs a compensatory pCO_2 increase (respiratory acidosis)
–as HCO_3 decreases (metabolic acidosis) there occurs a compensatory pCO_2 decrease (respiratory alkalosis)

Consequently, changes in pCO_2 reflect respiratory adjustments, while changes in HCO_3 reflect metabolic adjustments. *Compensation may be considered to be occurring when the more normal of the two values (pCO_2 and HCO_3) begins to change to stabilize the acid-base balance.*

Study the following examples and their interpretation:

pH = < 7.4 indicates an acidosis because the pH is less than 7.4
pCO_2 = > 45, ∴ a respiratory type acidosis occurs because change is in pCO_2
HCO_3^- = 22 to 28 (normal) acidosis uncompensated because HCO_3^- has not shifted to correct acid-base imbalance
∴ uncompensated respiratory acidosis (hypoventilation emphysema).

pH = 7.4 neutral
pCO_2 = > 45, ∴ respiratory type acidosis occurs because pCO_2 is primarily increased
HCO_3^- = > 28. Now risen secondarily to compensate and correct acid-base imbalance
∴ compensated respiratory acidosis.

pH = > 7.4 indicates an alkalosis because pH is greater than 7.4
pCO_2 = < 35, ∴ respiratory type because change is in pCO_2
HCO_3^- = 22 to 28 (normal) no change, consequently uncompensated.
∴ uncompensated respiratory alkalosis (hyperventilation).

pH = 7.4 neutral
pCO_2 = < 35, ∴ respiratory type alkalosis because Pco_2 is primarily down
HCO_3^- = < 22. Now fallen secondarily to compensate and correct acid-base imbalance
∴ compensated respiratory alkalosis.

pH = > 7.4 indicates alkalosis because pH above 7.4
pCO_2 = 35 to 45 (normal) no change, consequently uncompensated
HCO_3^- = > 28, ∴ metabolic type alkalosis because of primary change in HCO_3-
∴ uncompensated metabolic alkalosis (pyloric obstruction).

pH = 7.4 neutral
pCO_2 = > 45. Now risen secondarily to compensate and correct acid-base imbalance
HCO_3^- = > 28, ∴ metabolic type alkalosis
∴ compensated metabolic alkalosis.

pH = < 7.4 indicates acidosis because pH below 7.4
pCO_2 = 35 to 45 (normal) no change, consequently uncompensated
HCO_3^- = < 22, ∴ metabolic type acidosis because HCO_3^- is primarily down
∴ uncompensated metabolic acidosis (diabetes).

pH = 7.4 neutral

pCO_2 = <35. Now decreased secondarily to compensate and correct acid-base imbalance.

HCO_3^- = < 22, ∴ metabolic type acidosis because HCO_3^- primarily down

∴ compensated metabolic acidosis.

In summary:	HCO_3^-	pCO_2	pH
Metabolic acidosis	↓	⇣	⇣
Respiratory acidosis	⇡	↑	⇣
Metabolic alkalosis	↑	⇡	⇡
Respiratory alkalosis	⇣	↓	⇡

Clinical Applications

Metabolic acidosis may be caused by acid retention or alkali loss. Frequently this is called *primary alkali deficit*. Metabolic acidosis is the most frequent form of acidosis. Acid retention is caused by the pathophysiology of diabetes, starvation, renal failure, some diuretic drugs and the ingestion of ammonium or calcium chloride. Alkali loss occurs most frequently in the drainage of gastrointestinal fistulas or in chronic diarrheas.

Metabolic alkalosis follows alkali retention. Retention itself is uncommon but the ingestion of sodium bicarbonate for gastrointestinal complaints is not. Impaired renal function is about the only cause of alkali retention that can occur. Acid loss is another provoking factor leading to metabolic alkalosis. The only time the usual family physician will encounter this problem is when his patient continues vomiting acid gastric juice.

Respiratory acidosis is most frequently the result of a carbon dioxide excess. This problem is the one most frequently encountered in pulmonary disease and results from the impaired elimination of CO_2 from the lungs. All this is basically an alveolar hypoventilation leading to pO_2 decrease and a pCO_2 increase. Look for this state of affairs also in poliomyelitis and in the respiratory depression of drugs.

All respiratory acid-base problems are best defined by determining pCO_2. Too many compensatory factors are at work to rely on even the pH. When respiratory acidosis is uncompensated the picture is more apparent: increased pCO_2, increased CO_2 content and decreased pH. While the problem remains compensated, however, the pH tells nothing and the only reliable index is the pCO_2.

Remember the danger of giving oxygen in anoxic states. In anoxemia the respiratory center depends on the anoxia for stimulation. Oxygen may release the center from its "drive" and further depress respiration. The patient may be somewhat relieved from his anoxia only to accumulate more CO_2 in the blood. When the pCO_2 increased to 100 mm Hg and pH decreases to 7.2 the patient develops mental symptoms. If the pCO_2 further increases to 120 mm Hg and the pH drops to 7.1, the patient will sink into coma.

Think of respiratory alkalosis as a carbon dioxide deficit. This respiratory problem is the most frequent respiratory acid-base imbalance. Hyperventilation is the key disturbance. Hyperventilation washes out the CO_2. Again, pCO_2 is the only dependable factor, especially as long as the patient stays compensated. When compensation breaks the pH will increase.

In all acid-base problems the physiologic changes are complex and varied. Very seldom does one encounter acid-base problems as clear cut and simple deficiencies or excesses. Losses of body water, changes in total body content of electrolytes, osmotic imbalances and shifts between the various fluid compartments can cause treatment frustration. The big key in unraveling these problems is a persistent check of the pCO_2.

COMMON ANTIBIOTICS FOR RESPIRATORY INFECTIONS

Cough Mixtures

With Narcotic Content

The following proprietary cough mixtures contain narcotics.

Elixir terpen hydrate and codeine, 5 ml contains 85 mg terpen hydrate and 10 mg codeine.

Cheracol, 5 ml contains 11 mg codeine in a mixture of ammonium chloride, potassium guaiacolsulfonate, tartar emetic, chloroform, 3 percent alcohol, white pine and wild cherry. Dose: 5 to 15 ml every 2 to 4 hours.

Hycodan Syrup, 5 ml contains 1.5 mg homatropine and 5 mg hydrocodone bitartrate. Dose: 5 ml every 4 hours.

Syrup Calcidrine, 5 ml contains 10.8 mg codeine phosphate with a mixture of ephedrine, pentobarbital 4.2 mg, calcium iodide and 6 percent alcohol. Dose: 5 to 10 ml every 4 hours.

Non-narcotic

The following are considered non-narcotic cough mixtures generally depending on dextromethorphan for their antitussive effect which acts specifically on the cough reflex. These preparations are not as constipating as the above narcotic mixtures.

Cheracol-D, 5 ml contains 10 mg dextromethorphan instead of codeine in approximately the same basic ingredients as listed for Cheracol.

Elixir terpen hydrate and dextromethorphan HBr, 5 ml contains same ingredients as elixir terpen hydrate and codeine except the dextromethorphan has been substituted for the codeine.

Syrup Robitussin—DM, 5 ml contains 15 mg dextromethorphan in glyceryl guaiacolate and 1.4 percent alcohol. Dose: 5 ml every 6 to 8 hours.

With Expectorant Effect

Two cough mixtures which depend on their expectorant effect are:

Elixir Organidin, 5 ml has 60 mg iodinated glycerol. Dose: 5 ml every 4 hours.

Syrup Glyceryl Guaiacolate, 5 ml contains 100 mg glyceryl guaiacolate in 10 percent alcohol. Dose: 5 ml every 3 to 4 hours.

Nasal Vasoconstrictors

Neo-Synephrine HCl Intranasal. Active ingredient: phenylephrine HCl. Supplied in strengths of 0.125 percent, 0.25 percent, 0.5 percent and 1.0 percent in spray bottles.

Privine. Active ingredient: naphazoline HCl. Supplied in 0.5 percent spray bottles.

Gluco-Fedrin. Active ingredient: 1 percent ephedrine in chlorobutanol and menthol in aqueous dextrose. Used as a spray.

MALIGNANT TUMORS OF THE LUNG

Bronchogenic Tumors

Bronchogenic carcinoma is the commonest primary malignant tumor of the lung (Fig. 11-29). About 90 percent of the patients with bronchogenic carcinoma are males between 40 and 70. As to etiology, the magnitude of the effect of cigarette smoking far outweighs all other etiologic factors. Cytologic examination of the sputum or bronchial washings by an experienced cytopathologist should confirm the diagnosis in 60 to 70 percent of the cases.

The epidermoid or squamous type, is the most common of the bronchogenic carcinomas, accounting for about 50 percent of the primary malignant lesions of the lungs. It also has the best prognosis. The anaplastic (Fig. 11-30) or undifferentiated variety accounts for 30 percent and spreads the most rapidly. The incidence of adenocar-

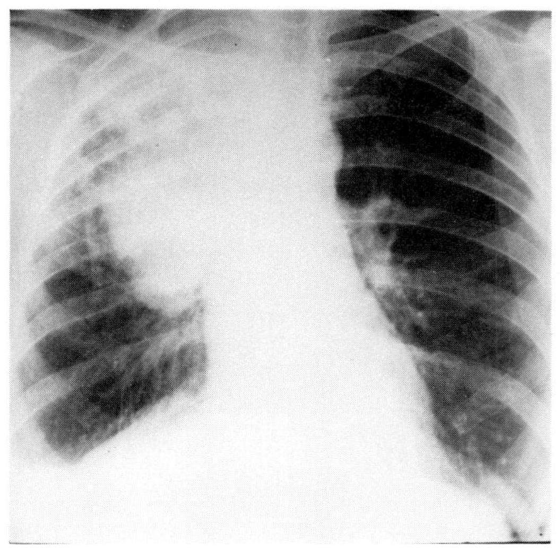

Figure 11-29. Bronchogenic cancer of the RUL.

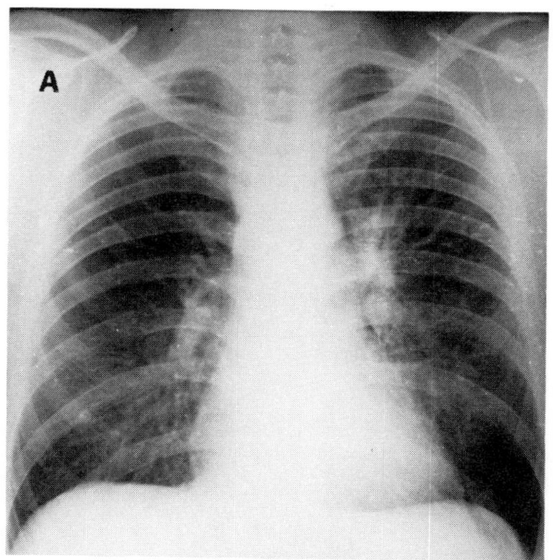

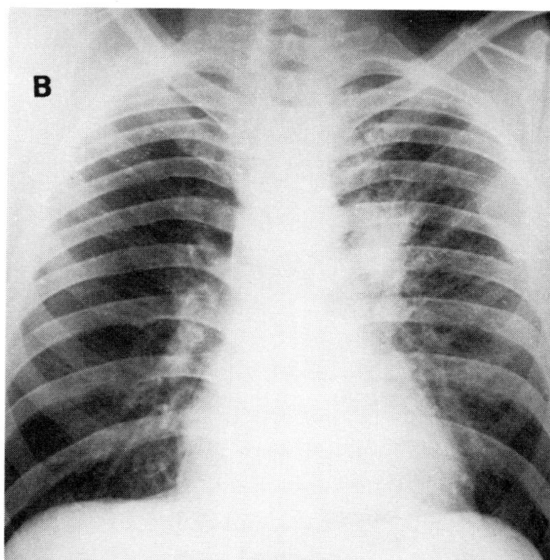

Figure 11-30. *A*, Anaplastic carcinoma of the left hilum; *B*, Within 4 weeks, the carcinoma has spread to the fifth rib and pleura.

cinoma is roughly about 20 percent of the primary malignant lesions and in prognosis lies somewhere between the least dangerous of the squamous and the most dangerous of the anaplastic carcinomas.

Bronchogenic carcinomas spread by three routes. The growth may invade all nearby structures including the mediastinum, ribs and pericardium. It may spread by the lymphatics to the hilum (Figs. 11-31 and 11-32), up the paraesophageal glands to the supraclavicular group. By the blood it spreads to the liver, the adrenals, brain, vertebraes and other organs.

Miscellaneous Tumors

Some tumors of the lung are accompanied by pneumothorax (Fig. 11-33).

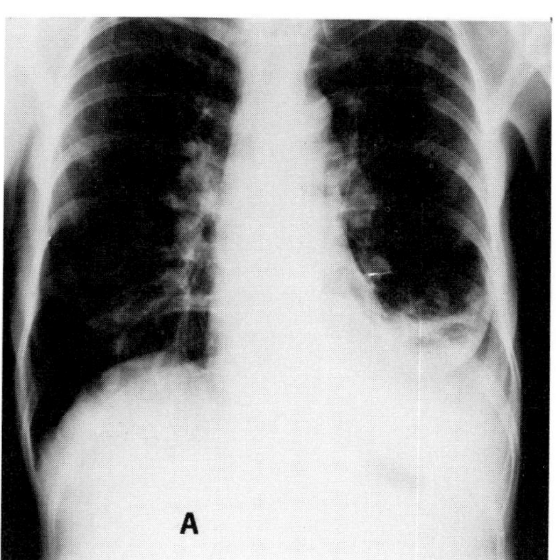

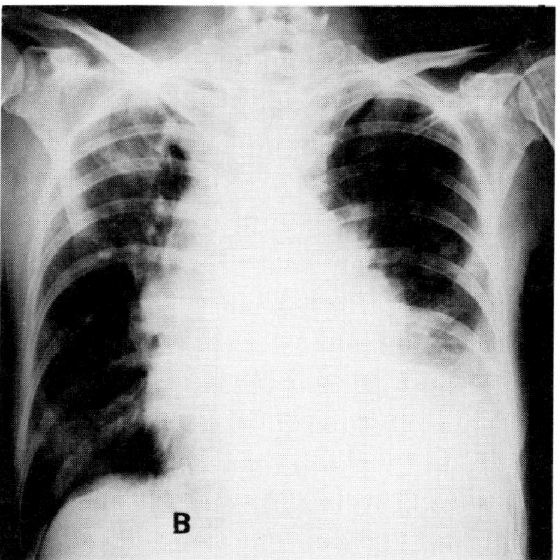

Figure 11-31. *A*, Lymphosarcoma in the lung; *B*, Same patient 4 weeks later. The patient died a few days after the second picture.

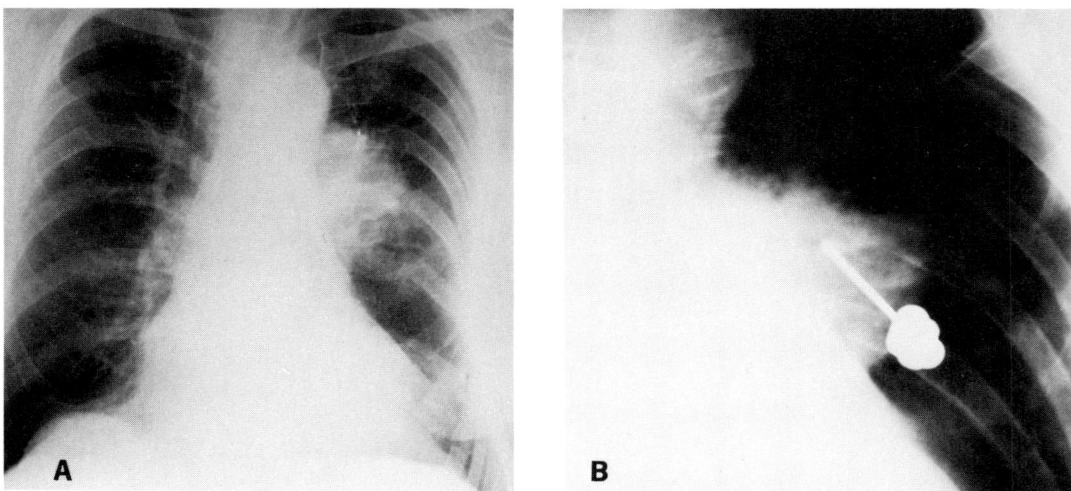

Figure 11-32. *A*, Primary bronchogenic carcinoma in the superior subsegment of the LLL. Streaky shadows radiating from the hilar mass shadow indicate lymphangitic spread. *B*, Lesion proven by needle biopsy.

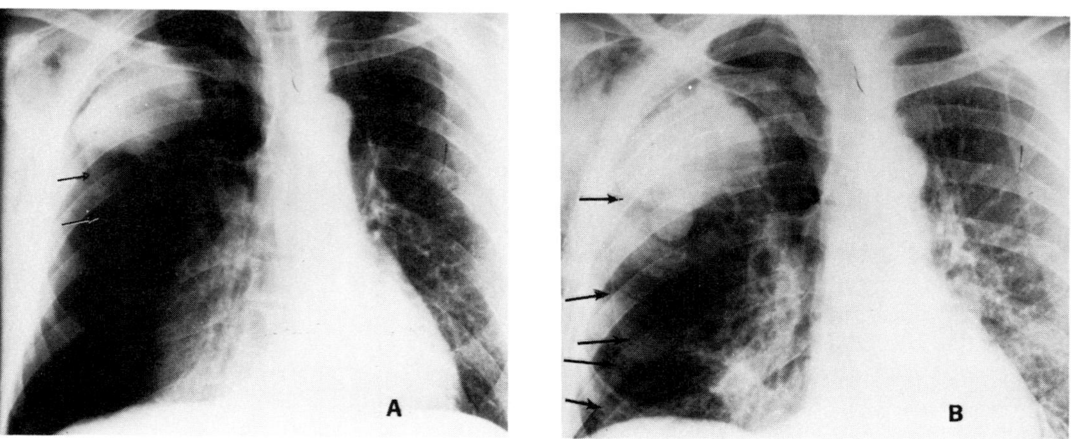

Figure 11-33. *A*, Carcinoma of the lung with 40 percent pneumothorax; *B*, Same patient, carcinoma of the lung with 15 percent pneumothorax.

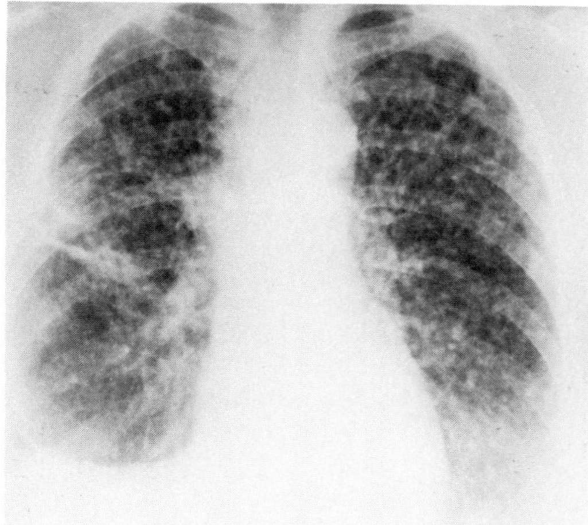

Figure 11-34. Reticular webbing seen in radiographic lymphangitic cancer.

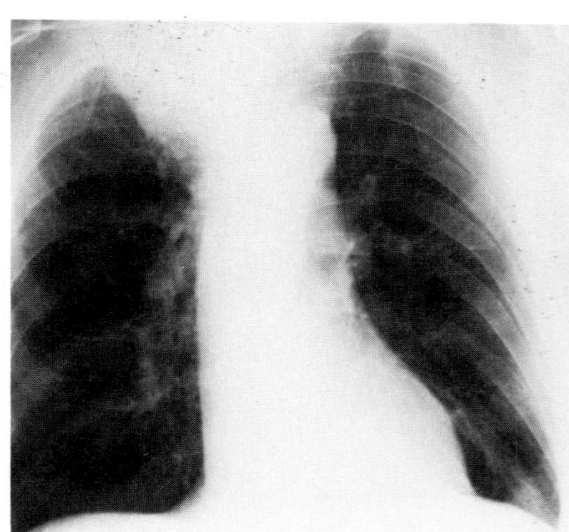

Figure 11-35. Pancoast's tumor. Note rib destruction.

Diffuse alveolar cell carcinoma must be differentiated from chronic hematogenous pulmonary tuberculosis and sarcoidosis of the lungs. The radiographic appearance of lymphangitic cancer is best described as that of a reticular webbing throughout both lung fields (Fig. 11-34).

Pancoast's syndrome is caused by a tumor in the pulmonary apex (Fig. 11-35). The tumor causes severe pain in the posterior part of the shoulder and axilla, which often shoots down the arm. It causes atrophy of the arm, Horner's syndrome and local destruction of bone.

An oat cell carcinoma of the RUL and hilus is illustrated in Figure 11-36. If the diagnosis of malignancy remains in doubt, the patient should be bronchoscoped and a biopsy of the lesion removed for microscopy. Bronchoscopy is essential in order to assess the extent of the growth and its operability if surgery is contemplated.

Cancer of the lung quite often is caused by metastases of a primary growth, the site often unknown. Metastatic nodules (Fig. 11-37) may be single or multiple. They usually are rounded and sharply circumscribed. Occasionally the nodules are quite large, so-called *cannon ball* metastases, often secondary to sarcoma or hypernephroma.

Diagnosis and Treatment

Symptoms of lung cancer are:

- –cough, or change in cough and appearance of sputum
- –weight loss
- –discomfort in the chest
- –unilateral wheezing
- –attacks of fever simulating viral pneumonitis, which further obscures the diagnosis

Remember:

- –The cough is usually out of proportion to the sputum produced.
- –about half of the patients with carcinoma will expectorate blood-streaked sputum and it is rarely a primary symptom.
- –A bad prognostic sign is a weight loss of more than 15 lb.
- –Severe pain and pleurisy usually indicates invasion into local tissue.
- –Indiscriminate use of antibiotics causes temporary improvement of symptoms only delaying a definitive diagnosis.

X-rays show some evidence of malignancy in 97 percent of the patients. In 3

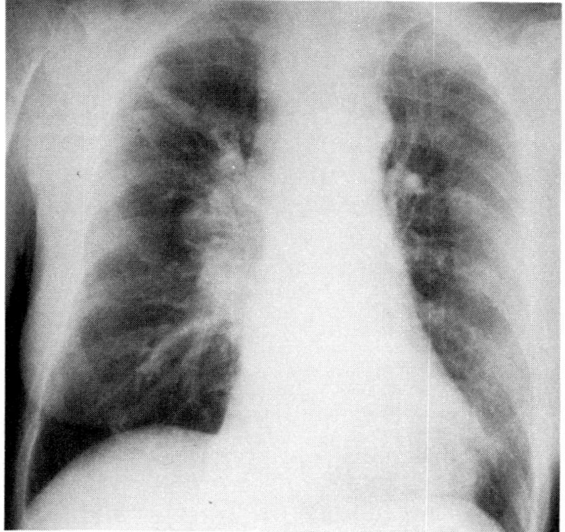

Figure 11-36. Oat cell carcinoma of the RUL and hilus.

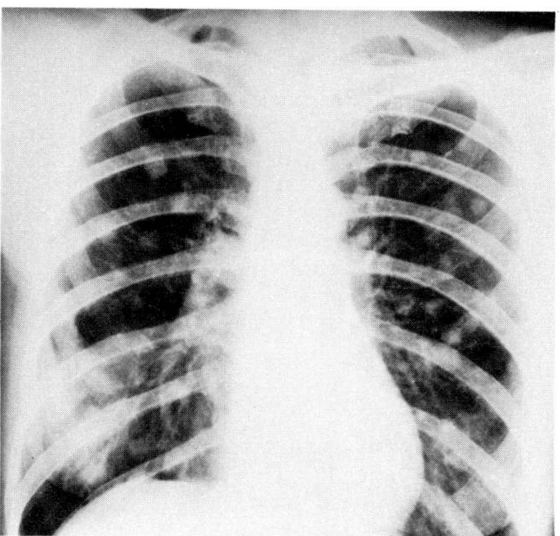

Figure 11-37. Metastatic cancer of the lung with multiple nodules; the primary site is unknown.

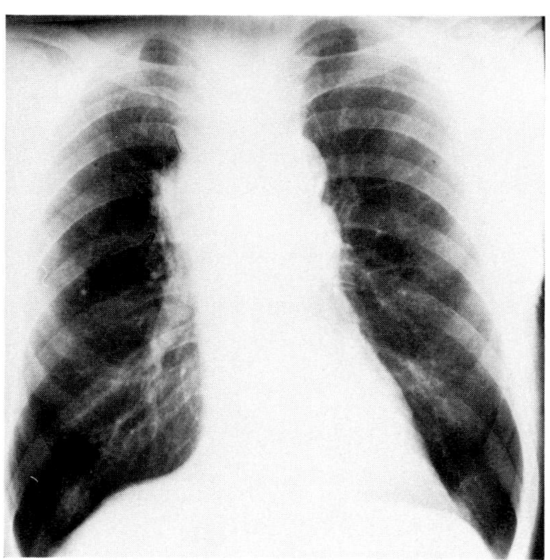

Figure 11-38. Epidermal carcinoma of the lung against the right mediastinum. A dry cough is the commonest early symptom. Recurrent hemoptysis may result from ulceration of blood vessels.

percent the lesions may be hidden behind the heart or engulfed in the mediastinum in some way (Fig. 11-38).

Bronchoscopy, supplying smears of secretion and material for biopsy, is one tool in establishing a diagnosis. However, only 25 percent of the tumors can be biopsied, but 30 percent can be diagnosed by studying the secretions collected directly or by saline washings. Because of the limitations in the use of biopsy, approximately a third of the patients with suspicious pulmonary lesions will need surgery without a positive cell or tissue diagnosis.

Rule out tuberculosis, pneumoconiosis, lipoid pneumonitis with granuloma formation, sarcoidosis, histoplasmosis, other fungus diseases, metastatic lesions from hypernephroma and ovarian or colonic cancers, adenomas and hamartoma.

Treatment is largely by surgical excision. If a patient has a surgically resectable pulmonary lesion but for one reason or another surgery is precluded, radiation therapy may be tried. There is little evidence, however, that radiation improves survival rates. Patients who have annoying symptoms, such as cough, hemoptysis, obstruction or pain may obtain some relief from radiation. Preoperative radiation is controversial and not recommended. One exception to this may be apical lung tumors.

PREVENTING POSTOPERATIVE PULMONARY ATELECTASIS

Have the patient treated for infected gums and sinusitis before being administered an anesthetic. Do not administer anesthesia to a patient with an acute respiratory infection except in an emergency.

Before general anesthesia order breathing exercises, postural drainage and perhaps antibiotics for those patients with chronic respiratory infections. Smoking increases the hazards of pulmonary atelectasis.

As soon as the anesthesia wears off, have the patient cough and change his position regularly.

PREVENTION OF LUNG DISEASE

Since cigarette smoking causes more lung disease than any other factor, it is important that you encourage, or demand, your patients to stop smoking.

"Why We Smoke"[8] is one of the best bits of antismoking propaganda I have found. Copy the article and give it to your patients. It has helped my patients.

REFERENCES

1. Mogabgab WS: Terminology of respiratory illness. *JAMA* 214:1715, 1970.
2. Unger JD, et al: Gram-negative pneumonia. *Radiology* 107:283–241, 1973.
3. Harris S: Influenza, ed 2. Baltimore: Williams & Wilkins Co., 1965.
4. Davey ML, Reid D: Relationship of air temperature to outbreaks of influenza. *Brit J Prev Soc Med* 26:28–32, 1972.
5. Amagrams: *JAMA* 220:1172, 1972.
6. Chronic Obstructive Pulmonary Disease: A Manual for Physicians, ed 2. Portland, Oregon: Oregon Thoracic Society, 1966.
7. Wang Kuang Chich: Intravenous sodium bicarbonate in severe status asthmaticus. *Chin Med J* 4:234–237, 1973.
8. Foster FP: Why we smoke. *Ca* 17:118, 1967.

GENERAL STUDY AIDS

Bukantz SC: Objective tests for bronchial asthma. *JAMA* 211:1706, 1970.

Cooper, Jr. OV: Arterial puncture simplified. *Res Staff Phys* 18:62–68, 1972.

Zelefsky MN: Inflammatory disease of the lung: a radiologic approach. *Hosp Med* 8:82–89, 1972.

Comroe, Jr, JH, Nadel JA: Screening tests for pulmonary function. *N Eng J Med* 282:1249, 1970.

Epstein RL: Sputum cellular makeup: a simple technique. From an unpublished paper presented as a scientific exhibit, AMA annual convention, San Francisco, Oct. 1, 1972.

Kaye D: Management of patients with pneumonia. *Drug Therapy* 1:65–71, 1971.

Lugliani R: Primary alveolar hypoventilation syndrome (Ondine's curse) failure of automatic control of ventilation. *Current Concepts Chest Dis* 12:1, 1972.

Kettel LJ, et al: Proper use of oxygen in the treatment of respiratory failure. *GP* 37:86–95, 1968.

Pierce JA: Office management of chronic obstructive pulmonary disease. *Clin Notes Resp Dis* 7:3–11, 1968.

Falliers CJ: Environmental and psychologic influences on allergic disease. *Postgrad Med* 46:127–132, 1969.

Itkin IH: Fundamentals of the treatment of asthma. *AFP* 4:82–90, 1971.

Goldsmith JR: Prevention of chronic lung disease. *Postgrad Med* 51:93–99, 1972.

CHAPTER 12

Gastrointestinal Diseases

INCIDENCE OF GASTROINTESTINAL DISEASES

Several studies have suggested the following, listed in order of their frequency, as the common diseases of the gastrointestinal tract: duodenal ulcer; esophagitis; cirrhosis; hiatal hernia; gastric ulcer; pancreatitis; biliary tract disease; viral hepatitis; diverticulosis and diverticulitis; carcinoma of the colon; ulcerative colitis; carcinoma of the stomach; regional enteritis; achalasia; nontropical sprue; carcinoma of the esophagus; carcinoma of the small bowel; familial Mediterranean fever.

MOUTH AND TONGUE COMPLAINTS

What to Look For

Conditions which occur in the mouth and tongue are listed under Differential Diagnosis later in this section.

Examining the Mouth

The experienced physician may be able to give the mouth a casual glance and recognize a variety of disease states. But even he will profit by making a step by step observation of the structures of the mouth. Certainly all beginning physicians would do well to study the gums, the tongue, the buccal mucosa, teeth, lips and the sublingual space separately.

First of all take a detailed history. Elicit all subjective symptoms. Find out when the symptoms started. Have the patient describe previous attacks. Question the patient regarding present medications. Find out if the patient has concurrent skin, genital or eye lesions.

Start your examination by observing the lips. Are they the proper color? Can the patient whistle? Suspect facial or 7th nerve damage in a patient who cannot pucker or whistle. How about the angles of the mouth? Is cheilosis present? Rhagades? Ulcers with or without evidence of cancer? Retract the lips with a tongue blade in order to inspect their inner surfaces.

Normally the exposed portion of the lips is dry; inside the line of closure they are moist. The color also varies from outside to inside: vermilion on the exposed mucous membrane and on the inside grayish red, the same color as the rest of the oral mucous membrane.

Next examine the teeth. Has the patient lost any teeth? What shape are the teeth? Is there notching? Tap each tooth for deep tenderness. What about caries? Are the teeth discolored? If so, from what?

The teeth cannot be evaluated without studying the gums, the source of their nourishment. Do the gum margins and the interdental papillae have a healthy color? Are they swollen? Retracted? Can you express pus from the gingival margins by light pressure with the tongue blade? Are the gums spongy? Do they bleed easily?

Is there a lead or bismuth line? Are there localized infections or tumors?

Inspect the buccal mucosa by retracting the cheek with a tongue blade. Is the orifice of the parotid duct swollen or red? Is the mucosa discolored in any way with melanin, leukoplakia, aphthous ulcers, Koplik's spots or by lichen planus? In health the buccal mucous membrane has an even grayish-red color. Just under the surface, and barely discernible with the eye, is a meshwork of tiny blood vessels. The gums should appear the same. The hard palate is a pale pink and gradually changes into the deeper pink of the soft palate and uvula.

And last of all, take a good look at the tongue both in the resting position and protrusion. The tongue is usually not furrowed except for a midline groove. Anteriorly it is covered with filiform, fungiform and circumvallate papillae. The filiform papillae give the tongue its gray-white coating. They are hairlike and most numerous. On the base of the tongue are the circumvallate papillae, a dozen large mushroomlike papillae arranged across the tongue in an inverted "V." The fungiform papillae are larger than the filiform among which they are randomly scattered but smaller than the circumvallate papillae. They occur more noticeably on the tip and sides of the tongue.

Have the patient move his tongue about, protruding it and touching the roof of his mouth. Assess its size, shape and mobility. Learn to use the tongue blade properly. Instruct the patient to keep the tip of his tongue loosely placed behind the lower teeth. Approach the tongue with the tongue blade in the left hand, allowing the right hand freedom to hold a flashlight or to pick up other instruments. Place the free end of the blade just over and behind the midpoint of the arched tongue. Gently press the arch downward and forward. Adjust the blade's placement until it appears to feel right to the patient. Too much pressure forces the tongue backward and causes gagging; too much pressure near the tip forces the arch backward and interferes with your observation of the pharynx and tonsils.

Do not hesitate to use a gloved finger to palpate any suspicious oral lesions. The feel of a lesion may give an entirely different impression of what is wrong. When palpating the tongue, instruct the patient to keep the tongue in his mouth behind the incisors in a relaxed position.

Inspection and palpation of the undersurface of the tongue may be as fruitful as the examination of the upper surface. A thorough examination will include palpation of the sublingual and submaxillary salivary glands.

Remember that five cranial nerves can be checked while examining the lips and mouth. Test the 5th cranial (trigeminal) while observing the alignment of the upper and lower incisors as the mouth is opened and shut. Paralysis of one pterygoid muscle causes deviation to the weak side. Palpate the tone of the masseter muscles. Check the 7th cranial (facial) by having the patient grimace, bare his teeth evenly, whistle or puff his cheeks. In each instance, only the unparalyzed side retracts. Observe the 9th and 10th (glossopharyngeal and vagus) by having the patient say "ah" while observing the soft palate and uvula. The uvula will deviate to the strong side. In the 12th cranial (hypoglossal), the protruding tongue deviates toward the weak side.

Lesion Biopsy

Biopsy of a lesion is essential for a definitive diagnosis and should be done on any mucosal ulceration that has persisted for 3 weeks or longer. Biopsy of superficial lesions can be safely performed by any doctor who has adequate facilities and knows the proper technique. Deeper and and more dangerous lesions may require biopsy by a surgeon in an operating room with the patient under general anesthesia.

Do an excisional biopsy if the lesion is small, superficial, accessible and probably benign. Remove the entire lesion as well as a small amount of the surrounding normal tissue.

Do an incisional biopsy to obtain a small portion of tissue for microscopic identification. This is preferred in most cases because it will give the therapist the time and the knowledge to plan proper therapeutic management.

If anesthesia is needed, infiltrate the area with 1 or 2 percent Xylocaine. Do not inject into the lesion but into the surrounding normal tissue. Use a scalpel and fine tissue forceps to obtain a small elliptic wedge-shaped specimen. Take the wedge of tissue from the edge of the lesion and include a small amount of normal tissue. Bleeding can often be stopped by gentle pressure. Occasionally a suture or two of fine catgut on a small curved needle are required. Do not handle the specimen. Place it immediately into a solution of 10 percent formalin. Label and describe the lesion for the pathologist.

Biopsy of a tumor lying under the skin is a little more involved. Infiltration of anesthesia is always needed. Incise the mucosa or skin and excise a wedge of the tumor with a scalpel. A biopsy punch may be used to free a small plug of tissue (Fig. 12-1). Perform the biopsy gently, causing as little disruption of the tissues as possible in order not to complicate definitive surgery.

Oral Cytology

Prepare a slide from the oral lesions that can be studied cytologically. However, if the lesion persists even with a negative cytology, do a biopsy. In some cases cytology may add useful information to a biopsy.

Check an oral lesion which appears benign. In this instance, the cytologic examination may aid in the differential diagnosis. Some physicians think oral cytology can detect suspicious or malignant cells regardless of the clinical appearance of the lesions; others believe that the procedure most accurately detects cancer only in red or ulcerated lesions. Leukoplakia is not detected by cytology; it is better to do a biopsy to verify leukoplakia lesions.

Check any oral lesion suggestive of clinical cancer. Biopsy is indicated, of course, but some patients may refuse a biopsy until a positive cytology is demonstrated.

Cytology is also useful in monitoring patients following treatment for oral cancer.

Oral pathologists generally provide a kit

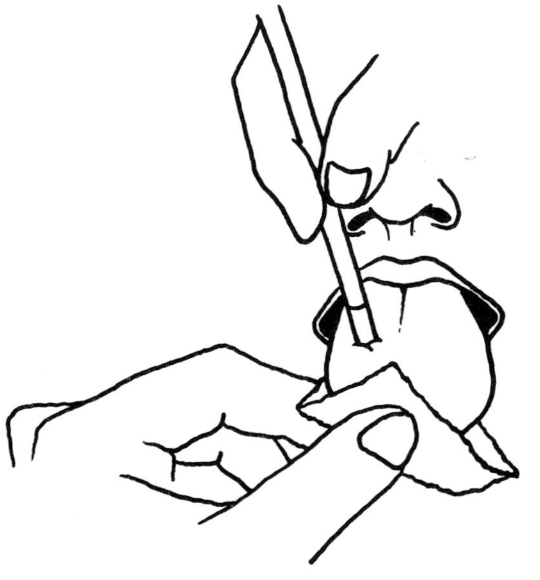

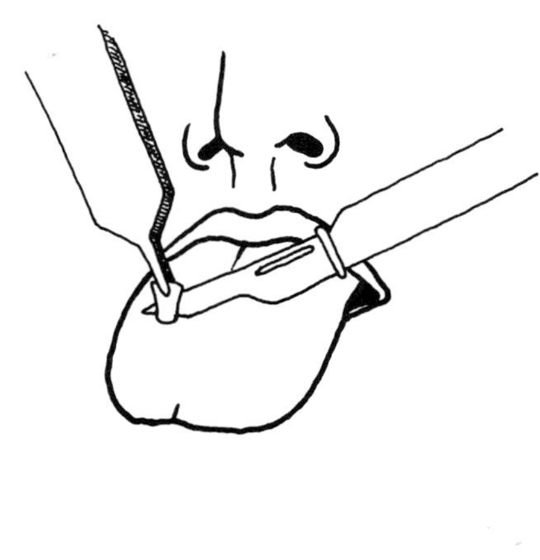

Figure 12-1. Biopsy punch: With a circular motion excise the core of the lesion or the entire lesion if it is small and then, with the aid of a thumb forceps, lift out the tissue core and free it from its bed.

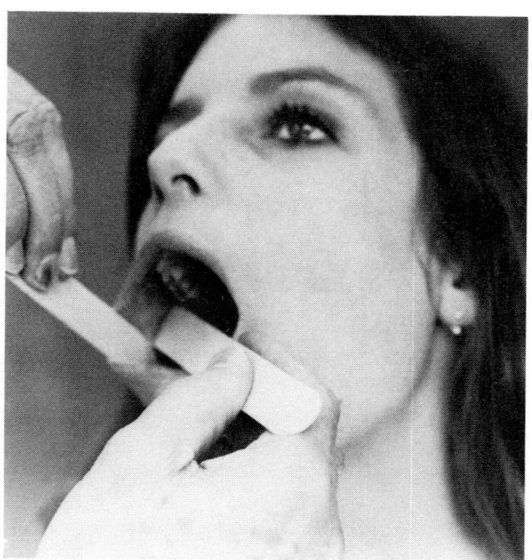

Figure 12-2. To take a cytologic smear, scrape the ulcer with a tongue blade.

and history form for cytology. The history form should be completed describing and identifying each lesion.

Remove debris from the lesion. Split a soaked tongue blade longitudinally providing a sharp edge for scraping (Fig. 12-2). Stroke across the lesion until a suitable amount of material has been collected on the free edge of the blade. Smear the collected cells onto a slide with frosted ends. Prepare two slides and label. Fix the slide by spraying with Aqua Net hair spray. Allow the slide to air dry and send it to the pathologist for Papanicolaou staining and study.

The final report will be: Negative for cancer, suspicious for cancer or positive for cancer.

False interpretation may follow a scanty smear, a smear of poor quality because debris was not removed from the lesion or a slide which was not fixed while the sample was still wet.

The Toluidine Blue Screening Test for Oral Cancer

Toluidine blue will not stain normal mucosa but will stain carcinoma in situ or invasive carcinoma. The test has been reported to be dependable in squamous and epidermoid carcinoma, melanoma, fibrosarcoma and lymphosarcoma. It is also positive in leukoplakia, lymphoid hyperplasia, lichen planus and traumatic ulcerations.

Use the test to:

- diagnose leukoplakic lesions and dysplasia
- differentiate traumatic and inflammatory ulcers
- determine the margins of resection prior to excision
- demonstrate small secondary, primary or satellite lesions adjacent to a larger lesion

Remember toluidine blue does not stain normal mucosa; therefore, the test is of no value in diagnosing tumors that do not involve the overlying mucous membrane.

Have the patient rinse his mouth with water and swallow several sips of it. Aspirate excess saliva with suction and apply 1 percent acetic acid with a cotton applicator. Remove any debris by suction. Paint a small amount of toluidine blue over the lesion and surrounding mucosa. Again have the patient rinse his mouth with water to clear away excess dye.

If the lesion stains, the test is positive. Biopsy should be done immediately on the stained areas and on lesions that do not take up the stain in order to document their precise nature. Staining results are controversial but the test is a valuable preliminary screening test.

Tongue cancer which is 2 cm or less in diameter and noninfiltrating can be cured by radiotherapy in a high percentage of cases. The rate of cure falls off as the degree of malignancy increases. The cure rate for one course of radiation for Stage T is about 55 percent and with further treatment of recurrences by re-irradiation the cure rate will rise to about 72 percent. In Stage T_4, however, further irradiation will only raise the percentage of cure from 20 percent to 25 percent. If the first course of radiation does not help, further treatment is practically hopeless.[1]

Differential Diagnosis

Recurrent Aphthous Ulcers (Canker Sores)

About one fifth of the population at one time or another suffers from the painful aphthous ulcers. One important differential point is that aphthous ulcers tend to occur *in* the mouth, i.e. on the buccal and labial mucosa, tongue, soft palate, lingual sulci, gingiva and pharynx. The ulcers produced are intensely painful and may persist from 5 to 30 days. The cause is unknown but minor trauma or minor respiratory infections often precede the appearance of the lesions. About 70 percent of patients will have one to three ulcers per attack. These ulcers have a fairly regular margin and are covered with a whitish-gray membrane.

Nearly everything has been used for treatment. Probably one of the best programs is the application of Declomycin (demethylchlortetracycline) on cotton-soaked pledgets directly on the lesions. An alternative course would be to hold a teaspoonful of Declomycin in the mouth near the lesion for 5 minutes four times daily. Restrict food or water ingestion for 1 hour following treatment.

Steroid ointment or lozenge applications have their boosters. Cortone (1.5 percent cortisone acetate) or Hydrozets (hydrocortisone acetate-antibiotic lozenge) applied four times a day for 5 to 7 days apparently reduces the healing time.

For pain relief, nothing seems any better than the local application of Dyclone (0.5 percent dyclonine hydrochloride). Applied just before a meal, it will be useful in reducing the pain associated with chewing.

Recurrent Herpes Simplex

Herpetic lesions are often confused with aphthous ulcers. Keep in mind that herpes simplex occurs most frequently on the mucocutaneous junction of the mouth or on the skin some distance from the mouth. They are frequently seen under the nose and are heaped up and crusted. Do not confuse these lesions with impetigo. The actual appearance of the lesion is often preceded by stinging and soreness about the site.

Treatment is symptomatic and supportive. Do not give or apply steroids because they may cause generalized complications. As with aphthous ulcers the application of a local anesthetic (Dyclone) is helpful. Prescribe a vitamin supplement.

Often overlooked is primary herpes simplex in children. The oral lesions are accompanied by tender submandibular adenopathy, fever, malaise, and anorexia. The disease occurs only once and disappears in 10 to 14 days. Both the local and generalized forms of herpes simplex are caused by the most troublesome virus of all, the H. simplex virus. For a specific diagnosis in either the local or generalized types of herpetic infections, order a viral culture of vesicle fluid or saliva. A quicker method which may be helpful would be the examination of a smear from the base of a vesicle for giant cells with large ballooned nuclei. Last of all, the patient will be sera positive for herpes antibodies in both the acute and convalescent stages.

Moniliasis (Thrush)

When this infection occurs in infants, the disease is called thrush; when it occurs in adults after taking antibiotics or steroids, it is called moniliasis. The lesions are not difficult to identify: white patches on the oral mucous membrane when scraped off leave a raw bleeding surface.

The lesions appear most often on the soft palate and oropharynx, but the lips and tongue may become involved, the gingival surface only rarely. Take a smear and gram stain. Look for budding cells and filaments of Candida albicans. If in doubt a culture will confirm the diagnosis.

Vincent's Angina

Fusospirochetal infection, trench mouth and necrotizing ulcerative gingivitis are other names for this condition. Think of this fusospirochetal infection when the gingivae are primarily infected. It is a local or general inflammation of the gum margins.

The first symptoms are pain and bleeding of the gums, especially after eating or brushing the teeth. Generally the patient has some prior and considerably local adenopathy. If untreated, severe local ulceration occurs.

To diagnose, take a smear and gram stain of the pseudomembrane. The common organisms found are gram-negative spirochetes (Borrelia vincentii) and Bacillus fusiformis. Do not bother about culturing.

Infectious Mononucleosis (Kissing Disease)

This disease is a communicable, systemic disease occurring mainly in teenagers and young adults. Systemic symptoms and findings include fever, fatigue, splenomegaly, general adenopathy and occasionally a maculopapular erythematous rash.

The local lesions in the mouth are generally centered about the tonsils, appearing as an exudative tonsillitis. The oral mucosa is sprinkled with small ulcers with red borders.

Base your diagnosis on blood findings: A lymphocytosis of over 65 percent which are more than 25 percent atypical. The Monospot test may be helpful but the serologic heterophile is confirmatory. The latter test remains positive for some time and may show a rise in titer when the patient has some other acute diseases.

Primary and Secondary Syphilis

The first sign of primary syphilis may be a chancre, an indurated ulcer with a smooth base. Common locations are the lips, tongue or tonsillar areas. No chancre appears on the external genitalia if the primary site is on the lip.

Darkfield examination of the serum from a lip chancre is not as diagnostic as is the serum from an ulcer on the genitalia. The difficulty arises in differentiating the spirochetes in oral flora from Treponema pallidum. Examine any lingual ulcer by drying and pressing it with a cotton sponge. Inspect it carefully. Palpate the surrounding and underlying tissue with gloved fingers. Remember that the pain from lingual lesions may be referred to the ear. The serologic test may not be positive for 3 to 4 weeks. The oral chancre heals in 7 to 10 days without scarring.

Oral lesions of secondary syphilis, condyloma latum, have a different appearance than the primary chancre. They are often described as mucous patches. If you look at the patch closely it appears to be a shallow erosion covered with a gray membrane. Palpate the lesion with a gloved finger; it will feel indurated and painless. Check the lumph glands; they are enlarged. This painless lesion most commonly appears on the oropharynx, but inspect the lips, buccal mucosa, palate and tongue also.

Herpangina

This Coxsackie virus A infection attacks the general oropharynx with erythema and vesicles which rupture and form shallow discrete 1 to 2 mm ulcers. The symptoms: sore throat and dysphagia which resolve in 2 to 4 days. Make the diagnosis from clinical signs and symptoms.

Leukoplakia (Smoker's Patch)

Don't call every white lesion in the mouth leukoplakia. Leukoplakia starts as small yellowish-white patches which in time coalesce and become leathery. At that time, they may ulcerate, crack and bleed. The tongue may appear to be covered with white paint which was aged and cracked. Try pressing a glass slide on the small early lesions. The leukoplakia will be seen displacing the papillae with their white lesions.

Don't guess as to which lesions will become leukoplakic; some will but many do not. The only safe course is to biopsy suspicious lesions, and the sooner the better. Around 5 percent will degenerate into squamous cell carcinoma.

Surgically remove all leukoplakia lesions when the pathologist verifies a precancerous change. If no precancerous changes are noted use vitamin A, 150,000 USP units twice daily, and supplemental vitamins B and C. Eliminate all sources of irritation, whether it be ill-fitting dentures or smoking. Keep the mouth clean and healthy and insist on regular check-ups. If there is no improvement within 3 months, consider prophylactic surgery.

There appears to be an association between tobacco and leukoplakia, for lesions appear adjacent to teeth stained by tobacco, and in areas where tobacco is retained by snuff users.

Inspect every leukoplakic lesion for Bowen's disease, a squamous cell carcinoma in situ or intraepidermal. Look for a dull red to brownish-red patch with a sharp irregular outline. Fortunately Bowen's disease shows no evidence of invading underlying tissue.

Lichen Planus

Learn to differentiate between leukoplakia and lichen planus. Mistakes are often made. Look for slightly raised lacy or linear white lines or small white papules. Very occasionally bullae or vesicles form. The buccal mucosa and tongue are the most commonly involved sites. Generally the lesions are asymptomatic. When you see an oral lesion of this type, check the flexor surfaces of the wrists and ankles. Finding an associated skin lesion may help confirm your opinion.

Lichen planus has no known cause but there is a strong emotional component because the disease invariably occurs in nervous individuals or in constant worriers.

Keep in mind that the disease has both an erosive and nonerosive form. The nonerosive white lesion is not often confused with other white oral lesions. In the erosive type, however, a biopsy is essential. Make an early and definite diagnosis. These apprehensive patients do not tolerate indecision when they suspect cancer.

In addition, the erosive form causes pain. There is no effective treatment. Order alkaline mouth washes such as sodium bicarbonate. Have a dentist remove all irritants. Dyclone 0.5 percent is an excellent topical anesthetic which the patient can use before eating. Consider a mild tranquilizer if anxiety is a problem. Fortunately only rarely does cancer complicate the disease.

Fordyce's Spots

These mucosal sebacious cysts are harmless isolated white or yellowish spots less than a millimeter in diameter. They are mentioned to avoid confusion with leukoplakia or lichen planus. They are most often seen on the buccal surface.

Koplik's Spots of Measles

Consider Koplik's spots in an ill child as the heralding spot for the exanthem of measles. Usually the redness of the rash first catches your attention, but on close inspection one can see a small white center. They first appear on the buccal membrane opposite the molars and forecast the rash of measles.

Parotid Duct Sign of Mumps

The orifice Stenson's duct opposite the second molar becomes red during acute parotitis or mumps.

Retention Cyst

This is an enlarged mucous gland caused by obstruction to its duct. Recognize them by the blue domed, translucent appearance.

Dental Ulcer

Do not mistake the simple dental ulcer for more serious lesions of tuberculosis, syphilis and carcinoma. Dental ulcers always occur on the sides or undersurface of the tongue. Most often they result from the irritation of an illfitting denture or a malplaced tooth. On inspection the ulcers may appear dangerous and simulate cancer for they may be indurated and possess the everted edges of carcinoma. Confusion in differential diagnosis will exist until lesions are biopsied.

Aspirin Burn

It is wise to question patients with oral ulcerations regarding their use of aspirin. Some people place aspirin tablets in the mucobuccal fold to relieve toothache. This habit will produce burns with macular white patches. Obviously, the only treatment in traumatic and burn ulcers is the removal of the irritants. They should heal within 2 weeks or a biopsy should be done.

Other Conditions

When you are confronted with mouth lesions and are unclear as to their origins, order a complete blood count. This may save the embarrassment of overlooking the early signs of leukemia, agranulocytosis, infectious mononucleosis and other systemic diseases.

Be aware of the following diseases: *Erythema multiforme* produces transient bullae that rupture, leaving painful eroded areas which heal in 1 to 3 weeks. The disease may follow or accompany a drug reaction or an upper respiratory infection. Biopsy if the lesion does not heal promptly to rule out *pemphigus*. This disease produces a painless lesion but one which may be fatal unless treated. Again the disease starts as a bullae that ruptures and leaves an eroded base. Biopsy. There are no specific diagnostic tests for *mucous membrane pemphigoid*. A biopsy will help rule out pemphigus and its chronic course will help rule out erythema multiforme. The clinical appearance is not characteristic but look for thick-walled bullae, which often rupture but still have overlying epithelium that causes an opaque yellow color.

TONGUE CONDITIONS. Geographic tongue, migratory glossitis, is a harmless, painless lesion of unknown etiology. The configuration changes constantly. Hairy tongue, also called furry or black tongue, often appears during treatment with antibiotics that inhibit the normal oral flora and permit the overgrowth of fungi such as Aspergillus niger or Candida albicans. In Strawberry tongue or raspberry tongue, the lingual papillae become swollen and red as a result of systemic toxins. It commonly occurs in scarlet fever. *Scrotal tongue* with congenital furrows is a harmless, inherited condition. The tongue appears to have a median raphe with deep transverse furrows. It must be distinguished from *syphilitic glossitis* in which the fissures are mainly longitudinal.

Dry tongue with longitudinal furrows is the most reliable sign of general dehydration. Remember that longitudinal furrows develop due to reduction in size of the tongue. This occurs, it is reported, whenever there is a loss of 3 L of extracellular fluid. Dry tongue with no loss of volume or furrowing may result from simple mouth breathing or from the more complicated Sjogren's syndrome. The latter disease, a form of arthritis, is accompanied by a lack of saliva (xerostomia). When you see a transiently *enlarged tongue* think of hematoma, abscess, angioneurotic edema, glossitis, stomatitis or cellulitis of the neck. A permanently enlarged tongue should remind you to examine the patient for mongolism, cretinism, adult myxedema, acromegly or amyloidosis. *Tremor of the tongue* is a characteristic of thyrotoxicosis. A coarser tremor often signifies nervousness, weakness, alcoholism, paresis or drug addiction. *Tongue tie* is a congenital shortening of the frenulum. If severe it restricts the movement of the tongue and may keep the tip from touching the roof of the mouth. Surgery is necessary to correct it.

Atrophic glossitis is recognized by dryness of the tongue, intermittent burning, paresthesia of taste and a progressively smaller tongue which becomes slick and glistening. Check the patient's blood count and order a test for hypo- or achlorhydria. Actually the best diagnostic measure is a therapeutic test with vitamin B_{12}. Atrophic glossitis is present not only in classic pernicious anemia but also in other macrocytic megaloblastic anemias associated with idiopathic gastritis, cirrhosis, vegetarian diets, fish tapeworm infestations, blind intestinal loops and postgastrectomy syndromes.

Pellagrous glossitis produces a red tongue. A patient with full bloom pellagra is seldom seen but, when a patient complains of a burning tongue aggravated by hot or spicy food, think of the possibility. Later, when the burning becomes constant, other signs and symptoms make the diagnosis secure, i.e. the 3 D's—diarrhea, dementia and dermatitis. A therapeutic test confirms the diagnosis: the oral administration of 100 mg of niacin will cause the disappearance of the erythema and burning within 24 hours.

In *riboflavin deficiency* (ariboflavinosis,

magenta cobblestone tongue) burning of the tongue is relatively mild as compared with the tongue of pellagra. Look for the reddened elevations that suggest cobblestones in appearance. Remember pellagra—red tongue; riboflavin—magenta tongue. A riboflavin deficiency attacks the corners of the mouth, causing cheilosis or angular stomatitis and the corners of the eyes and the nasolabial folds.

Again, burning of the tongue is the prominent symptom in *menopausal glossitis*. Inspect the tongue carefully and you will notice a slight atrophy of the lingual mucosa. Menopausal glossitis and senile vaginitis both stem from a common cause. The administration of estrogen will improve both.

TUMORS WHICH APPEAR IN THE MOUTH. Carcinoma may occur as an indurated ulcer or a warty growth. Retention cyst was described previously. A torus is a bony protuberance on the midline of the hard palate. It is of no clinical significance.

SCURVY. The usual early complaints made by patients with a vitamin C deficiency are soreness, swelling and bleeding gums. The first findings are capillary dilitation and congestion of the interdental papillae. From this site the lesion spreads, as the disease advances, to the gingival margins and finally to the alveolar mucous membrane.

Look first at the interdental papillae. Are they a deep blue-red color? Does the discoloration extend into the gum in places? Is there swelling? Collars of unhealthy tissue may surround the teeth; debris and organisms collect in the pockets along the gingival margin. Gum infections may predispose the patient to scurvy and/or accompany the disease. As the acuteness of the disease subsides, atrophy of the gum margins occur and teeth loosen and may fall out following bone changes.

Other general symptoms associated with vitamin C deficiency are ecchymosis around or near joints following slight trauma, hemarthroses, subperiosteal hemorrhages and perifollicular hyperkeratosis and hemorrhage. The disease responds to vitamin C. In a few cases, if anemia supervenes, folic acid may speed recovery.

DILANTIN GINGIVITIS. Many of your patients may need to take Dilantin for years to control epilepsy. Some of them will develop a hypertrophy of the gums. After hypertrophy develops, the gums become sore, swollen and bleed easily. The swelling and hypertrophy may so surround the teeth as to cover a large part of the enamel. Insist that these patients develop good habits of dental hygiene.

Preventing Dental Caries

The average child who reaches school age has many carious teeth. Prevention is important, and the family physician has a responsibility equal to that of immunization to his pediatric patients. Deciduous teeth begin to form during the third prenatal month and erupt about the fifth or sixth month after birth until 3 years of age. Permanent teeth take shape before birth too; they begin to erupt about the fifth year and continue to erupt until the patient is in his mid-20's.

The family physician's responsibility lies in:

- –prescribing a fluoride tablet to every expectant mother
- –supporting municipal fluoridation of water
- –educating parents and children to visiting their family dentist beginning around 2 to 2½ years.
- –prescribing extra dietary fluoride to the children under his care

The Council on Dental Therapeutics of the American Dental Association suggests the following dose schedule:

- –For children under 2 yr of age, order 1 fluoride (1 mg) tablet daily
- –For children between 2 and 3, give 1 fluoride tablet every other day
- –For children over 3 yr of age, give 1 tablet daily.

Do not give extra dietary fluoride when the drinking water exceeds 0.3 mg per day. Check with your Public Health Department for fluoride assay. (One quart of water with 1 PPM of fluoride contains about 1 mg of fluoride.) Excessive intake of fluorides may cause dental fluorosis.

Some fluoride products are Luride and Lozi tablets 0.5 and 1 mg tablets, Karidium (1 mg tablets) and Pediaflor drops (0.5 mg fluoride per ml).

Some multivitamins are combined with fluoride. The following are commonly prescribed multivitamin and fluoride preparations that come in both drops and chewable tablets (all drops have 0.5 mg fluoride in 0.6 ml and all chewable tablets 1 mg per tablet): Adeflor drops and chewable tablets; Vi-Daylin/FADC, Vi-Daylin/F drops, and Vi-Daylin-W/Fluoride chewable tablets; Decca-Vi-Flor drops and chewable tablets; and Poly-Vi-Flor drops and chewable tablets.

DYSPHAGIA

What to Look For

If your patient's problem is difficulty in swallowing consider any of the following: carcinoma, lower esophageal ring (Schatzki's ring), esophagitis and stricture, cardiospasm (achalasia), diffuse spasm, scleroderma, extrinsic compression from long spurs, mediastinal tumors or aberrant vessels (dysphagia lusoria); myasthenia gravis; amyotrophic lateral sclerosis; muscular dystrophies; incoordination of cricopharyngeal muscles; Zenker's diverticulum; inflammations and strictures; foreign bodies; cervical osteophytes; goiter; cervical nodes; psychoneurosis (globus hystericus); stroke; poliomyelitis; immunosuppressive medication (monilial esophagitis); or Plummer-Vinson syndrome (filamentous web in the upper esophagus.

General Symptoms

Distinguish between dysphagia and odynophagia. Dysphagia implies difficult swallowing which may or may not be associated with odynophagia or painful swallowing. The patient with dysphagia is able to tell where in his esophagus the difficulty is arising.

Ask the patient also whether he has equal trouble swallowing fluids and solids. In neuromuscular disabilities of the pharynx the patient has trouble passing fluids from the oropharynx into the esophagus. Aspiration and choking cause great disability. In esophageal dysphagias, the patient has trouble swallowing solids long before he has trouble with liquids. Does the patient have difficulty at the beginning, during, or after swallowing? Difficulty at the beginning points toward neuromuscular diseases. The symptom may be the first sign of a general neurologic or muscular malfunction.

Food, especially solids, which is difficult to pass through the esophagus, causes symptoms during or after swallowing. Carcinoma of the lower esophagus causes such dysphagia.

Other questions which you should ask are: exactly where the discomfort is located; whether the difficulty is intermittent, constant or progressive; whether the patient regurgitates acid stomach contents; whether the food is undigested and alkaline as in achalasia or diverticulum; whether pain accompanies the dysphagia; and whether the patient has any other disease.

Differential Diagnosis

Carcinoma of the Esophagus

The most frequently encountered malignant tumor is carcinoma. Because of its high

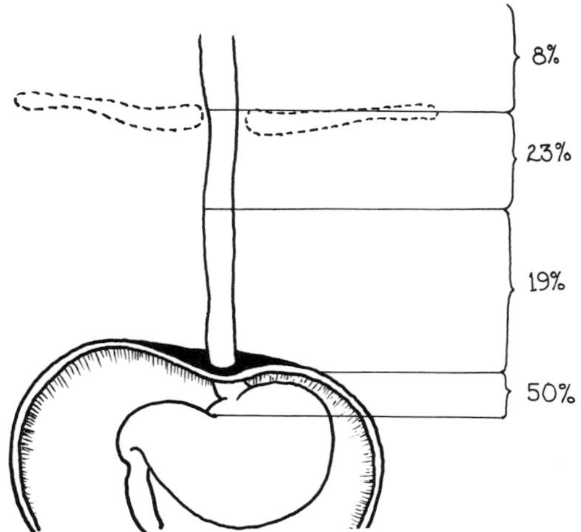

Figure 12-3. Common sites of carcinoma of the esophagus.

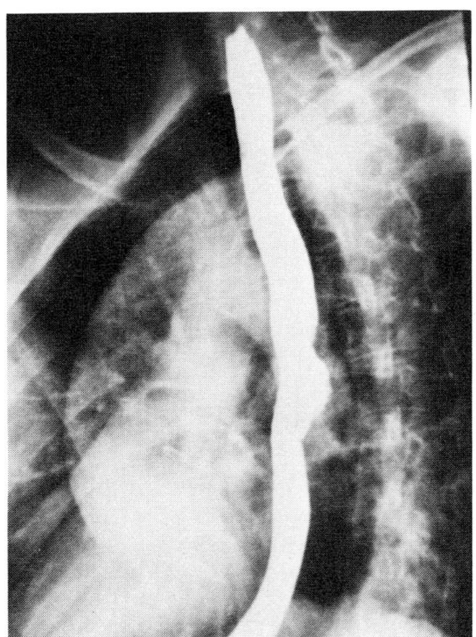

Figure 12-4. Carcinoma of the middle third of the thoracic esophagus.

mortality rate it is one of the most important afflictions of the esophagus. It may occur at any level but has sites of predilection (Fig. 12-3).

A detailed history reveals a characteristic series of events—a progressive dysphagia, first to solids, then soft foods and then to liquids. The duration of the disease is usually less than 6 months.

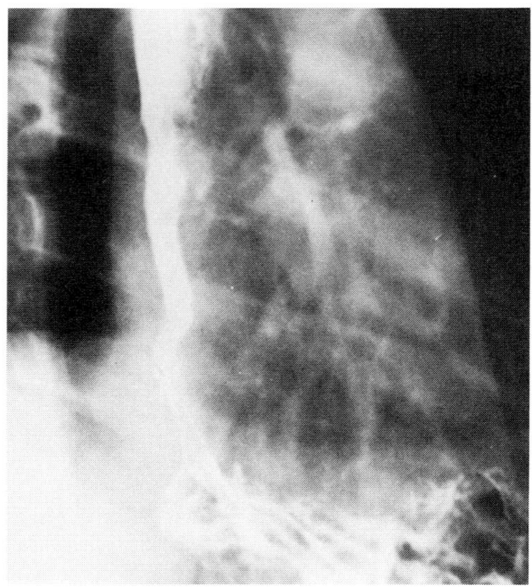

Figure 12-5. Narrowing of the lower third of the esophagus—possible carcinoma. Hiatal hernia.

Diagnosis is not difficult (Figs. 12-4 and 12-5). Start with a barium swallow. If the x-rays are inconclusive or negative, ask a consultant to do an esophagoscopy. Suggest that he collect secretions during the examination for later Papanicolaou smears. If no secretions are present, he should flush the esophagus with 20 ml sterile saline and then aspirate the fluid through the esophagoscope. Biopsy of any abnormal mucosa should be done at the same time. Remember that an area of esophagitis may surround the carcinoma and cause confusion in diagnosis.

Cardiospasm (Achalasia)

Cardiospasm is the second most frequent cause of esophageal obstruction. Look for a dilitation of the lower end of the esophagus as a result of a constant spastic contraction of the lower ring. There is no anatomic stenosis. The patient complains of dysphagia to solids or liquids and of regurgitation. Odynophagia is not common. Suspect cardiospasm when cardinal symptoms have been present for 6 to 12 months and when there is no history of the ingestion of a caustic which may have produced a cicatricial stricture.

Again a diagnosis depends in good measure on x-ray evidence of a dilated esophagus. The atony is manifest by an absence of primary and secondary peristalsis and the retention of barium. The distal end is tapered. Don't be surprised to find an esophageal dilitation of large size; occasionally the lower esophagus will hold 1 to 2 L. With the patient standing, the level of barium will gradually fall until the hydrostatic pressure will no longer force the fluid into the stomach. The level of barium will stabilize about 8 inches above the cardia.

To rule out carcinoma, esophagoscopic examination of the distal esophagus is essential. Again do washings for Papanicolaou stains and biopsies as indicated.

If there is doubt as to the nature of the lesion, special gastrointestinal laboratories are equipped to do special balloon-kymography studies with meckolyl. Manometry never records peristaltic waves but only simultaneous contractions throughout the esophageal tube.

In the immediate past, the conventional therapy for achalasia has been a trial of medical therapy and bougienage. Surgery has been held in reserve and has not been uniformly good. Misunderstanding of the part played by reflux esophagitis held back advances in surgery. Now with better techniques and a clearer understanding of the pathophysiology, direct surgical management is emerging as the treatment of choice. This will eliminate the short-term relief and perforation hazard of bougienage.

Lower Esophageal Ring (Schatzki's Ring)

This ringlike narrowing at the lower end of the esophagus causes intermittent dysphagia, usually over a number of years. The lumen must narrow to 13 mm in order for dysphagia to occur and, when it does, the patient's difficulty is with solid food, especially beef and bread.

Ask the patient to describe the last attack. Invariably it occurred when he was chewing hastily and swallowing rapidly and was under stress. Suddenly a piece of meat or a bolus of bread lodged above the ring.

Diagnosis can usually be made after a barium swallow. If the lower esophagus is dilated, the typical ring can be seen. If doubt exists, give a bread bolus with the barium to reproduce the symptoms.

Diffuse Spasm of the Esophagus

Swallowing normally is followed by a smooth peristaltic wave down the esophagus. In diffuse esophageal spasm, the peristaltic function is lost and swallowing invokes strong simultaneous and repetitive contractions throughout the esophagus. The gastroesophageal sphincter function remains normal.

Dysphagia to solids predominates. The patient complains of pain (odynophagia). Question the patient about the pain (Fig. 12-6): it occurs when the patient swallows but, in addition, the pain persists even when there is no attempt at swallowing. In some instances the pain awakens the patient from sleep.

When the patient is given a barium swallow, look for simultaneous bizarre, segmental contractions. If in doubt and a gastrointestinal laboratory is available, order balloon kymography. The test is positive in 60 percent of the cases if the mecholyl test is added. Manometry reveals what is anticipated—exaggerated, simultaneous repetitive contractions. A peristaltic wave

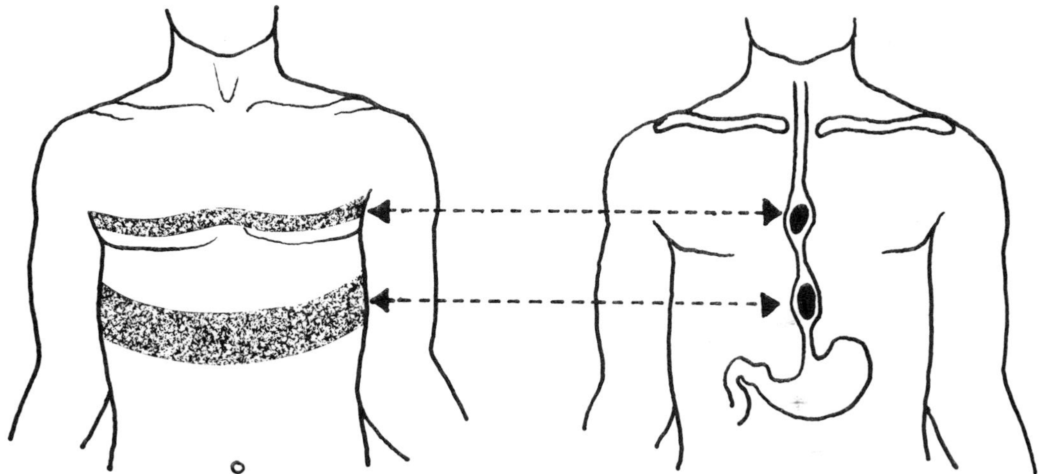

Figure 12-6. Esophageal pain may radiate around the chest at the same level of the lesions's spinal segmental distribution. The upper band corresponds to the T_4 spinal nerve, while the lower level corresponds to the distribution of the T_7 and T_8 spinal nerves. This must be kept in mind in the differential diagnosis.

should be seen sometime during the examination.

Esophageal Diverticula

A diverticulum is a hernia of the submucosa and mucosa between the fibers of the muscular wall. The size ranges from a small depression to a sac of considerable dimensions. The most common variety is the traction diverticulum (Fig. 12-7). These occur in the midportion of the esophagus at the crossing of the left bronchus. They are small and of little clinical importance.

Pharyngoesophageal diverticula (Zenker's) are the most important type and occur at the junction of the pharynx and esophagus (Fig. 12-8). Family physicians do not detect these diverticula until the sac becomes large enough to catch food. Patients complain of difficulty in swallowing, regurgitation and fullness in the lower neck or upper chest. When the trapped food finally comes up, the patient may report it appeared to be yesterday's meal totally undigested. Obviously the food is never acted upon by the gastric juices.

The patient may also become aware of gurgling in the neck during swallowing. When the hypopharynx becomes flooded with diverticular contents during the night, the patient reports aspiration and annoying coughing.

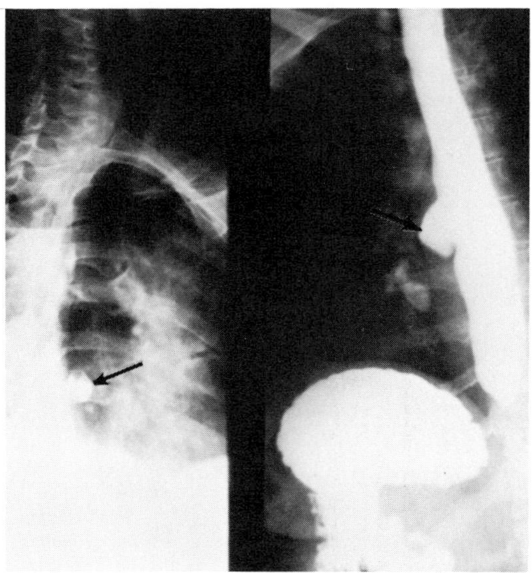

Figure 12-7. Two traction diverticula.

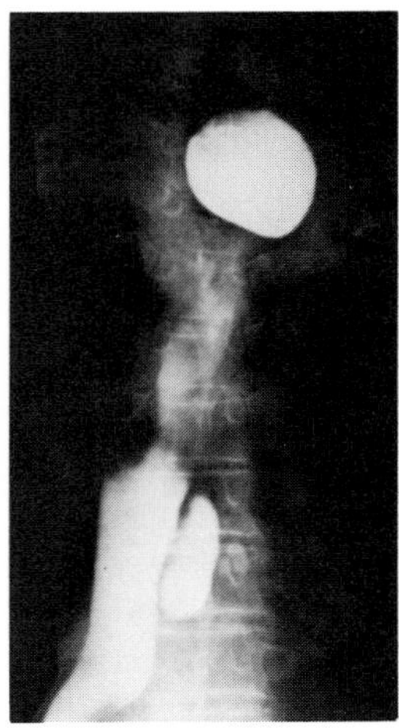

Figure 12-8. Moderate size Zenker's diverticulum. The patient also has a traction diverticulum of the middle esophagus.

Other minor forms of diverticula are the pressure traction diverticulum, which probably starts as a simple traction type and enlarges as the result of pressure from within, and pressure or pulsion diverticula. Again these often do not cause clinical symptoms unless they become inflamed. Then secondary spasm occurs. These diverticula may reach fairly large size and also cause food stagnation. They occur at both ends of the esophagus.

The most important diagnostic aid is the barium swallow. Multiple positioning under fluoroscopic control is important. Ordinarily, esophagoscopic examination is not reliable for detection but is important in the evaluation of the esophagus. Esophagitis can be most confusing.

Plummer-Vinson Syndrome

This syndrome occurs in postmenopausal women and is characterized by iron deficiency anemia; dysphagia, commonly the first and only complaint for many weeks; pharyngoesophagogastric mucosal atrophy and web; and occasionally hypopharyngeal carcinoma.

Dysphagia Lusoria

Several arterial anomalies may cause obstructive symptoms by pressing against the esophagus. An experienced radiologist can detect these extrinsic pressures by the configuration of the esophagus after a barium swallow.

Scleroderma

Dysphagia occasionally appears as a symptom of systemic disease. Ask the patient with dysphagia about arthritic symptoms, skin problems and Raynaud's phenomenon. Generally the diagnosis of scleroderma is made from other symptoms and the esophagus is investigated secondarily. Have the patient's esophagus checked by x-rays and an esophagoscopic examination. If the esophagus shows mucosal disease, a biopsy should be taken to confirm the diagnosis of scleroderma.

The barium x-ray study will confirm the presence of a dilated esophagus, impaired peristalsis and a widely patent esophageal sphincter allowing reflux. Because of the latter, esophagitis often complicates the picture.

Foreign Bodies

Managing foreign bodies in the pharynx and esophagus is a complicated problem. It is better for the family physician to call an esophagoscopist.

Usually a foreign body will pass down the gastrointestinal tract without difficulty. At most, the passage will cause a superficial erosion. Large objects may become impacted at one of the normal anatomic narrowings (Fig. 12-9). Objects stuck in the esophageal passage lead to complications, i.e. obstruction, inflammation, edema, spasm of the sphincters, periesophagitis, mediastinitis or empyema.

Prompt treatment is essential. Order an x-ray study. It will show the kind, size, shape and position of the object. A negative finding in a suspicious case is not conclusive and must be followed by esophagoscopy. The esophagoscopist should be prepared not only to make a diagnosis but also to remove the foreign body.

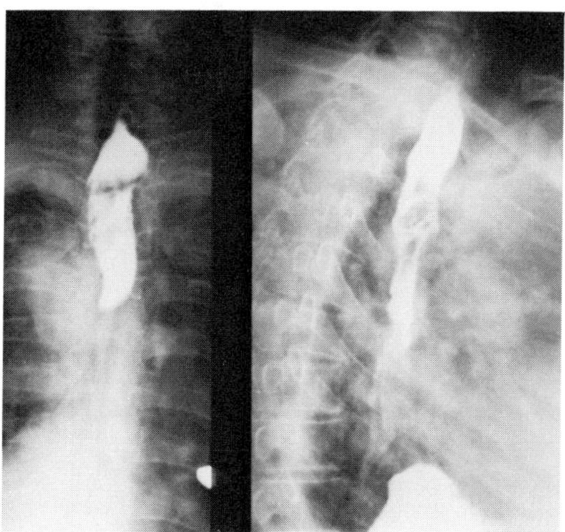

Figure 12-9. Particles of meat stuck in the esophagus.

Occasionally a patient may be unaware that he has swallowed something that could lodge in his throat. More often, though, a patient will complain of something in his throat when there is no evidence of such an occurrence. Family physicians often are uncertain how far to carry diagnostic studies in these situations. There are potential legal complications in every case.

Patients often relate having had a sudden painful scratch while eating with each swallow thereafter causing discomfort at the same spot. When a foreign body is present the patient may have these symptoms, but more likely he is bothered by salivation, regurgitation and gagging. Dysphagia is variable.

On the other hand, the absence of dysphagia does not assure that no foreign body is present. A careful history of the original incident will help: some odynophagia felt within the chest is almost always present at the start. If the object remains in the chest, the pain may disappear only to return if penetration and periesophagitis develops.

Corrosive Stricture

Single or multiple strictures follow the swallowing of a corrosive substance such as caustic soda, lye or boiling fluids accidentally or in an attempt at suicide. Many will die, but in those who live a stricture usually develops. The final result depends entirely on the depth and extent of the burn. The stricture may be soft or very rigid, incomplete or complete.

Do not be misled by an asymptomatic period that lasts for several weeks or even a year. The mouth lesions heal and the odynophagia disappears. In the meantime a cicatrix is forming and dysphagia begins. Perhaps a bolus will lodge in the throat and require emergency care.

X-ray films show the pathology and can serve as an invaluable record for later comparison. Esophagoscopy is important and permits biopsy and cytologic studies in an effort to recognize early malignant changes. The patient will need observation and treatment the rest of his life. Cases of this nature are best treated from the start by a specialist with experience in esophageal diseases.

Dafoe and Ross[2] have outlined their treatment aimed at preventing the formation of strictures. Esophagoscopy under general anesthesia is done within the first 48 hours if possible. If no esophageal burn is found in the esophagus, treatment is directed toward the oropharynx only. For lye burns, the patient swallows citric juices during the first 2 or 3 days. Small amounts of olive oil should be swallowed with a soft or liquid diet. If the esophagus is involved, a plastic tube is put into the stomach through a cervical esophagostomy or pharyngostomy. The tube is not removed for 2 to 3 months. Antibiotics are given for at least 2 weeks. In severe cases, steroids should be given for 2 to 3 months. If strictures form in spite of the medical treatment, Dafoe and Ross start visual dilatation at 2 week intervals. Occasionally, when the esophagus appears to be beyond successful dilatation, some help may be obtained by replacing the narrowed esophageal segment by a colon transplant.

INDIGESTION (DYSPEPSIA)

What to Look For

If your patient complains of indigestion look for the conditions listed under Differential Diagnosis later in this section.

How the Stomach Functions

The stomach is divided into an upper fundic area, a central area and a portion near the pylorus called the antrum. This is important because the distribution and characteristics of the stomach glands vary from area to area.

In the fundus the glands secrete mucus. The mucus serves as a protective coating for the surface cells of the stomach.

The glands in the central area produce hydrochloric acid (HCl), most of the enzymes and mucus. HCl is produced by the parietal cells. According to some estimates, the central portion of the stomach has 1 to 1½ billion parietal cells. If stimulated properly these cells can produce a cup (200 ml) of 0.17 normal hydrochloric acid per hour. The exact chemical reaction which produces HCl is not known but hydrogen and chlorine ions are secreted into the lumen while sodium and carbonate are carried away by the blood.

The most important of the enzymes, pepsin, is produced by its own special manufacturing structure, the chief cell. The special function of pepsin is to digest proteins. Pepsin in the presence of HCl can break up a proteinlike egg albumin with 500 amino acids into numerous fragments or peptides and prepare proteins for further digestion in the small intestine. If the stomach contents are neutral, such as occurs after taking an antacid, or if the stomach cannot produce HCl, pepsin is inactive and little protein digestion takes place.

The stomach lining produces other enzymes, some of which digest proteins in a neutral milieu. There is no enzyme secretion from the stomach walls which digests carbohydrates. There is, however, a gastric lipase that splits short or medium-length chain fatty acids. However, the total amount of intragastric digestion not attributable to either acid or pepsin is of minor importance.

The antrum glands secrete gastrin as well as mucus. Gastrin is a hormone which is secreted by the antrum of the stomach and goes into the blood stream. When it returns to the stomach it stimulates the parietal cells in the central area to secrete HCl.

The secretion of gastrin begins when the individual thinks of food or begins to enjoy its taste and, again, when food enters the stomach. This mechanism is determined in part by the stomach acidity. When food enters the stomach, it tends to neutralize the acidity of the gastric contents and mechanically stretches the antrum. This results in the production of gastrin which stimulates the acid-producing mechanisms. Once the gastric contents turn acid again following the secretion of HCl, gastrin production is turned off—one of the most effective feedback controls ever devised.

The gastric glands also contain argentaffin cells which secrete serotonin into the blood stream.

A close view of the gastric mucosa shows it is lined by columnar epithelium in which are pits or openings for the above described gastric glands. The columnar epithelium produces mucus as well as a variety of other active substances and controls the passage of various chemicals:

- –water and electrolytes pass into the stomach
- –hydrogen ions move out into the stomach but are prevented from reentering
- –large water-soluble molecules such as glucose are blocked from passage by the columnar epithelium
- –fat-soluble drugs from the lumen move into the tissues through the columnar cells
- –aspirin, which is water-soluble at low acidities, is blocked by the columnar cells (At high acidities, aspirin becomes fat-soluble and so can pass into the body tissues through the columnar cells)

While all this is going on the stomach is churning and storing the food. The two valves at each end of the stomach are complex mechanisms. The one at the upper end, where esophagus and stomach join, must prevent regurgitation of gastric contents but must open for swallowing, burping or vomiting. At the other end, the pyloric muscle helps to control the discharge of gastric contents. It prevents the dumping of unprepared food into the small intestine.

Finally, the stomach keeps us alive, not because of its digestive function but because of its effect on the blood. When the stomach is totally removed from a patient, he will die in 4 or 5 years of pernicious anemia. The physiology is complex, but in general it follows this plan:

- –The parietal cells of the stomach produce intrinsic factor (IF).
- –In the stomach and upper intestine, IF links up with vitamin B_{12} from ingested foodstuffs and passes the IF-B_{12} complex along into the lower intestine.
- –IF and vitamin B_{12} are reabsorbed together in the ileum by a special mechanism. This mechanism will not absorb free vitamin B_{12}.
- –If there is no IF production, either because the gastric mucosa is diseased or because the stomach has been removed, pernicious anemia results. Unless the patient is given vitamin B_{12} by injection he ultimately dies.

Testing in Indigestion

Tests for Gastric Secretions

SCREENING FOR ACID. The Diagnex blue test has been used long enough to prove its worth as a screening test for gastric acidity. The test is dependable: 95 percent accurate in identifying acid secretion and 97 percent accurate in identifying achlorhydrics.

Tell the patient to start the test immediately on arising without eating or drinking anything for breakfast. He is to start the test by urinating and discarding the urine. The patient then takes two tablets, one of caffeine and one of sodium benzoate, with a glass of water.

One hour later have the patient urinate into a container marked "control urine." At this time he opens the packet of azure

A, dissolves it in ¼ glass of water, stirs and drinks it. The granules do not dissolve well and the glass may need to be flushed with water. It is important that the patient swallows all the granules.

Two hours later: Have the patient urinate into a container marked "test urine."

The Squibb Company provides a color comparator block with two color standards. One represents a color intensity of 0.6 mg azure A and the other 0.3 mg. Instructions are enclosed.

If the color intensity of the test urine is equal to or exceeds that of 0.6 mg standard, the patient has secreted free gastric hydrochloric acid and the test is complete. The gastric contents must be pH 3 or less to produce a positive test.

Presumptive evidence of hypochlorhydria: the color of the test specimen falls between 0.6 mg and 0.3 mg.

Presumptive evidence of achlorhydria: the color of the test specimen falls below 0.3 mg.

If the test results are questionable or indicate achlorhydria, repeat the test using betazole for gastric stimulation. When indicated, a subcutaneous or intramuscular dose of 50 mg of betazole for a person weighing 100 to 250 pounds may be substituted for the orally given caffeine and sodium benzoate as stimulants to gastric secretion.

If the last test still produces a negative result for acidity, order an augmented betazole test after intubation.

The oral azure A test may give misleading results in renal or liver insufficiency or in a malabsorption syndrome.

ONE-HOUR BASAL SECRETION TEST. This test is made after an all night fast. A tube is passed and the residual gastric contents aspirated and examined. Then four 15-minute collections are made by continuous suction. The results are expressed in milliequivalents per hour.

The maximal acid output (MAO) is determined by studying acid secretion after the injection of histamine or betazole hydrochloride in 2 mg per kg doses. Betazole has fewer side effects and is as strongly stimulating as histamine. Pentapeptide, an analogue of gastrin in doses of 0.6 mg per kg, may be used also. There are not reported side effects and it is as stimulating as either histamine or betazole.

The most reliable and informative procedure is a 2 hour test. The initial hour measures basal acid production and the second hour's collection follows a maximal dose of betazole. Do a 2 or 3 hour test to help verify duodenal ulcer, gastric ulcer, gastritis, pernicious anemia or Zollinger-Ellison syndrome. This is the best test to determine achlorhydria, and indicates a failure of the gastric contents to fall below a pH of 6 after maximal stimulation.

If the test results indicate 50 mEq/L or more, the case is probably one of a hypersecretor and may help the physician decide on advising medical or surgical treatment.

Serum pepsinogen is being determined more frequently. If pepsinogen serum value is under 200 units it is conclusive evidence of gastric atrophy with associated achlorhydria.

INSULIN (HOLLANDER) TEST. Insulin to used to stimulate the parietal cells to produce acid, the chief cells to produce pepsin and the antrum to produce gastrin via the production of hypoglycemia and vagus stimulation. Secretory response occurs when the blood sugar falls to 50 percent or less of the fasting level. The response is abolished by vagotomy and is used at times to test the completeness of a vagotomy.

The tube must be correctly placed, especially after a gastrectomy. Specimens are collected as for the basic 1 hour secretion test. Blood sugar should be checked every half hour to confirm the proper level of hypoglycemia.

Vagal innervation is present if acid rises to 70 mEq/L above control values, when free acid is present in the fasting specimen, or to 10 mEq/L if control values show no free acid. If vagotomy is complete there is no rise.

Other Stomach Studies

GASTRIC. *Gastric cytology* is used in suspected cases of carcinoma of the stomach.

GASTROSCOPY AND BIOPSY. One way to determine if you are ordering too many gastroscopic examinations is to compare the number of positive and negative results obtained. If gastroscopy almost never turns up something positive, you are probably ordering the examination too often and in the wrong patients.

The most common reason for ordering a gastroscopic examination is in patients with gastrointestinal bleeding in whom the x-ray films are negative.

The second most common cause is to differentiate an inflammatory (benign) and neoplastic (malignant) ulcer.

Other indications are:

- investigation of an undiagnosed gastric complaint which cannot be diagnosed by other means
- determination of the extent of a lesion
- check up on previous surgery estimating the size of the stomal opening, the health of the mucosa, and the presence of marginal ulcers
- diagnosis of ulcerative lesions of the stomach and observe their response to therapy

Contraindications are:

- severe esophageal obstructions
- aneurysms
- recent corrosive poisoning
- hepatic cirrhosis with varices
- psychotic or uncooperative patients

Relative contraindications are:

- angina pectoris
- curvature of the spine and cervical arthritis
- acute infections about the mouth and pharynx
- cardiospasm
- any anatomic abnormalities of the mouth, teeth, pharynx or neck
- emphysema or other pulmonary diseases of significance
- mediastinal tumors and inflammation
- acute abdominal disease

Saline load (Hunt) is used for pyloric obstruction. Upper gastrointestinal x-ray studies are helpful.

EXTRAGASTRIC. Other extragastric studies usually required as indicated are:

- cholecystography
- small bowel x-ray study
- barium studies of the esophagus
- barium enema study of the colon
- esophagoscopy
- sigmoidscopy
- occasional psychiatric evaluation
- Bernstein acid perfusion for esophagitis, atypical angina pectoris and chest pain
- duodenal drainage for bile crystals in atypical cholelithiasis with negative x-ray
- liver biopsy for metastatic carcinoma, hepatitis, cirrhosis and diffuse liver disease
- small intestine biopsy for sprue, lymphoma and suspected Whipple's disease
- string test for obscure gastrointestinal bleeding
- small intestine intubation for identifying the source of gastrointestinal bleeding

When to Use Gastric Secretory Tests

After partial gastrectomy, a patient with a MAO greater than 8 mEq per hour has a 70 percent chance of developing a stomach ulcer.

After a vagotomy and drainage surgery, the MAO should fall to ½ of the preoperative level; after partial gastrectomy to about $^{1}/_{8}$; and after vagotomy and antrectomy to $^{1}/_{15}$ of the preoperative level. If postoperative secretory levels exceed these, surgery may have failed—vagotomy was incomplete or antrectomy or resection inadequate.

In Zollinger-Ellison tumor the basal secretion exceeds 60 percent of the MAO in 80 percent of the patients. The overnight secretion exceeds 1,000 ml with acid content greater than 100 mEq. The best test for diagnosing Zollinger-Ellison tumor, however, may be the serum gastrin.

Use gastric secretory tests when you suspect there is no acid as in severe atrophic gastritis or the gastric lesion of pernicious anemia. Gastric analysis by the tube-Toepfer method but without stimulation indicates about 40 percent of the normal persons are hypochlorhydric. When histamine stimulation is used the results are more dependable: 17 percent of normals were achlorhydric and only 21 percent hypochlorhydric. Consequently, gastric analysis as a screening test for stomach cancer is not effective.[3]

On suspicion of a very high acid, as in the Zollinger-Ellison syndrome, use gastric secretory tests. In this case an extremely large volume and a low pH of the basal collection is diagnostic even without gastric stimulation.

Patients with recurrent anastomotic ulcers who have previously undergone a gastric resection and vagotomy need the tests. The best type for this purpose is the Hollander or insulin test. The results will indicate whether the vagus is contributing to the acid secretion and whether a repeat vagotomy should be attempted. This is important, since there may be other reasons for the recurrent ulcer, such as retained antrum.

Remember the pH of gastric juice is not helpful in diagnosing duodenal or gastric ulcer but may be used preoperatively to help decide on the type of procedure to be performed. A maximal histamine stimulating test is helpful in determining whether a gastric ulcer is malignant.

The family physician should depend only on a gastric analysis that is done after a fluoroscopically placed radiopaque tube. Gastric secretions should be collected by hand suction. A ½ hour or 1 hour basal collection should be taken prior to stimulation. If the specimen has a pH of less than 5.0, adult pernicious anemia is not present. If the pH is 5.0 or higher and pernicious anemia is suspected, stimulation should be done. Normally the pH will drop more than one pH unit following stimulation.

After stimulation take fractions every 15 minutes for 1 hour following maximal histamine stimulation and 75 minutes following betazole. The pH of each 15 minute sample is determined by use of a pH meter.

Contraindications: Stimulatory agents should not be used in patients who have a history of coronary artery disease, asthma or allergies. Precede the injection of histamine with the administration of an antihistamine. Betazole stimulation produces less side effects than histamine when given in doses of less than 100 mg. Higher doses may be dangerous.

Differential Diagnosis

Duodenal Ulcer

Symptoms of a duodenal ulcer are:

- –pain located with one examining finger
- –dyspepsia (burning or gnawing)
- –pain is lessened by food, alkali and milk
- –pain is increased when the stomach is empty
- –pain commonly awakens the patient 2 to 4 hr after going to sleep
- –attacks of painful indigestion will last 5 to 7 days with lessening of pain between attacks
- –some drugs, orange juice, coffee and alcohol will increase the indigestion

Diagnosis is made by upper gastrointestinal x-ray studies followed by whatever other gastrointestinal studies that may be needed. Classic features of the duodenal ulcer are deformities of the duodenal bulb with a rounded, punched-out niche (Figs. 12-10 and 12-11). Deformity of the bulb is due to edema of the muscularis. This causes straightening of the wall near the ulcer, shortening of the lesser curve of the bulb, contracture of the greater curvature border and formation of incisura opposite the crater.

Medical treatment for duodenal ulcer has been simplified in recent years. The main therapeutic attack is neutralizing stomach acid by antacids taken hourly except at mealtime and when asleep. Check serum calcium levels 2 weeks after instituting therapy if the antacid contains calcium.

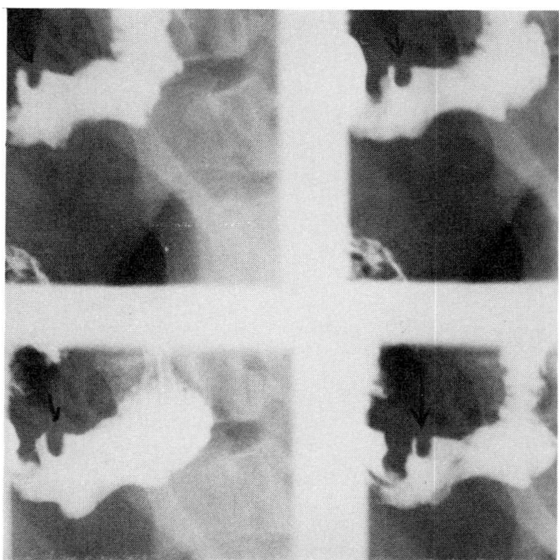

Figure 12-10. Deformity of the duodenal bulb with niche due to an ulcer.

Diet is not emphasized, but alcohol, aspirin, citric acids and coffee should be avoided. Smoking should be curtailed if not stopped.

Order anticholinergic agents at bedtime to suppress gastric acid secretion. To do any good, these agents must be given to the point of mouth dryness or vision blurring and then reduced by one increment and maintained at the tolerance level. Give sedatives or tranquilizers with anticholinergics at bedtime. They are clearly counterindicated in patients with glaucoma or prostatic hypertrophy with urinary retention. When ulcer pain has been absent from 4 to 6 weeks, all therapy should be stopped.

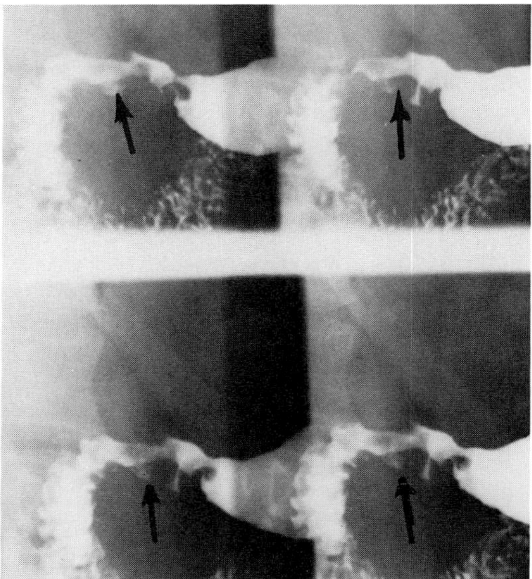

Figure 12-11. Deformities of the duodenal bulb with niche due to an ulcer.

PREVENTION OF RECURRENCE. To prevent recurrent attacks avoid the following:

- emotional conflicts or distress
- faulty and irregular eating habits
- emotional stress during meals
- large meals
- deleterious drugs: aspirin, steroids, antirheumatic drugs, antihypertensive drugs and anticoagulants
- smoking
- coffee

If drugs must be administered, order frequent feedings and antacids. If alcoholic beverages are used occasionally, they should be diluted and taken immediately before or after meals.

Most important in prevention is to instruct the patient to resume frequent small feedings and hourly antacids:

- when confronted with emotional stress
- during febrile illnesses
- preoperatively, even before teeth extractions
- if his history indicates his ulcer tends to recur at certain times of the year
- during work crises

Chronic Gastritis

Evidence suggests that chronic gastritis may be a progressive disease beginning as a superficial gastritis and developing very slowly into irreversible gastric atrophy. The cause has not been verified but drugs, chemicals, alcoholic beverages, allergens, spices, thermal injuries, infections and irradiation have been implicated. Look for emotional stresses as playing a part in the exacerbation of chronic gastritis if not the actual cause.

Zollinger-Ellison Syndrome

Like many other rare diseases, the family physician may never see this syndrome, but must keep its occurrence in mind in all ulcer cases refractory to medical and surgical treatment. The possibility of the syndrome arises when the physician orders a gastric secretory test and finds basal secretion volumes in excess of 100 ml/hr, acid secretions in excess of 10 mEq/L of HCl and poor increase in either test after maximum histamine stimulation.

X-rays are not often diagnostic but may show prominent gastric rugae and unusual small bowel patterns. In addition, look for multiple ulcers and ulcers in unusual positions.

Selenium scan and arteriography help detect the presence and location of pancreatic tumors. Verification of the diagnosis may have to be done at a medical center where serum gastrin immunoassay can be performed.[4]

Pyloric Ulcer

The classic symptoms of pyloric ulcer so well detailed in most textbooks mean little or nothing. This condition (Fig. 12-12) has no unique symptoms. Even at surgery the pathology is difficult to describe because the anatomic limits of the pylorus are vague. In addition about 30 percent of patients with pyloric ulcers have one or two other

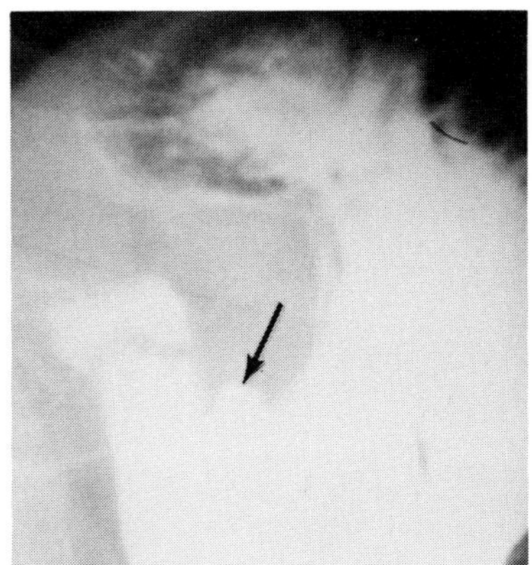

Figure 12-12. Benign gastric ulcer.

Table 12-1. Main Presenting Complaints of 75 Patients

Presenting Complaint	*No. of Patients*
Epigastric hunger pain with food relief	17
Sudden hemorrhage	17
Pain, heartburn, weight loss	12
Patternless abdominal pain	8
Pain after meals	7
Nausea, vomiting, gas	4
Crater discovered by chance	3
Vomiting only	2
Left upper quadrant pain	2
Sudden perforation	1
Heartburn only	1
Back pain only	1

Reprinted from Palmer ED: Pyloric ulcer. AFP 5:104, 1972, with permission.

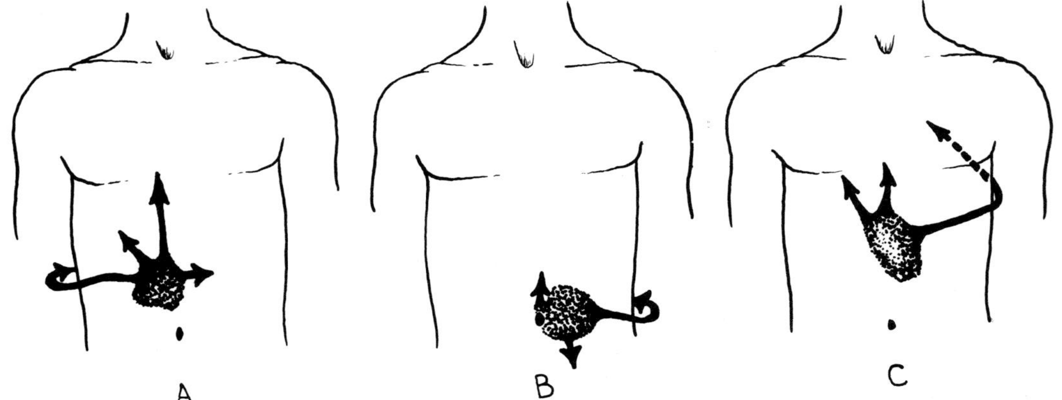

Figure 12-13. Peptic ulcer pain and its radiation: *A*, Nonperforating duodenal ulcer; *B*, Nonperforating jejunal ulcer; *C*, Nonperforating gastric ulcer.

Table 12-2. Complications Among 75 Patients

Complication	*No. of Patients*
Hemorrhage	32
Cicatricial pyloric obstruction	13
Perforation	3
Pylorocholedochal fistula	1
Penetration	1

Reprinted from Palmer ED: Pyloric ulcer. AFP 5:104, 1972, with permission.

ulcers. The main complaint of patients with pyloric ulcer usually is pain (Fig. 12-13). Other complaints are listed in Table 12-1.

About 20 percent of these patients come to surgery because of the high incidence of complications (Table 12-2). The surgical procedure is still debated: subtotal gastrectomy vs. vagotomy and pyloroplasty.

Diaphragmatic Hernia and Esophagitis

A diaphragmatic hernia is a protrusion of abdominal contents through an abnormal opening in the diaphragm (Fig. 12-14). The diaphragmatic opening occurs as a result of congenital absence of a portion of the diaphragm (Morgagni's and Bochdalek's hernia [Fig. 12-15]); enlargement of a normally occurring opening (Sliding hiatal hernia and paraesophageal hernia); or blunt or sharp trauma to the diaphragm.

CONGENITAL DIAPHRAGMATIC HERNIAS. BOCHDALEK DEFECT. The most common congenital hernia is the posterolateral Bochdalek defect. It accounts for 20 percent of all congenital diaphragmatic hernias and is present in 8.5 percent of stillbirths. It occurs once in every 1,500 to 2,200 births. The hernia occurs five times more frequently on the left than on the right. Severe respiratory distress, cyanosis and even death may occur in infants when the hernia is large if the defect is not repaired immediately. In the infant with respiratory distress, a chest film with or without a contrast medium is usually sufficient to establish the diagnosis. The family physician with the aid of a radiologist should be able to diagnose the defect and institute medical supportive measures until a surgeon familiar with the repair is contacted.

Insert a nasogastric tube to deflate the gas-filled loops of bowel and place the infant in a semi-Fowler position. If oxygen is needed, administer it by endotracheal tube. Oxygen by mask increases the amount of gastrointestinal gas.

Surgery for repair is a complicated procedure usually done through an abdominal or transthoracic incision. In addition an intercostal catheter is put into the pleural space and attached to a water-seal container for drainage.

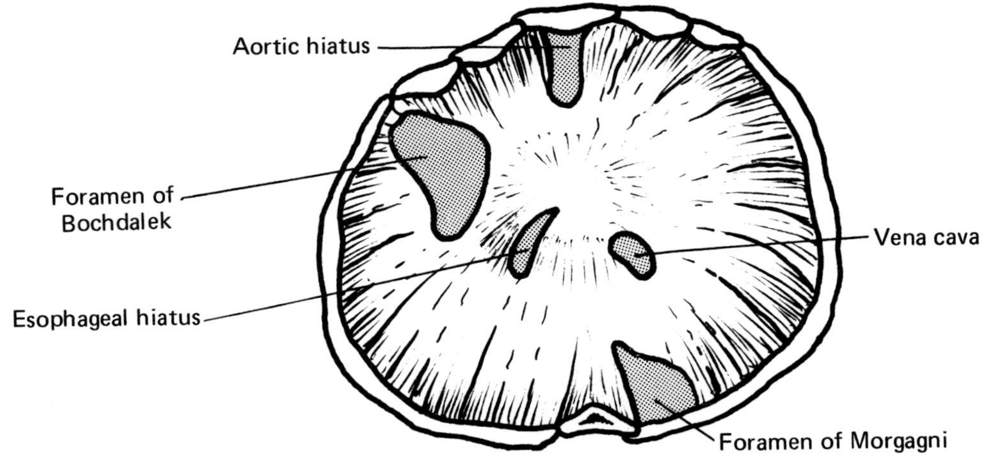

Figure 12-14. Cross section of the diaphragm with its normal apertures as viewed from the chest.

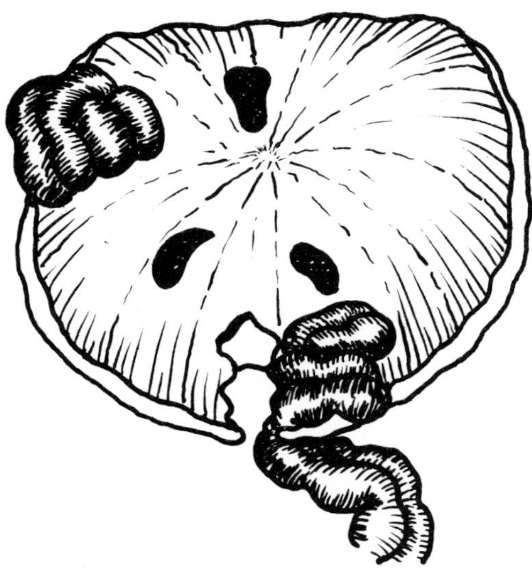

Figure 12-15. Hernias through the foramen of Morgagni (anterior) and the foramen of Bochdalek (posterior right).

In the older child or adult with a previously unrecognized Bochdalek's hernia the symptoms range from none to those of constipation, partial intestinal obstruction, chest pain, hematemesis or melena.

MORGAGNI'S HERNIA. About 3 percent of congenital hernias are of the subcostosternal or Morgagni variety. The defect is often asymptomatic and, if symptoms do occur, they are gastrointestinal in nature and in patients past 40 years of age.

Chest x-ray study reveals a mass in the right cardiophrenic angle. The lateral view of the chest locates the mass in the most anterior aspect of the diaphragm just under the sternum. Look for gas-filled loops of bowel in the same area. Unless the omentum occupies the hernial sac, a barium enema will be diagnostic. Advise repair of asymptomatic Morgagni's hernias because of the danger of bowel incarceration and obstruction. The repair is usually done by the abdominal approach.

HIATAL HERNIA. This represents the most common type of diaphragmatic hernia occurring in adult life (Fig. 12-16). It occurs most commonly in an obese middle-aged patient. The types of hiatal hernia are esophagogastric or sliding hernia, paraesophageal hernia and short esophagal type.

SLIDING TYPE. In the sliding variety the increased laxity of the hiatal opening allows the stomach, or a portion of it, to slide in and out of the thorax (Fig. 12-17). While the patient is standing or is propped up in bed, the hernia remains reduced. When the patient stoops or is recumbent, the stomach slides into the thorax (Fig. 12-18). Exposure of the distal esophagus to the continuous irritation of gastric secretions of low pH causes a peptic esophagitis. Consequently, the symptoms, when they occur, mimic other diseases such as peptic ulcer, chronic cholecystitis, or coronary artery disease. The typical symptoms are substernal or epigastric burning aggravated by lying down, bending or eating heavy meals and relieved by standing or by antacids. More than a half complain of heart burn, vomiting and regurgitation. Asymptomatic patients do not have reflux.

Because of the sliding nature of this hernia, x-rays should always be taken in the Trendelenberg position. The roentgenographic demonstration of the presence of gastroesophageal reflux is probably the most important single determination that can be done to evaluate the clinical significance of a hiatal hernia.

The acid perfusion test (Bernstein's) is a safe and effective test for esophagitis. Esophagitis may or may not be associated with hiatal hernia.

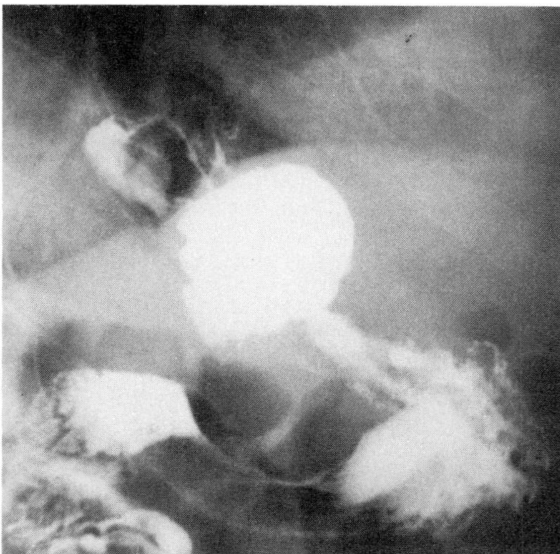

Figure 12-16. Hiatal hernia. Hernial sacs can best be identified above the diaphragm.

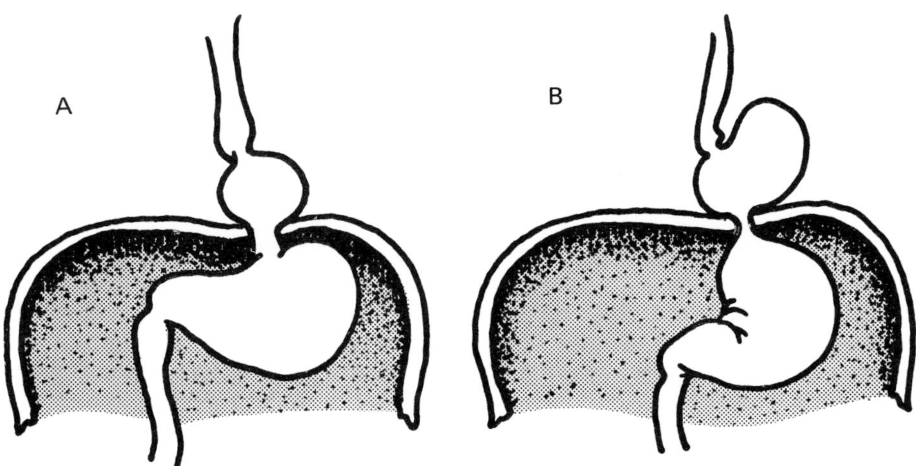

Figure 12-17. *A*, Pulsion type hiatal hernia (incompetent hiatus); *B*, Esophageal hiatal hernia with elevation of the esophagus.

Introduce a radiopaque gastric tube into the stomach of a fasting patient who is in an upright position. Aspirate the gastric contents. Withdraw the tube so that the distal opening is placed 30 to 35 cm from the incisor teeth. Anchor the tube over the patient's shoulder and connect it to a two-way infusion set. In the meantime procure a stand to hold two test solution bottles. One bottle of 0.9 percent sodium chloride or 5 percent dextrose and one of 0.1 normal hydrochloric acid. Place the stand and test solution behind the patient out of sight. Start the test by allowing the dextrose or saline solution to run at a rate of 100 to 120 drops per minute for 10 minutes. Then the hydrochloric acid test solution is allowed to run at the same rate for 15 minutes. If pain does not develop, increase the rate. Repeat the sequence if pain occurs.

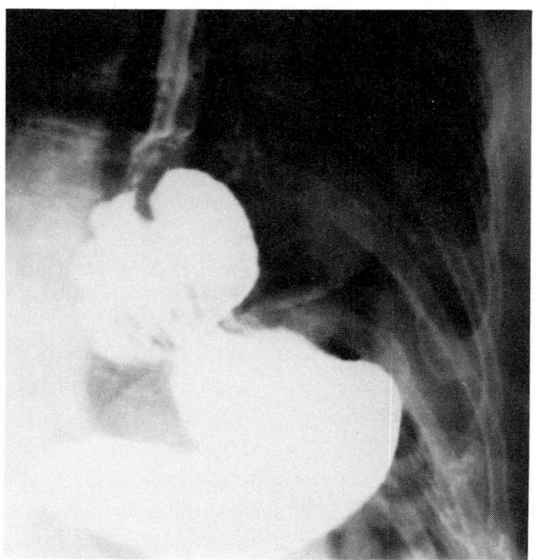

Figure 12-18. Large sliding hiatal hernia.

Interpretation of results: Negative if no heart burn or retrosternal pain develops during acid perfusion. Positive if there is a reduplication of the patient's complaint. False-positive if symptoms are produced which are entirely new and do not mimic the patient's complaints.

Production of abdominal pain will help localize the origin of pain. If abdominal pain continues, suspect gastric or duodenal disease. If abdominal pain is relieved by saline, suspect esophagitis.

The test is unreliable if pain is stimulated by both the saline and the hydrochloric acid.

Perfusion of autogenous gastric contents may result in a positive test when hydrochloric acid falls. Pain produced by the acid may be relieved by the perfusion of an antacid. A combination of the acid perfusion test and simultaneous measurement of intraesophageal pressure changes is a more efficient procedure in the diagnosis of esophagitis.

Even when the diagnosis is supported by radiologic findings and by a positive acid perfusion test, other studies may be necessary—esophagoscopy to confirm inflammatory changes, manometry to evaluate esophageal motor disturbances and localize the gastroesophageal junction and cytology to eliminate the suspicion of neoplasm.

The modern flexible, fiberoptic esophagoscope gives excellent visualization of the lower esophagus and herniated portions of the stomach. This instrument permits air inflation of the esophagus and stomach. This helps to demonstrate a small hernia. Remember that mild or moderate esophagitis is seldom shown by the mucosal relief of x-rays.

Paraesophageal Hernia. This type is relatively asymptomatic even when a large portion of the stomach is herniated into the chest cavity. Regurgitation is fairly common. In this variety the cardia of the stomach protrudes into the thorax through a defect in the diaphragm beside the esophageal opening, not through the hiatus, so esophagus and cardia are separated by a thin band (Fig. 12-19). Upper gastrointestinal series of barium x-rays usually demonstrate the esophageal hernia and separate the sliding type from the paraesophageal type. It is true, however, that more frequently than not the paraesophageal hernia is associated with a sliding component. The greatest difference is that esophagitis does not occur in paraesophageal hernia while it is the main complication in sliding esophageal hernia.

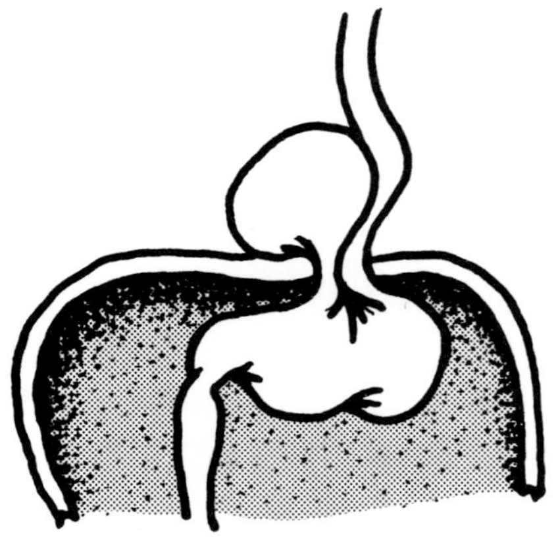

Figure 12-19. Paraesophageal hernia (esophagus in normal position).

Traumatic Diaphragmatic Hernia. If it is large it will compress the pulmonary tissue and produce dyspnea and respiratory distress. If the opening is small and the herniation of bowel is gradual, symptoms of partial obstruction occur, that is, cramping abdominal pain following meals.

Medical Management.[6] Most patients with symptomatic hiatal hernia respond to medical management.

First, attempt to reduce esophageal reflux by:

- urging the patient to avoid activities that increase intra-abdominal pressure
- helping the patient lose weight if overweight
- asking the patient to abandon the use of tight corsets or belts
- changing the patient's eating habits if esophagitis is present
- giving antacid therapy

Have the patient sleep with his head and chest elevated. If the patient has the funds, suggest an electrically controlled hospital type bed. The head of the bed may then be raised and lowered as needed. There are simpler and more inexpensive devices: a wedge-shaped piece of foam rubber placed under the patient's head and chest or a plywood adjustable support slipped between the box springs and the mattress. Eight inches will serve as the proper elevation.

The patient should avoid alcohol; coffee; Sanka; tea; cola; chocolate; aspirin products; orange, pineapple, tomato and grapefruit juices; carbonated beverages; and hot or cold liquids. Instruct the patient not to distend his stomach by overeating or by ingesting large meals and to refrain from liquids for 1 hour after meals. If any stenosis is present, the patient should eat only purées.

For antacid therapy order a nonabsorbable formula. Use 2 Albertabs, 5 Gelusil, Mylanta or Tums tablets or 1 ounce of liquid antacid after meals. If considerable esophagitis is present prescribe hourly doses of the antacid as long as the patient is awake.

Surgical Treatment. Indications for surgery are:

- –anemia from the prolonged chronic loss of blood
- –stricture of the esophagus
- –strangulation of the herniated stomach
- –persistent symptoms in spite of medical management
- –respiratory complications due to aspiration

Don't be misled by the optimistic attitude of the surgeon. Recurrence after surgery may be as high as 25 to 30 percent. Such a high recurrence rate indicates that surgeons still have something to learn about hiatal hernia repair. Some surgeons will merely repair the hiatal hernia. Others will perform a balanced operation—repair the hernia; do a bilateral vagotomy and pyloroplasty, thereby reducing the acid factor; do a restoration of the cardioesophageal angle; and correct any other associated diseases.

Preventing Recurrence. There are several predisposing factors to consider when attempting to prevent hiatal hernia or its recurrence after surgical repair or simply

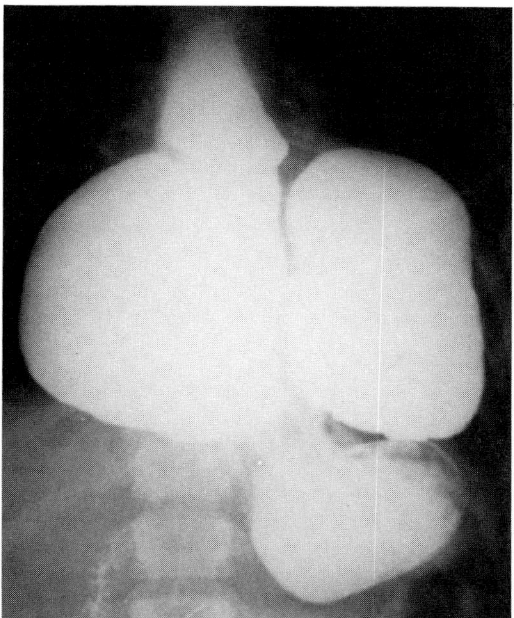

Figure 12-20. Diaphragmatic eventration in a child: left diaphragm with upside-down stomach.

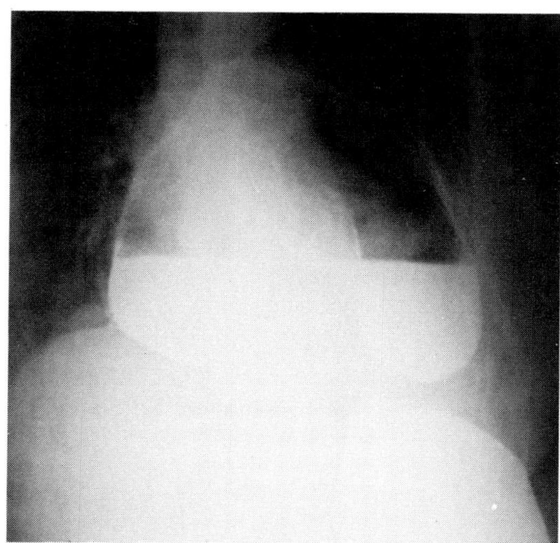

Figure 12-21. Intrathoracic stomach, upside down.

in preventing the complications of a diaphragmatic hernia.

Nothing much can be done to strengthen a lax or wide hiatal aperture (Figs. 12-20 and 12-21) in a patient born with such a defect, but considerably more can be done to decrease the intra-abdominal pressure that, with the lax opening, produces the hernia. Factors which increase intra-abdominal pressure are pregnancy, obesity, ascites, abdominal tumors, belching, regurgitation, vomiting and occupational strains.

Structural changes in the tissue around the hiatus may result from obesity, loss of muscle tone as in some systemic diseases, spasm of the esophagus and congenital shortening of the esophagus. A weakness also may be caused by gastric or esophageal surgery or even a vagotomy. Accidents, physical strain, overeating and aerophagia are other factors favoring the development of diaphragmatic hernias.

Cancer of the Stomach

An early symptom of cancer of the stomach is anorexia, perhaps better described as early appetite satiety. Do not be surprised if there are no symptoms until the disease is well advanced. Abdominal pain or discomfort may suggest peptic ulcer disease.

Be on the alert if a patient complains of a change in gastrointestinal symptoms. There is no reason that a patient with a long history of dyspepsia or of a proven ulcer cannot develop a cancer.

High risk patients are patients over 45 years of age, those with achlorhydria and those with unexplained occult blood in the stool or with an unexplained anemia (Fig. 12-22). The incidence of stomach cancer in patients with atrophic gastritis is significantly higher than normal and patients with pernicious anemia show a fivefold increase in the risk of cancer of the stmach. Patients with a history of gastric ulcer or polyps and those with a family history of gastrointestinal cancer are high risk patients.

Other findings are obstructive symptoms, anemia following chronic blood loss, unremitting back pain, weight loss, hypoproteinemia and abnormal liver function tests. Some findings represent a surgically incurable stomach lesion: a firm supraclavicular lymph node, an enlarged irregular liver margin and an enlarged anterior rectal mass (Blumer's shelf). All are distant metastases.

Diagnosis depends on x-ray studies that show filling defects, irregularity of either curvature and loss of normal distensibility and on gastric acid study. The absence of free acid after stimulation supports the diagnosis of gastric cancer. Cytologic studies on centrifuged gastric washings and gastroscopy are an aid to diagnosis. There are blind areas, however, in the stomach which the gastroscope cannot reach. Consult with a skilled endoscopist regarding the feasibility of gastroscopy. The difference between benign gastric ulcer and an ulcerated gastric neoplasm is small and confusing.

Interpretation is the most important and difficult aspect of endoscopy. But, by photography, interpretation can be made more reliable, since it allows the clinician time to study the record itself and to compare it with other photographic records.

Suspect gastric malignancy with the following:

- a lesion on the greater curvature, the fundus or in the prepyloric portion of the lesser curvature
- failure of a lesion of the stomach to heal within 3 wk
- presence of achlorydria as proven by a stimulted gastric analysis
- malignant cells in the gastric aspirate
- gastroscopic evidence of malignancy
- X-ray evidence of malignancy (Fig. 12-23)

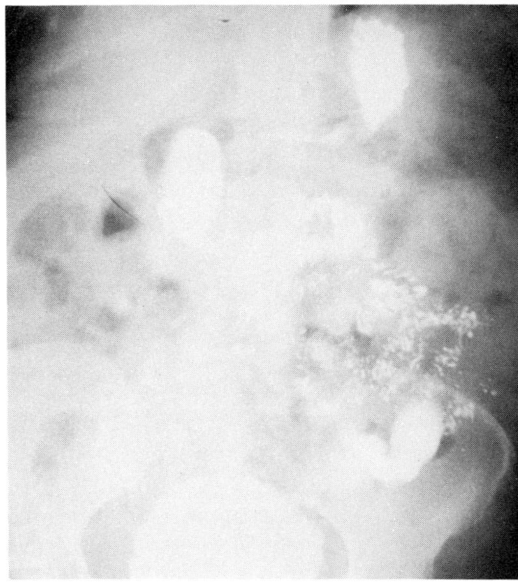

Figure 12-22. Leiomyoma of the stomach with bleeding.

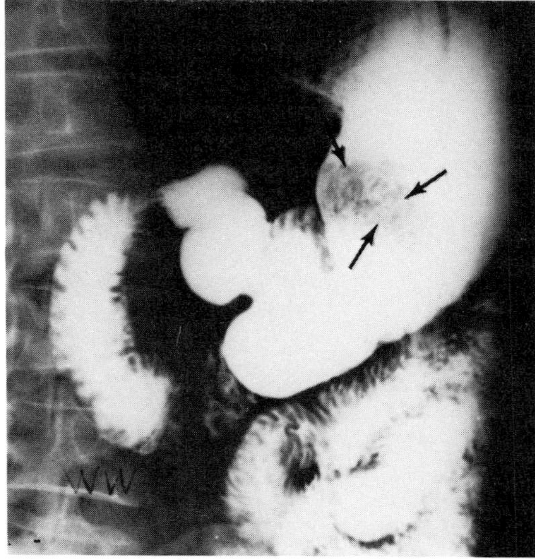

Figure 12-23. Carcinoma of the stomach and fibroids of the uterus.

There are no typical symptoms of gastric cancer but epigastric pain, loss of weight, anorexia and tiredness may herald the onset of gastric cancer.[7]

There is no known cure of cancer of the stomach except complete surgical excision of the cancer and its metastases. Although surgical removal of a stomach cancer does not appear a cure in more than 40 to 60 percent of the cases, comfort may be given to the patient for months by a combination of surgery, chemotherapy and supportive care.

Probably the best approach to a resectable lesion is by gastrectomy followed by either a Billroth I or Bilroth II repair.

Chemotherapy: 5-Fluorouracil (5-FU) given IV in 5 day courses. Dose: 10 to 15 mg per kg of body weight per day. After the first 5-day course, continue the 5-FU but on alternate days. Therapy should be guided by periodic blood counts.

Nonulcerative Diseases of the Duodenum

Duodenal peristalsis is inhibited much more easily than peristalsis in other parts of the gastrointestinal tract. Inhibitory impulses controlled by psychogenic factors can easily result in functional disease of the duodenum. This may explain why ordinary conditions such as slight obstruction or angulation produce disturbances in the propulsive capacity of the duodenum. Even reversed peristalsis has been noted fluoroscopically under normal and abnormal conditions. Look for functional disorders, duodenitis, diverticula, congenital anomalies, foreign bodies or tumors and polyps.

Great confusion exists as to the diagnosis and treatment of duodenal diseases. Symptoms are often confused with the symptoms of other gastrointestinal, biliary, hepatic and pancreatic diseases, both organic and functional. The differential diagnosis is often difficult and confusing. Occasionally the combined judgement of the family physician, roentgenologist, surgeon and even a psychiatrist is essential.

The family physician finds few if any physical signs associated with duodenal diseases. Cardinal symptoms relate to all duodenal diseases. The one diagnostic measure and a sine qua non is the barium meal fluorscopic and x-ray examination. This study must be made by an experienced roentgenologist with the patient examined in several positions. If necessary, the study should be repeated several times. X-ray examinations are the only way duodenal diseases can be differentiated from gastric and duodenal ulcers and gallbladder disease.

Duodenal Diverticula

Duodenal diverticula (Fig. 12-24) cause symptoms in about half the patients with the condition. The diverticula which cause symptoms are the ones that empty with difficulty because of their dependent position or because they have a narrow neck. Symptoms, when they do occur, are equally divided between digestive disturbances, such as indigestion and belching, and pain which is made worse rather than relieved by eating. In this way, the symptoms differ from the pain of an ulcer.

If the diverticulum empties easily, shows no 6 hour residue and is not tender on direct palpation, it is, in all probability, harmless. Leave it and reassure the patient.

If it retains barium, is placed dependently and is tender to pressure, try a modified ulcer regimen. If these measures fail and tenderness and signs of inflammation persist, consider surgical removal.

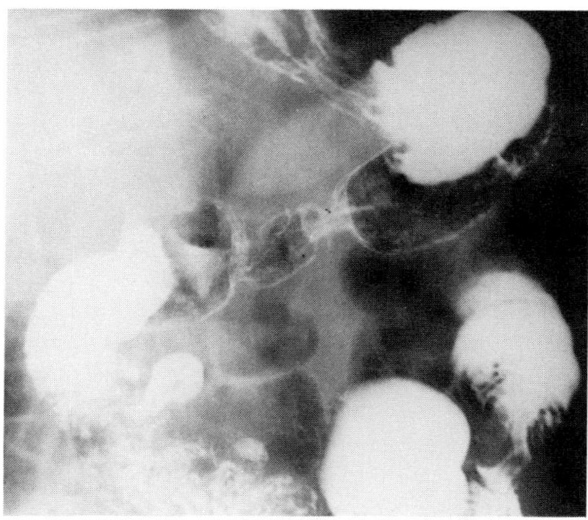

Figure 12-24. Multiple duodenal diverticula.

Obstruction

The most common cause of acute duodenal obstruction is angulation of the third or preaortic portion of the duodenum by the superior mesenteric vessels, congenital or acquired bands, anomalies of rotation, internal or external tumors or pancreatic diseases. As the duodenum fills, the angulation traps pancreatic, biliary, and gastric secretions causing a rapid dilitation of the stomach and duodenum proximal to the obstruction. The patient's signs and symptoms point toward high intestinal obstruction.

Unless the angulation of obstruction is relieved within the first 24 hours, the patient's condition runs rapidly downhill. If the problem is the superior mesenteric artery syndrome, put the patient in the head-down prone position and lavage with water at a temperature of 110° F. Relief is prompt.

A chronic duodenal obstruction can occur from the same causes as does the acute obstruction plus neurogenic stasis without any demonstrable organic factors. In organic obstruction, the vomiting and indigestion is constant and without periods of relief. In functional stasis, distress comes in attacks and often is associated with emotional disturbances or fatigue.

The prognosis depends on whether the stasis is caused by organic factors or by a functional affair. In the latter group, emotional help is all important. The family physician should deal vigorously with the anxiety even if an organic component is found.

Duodenal Fistulas

These are of the internal or external variety. The internal fistula is the result of an erosive process such as a gallstone ulcerating through the wall of the gallbladder into the duodenum. Except for rare cases, with spectacular symptoms, internal fistulas are not diagnosed until surgery or autopsy. External fistulas are most commonly caused by disruption of the duodenal stump following gastric surgery. There is no more serious complication in abdominal surgery except massive hemorrhage. It complicates a serious operation and develops, as a rule, within the first few postoperative days.

Duodenitis

No one is certain whether there is such a disease, but most surgeons and roentgenologists talk freely about the syndrome. It has no known etiology and the symptoms are easily confused with duodenal ulcer and gallbladder disease.

Roentgenologists describe a syndrome characterized by reduplication of the duodenal mucosal folds associated with an irritable and tender bulb. Occasionally, at surgery the preoperative diagnosis of a duodenal polyp is found to be erroneous and, in reality, the lesion will appear to be redundant mucosa partially obstructing the pylorus.

Tumors and Foreign Bodies

Primary tumors are polyps (Fig. 12-25), lipomas, adenocarcinomas and sarcomas. The sentinal symptom of a duodenal polyp is hemorrhage.

Foreign bodies in the duodenum are usually sharp objects such as pins, needles or fish bones. Watch the patient for a few hours to observe any progress of the object

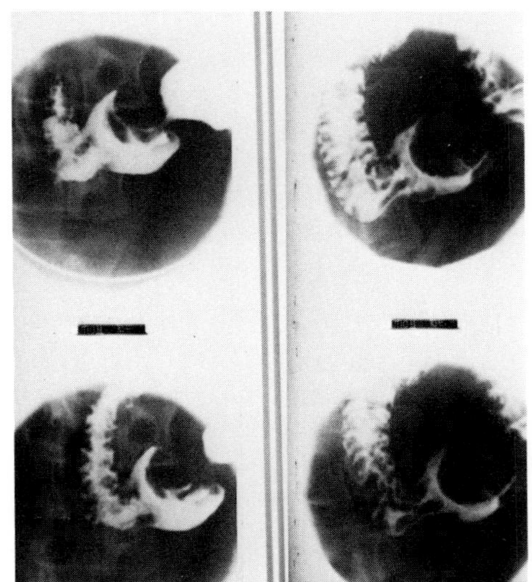

Figure 12-25. Benign prepyloric polyp herniating into the duodenum.

beyond the duodenum. As a rule, the object, even when sharp, is passed per rectum. Advise surgery if the object appears by x-ray film to remain in a fixed position in the duodenum.

Nervous Indigestion

The common symptoms of nervous indigestion or dyspepsia are seen in so many organic and functional lesions of the upper gastrointestinal tract and bile passages that great confusion occurs in diagnosis and therapy. Many patients are medically treated for years for a so-called nervous indigestion when they have had a surgically remediable organic lesion; others are subjected to surgical procedures when no organic lesions are present only to find their symptoms intensified and their neurosis deeper than previous to surgery.

The two most common mistakes in dealing with these patients are failure of the family physician, the roentgenologist and perhaps a surgeon to work together in studying the duodenum and failure to deal adequately with the underlying neurosis or a debilitating process in some other part of the body. Many of the patients in this group have deep-seated, often subconscious, problems that require the skill, patience and time of an experienced psychiatrist. The failure in surgical and medical therapy in these cases can be largely explained by the failure to recognize and deal with psychological factors. An anxiety neurosis is practically always an etiologic factor.

Some functional syndromes are:

- persistent bitter, metallic or burning sensation in the mouth without evidence of glossitis
- globus hystericus
- pyrosis or heartburn in the absence of gastroesophageal reflux and esophagitis
- symptomatic aerophagia (see later in this chapter)
- functional vomiting

If there is a persistent sensation in the mouth without evidence of a glossitis, exclude a suppurative focus in the mouth, sinuses and lungs. Check for an esophagitis and saliva contaminated with food or drugs.

Family physicians often spend the patient's time and money tracing down the ethereal symptoms of globus hystericus when simply listening to the patient would be more in order.

Pyrosis, or heartburn, in the absence of gastroesophageal reflux and esophagitis is a common functional complaint. There are no physical findings associated with functional heartburn and symptoms are more frequent after meals. Unlike esophagitis or hiatal hernia, there is usually no postural component and no history of relief with antacids.

Functional vomiting is a clinical diagnosis. The vomiting occurs soon after meals without prior nausea. The patient may resume eating after vomiting.

Do a rather complete gastrointestinal work-up. Remember the symptoms often can not be differentiated from organic disease. Both the family physician and his patient need the assurance that only a complete study can give.

Functional disorders of the gastrointestinal system tend to be recurrent or chronic. Most complications occur as a result of inaccurate diagnosis or of improper treatment. Refrain from suggesting that symptoms may be due to ulcer or gallbladder. In the neurotically inclined patient, such indecision and guesses lead the patient to believe he has a serious organic disease.

Functional Gastrointestinal Disorders

In all these functional disorders pay special attention to the patient's emotional problems. Start by investigating the impact of psychologic difficulties on the patient's illness. If you have no time for this investigation, seek the early cooperation of a psychiatrist.

As a family physician you should be able to take a psychologic history and know how and when to use a psychiatrist as a consultant. Psychological history-taking requires the collection of detailed information regarding the patient's emotional development and his ability to relate to those about him. From this a picture of his personality make-up and his psychologic needs will emerge. At this point, and with this information, make the decision as to whether to refer the patient to a psychiatrist.

Further responsibility of the family physician is to attempt to motivate the patient to see a psychiatrist. This requires that you be able to convince the patient that his emotional conflicts give rise to his anxieties and complicate his gastrointestinal symptoms.

In the *irritable bowel syndrome,* expect:

- –diarrhea alternating with constipation with one predominating
- –crampy abdominal pains
- –abdominal distention
- –bowel gas
- –borborygmi
- –ribbonlike stools
- –mucus stools
- –palpable bowel loops
- –spastic x-ray pattern

In treating the patient, give Lomotil, increase bulk in his diet and eliminate spicy foods, give Konsyl (psyllium seed), 1 to 2 tsp daily for nonirritating bulk, and check for lactase (milk) malabsorption and eliminate milk if indicated.

The patient with *atonic bowel* will show:

- –a long history of constipation with laxative abuse
- –atonic x-ray pattern
- –dilated rectum full of feces

Treatment includes increasing roughage in the diet and adding stool softeners and peristaltic stimulants such as Senokot or Dulcolax.

Intermittent dysphagia is dysphagia in anxious, high-strung patients without organic disease. Treatment consists of antispasmodics, bland diet and antacids.

Indications of Magenblase syndrome are:

- –trapped gastric and colonic gas producing angina-like symptoms
- –upper gastrointestinal series showing trapped air bubbles

Treatment consists of a modified ulcer diet, avoidance of excess coffee, alcohol, salicylates and spices, use of antacids and sedatives and three meals per day without overeating.

In *upper gastrointestinal dysfunction* the symptoms will be:

- –peptic ulcer-like, i.e. post prandial fullness, indigestion, epigastric fullness, belching, acid regurgitation and substernal discomfort
- –gastric hyperacidity

Treatment is the same as for the Magenblase syndrome.

In *biliary dyskinesia* the patient will have:

- –discomfort within ½ hr in the RUQ after meals
- –tender gallbladder
- –impaired gallbladder emptying after a fatty meal or cholecystokinin injection

Relief is obtained with sublingual nitroglycerin or antispasmodics or both.

The main symptom of *mucousy colitis* is diarrhea with excess mucus. This is a misnomer. Watch for ulcerative colitis.

In *rectal spasm* there is severe rectal pain in tense and anxious patients.

Treatment consists of the usual measures for lower bowel syndrome and occasional use of opium and belladonna suppositories.

Frequently Prescribed Medicines for Indigestion

Antacids

Examples of antacids and their characteristics follow.

Aluminum hydroxide gel. 1 ml is capable of neutralizing 10 to 15 ml of N/10 HC1. There is no acid rebound but it has constipating tendencies. Usually dispensed in suspension containing 320 mg of dried aluminum hydroxide gel per 5 ml. Example: Amphojel liquid and tablets. Dose: 1 or 2 tablets or tsp.

Aluminum phosphate gel is similar to aluminum hydroxide gel but is about half as effective as a neutralizer. Example: Phosphaljel. Dose: 15 to 30 ml.

Dihydroxyaluminum aminoacetate. Advantages claimed over aluminum hydroxide gel are questionable but it is more prompt and prolonged in action and is less constipating. It is usually dispensed as 500 mg tablets or 500 mg per 5 ml liquid. Example: Alzinox or Robalate tablets. Dose: 1 or 2 tablets or tsp.

Magnesium trisilicate. 1 g neutralizes 155 ml N/10 HCl in 4 hr. Large doses may cause diarrhea. Example: Magnesium trisilicate 0.5 g tablets. Dose: 2 to 8 tablets.

Some combinations of aluminum hydroxide and magnesium: Gelusil tablets and liquid. Each tablet or tsp contains 250 mg aluminum hydroxide and 500 mg magnesium trisilicate. Dose: 1 or 2 tablets or tsp. Maalox is the same as Gelusil with different proportion of the hydroxides of aluminum and magnesium. Dose: 1 or 2 tablets or tsp. Aludrox is still another combination of aluminum hydroxide and magnesium. Dose: 1 or 2 tablets or tsp.

Calcium Carbonate

One g neutralizes 210 ml of N/10 HCl. It releases carbon dioxide in the stomach and tends to be constipating. Examples: Tums and Dicarbosil. In the latter 400 mg calcium carbonate is mixed with 11 mg magnesium carbonate and 6 mg magnesium trisilicate per tablet. In Titralac calcium carbonate is mixed with glycine and comes both as a liquid or tablet. Dose: 1 or 2 tablets or tsp. (Note: glycine is thought to provide rapid buffering action.)

Defrothicants and Combinations

These agents contain simethicone, a defoaming agent plus antacids. Mylicon tablets. Dose: 1 tablet. Mylanta, a combination of simethicone plus magnesium hydroxide and aluminum hydroxide gel in chewable tablets and liquid. Dose: 1 or 2 tablets or tsp p.r.n. Silain Gel, a combination of simethicone, magnesium hydroxide and magnesium carbonate and aluminum hydroxide in tablets and liquid. Dose: 2 tablets or tsp after meals and at bedtime.

Anticholinergics

These preparations are usually given to inhibit gastric secretions, reduce acidity and decrease motility. They also exhibit some ganglionic blocking action; consequently, their use is debated. Side effects may vary, but patients can expect to experience some degree of mouth dryness, visual blurring, urinary hesitancy and constipation. Do not give to patients with glaucoma and be cautious in administrating anticholinergics to patients with pyloric or uninary tract obstructions.

Homatropine methylbromide. Example: Mesopin, 5 mg tablets and 2.5 mg per 5 ml elixir given 4 times daily. Also comes with phenobarbital 15 mg, Mesopin PB.

Methscopolamine bromide. Example: Pamine Bromide. 2.5 mg tablet and 1.25 mg per 5 ml syrup given 4 times daily. Also comes with phenobarbital 15 mg (Pamine with Phenobarbital).

Anisotropine methylbromide. Example: Valpin. 10 mg tablet and 10 mg per 5 ml elixir given 3 to 4 times daily. Also comes with Phenobarbital 8 mg, Valpin PB.

Methantheline bromide. Example: Banthine. 50 mg tablet given every 6 hr, then adjusted to need. Also comes with phenobarbital 15 mg, Banthine-Phenobarbital.

Propantheline bromide. Example: Pro-Banthine. 7.5 mg and 15 mg tablets given usually 15 mg with meals and 30 mg at bedtime. Also comes with phenobarbital 16 mg, Pro-Banthine with Phenobarbital.

Oxyphencyclimine. Example: Daricon. 10 mg tablets given twice a day because of prolonged action. Also comes with phenobarbital 15 mg, Daricon PB.

Mephenzolate methylbromide, said to have a specific action on the colon. Example: Cantil. 25 mg tablets given 3 times a day. Also comes with phenobarbital 16 mg, Cantil with Phenobarbital.

Anticholinergics with Tranquilizers

Milpath, a meprobamate and tridihexethyl combination. Dose: 1 tablet 3 times a day and 2 at bedtime.

Enarax, an oxyphencyclimine and hydroxyzine combination. Dose: 1 tablet 3 times daily.

Combid Spansules, an isopropamide and proclorperazine combination. Dose: 1 every 12 hr.

Librax capsules, an anticholinergic and chlordiazepoxide HCl combination. Dose: 1 or 2 capsules 4 times a day.

Digestants

Peptenzyme Elixir. 259 mg per 30 ml. Dose: 4 to 8 tsp. Also comes in tablets and powder.

Taka-Diastase, a diastatic enzyme which liquifies 450 times its weight of insoluble starch in 10 min. In tablets, capsules, powder and liquid. Dose: 5 to 15 gr.

Converzyme tablets, a combination of amylolytic, proteolytic, cellulolytic and lipolytic enzymes. Dose: 1 or 2 tablets with or after meals.

Entozyme tablets, a combination of pepsin, bile salts and pancreatin. Dose: 1 or 2 tablets after meals.

Donnazyme tablets are more than a simple digestant for they contain pancreatin, bile salts, pepsin, hyoscyamine sulfate, atropine, hyoscine and phenobarbital. Dose: 2 tablets after meals.

Hydrocholeretics

These are used for nonobstructive biliary stasis, bile insufficiency, postoperative management of biliary disease and as an adjunct in cholecystitis, cholangitis, and cholelithiasis in the absence of complete obstruction.

Dehydrocholic acid tablets, 250 mg tablets. Dose: 2 to 6 tablets. Cholan V tablets, same as above plus 5 mg homatropine MBr per tablet. Dose: 3 to 6 tablets. Cholan HMB contains a combination of dehydrocholic acid, homatropine MBr and 8 mg phenobarbital. Dose: 2 to 6 tablets.

Combined hydrocholeretic and choleretic preparations are used to produce an increased volume of bile as well as to stimulate the excretion of bile. Used mainly in chronic inflammatory diseases of the gallbladder, bile ducts and liver.

Triketol, 250 mg ketocholanic acid. Dose: 2 to 6 tablets. Ketochol, as above. Dose: 3 tablets. Oxsorbil capsules, a combination of dehydrocholic acid, desoxycholic acid, bile extract, oleic acid and polysorbate. Dose: 3 to 6 capsules.

Choleretic and/or cholagogue preparations are used to stimulate the excretion of bile by the liver (choleretic) and to promote the discharge of bile (cholagogue). Recommended for steatorrheas, biliary fistulas, chronic pancreatitis and fat indigestions.

Ox bile extract tablets in 195 mg and 325 mg tablets. Dose: one 325 mg tablet 3 times daily. Bilron Pulvules, bile salts and iron in 325 and 165 mg tablets. Dose: one or two 365 mg tablets 3 times daily.

ANOREXIA, NAUSEA AND VOMITING

General Considerations

Consider anorexia (lack of the desire for food) and nausea (a feeling of revulsion for food) and vomiting as different degrees of the same physiologic mechanisms. Actually, the idea may not be physiologically sound, but it provides an excellent clinical approach to understanding the underlying cause and treatment of anorexia, nausea and vomiting.

Anorexia, nausea and vomiting are the symptoms of a wide variety of diseases, from minor temporary disorders to major life-threatening disasters. To make the differential diagnosis more complex, other body systems beside the gastrointestinal tract cause identical symptoms.

Nausea infrequently appears as a lone symptom. Remember this when taking a history: the patient may have a different sensation than you believe him to have. Nausea is usually associated with salivation, sweating, tachycardia and later a bradycardia. Patients often describe the sensation as "in the back of the throat" or "just feel sick" or "sick at the stomach."

Nausea inhibits stomach activity: acid secretion dries up and the contractions cease. The droopy stomach hangs loose and resembles a bag. In contrast to the stomach, the duodenum increases in contractility, upsetting the smooth peristaltic gradient of the digestive tube. When this happens duodenal contents are regurgitated backward into the stomach. Vomiting is an intense nausea. The stimulus that produces a sick feeling will, when it occurs in greater strength, produce vomiting.

In the past, the causes of anorexia, nausea and vomiting have been classified as being either central or local. Other researchers have gone further, listing the causes as cerebromedullary, toxic, visceral, deficiencies and motion sickness. Forget all the classifications. Nausea and vomiting are symptoms so general and universal that attempting to classify them leads only to more confusion. Just understand that nearly any impact on the body can cause nausea and even vomiting. Occasionally, a family physician must come to grips with the differential diagnosis. Whenever the patient's chief complaint is nausea and vomiting, the diagnosis is made from accompanying signs and symptoms.

What to Look For

Do not overlook these common causes of anorexia, nausea and vomiting: food poisoning, obstruction of the bowel by hernia or adhesions, appendicitis, hypertensive crisis, intracranial lesions, congestive heart failure, upper gastrointestinal carcinomas, peptic ulcers, gastric outlet obstruction, alcoholism and pancreatitis, drugs, previous surgery with obstructive symptoms, functional bowel disorder, radiation, labyrinthitis, Meniere's syndrome, depression, migraine, central neuronitis, fecal impaction, stress and fear, neurosis and psychosis, anorexia nervosa, shock, pain, hypoxemia, hot weather, febrile diseases, uremia, liver failure, diabetic acidosis, allergy, general or local peritonitis, pregnancy and motion sickness.

Varieties of Vomiting

A significant hematemesis signals a serious emergency. If massive, death may be imminent. "Coffee ground" vomitus is a sign of gastric bleeding.

Projectile vomiting, even without blood, may herald an increase in intracranial pathology. This type of vomiting may occur without preceding nausea and be explosive in nature because of the suddenness of the impulse. Examine the patient for concussion, cerebral tumors or abscesses, meningitis, cerebral hemorrhage or even more simple diseases such as migraine. Do not fail to take the patient's blood pressure. Otherwise a serious hypertensive crisis may be overlooked.

The appearance of feculent vomitus warns of an obstruction. An obstruction at the gastric outlet produces a vomitus of less bile than that with acute cholecystitis or pancreatitis.

Remember that several hours of vomiting can produce dehydration and electrolyte imbalance. In the elderly this alone can be fatal. In the very young and the elderly, the risk of aspiration increases. Severe retching may produce a tear in the esophagus, the Mallory-Weiss syndrome. Other diseases dormant in the patient may suddenly be activated by severe vomiting, i.e. hernia and angina. Vomiting can produce serious complications; the patient may need to be treated as an emergency.

Nausea and Drugs

We live in a drug culture where drugs are available to anyone by prescription, over-the-counter, or by illegal means. Keep this possibility in mind when consulted by a patient with chronic recurrent nausea or vomiting. Be alert especially for the following drug ingestion: digitalis, alcohol, histamine, epinephrine, lidocaine hydrochloride (Xylocaine), nalidixic acid (NegGram), salicylates, mycins, carminatives as gentian, iron, quinine, indomethacin (Indocin), Sansert, diuretics, amphetamines, ammonium chloride, chloroquine (Aralen), codeine and aminophylline.

Disease in the Gastrointestinal Tract

In the gastrointestinal tract there are irritative and obstructive lesions too numerous to mention. Failure to recognize an obstruction can be disastrous. The triad of abdominal pain, vomiting and distention signifies an organic cause. Inspect the patient's abdomen for surgical scars and hernias. Postsurgical adhesions are the commonest cause of organic obstruction, hernia the second. If neither of these diseases are present, think next of gallstones.

The violence of the symptoms depends on whether the obstruction is high or low or partial or complete. In acute, complete obstruction, the bowel has no chance to accommodate to the sudden pressure and symptoms are intense. In chronic partial obstruction, the bowel may dilate and hypertrophy and by increased force keep intestinal contents moving.

Consider the possibility of *fecal impaction* in both the young and elderly when nausea and vomiting occur. Listen to the bowel sounds, not for just a moment but long enough to describe their location and pattern—the rushes and tinkles of organic disease.

When you have ruled out the obstructive lesions, think next of *acute appendicitis*. In the typical attack of appendicitis, however, pain precedes nausea and vomiting. This is axiomatic. But not all attacks are typical, especially in the elderly.

Peritoneal irritation causes nausea and vomiting through the viscerovisceral (peritoneovisceral) reflex. Stimuli arising in the peritoneum pass through the vagus and splanchnic afferent fibers to the medullary vomiting centers. Here, through synaptic connections, arise the efferent impulses which terminate in the pharynx, esophagus, cardia, stomach, diaphragm and abdominal muscles. This reflex can cause either ileus or vomiting.

Extragastrointestinal disease, operating through the same reflex, also causes nausea and vomiting. The genitourinary tract has a common autonomic nerve supply with the gastrointestinal tract; consequently, *chronic kidney disease* may cause severe anorexia. Of course, other factors may be partially responsible for symptoms, i.e. nitrogen retention, acidosis, nutritional deficiencies.

Another genitourinary problem which leads to nausea and vomiting is the *uremia* associated with prostatic obstruction. Look for a distended bladder and ask the patient when he urinated last and whether he has been dribbling. In addition, do a digital rectal examination. Along the same line but with the pathophysiology not clearly described are *diabetic acidosis, Addison's disease* and *thyrotoxicosis*.

Vertigo

Vertigo is associated with nausea and vomiting. Infections, allergies, trauma, thrombosis, hemorrhage and tumors of the internal and external ear, the eighth nerve and the brain stem nuclei cause vertigo with or without nausea and vomiting. Think of acute toxic labyrinthitis, vascular diseases and Meniere's syndrome. Lesions of the eighth nerve, however, cause a hearing loss while brainstem disease does not.

Vertigo is severe in acute *toxic labyrinthitis* but there is no tinnitus or hearing loss. The whirling reaches its climax in 24 to 48 hours and disappears in 3 to 6 weeks. During this time the patient's symptoms are aggravated by raising his head. He seeks to prevent the vertigo by lying in a horizontal position. Vascular spasm, a rupture of an artery or vein and concussion cause similiar symptoms. In *Meniere's syndrome*, the attack of vertigo may last hours but not days. The vertigo is intermittent but the tinnitis and hearing loss persist. (For more discussion of vertigo see Chapter 8).

The nausea and vomiting of *migraine* are not often difficult to recognize. Question the patient for the presence of a premonitory aura, localization of pain over one eye and nausea with vomiting. Peculiarly enough, some of these patients complain only of nausea and vomiting. Careful questioning may be necessary to identify the symptoms as migrainous in nature.

In the older patient with obscure nausea and vomiting, a careful examination of the heart, chest and blood pressure is essential. The usual symptoms of pulmonary edema, milder forms of heart failure or myocardial infarction may be hidden by an overriding nausea and vomiting.

No matter how secure you feel the diagnosis may be, always examine the patient's abdomen. Look for abdominal distention, a retrocecal appendix, pancreatitis and gallbladder disease. Remember Murphy's sign. Perform it by pressing the finger tips under the right costal margin in the area of the gallbladder. Ask the patient to inhale. As he does so the liver and gallbladder descend and, if the organs are inflamed, the finger pressure causes pain.

A careful history will usually lead to the proper diagnosis in cases of nausea and vomiting secondary to pregnancy, hot weather, motion sickness, hypoxemia, anorexia nervosa, stress, fear, depression, neurosis, psychosis, fasting or starvation.

Treatment

Antiemetic Agents

Emetrol, a mint flavored oral solution containing levulose, dextrose and orthophosphoric acid. Works directly on smooth muscle in proportion to amount taken. Prescribe for the nausea and vomiting of epidemic psychogenic vomiting, regurgitation in infants, nausea and vomiting of pregnancy and as an antiemetic for nausea caused by drugs. Free from toxicity. Dose: children, 5 to 10 ml; adults, 15 to 30 ml. Do not dilute the mixture or swallow fluids for 15 min before or after dose.

Gravatose, a chewable tablet containing dextrose, lactose, sucrose and fructose. Recommended for the relief of nausea and vomiting during the first trimester of pregnancy. Chew 1 or 2 tablets at bedtime, on arising and as needed.

Probutylin (procaine isobutyrate), a local anesthetic recommended for nausea and vomiting of pregnancy, postoperative nausea, pylorospasm, post alcoholic gastritis and gastroenteritis. Capsules 300 mg, 1 or 2 capsules or 5 to 10 ml 10 percent elixir. Do not use in patients with moderate to severe hypertension.

Antiemetic and Antivertigo Agents

Dramamine (dimenhydrinate). Use for motion sickness, labyrinthitis, Meniere's syndrome, hypertension, radiation sickness, postfenestration syndrome and migraine. Dose: adult oral, 50 to 100 mg every 4 hr; IM, 50 mg p.r.n.; IV, 50 mg in 10 ml sodium chloride, injected slowly over 2 min. Children orally or rectally, from age 6 to 8, 12.5 to 25 mg 2 or 3 times daily; age 8 to 12, 25 to 50 mg 3 times daily.

Marezine (cyclizine). Use for motion sickness, postoperative vomiting, vertigo, radiation sickness and psychologic vomiting. Use cautiously in pregnancy. Dose: Adult, 50 mg tablets 3 to 4 times daily; injection, 50 mg per 1 ml; suppositories, 50 to 100 mg.

Bonine chewable tablets (meclizine HCl). Use for most cases of nausea or dizziness. Use cautiously in pregnancy. Dose: Adult, chewable tablets, 25 mg 3 to 4 times daily.

Tigan (trimethobenzamide HCl). Use for most cases of nausea, vomiting and vertigo. Dose: adult, 250 mg capsules 3 to 4 times daily. Injection, 100 mg per ml. Children (30 to 90 lb), 100 mg capsules 3 to 4 times daily. Suppositories, 200 mg suppositories. For cautious use in pregnancy, order a 250 mg capsule at bedtime. If no sustained relief, add another capsule in morning. May increase to 3 to 4 times daily.

Torecan (thiethylperazine). Use more cautiously because of adverse effects. Do not use in pregnancy nor in children under 12. Review adverse reactions before use. Dose: Adults only. Tablets 10 mg; injection, 5 mg per ml; suppositories, 10 mg.

Vontrol (diphenidol). Consult literature before using. Limit use to hospitalized patients. Use in infants under 25 lb and in pregnancy is contraindicated. Dose: adults, 25 to 50 mg p.r.n. every 4 hr.

Antiemetic and Antivertigo Combinations

Dramaine-D, a combination of dimenhydrinate and 5 mg dextroamphetamine sulfate. Use in vertigo, nausea and vomiting of pregnancy; nonspecific causes; and motion sickness. Dose: adult, 1 tablet every 4 to 6 hr.

Antivert, 12.5 mg meclizine and 50 mg niacin. Use in many cases of vertigo and nausea. Dose: adult, 1 tablet or syrup 5 to 10 ml 3 times daily before meals.

Bonadoxin, 25 mg meclizine and 50 mg pyridoxine. May use in nausea and vomiting of pregnancy and in other causes of vomiting, nausea and vertigo. Dose: adult, 1 to 4 tablets daily; drops 3 ml from 1 to 4 times daily. For motion sickness, take 1 tablet 1 hour before beginning trip.

Bucladin Softabs, 50 mg buclizine HCl, 10 mg pyridoxine, 0.2 mg scopolamine, 0.05 mg atropine sulfate and 0.05 mg hyoscyamine sulfate. Prescribe 1 tablet for mild symptoms; for untreated patients or those with severe symptoms use 2 or even 3 tablets.

Tigacol, 100 mg trimethobenzamide, 50 mg nicotinyl alcohol. Not recommended for children. Dose: 1 to 2 capsules 3 times daily.

Bendectin, 10 mg doxylamine succinate, pyridoxine HCl and 10 mg dicyclomine HCl. May use in pregnancy. Dose: adults, 2 tablets at bedtime. In severe cases, repeat tablet in the morning and perhaps add a fourth in the afternoon.

Benacine, 25 mg diphenhydramine HCl, 0.325 mg hyoscine. Prescribe for motion sickness and parkinsonism. Dose: adults, 1 tablet 1 hr before departing, then one every 4 hr (3 tablets daily). In parkinsonism, 2 tablets every 4 hr.

FLATULENCE AND GASEOUS DISTENTION

What to Look For

Consider the following when your patient has excessive gas in the stomach and intestines: aerophagia, gallbladder disease, gastritis, peptic ulcers, gastric tumors and cancer, hiatal hernia, hypoacidity, malabsorption problems of meat, fats and carbohydrates, pancreatic insufficiency, intestinal hypomotility, hypermotility and hypopropulsivity, acute appendicitis, acute pancreatitis; diabetic acidosis; perinephric abscess; adhesions from abdominal surgery; ruptured viscus; strangulated hernia; ganglionic blocking agents; belladonna overdose; uremia; hypokalemia; abdominal aortic aneurysm; mesenteric vascular occlusion; ascariasis; and staphylococcal enterocolitis.

Differential Diagnosis of Flatulence and Gaseous Distention

Aerophagia

Swallowed air accounts for 65 to 70 percent of the gas in the gastrointestinal tract. Problems in diagnosis arise when a patient suddenly develops flatulence or in those in which flatulence is associated with other gastrointestinal symptoms suggesting organic disease. Air is introduced during eating, drinking, smoking, chewing gum, sipping, gulping hot food or eating rapidly.

Patients with abdominal distress often swallow air to induce belching in an attempt to bring relief. Studies show that such action leaves more gas in the stomach then was present before the attempt at relief.

A cycle may become established: anxiety—air swallowing—abdominal discomfort—more anxiety—more air swallowing—more abdominal discomfort. The cycle is broken temporarily when the patient belches. This leads the patient to believe that induced belching is his only means of relief.

Observe the patient while he is being interviewed and is under stress. Occasionally during pauses in the interview saliva collects and he can be seen air swallowing. Many patients appear to be anxious to demonstrate the explosive belch that follows the gulping of several swallows of air.

Swallowed air, if not eructated, passes through the intestine and accumulates in likely anatomic areas—the stomach (Mogenblase syndrome) and the splenic flexure. The transit time of gas from the stomach to ileum is 10 minutes and from stomach to rectum 20 minutes. The volume of intrinsically produced gas is 1,000 to 1,500 ml depending on the patient's diet and gastrointestinal motility.

Aerophagia is a troublesome and vexing symptom, complex both for the doctor and his patient. Gastroenterologists spend a substantial part of their time diagnosing and treating the vague, ill-defined symptoms of gaseous discomfort, bloating, eructation, borborygmus and flatulence. The symptoms associated with gas passing through the gastrointestinal tract are the most common functional disorders of this system.

Treatment is based on training the patient. Convince the patient that swallowing air for relief always leaves more gas than is belched back. Insist that the patient eat less hurriedly and under quiet circumstances. Instruct the air swallower to exhale before swallowing.

Establish proper drinking habits. Have the patient drink from a cup slowly and continuously while the glass or cup is tilted at an angle that keeps the upper lip covered with fluid. Drinking from a water fountain increases air swallowing.

Point out to the patient that each time he sighs, when under stress he will swallow air.

The patient often discovers that certain foods increase the gas. These should be eliminated from the diet as well as carbonated drinks, beer, certain gaseous vegetables as beans and cabbage and foods that contain unusual amounts of air such as milk shakes and sponge cake. During the sipping of hot liquids, patients often draw in air to cool the liquid.

Prescribe certain medications: Dimethicone (Silain Gel, Mylicon) given immediately after meals often gives relief. Dimethicone plus enzymes in the proprietary Phazyme may be tried. Anticholinergic drugs do not work well in aerophagia. If the drugs are given in sufficient doses to modify bowel motility, the accompanying dryness creates more aerophagia, delayed stomach emptying and more gastric distention. If definite emotional problems are involved, a tranquilizer or antidepressant given 1 hour before meals is useful in controlling stress and anxiety.

A new drug was recently reported[8] to have exceptional properties in relieving flatulent dyspepsia by speeding gastric emptying time and relaxing the duodenal cap. The drug: Metoclopramide (Maxolon by Beechan Research). The suggested dosage is 10 mg 3 times daily. For patients whose distress starts during eating or within 45 minutes following eating, administer the medication before meals. Otherwise give after meals. The only side effect in a few patients was drowsiness which may be relieved by cutting the dosage in half.

Activated charcoal is often prescribed but again the results are variable. The dosage: 2 capsules (each capsule containing 4 gr of activated charcoal) 4 times daily. Requa Manufacturing Company prepares an acceptable vegetable carbon product.

Organic Bowel Problems

Although the family physician's first thought should be aerophagia when patients complain of gas, he should be alert to the possibility of the many organic bowel problems. Nearly every gastrointestinal disease may produce gas as one of many symptoms. Cardiac symptoms accompanying gas distress are common and confusing. Large amounts of gas in the stomach and splenic flexure may press upon the heart and cause distress. On the other hand, gas may accumulate as a result of disturbed circulation. Gas in the bowel may cause pain or discomfort in the neck, chest, dyspnea and altered cardiac rate or rhythm. Before shifting the patient back and forth between a gastroenterologist and cardiologist, do a resting and exercise electrocardiogram, and carefully check patient's response to exercise and to nitroglycerin.

Intrinsic gas production may vary according to foodstuff ingestion and the bacterial flora of the bowel. Beans may increase gas production tenfold. In this case, the gas is mostly carbon dioxide and is formed by the action of anaerobic bacteria on the indigestible residue. Anaerobic bacteria also produces hydrogen, hydrogen sulfide and methane. Sixteen types of organisms account for 75 percent of all intestinal gas. In this way, 600 ml of gas is produced per day.

ALTERED MOTILITY. This is a frequent cause of gaseous distension. Both the hypermotility of stress and hypopropulsivity. Hypotonicity more commonly occurs in the elderly and symptoms begin ½ to 2 hours following a meal. Gas accumulates generally in likely bowel segments and can be found on examination or by x-ray film. For treatment try reducing carbohydrates and increasing motility by bethanechol chloride (Myocholine, Urecholine), 10 to 30 mg 3 to 4 times daily.

Hypermotility with an irritable bowel and large frothy stools can usually be diagnosed by giving the patient 300 mg of carmine red dye at breakfast. Then have the patient report how long it takes before the dye appears in the stool. In the normal patient, the dye appears within 12 to 18 hours. Fluoroscopic examination is also helpful in determining the degree of bowel activity. Again try simethicone products without or with Phazyme for treatment.

MALABSORPTION SYNDROME. This syndrome is caused by a deficiency of a disaccharide (sucrase, lactase or maltase) or a pancreatic insufficiency and may account for gas and diarrhea. Order a lactose tolerance test. A positive test is suggested by a flat curve or at least one with less than a 20 mg percent rise. For further confirmation, compare with a glucose tolerance test. If a true deficiency is present, the lactose tolerance curve will be flat while the glucose tolerance curve will be normal.

Stool specimens collected for 48 hours and examined for undigested meat fibers, starch or fat may be of help in spotting malabsorption problems. Normal fecal nitrogen is less than 2 g per day. In sprue and severe pancreatic deficiency there is a marked increase in fecal nitrogen.

Normal fecal fat is less than 6 g per 24 hours if averaged over 3 days with a diet including 100 g of fat per day. In chronic pancreatic disease, fecal fat will average more than 10 g per 24 hours. Staining a stool specimen with Sudan III stain may give a quick estimation of the quantity of fat in the stool. More than 3 globules per microscopic high dry field or globules larger than 75 μ indicate a fat malabsorption. Serum carotene is abnormal in steatorrhea unless therapy is successful. Normal is 70 to 290 μg per 100 ml. Mild depletion is 30 to 20 μg per 100 ml. Severe depletion occurs in quantities less than 30 μg. Do not confuse malabsorption syndromes with functional aerophagia nor with the intermittent diarrhea of spastic, irritable colon.

HYPOCHLORHYDRIA. Hypochlorhydria may cause an inordinate amount of gas and is often associated with gastritis, both specific (benign giant hypertrophic gastritis—Menetrier's disease) and nonspecific, and with adenomatous polyps and carcinoma of the stomach. In the latter, achlorhydria following histamine or betazole stimulation occurs in 50 percent of cases, hypochlorhydria in 25 percent and normal gastric acidity in 25 percent.

ACHLORHYDRIA. Achlorhydria occurs in persons with pernicious anemia as well as in some normal individuals: in 4 percent of children increasing to 30 percent of adults over age 60. Hypoacidity may be the reason the elderly suffer more gaseous distension. A low gastric acidity allows Bacteroides to increase and invade the small bowel where food fermentation produces voluminous gas.

A screening for achlorhydria can best be done with the Diagnex blue indication test. If the test is negative for free hydrochloric acid, do a gastric analysis with histamine or Histalog stimulation for verification.

If doubt exists as to whether the flatulence is caused by low gastric acidity, order a therapeutic trial with glutamic acid hydrochloride (Acidulin, Glutan H-C-L, Acidoride) capsules 1 to 2 meals and at bedtime if food is taken. Another suggestion, if the above fails, is a trial of an antibiotic to cut down the bacterial count. If no antibiotic sensitivity test is available, try tetracycline for 2 to 3 weeks.

Miscellaneous

There are other upper abdominal diseases that cause gas as one of several gastrointestinal symptoms. More detailed information will be found earlier in this chapter.

GASTRITIS. In early cases the diagnosis may be made with difficulty because x-rays are not always helpful. To be definite, gastroscopy and a mucosal biopsy may be necessary. Gastritis usually presents with an indigestion that occurs after meals, before breakfast, and is aggravated by orange juice, coffee, and carbohydrates. Look for a hypochromic microcytes anemia and occult blood in the stools because gastritis patients often bleed slowly. Gastric acidity varies from a hypochlorhydria in early cases to achlorhydria for advanced cases with complete mucosal atrophy.

ULCER. Patients with ulcers often complain of gas pains aggravated by spicy foods and an empty stomach. Typical symptoms are epigastric pain, 1 to 4 hours postprandially, with rhythmicity and periodicity and relieved by food and alkali. The symptoms are similar whether the ulcer is gastric, pyloric, duodenal or stomal. The patient's gas pains are relieved by antacids and the elimination of alcohol, caffeine and spices. The term gas pains is an interpretative one but seems the best the patient can come up with to describe the symptoms of burning and gaseous acidic eructations. No crater can be demonstrated by x-ray in 25 percent of the ulcer patients. Again, do a gastroscopic examination if symptoms are severe. Always check the history for the ingestion of steroids or salicylates. Duodenal ulcer is never present with untreated ulcerative colitis, carcinoma of the stomach, pernicious anemia, pregnancy nor an achlorhydria of any type.

GASTRIC TUMORS. The symptoms of these conditions, adenomatous polyps and carcinoma, are not always distinguishable from ulcers. Therefore any gastric ulcer, especially of the antrum, should be investigated. Obtain a gastroscopic examination on all antral ulcers or on any gastric ulcer that does not heal in 3 to 4 weeks. Exfoliative cytology is positive in 80 percent of the patients; false positive in less than 2 percent. Do periodic prophylactic screening in all high-risk patients, especially those with pernicious anemia, gastric atrophy and gastric polyps.

HIATAL HERNIA. A hiatal hernia (Fig. 12-26) may be missed unless the family physician specifically requests the radiologist to search for one. In the commonest type, the sliding hernia, the hiatal ring is enlarged and the gastric cardia slides into the thorax, especially in the supine or head

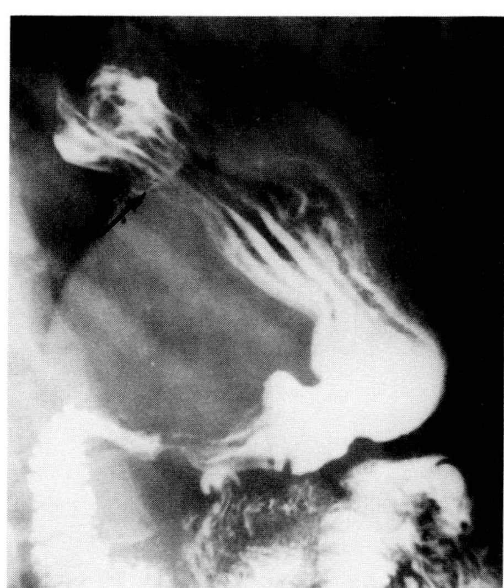

Figure 12-26. Fixed hiatal hernia seen on erect abdominal film.

down position. The latter posture should be employed for x-ray examinations. An important historical clue: discomfort when lying down, relief when sitting up. The discomfort sometimes resembles angina pectoris but is not relieved by nitroglycerin.

GALLBLADDER DISEASE. Cholecystitis and cholelithiasis occur typically in the fat and flatulent female. If the gas is associated with pain in the right upper quadrant, the diagnosis becomes more likely. A cholecystogram may verify the diagnosis. If the gallbladder does not opacify repeat the study with a double dose of dye. If opacification still does not occur either do an intravenous cholecystogram or, as many surgeons, a cholecystectomy.

Drugs

Ganglionic blocking agents such as hexamethonium frequently used for control of hypertension can cause gaseous abdominal distention. Associated findings are elevated supine blood pressure, falling on standing; dizziness and light headedness; mydriatic pupils; blurred vision; and constipation.

Belladonna overdose will cause mild abdominal distention. Belladonna poisoning is not hard to recognize: dry mouth; blurring of vision; dilated pupils; rapid pulse and palpitation; warm and dry skin with a flush on the face, neck and upper part of the trunk.

Other Causes

Gastrointestinal symptoms are also commonly seen following surgery on the upper gastrointestinal tract or the gallbladder, during prolonged antibiotic therapy and during convalescence.

Patients with lower bowel disorders often first complain of gas or abdominal distention. If associated with a change in bowel habits, recommend a complete gastrointestinal work-up. In the elderly think of a possible malignancy or a partial diverticular obstruction; in the young, a beginning ulcerative colitis.

The complaints of the elderly with an obstruction are bloating, crampy pains, the feeling of fullness, constipation with intermittent diarrhea and rectal bleeding. Remember to obtain a flat film of the abdomen or a barium enema before ordering a gastrointestinal series.

Gradual gaseous abdominal distention occurs in a number of other conditions with which the family physician should be alert: diabetic acidosis, perinephric abscess, strangulated hernia, tumors, uremia, hypokalemia and typhoid fever. Sudden gaseous distention may occur in the course of: acute pancreatitis, acute appendicitis, abdominal surgery, ruptured viscus, adhesions, volvulus, intussusception, bleeding abdominal aortic aneurysm, mesenteric vascular occlusion, toxic megacolon, ascariasis and staphylococcal enterocolitis.

CONSTIPATION

What to Look For

If constipation is of sudden onset consider intestinal obstruction, mesenteric vascular occlusion or pyloric stenosis.

If the onset is gradual think of colonic diverticula, lymphogranuloma venereum, pelvic tumor, Hirschsprung's disease, tabes dorsalis, porphyria, myxedema, hyperparathyroidism, hypokalemia, parkinsonism, lead colic, spastic constipation, opiates, ganglionic blocking agents, emphysema, cauda equina tumor or depressive psychosis.

The following conditions may be present in either sudden or gradual onset: carcinoma of colon, abdominal inflammatory disease, anal narrowing or inflammation and dehydration.

The commonest causes of bowel habit changes are from variations in diet, weather, mood, activity or even barometric pressure. Regularity and daily elimination are not vital to good health. Probably not half the population has daily elimination. A fair percentage have elimination once or twice a week or even less than weekly and remain in good health. And there are others who have total irregularity either at intervals of months, weeks, days or all the time.

The autointoxication school is dead. There is no recognized toxemia from intestinal stagnation that contributes to arthritis, hypertension, hypotension, coronary disease, etc.

When a patient says he is constipated and needs a laxative, he usually means he doesn't have daily stools and thinks he should. Obviously, the importance of preventing fecal impaction in patients who are suddenly at rest and taking constipating medication is certainly real and valid. But, beside incidents of this kind, the family physician should be correct with the patient and simply explain his normality. Admittedly this takes more time than prescribing a laxative, but it is the only honest and scientific approach. However, changes in stool color and consistency and bowel habits should be investigated.

Retraining the Laxative-Dependent Patient

The family physician, to successfully treat the laxative dependent patient, must recognize the basic causes of the patient's problem. The etiology is complex but is tied in with the patient's misconception of the need for a daily bowel movement if he wishes to stay healthy. Conditioning to this belief starts in early childhood by parental teaching. This belief is reinforced by press, radio and television advertising. Other factors that promote constipation may be as simple as the lack of privacy, a busy schedule and postponement of the defecation urge.

Begin by counselling the patient, dispelling misconceptions and establishing new habit patterns. Urge the patient to establish a regular time for defecation. If possible have him sit on the toilet for 15 min daily or 30 min. after breakfast without straining. Instruct him to heed any and all urges to defecate. Encourage exercise suitable to the patient's age and conditioning. Increase water intake to 6 glasses of water daily.

Most physicians encourage the eating of bulk foods, i.e. raw vegetables, cooked cabbage or celery, whole grain cereals or breads, stewed or dried fruit, fruit juices and fresh unpeeled fruit. If increasing food bulk is impractical or is intolerable to the patient, prescribe a bulk-producing agent such as Metamucil, Mucilos, Effersyllium, Cellothyl, Cologel and Hydrolose. A proper water intake is essential for the successful use of these agents. Otherwise they may actually increase the patient's constipation.

Occasionally a stool softener or lubricant is necessary. The following are suggested: Colace, Surfak or Kondremul.

Be certain the patient has no impaction to begin with. If an impaction is present, remove it digitally or with a Fleet's regular or mineral oil enema. Resort to laxatives for an emergency basis and only for short periods. Be patient. Retraining may take from 3 to 12 months.

The California Medical Association presents the following tips to the general public in its patient education material. The tips are good for family physicians to use in patient education.

Laxatives: Use Them Rarely—If at All*

The laxative is probably the most overused commodity in the family medicine chest. Many people believe that if they do not have a daily bowel movement they must help nature along with a laxative, an enema, or a suppository. In addition, there is widespread misinformation about the bowel inevitably becoming sluggish after age 35, and too many people believe that a daily laxative must be standard procedure for them in order to "keep regular." The truth is that there is nothing sacred about a daily bowel movement. Some people normally have a movement only once in two or three days, or even only once a week. These people are not constipated. A person is considered constipated only if his *customary* pattern of bowel action is disrupted.

Often this change in habitual bowel movement is only temporary. It can be brought on by travel, change of diet, emotional tension, or as a side effect of certain medications. In such cases, it is much wiser to be patient than to rush into self-treatment. Normal bowel action usually returns with no treatment and with no ill effects, except a slight feeling of discomfort. If the usual rhythm of bowel action does not return after a week's time, the condition can be considered a true constipation and your doctor can guide you in treating it. First, he will want to make sure that your bowel action is not being blocked by a growth in the colon or the rectum. In most cases of constipation, such a growth is not found. Often the bowel trouble has been carried from childhood into the adult years, the result of overemphasis on regular bowel movement during the early years. In other cases, it may result from overreliance on laxatives which need never have been taken and sometimes it is caused by lack of enough bulk in the diet.

Although most of the common laxatives can be obtained without a prescription, many of them can produce undesirable side effects, and consequently they should be taken only under medical supervision. Some laxatives, such as milk of magnesia and Epsom salts, act by drawing fluid into the bowel so that its contents move along more readily. These are among the most harmless of laxatives. Others, such as castor oil and cascara, act by irritating the bowel. In doing so, they may also cause irritation of the kidneys and produce skin eruption. Substances such a mineral oil and liquid petrolatum produce results by making the content of

---

*Reprinted from Laxatives: Use Them Rarely—If at All. Health Tips 176, Calif. Med. Assoc., 693 Sutter St., San Francisco, Calif., 1972, with permission.

the bowel oily. If such laxatives are taken by adults very occasionally, they are harmless—but if they are taken regularly, they can interfere with the absorption of certain vitamins, and may cause inflammation of the lower part of the rectum. If the constipation is caused by lack of bulk in the diet, bulk-producing laxatives such as psyllium seed or agar may be used. However, fruits and vegetables in the diet can accomplish the same objectives more naturally.

Both enemas and suppositories can be used safely if they are used *only occasionally*. Plain water should be used in the enema, and it should be applied in small amounts and under very low pressure. The "high colonic" is useless and can be dangerous. Even mild suppositories, if used repeatedly, can be harmful. If there is pain in the abdomen, never use a strong laxative or an enema. The pain may be caused by an inflamed appendix or a bowel obstruction, and these conditions can be made more severe by irritation.

Diagnostic Aids

Barium Enema

X-ray examination is the most reliable tool in diagnosing colon diseases. But the examination is expensive, uncomfortable and time-consuming. The load such a test would place on existing x-ray resources renders it impractical as a routine diagnostic procedure.

SELECTION OF PATIENTS FOR SCREENING. Gregor[10] studied the practicality of selecting a higher-risk group for x-ray screening. His conclusion is that the healthy patient over 40 who has at least one positive reaction to a stool test (a modified guaiac test for occult blood) deserves a barium enema examination. This examination should be given even if the patient is not on a meat-free diet and even though the reaction is only weakly positive. Colon carcinoma is too common to allow the luxury of discarding even a weak clue.

A single specimen or stool obtained on the examiner's glove is not reliable. Only 2 of his 8 patients with cancer had uniformly positive reactions. The remaining 6 had negative reactions in at least 1 of 3 tested specimens, and some patients even had 2 negative reactions in 3 specimens submitted.

Gregor realized that the chore of checking large numbers of stools in a doctor's office was not feasible. Consequently, Laboratory Diagnostic Co., Roselle, N.J., prepared Hemoccult Slides to enable the patient to collect specimens at home. The slides are made of special guaiac impregnated paper. Because it is necessary to protect the paper from direct sunlight or other sources of ultraviolet light, the slide comes inserted in a small cardboard envelope. Collection instructions are printed on the envelope container. He is requested to prepare the stools on 3 separate days, and thus he submits for testing six separate slides.

Gregor submits the results of 2000 examinations performed on asymptomatic patients. During the 2000 examinations he found 7 patients with invasive carcinoma of the colon. All 7 patients had positive tests for occult blood in at least 1 of 3 stool specimens.

In 33 other patients who had a positive reaction for occult blood, the following was found:

Diverticulosis	4 cases
Diverticulitis	2 cases
Irritable colon	1 case
Hemorrhoids	4 cases
Carcinoma	2 cases
Duodenal ulcer	2 cases
No pathology	18 cases

In another study[10] of 556 patients, and by the use of the special guaiac impregnated slides, 5 silent colon cancers were detected.

The special diet recommended by Gregor,[10] and to start 24 hours before the patient examines the first stool, is as follows:

- –eat no meat, fish or chicken
- –eat plenty of vegetables, both raw and cooked
- –eat plenty of fruit, especially prunes, grapes, plums and apples
- –eat moderate amounts of peanuts and popcorn
- –use All-Bran as a daily cereal

PREPARATION OF PATIENTS FOR BARIUM ENEMA EXAMINATIONS.[11] The quality of colon examinations has improved and the number of repeat examinations have been reduced by following a liquid diet and hydration program preceding the x-ray study.

Preparation begins at lunch the day preceding the examination. Lunch may include clear broth, white chicken meat sandwich (no butter, lettuce or other additives) or two hard boiled eggs, strained fruit juices, jello or gelatin (not containing fruits or nuts), coffee or tea (without milk or cream) and carbonated beverages.

1:00 PM Patient to drink one full glass or more of water.
3:00 PM Patient to drink one full glass or more of water.
5:00 PM Patient's supper to follow the same rules as for lunch.
7:00 PM Patient to drink one full glass or more of water.
8:00 PM Patient to drink one full glass or more of water.
10:00 PM Patient to take 4 Dulcolax tablets with one full glass or more of water.

The following morning, the patient should skip breakfast except for coffee or tea without milk or cream and strained fruit juice.

7:00 AM Patient to drink one and one half glasses of water and insert the Dulcolax suppository into his rectum.

The patient then may report for examination after complete defecation.

LIMITATIONS. Improper bowel cleansing prior to the examination will limit the effectiveness of the barium enema examination. Inability of the patient to retain the barium causes suspicion of an obstruction. Attempt to fill the entire colon by filling the terminal ileum and/or the appendix.

Haustra may, at times, cause radiologic evidence of obstruction. The small mucosal abnormalities of ulcerative colitis cannot be demonstrated without clear postevacuation films and overlapping parts of the colon are difficult to distinguish.

The barium meal method is not recommended for diagnosing organic lesions of the colon. If it is used for studying an irritable colon, be certain there is no colonic obstruction.

Proctosigmoidoscopy

Contrary to what most family physicians have been taught proctosigmoidoscopy leaves something to be desired in searching for carcinoma of the colon. Some researchers have stated that proctosigmoidoscopy is of no practical value in the diagnosis of cancer in the routine patient. Others have pointed out the hazards of the examination, i.e. 1 out of every 1430 proctosigmoidoscopic examinations will result in a perforation of the rectum or sigmoid. The mortality rate associated with the examination is approximately 1 to 10,000 examinations.

Bolt[12] sees little justification for routine proctosigmoidoscopy examinations in patients under 40 years of age. In 1962, a group of investigators reported that proctosigmoidoscopy examinations detected 13 percent of carcinomas in the first 8 cm; 43 percent more in the next 7 cm; another 10 percent in the following 5 cm; and in the last 5 cm another 5 percent. This makes a total of 70 percent below 25 cm and 29 percent above the 25 cm mark. But, in light of the fact that cancer of the rectum and colon is the most common internal cancer and that 70 percent occur within reach of the sigmoidoscope, proctosigmoidoscopies should be routine.[13]

In any event, a family physician should be able to perform a proctosigmoidoscopy examination quickly, effectively and with a minimum of pain on:

–asymptomatic patients over 40 years of age during routine examinations
–symptomatic patients at any age
–any middle-aged patient with a change in bowel habits
–follow-up examinations of patients who have had adenomas, adenocarcinomas or ulcerative colitis

Symptomatic patients are those with bleeding, increasing flatus, tenesmus, intermittent diarrhea and constipation.

Contraindications are:

- –an unwilling or uncooperative patient
- –an anal problem that hinders or obstructs a digital examination
- –acute infections of the anus, rectum or pelvis
- –during a massive hemorrhage
- –serious heart or cerebral vascular disease

PREPARATION OF THE PATIENT FOR PROCTOSIGMOIDOSCOPY. Explain to the patient the need for the examination. Do not force a proctosigmoidoscopy on any unwilling patient. Explain that the examination requires the insertion of a smooth tube into the rectum to examine the inside of the colon.

Ask the patient to eat lightly of bland foods the night before the examination and have the same kind of breakfast the morning of the examination.

If the patient has regular AM bowel movements, all he needs is an enema following this movement. The enema should be lukewarm tap water or a disposable enema. If he is irregular, instruct him to take an enema the night before and again about 2 hours before the examination.

If the patient is ordinarily constipated, instruct him to take 2 to 4 tbsp of milk of magnesia at bedtime the night before the examination. Then have him take an enema following the next morning's bowel movement or 2 hours prior to the examination.

In patients who are weak or feeble and unable to take an enema, a Dulcolax suppository may be tried in place of the enema.

ROUTINE EQUIPMENT. The sigmoidoscope is 25 cm long and ⅝ in in diameter with air insufflation equipment and lighting. The Welch Allyn sigmoidoscope is an old standby, although the new fiber optic type is becoming popular. Disposable plastic sigmoidoscopes are available but are somewhat expensive considering the cost of the permanent handle. They are more awkward to use and sometimes fit with difficulty into the handle.

Use gloves, a lubricant jelly such as KY and water or motor suction. Use long cotton swabs if suction is not available.

STEPS IN THE EXAMINATION. Patient positions for proctosigmoidoscopy are illustrated in Figure 12-27. Any of these positions are permitted, but the position in Figure 12-27C makes the examination easier for both the patient and the physician. First examine the patient digitally. This will help relax the anal sphincters and lubricate the orifice. With the finger sweep the anal walls. The muscles should be palpated between the examining finger and the thumb. In the male, palpate the prostate and seminal vesicles.

Insert the lubricated sigmoidoscope into the anus with the point toward the patient's umbilicus (Fig. 12-28A). Have the patient aid in the insertion by gently straining down over the scope's obturator. A definite muscle release can be felt at about the 2 cm level when the scope enters the large ampulla. Remove the obturator. Direct observation of the canal should guide further insertion.

Continue inserting the scope as the interior colon lights up, insufflating modest amounts of air as needed to help guide the scope through the lumen. Too much air will cause cramping. As the instrument passes through the ampulla direct it toward the sacrum by pulling down the proximal end of the scope (Fig 12-28B). The anal muscle, reinforced by the examiner's fixed thumb, serves as a fulcrum.

As the distal end of the scope approaches the sacrum, again change direction by pushing the proximal end of the scope upward (Fig. 12-28C), following the angulation of the bowel.

The rectosigmoid junction is reached at 8 to 10 in (Fig. 12-28D). An unskilled operator should abandon the examination at this point, if he cannot continue without unusual pain to the patient. After all, a good look at 15 cm of colon is better than digital examination alone. With a little practice, however, most physicians can learn to follow the colon to the 25 cm mark. The wise physician will continue to distract the patient by con-

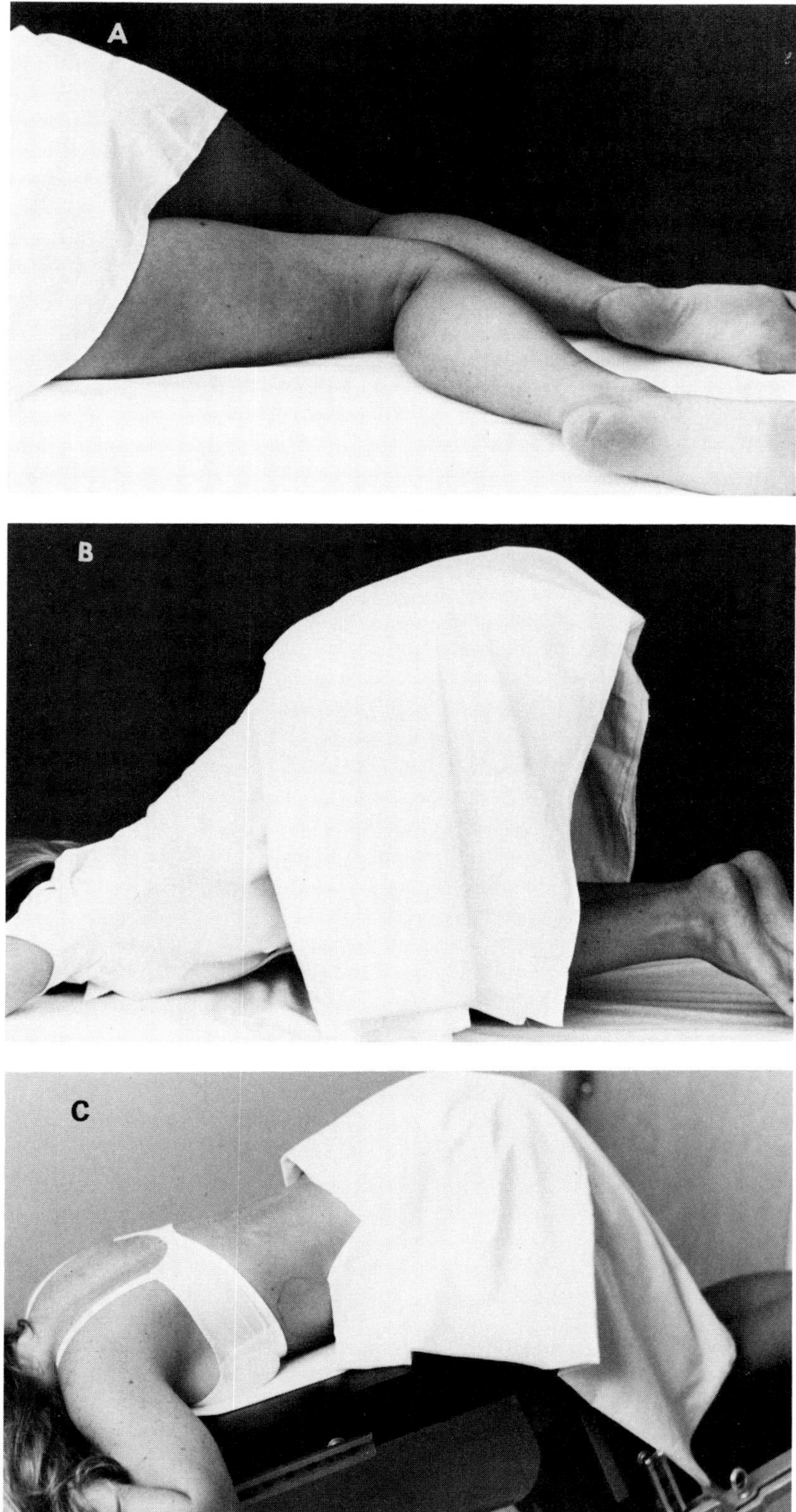

Figure 12-27. Positions for protosigmoidoscopy: *A*, Sims' position (left lateral prone); *B*, Knee-chest position; *C*, Proper position on a proctoscopic table.

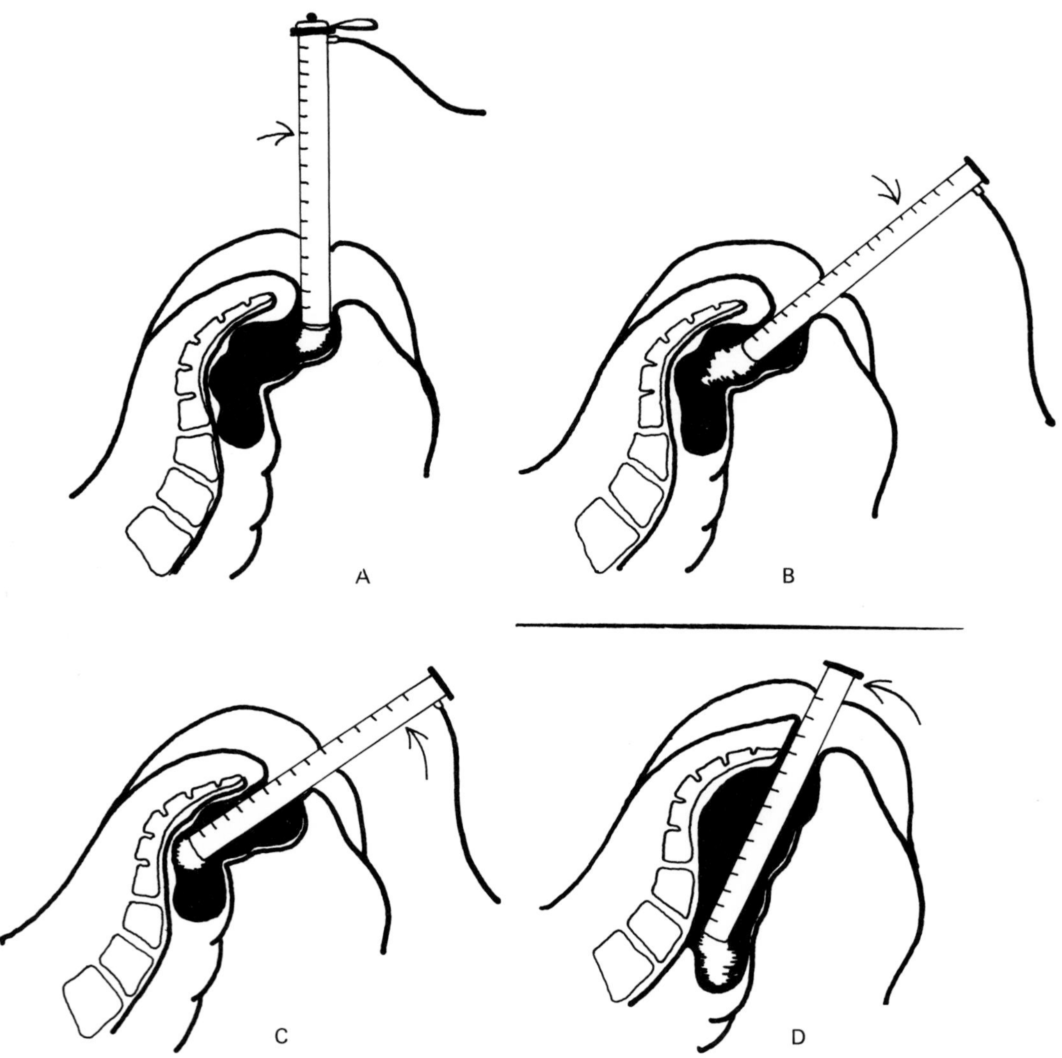

Figure 12-28. Sigmoidoscopic examination. *A,* The lubricated sigmoidoscope is introduced into the anus and pointed towards the patient's umbilicus; *B,* As the interior colon lights up, gradually lower the distal end of the scope; *C,* The distal end of the scope is elevated as the proximal end slips over the hump of the sacrum; *D,* As the scope passes the sacrum and falls to the patient's left side, the proximal end of the scope falls into the sigmoid.

stant reassurance. Occasionally instructing the patient to pant will facilitate further insertion.

The most fruitful observation occurs while the scope is being withdrawn. More air can be insufflated at this time, forcing the lumen to open and allowing polyps to be more easily seen. With the anal muscle acting as a fulcrum, the scope can be swept around 360° observing all parts of the interior colon. Remember the scope can be advanced, withdrawn or even used to push folds of mucosa out of the observer's line of vision.

When the maximal depth is reached, certain studies can be carried out, i.e., aspiration for parasitologic study and culture. If the examiner is experienced, he may remove polyps, cauterize and biopsy. Finally, when indicated, take scrapings of the skin, culture for fungus and NIH smears, biopsy and explore any fistulous tracts.

To complete the examination, minimize the patient's distress by cleaning the anus and perianal skin, draping and allowing the patient to rest if he desires. To prevent snycope, instruct the patient to rise slowly.

Complications are bleeding, tearing and perforation by scope, biopsy or cautery.

Polyps

The term *polyp* is applied in a clinical sense and refers to the appearance of a lesion protruding into the bowel. No specific histologic diagnosis is implied.

Polyps are the most common pathologic process found by proctosigmoidoscopy examinations. Some studies suggest an incidence as high as 12.5 percent. Their characteristic features should be described and recorded: size, location, shape and bleeding tendency.

Although it is a questionable deduction, some physicians relate size to malignancy: if the polyp is less than 0.5 cm, there is only a remote possibility of malignancy; from 0.5 cm to 1.5 cm an incidence of 6 percent exists; and polyps larger than 1.5 cm vary but there is an overall incidence of 18 percent.

Note the location by cm in depth and by the anatomic terms: anterior or posterior and right or left.

State whether the polyps are pedunculated, sessile or ulcerated and whether a bleeding tendency exists in the polyp.

Types

Adenomas account for 90 percent of all polyps in the colon. They are pedunculated and freely movable, signs of benignancy.

Villous or *papillary adenomas* account for 5 percent. They are irregular and have deep clefts in which barium can be trapped. They are most often sessile and may surround the bowel. These lesions are more likely to produce a diarrhea than a constipation. The incidence of invasion and malignancy is much higher than with simple adenomas.

Polypoid cancer. Adenocarcinoma is more likely to be flat and sessile or merely an ulceration, but occasionally it occurs as a polyp. If more than one polyp is present, the incidence of cancer is higher. Look for a large fixed base.

Lipomas are more commonly found in older women in the right colon.

Juvenile polyps are found in children and adults under 25 years of age and primarily in the left colon. They may bleed but are seldom malignant.

Carcinoid tumors again are found in the region of the appendix or rectum in the young or middle aged. These tumors arise in the submucosa and, as they grow, protrude into the lumen. Small ones rarely metastasize.

Hereditary polyps include the more common familial polyposis associated with anal bleeding and diarrhea. A prophylactic colectomy is usually required. All members of the family should be investigated. Other familial syndromes are the polyposis associated with osteomas of the facial bones and the Peutz-Jeghers polyposis with mucocutaneous melanin pigmentation around the mouth and buccal mucosa.

Do not forget the secondary growths —leiomyomas, lymphomas, lymphangiomas, etc.

What to Do

Polyps found with the sigmoidoscope should be removed through the scope.

Polyps found by barium enema examination and located higher than can be reached by the scope, if removed, must be done so by laparotomy. Therefore, the risk of cancer in the polyp must be greater than the hazards of surgical excision.

In asymptomatic polyps, verify the diagnosis by at least two barium enema examinations before doing a laparotomy.

A laparotomy is mandatory for all polyps which bleed, intusscept, ulcerate, double their size in 6 to 12 months or appear villous in character.

Do not hesitate to advise laparotomy in healthy young or middle-aged patients. In older patients who have polyps less than 1.2 cm and pedunculated, follow by serial x-rays as these polyps have a malignancy rate of less than 1 percent, a lesser rate of mortality than the hazards of a laparotomy in a high-risk patient.

Recently the adenomatous polyp has lost some of its significance as a premalignant lesion. The papillary or villous adenoma still is considered a hazard. Its change to cancer is not frequent, but many papillary adenomas will be found to contain a cancerous foci with invasive ability. In some cases, it may be well to follow certain patients with small tumors. But the only way to establish a definite diagnosis and exclude the presence of cancer is by biopsy.

High-Risk Patients

High-risk patients are those who have had ulcerative colitis, those who have had benign polyps or a previous cancer and those born into families with hereditable familial disease. Patients with benign polyps or a previous cancer are particularly susceptible to a recurrence.

Cancer of the Colon

In a Naval Hospital study,[14] colon cancer symptoms listed in order of frequency were:

- change in bowel habits in 65 percent, including persistent constipation or alternating constipation and diarrhea and the increased use of laxatives
- abdominal pain in 60 percent, i.e. gas, indigestion, dyspepsia, vague abdominal discomfort, abdominal cramps or vague indefinite pain simulating peptic ulcer or gall bladder disease
- rectal bleeding in 45 percent
- weight loss in 30 percent

Although not reported in the Naval Hospital study, other symptoms to look for are weakness, fatigue, anemia of unexplained origin and a sense of incomplete evacuation. Port-wine or mahogany red discharge occurs if the right colon is cancerous and bright red if the cancer is in the left colon. Bloody mucus is always a bad sign. In a patient over 40 years of age, never ascribe bleeding to hemorrhoids unless cancer has been ruled out.

The same Naval study reported the following physical findings in the individuals studied:

- abdominal mass in 25 percent
- rectal mass in 15 percent
- hepatomegaly in 28 percent
- benign rectal polyp in 10 percent
- metastatic lesions in 20 percent
- obstruction in 8 percent
- perforation in 3.5 percent

Some symptoms and signs differentiating right and left colorectal carcinona are: right colon cancer: occult blood in stools, anemia, symptoms somewhat suggestive of gallbladder disease and sentinel polyp; left colon cancer: bright blood in stools, obstructive symptoms, sentinel polyps and hemorrhoids and small colites of stools.

Percentages of a positive diagnostic study were as follows:

- barium enema in 92 percent
- biopsy in 87 percent
- proctosigmoidoscopy in 60 percent
- stool guaiac in 45 percent
- anemia of less than 11 g in 27 percent
- digital examination in 15 percent

Examinations of practical value in detecting cancer of the rectum and colon are digital examination, proctosigmoidoscopy (see previously in this chapter) and barium enema with contrast (Figs. 12-29 and 12-30) (see previously in this chapter). In digital examination, separate the buttocks for thorough inspection of all perianal tissue. Insert your index finger into the anus and palpate the anal muscles and tissues between your index finger and thumb. Continue the examination the full circumference of the anal ring. Carefully check the blind pouch in the presacral area of the rectum. Include a check of the prostate.

In acute obstructive cases, a preliminary decompression (colostomy) may be advisable. Later a definitive resection is done. Occasionally a resection can be done even in the presence of obstruction. Without an obstruction, a definitive resection is done as quickly as possible.

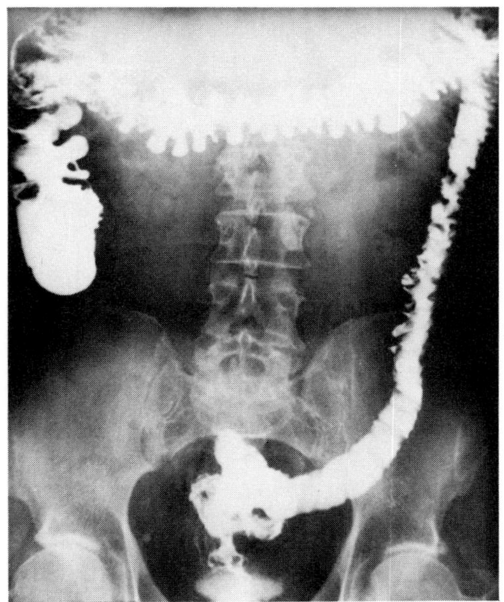

Figure 12-29. Carcinoma of the rectum with diverticulosis.

Some postoperative complications following adequate pelvic resection are difficult micturation (sometimes permanent), inability to obtain erection and/or ejaculation, late wound infections, necrosis of the colostomy and leakage of the anastomosis.

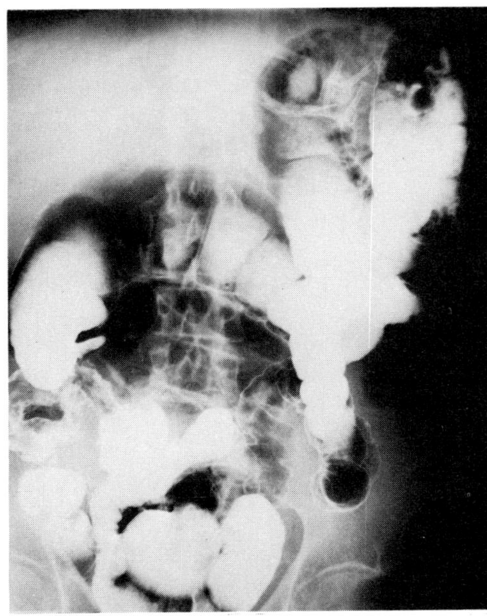

Figure 12-30. Carcinoma of the cecum.

Common Type Laxatives

Saline laxatives increase the liquid in the colon and purge it by distending the colon with fluid. Examples: Fleets Phospho-Soda, 5 to 20 ml.

Irritants and stimulants increase intestinal tract motor activity. Examples: Castor Oil, 15 ml; Neoloid, 10 to 20 ml; Senokot, 2 tablets, 5 ml or 1 suppository or syrup, 10 to 15 ml; Dulcolax, 5 mg tablets (act in 1 to 6 hr) or 10 mg suppositories (act in 15 to 60 min).

Bulk-producing laxatives absorb water and add bulk to the stool. Obviously they should be given with water. Examples: Effergel, 5 mg a.m. and p.m.; Metamucil, 5 ml.

Fecal softeners wetting agents penetrate and soften the fecal mass. Examples: Colace, syrup 5 ml or 1 to 4 capsules; Dialose, 1 capsule t.i.d.; Peri-Colace, 1 to 2 caps at bedtime.

Emollient laxatives lubricate the gastrointestinal tract and soften fecal matter. Examples: Petrogalar in mineral oil, 1 to 2 T or with cascara; Fleets oil retention enema; Agoral, ½ to 1 T at bedtime.

Enemas

Enemas should be administered with the patient lying on his left side and the enema bag approximately 2 feet above the level of the rectum. If the hydrostatic pressure is much greater than 2 feet of water, the patient will have difficulty in retaining the fluid. The enema material should be introduced slowly, interrupting the flow as needed to prevent cramps. This may take as long as 10 to 20 minutes for 500 ml of fluid. When finished, turn the patient to his right to enforce flow throughout the colon. Have the patient attempt to evacuate the fluid after resting for 5 minutes on the right side.

In general, either warm tap water or warm saline enemas are preferred. The packaged enemas have practical advantages but should be used with caution. The hypertonic phosphate salts are irritating and stimulate the colon to produce large amounts of mucus. They may also give rise to sodium retention. Limit their use to a single administration. If further cleansing is necessary, fill the empty squeeze bottle with warm tap water and reuse.

DIARRHEA

What to Look For

Diarrhea can be characterized as acute or chronic. Under acute diarrhea are conditions caused by bacteria, viruses and parasites as well as heavy metal poisoning, plants and seafood poisoning and food idiosyncrasies. Chronic diarrhea may be caused by functional colonopathy, malabsorption syndromes and inflammatory bowel disease. These conditions are given in more detail on the following pages. Other disease states which cause diarrhea as a side-effect are listed at the end of this section.

Acute Diarrheas

Bacterial, Viral and Parasitic Diseases

VIRAL GASTROENTERITIS. This is the most common cause of the acute diarrheas. Some 60 enteroviruses are involved in the etiology. The first symptom is explosive vomiting at 10 to 30 minute intervals. The patient will complain of influenza-like myalgia and malaise.

Because of variations in type of pain, gastroenteritis is occasionally confused with appendicitis, cholecystitis, diverticulitis and even bowel obstruction. The development of diarrhea and the absence of spot tenderness will help differentiate acute gastroenteritis from other conditions causing abdominal pain.

Gastroenteritis is generally a self-limiting disease. Only supportive measures are necessary: heat to the abdomen, bed rest and oral fluids (intravenous fluids if necessary). Unless unduly severe do not stop the vomiting and diarrhea during the first 24 hours. For an otherwise healthy adult, a saline laxative is effective in bringing about a recovery within 24 hours.

Diagnosis is made by exclusion. Leukopenia suggests a viral infection.

STAPHYLOCOCCUS ENTERITIS. Food poisoning is most often caused by staphylococcus. It is the common type of bacterial food poisoning. The disease is commonly confused with upset stomach, influenza or plain indigestion. Outbreaks of food poisoning are explosive; consequently, the timing of new cases aids in the diagnosis. Common foods involved are pies, pastries, custards, pork, milk and cheese.

To diagnose, find the bacteria in suspected food. Suspect the food that has been kept warm for several hours before being served. Symptoms appear within 3 hours after eating, the time being dependent on the amount of enterotoxin ingested. The first symptoms are salivation, nausea, vomiting and retching, followed by cramping, diarrhea and prostration. Symptoms begin to subside in 5 to 6 hours.

Control of food poisoning depends on proper methods of sanitation. Pasteurization of milk and chlorination of water have eliminated major sources of infection; now attention should be directed to controlling food preparation and delivery. Many foods which cause food poisoning receive no terminal sterilization except that which is incidental to the cooking process. Staphylococcus toxin is thermostable; symptoms can be produced without live bacteria. In addition, foods cooked in public institutions and restaurants are exposed to many different handlers who are often unaware of or indifferent to the most elementary sanitary techniques. Frequently, staphylococcus are introduced to food from lesions on the skin of the food handlers.

Most food poisoning victims receive little treatment because the disease is often mild; consequently, many outbreaks go unreported. Many agencies and commercial establishments want to avoid unfavorable publicity or suits for personal injury. This negligence is unfortunate because reporting of even one outbreak makes public institutions and restaurants more conscious of the dangers of poor sanitary conditions.

SALMONELLA INFECTIONS. TYPHOID FEVER. Salmonella typhosa causes typhoid fever. When typhoid fever is suspected, consider the following diagnostic aids:

- –First week: blood culture positive in 90 percent of patients
- –Second week: urine culture positive in 30 percent
- –Third week: feces culture positive in 50 percent (Later the culture may be as high as 90 percent dependable.)
- –Fourth week: Widal agglutination positive in 100 percent
- –Decreased white blood count

Paratyphoid Fever. Other Salmonella infections (gram-negative) are exemplified by paratyphoid fever. This is one of a variety of syndromes caused by Salmonella strain of organisms. Check for these infections in cases of diarrhea with fever. Stool specimens collected by anal swab through a scope and cultured on Salmonella—Shigella agar plates are effective aids to diagnosis. Consider running a blood culture and agglutination tests after 2 or 3 weeks. Again, blood counts are low.

Food Infection. Salmonella, too, has long been associated with food infection. The onset of symptoms varies from 7 to 72 hours after contaminated food has been eaten. The first symptoms are headache and chills followed by abdominal cramps and a persistent, foul-smelling diarrhea.

Sources of poisoning include meat from cold slaughter or sick animals, raw or improperly pasteurized milk, frozen eggs or egg powder products, foods contaminated by flies or sick rats. By-products of the meat packing industries, such as bone meal, fertilizer and pet foods, may be a source of salmonellosis. Sanitation is the key to control. Meat and eggs should be adequately cooked; water and milk supplies controlled and fresh foods handled properly.

Caused by Pet Turtles. Don't overlook another frequent cause of salmonellosis—the popular little turtle so often given to children as pets. It can be identified as the baby green turtle or the red-eared turtle (a red patch over each ear). Most physicians underrate its danger; however, in one survey in Connecticut, these turtles accounted for 30 percent of the salmonellosis cases.

The organisms are transferred from the turtle itself or the water in which it is kept to the hands of the child and then into his mouth. The incubation period is about 3 days. Symptoms are similar to any gastroenteritis and it finally runs its course. A greater danger exists for those who have sickle-cell anemia. In these cases all kinds of localized infections occur.

Traveler's Diarrhea. This annoying syndrome typically lasts 2 to 3 days and is characterized by diarrhea, abdominal cramps, fever, nausea and vomiting. Once a specific organism is isolated, however, the diagnosis of traveler's diarrhea is dropped and the disease becomes shigellosis, salmonellosis, amebiasis, etc.

Little is known of the etiology and much of that is mixed with myths and unsubstantiated observations. In the past, gastroenterologists put heavy blame on Giardia lamblia. The ordinary tourist, along with many doctors, continue to blame a change in drinking water or drinking water contaminated by Escherichia coli (Fig. 12-31).

There is some recent evidence that a new toxin-producing coliform organism may be responsible for traveler's diarrhea. If so, new techniques of isolation must be developed. If the disease is not due to new organisms, consideration should be given to the development of an imbalance among the intestinal bacteria after the introduction of serotypes of E. coli.

A substantial and reliable program of prevention has not developed. Most family

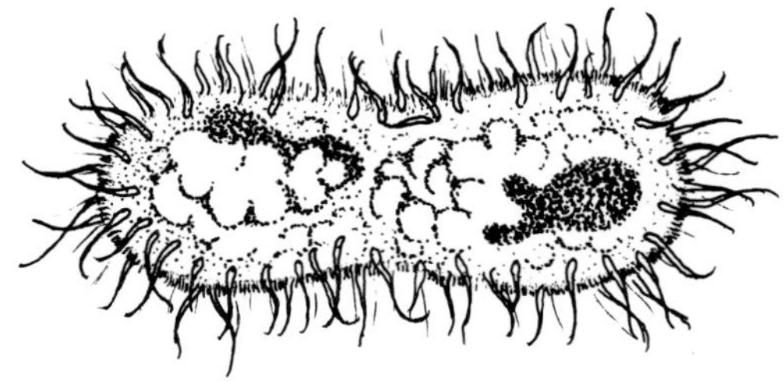

Figure 12-31. Escherichia coli. Most strains have flagella and are motile.

physicians give free-wheeling advice either based on hearsay or their own unfortunate experience. The two widely prescribed medications for prevention are Entero-Vioform (iodochlorhydroxyquin), Strepotriad (a streptomycin-triple sulfa preparation) or a sulfa-neomycin widely used in Europe. The research that has been done indicates there is no difference in the incidence of diarrhea between those who take prophylactic medication and those who do not.

Some of the Olympic teams who went to Mexico City in 1968 followed a prophylactic program. They washed their hands with hexachlorophene soap after going to the bathroom, took prophylactic Strepotriad and avoided salads and fruits. Probably the best advice a family physician can give to a traveler is to avoid all uncooked vegetables and fruits and use boiled water in all areas where coliform organisms are known to contaminate the water supply. Also, good hot tap water exceeds pasteurizing temperature and would appear to be safe.

For treatment various combinations of Lomotil and paregoric are suggested.

Shigella Infections. Bacillary dysentery caused by the Shigella group of organisms causes copious alkaline and inoffensive mucopurulent stools. Make a presumptive diagnosis on the basis of an abrupt onset of fever, bloody diarrhea and/or mucus, pain, tenesmus and tenderness. If you find pus in the stool, think of bacillary dysentery. Again, stool specimens collected on a swab through a scope and cultured on a Salmonella-Shigella agar plate offer the soundest method of diagnosis. Agglutination tests may be positive after the sixth day.

Cholera. In some parts of the world the disease caused by Vibrio cholerae is endemic. Physicians in these areas must be alert to the sudden abdominal cramps, the vomiting and the diarrhea (rice-water stools) that usher in this disease. Dehydration and electrolyte imbalance occur rapidly and the patient may collapse and die. Prompt attention to these complications is the key to treatment.

PARASITIC DISEASES. Parasitic diseases are numerous and their incidence depends somewhat on geographic location. *Amebiasis* caused by Entamoeba histolytica provokes vague gastrointestinal symptoms with an intermittent diarrhea of offensive, acid stools. Sigmoidoscopic examination (see previously) allows the examiner to observe the bowel mucosa and to collect ulcer exudate for examination. Material gently scraped from the floor of an ulcer will almost invariably reveal trophozoites. A fresh stool specimen is essential for the diagnosis (Fig. 12-32). Occasionally a therapeutic trial is necessary when suspicion is high.

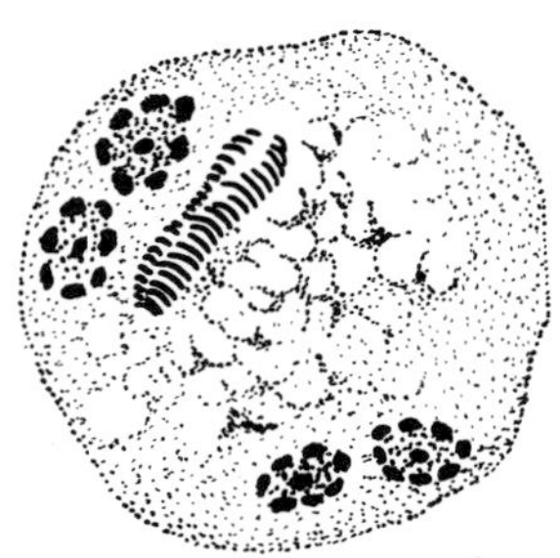

Figure 12-32. In intestinal amebiasis, Entamoeba histolytica will be found in the first stool specimen in 80 percent of the patients.

Other parasitic diseases suspected by eosinophilia and verified by finding ova or larvae in a fresh, warm stool specimen are:

- –hookworm disease of small bowel (Ancylostoma duodenale, Necator americanus)
- –strongyloidosis (Strongyloides stercoralis, threadworm)
- –ascariasis (Ascaris lumbricoide, roundworm)
- –trichuriasis (Trichuris trichiuria; whipworm)
- –fish, beef or dwarf tapeworm (cestodiasis, tapeworm) A search of the stools may reveal proglottides and/or the scolices as well as ova.

Trichinosis. This disease, caused by the ingestion of trichinella spiralis, probably is more common than suspected. A skin test and an eosinophilia is an aid to diagnosis. Trichinosis resembles food poisoning in that it can simultaneously affect many people who have eaten the same food. Since only about 70 percent of the pork raised in this country is under sanitary scrutiny, there remains a large supply that may carry live parasites. The cysts do not calcify in pork and are almost invisible to the eye. They are not searched for during government meat inspections.

If meat is heavily infested, an invasion of the intestinal mucosa occurs 1 to 4 days after ingestion. The local irritation results in nausea, vomiting and diarrhea. By the seventh day migration of the larvae produces muscular weakness, stiffness and pain accompanied by remittent fever. Edema is the next most common finding. If the parasite can be demonstrated in the suspected meat while the patient is still having gastrointestinal symptoms, the administration of an anthelmintic will remove some adult worms. No drug is effective against the larvae.

Echinococcosis caused by the larval stage of the tapeworm, Echinococcus granulosus, is best diagnosed by a skin test plus eosinophilic count.

FLAGELLATES. Giardia lamblia can be found swimming in a fresh warm stool specimen. Atrabrine is the treatment of choice.

SCHISTOSOMIASIS. The world's most serious parasitic disease is schistosomiasis (bilharziasis) the blood flukes. The disease is most common in Asia, Africa and tropical America. Ova are found in both the feces and urine.

PINWORM INFESTATION. A very common pinworm infestation of children is oxyuriasis. The adult pinworms (Enterobius vermicularis) lay their eggs about the anus at night, causing anal itching and insomnia. They can often be seen with the aid of a flashlight when searched for in the early morning while the room is still dark. Look for short, undulating hairlike objects. Their movement is what will attract your attention.

To diagnose pinworm infestation collect the ova from the anus by the following technique. Have the parents inspect the child's anus immediately after awakening in the morning. Do not bathe the child prior to taking the specimen. The child should lie across the bed face down or on one side with knees drawn up and fully relaxed. One parent should gently spread the buttocks so the rectal opening is well exposed. The other parent should handle the flashlight. They should gaze at the anus, taking their time to inspect the area for any hairlike movement. The sight of a large hair undulating slowly helps differentiate a pinworm from hair or sticky bowel mucus. This alone could verify the diagnosis.

If no pinworms are seen, the parents should proceed as follows. A strip of transparent tape about 3 inches in length is placed sticky side horizontally across the rectal opening. Instruct them to press the tape against the rectal opening with a wooden tongue depressor or a blunt teaspoon handle so that thorough and repeated contact is made at several points with the skin surface immediately next to the rectal opening. Contact with areas several inches away from the anus is of no value. Then the tape should be spread, sticky side down, without wrinkling on one of the glass slides. The area of tape that touched the rectal area should be in the center of the glass slide. The procedure should be repeated using a second slide. Both slides should be returned to your office in an envelope. Each envelope should be plainly marked with the patient's name and telephone number.

The parents should scrub their hands and fingernails carefully after making the slides. Adults in the family should perform their own tests immediately upon arising and before bathing by assuming a squatting position over a small mirror.

Heavy Metal Poisoning

Heavy metals may be ingested accidentally or with suicidal or homicidal intent. In treating poisonings by any of the subsequent chemicals give consideration to early lavage, sedation, morphine for pain, intramuscular injections of dimercaprol (BAL) and correction of fluid and electrolyte deficits.

ARSENIC. Symptoms begin within 10 minutes after ingestion—dryness of throat, abdominal pain, vomiting, diarrhea and tenesmus with mucus and blood. Lavage with sodium bicarbonate solution.

LEAD. Symptoms occur within 30 minutes. A frequent cause is accidental use of insecticide powder in the preparation of food. Lavage with sodium bicarbonate solution. In chronic lead colic, administer 5 percent calcium chloride intravenously or the newer EDTA (calcium disodium resenate).

SODIUM FLUORIDE. Symptoms occur within a few minutes to 2 hours following ingestion of the white powder often used in food institutions to exterminate cockroaches. It is often mistaken for baking soda or flour. Emergency home treatment is ingestion of milk. Lavage with lime water.

MERCURY. Symptoms begin 2 to 30 minutes after ingestion of bichloride of mercury. First symptoms include the sensation of an astringent metallic taste, salivation, thirst, vomiting, abdominal pain and, later, a water diarrhea. Lavage with a solution of sodium formaldehydesulfoxylate followed by 4 percent sodium bicarbonate twice daily and later 2 percent colonic irrigations of sodium acetate twice daily.

OTHER FOOD SOURCES. Other food sources of poisoning with resulting diarrhea include *cadmium* following storage of acid foods such as citrus juices in cadmium-plated utensils and *antimony* dissolved by citrus acid from the antimony used as a binder between enamel and metal in older cooking utensils.

Plants and Seafoods

MUSHROOMS. Two or three of these white or yellow toadstools, Amanita phalloides, are sufficient to cause illness or death. More than half of those poisoned die. Illness occurs within 6 to 15 hours. Gastric irritation causes trauma, vomiting, diarrhea and abdominal cramps. Liver damage produces jaundice and shock. There is kidney damage and acute renal failure. Treatment consists of immediate gastric lavage, castor oil, rest, opiates, adequate fluid replacement and strychnine for collapse.

Although the muscaria type mushroom causes rapid symptoms the prognosis is more favorable. Symptoms are due to stimulation of the autonomic nervous system, i.e. nausea, vomiting, diarrhea, perspiration, lacrimation, salivation, pinpoint pupils, bradycardia, and rarely convulsions. The antidote is atropine.

SHELLFISH. Shellfish which have fed on Gonyaulax cause the poisoning. These include mussels, clams and crabs. The neurotoxin is not destroyed by cooking. Shellfish poisoning resembles curare poisoning, i.e. paralysis of different groups of muscles, especially those of respiration. Other symptoms are trembling about the lips and weakness of neck muscles. Treatment is similar to curare poisoning: prostigmine methylsulfate, 1 ml of 1:4000 solution intravenously and respiratory aid.

MISCELLANEOUS. Other plant poisoning includes *ergotism* from eating rye meal or bread prepared from rye contaminated with the fungus, Claviceps purpurea. Besides gastrointestinal symptoms, the patient suffers from headache, giddiness, painful cramps in the extremities and itching of skin. Treatment is supportive and symptomatic. Gangrene of the fingers, toes, ears and nose occasionally occur in severe poisoning.

For poisoning by *water hemlock,* Cicuta virosa, treat by lavage, castor oil and sedation. *Rhubarb Leaves* and some other leaves with oxalic acid are poisonous. Treatment is lavage and castor oil. *Raw sprouted potatoes* cause poisoning. Treatment is lavage, castor oil and supportive and symptomatic adjustment of fluid and electrolytes. There are various other food idiosyncrasies.

Patients do not always react to a food to which they may be allergic; consequently, food allergies are difficult to diagnose and manage. Symptoms include belching, nausea, epigastric discomfort and constipation, or a constipation alternating with diarrhea. Spasm of the colon causes abdominal pain. A diarrheal stool filled with mucus and eosinophiles is common. To diagnose, prescribe elimination diets or ask the patient to keep a food diary. A history of previous individual or familial allergy is helpful.

Treatment consists in eliminating the food from the diet or desensitization. Epinephrine given intramuscularly controls acute symptoms effectively.

Chronic Diarrhea

Functional Colonopathy

The new name for the symptom-complex associated with an irritable colon is functional colonopathy. It is possibly the most common of the noninfectious diarrheal diseases. Such a patient is not difficult to spot for he appears to have a nervous and anxious personality. When you check into his history you find a long-standing but intermittent diarrhea without weight loss or emaciation.

Check the stool. If it contains a large amount of mucus and the patient has abdominal cramps, refer to the constellation of symptoms as *mucous colitis*. The chief complaints in *spastic colitis* are pain and constipation. There is little or no cramping in *nervous diarrhea*. Obviously, because of the functional nature of these problems, there is considerable overlapping of symptoms and findings.

Malabsorption Syndromes

NONTROPICAL SPRUE. Inheritable nontropical sprue (gluten enteropathy) causes diarrhea, steatorrhea, malnutrition and weight loss. The small bowel is unable to handle the grain protein gluten. This interferes with the absorption of other foods and causes the symptoms. The small bowel mucosa undergoes degenerative changes.

The disease must be differentiated from the diarrhea following vagotomy and pyloroplasty, gastric, or pancreatic surgery and diabetic visceral neuropathy.

Laboratory tests include 72 hour stool fat test, low serum carotene, d-xylose absorption and excretion, glucose tolerance, x-ray of small bowel, biopsy of bowel and therapeutic trial of gluten restriction.

MILK (LACTOSE) INTOLERANCE. This is caused by a hereditary or acquired lactase deficiency. The disease is often associated with other enzyme deficiencies. Consider them all diffuse mucosal diseases of the small bowel. Oral and intraduodenal lactose tolerance test and stool examinations help to verify the diagnosis.

GASTROINTESTINAL SURGERY. POSTGASTRECTOMY AND POSTVAGOTOMY DIARRHEAS. Medical treatment is usually unsatisfactory in these cases. The best prevention is care in selection of the patients on whom to perform the procedures. If necessary, revert to surgery for treatment: convert a Billroth II to a Billroth I and reverse the afferent loop or increase the size of the gastric reservoir.

ILEAL RESECTIONS. Resections cause a bile salt malabsorption with a resulting diarrhea. Cholestyramine preparations (Cuemid or Questran) alleviate the symptoms.

OTHER RESECTIONS OF THE SMALL BOWEL. These may take their toll. Stool texture and odor vary with the height of the resection. Profuse and watery stools occur with low resections, and bulky, foul-smelling stools with steatorrhea occur after high resections. Depending on the type of resection, other findings associated with bowel resection are:

- –decreased glucose absorption as determined by a glucose tolerance test (in jejunal resections)
- –decreased folic acid absorption (in jejunal resection)
- –increased fecal fat
- –vitamin B_{12} deficiency (resection of the terminal ileum) and
- –many other deficiencies: calcium, magnesium, vitamin D and K, potassium and protein

Inflammatory Bowel Diseases

Chronic ulcerative colitis and Crohn's disease occur with the same annoying symptoms—frequent stools and abdominal cramping.

CROHN'S DISEASE. This granulomatous colitis is a chronic cicatrizing enteritis of unknown cause. In about half the patients the intestinal lesions are limited to the terminal ileum and the ileocecal valve (Fig. 12-33). The disease process may be a single lesion in the small intestine, the colon or even the stomach or it may involve several areas in an extensive disease process.

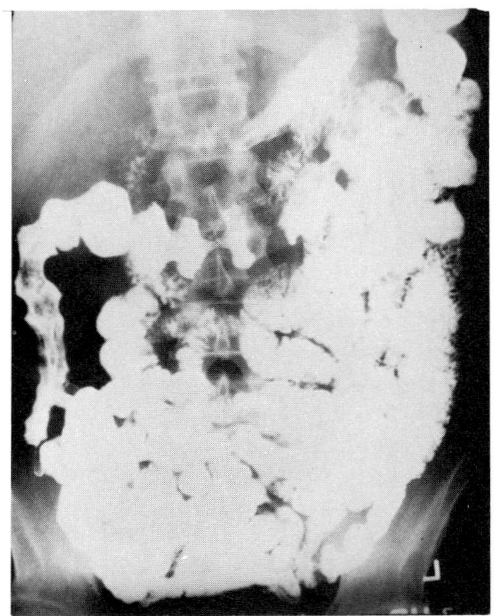

Figure 12-33. Granulomatous colitis with minimal involvement of the distal ileum. The ascending and proximal portion of the transverse colon appear to be free of disease.

Crohn's disease first involves the submucosa causing fibrosis, granulomas, lymphatic obstruction and regional adenitis. It is probably the most common cause of fever of unknown origin resulting from gastrointestinal disease.

ULCERATIVE COLITIS. This condition is usually limited to the colon (Fig. 12-34). The disease, contrary to granulomatous colitis, begins in the mucosa as a crypt abscess. This infection causes mucosal edema (Fig. 12-35), vasculitis and necrosis.

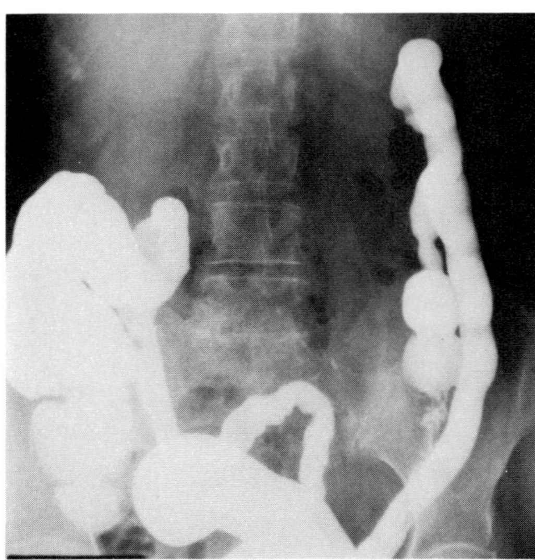

Figure 12-34. Ulcerative colitis.

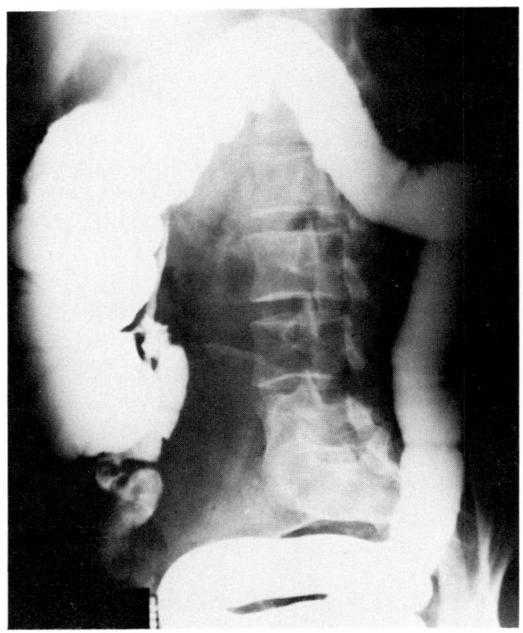

Figure 12-35. Burned out ulcerative colitis. Note loss of normal haustral and mucosal pattern.

To diagnose these diseases do a:

- –history and physical examination including a sigmoidoscopic examination with smears for parasites
- –barium enema
- –gastrointestinal series of x-rays with hourly studies of the small bowel
- –chest x-ray
- –intravenous pyelogram
- –routine blood and urine studies
- –check stools for occult blood and ova and parasites and culture
- –electrolytes including calcium
- –serum electrophoresis

To understand the variety and extent of the malabsorption problem check:

- –d-xylose for carbohydrate absorption
- –Schilling's test for vitamin B_{12} absorption
- –glucose tolerance test for carbohydrate absorption

–serum carotene for fat absorption
–72-hour fecal fat study for fat absorption
–72-hour stool nitrogen for protein absorption

DIFFERENCES BETWEEN ULCERATIVE AND GRANULOMATOUS COLITIS. Ulcerative colitis is often associated with pseudopolyps, perforation in toxic megacolon, rectal bleeding and a 3 to 10 percent incidence of carcinoma (Fig. 12-36). Granulomatous colitis, on the other hand, is more frequently related to malabsorption problems, fistulas, strictures, and small bowel disease. Ulcerative colitis is more frequently a disease of the descending colon and rectum; granulomatous colitis is a disease of the cecum and ascending colon.

Sites of granulomatous disease in 100 patients:*

Terminal ileum	91
Ascending colon	38
Transverse and descending colon	19
Upper and midileum	16
Sigmoid and rectum	13
Jejunum	7
Duodenum	5

The family physician should attempt to distinguish between the two diseases because ulcerative colitis has a poor prognosis, a greater incidence of carcinoma and needs surgery more frequently. Generally, history, physical examination and x-ray studies are enough to make the distinction but sometimes a biopsy or a laparotomy must be done.

The incidence of complications in ulcerative colitis is 20 to 25 percent. Death occurs in 5 to 7 percent of the patients. The major complication of ulcerative colitis is progression of the disease (Fig. 12-37). Toxic megacolon, pseudopolyposis, carcinoma and perforation are complications that require immediate surgical intervention.

TREATMENT. DIET. If granulomatous strictures are present, prescribe a low fiber diet to prevent obstruction. During severe

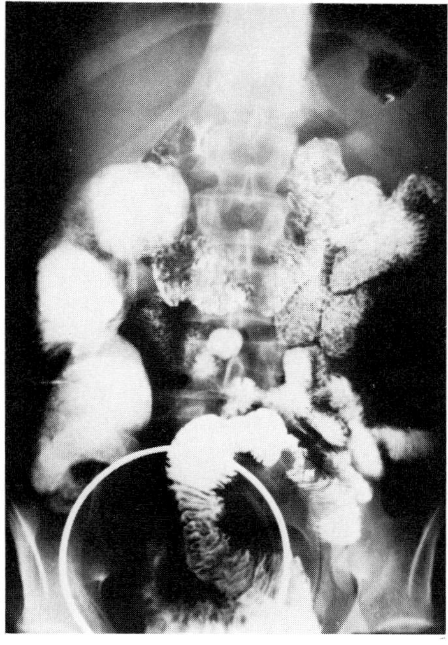

Figure 12-36. X-ray of a 40 year old male with 20 years of ulcerative colitis. The plate reveals an extensive carcinoma of the neck of the sigmoid and of the transverse colon. Two feet of the distal ilium are involved secondary to mesenteric metastatic lesions. Findings were proven at surgery.

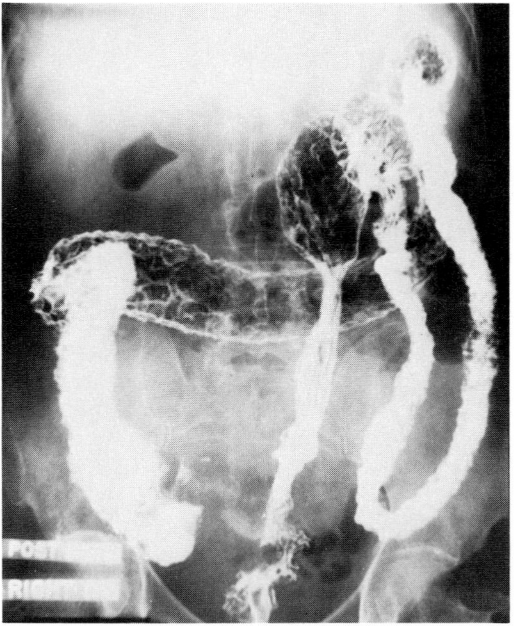

Figure 12-37. This patient had ulcerative colitis for 6 years. Note regression and progression. Pseudopolypoid changes on plain film can make diagnosis of pseudopolyposis.

*Reprinted from Ruffin J: Management of Ileocolitis. Consultant May:31, 1971, with permission.

exacerbations, use a soft diet. If toxic megacolon develops, insert a nasogastric tube. Many times frequent small feedings of a normal diet are preferable and more likely to maintain good nutrition. Keep it high in protein and vitamins and low in residue. Symptoms, when severe, may be relieved by 3 to 5 days of bowel rest while the patient is sustained by parenteral feeding. Remember that half of these patients have milk intolerance and a few others either gluten or fat intolerance. Careful observation of stools and the patient's symptoms may establish the presence of these intolerances.

REST. Both physical and mental rest should be prescribed as needed, but prolonged bed rest is not warranted. For acute or chronic heavy loss of fluids, assay and then balance electrolytes and water. Do this intravenously.

DRUG THERAPY. *For severe diarrhea and cramps:* Lomotil (diphenoxylate), which is not addicting, or codeine and deodorized tincture of opium, which are: Dose of Lomotil, 2.5 to 5 mg every 4 hours. Dose of Paregoric, 5 to 15 ml every 4 hours as needed. Dose of deodorized tincture of opium, 8 to 12 drops after each loose stool.

For anemia: If unable to tolerate plain ferrous sulfate tablets, try a liquid preparation such as Fer-In-Sol. Occasionally parenteral iron is needed (intramuscular iron dextran 4 ml daily in divided doses for 1 week).

For immunosuppressive therapy: Consider Purinethol (6-mercaptopurine) and Imuran (azathioprine) 50 to 150 mg daily.

For antibotic therapy: Use of antibiotics is debated, but Azulfidine (salicylazosulfapyridine) is a popular choice. Dose 4 g per day. When Azulfidine is not tolerated, try Gantrisin. 4 g per day, or tetracycline. The antibiotic Azulfidine appears to be useful when given intermittently, i.e. 2 weeks of medication alternating with 1 week of rest.

For intractable diarrhea due to inability to absorb or metabolize bile salts: Cuemid (cholestyramine resin).

For sedation: Phenobarbital 15 to 30 mg 4 times daily; Valium (diazepam) 2 to 5 mg 4 times daily; or Elavil (amitriptyline) 10 to 25 mg 3 times daily.

For weight gain and general nutrition: Dianabol (methandrostenolone) 5 to 10 mg twice a day. Injections of Plebex or Novogran and B_{12} 100 to 1000 meg once a month.

For steroid therapy: Indications for use of steroids are controversial, but most physicians believe they should be used when systemic symptoms are present. Consider local steroid treatment in ulcerative cloitis.

Many agree that when steroids are used, treatment should begin with high dosages (40 to 80 mg prednisone). Within 10 days, on evidence of remission, gradually reduce dose to 15 to 20 mg over a period of 4 weeks. Further reduce the dosage even more slowly, 5 mg per month. If the patient cannot be maintained on less than 20 mg per day, steroids should be abandoned. There is some evidence that the full dose given at 8 A.M. will minimize adrenal suppression. Try patients with ulcerative colitis on hydrocortisone enemas (Cortenema 100 mg) or Medrol Enpak (40 mg methylprednisolone) or suppositories (Cort-dome acetate, high potency).

Remember the side effects of steroids

–emotional problems
–disturbed electrolytes
–genitourinary, tuberculosus and mycotic infection
–osteoporosis
–growth retardation
–delayed menarche
–cataracts
–slow wound healing
–peptic ulceration

A recent report[15] from London suggests that an effective therapeutic scheme for Crohn's disease involved the use of prednisolone until maximum remission was achieved. At that point the patients were given azathioprine 2 mg per kg daily and the prednisolone was gradually reduced. On this program the azathioprine tended to maintain the improvement brought about by the steroid for at least 6 months. Others in the study who received only the steroid rapidly reverted to their previous symptoms.

SURGERY. Indications for surgery are:

- –perforation or threat of perforation with megacolon
- –obstruction due to strictures
- –chronic blood loss
- –malignancy
- –intra-abdominal or rectal fistulas
- –abscesses
- –decline in general condition with anemia, increased sedimentation rate, low serum protein and loss of weight
- –retarded physical and mental growth in the young
- –any sign of cirrhosis, pseudopolyp formation, arthritis, iridocyclitis, carbuncles or pyoderma

The surgical procedure of choice is debated between conservative gastroenterologists and radical surgeons. Opinions vary from resection of the diseased area with end-to-end anastomosis in granulomatous disease to total colectomy with ileorectal anastomosis or permenant colostomy in ulcerative colitis.

Disease States Associated with Diarrhea

- –thyrotoxicosis with hypermotility
- –adrenal cortical insufficiency, particularly after hemorrhage, surgical excision or withdrawal of steroid therapy
- –pernicious anemia
- –hypoparathyroidism with hypocalcemia
- –carcinoid tumor with release of large quantities of serotonin and other agents
- –tuberculosis
- –intestinal lipodystrophy (Whipple's disease) a syndrome accompanied by polyarthritis, polyserositis and a chronic diarrhea
- –alimentary tract fistulas following gastric surgery or as a complication of gallstones
- –Zollinger-Ellison syndrome with the secretion of large amounts of acid fluid
- –fibrocystic disease of pancreatic insufficiency. Diagnosis depends on a positive genetic history plus biopsy of the rectal mucosa and increased sodium chloride in the patient's perspiration.
- –pellagra, especially that caused by alcoholism and general malnutrition
- –chronic pancreatitis with intermittent abdominal pain and loose, frothy, foul stools which float on water. The disease may occur in patients with alcoholism or in those who suffer from cholelithiasis. Serum amylase increases within 8 hours after onset. X-ray evidence of pancreatic calcifications help to establish the diagnosis. Chronic inflammation of the pancreas, with the resulting fibrosis, leads to pancreatic insufficiency with malabsorption and diarrhea.
- –diabetes mellitus

Other Useful Remedies for Diarrhea

Antidiarrhetics are intended to allay inflammation by coating the mucous membrane of the intestinal tract, inactivate toxic products and modify the intestinal flora.

Bismuth salts.
Milk of bismuth, 1 to 3 tsp.
Bismuth subcarbonate, 1 g PRN-bland protective and astringent.

Opiate. After initial stimulation, the opiates sedate the large bowel.
Tincture of opium (Laudanum), 0.6 ml
Camphorated tincture of opium (Paregoric), 4 ml. Good for children for the dose is large and noncritical.

Lomotil. Related to merperidine, inhibits smooth muscle of bowel.
Lomotil, 2.5 mg.

Kaolin and pectin.
Kaopectate, 5 ml for infants to 45 ml for adults. Over 12 yr, 4 tbsp; 6 to 12, 2–4 tbsp; 3 to 6, 1 to 2 tbsp. May be used after each loose bowel movement. Occasionally 5 ml given every 15 min for 6 doses will stop a diarrhea.
Pectocel, 2 to 5 tbsp.

Kaolin, pectin and bismuth.
K.B.P., 2 to 4 tsp.

Kaolin, pectin, bismuth and paregoric
Mul-Sed, 1/2 to 1 tbsp

Kaolin, pectin and paregoric
Parepectolin 1 to 2 tbsp.
Pecto-Kalin Forte 1 to 2 tbsp.

Bacterial cultures. Lactobacillus acidophilus to modify intestinal flora.
Neo-cultol (USUC), 1 to 2 tsp.
Pectin, attapulgite, polymyxin B, dehydrostreptomycin.
Polymagma, 2 tablets after each loose bowel movement. Suspension, 20 ml 3 to 4 times daily. For older infants and children, 10 ml 3 times daily.

MELENA AND HEMATEMESIS

What to Look for

Consider simulated melena caused by charcoal, iron sulfate, bismuth, bilberries, black cherries or beets.

Other causes to be considered are: hemoptysis, epistaxis, esophageal varices, hiatal hernia, gastritis, gastric carcinoma, gastric ulcer, duodenal ulcer, salicylate and anticoagulation therapy, duodenal diverticulum, intestinal polyps, contusions from external trauma, thrombosis of mesenteric veins, embolism of superior mesenteric artery, hemorrhoids, anal fissure, anal fistula, polyps and benign tumors of colon and rectum, carcinoma of colon and rectum, proctitis, ulcers from tuberculosis or syphilis, intussusception, bacillary dysentery, ulcerative colitis, diverticulitis, actinomycosis, poisons, purgatives, fecal impaction, infestations with Oxyuris vermicularis, amebiasis or Meckel's diverticulum.

Miscellaneous causes not directly related to gastrointestinal problems are: uremia, shock, leukemia, typhoid fever, cholera, yellow fever, relapsing fever, leptospirosis, scurvy, vitamin K deficiency, thrombocytopenia, pseudoxanthoma elasticum, Schönlein-Henock purpura and defibrination.

General Considerations

Hematemesis occurs following a hemorrhage from a site above the ligament of Treitz. *Melena without hematemesis* usually indicates bleeding below the pylorus but not invariably so.

The color of the blood, whether bright red or tarry, depends more on the time the blood remains in the gastrointestinal tract than the level from which the bleeding originated. As a general rule, however, bright red blood usually comes from low in the gastrointestinal tract. The passage of a tarry stool does not always indicate a massive gastrointestinal hemorrhage. The ingestion of 50 ml of blood has been known to produce a tarry stool. Tarry stools may persist 3 to 5 days and occult blood 2 to 3 weeks following the single ingestion of blood. Consequently occult blood does not always indicate continuing hemorrhage.

Don't estimate the quantity of blood loss by the appearance of the vomitus. A considerable amount of blood passes into the lower tract; on the other hand, that which is vomited is diluted with gastric contents.

Remember the rapid loss of small amounts of blood may produce shocklike symptoms more quickly than the gradual loss of large amounts of blood. The pulse rate is not an infallible indicator of the amount of hemorrhage. Don't be misled by hemoglobin determinations. One study has shown the lowest values occur 6 to 48 hours after hemorrhage and as a result of dilution of the blood by tissue fluid. After 2 hours the change in plasma volume is more accurately reflected by the hematocrit.

Check the blood urea nitrogen. It is a valuable test in judging the severity of upper gastrointestinal tract hemorrhage. A rise in the BUN of less than 30 mg percent is a favorable sign; a rise to 50 mg percent is more guarded. One study indicated a 33 percent mortality range, and a rise to 70 mg percent increased the mortality to 66 percent. Search for preexisting renal disease if the BUN is above 100 mg percent. Use the BUN elevation to help differentiate upper from lower gastrointestinal tract hemorrhage. Azotemia does not appear following a hemorrhage from the colon. Subsequent to a single hemorrhage, the BUN begins to increase within a few hours, reaches a peak within 24 hours and drops to normal by the third day.

Don't be misled by suppositions: With previously known gastrointestinal lesions,

40 percent of the patients bleed from a different site. In addition to the main cause of bleeding, 50 percent of patients have an additional disease that could cause bleeding.

In one recent study of nearly 100 patients with massive upper GI bleeding, the bleeding site was located in all but 8 cases by emergency endoscopy. X-ray examination provided identical results in 41 percent. If a trained endoscopist is available, family physicians should give thought to seeking consultation with him as an aid in diagnosis.[32]

Unusual Diseases That Cause GI Bleeding

Small Bowel Tumors

The ratio of malignant to benign tumors of the small bowel is in the order of 2:1. A palpable mass nearly always indicates a malignant tumor. If the mass is tender, suspect a lymphoma. Peculiarly enough, tumors found incidentally at operation are nearly always benign. There are about 35 small bowel tumors ranging from benign to malignant. There are two which should not be difficult to diagnose providing you remember their association with observable external findings.

PEUTZ-JEGHER'S SYNDROME. This is a familial disease that produces brown and black spots on mucocutaneous tissue plus gastrointestinal polyps. To check for spots inspect the nasal mucous membrane where freckles do not occur. Be suspicious of the appearance of a brown spot on the lips.

POLYPS ASSOCIATED WITH OSTEOMAS OR SOFT CUTANEOUS TUMORS. Other polyps of the small as well as the large bowel are associated with osteomas or soft subcutaneous tumors. Symptoms are confusing and consist of vague intermittent abdominal cramps, anorexia and weight loss. Occult blood in the stools and anemia calls for a complete gastrointestinal work-up. Even with the most meticulously performed small bowel study 50 percent of the cases will be missed. If no cause for occult blood in the stools can be found in a patient with vague abdominal cramps, a laparotomy is justified. By this means most benign lesions can be cured. Malignant lesions, on the contrary, are cured in only about 50 percent of the patients. If small bowel lesions are diagnosed within 6 months after the first symptoms, surgery is more successful.

Diverticulosis of the Colon

Bleeding from diverticulosis is probably the most common cause of massive large bowel hemorrhage. Reports indicate that 5 to 30 percent of the patients with diverticulosis will show gross or occult blood in their stools.

Workers at the Massachusetts General Hospital recently reported that with the aid of mesenteric arteriography on 15 patients bleeding massively from colonic diverticular disease, the bleeding site was pinpointed in all 15 cases. About half the patients were treated successfully by vasoconstriction drugs per selective mesenteric arterial infusion.[16]

When massive red or maroon stools occur from diverticular bleeding, support the patient medically with bed rest, sedation and blood transfusions. Adams[17] however, suggests performing an emergency barium enema as a treatment modality. Failure to respond to the barium tamponade suggests the need for emergency colectomy. Older physicians have controlled the minor episodes of diverticular bleeding by administering a barium meal once or twice a week before breakfast. No harm has come from this treatment except mild constipation. A reduction in the dose will relieve this side effect.

Hiatal Hernia

No one knows the occurrence rate of hiatal hernias; figures vary from institution to institution. The incidence will not be known until radiologists accept a common definition and a common description of the esophagogastric junction. The size of the hernia has little to do with the severity of symptoms. Often the hernia is not clinically significant. Symptoms are more likely to be associated with the type of hernia (sliding or paraesophageal) and the degree of esophagitis caused by reflux gastric acid.

In sliding hiatal hernia, symptoms are similar to peptic ulcer disease. They are heartburn, sour eructations, postural regurgitation, dysphagia and aerophagia. The persistence of postural regurgitation into the esophagus is diagnostic of a sliding hiatal hernia. Bleeding tends to be slow and occult.

In the paraesophageal type hernia, symptoms are related to the hernia's size and the extent of gastritis with or without ulceration. Do not confuse the symptoms with other diseases—angina pectoris, cholelithiasis, peptic ulcer, other esophageal diseases and other causes for gastrointestinal bleeding.

The pressure of the hernial mass on the lungs may cause dyspnea resembling lung or heart disease. Walking about for a few minutes will often relieve the pain and belching.

Treatment generally is medical; only 5 to 10 percent may need surgery. Treat the patient as follows: weight reduction, bland diet, liberal antacids, elevation of the head of the bed and anticholinergic agents. If symptomatic esophagitis is verified by esophagoscopy and medical management brings no relief in 4 to 6 weeks, recommend surgical repair.

Because of the size of paraesophageal hernias and their tendency to bleed, advise surgical repair on almost all paraesophageal hernias. Recommend a vagotomy and pyloroplasty at the same time if the patient has duodenal ulcer disease.

Gastroenterologists recommend a complete work-up preliminary to surgery: barium studies, esophagoscopy, pH determinations, esophageal motility studies and cinefluorography. I have been recommending surgical repair on the basis of symptoms, barium studies, Bernstein test and occasionally esophagoscopy for years with satisfactory results.

Esophagitis

An extra word regarding simple, uncomplicated esophagitis. A reflux of peptic acid juice into the esophagus causes pain or a burning sensation. A weak valve at the lower end of the esophagus or a hiatal hernia are common causes of peptic esophagitis.

Paroxysmal pain on swallowing is a constant symptom of the acute disease. Usually the discomfort is substernal, but it may radiate to the back. When the esophagus is quiet, pain may nearly disappear but often a dull discomfort persists.

The family physician can better counsel his patients if he understands the pathophysiology of esophagitis: Starting with simple erythema the process advances to superficial ulceration, deep ulceration, transmural fibrosis, stricture and finally the short esophagus. This pathology causes obstruction, dysphagia, severe substernal pain and either occult or overt hemorrhage.

Order a Bernstein test. A positive test is pathognomonic of esophagitis. Swallowing foreign bodies, spicy foods or alcohol or smoking cigarettes aggravate acute esophagitis. Occasionally esophagitis follows an acute infectious disease.

Treatment is medical. Reduce the acidity of the patient's stomach contents by recommending the avoidance of alcohol, coffee, meat broths, concentrated sweets and spicy foods. When the patient has dysphagia, suggest only bland foods. Have the patient avoid overeating, especially at dinner. Suggest frequent small feedings because they help absorb acid.

Neutralize the patient's excess acid by giving 1 to 2 tbsp of antacids after meals and at bedtime. Maalox, Mylanta, Amphogel, Gelusil or Silain Gel are frequently used proprietaries. Instruct the patient to avoid belching and drinking carbonated beverages.

Mechanical aids that will help keep the stomach contents down are elevation of the head of the bed 4 to 6 in, avoidance of tight belts and girdles, weight loss to provide more stomach space, avoidance of heavy lifting and straining such as from constipation and coughing. Have the patient continue to sit or stand when his stomach is full and to avoid swallowing air (see earlier in this chapter) or gulping his food.

Avoid prescribing belladonna preparations which weaken valve action. Do not allow the patient to use aspirin preparations. Do prescribe Compazine or Dramamine for nausea; bismuth subcarbonate, 1 to 2 tsp hourly, for severe acidity; and Xylocaine Viscous, 1 tsp on the back of the tongue, or Oxaine, 1 to 2 tsp hourly, p.r.n. but no oftener.

Rare Diseases

Rare diseases account for about 10 percent of all gastrointestinal hemorrhages. The other 90 percent are generally due to the common gastrointestinal diseases. A number of the uncommon 10 percent are associated with skin lesions. Recognition of the visible skin findings will tip you off to the invisible lesions of the digestive tract.

Intestinal polyposis. (Peutz-Jeghers syndrome) is inherited by simple dominance. Pigmentation around the lips and buccal mucosa appears as small brown to bluish spots. The spots appear soon after birth. X-ray and sigmoidoscopic examination reveals intestinal polyps. The polyps, however, are found more commonly in the small intestine. The polyps rarely terminate in cancer.

Gardner's syndrome is another disease inherited by simple dominance. The skin lesions appear as multiple sebaceous cysts, fibromas, lipomas, etc. They appear before the polyps in the colon and rectum appear.

Hereditary hemorrhagic telangiectasia (Rendu-Osler-Weber disease, ROW) is another hereditary disease passed on by the laws of simple dominance. Bleeding occurs in approximately 89 percent of the victims. The nose is the most common site of bleeding. The basic lesion is a capillary arteriovenous communication. Look for the lesions on the tongue, lips, buccal mucosa and rectum. They are characteristic of the disease.

Pseudoxanthoma elasticum is a disease of the elastic tissue of the skin, eyes and cardiovascular system. Elastic tissue becomes calcified. Of the lesions, 75 percent of the lesions occur with ocular manifestations, 25 percent with vascular problems and 15 percent with gastrointestinal lesions. The patients develop loose and aging skin long before their time. Flat yellow plaques make their appearance on the skin of the neck, axillae and thighs. Roentgenography reveals calcified arteries. On ophthalmoscopic examination look for angioid streaks in the retina. You may mistake the lesions on the tongue for leukoplakia. Inspect the skin of the neck. It may appear as the skin of a plucked chicken.

Blue nevus on the skin is associated with angiomas of the gastrointestinal tract. Bean[19] named the disease blue rubber-bleb nevus. The nevi appear like rubber nipples and are compressible.

Neurofibromatosis (Recklinghausen's disease) is a hereditary disease. The skin may have from a few to many fleshy tumors along nerve trunks. The more noticeable signs, however, are the cafe-au-lait spots of pigmentation. If three or more cafe-au-lait spots are present, search for neurofibromas. Gastrointestinal hemorrhages occur from similar lesions in the digestive tract which become ulcerated. In patients in which the bleeding point cannot be located, search the skin for cafe-au-lait spots.

Cutis hyperelastica (Ehlers-Danlos syndrome) is a congenital or familial condition characterized by cutaneous fragility. This fragility is the primary cause of pseudotumors, hyperelasticity of the skin and hyperflexibility of the joints. It is a hereditable disease of the connective tissue. The disease can cause chronic bleeding from the digestive tract because of tissue friability. When hard stools are passed the underlying anal tissue stretches and causes splitting of the anal mucosa with a resulting hemorrhage. Bowel ruptures and perforations have been known to occur.

Others of the uncommon 10 percent of gastrointestinal hemorrhages occur with skin problems often associated with gastrointestinal bleeding or tumors. They are hematologic diseases such as Schonlein-Henoch purpura and polycythemia vera plus Hodgkin's disease, amyloidosis, Raynaud's phenomenon, Kaposi's sarcoma, calcinosis, scurvy, carcinoid syndrome, acanthosis nigricans and skin metastases.

ABDOMINAL PAIN

What to Look For

Conditions may range from bowel obstruction, renal failure, gynecologic problems, ulcers, etc. These are described in detail in this section. In examining a patient who has pain of the abdomen consider any of the following: gallbladder disease, pancreatitis, pneumonia, peptic ulcers, gastritis, renal tumor, hydronephrosis, splenic flexure syndrome, regional enteritis, diverticulitis, ulcerative colitis, renal calculi, renal infarction, testicular torsion, complications of pregnancy or ectopic pregnancy, endometriosis, ovarian pathology, pelvic inflammatory disease, functional pain caused by anxiety, depression and neurosis aneurysm, appendicitis, mesenteric adenitis, splenic rupture or infarction, obstructed or perforated bowel, bacterial enteritis, amebic abscess, mittelschmerz, distended or ruptured bladder, viral hepatitis, acute cholangitis, congestive heart failure and systemic lupus erythematosis.

Examinations

Medical History in Cases of Abdominal Pain

The medical history obtained from a patient with abdominal pain is your most rewarding diagnostic tool. Each pain-producing disease has its characteristic symptoms. It only remains for the family physician to seek them out by intensive questioning. Effective history taking will save time, expense and the performance of dangerous tests.

An acute condition within the abdomen is considered an emergency and treatment should be prompt. But more errors are made by failure to question and examine the patient than from the delay caused by careful analysis of the patient's problem.

Have the patient describe the pain in his own words and, if possible, while the pain is occurring. Ask the patient to point out the exact location of the pain (Fig. 12-38). Pain behind the sternum at the level of the xiphoid or suprasternal notch suggests dis-

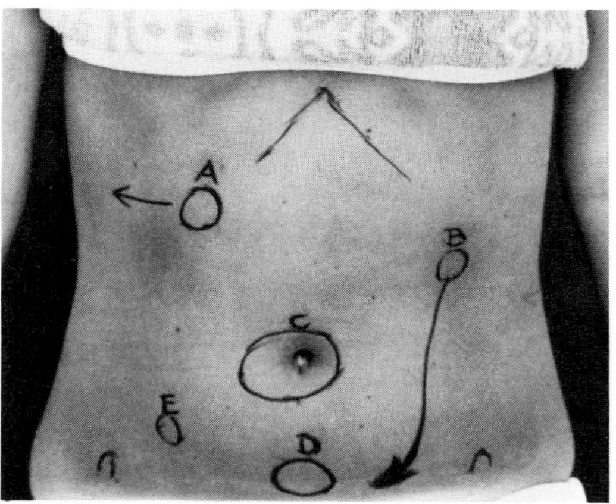

Figure 12-38. Locations of abdominal colic: *A*, Gallstone colic and its radiation; *B*, Renal colic and its radiation, *C*, Small bowel colic; *D*, Large bowel colic; *E*, Appendicular colic.

ease of the esophagus while high epigastric pain indicates diseases of the stomach and duodenum. Diseases of the gallbladder and extra hepatic biliary ducts cause pain in the high epigastrium and in the right side of the back; pancreatic diseases cause high epigastric pain but in the left back. Hepatic discomfort occurs in the epigastrium, colon pain below the umbilicus and rectosigmoid pain in the low abdomen just above the symphysis.

In general, the location of pain is associated with the site of tenderness but not always. Early, the pain of appendicitis is in the epigastrium but tenderness is in the lower right quadrant. Splenic pain is often in the left shoulder but tenderness is in the upper left quadrant.

Ask the patient to describe the size of the painful area. Colon disease produces a rather diffuse abdominal pain while the agony of a peptic ulcer produces a localized pain to which the patient can point.

Abdominal pain may be continuous, intermittent, pulsating or wavelike in intensity. Gallbladder colic is intensified by eating. Peptic ulcer pain recurs a few hours after eating. It is also relieved by alkali, food and milk. Pancreatic pain is not specifically related to meals. Burning pain may arise from the mucous membrane of the upper gastrointestinal tract.

Establish the date when the discomfort

started. This date can be important in evaluating abdominal pain. Obviously, a pain suffered over many years without complications is likely to be functional. If the patient's age is more than 40 and his pain is of short duration, check out the gastrointestinal tract for carcinoma. Remember that most abdominal pain can be aggravated by specific factors. Use this characteristic as a diagnostic aid. Ask the patient if he knows what brings the pain on. Coughing or sneezing will intensify spinal root lesions. Disease in the lower colon is related to defecation while disease of the gallbladder is provoked by ingestion of some offending food. Stress or exercise often provokes angina.

What the patient does to relieve the pain is an important consideration. The intensity of the pain can often be judged by the strength of the analgesia needed for relief. For instance, gallbladder pain is relieved by an ordinary dose of Demerol (meperidine hydrochloride). The same dose would give little relief in acute pancreatitis. Ulcer pain subsides after ingesting milk, food or an alkali. Peculiarly enough, pressure on the abdomen may reduce the pain of a pancreatic cyst or tumor.

The patient may assume certain characteristic positions during an attack of pain:

- biliary colic causes writhing about in search of a position to relieve the pain
- pancreatic pain causes the patient to walk about stooped with his hand pressed against his abdomen; he may also sit up or lean forward
- hiatal hernia may be relieved by sitting up or walking about
- peritonitis causes the patient to freeze; he changes his position with greatest caution doing most of the work with his arms and his facial expression is one of anguish
- gut pain causes the patient to writhe intermittently; when he does lie still it is usually in a jack-knife position
- in psoas irritation by appendicitis or perinephritic abscess the patient lies with his thigh flexed at the hip and will only reluctantly extend his leg

Evalute the intensity of the patient's pain. It is difficult for the patient to express objectively the degree of pain. Some patients with low intensity pain will complain bitterly more because of the persistence of the pain than because of its severity. While taking the history and doing the examination the wise physician will look for any diminution of the pain while the patient is distracted. It may be enlightening to ask the patient to compare the pain to the most intense pain he has ever had. Do this by asking the patient to judge the degree of pain using the figure 10 to represent his most severe pain. Ascertain the patient's pain threshold by observing his reaction to painful stimuli. Provide the stimulus by fingertip pressure in the soft notch just below the earlobes. In a patient with low pain tolerance, the slightest pressure causes the patient to wince and complain. Others with high tolerance will barely flinch as the examiner's fingers poke his neck.

In order not to cause confusion and delay in making the diagnosis, do not administer analgesic until the nature, location and intensity of the pain are clearly understood. This may well mean delaying narcotic administration until after a surgical consultation. Most patients will tolerate some delay when they recognize they are constantly being observed and repeatedly examined. Stay at the patient's bedside until a presumptive diagnosis is made.

General Examination

The simple topographic divisions of the abdomen are illustrated in Figure 12-39.

Make the patient as comfortable as possible for the examination. Cover the breasts of a female patient with a towel and the lower extremities with a sheet. Raise the head and knees slightly in the elderly, thus producing more abdominal relaxation.

Place your right hand on the patient's abdomen and lightly palpate to the depth of 1 cm (Fig. 12-40A). Search the entire abdomen for signs of pathology. Whenever a patient tenses the abdominal wall because of ticklishness, ask her to place her hand light-

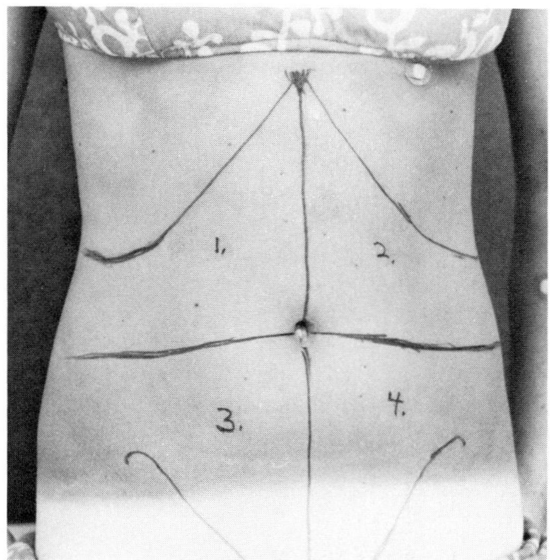

Figure 12-39. Topographic divisions of the abdomen: *1*, Right upper quadrant (RUQ); *2*, Left upper quadrant (LUQ); *3*, Right lower quadrant (RLQ), and 4, Left lower quadrant (LLQ).

ly on your examining hand and follow your movements (Fig. 12-40B).

Continue the examination by deep abdominal palaption with your single examining hand. Place your entire hand on the patient's abdomen (Fig. 12-41). Slant your fingers to a depth of 4 to 5 cm. Sensations are received through your fingerpads. In light palpation her abdomen should not depress more than 1 cm deep.

For reinforced palpation of the abdomen, place your right hand on her abdomen as in the single hand method; then reinforce your terminal interphalangeal joint with the pressure of your left hand (Fig. 12-42). This allows the examiner to receive more tactile sensations through the fingerpads of the right hand. Again palpate to the depth of 4 to 5 cm.

Gently push the fingers of your right hand under the rib margin to palpate the liver and right kidney. While the patient takes a deep breath percuss in the right costovertebral angle with your left hand (Fig. 12-43). The fingers of your right hand can sense the ballottement of her right kidney or its lower pole.

In the percussion test for acute hepatitis and acute cholecystitis, place your left hand in her lower right anterolateral ribs and strike with your right hand (Fig. 12-44). This elicits pain in liver and gallbladder disease.

Use Middleton's method for palpation of the spleen (Fig. 12-45). Have the patient place her fist under her eleventh rib to force the thorax upward. Curl your fingers under the patient's ribs and palpate for the splenic margin when the patient takes a deep breath.

Areas of abdominal hyperesthesia help distinguish cholecystitis from appendicitis. When the disease is appendicitis, the triangular area of hyperesthesia lies below the umbilicus. When the triangular area of abdominal hyperesthesia lies above the umbilicus, the diagnosis is more likely to be cholecystitis than appendicitis.

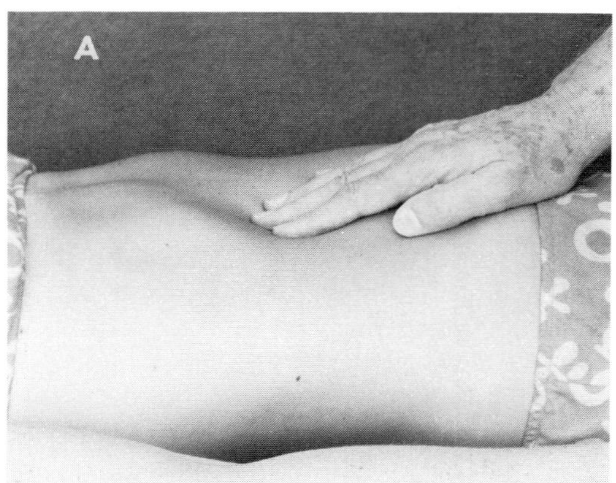

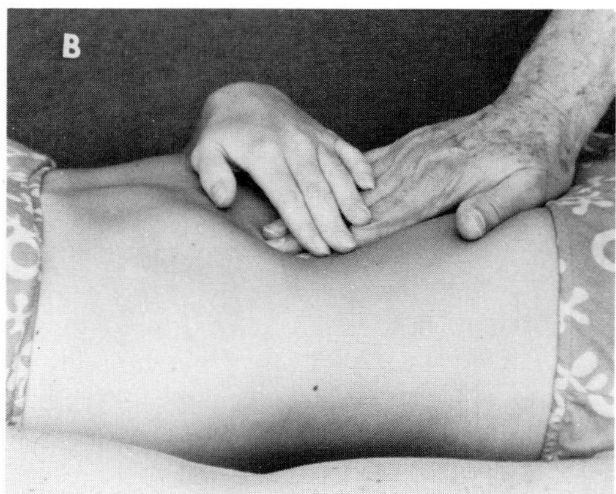

Figure 12-40. *A*, Light palpation; *B*, If the patient has a ticklish abdomen, ask her to place her left hand lightly on your examining hand and follow your movements.

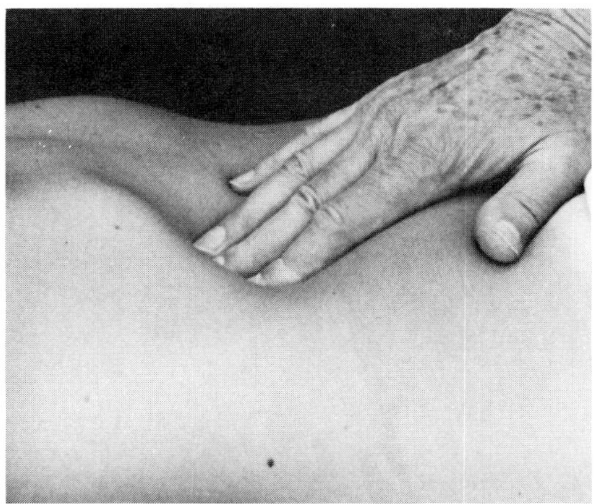

Figure 12-41. Deep abdominal palpation with the single examining hand.

Examination in an Acute Abdominal Condition

Check for rebound tenderness in the patient with an acute condition in the abdomen. Place your examining hand on her abdomen as you did in light palpation (Fig. 12-46) but apply deep pressure into the abdominal tissues and then suddenly withdraw your hand. This action causes pain in the area of disease and indicates peritoneal irritation. Before attempting this maneuver warn the patient of possible pain.

In cases of suspected trauma the abdomen should be examined every half hour by the same person. Delay surgery if early signs subside and check for muscular rigidity.

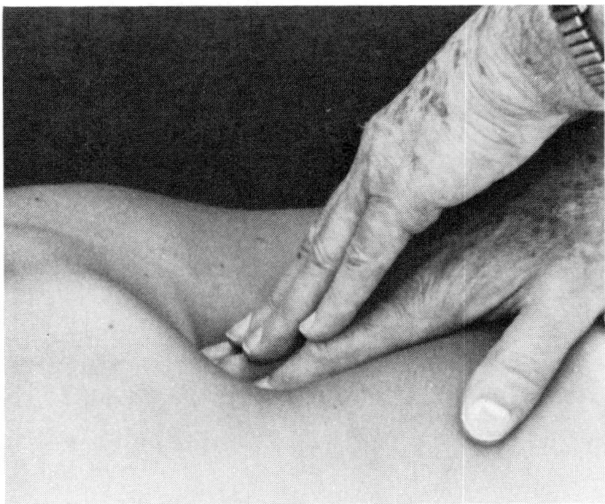

Figure 12-42. Reinforced palpation of the abdomen.

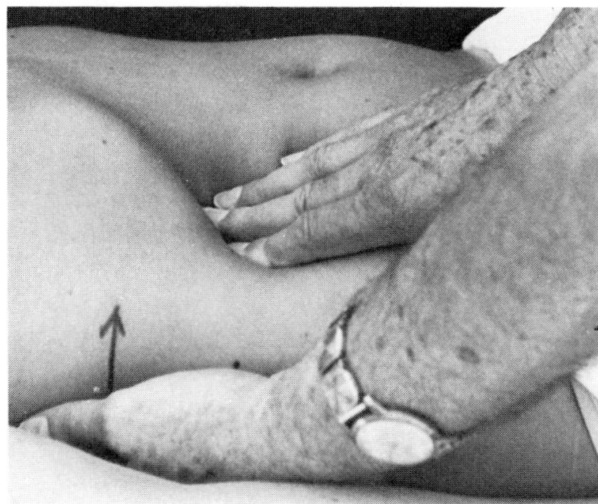

Figure 12-43. Palpation of the liver and right kidney.

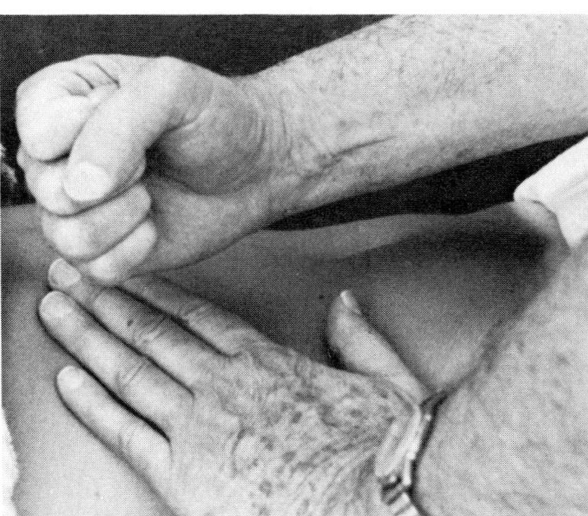

Figure 12-44. Percussion test for acute hepatitis and acute cholecystitis.

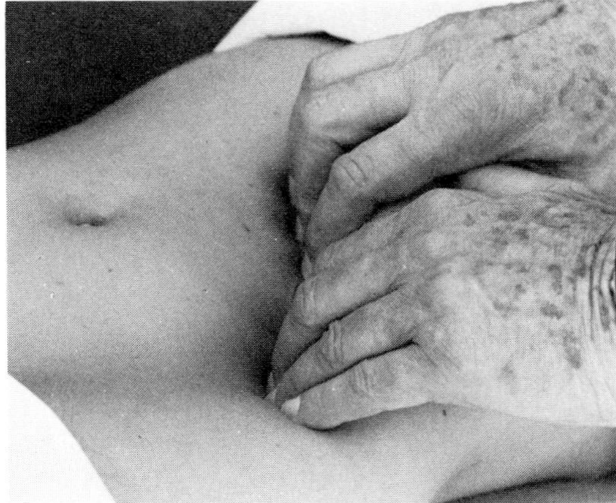

Figure 12-45. Middleton's method of palpation of the spleen.

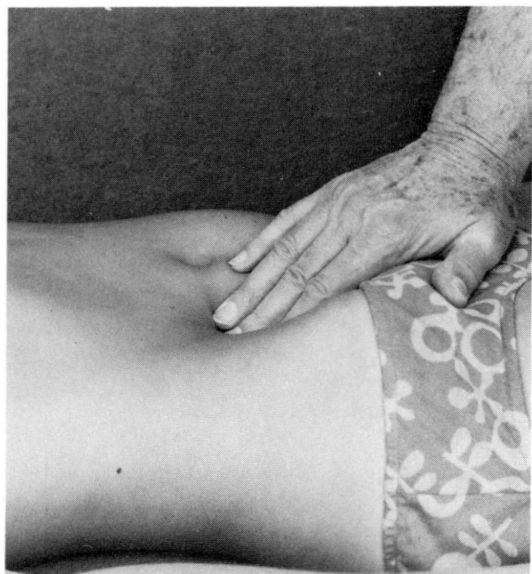

Figure 12-46. Check for rebound tenderness.

The patient with peritonitis lies perfectly quiet; he changes his position with the greatest caution. Localized tenderness is another sign of early peritonitis. Signs of late peritonitis are vomiting and abdominal distention (Fig. 12-47). Think of a ruptured hollow viscus, including an injury to the kidney.

Causes of Pain in the Right Side

An acronym helps the physician recall the diseases that cause pain in the right side of the abdomen. The acronym is *NABISCO*

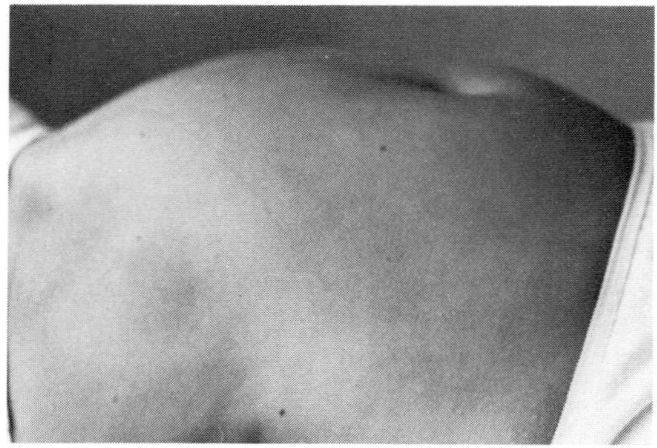

Figure 12-47. Late sign of peritonitis is abdominal distention.

Nephritides
Appendicitis
Biliary and hepatic diseases
Intestinal diseases
Spasms of pylorus secondary to other conditions
Constipation, primary or secondary to diseases of the colon or chest
Ovarian, tube and other gynecologic diseases

Differential Diagnosis

Appendicitis

The mortality rate for appendicitis has been low during the past decade. The decreased death rate from appendicitis is due to earlier recognition, improvements in surgical techniques and anesthesia, the use of antibiotics and postoperative intensive care units.

Fatalities from appendicitis are kept low when the patient is treated before complications such as peritonitis arise. The death rate increases rapidly with delay in seeking treatment. Some surgeons believe they can wait 48 hours after the onset of pain before rupture is likely but this is not always true.

DIAGNOSIS. About 50 percent of the patients with appendicitis, who consult their family physician, have the typical textbook signs. Therefore, the physician should be very careful in his examination and diagnosis.

The use of the acronymn *PETER* is

Pain
Emesis
Tenderness
Elevation of temperature
Rigidity

Pain in the lower right quadrant is aggravated by coughing. Early in appendicitis, when the patient is asked to locate the pain, she will put her hand over the epigastrium (Fig. 12-48A). Later in the course of acute appendicitis the patient points to the right lower quadrant (Fig. 12-48B). The change from a diffuse epigastric distress to a colicky pain in the right lower quadrant within 24

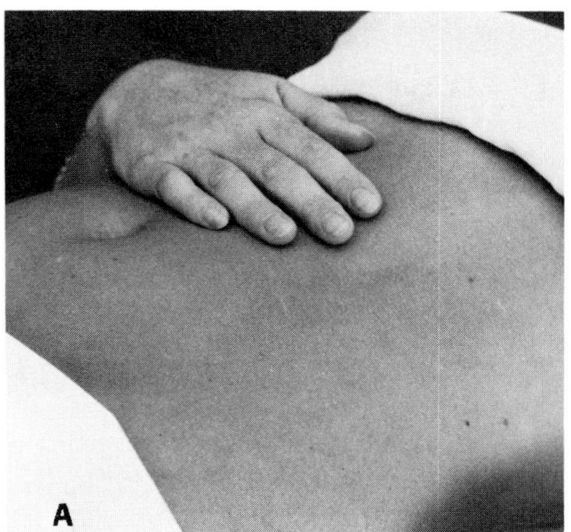

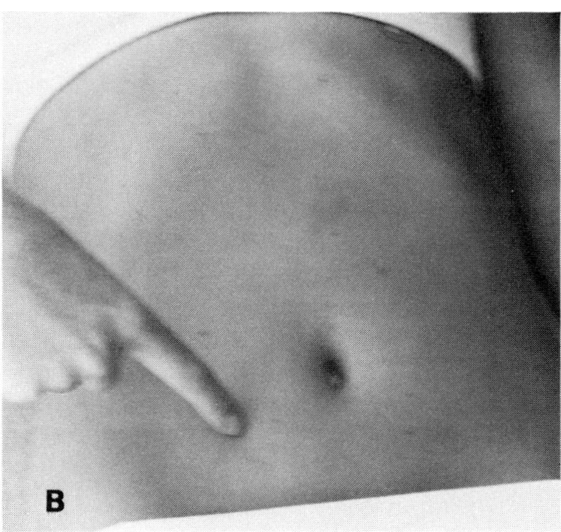

Figure 12-48. *A*, The patient initially places her hand over her epigastrium to locate the pain; *B*, Later in the course of acute appendicitis the patient points to the right lower quadrant.

hours is typical of acute appendicitis. In pregnancy an enlarged uterus temporarily displaces the appendix and causes pain in the midabdomen or flank. Pain in the right lower quadrant during pregnancy is more often due to tensing and stretching of the round ligament. If during pregnancy, however, all other signs and symptoms of appendicitis are present, do not hesitate to advise surgical treatment.

Emesis (nausea and vomiting) is not invariably present in an attack of appendicitis.

Point *tenderness* is found over McBurney's point (Fig. 12-49) and later there is rebound tenderness (see previous section). There can be variation in the type and intensity of palpable tenderness. An inflamed appendix located deep in the pelvis may cause little tenderness in the usual location. The tenderness from a retrocecal (Fig. 12-50) or retroileal appendicitis may be in the flank or loin. Do a rectal examination. Tenderness in the pouch of Douglas may be the first sign of peritonitis when the appendix is in the pelvis. An indication that the patient's appendix may have already ruptured, creating an elusive calm, is when examination shows that tenderness in McBurney's point is minimal.

Elevation of a temperature which is characteristically low is another sign. However do not be misled by the patient's temperature. A higher fever than expected may

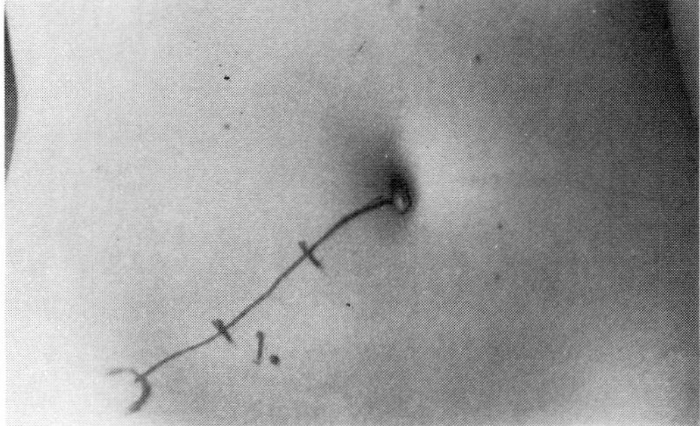

Figure 12-49. McBurney's point: The point is located one third the distance to the umbilicus on a line drawn from the anterior superior iliac spine to the umbilicus. The location of tenderness varies with the position of the appendix.

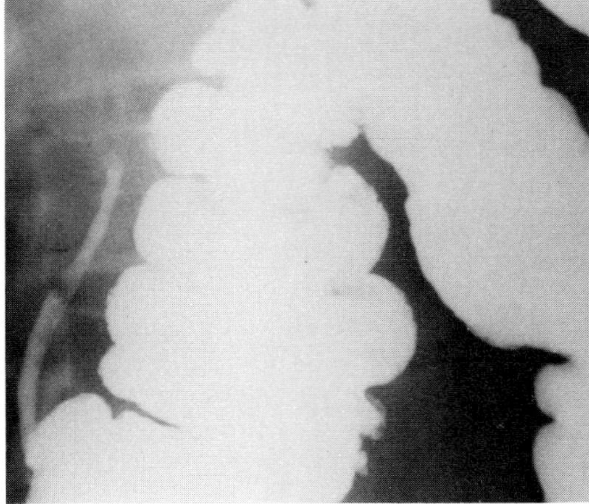

Figure 12-50. Oblique AP view of retrocecal appendix.

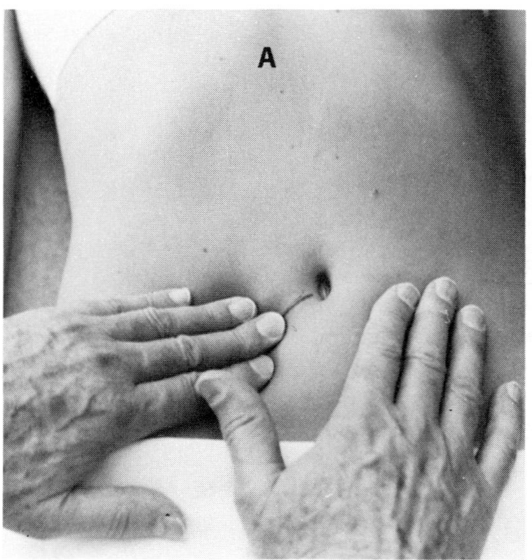

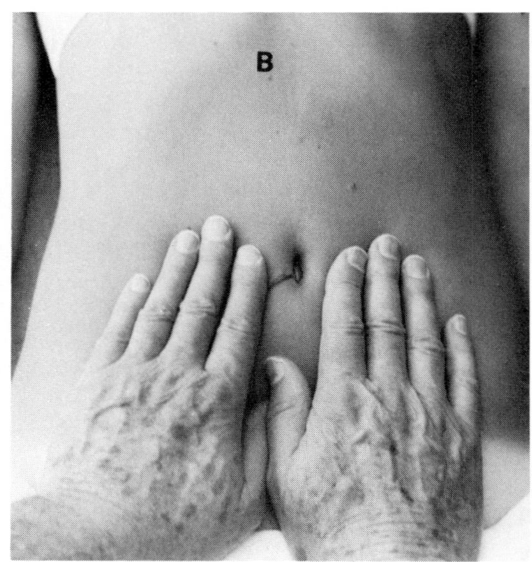

Figure 12-51. A, Place your finger tips on each recti and palpate for resistance; *B*, Check for right rectus rigidity.

indicate that an abscess is forming or a peritonitis is spreading. On the other hand, a gangrenous appendicitis may develop without any fever.

Rigidity of the abdominal muscles is indicative of appendicitis. Take into account the peritoneal gutters through which pus may travel to a distant site. Fluid from a ruptured appendix may spread upward to the suprahepatic or infrahepatic spaces. The gutters may also contain corrosive fluid if a perforated ulcer spreads down the right pericolic gutter to produce intense pain and muscle spasm in the right lower quadrant. Check for muscular resistance. Place your fingertips on each recti and palpate for the resistance of both muscles (Fig. 12-51A). Do not confuse muscular resistance with right rectus rigidity. To check for right rectus rigidity, place the palms of your hands rather than your fingertips on the bellies of the recti (Fig. 12-51B). Sense the tenseness in the right rectus if an inflammatory process underlies its belly. The left rectus remains relaxed.

Order a white and differential blood count. The usual blood picture is an increased white blood count (12,000 to 14,000 cu mm) with a shift to the left in acute catarrhal stage and a higher and more rapid rise with suppuration or perforation.

Flat and upright roentgenography will rule out fecal distention and, in children, an enema with a 30 minute wait relieves a constipation. In questionable cases a barium enema is advisable before surgery. If the barium fills the appendix it is not inflamed.

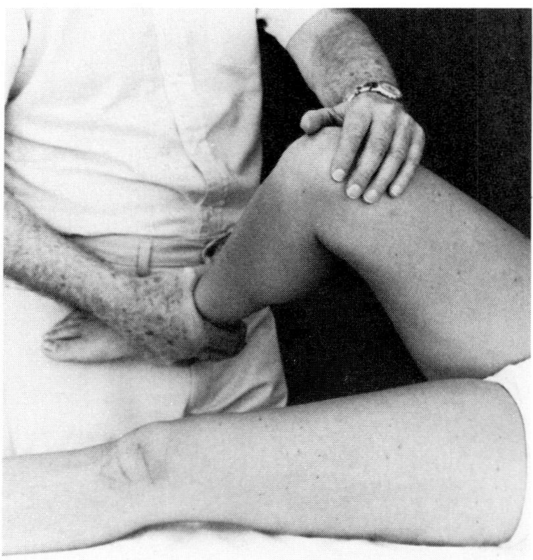

Figure 12-52. Obturator test for inflammation or abscess in the pelvis. Flex the patient's right knee to 90°. Immobilize the ankle and push the knee medially for external rotation and pull it laterally for lateral rotation. Alternate movements cause pain if the obturator muscle is irritated.

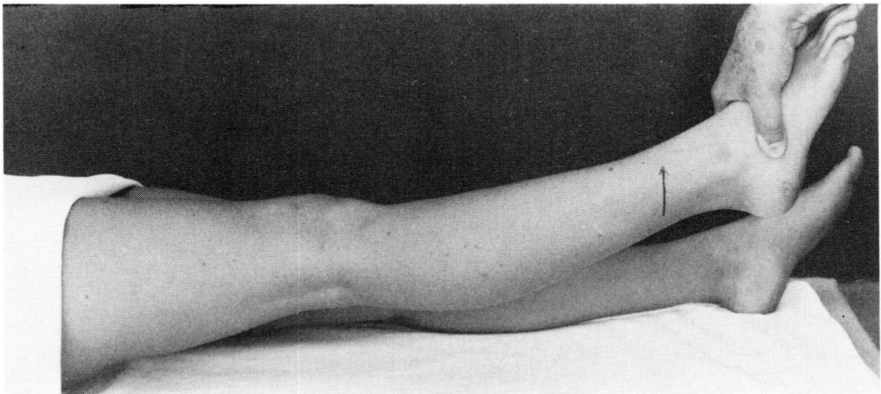

Figure 12-53. Iliopsoas test for appendicitis or other irritations to the iliopsoas muscle. Ask the patient to lift her extended leg against pressure. Pain in the pelvis is considered a positive test.

Roetgenography may also be helpful in detecting free air in the abdominal cavity which, in turn, indicates an intestinal perforation or air-fluid levels within the bowel that suggest intestinal obstruction. Gallstones may sometimes be visualized as well as pancreatic calcifications.

Rotate the patient's thigh internally and if the inflamed appendix is near the obturator internus muscle the maneuver will cause pain (positive obturator sign) (Fig. 12-52). Have the patient attempt to straight leg raise against resistance. If pain is produced, the appendix is near the psoas muscle (positive psoas sign) (Fig. 12-53). Percuss the left iliac fossa while the patient coughs. This will usually produce pain in the area of the inflamed appendix (Roving's sign).

IN CHILDREN. Diagnosis is difficult and often made too late in children under 5 years. Perforation in this age group occurs in 65 to 70 percent of the individuals. In addition, perforation can occur in a very short time—sometimes within 6 hours. Some complicating factors are rapid course of the disease, inability to obtain an accurate history of symptoms and frequent association with URI and gastroenteritis.

IN THE AGING. In those over 60 years of age, the appendix perforates in more than 60 percent of the patients before surgery. The onset of appendicitis is insidious in the elderly and the severity of the disease is not in proportion to the symptoms. The atypic cause of perforation in the aged is inability to perceive somatic pain, reluctance to seek medical care, poor resistance to infection, senile vascular changes in the appendix and senility.

Complications are perforation with abscess formation or generalized peritonitis; secondary abscess in the pelvis or diaphragmatic spaces following peritonitis; organic small bowel obstruction secondary to fibrinous adhesions; and wound infection following a perforated appendix. Pylephlebitis of mesenteric veins is rare.

ACUTE DIVERTICULITIS. A disease that is easy to confuse with appendicitis is acute diverticulitis of the ileocecal region. Its peak incidence is in patients between 35 and 45 years of age. This disease accounts for 15 to 20 percent of the operations for diverticulitis of the colon (Fig. 12-54). The

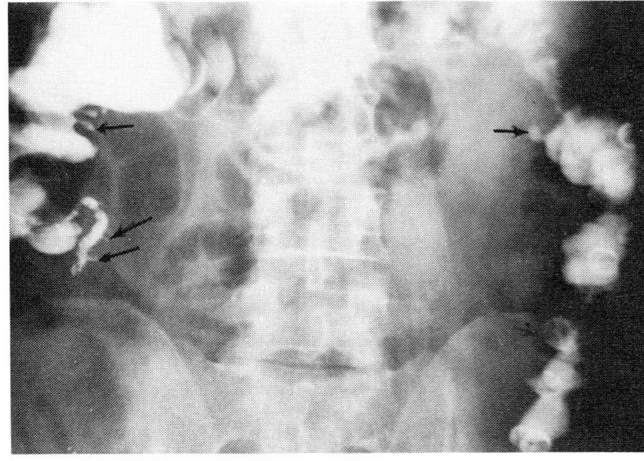

Figure 12-54. Diverticulosis of the appendix; the patient also has a duodenal tic and diverticulosis of the colon.

origin of diverticula is not clear; some believe they may be congenital. Cecal diverticula appear to be anatomically different than the usual diverticula because their walls are composed of all the layers of the intestine.

Except for a longer and more recurrent illness, symptoms and findings resemble appendicitis. Surgery is the treatment of choice and may vary from a single excision of the diverticula to right hemicolectomy when inspection does not dispel doubts of a malignancy.

Gallbladder Disease

Like acute appendicitis the pain of acute cholecystitis may begin in the epigastrium but, unlike appendicitis, the pain soon becomes localized in the right upper quadrant. Further, the pain may radiate to a point below the tip of the right scapula or even upward to the shoulder.

Elicit Murphy's sign. Murphy's sign is positive if respiratory arrest occurs because of pain. Remember this sign can also be positive in subphrenic ulcer irritation and right pyelonephritis. Fist percussion elicits pain, but it also does so when hepatitis is present. As gallbladder disease progresses, palpate gently for an exquisitely tender globular mass under the border of the liver. Abdominal muscles do not become rigid unless peritonitis is present.

Gallbladder disease occurs more frequently in the older person; however, the family physician must be alert to the possibility of its occurrence in young girls and in the pregnant woman. Women with the disease outnumber men 3 to 1. Most acute attacks of gallbladder disease and its ducts are preceded by a history of gaseous indigestion—a feeling of fullness or bloating after meals, vague abdominal discomfort, belching and flatulence. The patient often relates the symptoms to the ingestion of fatty or cabbagelike foods.

The family physician should not only be able to point to the gallbladder and its ducts as the site of a disease but also be able to differentiate between the ailments which affect this organ. This can best be done by

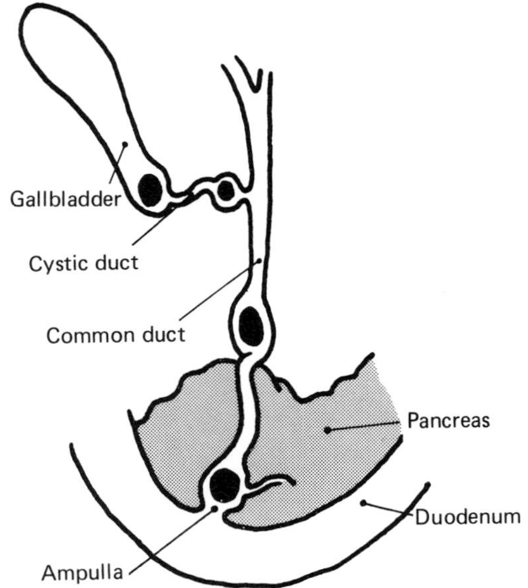

Figure 12-55. Sites of calculi obstruction in the biliary tree.

x-ray studies with or without the oral or intravenous use of dye and with or without complimentary laminography.

Cholangiography may also be performed at surgery before exploration of the bile ducts in patients who have gallbladder stones and are suspected of having choledocholithiasis as well (Fig. 12-55). It may also be performed after surgery to ensure all stones have been removed before closing the abdomen. If doubt remains, the procedure may also be done postoperatively before removing the T-tube. In the latter instances, cholangiography is performed by instilling contrast material through the intraductal drainage tube.

Percutaneous transhepatic cholangiography (Fig. 12-56) is often of great value in obscure problems. Not only is it used to demonstrate the nature of the lesion but also to show its site and how much unaffected duct remains. Peritoneoscopic examinations and cholangiography are being done more frequently in obstructive lesions of the bile ducts.

TYPES. Attempt to differentiate the following gallbladder problems. The family doctor is dependent on radiologic studies of one sort or another in differentiating these diseases.

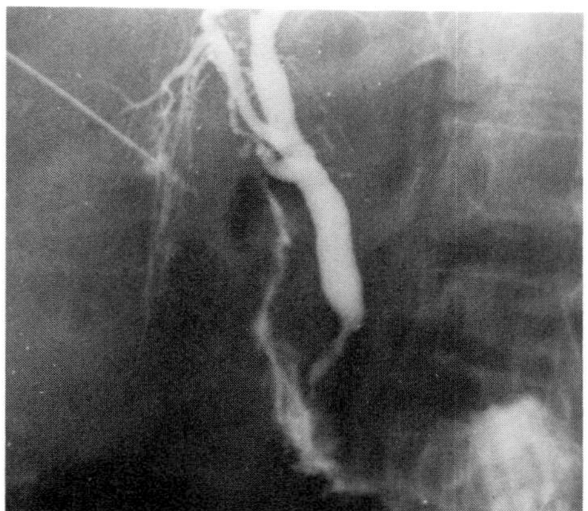

Figure 12-56. Transphepatic cholangiography.

ACUTE CHOLECYSTITIS. In acute cases the gallbladder will fail to visualize by cholecystography. An intravenous cholangiogram may be helpful in demonstrating cystic duct obstruction. In the latter there is opacification of the ducts but not of the gallbladder. A flat film of the abdomen may show stones, calcification of the gallbladder, gas in the biliary ducts, gas in the gallbladder and a local or general ileus. Cholecystography may be helpful.

CHRONIC CALCULUS CHOLECYSTITIS. A plain film of the abdomen may show opaque gallbladder calculi (Fig. 12-57). Translucent stones may be demonstrated by oral cholecystography if the film can delineate the gallbladder and there is no obstruction at the neck of the gallbladder. The likelihood of gallbladder disease is nearly always assured when the gallbladder fails to opacify with repeated and reinforced oral cholecystography. The consensus is that 90 to 95 percent of these patients will have gallstones. Should verification be needed, order an intravenous cholecystogram. This will show the gallbladder and its stones as well as stones in the duct.

CHRONIC NONCALCULUS CHOLECYSTITIS. If intestinal absorption and liver function are normal, nonvisualization of the gallbladder after orally administered dye can be taken as evidence of chronic disease of the gallbladder. Stones may be present, however.

CHOLESTEROLOSIS (STRAWBERRY GALLBLADDER). In this condition, because of the accumulation of cholesterol, oral dye will hyperconcentrate. Another characteristic is an exaggerated contraction of the gallbladder with complete or almost complete emptying within 30 minutes after the ingestion of a fatty meal. Single or multiple polypoid excrescences projecting into the

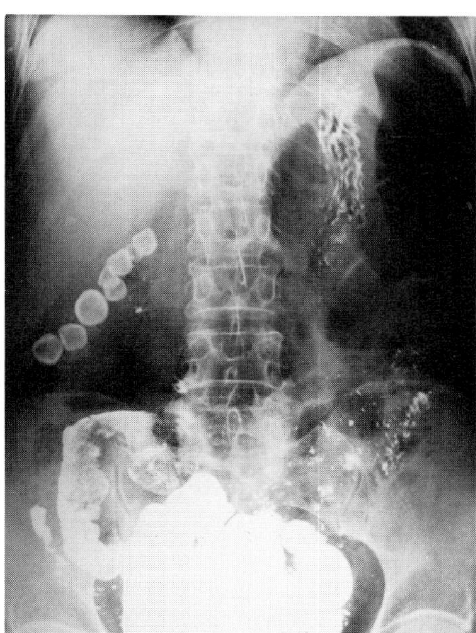

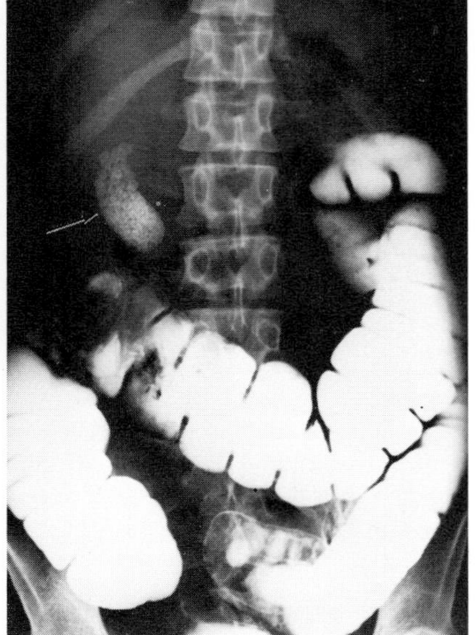

Figure 12-57. Gallstones.

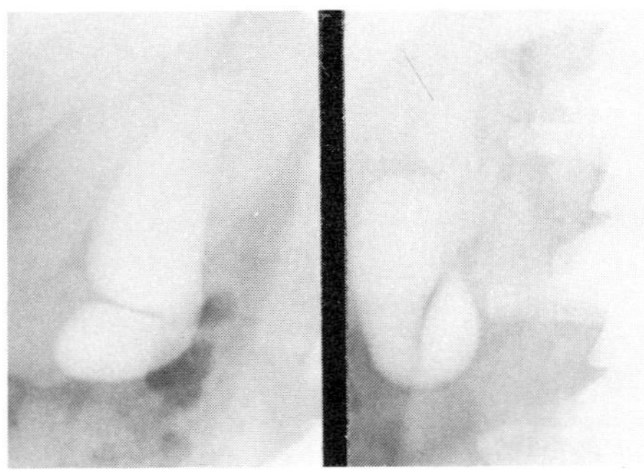

Figure 12-58. Gallbladder with phrygian caps.

lumen may be visualized. Cholesterol stones are frequently seen.

ADENOMYOMATOSIS. Order one oral cholecystogram with a fatty meal. Look for intraluminal or extraluminal tumorlike thickenings in the fundus of the gallbladder. On the film taken after the fatty meal, look for a chain of beadlike opacities at the periphery of the gallbladder, which represent diverticula filled with dye. If the thickening occurs in only one area of the gallbladder, the contracted gallbladder may appear irregular, similar to a phrygian cap (Fig. 12-58). The difference is that in adenomyomatosis the cap will not change its appearance as does a phrygian cap when it contracts.

BENIGN TUMORS. Ordinarily, if the gallbladder fails to visualize following oral cholecystography, it is because of chronic cholecystic changes or occlusion of the cystic duct by tumor. If the gallbladder does visualize and you suspect a tumor, look for a fixed filling defect that cannot be differentiated from other gallbladder problems.

CHOLEDOCHOLITHIASIS. In 15 to 25 percent of the patients opaque calculi can be seen near the extrahepatic bile ducts on a plain film of the abdomen. Oral or intravenous cholangiography may demonstrate stones within the bile ducts, but usually complimentary laminography is needed. If the patient is jaundiced or has liver impairment a percutaneous transhepatic cholangiogram is a valuable method of visualizing intraductal calculi. Cholangiography may be done during surgery either before exploring the ducts or after calculi removal to verify the removal of all stones. A dye can be introduced into the T-tube at any time before its removal to detect any residual stones or strictures.

STRICTURE. The most common cause of bile duct stricture is operative trauma during a cholecystectomy. It may occur secondary to other causes, i.e. cholangitis, pancreatitis, duodenal ulcer, inflammation due to bile leakage and drainage tube irritation and choledocholithiasis. Diagnosis of a stricture is best made by percutaneous transhepatic cholangiography.

CANCER. Liver complications usually preclude any effective findings by oral or intravenous cholangiography. A percutaneous transhepatic, operative or peritoneoscopic cholangiogram is necessary. These, of course, only show an obstructive lesion in the ducts.

EXAMINATION. Order a fatty noon meal on the day prior to examination and a fat free supper at 6:00 PM followed by 3 to 5 g Cholografin.

Take the first scout film 12 to 14 hours after ingestion of dye and repeat until gallbladder is visualized. Films taken while the patient is erect may show a translucent band across the gallbladder (Fig. 12-59). This is a stratification of small stones floating on the bile in a partially filled gallbladder.

Visualization of the gallbladder may recur 1 to 4 hours after the administration of intravenous Cholografin (Biligrafin). Visualization of biliary passages are best seen 15 to 45 minutes postinjection.

Nonvisualization of the gallbladder may be caused by any of the following:

- errors in technic
- vomiting, diarrhea or nonabsorption
- decreased liver function
- duct obstruction
- cholecystitis
- empyema of the gallbladder
- jaundice
- calculi packed gallbladder
- congenital absence of the gallbladder
- gallbladder stones with infection
- biliary dyskinesia
- any organic disease of the gallbladder
- pregnancy

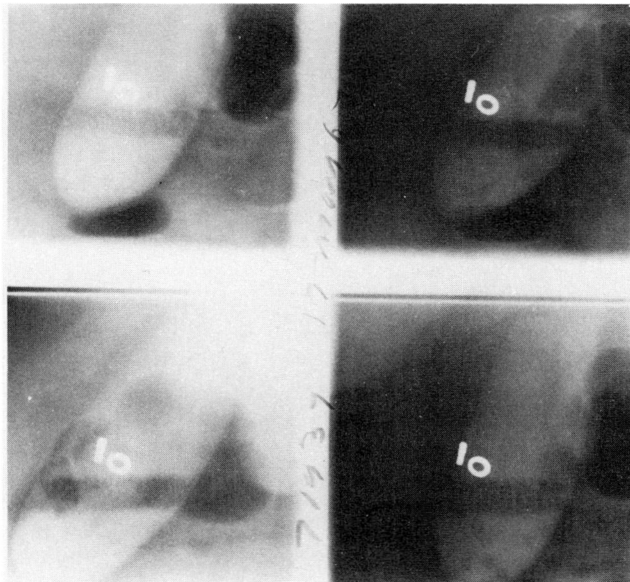

Figure 12-59. In erect view there is a translucent band across the gallbladder which represents a layer of small nonopaque calculi.

Shadows simulating biliary calculi may be caused by:

- –renal stones
- –calcified costal cartilages and lymph glands
- –fecalith and foreign material in the colon
- –empyema of the gallbladder
- –vertebral transverse processes
- –calculi in other organs

PREVENTION OF RETAINED OR REFORMED STONES. Surgeons do not like to acknowledge that as high as 49 percent of patients undergoing cholecystectomy will have retained stones and 20 percent of patients undergoing choledocholithotomy without operative cholangiography will also have overlooked stones. In addition, about 1 percent of all patients undergoing a cholecystectomy will reform stones in the bile ducts. Consequently, the potential for residual stones may amount to 7 percent. Of this 7 percent, from 30 to 83 percent will require reoperation.

Operative cholangiography is becoming the best method to detect retained stones. The study also establishes a base record which can be compared with future cholangiograms in patients with complaints following a cholecystectomy. Shore[20] reports that routine operative cholangiography will lead to the discovery of unsuspected stones in 2.4 percent of patients undergoing cholecystectomy. He advises performing an operative cholangiogram during every cholecystectomy.

He further points out that the classic indications for common duct exploration leads to unnecessary choledochotomy in more than 50 percent of the patients. This error cannot be completely corrected by the usual operative cholangiography. The new approach—completion cholangiography with television-fluoroscopy—will virtually eliminate false negative reports. The procedure involves the application of the image intensifier with television monitor and a 70 by 70 mm roll film camera. This gives the advantages of fluoroscopy and spot film technique with high resolution.

Shore also advocates the use of the flexible fibrotic choledochoscope for biliary tree endoscopy. Routine use of this scope performed through the choledochotomy incision following exploration but before completion cholangiography led to the detection of overlooked stones in 22 percent of the patients. With these new aids a sixfold decrease in the incidence of retained stones can be expected.

INDICATIONS FOR SURGERY. Indicative are the following:

- frequently recurring biliary colic without jaundice and with or without enlargement of the gallbladder
- enlargement of the gallbladder
- painful jaundice suggesting stones in the common duct
- gallbladder empyema
- acute right upper quadrant peritonitis
- abscess in right upper quadrant
- pain persisting after the passing of a stone or stones
- biliary fistulas
- undiagnosed jaundice with an enlarged gallbladder suggesting common duct obstruction or malignancy
- gangrenous cholecystitis
- wounds involving the gallbladder

SILENT STONES. Half the patients with asymptomatic gallstones will develop one of the following complications within 8 to 10 years: carcinoma of the gallbladder in 2 to 3 percent of patients under 70 yr, acute cholecystitis or common duct stones with liver, pancreas and biliary involvement.

These complications will cause death in about 5.6 percent of patients with silent stones if the stones are not removed. On the other hand, the risk of surgery is equal to the risk of cancer. Gallbladder surgery is commonly done but is among the most hazardous. The risk of emergency biliary surgery is about 1.5 percent. This is about three times greater than elective surgery. The surgical risk decreases to 0.3 percent in patients under 40 years of age.

Advise surgery in healthy patients under 40 years of age if competent surgical care is available. One attack of biliary colic justifies removal of gallstones along with the gallbladder.

Explore the common duct under the following conditions: an enlarged cystic duct, a patient with a history of jaundice and/or fever and pain, an enlarged or thickened common duct, a contracted gallbladder with stones or enlarged head of pancreas.

In older patients a cholecystectomy requires 15 days of hospitalization while the patient with a cholecystectomy plus common duct exploration requires 20 days. A high percentage of older patients will have arteriosclerotic heart disease and are in danger of a myocardial infarction following surgery.[21]

ORAL THERAPY. Danziger and coworkers[22] report that feeding chenodeoxycholic acid (a primary bile acid) to seven women with cholesterol stones caused shrinkage or complete dissolution of the stones in four patients after 6 to 22 months of therapy. The study concludes, however, that at the present time, elective cholecystectomy remains the method of choice in the management of gallstones.

Acute Pancreatitis

A history of alcoholism or biliary tract disease should direct your attention to possible pancreatitis. Three symptoms always occur in 95 percent of the patients: nausea, vomiting and abdominal pain. In addition, three signs point out the possibility of pancreatitis: epigastric tenderness, epigastric distention and shock. An acute condition of the abdomen plus shock is virtually limited to abdominal aortic aneurysm, acute hemorrhagic pancreatitis and, in a woman, a ruptured ectopic pregnancy.

Without warning, the patient is seized with excruciating epigastric pain, severe enough to cause collapse. The pain may radiate to the lumbar area, to the left shoulder and especially to the right lower quadrant. Usually the patient assumes a sitting position, leaning forward to lessen the pain. The pain is severe and not relieved by morphine. Retching and vomiting are severe.

Some tenderness is present in the epigastrium but muscle rigidity is absent. Do not be surprised at the disparity of the severity of the symptoms and the absence of definite findings in the abdomen.

Within 2 or 3 days a blue-green ecchymoses appears in the flanks (Turner's sign) or a bluish discoloration about the umbilicus (Cullen's sign).

The most helpful laboratory finding, when it occurs, is an elevated serum amylase. This enzyme begins to increase in 3 to 6 hours, rises to over 250 Somogyi units within 8 hours in 75 percent of patients. It reaches maximum in 20 to 30 hours and may persist 48 to 72 hours. The increase may be up to 40 times normal. The level should be at least 500 Somogyi units per 100 ml to be significant in acute pancreatitis; however, more than 10 percent of patients with acute pancreatitis may have normal values even when dying. Similar high values may occur in obstruction of the pancreatic duct; these tend to fall after a few days. An elevated serum amylase can also occur in acute cholecystitis, perforated peptic ulcer, intestinal obstruction and mesenteric thrombosis. Therefore, do not be misled by an elevated amylase.

Serum lipase increases in 50 percent of cases and may remain elevated as long as 14 days after amylase returns to normal. Run a lipase whenever doing an amylase since the amylase may have already returned to normal.

Increased urinary amylase follows the serum changes by a time lag of 6 to 10 hours. Sometimes the increased urine levels are higher and of longer duration than serum levels.

Serum calcium will decrease in 1 to 9 days after onset as a result of binding to soap in fat necrosis. The decrease occurs after serum amylase and lipase levels have become normal. Hypocalcemia, if untreated, can lead to tetanus and death. Glycosuria with mild increase in blood sugar may occur in 25 percent of the patients. Glycosuria in a nondiabetic patient is a simple yet excellent confirmatory test.

One half to 2 L of cloudy, bloody or prune juice ascites may develop. The ascitic fluid will contain higher values of amylase than the serum. Bile will not be found in the ascites as is the case in perforated ulcer. A gram stain of the fluid will not show bacteria unlike the ascites in intestinal infarction. In all cases wherein the diagnosis is in doubt, a peritoneal tap should be done. A hemorrhagic peritoneal fluid with a high amylase (above 7800 Somogyi units) is pathognomonic of acute hemorrhagic pancreatitis. An x-ray study for free air beneath the diaphragm should precede the tap.

X-ray studies may help by providing three clues: gallstones, calcification of the pancreas and the sentinel loop. The sentinel loop is a gas-filled loop of bowel contiguous to the inflamed pancreas isolated in the lesser peritoneal cavity. Recently authorities have begun to rely on intravenous cholangiograms to differentiate cholecystitis from pancreatitis. If the bile duct opacifies and the gallbladder does not, suspect a cystic duct stone; if both the duct and the gallbladder opacify, suspect pancreatitis.

As a rule, surgery is indicated only when pancreatitis is associated with cholelithiasis.

Most surgeons will advise a careful surgical exploration of the gallbladder, pancreas and common duct if pancreatitis recurs. Prolonged drainage of the common bile duct with or without sphincterotomy must then be considered.

Pancreatitis may be the initial disease of biliary tract pathology without any previous clinical or roentgenologic evidence of gallstone disease. Consequently, in all attacks of pancreatitis, all efforts should be made to demonstrate biliary pathology. In suspected cases and in spite of repeated negative x-ray studies, surgical exploration is indicated. Stones may not be found unless the bile is aspirated and filtered for tiny stones. Relief is prompt.[23]

MEDICAL MANAGEMENT. Give Demerol 100 to 200 mg whenever necessary to give relief. Morphine sulfate causes spasm of the sphincter of Oddi and should be avoided. Treat shock. Banthine, 50 mg, or Pro-Banthine, 30 mg, given parenterally every 8 to 12 hours reduces pancreatic secretion and inhibits the secretin mechanism. Give antibiotics prophylactically to combat septic complications of pancreatic necrosis. Use nasogastric aspiration with proper electrolyte and fluid replacement plus added vitamin B complex, ascorbic acid, vitamin K and, if needed, 1 g of calcium gluconate daily. Watch for hyperglycemia and treat appropriately.

About the best program of prevention is the absolute abstinence of alcohol beverages, small feedings, maintenance of normal weight and a rather bland diet.

Perforation of a Peptic Ulcer

The symptoms of a perforated ulcer may simulate those of acute appendicitis because the spill of gastric contents collects in the right peritoneal gutter. The history of dull epigastric pain occurring 3 to 4 hours after meals and relieved by food or alkali is often helpful in recognizing a perforation. Occasionally there are no prior symptoms of indigestion.

Surgeons recognize three stages. *Stage of prostration*—sudden excruciating pain in epigastrium and shock symptoms. *Stage of reaction*—a brief respite which may confuse an inexperienced physician. Peritonitis causes a boardlike rigidity of the abdominal muscles. Free fluid collects in the abdominal cavity. Pain occurs in both shoulders as a result of irritation of both diaphragms. *Stage of frank peritonitis*—ileus distends the abdomen. Vomiting resumes and increases in intensity. Rigidity may lessen in later stages. The patient develops facies hippocratica because of dehydration. If perforation is untreated death is likely to occur in 3 days.

An x-ray of the abdomen may show the one solid objective sign of perforation —free air in the abdominal cavity. Routine films for acute problems of the abdomen which suggest surgery are: recumbent A-P view of abdomen, erect A-P view of abdomen or lateral decubitus if erect film is not possible and P-A film of chest for subdiaphragmatic areas. The latter is useful in excluding pneumonia with referred pain to the abdomen and also in detecting small amounts of free subdiaphragmatic air. Roentgenography may be more helpful if the patient can sit or stand for about 15 minutes prior to the examination.

Treatment for a perforated peptic ulcer is surgical repair.

Bowel Obstruction

Spasmodic pain associated with loud peristaltic sounds (borborygmi) occur from the start. In functional (adynamic) ileus a silent abdomen is usually present on auscultation. The higher the obstruction the sooner and more intense the characteristic vomiting. Bile-stained vomitus indicates an obstruction distal to the second portion of the duodenum. Fecal vomiting is the result of a low obstruction. Constipation is constant. Insert a nasogastric tube (Levine) and look for indirect signs of intestinal obstruction. Progressive changes in the amount and character of the aspirated fluid give valuable diagnostic information.

A scout film of the abdomen is essential for diagnosis and is most helpful if done serially. The stepladder pattern of the distended loops of small bowel and the absence of air in the large bowel is characteristic of an organic ileus of the small bowel.

In large bowel obstruction, the distention of both small and large bowels associated with a sharp cutoff of the colon at the site of obstruction is diagnostic. In functional ileus there is a diffuse distention of all elements of the gastrointestinal tract. Ureteral calculi may result in bowel obstruction.

The only contraindications to barium enema examinations in large bowel obstructions are poor general conditions of the patient and suspected colon perforations (Fig. 12-60). Water-soluble media (Gastrografin) may be used in checking the upper gastrointestinal tract.

Common causes of obstruction are:

- adhesions from previous surgery ($^1/_3$ of obstructions)
- incarcerated hernias ($^1/_4$ of obstructions)
- volvulus (cecum and sigmoid)
- intussusception
- tumors
- ascariasis
- stenosis
- foreign bodies
- mesenteric vascular occlusion
- gallstone ileus

The cause of obstruction is often not determined until surgery. Intussusception is the commonest cause of intestinal obstruction in infants. The enfolding sleeve of bowel points down the gastrointestinal tract (Fig. 12-61). The usual locations of the ten-

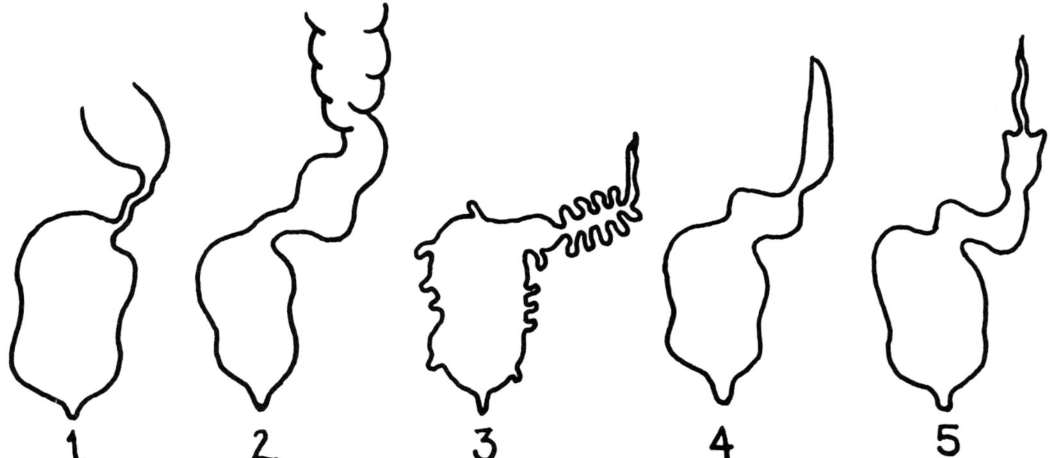

Figure 12-60. Types of obstructions found during barium enema examination: *1*, Volvulus; *2*, Intussusception; *3*, Diverticulitis; *4*, Spasm; *5*, Cacinomatous shelf.

der palpable masses follow the course of the colon. The patient passes mucus and blood from the anus. Order a barium enema examination. It will help in the differential diagnosis.

Intussusception in adults is associated with a malignancy in 24 percent of patients with small bowel intussusception and 54 percent of patients with large bowel intussusception. Almost any local pathology —benign, malignant or inflammatory, including a Meckel's diverticulum—can start an invagination.

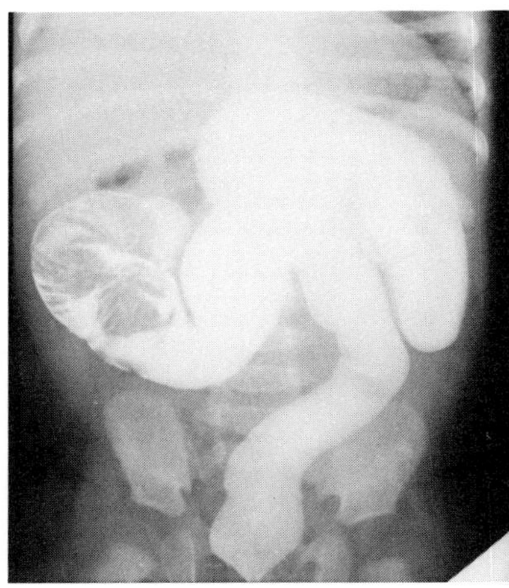

Figure 12-61. Intussusception.

In small bowel intussusception a generous amount of bowel should be excised rather than manual reduction of the intussusception and an attempt to anastamose the edematous bowel edges. In the ileocolic or ileocecal—colic type, a right hemicolectomy should be done. In a descending colon intussusception with obstruction, excise the entire intussusception.

CARCINOMA OF THE LARGE BOWEL. One of the causes of obstruction in elderly patients is carcinoma (Fig. 12-62). It may occur without weight loss, anorexia or a change in bowel habits.

VOLVULUS. This can best be verified by a barium enema. It is a torsion of the gut upon itself. The blood supply is occluded and obstruction results. The site is usually in the cecum or sigmoid (Figs. 12-63 and 12-64). Examine the abdomen for a tender knotted mass.

HERNIAS. In order of incidence hernias are indirect, direct, ventral or incisional, femoral, umbilical and esophageal.

INDIRECT INGUINAL HERNIA. This hernia produces a soft swelling at the site of the internal ring. It increases in size on standing, straining or coughing and it disappears with gentle pressure or when the patient reclines. Of significance is an expansible impulse on coughing, sneezing or straining.

At times small hernias are better observed by inspection than discovered by palpation.

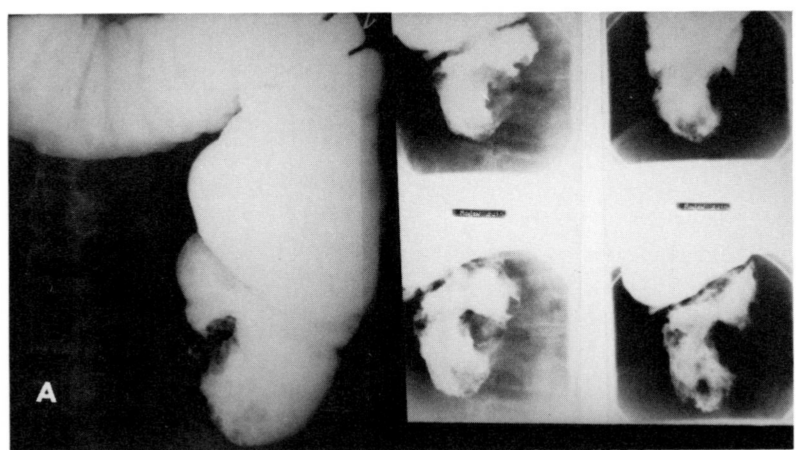

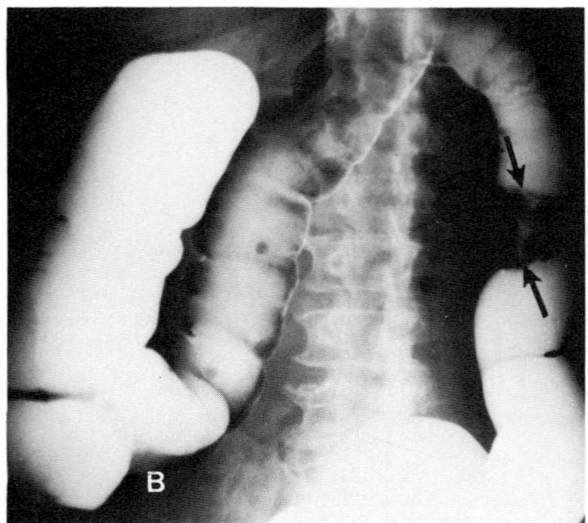

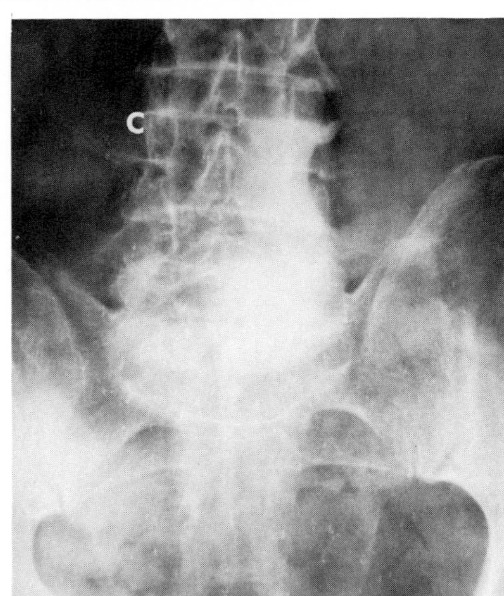

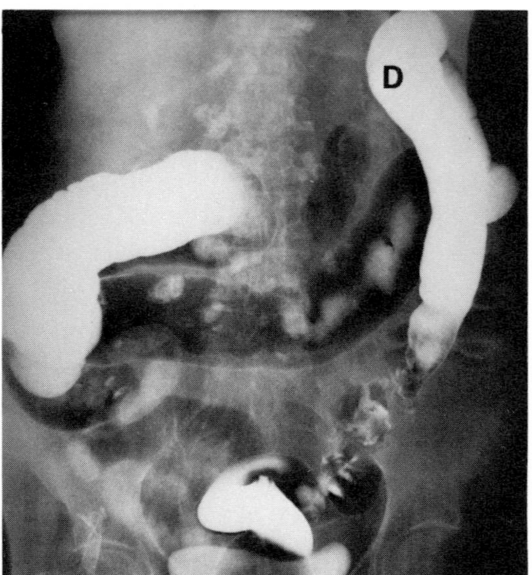

Figure 12-62. *A*, Cancer of the cecum. In the right half of the colon, particularly in the cecum, the bulky adenocarcinoma is the type which predominates. A most important clinical evidence of the disease is blood in the stools. *B*, Napkin ring carcinoma of the descending colon. *C*, Osteoblastic metastases of L_4 and L_5 from carcinoma of the colon. *D*, Cancer of the sigmoid. The number of cancers in the rectum and sigmoid account for well over half the total number of carcinomas of the colon.

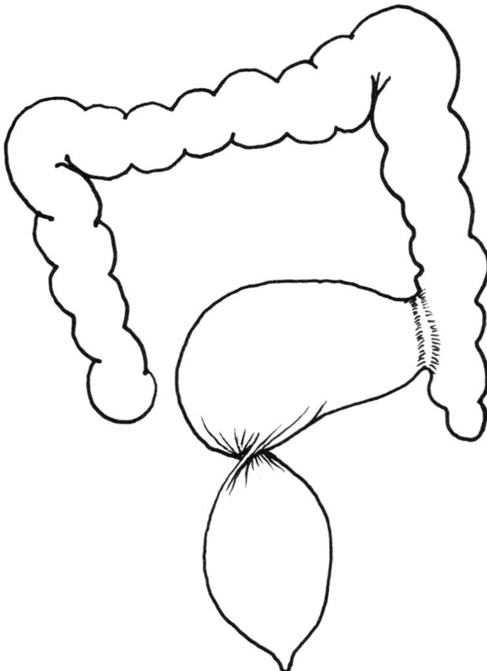

Figure 12-63. Volvulus of the sigmoid colon showing the distended sigmoid out of pelvis and the cork-screw twist with beaked lower segment.

This is particularly true in women or children. To elicit the expansible impulse produced by coughing, use the right index finger for the right side and the left index finger for the left inguinal ring. In men, invaginate the scrotum and pass the exploring finger upward and laterally into the inguinal canal. Do the examination with the patient standing. While the finger is in the inguinal canal, have the patient cough and estimate the size and descent of the hernial sac.

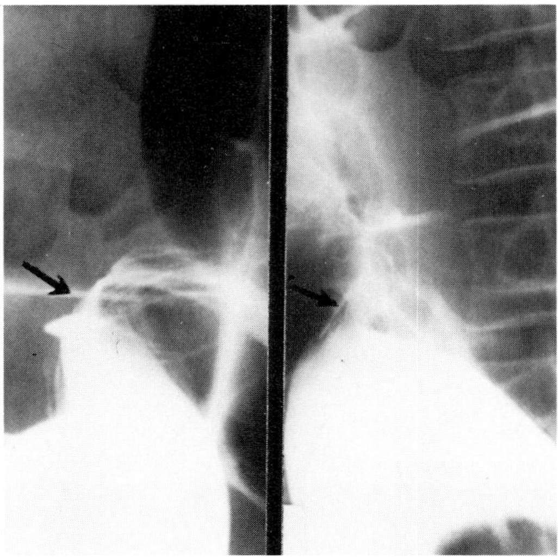

Figure 12-64. Sigmoid volvulus with marked distention of the large and small bowel.

The best technique in examining women is to place two fingers over the external inguinal ring and attempt to feel the presence or absence of an expansible cough impulse. If still in doubt, try the load test. Request the patient to lift a heavy object with legs spread and knees and hips flexed. If there is a hernial sac, a protrusion will be seen immediately.

The size of an external inguinal ring has little correlation with the future development of a hernia. In healthy males, the external ring may admit the index finger and even attain a 2 cm size without greatly increasing the risk of a hernia.

To distinguish inguinal from femoral hernias, first locate the inguinal ligament. If the hernial sac emerges above the ligament, the hernia is an inguinal one. If it emerges below the ligament, the hernia is of the femoral variety.

An inflamed hernia is one in which some part or parts (the peritoneal sac, its contents or both) are sites of an infective process. The hernial mass is red, hot and tender. It becomes irreducible. General physical symptoms will develop such as vomiting, colic, fever and tachycardia. Try palliative measures for a short time only. If the condition persists as long as 12 hours, surgery is imperative.

An incarcerated or irreducible hernia is one in which the sac and its contents cannot be replaced within the abdominal cavity. Perform or arrange for surgical repair.

Obstructed hernia is one in which the lumen of the herniated intestine is occluded. Recommend surgery if palliative measures are ineffective.

In strangulated hernia the hernial contents are constricted and the blood supply is obstructed and ultimately arrested. The hernia is irreducible, tense and extremely tender. The pain of the hernia is referred to the umbilicus. Vomiting occurs early, the vomitus changing from bilious to a fecal quality. Surgery is imperative.

Correct physiologic and chemical imbalances and administer an antibiotic prior to surgery. Insert a tube for gastric lavage and leave the tube in situ during the operation.

In strangulation of less than a half hour duration attempt gentle manual reduction for no more than 10 minutes. Auscult the abdomen before and after reduction. Normal bowel sounds will follow successful reduction.

Davis and Jackson[24] report that 22.5 percent of all colon cancers seen in an 8 year period were associated with an inguinal hernia of recent origin, a recent recurrence of an inguinal hernia or recent symptoms. They suggest that a search be made for bowel cancer in all patients over 55 years of age before hernia repair. This should include both sigmoidoscopy and a barium enema.

Direct Inguinal Hernia. Direct inguinal hernias, as a rule, are asymptomatic. The patient frequently discovers the hernia while viewing himself in a mirror. The mass reduces instantly when the patient lies down and reappears on straining in the recumbent position or on rising.

Explore for a direct hernia close to the tubercle of the os pubis near the lateral border of the rectus muscle. To differentiate from the indirect, reduce the hernia and insert the index finger of your left hand into the patient's left inguinal ring by invaginating a portion of the scrotal skin. Check for an expansible impulse. Then compress the inguinal canal with the third and fourth fingers of the right hand medial to the deep inguinal ring. Instruct the patient to cough again and, if an impulse is now felt with the tip of the right index finger, a direct inguinal hernia is present.

In the thumb-test to differentiate indirect from direct inguinal hernia, reduce the hernia and place the ball of your thumb over the internal ring half way between the anterior superior spine and the symphysis pubis. Ask the patient to cough and observe whether the hernia protrudes. If the hernia protrudes, it is direct; if your thumb prohibits protrusion, the hernia is indirect.

Unusual Varieties. An indirect and direct inguinal hernia may coexist. *Sliding hernia* is the term applied to the herniation of a viscus such as the cecum or sigmoid into the internal ring. This is produced by a loosening of the parietal peritoneum which invaginates into the ring and may become a part of the sac wall. A hernia of the urinary bladder may protrude into the sac. *Littre's hernia* is a hernia containing Meckel's diverticulum. *Maydl's hernia* refers to a loop of bowel that passes into the hernial sac, coils back into the abdominal cavity and then returns again to the sac in a "W" formation. *Richter's hernia* contains only a segment of the circumference of the intestine.

Recurrent Inguinal Hernia. Many surgeons do not realize they are curing less than 44 percent of the patients they operate on. However, family physicians who follow patients longer than surgeons have a better realization of the recurrence rate.

There are no patient profiles that will predict a recurrence. Follow-up studies indicate that a recurrence localized to the pubic tubercle is best treated by repairs of the defect only; a recurrence through the floor by use of Cooper's ligament; and a recurrence at the internal ring is poorly treated by repair of the ring only.[25]

Some surgical factors that cause a recurrence of inguinal hernia are:

–poor hemostasis during surgery
–postoperative infection
–excessive tissue tension during repair
–poor suturing technique
–ligating the hernial sac too low
–inadequate closure of fascial defect
–failure to recognize and properly repair a sliding hernia and/or associated direct or femoral hernias
–poor control of chronic cough or constipation
–poor choice of operative procedure

Should bilateral repair be done in one operation? The answer is yes, providing the first repair takes no more than 1½ hour, no infection is encountered in the first side, the bowel is not open and the first and most important hernia, which should be done first, is not unusually large. If one side is so large that increased peritoneal tension will result when the first side is repaired, postpone the second repair.

INFANT HERNIAS. Hernias in infants strangulate and display all the complications of adult hernias. About 50 percent of infant inguinal hernias are bilateral or potentially bilateral. Inguinal hernias in infants are more frequently associated with undescended testicles.

Hernias in infants do not close spontaneously and a truss will not cure infant hernias. Repair inguinal hernias in infants early. With proper anesthesia infants are good surgical risks and develop few complications.

To check for the water-silk sign in an infant, place the infant in a supine position. Place your middle finger over his inguinal canal and move your finger back and forth over the canal, moving it from below to above the canal and crossing it at right angles. Palpate for increased thickness and a sensation of silky surfaces sliding over each other.

PROBLEMS FOLLOWING MASSIVE BOWEL RESECTIONS. Some types of obstructive lesions, including hernia repair, will require massive bowel resections. The family physician, who will be the patient's counsellor in the following years, should understand the patient's postoperative problems. The small bowel has the mean length of 22½ feet, and the patient can live comfortably with a loss of ⅓ of this or approximately 7 feet. Resection of ½ is the upper limit of safety. A few cases have withstood a greater loss but with poorer results.

Electrolyte and fluid loss is particularly massive following surgery. These losses must be replaced by the proper fluids as determined by electrolyte measurements and urinary output. An attempt to maintain urinary output between 1,000 and 1,500 ml per day appears desirable. Intravenous vitamins appear helpful. To avoid sudden electrolyte imbalance, check serum potassium, calcium and magnesium from time to time throughout the patient's lifetime.

Unrelenting diarrhea to the extent of 10 L per day for 7 days not only causes metabolic problems but also severe rectal and anal irritation. All kinds of malabsorption syndromes ensue, i.e. fat, protein, carbohydrate and calcium depletion.

After the rate of intestinal absorption slows down, the family physician must find the regimen that fits the patient's emotional and physical needs. Peculiarly enough, most of these patients end up with a gastric hypersecretion and fecal acidity. Vagotomy and antrectomy or vagotomy and pyloroplasty or even a reversal of a jejunal segment may make the patient's life tolerable.

POSTOPERATIVE CHECK-UPS IN CANCER OF THE BOWEL. Remember than an individual who has had one malignant growth of the colon is more likely to develop a second lesion than a patient who has never had cancer of the colon. If you discover one lesion, reexamine the bowel by another method to seek further tumors. If it is impossible to do so before surgery, examine during surgery. Tumors can be missed even by careful palpation of the colon.

See that all patients who have had a resection of the bowel for cancer are regularly reexamined the rest of their lives at 6 to 12 month intervals. Start the first examination 3 to 6 months postoperatively for purposes of establishing a base line.

Questionable areas should be reexamined in order to rule out artifacts or spasms. Compare x-rays with previous films to detect early changes (Fig. 12-65). If any x-ray is questionable, follow-up examinations should be done within 1 to 2 months.

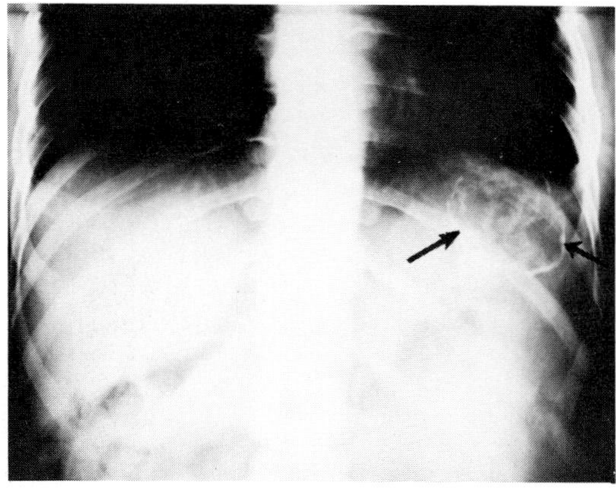

Figure 12-65. Splenic cyst from an old hemorrhage during surgery.

Renal Conditions

RENAL CALCULI. Each year in the United States, 1 in every 1000 persons requires hospitalization for kidney stones. Even in so common an ailment, no sound theory as to the primary cause of the origin and growth of a stone has evolved. But with an understanding of certain facts, the family physician can provide effective therapy in about 90 percent of these patients.

The commonest type of urinary stone in the United States is composed of calcium oxalate and phosphate. In more than half the cases stones are mixtures of calcium, oxalate, ammonium and magnesium phosphate and carbonates. Most statistics indicate that uric acid stones represent about 4 percent and cystine stones less than 1 percent of the total incidence.

The family physician should insist that every stone recovered or passed be analyzed. Knowledge of a stone's composition, and especially of its core, is invaluable information. In some areas where laboratories are not research oriented, stones should be sent out for detailed analysis by polarization microscopy and x-ray powder defraction. Often uric acid crystals serve as a small nidus upon which other minerals deposit. As the process continues, the usual chemical analysis will be misleading, for it will fail to detect the small but critically important uric acid deposit.

DIAGNOSIS. A sudden unilateral abdominal pain begins in the flank, the low back or lower abdomen and radiates to the groin, urethral meatus or the testicles or vulva. The pain is severe and has a tendency to wax and wave. There is accompanying nausea, vomiting, sweating and weakness. Transient hematuria, gross or miscroscopic, is often present. On occasion, hematuria may be the only finding. Generally, stone disease may be assumed to be present when a stone has been collected or when one or more radiodensities or suspicious radiolucencies are visualized by intravenous pyelography and shown to be within the kidney or urinary tract (Figs. 12-66 and 12-67).

Some historical findings that suggest stones are symptoms of hyperparathyroidism in the patient or his family, sarcoidosis, uric acid disorders, familial cystinuria or stones during childhood and a family history of weakness, stunted growth, bone disease or the stones of renal tubular disease.

Laboratory studies provide the most useful information regarding the etiology of stones. (See Fig. 12-68 for variety of crystals.) Long term preventive care in which

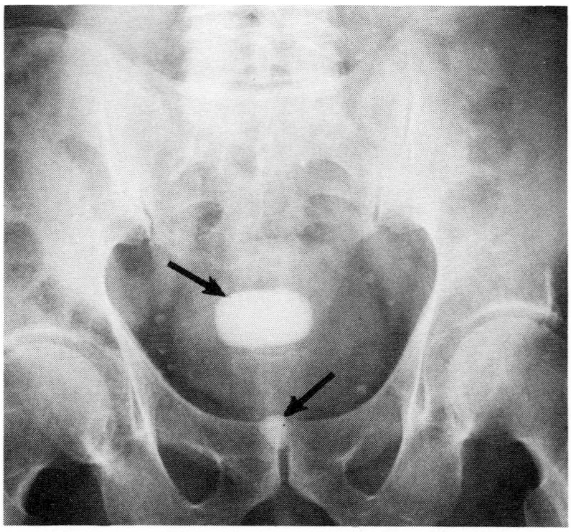

Figure 12-66. Right ureter partially obstructed by vesicle calculus (see circle). The ureter narrows in three places: immediately after leaving the renal pelvis, at the junction of the lower with the middle third and just before entering the bladder.

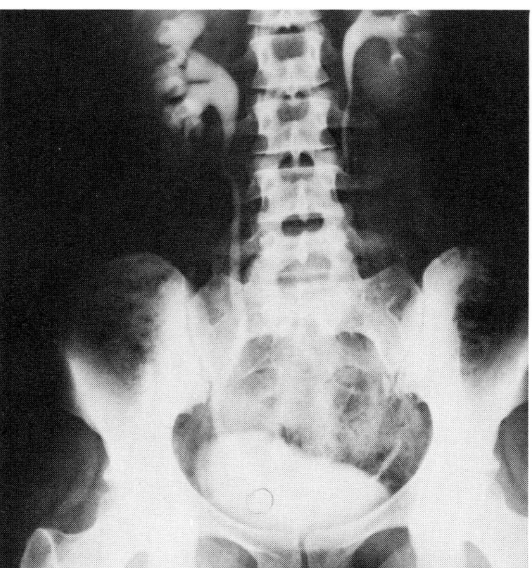

Figure 12-67. Two large bladder calculi, one near the urethral outlet.

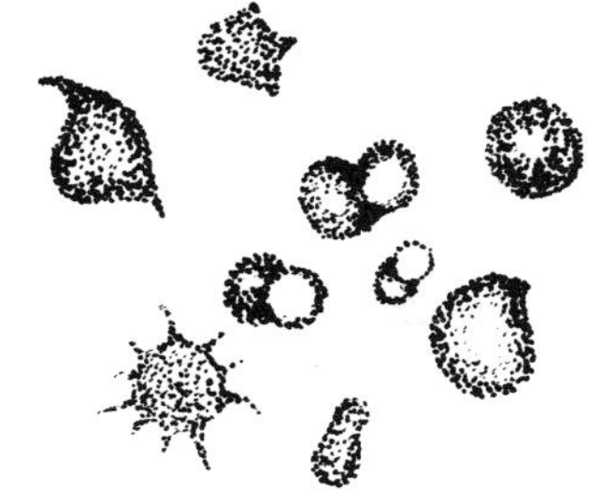

Ammonium urate crystals

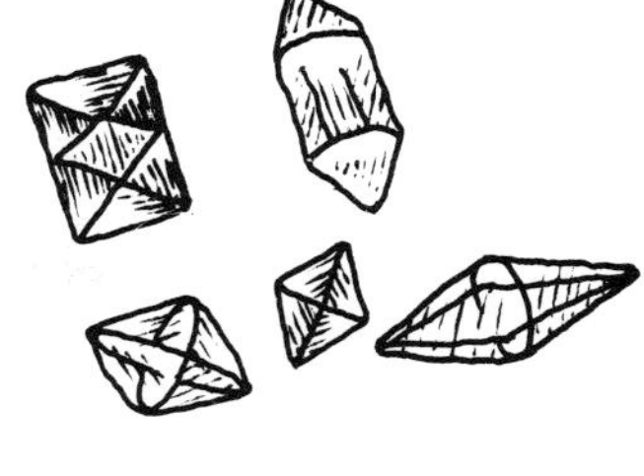

Calcium oxalate crystals

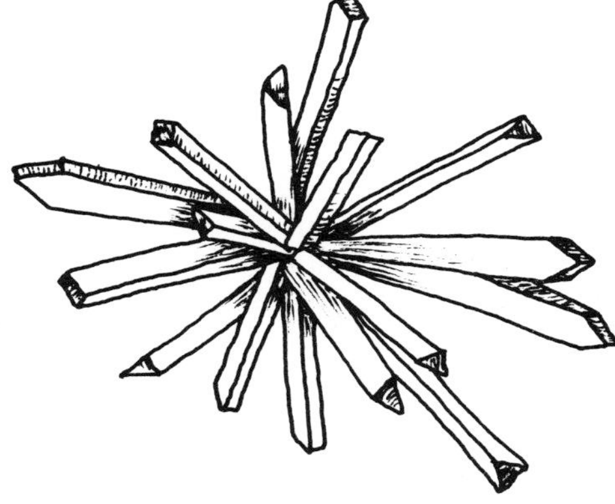

Calcium phosphate crystals

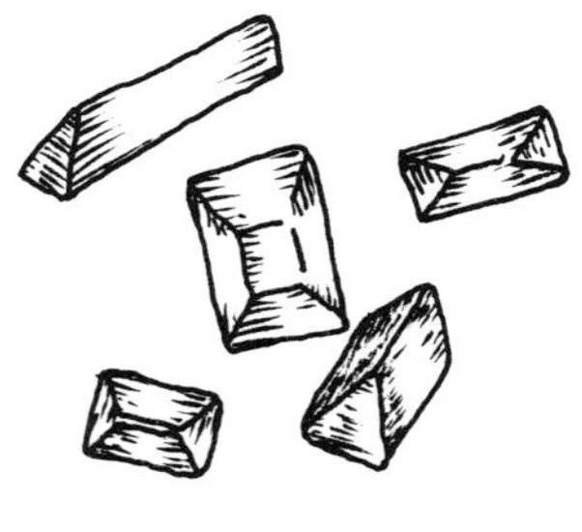

Triple phosphate crystals

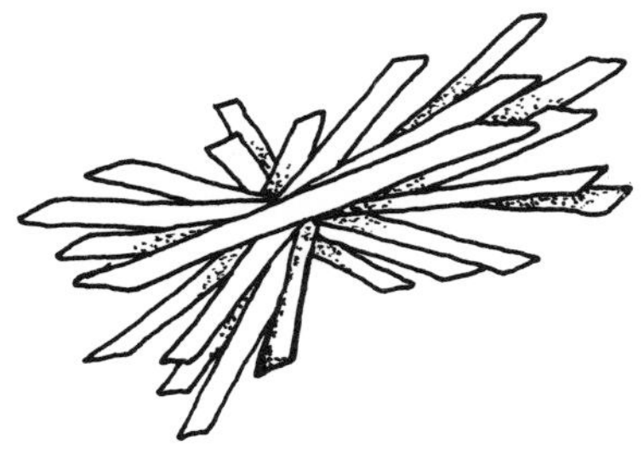

Sodium urate crystals

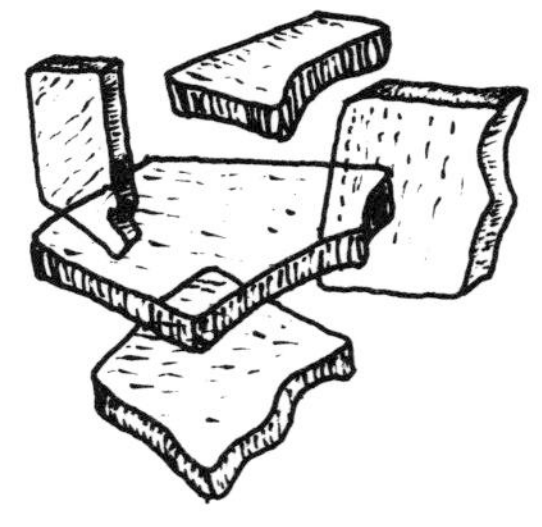

Uric acid crystals

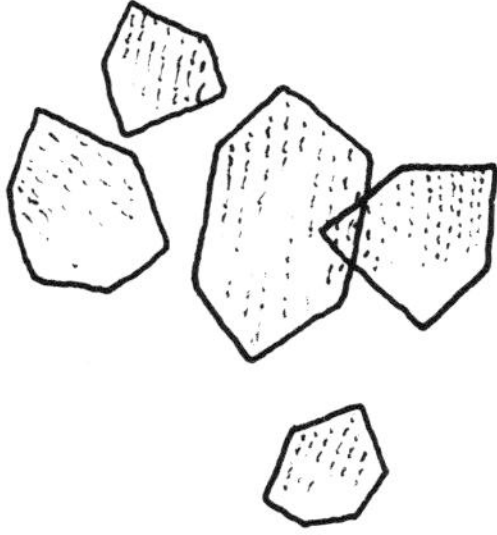

Cystine crystals

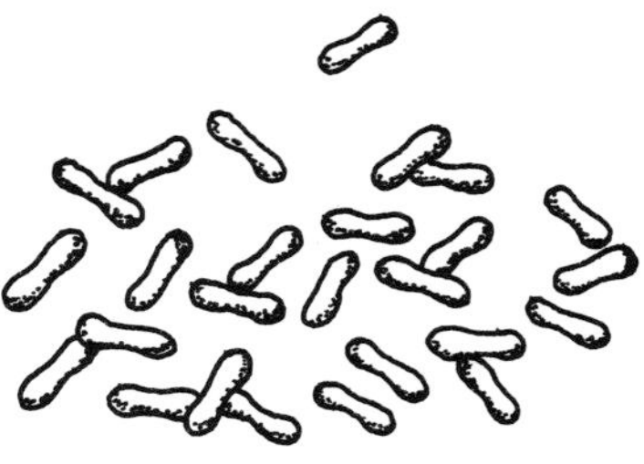

Calcium carbonate crystals

Figure 12-68.

the family physician should be skilled is based on laboratory findings. If the analysis of stones recovered can be properly performed, the physician's job becomes much simpler and expensive laboratory work can be avoided.

Cystine stones occur only in cystinuric patients. The urine of these patients contains 10 to 15 times more cystine than does normal urine. *Uric acid stones* form only in persons whose urine is more often and for longer periods acidic or contains greater than normal amounts of uric acid. Uric acid is highly insoluble when urine pH is below 6.5. *Ammonium magnesium calcium phosphate stones* are seen only in persons with ammoniacal urine of alkaline character due to infection with urea splitting organisms. Persons who excrete more calcium than normal in their urine have a far higher incidence of *calcium oxalate phosphate stones* than do those who excrete normal amounts of calcium.

Therefore, the problem of diagnosing the metabolic disorder causing any specific stone becomes more complex when the chemical make-up of the stone is unknown.

Order a blood serum and a 24 hour urine calcium test. If both are normal, do not proceed with further calcium metabolism investigation unless the history or physical examination is highly suggestive. When hypercalcemia is discovered, think of hyperparathyroidism or sarcoidosis. These two conditions are the only diseases in which hypercalcemia and renal stones are associated. Repeat the serum calcium determination three times.

Attempt to exclude sarcoidosis either by clinical and laboratory examination or by therapeutic trial with an adrenal glucocorticoid. If the hypercalcemia fails to respond quickly and completely to this therapy, make the diagnosis of hyperparathyroidism. If renal insufficiency is present with hypercalcemia, the diagnosis is more complex because a failing glomerular filtration rate causes a low calcium concentration masking hyperparathyroidism. Pay no great concern to this problem because a parathyroidectomy is indicated in either event. If no hypercalcemia is found but only hypercalciuria, think again of sarcoidosis, hyperthyroidism, renal tubular acidosis and idiopathic hypercalciuria.

Proceed to rule out sarcoidosis and hyperthyroidism in the usual fashion. If these diseases are not present and hypercalciuria persists in the absence of hypercalcemia, renal tubular acidosis or idiopathic hypercalciuria do exist.

Rule out renal tubular acidosis by the ammonium chloride loading procedure. Administer nonenteric coated ammonium chloride, 100 mg/kg by mouth. Follow this loading dose by collecting urine samples every 2 hours for 3 doses or a total of 6 hours. Determine the pH with nitrazine paper. Do not depend on litmus. In a normal person the pH will fall below 5.5 or even to 4.6. If the urine falls below a pH of 5.25, renal tubular acidosis is excluded. In this event, make the provisional diagnosis of idiopathic hypercalciuria. One clue to the latter diagnosis is the degree of hypercalciuria. Idiopathic hypercalciuria is nearly assured if calcium excretion is 400 mg per day. Other laboratory findings which suggest renal tubular acidosis are hyperchloremic acidosis, hypophosphatemia, unexplained hypokalemia, hypercalciuria, elevated alkaline phosphatase and evidence of osteomalacia.

The next most common stone is composed of uric acid crystals. Again, its diagnosis is assured on finding urate stones. If the composition of the stones is not known, make the presumptive diagnosis on the laboratory findings of hyperuricemia and/or hyperuricosuria. If highly suspicious of urate stones and the first blood and urine checks are within normal, recheck the findings at least two more times. Sporadic elevations of uric acid should be considered a clue to the diagnosis.

The diagnosis of cystinuria is made by screening the urine of suspects with the nitroprusside test. If positive, measure the urinary cystine excretion to establish the diagnosis.

The most complex problem relates to the coexistence of a urinary tract infection with stones. Some bacteria convert urea to ammonia, thus alkalinizing the urine. Alkaline urine in the presence of ammonia tends to precipitate out magnesium ammonium phosphate either on preexisting stones or as new stones. Adding to the puzzle: stones make eradication of the infection nearly impossible. What comes first then, infection or stone, is a difficult decision. Generally, a physician is correct in considering a urea-splitting infection as perpetuating rather than initiating stone formation. One must keep in mind, however, that finding pure magnesium ammonium phosphate stones may be due to urea-splitting bacteria. The finding of an alkaline urine with significant amounts of ammonium is chemical evidence of urea-splitting infection.

TREATMENT. The treatment of acute renal colic depends on where the stone lies in the genitourinary tract and to what size it has grown. Give the patient medical support, including pain relief for a reasonable time, as long as the kidney substance is not being damaged. A surprising number of stones will either pass or quiet down without surgical intervention. The surgical procedure for an individual case should be left to a urologic consultant. The tedious job of organizing a long term plan of prevention of subsequent stone formation generally falls to the family physician.

Calcium stones. Force fluids up to 3000 to 4000 ml daily. Obviously the more diluted the urine, the less the chances of precipitation. This intake is difficult for a patient to maintain over a long period. Continue the diuresis 24 hours per day. There is no point in pushing urinary flow for only two-thirds of the 24 hours.

Order a low-calcium and low-vitamin diet. Limit milk, cheese and other milk products to 2 cups of milk daily. Reduce the patient's intake of beet greens, collards, dandelion greens, kale, spinach, turnip greens, salmon or sardines.

Consider the use of sodium phytate which forms an unabsorbable complex with calcium. To compensate for the low calcium content of the diet, increase the protein intake since protein is believed to promote calcium deposition in the bones.

Acid-ash foods, which lower the pH of the urine, may help keep the calcium in solution. Diets of high protein content yield sulfuric and phosphoric acids and acidify the urine. Thus foods that do not taste acid such as meat, fish, eggs, milk and cereal lower the pH of the urine. The objective is to keep the pH of the urine at 5 to 6. Do not allow the patient to use products high in baking powder or soda.

Calcium-oxalate stones. Force fluids. Avoid foods high in calcium and oxalate such as asparagus, beet greens, spinach, sorrel, dandelion greens, cranberries, figs, gooseberries, plums, rhubarb, raspberries, black tea, chocolate, cocoa, coffee, gelatin and pepper. Oranges, pineapples, strawberries, beans, brussel sprouts, potatoes, tomatoes and beets should not be eaten more than once daily. But no matter how strict the diet, oxalate stones may continue to form.

Gershoff and Prien[26] in 1967 reported some success with daily administration of magnesium 200 mg and pyridoxine 10 mg on patients with recurring calcium-oxalate stones.

Oxalate stones are the type of concretions almost invariably found in hyperparathyroidism, renal tubular acidosis (hyperchloremic acidosis), sarcoidosis, vitamin D intoxication, Cushing's disease, neoplastic hypercalcemic diseases, and most frequently the so-called idiopathic hypercalciuric patients. Consequently, these conditions should be corrected by removal of a parathyroid adenoma, correction of Cushing's disease or control of sarcoidosis or the hyperchloremic acidosis.

Try phosphate salts: Neutra-Phos or K-Phos. Order from 0.3 to 0.5 g 3 times a day after meals. Occasionally a patient needs 2 to 2.5 g of phosphorus per day to achive results. Reports suggest that thiazides will reduce urinary output of calcium by ⅓ or more. At this level some patients will stop making stones.

Calcium-phosphate stones. Force fluids and use a low-calcium, low-phosphate diet. Foods high in phosphate are milk, milk products, eggs, organ meats (liver, kidneys, etc.), sardines, fish, roe, whole wheat bread and cereals, wheat germ, brown or wild rice, oatmeal and bran. Reasonable amounts of beans, nuts and meat in general are allowed.

Uric acid stones. Force fluids. Keep the urine alkaline so that the uric acid will remain in solution. The goal: 24 hour pH maintenance of 7 or 8. A high-alkaline diet consists of vegetables and fruits (except plums, prunes, cranberries and corn) and restricted intake of meat, fish, poultry, eggs, milk and cereals. Prescribe Polycitra, 15 ml after meals and at bedtime will usually keep the urine alkaline around the clock. Others will need 25 or 30 ml per dose.

If urinary alkalization alone is inadequate, restrict overall protein intake to 1 g per kg of body weight with restriction of purine intake. Use allopurinol for dissolution of large uric acid stones: Zyloprim 100 to 300 mg per day. Increase by 1 tablet per day until uric acid levels reach 6 mg/100 ml. There is some evidence that allopurinol may precipitate an acute attack of gout. Accordingly maintenance doses of colchicine should be given prophylactically when allopurinol is begun. The maximum recommended dose of allopurinol is 800 mg daily.

Cystine stones. Force fluids and use a high-alkaline diet (to keep the pH above 7), low in methionine and cystine. Give alkalizing agents such as Polycitra. When sizable stones of cystine are present, try D-Penicillamine 250 mg 3 times a day 30 min before meals. Use this drug to dissolve a large cystine stone but limit its use to short intervals.

Ammonium magnesium phosphate stones. Force fluids. Order large doses of antibiotics to which the organism is sensitive and continue for at least 2 weeks. Some continue long-term antibiotic therapy hoping to keep the organism population low and unable to produce too much ammonia. Although a high ammonia content and alkaline urine are main factors in promoting precipitation of ammonium magnesium phosphate, it is nearly impossible to acidify the urine in the presence of a virulent proteus infection.

ACUTE PYELONEPHRITIS. Acute pyelonephritis produces pain in one of the upper abdominal quadrants. It is an acute bacterial infection of the kidney pelvis and parenchyma. At first the pain is severe and may be accompanied by vomiting. Costovertebral angle tenderness is usually present and can be elicited by gentle percussion of the angle. Place one hand around the flank with the fingertip in the costovertebral angle. Cover the anterior aspect of the abdomen with your other hand. Tell the patient what you are about to do, and percuss the kidney with your fingers in the costovertebral angle. With this technique ballotte the kidney or its lower pole. Determine if there is tenderness in the costovertebral angle or enlargement of the kidney.

Acute pyelonephritis may be preceded by variable degrees of frequency and dysuria. This history is inconstant, however, and in many cases the disease starts with sudden fever, chills and flank pain without preceding lower tract symptoms.

The temperature may be the highest found in adults and may reach 103° to 104° F. If associated with a gram-negative septicemia the blood pressure may be low and the patient may show evidence of shock. Patients appear acutely ill with a flushed face and may move about during the examination attempting to find a comfortable position.

Verify the diagnosis by checking the urine. Bacteria are easily found on a gram stain of the sediment. White blood cells may fill the field. Most organisms that cause acute peylonephritis can be cultured readily in 24 hours. Culture the urine in all cases and order a sensitivity study. Generally the quantitative colony count will be above 100,000 per ml of urine.

The diagnosis of a urinary tract infection is untenable without a positive quantitative culture or gram stain of bacteria on unspun urine. Pyuria is a good index of urinary tract infection; however, bacilluria can occur without pyuria and pyuria can occur without urinary tract infection. Consider 6 to 10 white cells per high-power field suspicious; over 10 cells per field is definitely abnormal.

X-rays of the abdomen are of little use unless hydronephrosis is also present. An intravenous pyelogram is also of little value in making the diagnosis. In the acutely ill patient intravenous pylography is not recommended because of the dehydration required for this test. If the right kidney is involved, consider a cholecystogram to rule out gallbladder disease.

For the first attack of pyelonephritis, order a bactericidal drug such as ampicillin to be taken for 10 days. Then switch to a bacteriostatic drug such as Gantrisin or Furadantin for a second or third week of treatment. Consider this a minimal course even if the patient is symptom free in 48 hours.

By far the most common organism in urinary tract infection is Escherichia coli. But species of Enterobacter, Proteus, Pseudomonas, enterococci and Klebsiella can also be pathogenic organisms.

E. coli infection usually occurs in an acid urine. Consequently alkalinization with 3.0 g each of sodium citrate and sodium bicarbonate every 2 hours until the urine is alkaline is necessary. Then reduce the dose to maintenance levels. A better and more pleasant way is to give Polycitra 15 to 30 ml after meals and at bedtime.

HYDRONEPHROSIS. Hydronephrosis implies obstruction of the urinary tract which produces dilatation of the renal pelvis. It may be congenital or acquired and may occur in one or both kidneys. Renal function is frequently impaired. If both kidneys are involved, renal failure may develop without separate symptoms. If one kidney is involved, complete destruction of the kidney may occur without symptoms, the healthy kidney taking over the function of the diseased one.

Usually the patient develops some abdominal pain which is often described as dull or colicky in nature and located in the abdomen or groin. Most often a mass is found in the upper abdominal quadrants. Masses are movable, smooth and tender on palpation. The absence of a mass does not exclude hydronephrosis. Fist percussion over the costovertebral angle will elicit intense, deep-seated pain. One must be particularly careful to rule out a hydronephrosis in patients complaining of a backache, especially when relieved by lying down. In acute hydronephrosis secondary to blockage by a stone, nausea and vomiting may add confusing symptoms. In chronic or slowly progressive hydronephrosis, symptoms may simulate gastrointestinal diseases such as ulcers, gallbladder disease, pylorospasm and spastic colon.

Hydronephrosis is caused by any impediment to the flow of urine. Congenital anomalies include various types of stenosis-aberrant ureteropelvic junctions, aberrant vascular formations, renal anomalies, reflux or regurgitation of urine into the ureters and pelvis during micturition and vesical neck contractures.

Acquired causes are tumors, strictures, calculi, prostatic obstruction, repeated pyelonephritis, foreign bodies, neurologic disorders producing neurogenic bladder, intra-abdominal and retroperitoneal lesions which are the result of infections, fibrosis, tumors or trauma, and a nephroptosis.

In diagnosis give little weight to the urinary examination. Findings depend on the nature of the obstruction, its location and the degree of infection. There is nothing pathognomonic to be found.

Diagnosis depends in good measure on roentgenography and particularly on the intravenous pyelogram. This examination will demonstrate the degree of dilatation and obstruction. Normally, within 20 minutes after injection of radiopaque dye, the renal pelvis should be empty. Estimate the extent of the obstruction by the amount of dye remaining after 20 minutes. When there is no function by this excretory study, consider requesting a retrograde pyeloureterogram. This will nearly always outline the dilatation and source of obstruction.

If intermittent hydronephrosis is present, excretory studies may be normal. To put pressure on the upper urinary tract, order a micturition cystouethrogram by either conventional x-ray or the cinefluorographic method utilizing image intensification. In any event, a complete diagnosis will usually require an intravenous pyelogram, cystoscopy, micturating cystogram or retrograde pyelogram to exclude any structural disorders that require surgical treatment.

The first step in treatment is to surgically relieve any obstruction. Eradication of infection usually requires months of treatment by a culture-proven effective antibiotic. It is reasonable to start with 6 months continuous treatment changing the antibiotics every

2 weeks or as indicated by sensitivity studies. The objective is to produce a urine that is sterile and free of excess leukocytes. Thereafter the urine must be cultured at regular intervals and treatment started as required. (See Chapter 9 for details of antibiotic therapy.)

In renal failure, the dose of antibiotic may be halved. Renal failure may be precipitated by an acute infection and antibiotic treatment may enduce a remission. Correcting electrolyte imbalances may bring surprising relief as well.

Dissecting Aneurysms

Discussion of acute abdominal pain is incomplete without calling attention to abdominal aneurysms—dissecting or otherwise. In men over 40 years, the most common cause is a long-standing hypertension which has caused a degenerative necrosis in the aortic media and finally an intimal tear. The disease kills half the patients with the rare mesodermal defect of arachnodactyly (Marfan's syndrome).

Aneurysms commonly occur at the base of the aorta where blood extravasates into the media of the aorta, splitting the layers in its downward course. Consequently, the pain may begin in the thorax radiating to the patient's neck and only later occurring in the abdomen. At other times, abdominal pain is the first symptom.

The pain of an abdominal aneurysm is in the epigastrium and is associated with an involuntary muscle rigidity. It may suggest myocardial infarction in its sudden, crushing and tearing intensity. As the spinal cord is torn from its blood supply, numbness and even hemiplegia may result. The differences in the pulses may be the most diagnostic sign as to what is occurring.

On physical examination look for:

- –an anterior mediastinal mass or widening if the aneurysm is located in the ascending mediastinum
- –a tracheal tug synchronous with the pulse if the aneurysm is located in the arch
- –pulsations in the suprasternal or supraclavicular area
- –a palpable abdominal mass at the level of or above the umbilicus
- –a bruit at or near the mass (although this is not confirmatory of either the presence or absence of an aneurysm)
- –pulse differentials, especially in the popliteal areas where more aneurysms may be found

Take x-rays of the chest and abdomen. They may be diagnostic when they show widening of the aorta or when calcific plaques in the intima are widely separated from the outer border of the aortic wall. Aneurysms are often much larger than they appear on an x-ray film because of laminated clots within the lesion. These thrombi may even mask the lesion completely and give a relatively normal appearance to the dye column. However, such findings are uncommon and roentgenography remains your greatest single aid in diagnosis (Fig. 12-69).

Although arteriographic studies are not usually necessary to make the diagnosis,

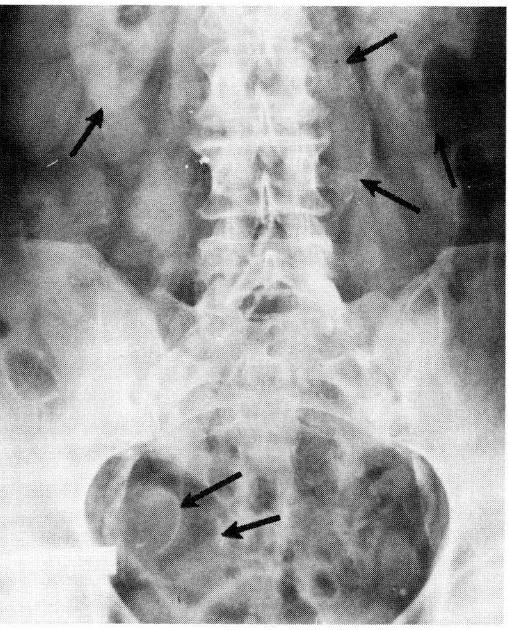

Figure 12-69. A patient with malignant hypertension. Two egg-shell aneurysms are seen in the pelvis and a contracted kidney on the right side. A large aortic abdominal aneuryom is outlined in the lumbar area.

they are often of help in outlining the extent of the lesion. In thoracic aneurysms, angiography is routinely done to differentiate aneurysms from other mass lesions. It is also of great help in confirming or excluding concomitant dissection of the aorta.

In time, aneurysms increase in size and eventually rupture. The rupture may occur through the external wall or, if high in the thorax, dissect back into the pericardium. In about 10 percent of the patients the dissection breaks back into the aortic lumen and becomes for the time being asymptomatic. The only prevention of a disastrous rupture is early detection and excision of all aortic aneurysms, particularly those located in the abdomen.

Mesenteric Vascular Occlusion

The superior mesenteric artery or vein becomes involved by either embolism or thrombosis (Fig. 12-70). Arterial occlusion produces the typical clinical picture; venous thrombosis is often atypical.

Incomplete obstruction of the artery may initially simulate an abdominal angina with postprandial pain, anorexia and weight loss. The pain is intermittent and begins a few minutes after eating and lasts from 20 minutes to 2 or 3 hours. Anorexia occurs from the patient's fear of eating and consequently he loses weight. The pain is relieved by fasting, ingestion of small meals, vomiting and flexion of knees on the abdomen. The location of the pain is in the general area of the epigastrium or in the periumbilical area. The finding of a short systolic bruit near the umbilicus resulting from a stenosed artery should be the clue in diagnosis. Atherosclerosis is the common cause.

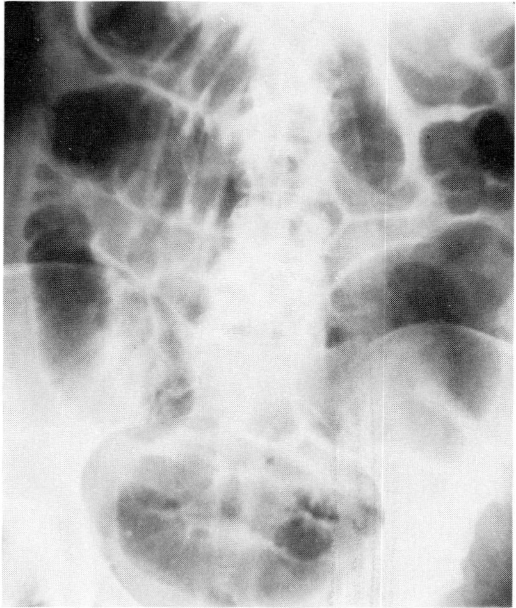

Figure 12-70. Superior mesenteric artery thrombosis with small bowel infarction.

The diagnosis is made following exclusion of other abdominal diseases and the performance of aortography. Visualization of the celiac artery and superior mesenteric artery at their origins will indicate partial occlusion of these vessels. Striking enlargement and tortuosity of the inferior mesenteric artery suggests occlusion of the superior mesenteric. This can be partially resolved by examining films taken in the lateral position as well as the standard A-P projections.

Sudden occlusion of the mesenteric blood vessels is a different matter, and the ischemic necrosis produced threatens the patient's life. Initially the abdominal pain is colicky but soon becomes continuous and is out of proportion to the meager findings of the abdominal examination. The pain becomes generalized, the patient begins vomiting and becomes distended, simulating the symptoms of intestinal obstruction. Narcotics give little relief.

Flat and upright x-rays of the abdomen are never normal but are not diagnostically reliable. Most commonly, they suggest paralytic ileus with gaseous distention of both small and large intestines. As with partial obstruction, aortography with the patient in the lateral position is the best diagnostic investigation. Except for autopsies, surgical exploration of the abdomen is the only way to confirm the diagnosis of acute mesenteric vascular occlusion.

Gynecologic Problems

ENDOMETRIOSIS. The symptoms of endometriosis can best be described as an acquired dysmenorrhea. You should be suspicious of endometriosis in all young women who have developed dysmenorrhea after having menstruated painlessly several years or whose dysmenorrhea grew worse as she became older. Often the pain causes an intense desire to defecate, but more often the patient describes the pains as though her intestines were in spasm. Pains may occur principally during menstruation or may be more or less constant.

In addition, menstrual flow is increased. If you ask you will find the patient has considerable dyspareunia. Fifty percent of the women with endometriosis appear to be sterile and the other 50 percent become pregnant without difficulty.

A careful and detailed history is the best evidence of endometriosis, but the diagnosis is strengthened by finding shotty and nodular small masses in the posterior cul-de-sac and on the uterosacral ligaments. You will find these irregular indentations painful to palpation. When the disease has been present for some time, the interal genitalia lose their mobility and the pelvic organs feel as though they are frozen.

Don't look for much help with roentgenography except in ruling out other diseases. A hysterosalpingography will only establish tubal patency. Endometriosis does not often close the tubes; consequently, the examination may be helpful in ruling out salpingitis.

Culdoscopic examinations are dangerous unless the uterine fundus is anteverted. In 60 percent of the patients the fundus is not only retroverted but adherent. Abdominal peritoneoscopy is safer but not always fruitful. Likewise dilatation and curettage provide little help diagnostically.

A therapeutic trial with birth control pills or stilbestrol to block ovulation is more helpful but has its drawbacks. Diethylstilbestrol, 5 mg daily for 20 days, may block ovulation and prevent the pain of endometriosis. Once the likelihood of endometriosis seems reasonably established, increasing the dose of birth control pills or Diethylstilbestrol to the amount necessary to eliminate menstruation has beneficial effects. In this event, prescribe the pills daily, increasing the dose as necessary to stop any menstrual spotting.

An adherent ovarian cyst presents a diagnostic problem. Rarely should an enlarged ovary be observed for more than 6 to 8 weeks before doing a laparotomy even though there is reasonable certainty that the mass is an endometrial cyst. There is too much danger of a concomitant carcinoma.

ACUTE SALPINGITIS. In acute gonorrheal salpingitis the entire tube becomes red and swollen. As the acute process subsides the fimbria close. If untreated, the tube and surrounding structures become one mass—a pyosalpinx. As time goes on the exudate becomes watery—a hydrosalpinx. Both tubes are involved to one degree or another. Similar pathology is caused by Streptococci, staphylococci and tubercle bacilli. The usual symptoms are pain in the lower quadrants of the abdomen, backache and a variety of menstrual complaints plus a vaginal discharge.

Attempt to differentiate acute salpingitis from acute appendicitis because the latter is an acute condition requiring surgery. Treat acute salpingitis with antibiotics and bed rest in the Fowler's position.

Make the diagnosis on clinical grounds. Acute salpingitis follows a history of a primary infection with dysuria, vaginal burning and discharge. Acute appendicitis is more typically a gastrointestinal disease with nausea, vomiting and generalized abdominal pain localizing under McBurney's point. Muscle spasm and tenderness are more localized in appendicitis with rebound tenderness being referred to McBurney's point.

In this connection, remember the inconstancy and unreliability of McBurney's point in diagnosing appendicitis. Actually, tenderness and spasm at McBurney's point occurs only when the appendix happens to be beneath it. Absence of this sign does not minimize in the slightest the chance that a particular case is one of appendicitis. When the appendix lies on the pelvic brim or in the pelvis the only tenderness detected may be that found on pelvic or rectal examination.

To diagnose any acute condition of the abdomen without doing a rectal or pelvic examination is unforgivable. Bilateral tenderness on pelvic examination is the most reliable differential point. Movement of the uterus and cervix is extremely painful. If you feel a painful mass in one or both lateral fornices, the diagnosis of pyosalpinx with peritonitis is probable. But in a few cases, you will find it impossible to be certain whether one is dealing with an abscess arising from the tubes or from an appendix lying over the pelvic brim.

The laboratory provides little aid in acute conditions unless there is time for cultures and blood smears. Both conditions have varying degrees of leukocytosis. In gonococcal infections, gram stains from involved sites such as the urethra and cervix may help spot a case of gonorrheal salpingitis, but smears can become negative within hours after instituting antibiotic therapy. Bacterial cultures are more dependable in women if the pus is incubated in 10 percent carbon dioxide on special chocolate agar.

ECTOPIC PREGNANCY. Ectopic pregnancy is mentioned here as a cause of abdominal pain because its occurrence should be considered in every painful female abdomen. Culdocentesis is a simple and reliable diagnostic aid which should be done in every patient suspected of having an ectopic pregnancy (See Chapter 2).

TORSION OF OVARIAN CYST. There are a variety of ovarian tumors; about 95 percent of them are cystic and most of them are benign. *Simple follicular cysts* are multiple, usually bilateral, small in size and consist of unruptured graafian follicles from which the ova have disappeared. *Serous cysts* usually are unilocular pedunculated and benign. Ordinarily they are moderate in size but may attain enormous dimensions. *Corpus luteum cysts* generally are single, unilateral and seldom become larger than 8 cm in diameter. They are benign. *Endometrial cysts* (chocolate cyst, endometriosis) may be multiple, unilateral or bilateral. They have no pedicle but may rupture, allowing endometrial implants to escape and spread throughout the pelvis. *Dermoid cysts* are unilateral, congenital, spherical and measure from 15 to 20 cm in diameter. The contents are usually a combination of hair, teeth, bone or sebacious matter. *Cystadenomas* (pseudomucinous cysts) are multiple, uni-or bilateral and grow to huge proportions. They are usually benign. If they rupture into the abdomen their contents become implanted on abdominal organs and produce pseudomyxoma peritonei.

Papillary cystadenomas may grow large and are potentially malignant. They are multilocular and thick walled. A leakage of its contents into the abdomen will produce secondary growths throughout the peritoneal cavity. *Cystic carcinomas* of the ovary may be primary or a degenerative stage of the above papillary cystodenoma. They are adenocarcinomatous, have a rapid growth and cause early ascites. Pain is a common symptom. *Krukenberg's tumors* are secondary carcinomas, the stomach being the usual primary site. *Parovarian cysts* are unilocular and unilateral and grow between the leaves of the broad ligament. The cyst is embedded and displaces the uterus and even the ureter.

Solid tumors are rare. *Fibromas* attain moderate size, 12 to 15 cm in diameter. Their wall is smooth and they develop a pedicle. They tend to become malignant. Sarcoma of the ovary is rare and commonly bilateral. This type metastasizes slowly. *Granulosa cell tumors* are semicystic, usually unilateral, small in size and well encapsulated. They are probably benign. In elderly women, granulosa cell tumors stimulate the endometrium and produce uterine bleeding. In children they give rise to precocious sexual development.

When a fluctuating, nontender, small spheroidal mass is felt in the region of the ovary the bimanual examination is diagnostic for ovarian tumors. But when the cyst enlarges and emerges from the pelvis and into the abdomen, no pelvic signs are present. An attempt must be made to distinguish it from other abdominal enlargements.

The largest cysts simulate ascites. Those that extend just above the pelvic brim are always in the midline and resemble a distended bladder. Persistence of the mass after catheterization suggests ovarian cyst, pregnancy or a fibroid uterus.

On examination of the abdomen, look for

three distinguishing signs: (1) When the patient is in supine position, the tympanitic intestines are pushed into the upper abdomen. Consequently the examiner will find two notes on percussion: dullness over the lower abdomen and a tympanitic note over the upper abdomen. (2) On careful inspection, the abdominal profile reveals two curves with a convexity in the lower abdomen. (3) The ruler test. Place a ruler transversely across the abdomen below the umbilicus. The ruler moves visibly with each abdominal pulsation when a cyst is present. With ascitic fluid, the aortic pulsation is not transmitted.

The most common complication of ovarian cysts and one that causes symptoms of an acute abdominal condition is torsion of the pedicle. Torsion first produces interference with the venous return, which in turn results in intense engorgement of the cyst and hemorrhage into its substance. If untreated, thrombosis of nearby vessels occurs followed shortly by necrosis and gangrene of the cyst. General peritonitis eventually occurs. The symptoms are sudden pain, vomiting, abdominal rigidity, distention, moderate shock and dysuria. Fever and leukocytosis may be confusing signs.

Other less frequent and spectacular complications of ovarian cysts are infection, rupture, ureteral obstruction and intestinal obstructions when the cysts become adherent to intestinal loops.

Porphyrias

Information about the porphyrias has increased in recent years and, although the disease is rare, it must often be considered in differential diagnosis. In order of frequency the porphyrias are acute intermittent porphyria, porphyria cutanea tarda hereditaria, porphyria cutanea tarda symptomatica, congenital porphyria and erythropoietic protoporphyria. They are all inheritable diseases except for porphyria cutanea tarda symptomatica. Look for this kind of porphyria in association with hepatic cirrhosis. The symptoms appear only in the skin.

Acute intermittent porphyria, as the name implies, is characterized by attacks of mental, abdominal and neurologic (MAN) symptoms and is often triggered by the ingestion of barbiturates. Mental symptoms are those of acute psychiatric disorders such as anxiety, depression, confusion, hallucinations and delusions. Abdominal pain may be confused with acute diseases that require surgery; consequently, the abdomen may be marked by several surgical scars. Neurologic symptoms suggest peripheral neuropathy.

Recognize *porphyria cutanea tarda hereditaria* by the skin lesions. Acute lesions are related to sunlight exposure and are photosensitive. They may range from simple erythema to large bullae. These patients may have some of the same symptoms as the patient with acute intermittent porphyria.

Look for *congenital porphyria* (erythropoietic) in children under 6 years. It can be detected in infants. Red discoloration of the teeth by deposited porphyrins is practically diagnostic. Parents resort to extraordinary measures to avoid sunlight. Anemia is another common finding.

Make laboratory checks in all patients with the following problems: skin rashes provoked by sunlight, acute abdominal pain with obscure etiology, peripheral neuropathy with obscure etiology, acute psychiatric problems and congenital anemia in a child with a rash.

Check the urine for porphobilinogen, uroporphyrin and coproporphyrin in suspected acute intermittent, cutanea symptomatica and congenital porphyria. Check the stools for coproporphyrin and protoporphyrin for cutanea tarda or erythropoietic protoporphyria. Most laboratories will understand if you ask for a check on the urine and fecal porphyrins.

JAUNDICE

What to Look For

In the jaundiced patient search for acute hepatitis (infectious hepatitis or serum hepatitis), steatosis, portal fibrosis, rotor syndrome, Dubin-Johnson syndrome, Gilbert's disease, hemolytic jaundice, neonatal jaundice (Crigler-Najjar type or physiologic jaundice of the newborn), cirrhosis (primary or alcoholic), metastatic disease, obstructive jaundice caused by cancer, stricture or stones, breast milk jaundice, Lucey-Driscoll syndrome, intravascular hemolysis, post-portacaval shunt, alcoholic steatonecrosis, Hodgkin's disease, recurrent jaundice of pregnancy, sclerosing cholangitis, benign recurrent intrahepatic cholestasis or hepatoxic drugs.

Commonly Used Drugs that May Cause Jaundice or Liver Damage

HYPOGLYCEMIC DRUGS. Dymelor, Diabinese, Tolinase and Orinase.

PSYCHOPHARMACOLOGIC DRUGS. *Phenothiazines:* Thorazine, Combid, Compazine, Eskatrol, Sparine, Phenergan, Mellaril and Stelazine. *Monomine oxidase inhibitors:* Marplan and Nardil. *Others:* Elavil, Triavil, Etrafon, Librax, Librium, Pertofran, Norpramin, Levanil, Tofranil, Miltown, Equanil, Aventyl HCL, Serax, Temaril and Trilafon.

ANTI-THYROID DRUGS. Tapazole, propylthiouracil and thiouracil.

ANTI-ARTHRITIS DRUGS. Zyloprim, gold, Indocin, Butazolidin, Sterazolidin and Benemid.

ANTIBIOTICS. Aureomycin, Ilosone, Fulvicin-U/F, Grifulvin V, Grisactin, Albamycin, Prostaphlin, penicillin, streptomycin, tetracyclines, Cyclamycin and TAO.

ANTI-CONVULSANT DRUGS. Paraflex, Valium, Dilantin, Mesantoin, Paradione, Phenurone, phenobarbital and Tridione.

CHEMOTHERAPEUTIC DRUGS FOR INFECTIONS. Isoniazid, nitrofurantoin, PAS, Atabrine HCL, and sulfonamides.

HORMONAL AND METABOLIC DRUGS. *Androgens and anabolic agents:* Halotestin, Ora-Testryl, Dianabol, methyltestosterone, Nilevar, Norlutin and Androyd. *Estrogen and progestational agents:* All natural estrogens and progestins, diethylstilbestrol, Enovid, Norenyl, Ortho-Novum and Ovulen.

MISCELLANEOUS. Aldoclor, Diupres, Diuril, Cholografin, Telepaque, Aldomet, Aldoril, Sansert, Nicotinic acid and Hedulin.

Cholestasis

Intrahepatic cholestasis is a failure of the liver to secrete conjugated bilirubin into the bile canaliculus. Obstructive lesions in the cholangioles, ductules or interseptal bile ducts also cause cholestasis by some yet unknown inflammatory mechanism.

Extrahepatic cholestasis results from blockage of bile flow by obstructions in the major bile ducts. Extrahepatic complications of cholestasis are skin changes such as pruritus, xanthomas, pigmentation and infections; hypoprothrombinemia and blood clotting problems; and, the most serious of all, renal disease from toxic factors and even from the contrast media given to a patient with obstructive jaundice.

Examining the Liver, Gallbladder and Spleen

See Figure 12-71 for instructions.

Liver Function Tests

X-ray and endoscopy studies are more important than the laboratory in clinical diseases of the digestive tube but the converse is true in diseases of the liver and pancreas.

TOTAL SERUM BILIRUBIN. There are two types of bilirubin: unconjugated indirect and conjugated direct. Direct and indirect bilirubin are terms referring to the method of measuring conjugated and unconjugated bilirubin. After determining the direct, conjugated bilirubin, alcohol is added to the sample and the total serum bilirubin is determined. The amount of direct bilirubin is then subtracted from the total giving the amount of indirect, unconjugated serum bilirubin.

Bilirubin that comes from red blood cell breakdown and has not been conjugated in the liver is unconjugated indirect bilirubin. Bilirubin that has been conjugated by the liver cells to bilirubin diglucuronide is conjugated direct bilirubin. This bilirubin is then excreted via the biliary ducts into the duodenum.

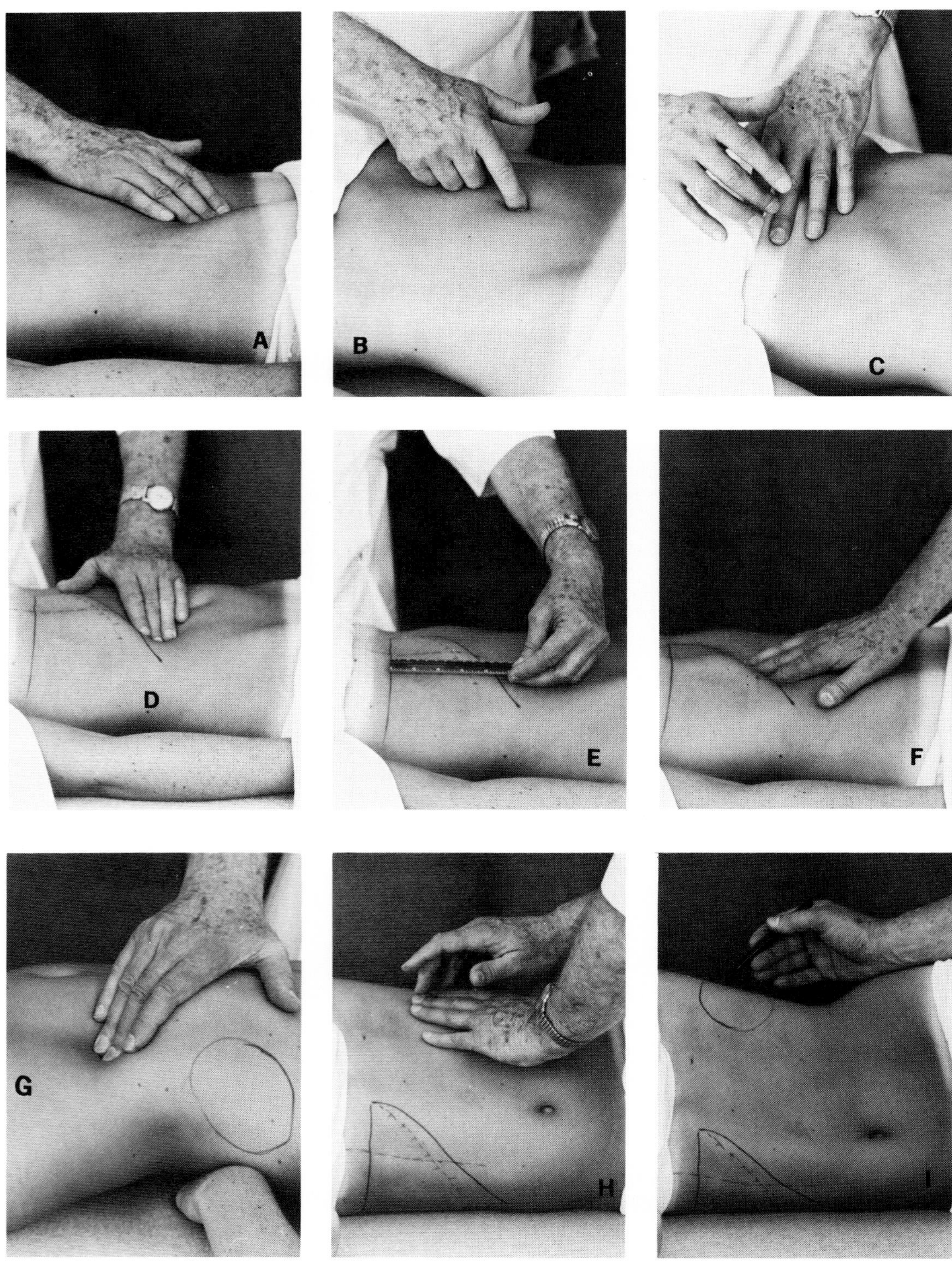

Figure 12-71. (See facing page for legend.)

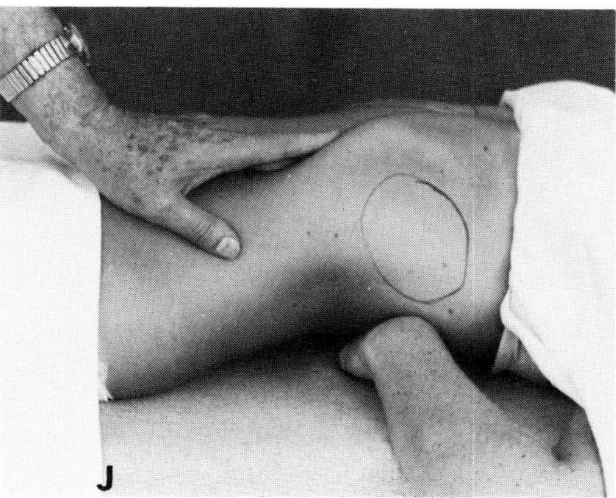

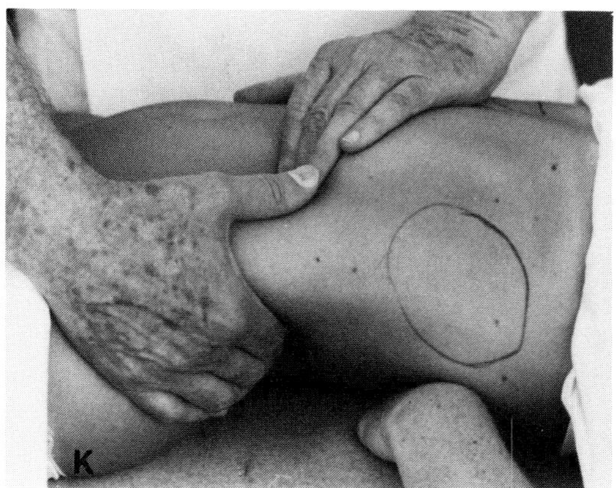

Figure 12-71. *A*, Start the examination by palpating the lower right quadrant of the patient's abdomen for tumors, local tenderness, muscular guarding and rigidity. Continue by repeating the examination in her lower left quadrant. *B*, Evidence of abdominal malignancies often appear first in or about the umbilicus. Palpate the depression for any tumors. *C*, Locate the superior margin of her liver by percussion and mark the boundary in the midclavicular line. Proceed downward until percussion indicates the inferior border of her liver. *D*, Palpate the lower border of the liver during both inspiration and expiration. *E*, Measure the liver size on both the midclavicular and midsternal lines. Normal measurements on the midclavicular line of an adult is 15 ± 2 and in the midsternal the line is 4 ± 2. *F*, Attempt to palpate the gallbladder on the upper right quadrant. Usually an enlarged gallbladder not only is tender but also can be palpated below the liver margin. *G*, Attempt to palpate her spleen before and during inspiration. *H*, Percuss the area of dullness at rest and on inspiration. *I*, The patient should be on her right side in order to differentiate an enlarged left lobe of the liver and spleen. In questionable cases, outlining the spleen with a grease pencil will help with identification as the patient is examined in different positions. *J*, Finally have the patient put her fist under her lower ribs to push her spleen upward and outward. Often the spleen can be felt enlarging downward and medially. *K*, The lower pole of the spleen can often be palpated only when the patient takes a deep breath.

The upper limits of normal are:

Total serum bilirubin—1.5 mg/100 ml serum
Direct reacting (conjugated)—0.25 ml/100 ml of serum
Indirect (unconjugated) is 1.25 mg/100 ml of serum

An increase in the total serum bilirubin points to one of the following:

- overproduction of bilirubin from excessive red blood cell breakdown
- decreased uptake of unconjugated bilirubin by the liver, allowing it to accumulate in the blood
- decreased excretion of conjugated bilirubin from the liver into the bile ducts
- regurgitation of conjugated bilirubin from liver into the blood stream as in hepatitis

If either of the first two pathophysiologic processes occur, the increase is in unconjugated indirect bilirubin. If either of the latter two processes occur, the serum bilirubin increase causes a direct conjugated hyperbilirubinemia.

Determining the direct-indirect bilirubin ratio is helpful. In hepatitis, cancer or hepatic congestion, the direct-reacting conjugated bilirubin may rise *before* the total serum bilirubin and persist for a longer period of time. In the physiologic jaundice of the newborn; in post-hepatitis hyperbilirubinemia; in rarer diseases such as Gilbert's disease, Crigler-Najjar syndrome and Lucey-Driscoll syndrome; intravascular hemolysis and following postcaval shunt the hyperbilirubinemia is of the indirect unconjugated type. To be significant the amount should exceed 1.2 mg per 100 ml of serum. Direct bilirubin should never be more than 20 percent of the total bilirubin.

Usually both the direct and indirect serum bilirubins are elevated in the jaundiced patient; consequently, the values are not of much significance in differential diagnosis. Check both, however, for 1 to 2 percent of jaundiced patients have either hemolytic disease of Gilbert's syndrome. If the patient's jaundice is due to indirect bilirubin, order a hemoglobin and reticulocyte count. If these are within normal limits, you can be sure the patient has Gilbert's syndrome. If the hemoglobin is low and the reticulocyte count high, the patient has hemolytic anemia.

Very high (30 to 40 mg percent) total bilirubin occurs in obstructive jaundice and when other conditions are superimposed on an already diseased liver. Look for renal disease or some type of hemolysis in addition to the liver problem.

Check for a fluctuating or nonfluctuating level of serum bilirubin. The pattern of fluctuation is important. Frequently a stone exhibits a changing serum level of bilirubin, while a cancer exhibits a persistent elevation. Rarely does an obstruction either from cancer or stone produce elevations higher than 15 to 25 mg percent. In obstruction, the kidney has a way of excreting enough bilirubin to maintain some balance between production and excretion. Viral hepatitis is more likely to produce the high levels of 40 mg percent.

BILIRUBIN IN THE URINE. Testing for bilirubin in the urine is inexpensive and easy to do. When positive, it indicates hepatic disease. Patients frequently observe a dark urine 2 or 3 days before their skin becomes discolored. Inspection of the urine may be all that is needed when the urine is deep yellow or reddish brown in color.

Bilirubin is present in the urine of 98 percent of patients who are jaundiced. Its absence is probably more important, for it implies hemolytic anemia or Gilbert's syndrome.

Shake the urine in a test tube. A yellow to brown foam indicates the presence of conjugated bilirubin. This rather imprecise determination is a useful bedside screening check.

The Ictotest is an easy but more precise diazo dye method. It is performed by dipping a strip of fiter paper into a specimen of fresh urine. If the test is negative in the presence of jaundice (acholuric jaundice) it suggests the presence of unconjugated indirect hyperbilirubinemia. Remember unconjugated bilirubin is never excreted in urine.

URINE UROBILINOGEN. After bilirubin is conjugated by hepatic cells and excreted into the duodenum, bacteria reduce it to urobilinogen. Intestinal bilirubin is not reabsorbed but urobilinogen is. Most of this reabsorbed urobilinogen is taken up again by the liver and again excreted by the liver as bile. Some of the urobilinogen escapes the liver and is excreted in the urine as urine urobilinogen.

Urobilinogen is apt to appear in the urine, and in greater quantities, early in the afternoon. Consequently, order the urine collected between 1 and 3 PM. The report will be given in Ehrlich units. Normal is 1 unit or less. If serial dilutions of the urine were requested, normal excretion is less than 1:20.

Total disappearance of urobilinogen from the urine indicates complete obstruction to the flow of bile. If any urobilinogen is present, it is evident that some bile is entering the intestine. If bile duct obstruction does exist, it is only partial.

Other causes for a decrease in urobilinogen are:

- –improperly timed urine collection
- –poor urine collection
- –acidic urine
- –renal insufficiency
- –decreased bilirubin production occurring in some types of anemia
- –diarrheas (because of the decreased transit time)
- –bowel sterilization during antibiotic therapy (because of the lack of organism to convert bilirubin to urobilinogen)
- –obstruction to the flow of bilirubin into the duodenum (by intrahepatic causes or by cancerous obstruction of the extrahepatic biliary tree)

Urinary urobilinogen is increased following:

- –excess bilirubin formation

- –constipation because of prolonged transit time
- –liver dysfunction causing a decreased pickup of urobilinogen by the liver, thereby shunting more to the kidneys for excretion
- –conditions in which more than normal numbers of bacteria are present in the bowel, increasing the production and absorption of urobilinogen

Total disappearance of urinary urobilinogen indicates complete obstruction to the flow of bile as in cancer. An increase in urine urobilinogen indicates hepatocellular damage unless it can be accounted for by increased blood destruction.

SERUM ALKALINE PHOSPHATASE. In actuality, serum alkaline phosphatase (SAP) is a group of enzymes. Of these enzymes, 40 to 70 percent originate in bone and the rest from liver, intestine and placenta. They have a half-life of seven days. Consequently, the amount present in the serum at any time represents a balance between input and degradation. The function of SAP is not known.

Use the test to detect early interhepatic or extrahepatic obstruction. Highest levels occur in extrahepatic biliary obstruction such as cancer, stones and stricture of the bile ducts. Smaller and less constant levels are obtained in viral hepatitis and cirrhosis.

In both primary or secondary hepatic malignancy, SAP is of particular value, occasionally being the only abnormal function test. Any space-occupying lesion will cause an elevation of SAP. This elevation occurs in a wide variety of diseases such as hepatic abscess, amyloidosis, leukemia, sarcoidosis and hepatoma.

Avoid a tight interpretation of any SAP elevation. A variety of diseases cause some elevation. Think of it in this way: very high values favor a diagnosis of extrahepatic obstruction but, even more important, low values are against it.

One way to overcome this nonspecificity is to order a serum leucine aminopeptidase (LAP) and a 5′ nucleotidase. Neither of these are derived from bone. Consequently, if these are elevated the enzyme is from some other source than bone, the most likely being liver. Therefore, if SAP, LAP and 5′ nucleotidase are all elevated, depend on at least some of the SAP as coming from hepatic disease. On the other hand, a normal LAP and 5′ nucleotidase with some elevation of SAP does not rule out liver disease.

It is most important to remember that in hepatocellular damage the level of SAP is rarely above 10 Bodansky units. In obstructive jaundice the level may be 10 times that figure.

Alkaline phosphatase values:

Normal value depends on method used.
Mild increase—2 times the normal upper limits
Moderate increase—2 to 4 times the normal upper limits
Marked increase—5 times the normal upper limits

SERUM TRANSAMINASES: Serum glutamic oxaloacetic transaminase (SGOT) is present in large quantities in liver, heart, kidney and skeletal muscle. If any acute destruction of these tissues occurs, SGOT is released and may go up from a normal 20 units per ml or less to 2,000 units or more, especially in liver cell destruction. Normal value for SGOT is 20 ± 7.

The particular value of a SGOT assay lies in its early elevation in acute hepatitis. Look for the highest values in early hepatitis, then a falling off as soon as jaundice develops.

Serum glutamic pyruvic transaminase (SGPT) occurs in the same tissue as does SGOT, but there is a higher proportion in the liver. An increase in SGPT is more specific for acute liver disease. Normal values are 7 to 25 units per ml.

Use the transaminases for:

- –early diagnosis of anicteric or preicteric viral hepatitis
- –checking on suspected relapses during convalescence
- –assessing the activity of persistent or chronic hepatitis
- –checking on early drug toxicity
- –searching the liver for infiltrative diseases

As an example: Transaminase value of over 1,000 indicates an acute hepatic disease and is evidence against extrahepatic obstruction. Values between 400 and 1,000 are only suggestive. Those below 400 units are not useful in the differential diagnosis of liver disease. Myocardial infarction causes a greater rise in SGOT than SGPT. Interpret any SGOT elevation carefully.

Transaminase values:

Normal—less than 40 Karmen units/ml
Mild increase—up to 250 Karmen units/ml
Moderate increase—250 to 500 Karmen units/ml
Marked increase—above 500 Karmen units/ml

PROTHROMBIN TIME AND ITS RESPONSE TO VITAMIN K. Prothrombin is necessary for blood coagulation. It is synthesized in the liver. Certain factors such as thromboplastin, calcium, activating factors and vitamin K are needed for its synthesis and conversion to thrombin.

Vitamin K is absorbed from the bowel only if bile salts are present. If bile production and excretion is shut off, as in biliary obstruction, vitamin K is wasted; none circulates to the liver and the conversion of prothrombin to thrombin is delayed. Other factors which may diminish vitamin K absorption are starvation, long continued parenteral nutrition and antibiotic administration which sterilizes the bowel.

Prothrombin time (PT) measures the conversion rate of prothrombin to thrombin. You will not be able to tell whether liver damage or other factors account for a prolonged PT unless parenteral vitamin K is given 24 hours before the PT is determined. Use phytonadione (K-1) (AquaMEPHYTON, Konakion, Mephyton) IV or IM. With the administration of vitamin K the liver has direct access to the vitamin and is no longer dependent on bowel absorption for the production and conversion of prothrombin to thrombin. Consequently, if you are using PT for a check on liver function, always give the patient 5 to 15 mg of vitamin K before checking the PT. If you are using the PT for evaluation of the patient's bleeding mechanism, the vitamin K is unnecessary.

Do not use PT as an index of liver disease because only about 10 percent of the liver cells participate in prothrombin synthesis. Use the PT to differentiate between parenchymal liver disease and extrahepatic obstructive jaundice. Check the PT first without vitamin K and then 24 hours after administering vitamin K. If a low prothrombin becomes normal after the administration of vitamin K, the liver is functioning normally, at least in response to prothrombin production. A failure to respond is good evidence of parenchymal liver disease.

Use the PT to determine prognosis. If it is below 40 percent despite vitamin K, the prognosis is poor. There is likely to be considerable necrosis. In addition, a PT greater than 4 seconds above control with no response to vitamin K signifies a poor prognosis in alcoholic cirrhosis.

Prothrombin values:

Normal—100% of control
Mild decrease—Down to 60%
Moderate decrease—65 to 45%
Marked decrease—less than 45%

SERUM PROTEINS. Albumin and alpha and beta globulin are synthesized in the liver; gamma globulin is probably synthesized in the reticuloendothelial tissue (RES). Albumin is 55 to 65 percent of the total serum protein, alpha globulin 9 to 14 percent, beta globulin 9 to 15 percent and gamma globulin 12 to 14 percent.

Liver damage causes a decrease in the protein substances synthesized within the liver, mainly albumin (Fig. 12-72). For some unexplained reason, gamma globulin from the RES is increased. The most consistent change of the two is an increase in the gamma globulin. These changes may reverse the usual albumin:globulin ratio. The ratio is of no great clinical importance but is usually recorded.

In portal cirrhosis albumin is reduced and gamma globulin increased. In biliary cirrhosis secondary to obstructive jaundice, alpha-2 and beta globulin are increased

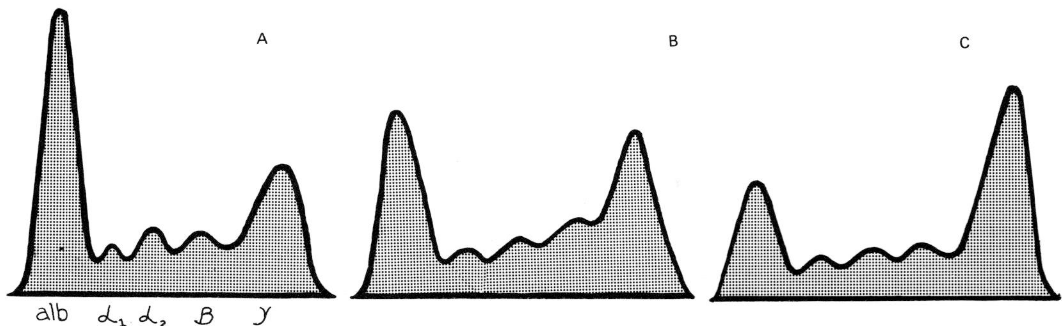

Figure 12-72. Plasma protein electrophoretic patterns: *A*, Normal; *B*, In viral hepatitis; *C*, In cirrhosis of the liver.

while gamma globulin remains low. In chronic or subacute hepatitis, hyperglobulinemia is the rule.

Do not depend on the serum proteins for diagnosis, but use the changing values to assess the course of the disease. Changes in serum proteins occur late in liver disease and, therefore, are not sensitive indications of acute liver damage.

Serum protein albumin values:

Normal values—4.2±0.4 g %
Mild depression—3.5 g %
Moderate depression—3.4 to 2.8 g %
Marked depression—less than 2.8 g %

Serum protein globulin values:

Normal values—3.2 ± 0.4 g %
Mild increase—to 4.0 g %
Moderate increase—4.1 to 5.0 g %
Marked increase—5.0 or more g %

BROMSULPHALEIN (BSP) RETENTION TEST. Bromsulphalein (BSP) is removed from the circulation by the parenchymal liver cells and excreted in the bile. In a normal person this occurs at a regular rate. Any delay in the excretory rate indicates a failure of the liver cells to pick up, conjugate and excrete the dye, thus providing an assessment of liver cell function. Other factors which may influence the rate of excretion are starvation, administration of Telepaque, fever, late pregnancy, obesity and age.

Administer the test using the following criteria. Have the patient fast. Give BSP IV, 5 mg per kg of body weight. The normal liver will remove all but 5 percent from the circulation within 45 minutes.

Consider the BSP test as the most useful single test of liver function. It is highly sensitive in uncovering early or mild hepatic disease. Abnormal BSP retention will occur in more than 80 percent of cases of hepatitis, cirrhosis, extrahepatic obstruction, metastatic disease and chronic passive congestion. As to the last, retention of 30 percent or more may be seen in cardiac decompensation.

Use the test to determine if liver damage is present. Do not use the test if the patient is jaundiced because jaundice is prima facie evidence of liver damage. Do not depend on the test to differentiate the types of liver-biliary dysfunction.

INDICATIONS FOR LIVER FUNCTION TESTS. Indications are jaundice, fatty or clay-colored stools, hyperthyroidism, alcoholism, dark stools, dark urine, hemorrhagic diathesis, splenomegaly, pruritus, flatulence, anorexia or nausea and vomiting.

Other Tests in Differential Diagnosis

GASTROINTESTINAL X-RAY SERIES. These have limited value in the differential diagnosis. The most helpful sign is a linear mass across the duodenal bulb. This obstructive sign is caused by a dilated bile duct. In complete obstruction the duct may dilate 2 or more cm. If the sign is present it indicates an obstruction somewhere near the ampulla of Vater.

FLAT PLATE OF THE ABDOMEN. The flat plate should be taken because 10 to 15 percent of gallstones are calcified and will be radiopaque.

FLOCCULATION TESTS. The tests are becoming obsolete; they are being replaced by the enzymes and serum protein determinations. Ordinarily they are positive in acute hepatitis and active cirrhosis but negative in obstructive jaundice. But they are positive in many other diseases such as malaria, kala-azar, collagen diseases and myeloma.

ICTERIC INDEX. Generally this is considered obsolete.

CORTISONE TEST. This produces too many false-positives and negatives. Most consider it too undependable.

FECAL UROBILINOGEN. It may be useful in certain circumstances but it is not a practical test. Most laboratories do not have a special laboratory to do fecal studies.

CHOLESTEROL DETERMINATION. Although it is not of diagnostic importance, a cholesterol determination is usually done. High levels (450) suggest prolonged canalicular or main bile duct obstruction.

HEPATITIS-ASSOCIATED ANTIGEN (HAA) (AUSTRALIAN ANTIGEN). The appearance of HAA in serum may antedate a rise in SGOT in anicteric viral hepatitis. Some reports indicate it may be the most sensitive index of early viral hepatitis. The test may also be of value in screening out potentially infectious blood donors.

Do the tests if the laboratory facilities are available. Perhaps your local blood bank will do the test for you. When it is positive, depend upon it for it occurs only with viral hepatitis type B (serum) hepatitis and not with type A (infectious). There is still much more to learn concerning the use of the test.

LIVER BIOPSY. Do a liver biopsy only if you suspect primary liver disease. In jaundice, a biopsy can be hazardous because it may cause bile peritonitis, particularly if the patient has cholestasis. Weigh the events carefully. In addition, pathologists experience some difficulty in differentiating extrahepatic obstruction from drug jaundice, stones and the various odd causes of jaundice. Use the biopsy procedure more freely in differentiating nonjaundiced liver diseases.

TRANSHEPATIC CHOLANGIOGRAM. If facilities are available, do a liver biopsy following a transhepatic cholangiogram. An unsuccessful cholangiogram usually indicates the patient does not have extrahepatic obstruction. A biopsy can then be done with little risk. The test, however, best be done only if surgery is contemplated. Visualize the precise site of obstruction with the test. This shortens the operative time.

Transhepatic cholangiography is done by passing a flexible needle deep into the liver substance with the objective of striking a dilated bile duct. Whether the strike is successful is usually determined by whether bile is aspirated and by the injection of a contrast medium under fluoroscopic control. When a mechanical obstruction is present, there is about a 55 percent chance of hitting a dilated duct. If the ducts are of normal size, most frequently they canot be tapped. The needle should be left in to decompress the biliary system. Corrective surgery should be done within 3 to 6 hours to provide drainage. This will prevent bile peritonitis.

ANTIMITOCHONDRIAL ANTIBODIES. These antibodies are present in nearly all patients with primary biliary cirrhosis. It is almost always negative in extrahepatic biliary obstruction. Therefore, a positive test indicates the need for medical treatment, not surgery. The use of the test is debated. Some doctors put more reliance on it than others. Possibly the wisest course would be to postpone surgery temporarily if the test is positive and await more definitive signs.

CHOLECYSTOGRAM. This very seldom aids in the differential diagnosis of jaundice. If the serum bilirubin is above 3 mg percent, the contrast media is not picked up by the liver cells.

LIVER SCANNING WITH RADIOACTIVE ROSE BENGAL. Scanning may exhibit a dilated common duct or full bladder. Rose bengal is injected intravenously. Then a 30 minute scan is done. Repeat the scan 24 hours later, using exactly the same scanning settings. If there is more than a 50 percent reduction in radioactivity, a nonsurgical condition is present. If there is no reduction, a surgically correctable lesion may be present.

Steps in Differential Diagnosis

Perform a complete history and physical examination. Order a complete blood count and the usual liver panel (direct and indirect bilirubin, SGOT, SGPT, alkaline phosphatase, prothrombin time and serum proteins). Check the stool for color and occult blood. If the patient is having chills and fever, order a blood culture.

If the diagnosis is not clear, proceed with a flat plate of the abdomen and possibly a barium meal, rose bengal scan of liver which is repeated in 24 hours, hepatitis-associated antigen test and antimitochondrial antibody test. Continue to recheck blood chemistry and reexamine the patient every 3 to 4 days.

If the diagnosis is still in doubt consider liver biopsy, transhepatic cholangiography and laparotomy.

Surgery in Jaundiced Conditions

Proceed with surgery if the following are present:

- patient's history suggests mechanical obstruction
- liver is smooth but enlarged
- patient is not confused
- there is no ascitis
- alkaline phosphatase is two to three times the upper limit of normal
- SGOT or SGPT is less than 300 units
- prothrombin time is normal

Otherwise, observe the patient for awhile. Do not be afraid to wait a reasonable time, especially if the time is being used for definitive testing. Leevy[28] reports that in jaundiced patients who refused surgery and were followed by a series of precutaneous liver biopsies, biliary cirrhosis did not develop for 2 to 3 months even in complete obstruction.

There is one exception to a wait and see attitude—the diabetic patient. These patients do not tolerate a cholangitis; mortality is high. Seek surgical consultation within a few hours of the onset of a definite cholangitis.

While Awaiting Surgery

If the patient has chills, fever and leukocytosis, do a blood culture and treat with antibiotics. Give daily vitamin K. Support the patient with intravenous fluids and consider giving steroids.

If the diagnosis is not clear after a week or two of medical observation and repeated laboratory testing, ask for surgical consultation. The time will be near for an exploratory laparotomy. The surgical objective should be more than a biopsy or an exploration of the bile ducts. If needed, the surgeon should plan to do an operative or T-tube cholangiogram and any reparative procedure needed.

On opening the abdomen, look first for an enlarged gallbladder and common bile duct. If they are enlarged the diagnosis is clear —obstruction is present. On the other hand, if no dilitation of either organ is found, operative cholangiography is the quickest way to establish a diagnosis. The cholangiogram should be done through the gallbladder. When completed it should show the duct from the duodenum to the bifurcation of the common duct. If bile flows freely into the duodenum and the duct is normal size, take a biopsy and close the abdomen.

Acute Hepatitis

There are two forms of hepatitis, both probably viral in origin: Infectious hepatitis (IH, type A hepatitis) and serum hepatitis (SH, type B hepatitis). Contrary to what a generation of physicians believed, both may be transmitted by either the fecal-oral route or injection. Contaminated hypodermic needles and transfusions account for most cases of serum hepatitis.

Is there any way for you to be certain which variety the patient has? Probably not except for what you can deduct from the history. If the patient is one of a number of patients following an epidemic, it is reasonable to assume a common causative agent.

There are no laboratory tests that will differentiate the individual case. The hepatitis-associated antigen (HAA), the Australian antigen, is only associated with serum hepatitis, but it is associated with serum hepatitis by inoculation or contact. And in those patients who are negative HAA, the diagnosis may be either serum hepatitis, in which HAA is no longer present, or infectious hepatitis.

The discussion is more than academic. Gamma globulin may be given, with a reasonable expectation of preventing or ameliorating the disease, to contacts of those with infectious or type A. Gamma globulin is useless in preventing or dampening the effects of serum hepatitis. In the future, the distinction may be even more important. Krugman and fellow workers[29] reported success in preventing serum hepatitis with a specific hepatitis B immune serum globulin. They believed their serum to be 70 percent effective. This is not available for use.

Prophylactic Gamma Globulin

All members of the infected patient's household should receive gamma globulin when the case is one of suspected infectious hepatitis. Playmates who have been in close contact with the infected child should be injected but this does not include all classmates. Also treat prophylactically contacts who have been living in the patient's household up to 2 weeks before the overt disease because infectious hepatitis virus has been excreted in the stool up to 2 to 3 weeks before clinical symptoms.

Do not give gamma globulin to contacts who have a definite serum hepatitis, casual office or factory contacts, schoolmates, pregnant women unless their contact has been close and continuous as a household member or hospital personnel who have been exposed. Isolation techniques have reduced the risk to minimum in the latter.

When the decision is made to give prophylactic gamma globulin, administer 0.01 to 0.02 ml per pound intramuscularly. The prophylactic value decreases with each day following exposure. Larger doses will not give greater protection. But they may have a longer lasting effect in cases where the patient anticipates long-continued exposure.

Warn the patient that the injection may be painful, the injection site may be red and warm, he may feel fluish and the serum may not prevent the disease but only lighten it.

Treatment

There is no certainty that rest is all important but, as in other viral diseases, rest would appear to be a wise suggestion.

A high protein diet is reported to have cut the duration of the acute illness by 20 percent, if the patient can tolerate it. In the rare patient with an encephalopathy, restrict proteins.

The administration of steroids is debatable. Most physicians do not recommend steroids for the routine treatment of hepatitis.

In summary, do not become overly concerned and create anxieties over remote dangers.

Fulminant hepatitis occurs in about 4 out of every 1,000 cases of infectious hepatitis and in 100 out of 1,000 cases of hospitalized patients with serum hepatitis. In these severe cases, treatment is still only symptomatic. Obviously, when encephalopathy develops not only restrict proteins but also give oral neomycin to reduce organisms that produce nitrogen. Consider steroid therapy. In a life-saving situation, try drastic measures—exchange transfusion and plasmapheresis.

The patient with chronic hepatitis appears more likely to benefit from treatment than does the acute sufferer. Winkelman and coworkers[30] reported that 15 out of 18 patients with chronic hepatitis treated with 100 mg of azathioprine and 20 to 40 mg of prednisone daily improved. Liver function returned to normal in 7 days and autoantibodies disappeared in 2.

Prognosis

After oral infection the death rate continues to be less than 4 per 1,000. Expect a mortality rate of 0.5 to 3.0 percent in cases of serum hepatitis following transmittal of the virus by needle among drug addicts. The mortality rate of transfusion hepatitis is around 10 percent of jaundiced patients and 2 to 5 percent of all patients.

If the disease is severe enough to cause encephalopathy, the mortality rate is 62 percent in children of 1 to 14 years, 74 percent in individuals of 15 to 44 years and 90 percent in those 45 and over. For patients in deep coma, the figures are 66, 78 and 98 percent respectively.

Prevention by the Family Physician

Use every precaution in giving injections to patients. Use disposable syringes and needles.

Instruct nurses and paramedical personnel to take care in preventing accidental injections to themselves. They run a greater risk than others. Care in handling and disposing applies to all needles, not only to those used on jaundiced patients. See that gloves are worn by all who may soil their hands with blood.

For intravenous therapy use sedimented red cells and/or lactated Ringers as much as possible. The highest number of transfusion reactions occur with the administration of fibrinogen or pooled plasma. Remember, there is no reason to give prophylactic gamma globulin for posttransfusion hepatitis. Screening blood donors for Australian antigen should detect $^{1}/_{4}$ to $^{1}/_{3}$ of the carriers.

Report all cases of acute hepatitis. This is an effective control technique if doctors would report more than 10 percent of their cases. Reporting is grossly neglected. A registry of donors of infected blood, if implemented, would virtually eliminate posttransfusion hepatitis.

Give gamma globulin to patients traveling to Africa, Asia, Central and South America, rural Mexico, the Philippines and South Pacific islands. Gamma globulin is unnecessary for those persons going to countries with good sanitation if they are staying only 2 to 3 weeks. The PHS Advisory Committee on Immunization Practices suggests the following: give travelers who will be in the above named countries for 1 to 2 months 0.01 ml of gamma globulin per pound of weight and give travelers who plan on extended stays of 3 to 6 months or who are to take up residence in the affected areas 0.5 ml gamma globulin per pound of weight. Advise the patient to have the dose repeated every 4 months.

Alcoholic Cirrhosis

The newest steps in treating cirrhosis include earlier detection of liver injury and prevention of cirrhosis and reversible liver insufficiency. All this depends on early detection in high risk patients. There is no higher risk group than the alcoholic patients; 10 to 30 percent of alcoholics develop cirrhosis. In addition, 65 percent of drinkers who consume enough alcohol to neglect their nutrition have histologic evidence of liver damage.

Recognition of Early Liver Damage

Attempt to establish the diagnosis of alcoholism by history and physical examination. This is not always easy. Frequently the clue will come from friends, coworkers or other members of the family. If you cannot find out in any other way, send the patient to the laboratory when he least suspects a check up. Ask for whatever test you want but also have his blood alcohol level checked. If the blood level is up, at least the patient and you can begin to talk about his real problem.

During the physical examination measure the liver in centimeters. It is now passé to describe liver size by fingers or anatomic landmarks. The adult liver should be no larger than 15 ± 2 cm at the midclavicular line and 4 cm ± 2 in the midline. The measurement is made by palpation and percussion, using relative rather than absolute dullness for liver size. Every alcoholic should have this measurement made and recorded.

The liver may appear to vary in size from visit to visit. Remember the patient's relaxation changes and your perceptivity changes, too, from time to time. The actual centimeter measurements do not change except in response to the progression of the disease. Be careful: the lower margin of the liver has a thin edge and may extend below the costal margin area yet be inpalpable and a small liver may be difficult to detect.

Palpate for a blunt edge or an irregular surface. Consider an irregular or nodular liver as cancerous until proven otherwise. Other possibilities are regenerating nodules of postnecrotic cirrhosis or congenital cystic disease. A liver enlarged more than 3 to 4 fingers below the costal margin usually indicates some disease besides hepatitis. A small or normal size liver in the presence of jaundice of 2 or 3 weeks duration practically eliminates the possibility of obstructive jaundice. Think of cirrhosis or cancer when the liver is hard and of inflammation or congestion when the liver is soft.

While checking liver size (see Fig. 12-71), do not neglect to palpate for an enlarged gallbladder and spleen.

Other signs and symptoms are:

- multiple spider angiomas, usually seen on the upper extremities, chest and neck (The finding is not very helpful.)
- glossitis and atrophy of the fungiform or filiform papillae may be clinical evidence of a deficiency of iron, protein, nicotinic acid, riboflavin, folic acid, vitamin B6, vitamin B12 or biotin
- anemia
- plane xanthomas of the palmar creases
- ascitis with or without dependent edema
- Dupuytren's contracture
- enlargement of parotids
- gynecomastia
- testicular atrophy
- clubbing of fingers
- palmar erythemia
- pale stools
- friction rub over liver

Most textbooks describe decreasing body and pectoral hair as a characteristic of cirrhosis. However, a study done at the University of California at Irvine by Smith[31] seems to disprove this old belief. In a study of 50 men with cirrhosis, none developed this sign nor did their hair decrease as the disease progressed.

Plane xanthomas of the palmar creases are rare but helpful when they do occur. Tuberous xanthomas occur in the tendons or tendon sheaths; xanthelasma beneath the eyes. Xanthomas may disappear or fade when terminal liver failure occurs because the liver fails to produce cholesterol.

Laboratory Aids

The bromsulphalein (BSP) is being replaced by the indocyanine green (ICG) clearance test utilizing dichromatic ear densitometry. This test can detect mild liver damage even before symptoms develop. Use the test to assay the extent of liver damage and to detect small changes either for the better or for the worse.

The test is performed by injecting a measured amount of indocyanine green (ICG) intravenously. Two photocells are clipped to the patient's ear. The photocells are connected to a densitometer and a graphic recorder. The photocells detect the appearance and disappearance of the dye in the capillaries of the earlobe. The recorded curve is then compared with a normal curve and evaluated.

If 5.0 mg/kg of dye is used, maximum, clearance occurs at the rate of 22 to 25 percent per minute. This figure detects minimal changes in liver function. Plot a comparison of repeated determinations. In this way follow the regeneration or degeneration of the liver.

The ethanol tolerance test determines ethanol-oxidizing capacity, index of the susceptibility to tissue injury. The standard test consists of administering 1.0 g/kg of ethanol in 1,000 ml of half normal saline over a 1 hour period. Serum ethanol, lactate and glucose are measured before the infusion, upon completion and 1, 2, 3 and 4 hours afterward.

Patterns of ethanol tolerance have been worked out for normal patients, alcoholics with mild hepatitis and alcoholics with cirrhosis. Basically, the observations permit detection of patients who are developing other clinical abnormalities such as acute hypoglycemia after alcohol intake.

Other laboratory tests which will enable you to evaluate the patient will be

–serum protein electrophoresis
–assay of circulating folic acid, vitamin B6 and thiamine
–studies of electrolytes in patients with ascitis or renal dysfunction
–coagulation work-up
–endocrinologic study in patients with hypogonadism
–other specialized tests to detect and plan treatment for major complications

The latter includes celiac angiography, splenoportography or hepatic portography for esophageal varices and catheterization of the umbilical-portal vein in patients with bleeding tendencies.

Preventive and Therapeutic Programs

The treatment of alcoholism is basic in treating cirrhosis. In early cirrhosis, controlling alcoholism may be all that is necessary to arrest or even cure liver disease. The prognosis for an alcoholic with cirrhosis is most influenced by his future drinking habits. The prognosis is poor with continued heavy drinking, improved with reduction and best with abstinence.

The treatment of alcoholism is multifaceted and includes physical, psychologic and social support.

Some physical aids might include the establishment of regular meals, tranquilizers and cooperation with Alcoholics Anonymous. If the patient's alcohol ingestion cannot be controlled, he should be encouraged to eat when no alcohol is present in blood or tissues to prevent malabsorption of certain vitamins and minerals. Give food or antacids before or after alcohol consumption to prevent ulcerative disease.

Fatty liver is one of the first changes to occur in the liver structure which is reversible. One-third of all alcoholics have some degree of fatty infiltration without fibrosis. Recognize this change by the tests already described and institute treatment. Order a high-protein diet, correct deficiencies and prescribe androgenic-anabolic steroids. If the patient stops drinking, fatty liver will disappear in 40 days and even sooner with more intensive treatment.

Alcoholic hepatitis may be the first basic change leading directly to cirrhosis. Usually, however, the liver damage involves both fatty infiltration and liver cell necrosis. The latter fluctuates with the patient's alcoholic intake. Treatment consists of as high a protein diet as the patient can tolerate without inducing an encephalopathy, parenteral vitamins, the correction of all deficiencies including anemia, hypoalbuminemia and hypoglycemia. Place emphasis on the need for folic acid, the one most important deficiency in this complication. There is a deficiency of this nutriment in over 60 percent of alcoholic patients with liver disease.

Whenever you diagnose cirrhosis, hospitalize the patient, and keep him there until all evidence of fatty liver and active hepatic cell damage has disappeared. The basic program will include as much protein as tolerated and the same vitamin supplement as outlined under alcoholic hepatitis.

Any special treatment will be directed toward the complications of cirrhosis.

FOR ASCITES. Restrict sodium intake and give potassium supplement. Even on a 200 mg sodium diet, it takes the patient nearly 2 weeks to accumulate a L of extracellular fluid. To combat a hyponatremia, you may find it necessary to limit fluid intake to 1,000 to 1,200 ml per day.

If hypoalbuminemia is present, give salt-poor albumin.

Test diuretic therapy. Cautiously give diuretics for 10 days while monitoring urinary sodium excretion and plasma potassium level. If serum bilirubin is 4 mg per 100 ml or less and other tests are only slightly off, the administration of a diuretic is usually safe. The best program is an intermittent one. Continue the diuretic until the patient loses 3 pounds and then wait 2 to 3 days before continuing. The best diuretic to prescribe as a basic one is Aldactone (spironolactone) 100 mg daily in divided doses. Give other stronger diuretics such as a thiazide or furosemide intermittently as needed. Remember it is better to leave a little ascitic fluid than to try for the last drop. Weigh the patient twice daily and adjust the dose of diuretic appropriately. Gradually increase the sodium restriction to an amount the patient will willingly follow. It will take 4 to 5 days to adjust the balance between diuretic dose and sodium restriction to maintain the patient's weight.

If SGOT, SGPT, LDH and serum bilirubin are elevated and if the patient is semicomatose, diuretics may not be needed and may actually make the patient worse.

Diagnosis of Minimal Abdominal Ascites. The finding of as little as 120 ml of ascitic fluid in the peritoneal cavity is possible by the "puddling" technique. Have the patient lie prone for 5 minutes; then instruct her to get on all-fours so that her midabdomen hangs. Fluid accumulates in the most dependent part of the abdomen. Hold the stethoscope bowl over the most dependent part of the abdomen with one hand while the other hand flicks (light percussion) the patient's flank (Fig. 12-73). Gradually move the stethoscope toward the opposite flank. When a fluid level is reached, the intensity and character of the percussion note changes.

To verify, have the patient sit up. Continue to hold the stethoscope over what was the dependent part of the abdomen while repeating the flicking maneuver. If the percussion note becomes loud and clear, the initial impression is substantiated.

Other Causes of Ascites. Portal cirrhosis, Budd-Chiari syndrome, portal vein thrombosis, primary carcinoma of liver, metastic liver disease, hepatic tertiary syphilis, Wilson's disease, hemochromatosis, Meig's syndrome, nephrotic syndrome, tuberculous peritonitis, Hodgkin's disease, cancer of the peritoneum, beriberi, congestive heart failure, pseudomyxoma peritonei, Gaucher's disease, acute pancreatitis, chronic constrictive percarditis and gonococcal pelvic inflammatory disease.

FOR ESOPHAGEAL VARICES. (Fig. 12-74) If there is bleeding consider balloon tamponade with or without posterior pituitary extract. Use fresh whole blood when available. Otherwise order corrected banked blood. Prescribe androgenic-anabolic steroids to patients with a bleeding tendency if vitamin K doesn't help. Seek consultation regarding surgical decompression in selected cases.

FOR ENCEPHALOPATHY. Restrict protein. In severe cases, eliminate protein

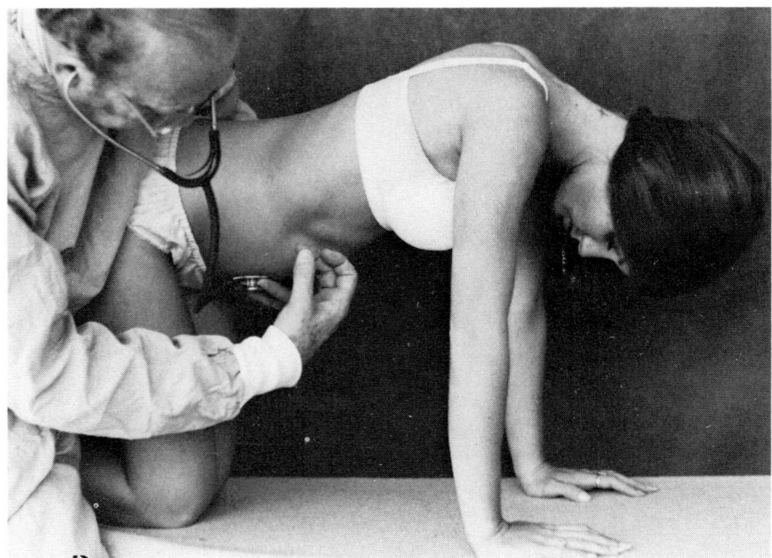

Figure 12-73. Listen for the puddle sign. The principle: the flicking sound is damped by fluid and flicking is transmitted better through gas in the bowels.

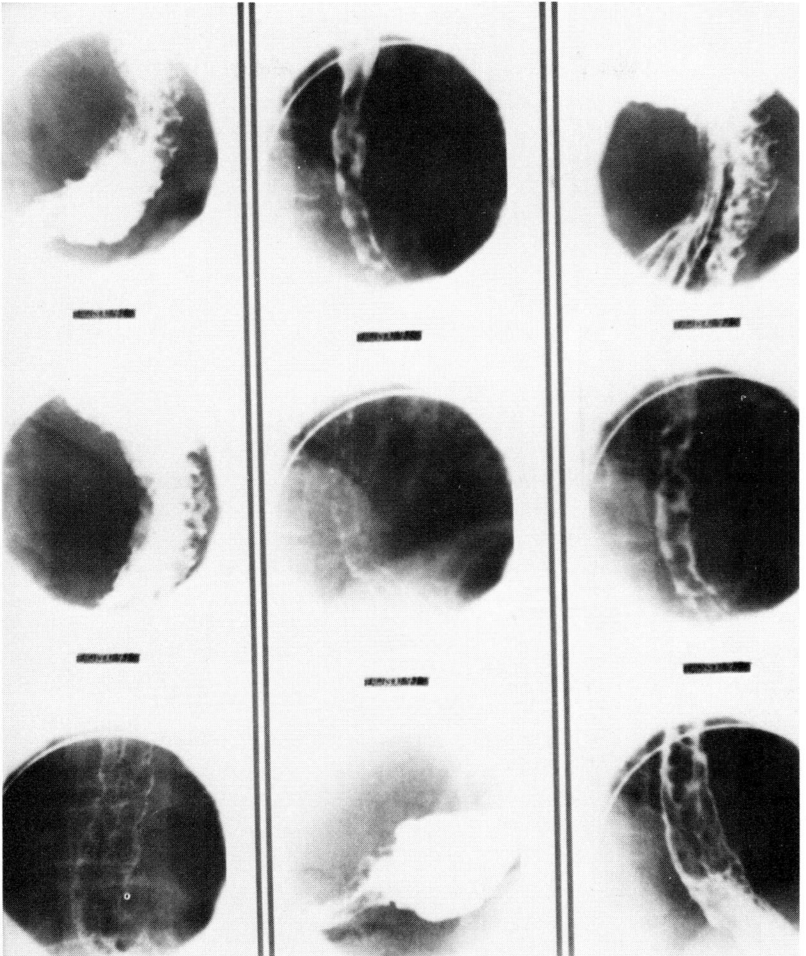

Figure 12-74. Esophageal varices. The patient also has hepatomegaly, gallstones and splenomegaly, and probably cirrhosis.

for a short time. If all protein is stopped, give 1,600 calories daily either as glucose drinks or as 20 percent glucose through a gastric drip. You can give 20 to 40 percent dextrose via the antecubital or femoral veins into the superior or inferior vena cava. Because the small veins will thrombose if high dextrose concentrations are given, an alternative might be 10 percent levulose.

As the patient recovers, add 20 g protein increments on alternate days. Divide the protein into meals. The limit of tolerance is 40 to 60 g per day, but it may be needed to control encephalopathy. Protein restriction is needed only in patients with signs of coma; other patients with liver disease may benefit by a high-protein diet.

Prescribe neomycin or a broad spectrum antibiotic or lactulose to reduce the number of intestinal bacteria which produce ammonia. Neomycin is safer than other antibiotics because little is absorbed from the bowel. Occasionally some does get into the circulation and cause decreased hearing. In acute cases, give 6 g daily in divided doses. For long term therapy reduce the dose to 3 or 4 g daily.

Give as little sedatives and narcotics as possible. Morphine and paraldehyde are absolutely counterindicated. If something must be given, try half the usual dose of butabarbital or an antihistamine.

There are two bedside tests for impending coma. One test is based on the patient's inability to orientate in space and is detected by his failure to copy a five pointed match star (Fig. 12-75).

The second test is the flapping tremor. The tremor is elicited by attempting dorsiflexion of the wrist while the arms are outstretched and the fingers separated. The tremor is absent at rest and lessened by intentional movement. The hand flaps quickly downward when the arms are outstretched and returns slowly to place.

Be certain to differentiate between subdural hematoma, vitamin deficiency encephalopathy and delirium tremens.

Finally, if the above measures succeed in prolonging life, the patient becomes more susceptible to hepatoma. For this, nothing short of a liver transplant will help.

Portal Hypertension

The syndrome of portal hypertension occurs as a result of partial obstruction to the portal vein. The obstruction may occur subhepatic (before the blood reaches the liver), intrahepatic (within the liver) or suprahepatic (after the blood leaves the liver). The obstruction creates splenomegaly and evidence of collateral venous circulation. It is often accompanied by hepatomegaly and ascites. The collateral venous circulation is most often found in the lower esophagus as varices but also on the abdominal wall and in the anus as hemorrhoids.

Most frequently but not invariably, portal hypertension is associated with hepatic cirrhosis. Suspect portal hypertension whenever a patient has a gastrointestinal hemorrhage, a history of liver disease, esophageal varices or liver disease (Banti's syndrome).

Subhepatic portal hypertension occurs in no more than 20 percent of cases. It occurs more often in children and the young. The cause is disputed but probably follows inflammation, phlebitis and thrombosis of the portal and/or splenic veins. In the rare instance when only the splenic vein is involved, consider a splenectomy. Usually it is curative. In subhepatic portal hypertension the liver is normal.

Suprahepatic portal hypertension (cardiac cirrhosis) is the train of events that follows chronic passive congestion of right heart failure, constrictive pericarditis, com-

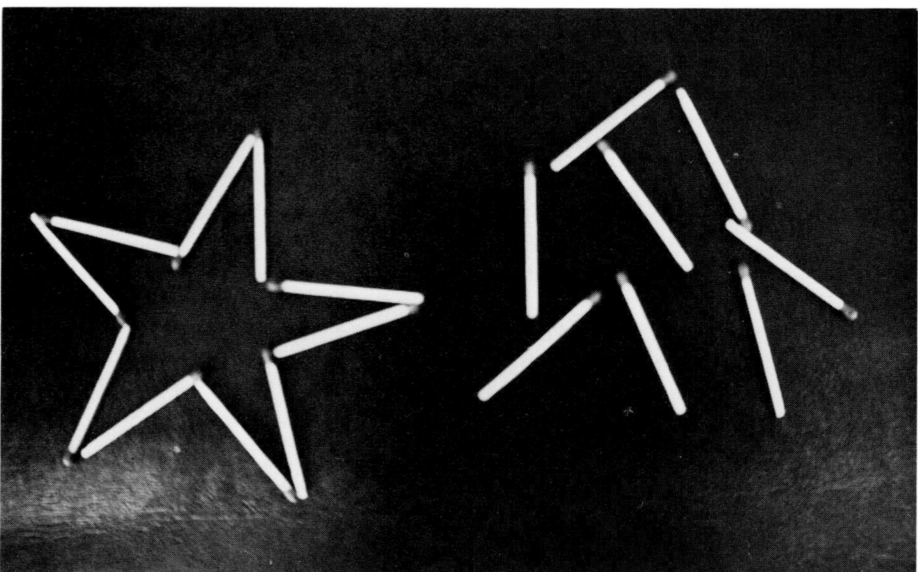

Figure 12-75. The patient's inability to assemble a matchstick star may signal approaching coma.

pression of the inferior vena cava or destruction of the hepatic veins. The last is referred to as the Budd-Chiari syndrome and follows an obliterating thrombosis of the hepatic veins. Look for an immediate appearance of large esophageal varicosities and ascites. The disease is so acute and the portal pressure so high that little or nothing can be done. If you can diagnose the syndrome be prepared for the patient's death.

Intrahepatic portal hypertension is the common syndrome and most frequently associated with hepatic cirrhosis. In this country, 80 percent of cases of portal hypertension is caused by intrahepatic pathology, most notably Laennec's cirrhosis. A few cases of necrotic hepatitis can apparently cause portal hypertension by other than the cirrhotic route.

Esophageal varicosities are the most consistent findings in portal hypertension. They are associated with ascites frequently, but also with jaundice and coma commonly. Some report spider angiomas in as high as 70 percent of the patients. A palpable spleen and some type of hemorrhage accompany 50 percent of esophageal varices.

The outlook without treatment is a dreary one indeed whenever you find unequivocal varices. A third will die of hemorrhage, another third from hepatic failure and the last third from conditions associated with hepatic failure.

On discovery of any of the major symptoms of liver disease, consider the possibility of portal hypertension. The signs and symptoms of liver disease have already been reviewed. If no liver disease is present look for the subhepatic type of portal hypertension whenever you find distention of the abdominal veins, a palpable spleen or a caput medusae (a rare venous rosette about the navel). The abdominal veins become dilated between the navel and the lower thorax. They will contain blood flowing upward in the normal direction.

An attack of hematemesis should always lead you to suspect portal hypertension even in the absence of other gross symptoms. Other rather vague findings on a general examination are complaints of unexplained weight gain or an enlarging abdomen in spite of wasting of the face and extremities, a change in skin color or an enlarged spleen or liver, which the patient interprets as a mass in the abdomen.

In suprahepatic portal hypertension the physical examination reveals splenomegaly, hepatomegaly and ascites. Do not confuse suprahepatic obstruction with the more common cardiac failure. Both conditions may have pleural effusion, hepatomegaly, ascites and edema of the ankles. A distinguishing feature is the absence of dyspnea in portal obstruction. Ascites with suprahepatic portal hypertension is so variably present that its absence casts doubt on the diagnosis even in the presence of a large spleen and liver and esophageal varices.

Ascites in intrahepatic hypertension may or may not be present, but has a more constant association with portal cirrhosis. And last of all, if you find ascites in what you believe to be a subhepatic portal vein obstruction, your diagnosis is probably wrong.

Of course the spleen is nearly always enlarged even in the absence of hepatomegaly. Remember, however, that the spleen usually enlarges two or three times its normal size before it is palpable. One can never be certain of splenomegaly by percussion, palpation or indeed by x-ray films following pneumoperitoneum.

The absence or presence of jaundice depends more on the state of the liver than on the duration and severity of portal hypertension.

X-ray and Laboratory Aids

Infer portal hypertension when esophageal varices are seen by fluoroscopic or x-ray examination. Early in the disease, repeated examinations may be needed before varices can be demonstrated. Splenoportography is a radiologic examination of great value in locating the site of obstruction. Esophagoscopy can also be used to diagnose varices and locate the site of bleeding.

The most helpful laboratory aids have been reviewed but give special attention to the bromsulphalein clearance, an excellent

Table 12-3. Assessing the Risk in Surgery

	Operative Mortality		
Signs	*Less than 10%*	*Less than 16%*	*54%*
Bilirubin	Under 2	2–3	Above 3
Albumin	Above 3.5	3–3.5	Under 3
Ascites	0	Easily controlled	Not easily controlled
Encephalopathy	0	Minimal	Advanced
Nutrition	Good	Good	Poor
RISK	Good	Moderate	Poor

test to detect liver damage when the disease is not obvious by jaundice; prothrombin assay and its response to vitamin K, again an excellent test in differentiating the cause of jaundice when positive; the SGOT and SGPT in reflecting the course of the disease rather than the cause; serum alkaline phosphatase, the higher levels pointing toward obstructive jaundice; and protein electrophoresis in detecting advanced stages of liver disease.

Something extra should be said about liver biopsy in portal cirrhosis. Because of possible bleeding from the puncture site, some physicians question its use. To overcome this hazard, do not do a puncture biopsy unless the prothrombin time is in excess of 50 percent. Although the biopsy tells little about the function of the liver, it is indeed helpful in distinguishing between intrahepatic and extrahepatic biliary obstruction, determining the presence and nature of cirrhosis, discovering the presence or absence of hepatitis and occasionally whether a tumor is present.

Treatment

The cause of the cirrhosis usually determines the outcome and benefit of the surgical correction of portal hypertension. Surgery can accomplish two objectives: remove the danger of hemorrhage from esophageal varices and relieve the portal hypertension. Keep in mind when advising surgical consultation that portal hypertension can persist even though the cirrhotic process may have become stable. Under this circumstance, shunting will reduce the hazard of hemorrhage and save the patient's life. With a patient who drinks and has advanced cirrhosis little can be accomplished by relieving portal hypertension. These patients will die shortly of hepatic failure if they escape a hemorrhage. When a cirrhotic process gets under way, it will continue even though the patient changes his ways.

Thorn[33] proposes the criteria in Table 12-3 for assessing the risk of surgery:

With maximum medical treatment, it is possible at times to change poor or moderate surgical risks into a better risk. This, however, is an expensive and time consuming endeavor and may take 2 to 3 months of hospitalization.

REFERENCES

1. Saxena VS: Cancer of the tongue: local control of the primary. *Ca* 26:788–794, 1970.
2. Dafoe CS, Ross CA: Acute corrosive esophagitis. *Thorax* 24:291, 1969.
3. Selbertson VA, Knotterud GL: Gastric analysis as a screening measure for cancer of the stomach. *Ca Cancer J Clin* 17:115–117, 1967.
4. Patterson M: The diagnosis of the Zollinger-Ellison syndrome. *Am J Gastrenterol* 54:470–479, 1970.
5. Palmer ED: Pyloric ulcer. *AFP* 5:104, 1972.
6. Wallace DP: Instructions for the treatment of esophagitis. (Unpublished but used by the Santa Monica Hospital Medical Center.)

7. Moyer CA, et al: Surgery, Principles and Practice (3rd edition). J B Lippincott Company. p 788 from McGlone FB and Robertson DW. Diagnostic accuracy of gastric ulcer. *Gastroenterology* 25:603–613, 1953.
8. Johnson AG: Flatulent dyspepsia drug. *Br Med J* 2:25, 1971.
9. Laxatives: Use Them Rarely—If at All. Health Tips 176, Calif Med Assoc, 1972.
10. Gregor DH: Diagnosis of large-bowel cancer in the asymptomatic patient. *Ca* 19:330–337, 1969.
11. Patient direction memo used at Santa Monica Hospital Medical Center, Santa Monica, Ca.
12. Bolt RJ: Routine sigmoidoscopics expose patients to some risks. *JAMA* 215:867, 1971.
13. Wilson JP, Letton AH: Routine sigmoidoscopy—an evaluation. *Ca* 17:113–114, 1967.
14. Lukash WM, et al: Cure colon cancer. *Mod Med* 39:99, 1971.
15. Willoughby JM, et al: Controlled trial of azathioprine in Crohn's disease. *Lancet* 2:944–7, 1971.
16. Baum S, et al: Angiographic management diverticular hemorrhage. *N Eng J Med* 228:1269–1271, 1973.
17. Adams JT: Therapeutic barium enema for diverticular bleeding. *Arch Surg* 00:457, 1970.
18. McHardy G, et al: Hiatal hernia and erosive esophagitis. *GP* 1:85–98, 1969.
19. Bean B: Vascular spiders and related skin conditions. *Calif Med* 114:1–6, 1971.
20. Shore JM: The prevention of residual biliary calculi. *Calif Med* 114:1, 1971.
21. Steiger E, et al: Cholecystectomy in the aged. *Ann Surg* 174:142–144, 1971.
22. Danziger RG, et al: Dissolution of cholesterol gallstones by chenodeoxycholic acid. *N Eng J of Med* 286:1–8, 1972.
23. Pfeffermann R, Luttwak EM: Gallstone-pancreatitis: Exploration of biliary system in pancreatitis of undetermined origin. *Arch Surg* 103: 484–486, 1971.
24. Davis WC, Jackson FC: Inguinal hernia and colon carcinoma. *Ca* 18:143–145, 1968.
25. Thieme ET: Recurrent inguinal hernia. *Arch Surg* 103:238–241, 1971.
26. Gershoff SN, Prien EL: Effect of daily MgO and Vitamin B_6 administration to patients with recurring calcium oxalate kidney stones. *Am J Clin Nutr* 20:393, 1967.
27. Lee GR: The porphyrias, diagnosis by simple laboratory methods. *Med Sc* May:36–40, 1964.
28. A roundtable discussion. Jaundice: pinpointing the curable cause. *Patient Care* 6:22, 1972.
29. Krugman S, et al: Viral hepatitis, type B (MS-2 strain) prevention with specific hepatitis B immune serum blobulin. *JAMA* 218:11, 1971.
30. Winkelman E, et al. Cleveland Clinic Foundation as reviewed in *AFP* 3:107, 1971.
31. Smith B: Pectoral hair in cirrhosis. *Amer J Gastroenterol* 55:387–390, 1971.
32. Knoblauch M, et al: Emergency endoscopy in acute upper gastrointestinal hemorrhage. *Schweiz Med Wochenschr* 103:731–733, 1973.
33. Thorn G: Lecture at the Thirteenth VSC Postgraduate Refresher Course, Honolulu, Hawaii, 1970.

GENERAL STUDY AIDS

Medak, McGrew, Burkalow and Trecke: Atlas of Oral Cytology. Public Health Service Publication No. 1949 ($4.75). Order from U.S. Govt. Printing Office, Washington, D.C. 20402.

Marks C: Diaphragmatic hernia. *Med Times* 97:145–158, 1969.

Berk JE: Management of uncomplicated duodenal ulcer. *AFP* 1:101–110, 1970.

Ingelfinger FJ: Gastric function. *Nutr Today* 6:2–10, 1971.

Shatz B, Barre AE: Medical and surgical aspects of hiatus hernia. *JAMA* 214:125, 1970.

Fromm H, et al: Granulomatous bowel (Crohn's) disease. *Arch Intern Med* 128:739–745, 1971.

Clinician-2: Liver disease. Booklet published by Medcome learning systems, 2 Hammarskjold Plaza, NY 10017, and Searle and Co, 1971.

CHAPTER 13

Principles of Cancer Detection

The cancer detection examination is no more than a regular physical examination with emphasis given to certain detection techniques. The American Cancer Society's *seven danger signals* are criteria the family physician as well as his patient should remember. They are:

- –any sore that does not heal
- –a lump or thickening in the breast or elsewhere
- –unusual bleeding or discharge
- –any change in a wart or mole
- –persistent indigestion or difficulty in swallowing
- –persistent hoarseness or cough
- –any change in normal bowel habits

These danger signals and what they represent have been discussed in detail in previous chapters pertaining to specific parts or functions of the body. Use the Table of Contents or Index to find these subjects.

In your search for cancer, give emphasis to the following:

- –Papanicolaou cervical smear
- –sigmoidoscopic examination
- –stool test for blood
- –barium enema
- –gastrointestinal series of x-rays
- –x-ray of the chest
- –mammography

Cancer of the colon and rectum is the most common internal cancer of the body, (see Chapter 12), ranking ahead of cancers of the breast, cervix or lung. Rather than looking for textbook signs and symptoms of cancer of the colon, look for:

- –slight blood spotting or streaking or a little mucous or watery seepage or no blood at all
- –slight abdominal discomfort
- –recent change in bowel habits
- –slight tenderness localized over the course of the colon

These symptoms should suggest cancer even in the presence of hemorrhoids.

A digital examination can only reach to the 9 cm level and is inadequate in detecting lesions less than 2 to 3 cm in diameter, pedunculated polyps or soft villus adenomas. *Sigmoidoscopic examination* performed under proper conditions with the bowel thoroughly clean, should visualize practically all lesions 2 mm or larger of the rectum and lower sigmoid colon.

A stool test for blood is a necessary test. And a *barium enema* is indicated in all patients with blood positive stools whether the sigmoidoscopic examination is negative or positive. Don't forget to do a barium enema bowel study when a polyp is found by sigmoidoscopic examination because the chance of lesions higher in the bowel is increased. If the colon is not too redundant nor reduplicated and is free of all fecal matter and decompressed, a radiologist with good equipment should be able to detect any lesion of the colon that is 5 mm or larger.

A *gastrointestinal series of x-rays* is mandatory on all hypochlorhydric patients.

Further information on *roentgenography of the chest* is given in Chapter 11.

The percentage of 5 year survivals in cancer of the cervix decreases from 70 in stage I to only 6.7 in stage IV. Therefore it is of vital importance to detect this cancer early. Regular *Papanicolaou smears* are extremely helpful in diagnosing cancer. Studies have also confirmed that there is a better than 75 percent accuracy rate in detecting endometrial adenocarcinoma with the Pap smear; however, a high percentage of the latter cases are also symptomatic.

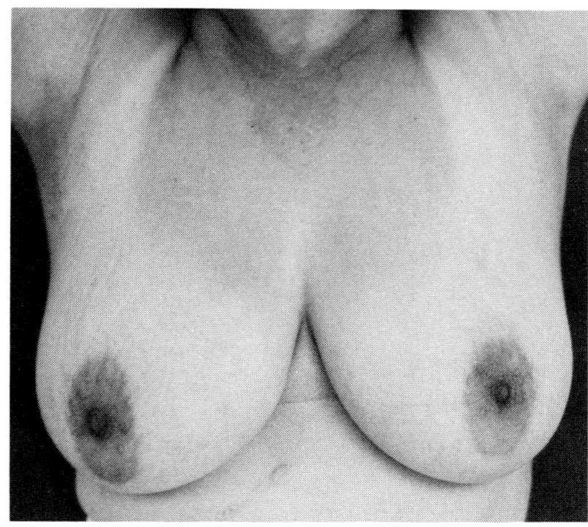

Figure 13-1. The patient tenses her pectoral muscles for inspection.

DETECTION OF BREAST CANCER

Breast Examination

Start your inspection of the patient's breasts with the patient in an upright position. Her arms should be at rest initially and then elevated. Ask her to tense her pectoral muscles (Fig. 13-1) by pressing her palms together or by pressing her hands on her hips.

Next, inspect her breasts for changes in contour, dimpling or nipple retraction. Examine her with her arms elevated first. Then have her lean forward (Fig. 13-2) while you inspect the skin for dimpling or nipple retraction. Palpate the axilla for enlarged nodes (Fig. 13-3). While you are doing this the patient should rest her forearm on yours.

Ask the patient to lie back in the supine position with a pillow under her back at chest level. Palpate her breasts for tumors (Fig. 13-4). Milk the nipples (Fig. 13-5) to express possible blood in secretions for cytologic study when questionable.

Teach the patient to inspect her own breasts. Have her lie supine with one hand

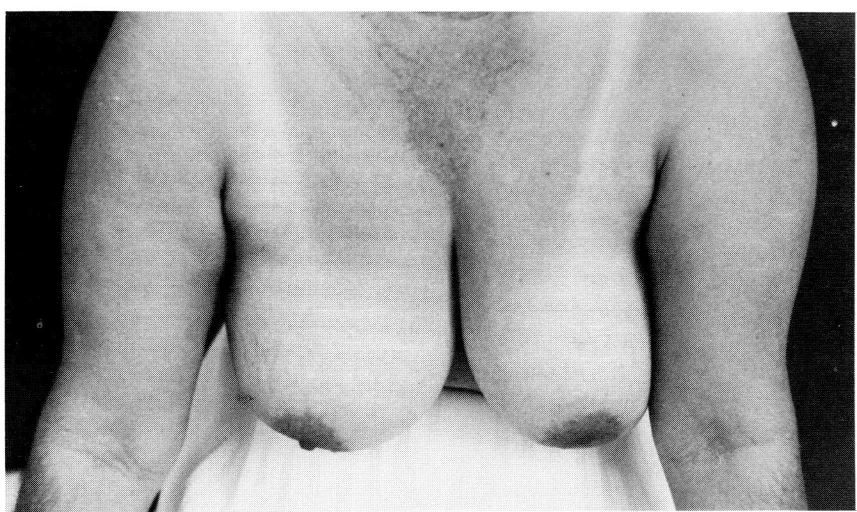

Figure 13-2. The patient leans forward for inspection of the skin for retraction.

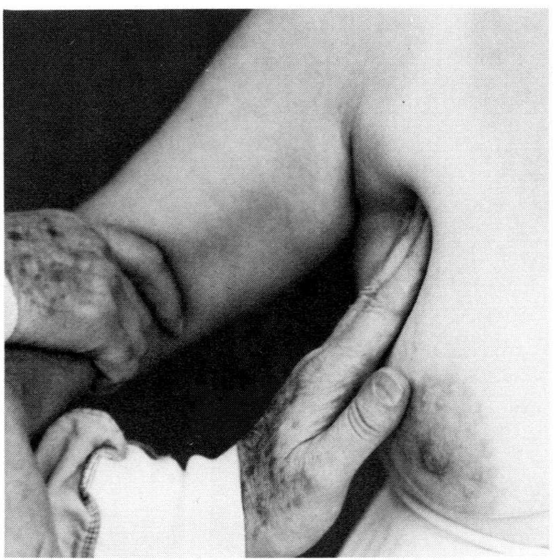

Figure 13-3. While the patient rests her forearm on your arm, palpate the axilla for enlarged nodes.

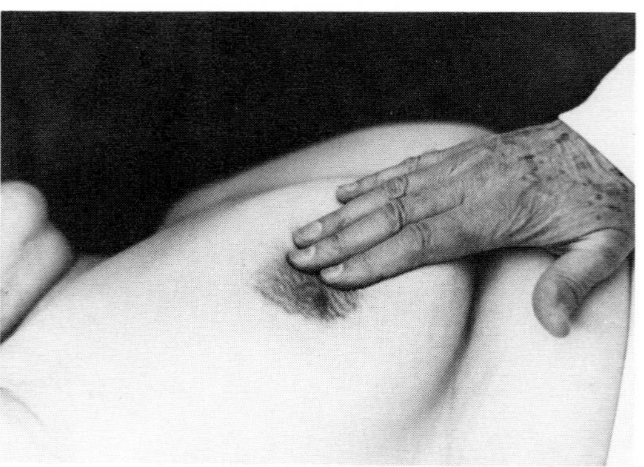

Figure 13-4. Palpate her breasts for tumors.

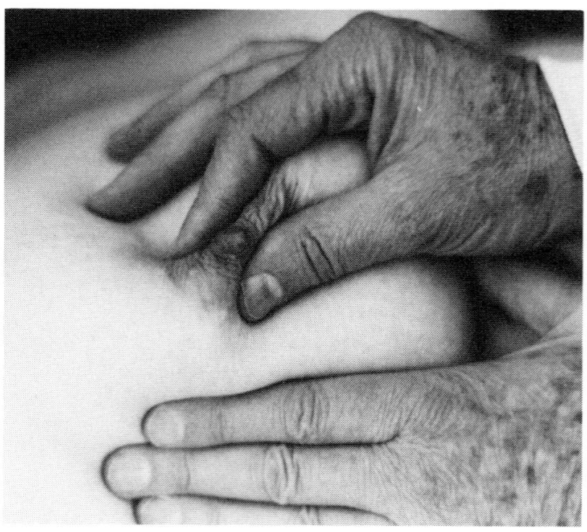

Figure 13-5. Milk the nipple to express secretions.

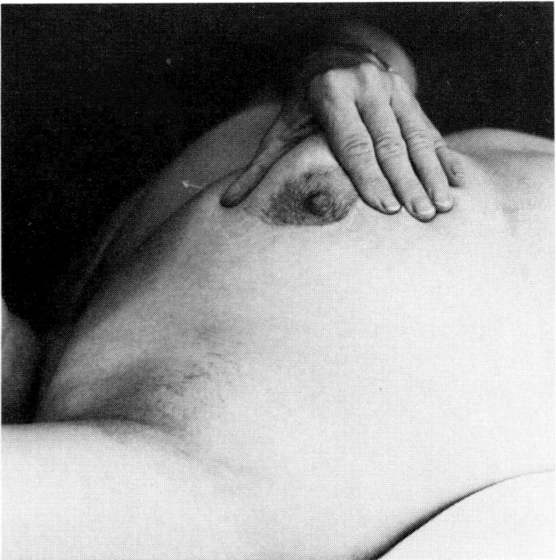

Figure 13-6. The patient should learn to inspect her own breasts.

behind her head and a pillow under her back. Have her feel her breast with her opposite hand with flattened fingers (Fig. 13-6). Tell her to go from quadrant to quadrant. Emphasize the light touch. Have her repeat the procedure while sitting up, still keeping her hand behind her head.

Needle Aspiration of Breast Cysts

Cysts of the breast are variable. They may be single or multiple. The mass is round and smooth and is movable. Aspirate the cyst or cysts for further study.

Anesthetize the area over the tumor with 1 percent lidocaine. Fasten the cyst between the second and third fingers of your free hand while tapping the cyst with the syringe (Fig. 13-7). Aspirate every drop of fluid from the cyst.

Mammography

Mammography is a debatable routine measure because 15 to 20 percent of the false-positives or negatives must be recognized as positive.

However, mammography should be routine in the woman who has had a mastectomy for carcinoma of one breast. Recent mammographic studies indicate that ap-

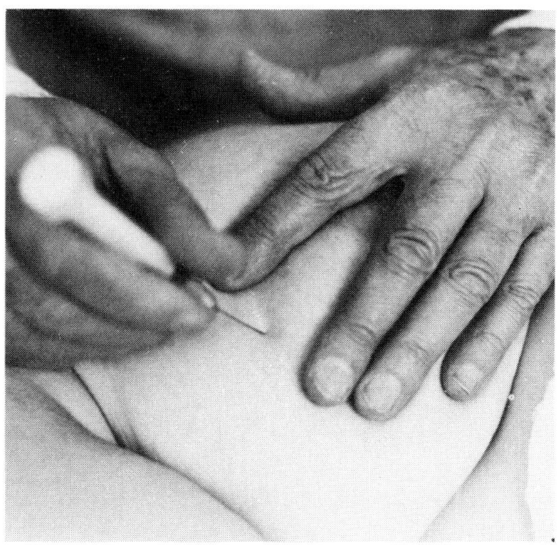

Figure 13-7. Tap the cyst while it is fastened between the second and third fingers of your free hand.

proximately 3 percent of all patients with cancer of the breast when first seen by the family physician have simultaneous bilateral primary carcinoma. This makes somewhat of a case in favor of doing mammograms when the patient is first seen. Another recent use of roentgenology is in helping the pathologist choose the proper area for pathologic examinations when taking a surgical biopsy or specimen.

In benign conditions such as fibrocystic disease, repeated mammography may help detect an early cancer. The use of mammography in high-risk patients results in an earlier finding of cancer in more patients and an earlier finding of localized cancer. If a suspected diagnosis is not obvious by mammography of one breast, do mammography on the opposite breast.

Some patients are not suitable for operative procedures. Mammography may aid in planning hormonal therapy or chemotherapy for these patients and in checking progress from time to time.

Postoperative roentgenology may aid in determining whether the cancer has been completely removed. The pathologist may use the x-ray examination to help determine the exact area for pathologic study.

Appendices

APPENDIX 1

Prevention of Malpractice Claims

The key to prevention of malpractice claims lies in maintaining current, accurate, adequate and legible records. Consent forms are part of your records. Be certain they are properly and legally executed. The patient must be informed as to hazards and prognosis in order to give his *informed consent*. Some patients will not understand unless procedures are explained to them as you would to a child.

Arrive at an understanding in advance as to your professional fees and do only those procedures which you are competent to perform. Be certain the pathology or symptoms warrant the procedure and document the pathology in writing. If you have any questions, seek capable consultation. If something unforeseen does happen or if complications do occur, explain it carefully in writing.

When a patient brings up the treatment or conduct of another physician, medical ethics require that you conduct the conversation as though the second doctor were present and hearing all that is said.

Be kind and sympathetic. Patients who have been grossly mistreated often stop legal action because of a physician's empathy. Remember you are not infallible. Be humble but confident. Answer to the best of your ability the questions of unhappy patients.

There will be patients with whom you are incompatible. Don't wear down your nerves or those of your patient by attempting to force a comfortable physician-patient relationship. Talk it over with the patient matter-of-factly. He may not relate to your method of practice; if so, sever the relationship as quickly and easily as possible. However, if the patient has a continuing problem, he must be given reasonable time to seek medical advice elsewhere. If the patient is unusually belligerent, sever your relationship with him by documented correspondence.

The emergency room can be a source of litigation because family physicians often have no on-going relationship with emergency room patients. Be certain the ER record is filled out completely. If the present ER recording system is inadequate, seek administrative help in providing an adequate record. Emergency room supervisors now are devising ER records that give the patient a signed carbon copy of the written follow-up instructions. Then if the patient loses his copy or throws it away, it's his neglect, not yours or the hospital's.

Remember, you assume *total* responsibility the moment you undertake to diagnose and treat a patient. Even though the patient arrives in an emergency situation, your responsibility to his total health is not lessened. Do not cut corners, no matter how medically logical it may seem at the time. What does this mean?

- –You will perform an adequate physical examination on the injured patient.
- –You will follow up on all signs and symptoms of illness offered by the patient.

- –You will make every effort to diagnose any medical condition brought to your attention. (The law expects you as a physician to be able to translate even vague complaints into diagnostic leads.)
- –You will ensure that the patient seeks out and obtains continuous and proper therapy after your emergency treatment.
- –You will inform the patient of the consequences should he fail to obtain the proper diagnostic follow-up.

You may transfer the patient to another physician with his consent. The patient's request for such a transfer or his desire to return to his family physician constitutes such a consent. But the burden of proof remains on you to show you were not negligent in seeing that the patient was given that opportunity. In most areas of the United States you can no longer claim that no true doctor-patient relationship existed even if the contact was a one-time insurance examination or a camp check-up.

CONFIDENTIALITY

Requests for patient information usually come from one of the following: relatives (patients, sponsors and others), insurance carriers for sickness benefits, employers to verify absences, schools for pupil records, police in emergency situations, Internal Revenue Service, and the inquisitive.

Unfortunately there are no fixed rules of confidentiality. Neither state laws nor the code of medical ethics helps much in specific cases. Court decisions are often split decisions, changing from state to state and from day to day. So, unless you feel a powerful moral obligation to disclose without the patient's consent, don't do so if you want to stay out of court. If you are in doubt, do not disclose. You may later find disclosure would be to the patient's best interest. Fortunately, your hard-nose stance can be altered. You have taken a reversible decision. But, if you have divulged confidential information, there is no retraction.

Think of the patient's records as belonging to him and, if you do so, although there are exceptions, you will make few mistakes. If needed, discuss the pros and cons of disclosure with the patient.

Family physicians do not like to be "taken" any more than others. They resent being asked by a patient to aid in defrauding an insurance company or in avoiding the military draft. So far there is no ethical way you can inform either without the patient's consent.

In the following states there are no legally protected patient-doctor privileges:

Alabama	Massachusetts
Connecticut	New Hampshire
Delaware	New Jersey
Florida	Rhode Island
Georgia	South Carolina
Kentucky	Tennessee
Maine	Texas
Maryland	Vermont

At this writing, in the other 34 states you don't have to reveal in court what you have learned during the doctor-patient relationship.

Occasionally the patient's right to privacy may conflict with your own legal obligations such as when the Public Health Department demands reports. Outright refusal to report in such instances will put you in a legally untenable position. If a full discussion with the patient does not put his mind at ease regarding the harmlessness of the report, perhaps a discussion with the public health officer will get you off the hook. Suggest a delayed report, if nothing else.

No matter what you do, when the law is not involved, get written authorization from the patient before divulging information. Adhere to this rule even when requests come from other doctors. Unless the physician to whom you are referring the patient sends a signed release of information, contact the patient and ask for authorization. If this is not convenient, write the physician and ask him to send you the patient authorization. Then, when you do send a patient's record to a third party, photocopy what was sent and make a note of the authorization in your records.

Although a patient has a third party contract, the agreement is between the two of them. The contract does not authorize you to disclose any of your records to the third party. Your receptionist can solve this by having the patient sign a blanket authorization listing to whom reports can be sent.

It has been comforting to me to know that patients do not need to tell everything about their entire lives and that of their forebearers. If the patient wishes, and you are in agreement, he can limit his authorization to pertinent matters. If this was more commonly recognized, it could put a crimp on the habit of sending commercial photographers to photograph the complete medical, family and past history of individuals.

In refusing to disclose information, be certain you are not denying your patient needed benefits or are not placing obstacles in his path. You may be right, but you may be straining your relationship with your patient.

How about information concerning parents and their children? Minors can now contract independently for medical services. This especially applies to minors with VD. Most states now permit you to treat patients as young as 16 for VD without informing their parents. But you will be wise to counsel the minor and suggest he inform his parents or allow you to do so if the parents' behavior warrants such information.

Confidentiality of husband-wife information is another area of which physicians generally are unaware. Husbands and wives cannot be treated as one in privileged communications matters. A husband or wife can demand that privileged information not be given to the spouse without his written consent.

The police have a right to information during an emergency only. This has been interpreted to mean while the patient is in the emergency room. Later in the hospital, if the police seek more information, delay disclosure until the patient gives his authorization or the police obtain a court order.

The same pertains to the IRS. You need not budge until a court order is obtained. Even court orders need not be heeded without a due interval. If you and your patient feel strongly about the disclosure, ask an attorney to appeal the order.

Occasionally problems occur over sending a copy of your medical records to a school to which a patient is seeking admission. Although the patient is willing, the wise course is to seek his authorization. He may prefer to send a restricted report that would delete information not pertinent to his pursuing academic goals. And, if at all possible, send the information to a physician in the health service rather than to a registrar where the information is open to all personnel.

SOME COMMON MALPRACTICE CLAIMS

The following are some common malpractice claims. It is wise for the physician to familiarize himself with the list.

- –Missed diagnosis
- –Failure to use roentgenology
- –Overdose of medication
- –Too tight a cast
- –Unsuccessful reduction of fracture or dislocation
- –Foreign objects left in patient during surgery
- –Unauthorized surgery
- –Unsightly scars from surgery
- –Improper suturing
- –Lack of informed consent
- –Infiltration of medicine during IV therapy
- –Surgical complications
- –Adverse drug reaction
- –Nerve injury following injections
- –Childhood deaths following poisoning or insect bites because of delayed or inadequate treatment
- –Nerve and muscle damage following use of restraints
- –Complications of cesarean section
- –Improper treatment
- –Denial of abortion following rubella exposure
- –Delay in reporting PAP results
- –Failure of fallopian tube ligation or resection

- –Complications of transfusions
- –Failure to remove barium after x-ray examination
- –Failure to repeat x-ray studies when needed
- –Cardiac arrest during tonsillectomy resulting in brain damage
- –Commitment for psychiatric care based on mistaken diagnosis
- –Delay in obtaining bronchoscopic removal of a foreign object in infant's lungs
- –Damage to nerve root following spinal anesthesia
- –Failure to test for phenylketonuria (in some states)

CONTRIBUTORY NEGLIGENCE

The legal definition of contributory negligence is "conduct on the part of the plaintiff, contributing as a legal cause to the harm he has suffered, which falls below the standard to which he is required to conform for his own protection." In other words, part of the patient's disability is his own fault.

In most states, negligence by the patient, if it occurs at the same time as negligence by the physician, precludes the patient from collecting any damages. An example: When a patient is requested to return for care and fails to do so, he is contributing to negligence and obviously cannot collect damages from the physician when his condition does not improve.

Physicians often seek refuge in contributory negligence. But they would do well to remember that the average intelligent rational patient may lose all of his rationality and some of his sense when he becomes ill. In addition, patients are frequently sedated or mentally or psychologically incapacitated during an illness. In determining whether a patient can be considered as contributing to his disability, his physical and emotional condition at the time must be evaluated. Therefore, the physician may not have a defense to a negligence charge simply because the patient disobeyed his orders. This is particularly true if the patient is not entirely dependable.

THE LIABILITY OF MISDIAGNOSIS

Generally a misdiagnosis is not actionable unless you do not use due care in determining the diagnosis. An instance of this is if the patient's symptoms warrant the performance of specific x-rays and laboratory tests and you did not do them or if you fail to use standard tests.

If you base your diagnosis on standard tests, usually you will not be held liable, even if your diagnosis is wrong. If you know, however, that the tests or their results are highly suspicious, you are obligated to solve any discrepancies. You may be liable if you do not pursue *further* examination when x-ray films indicate a problem exists.

A misdiagnosis does not present a liability unless the delay caused by the incorrect diagnosis causes damage. There must be some "causal connection" between the failure to diagnose and later damage. If no recovery was possible with the correct diagnosis, then a misdiagnosis is not actionable. And, if you have misdiagnosed the patient's illness, there is no liability if the treatment is right, even if given for the wrong reasons.

APPENDIX 2

*Family Practice Library**

FAMILY PRACTICE TEXTBOOKS

Eimerl TS, Laidlaw J: *Handbook for Research in General Practice,* ed. 2 Baltimore: Williams & Wilkins, 1969, $7.75.
Geyman JP: *The Modern Family Doctor and Changing Medical Practice.* New York: Appleton-Century-Crofts, 1971, $8.95.

ADOLESCENT MEDICINE

Daniel Jr, WA: *The Adolescent Patient.* St. Louis: C.V. Mosby, 1970, $20.50.
Gallagher, JR: *Medical Care of the Adolescent,* ed 2. New York: Appleton-Century-Crofts, 1966, $17.40.

COMMUNICABLE DISEASES

Brown WJ et al: *Syphilis and Other Venereal Diseases.* Cambridge: Harvard University Press, 1970, $8.00.
Committee on Infectious Diseases, American Academy of Pediatrics. Report of the Committee on Infectious Diseases, ed 16. Evanston: American Academy of Pediatrics, 1970, $2.00.

EMERGENCY CARE

Blakemore WS, Fitts WT: *Management of the Injured Patient.* New York: Harper and Row, 1969, $14.50.
Flint Jr, T, Cain HD: *Emergency Treatment and Management,* ed 4. Philadelphia: W.B. Saunders, 1970, $11.50.
Dreisbach RH: *Handbook of Poisoning: Diagnosis and Treatment,* ed 7. Los Altos: Lange Medical Publications, 1971, $6.00
Varga C: *Handbook of Pediatric Medical Emergencies,* ed 4. St. Louis: C.V. Mosby, 1968, $19.75.

FAMILY COUNSELING AND FAMILY DYNAMICS

Bell NW, Vogel EF (eds): *A Modern Introduction to the Family,* ed 2. New York: Macmillan, 1968, $11.50.
Satir VM: *Conjoint Family Therapy,* ed 2. Palo Alto: Science and Behavior Books, 1967, $5.95.

GENETIC COUNSELING

Gellis S, Finegold M: *Atlas of Mental Retardation Syndromes.* Washington: Superintendent of Documents, U. S. Government Printing Office, #1968-0-310-072, 1968, $5.50.
Valentine GH: *Chromosome Disorders: An Introduction for Clinicians,* ed 2. Philadelphia: J. B. Lippincott, 1970, $8.00.

*Reprinted from Lawrence DA: Selected recent books of interest to the practicing family physician. Calif Acad Gen Pract 23:11–14, 1972, with permission.

GERIATRICS AND THANATOLOGY

Anderson WF: *Practical Management of the Elderly,* ed 2. Philadelphia: F. A. Davis, 1971, $12.50.

Cowdry EV, Steinberg FU: *The Care of the Geriatric Patient.* St. Louis: C. V. Mosby, 1971, $22.75.

Kubler-Ross E: *On Death and Dying.* New York: Macmillan, 1970, $1.95.

Pearson L (ed): *Death and Dying: Current Issues in the Treatment of the Dying Person.* Cleveland: The Press of Case Western Reserve University, 1969, $6.95.

INDUSTRIAL MEDICINE

Mayers MR: *Occupational Health: Hazards of the Work Environment.* Baltimore: Williams & Wilkins, 1969, $17.50.

Adams RM: *Occupational Contact Dermatitis.* Philadelphia: J. B. Lippincott, 1969, $16.50.

INTERVIEWING TECHNIQUES

Browne K, Freeling P: *The Doctor-Patient Relationship.* Baltimore: Williams & Wilkins, 1967, $4.25.

Castelnuovo-Tedesco P: *The Twenty-Minute Hour.* Boston: Little, Brown, 1965, $8.50.

Lewin K: *Brief Encounters: Brief Psychotherapy.* St. Louis: W. H. Green, 1970, $15.00.

Harris TA: *I'm OK; You're OK: A Practical Guide to Transactional Analysis.* New York: Harper and Row, 1969, $5.95.

Chapman AH: *The Physician's Guide to the Management of Emotional Problems.* Philadelphia: J. B. Lippincott, 1969, $11.00.

Froelich RE, Bishop FM: *Medical Interviewing: A Programmed Manual,* ed. 2. St. Louis: C. V. Mosby, 1972, $5.35.

LEGAL MEDICINE AND MEDICAL ETHICS

Moritz AR, and Morris RC: *Handbook of Legal Medicine,* ed 3. St. Louis: C. V. Mosby, 1970, $9.50.

Torrey EF: *Ethical Issues in Medicine: The Role of the Physician in Today's Society.* Boston: Little, Brown, 1968, $9.50.

MARITAL AND SEXUAL COUNSELING

Klemer RH: *Counseling in Marital and Sexual Problems*—A Physician's Handbook. Baltimore: Williams & Wilkins, 1965, $11.00.

Lederer WJ, Jackson DD: *The Mirages of Marriage.* New York: W. W. Norton, 1968, $10.00.

Calderone MS (ed): *Manual of Family Planning and Contraceptive Practice* ed. 2. Baltimore: Williams & Wilkins, 1970, $14.50.

Bing E: *Six Practical Lessons for an Easier Childbirth.* New York: Bantam Books, 1969, $1.00.

OFFICE GYNECOLOGY

Greenhill JP: *Office Gynecology,* ed 9. Chicago: Year Book Medical Publishers, 1971, $21.50.

OFFICE MEDICAL RECORDS

Bjorn JC, Cross HD: *The Problem-Oriented Private Practice of Medicine.* Chicago: Modern Hospital Press, 1970, $2.75.

Sharp CL: *Presymptomatic Detection and Early Diagnosis,* ed 2. Baltimore: Williams & Wilkins, 1968, $19.00.

Weed LL: *Medical Records, Medical Education and Patient Care.* Chicago: Year Book Medical Publishers, 1970, $10.95.

ORTHOPEDIC SURGERY AND SPORTS MEDICINE

Kraus H: *Clinical Treatment of Back and Neck Pain.* New York: McGraw-Hill, 1970, $13.00.

O'Donoghue DH: *Treatment of Injuries to Athletes,* ed 2. Philadelphia: W. B. Saunders, 1970, $22.00.

Flatt AE: *Care of the Rheumatoid Hand,* ed 2. St. Louis: C. V. Mosby, 1968, $16.50.

PEDIATRICS

Bakwin H, Bakwin RM: *Clinical Management of Behavior Disorders in Children,* ed 4. Philadelphia: W. B. Saunders, 1972, $17.50.

Green M, Richmond JB: *Pediatric Diagnosis,* ed 3. Philadelphia: W. B. Saunders, 1968, $15.00.

Schaffer AJ, Avery M: *Diseases of the Newborn,* ed 3. Philadelphia: W. B. Saunders, 1971, $27.50.

PRESCRIPTION MEDICINES

Council on Drugs, American Medical Association. AMA Drug Evaluations. Chicago: American Medical Association, 1971, $15.00.

Burack R: *The New Handbook of Prescription Drugs,* ed 2. New York: Ballantine Books, 1970, $1.25.

SURGERY

Ferguson LK: *Surgery of the Ambulatory Patient,* ed 4. Philadelphia: J. B. Lippincott, 1966, $17.00.

Cope Z: *The Early Diagnosis of the Acute Abdomen,* ed 14. New York: Oxford University Press, 1972, $6.95.

GENERAL REFERENCES

Stearns S, Ratcliff W: An integrated health-science core library for physicians, nurses and allied health practitioners in community hospitals. *N Eng J Med* 283: 1489–1498, 1970.

Brandon N: Selected lists of books and journals for the small medical library. *Bull Med Library Assoc* 57:130–150, 1969.

APPENDIX 3

*Reading List in Sex Education for Teenagers**

Calderone: *Married Teenager*. New York: SIECUS (Sex Information and Education Council U.S.).

Duvall EM: *Love and the Facts of Life*. New York: Association Press, 1963.

Duvall EM: *Why Wait Till Marriage*. New York: Association Press, 1965.

Duvall EM, Hill R: *When You Marry*. New York: Association Press, 1962.

Johnson EW: *Sex and Love in Plain Language*. Philadelphia: J.B. Lippincott.

Johnson: *Masturbation*. New York: SIECUS (Sex Information and Education Council U.S.).

Johnson WR, Belzer EG: *Human Sexual Behavior and Sex Education*. Philadelphia: Lea and Febiger, 1973.

Kirkendall: *Sex Education*. New York: SIECUS (Sex Information and Education Council U.S.).

Kirkendall LA: *Too Young to Marry*. Pamphlet #236. New York: Public Affairs Committee Inc.

Kirkendall LA, Osborne RF: *Dating Tips for Teens*. Chicago: Science Research Associates.

Levinson F, Kelly GL: *What Teenagers Want to Know*. Chicago: Budlong Press.

Mace D: *What Makes a Marriage Happy*. Pamphlet #290. New York: Public Affairs Committee Inc.

Semmens JP, Krantz: *Adolescent Experience – A Counseling Guide to Social and Sexual Behavior*. New York: Macmillan, 1970.

Semmens JP, Lamers W: *Teenage Pregnancy*. Springfield: Charles C Thomas, 1968.

Semmens JP, Semmens FJ: Sex education of the adolescent female. *Pediatr Clin N Am* Vol. 19, 1972.

Sociology I—Teachers Guide for Family Living Instruction. Hayward, Ca: Hayward Unified School District.

*Adapted from Semmens JP: Patient Care 2:39, 1968.

APPENDIX 4

Diets

TABLE A. SALT AND CALORIES IN COMMON FOODS*

Low in Salt	*Usual Serving*	*Salt Units*†	*Cal*
MEAT, EGGS AND SUBSTITUTES			
Beef ground	1 med patty (3 oz)	1	225
Beef, lean (steak or roast)	1 large piece (3 oz)	2½	225
Chicken or turkey	¼ fryer (3 oz) or 2 large slices	1	225
Egg	1	1	75
Fish, fresh or frozen (no breading)	1 med piece (3 oz)	1	225
Lamb, fresh	1 med piece (3 oz)	2	225
Liver, heart, kidney	1 large slice (3 oz)	1	225
Peanut butter	2 tbs	1	190
Pork, fresh (chop or steak)	1 piece (3 oz)	1	225
Veal, fresh	1 large slice (3 oz)	3	225
Avoid: High in salt, calories, or both			
Bacon	2 slices	2	90
Bologna, salami, all lunch meat	3 slices	10	225
Canned and potted meats	1 slice (3 oz)	20	274
Frankfurters	3 med	11	225
Ham hocks, salt pork	1 piece	18	395
Sausage, all kinds	2 med patties (3 oz)	19	476
Tuna fish	¼ cup (2 oz)	8	144
MILK AND CHEESE			
Cheese, cheddar	1½ slices (1½ oz)	6	113
Cheese, cottage	½ cup	5	150
Milk, evaporated canned	½ cup	2¼	170
Milk, powdered skim	1/3 cup	3½	80
Milk, skim	1 cup	2¼	90
Milk, whole	1 cup	2¼	170
Avoid: High in salt			
Buttermilk	1 cup	6	90
Cheese, American	1 slice (1 oz)	8	75
Cheese, Velveeta	1 oz	8	90
Cheese, other	1 oz	7–10	75–90

*Reprinted from Flowers, Jr, CE: How to persuade pregnant women to diet.
†One salt unit equals 50 mg of sodium.

TABLE A—*Continued*

Low in Salt	*Usual Serving*	*Salt Units†*	*Cal*
VEGETABLES			
All fresh and frozen vegetables and canned tomatoes			
Beans and peas, dried	½ cup	0	70
Cauliflower, cabbage, okra	1 cup	0	30
Celery (limit: 11 servings per day)	1 stalk	2	2
Corn, fresh or frozen	⅓ cup	0	70
Green beans, fresh or frozen	½ cup	0	30
Green peas, carrots, fresh or frozen	½ cup	0	35
Lettuce	1 cup	0	15
Mustard, turnip, and collard greens	1 cup	0	30
Potato, sweet	¼ cup	0	70
Potato, white	1 small or ½ cup	0	70
Squash, summer	1 cup	0	30
Squash, winter	½ cup	0	35
Tomato, canned	½ cup	2	19
Tomato, fresh	1 med	0	30
Turnips, beets	½ cup	0	35
Avoid: High in salt			
All canned vegetables except tomatoes			
Beets, canned	½ cup	5	20
Green peas, canned	½ cup	4	35
Lima beans, canned	½ cup	5	70
Olives	5	12	35
Pickles, all kinds	1 med	14	15–30
Pork and beans	½ cup	9	125
Sauerkraut	½ cup	12	20
Soups, canned and powdered	2/3 cup (5 oz)	10	70
FRUITS, FRESH			
All low in salt			
Apple	1 med	0	40
Banana	½	0	40
Canteloupe	¼	0	40
Grapefruit	½ or ½ cup juice	0	40
Grapes	12	0	40
Lemon	1 med	0	40
Orange	1 small or ½ cup juice	0	40
Peach	1 med	0	40
Pear	1 small	0	40
Raisins	2 tbs	0	40
Strawberries	1 cup	0	40
Tangerine	1 large	0	40
BREAD, CEREALS, AND SUBSTITUTES			
Biscuit	1 small	2½	70
Bread, white or whole wheat	1 slice	2½	70
Cereals, cooked	½ cup	0	70
Cereals, dry (puffed rice, wheat, shredded wheat)	¾ cup	0	70
Corn bread	1½-in	3	70
Grits, rice, spaghetti	½ cup	0	70
Tortilla, corn	2 6-in	2	70
Tortilla, flour	1 med	2½	70

†One salt unit equals 50 mg of sodium.

TABLE A—*Continued*

Low in Salt	*Usual Serving*	*Salt Units*†	*Cal*
BREADS, CEREALS, AND SUBSTITUTES—Continued			
Avoid: High in salt			
Cereals, dry (cornflakes)	¾ cup	9	70
Cereals, dry (all others)	¾ cup	9–12	70
Crackers, all kinds: saltines, soda, Ritz	4–6	3–5	80–170
Doughnut, sweet roll	1	2½	135
Pancakes	2 med	5	120
Potato chips, Fritos	12	3	110
FATS			
Butter	1 tsp	1	45
Cooking oil	1 tsp	0	45
Lard	1 tsp	0	45
Margarine	1 tsp	1	45
Mayonnaise	1 tsp	1	45
DESSERTS			
Avoid: High in salt and calories			
Cake	2-in section	5	370
Candy bar	1	3–4	175
Cookies	4	7	480
Ice cream	½ cup	2	155
Jell-O	½ cup	5	95
Pie	1/7	2	200–300
SEASONINGS AND MISCELLANEOUS			
Chili sauce	1 tbs	0	0
Garlic, powdered, fresh	as desired	0	0
Onion, fresh	1 tbs	0	0
Pepper, black	as desired	0	0
Pepper, green	1 med	0	15
Vinegar	1 tbs	0	0
Avoid: high in salt, calories, or both			
Accent	½ tsp	6	0
Baking powder and soda	½ tsp	10	0
Catsup	2 tsp	5	17
Mustard	2 tsp	5	17
Seasoned meat tenderizer	½ tsp	5	0
Seasoning salts (celery, onion, garlic)	½ tsp	12	0
Sugar	2 tsp	0	30

†One salt unit equals 50 mg of sodium.

TABLE B. TYPICAL DAY'S DIET FOR A PREGNANT WOMAN*

	Salt Units†	*Cal*
Breakfast		
Citrus juice or fruit (1 cup, orange)	0	80
Egg (1 poached)	1	75
Cereal or bread (1 slice, toasted)	2½	70
Fat (1 tsp margarine)	1	45
Milk (1 cup)	2¼	170
Other beverage (1 cup black coffee)	0	0
Lunch		
Meat dish (1 3-oz hamburger patty)	1	225
Vegetable salad (1 serving lettuce and tomato salad)	0	15
Bread (2 slices)	5	140
Fat (1 tsp margarine)	1	45
Beverage (1 cup tea without cream or sugar)	0	0
Snack		
Fruit (1 med apple)	0	40
Milk (1 cup)	2¼	170
Dinner		
Meat dish (¼ baked chicken)	2	225
Vegetable, green or yellow (1½ cup, carrots)	0	35
Cereal or substitute (½ cup rice)	0	70
Bread (1 serving corn bread)	3	70
Fat (1 tsp margarine)	1	45
Snack		
Fruit (12 grapes)	0	40
Milk (1 cup)	2¼	170
Daily allowance of salt for seasoning (¼ tsp placed in saltshaker each day)	12	0
	36¼	1730

*Reprinted from Flowers, Jr, CE: How to persuade pregnant women to diet. Consultant July–Aug. 1967, p. 20–22, with permission.

†One salt unit equals 50 mg of sodium.

TABLE C. DIET IN UREMIA (Seven Day Menus)*

	Day One	*Day Two*	*Day Three*	*Day Four*
BREAKFAST	⅓ cup drained canned grapefruit sections with 1 maraschino cherry 1⅓ cups puffed rice 1 slice salt-free toast 1 tsp salt-free margarine 1 tsp apple jelly ½ cup milk 3½ tsp sugar 1 cup coffee	½ cup low-potassium orange drink 1 fried egg† 1 slice salt-free toast 2 tsp salt-free margarine 1 tbsp apple jelly 1 tbsp half-and-half 3½ tsp sugar 1 cup coffee	2 drained canned figs 1 scrambled egg† 1 slice salt-free toast 2 tsp salt-free margarine 1 tbsp jelly 3½ tsp sugar 1 cup coffee	⅓ cup drained canned grapefruit sections 1 scrambled egg† 1 slice salt-free toast 2 tsp salt-free margarine 1 tbsp grape jelly 3½ tsp sugar 1 cup coffee
DINNER	1 deviled egg† ¼ cup buttered potatoes† ½ cup lettuce with 2 tbsp salt-free mayonnaise 2 drained canned pear halves with 1 tbsp grape jelly in center 1 serving instant chocolate ice cream ½ cup Kool-Aid	1 English muffin ⅔ cup sautéed spiced apples ½ cup drained buttered wax beans† 1 tsp salt-free margarine 1 tbsp honey ⅓ cup drained fruit cocktail ½ cup milk	1 cup vegetable rice soup ½ cup lettuce with salt-free croutons, 2 tbsp salt-free mayonnaise and ¼ chopped egg† 1 drained canned peach half ½ slice salt-free bread 2 tsp salt-free margarine 1 tbsp jelly 1 iced cupcake ½ cup milk	1 serving stuffed green pepper with tomato sauce ¼ cup drained buttered carrots† 2 slices drained canned pineapple with 1 tbsp salt-free mayonnaise 1 strawberry tart with 1 tbsp whipped topping ½ cup cranberry juice
SUPPER	Omelet (1 egg)† ½ cup drained buttered green beans† ½ med cucumber with 1 tbsp vinegar and 1 tbsp oil ¼ cup drained frozen strawberries with 2 tsp powdered sugar 3½ tsp sugar 1 cup tea	1 sliced hard-cooked egg† ⅓ cup drained buttered asparagus† 1 small sweet potato with 21 miniature marshmallows ½ slice salt-free bread 1 tsp salt-free margarine 1 tbsp apple jelly 2 drained canned apricot halves 1 serving instant strawberry ice cream 3½ tsp sugar 1 cup tea	Omelet (1 egg)† ¼ cup drained buttered cabbage† ¼ cup drained buttered tomatoes† 1 corn pone 2 tsp salt-free margarine 1 tbsp grape jelly 4 spicy cut-out cookies 2 drained canned pear halves 3½ tsp sugar 1 cup tea	1 poached egg† ¼ cup buttered mashed potatoes† ½ cup chopped lettuce with 2 tbsp salt-free mayonnaise 3 tbsp cranberry sauce 2 Scotch shortbreads 3½ tsp sugar 1 cup tea
EVENING SNACK	2 drained canned peach halves 3 ginger cookies	1 serving peach crisp 1 slice salt-free bread 2 tsp salt-free margarine	1 slice drained canned pineapple with 42 miniature marshmallows 4 Scotch shortbreads	1⅓ cups puffed rice 3½ tsp sugar ½ cup milk

	Day Five	*Day Six*	*Day Seven*
BREAKFAST	2 drained canned purple plums 2 cornmeal griddle cakes 2 tsp salt-free margarine 2 tbsp syrup ½ cup milk 3½ tsp sugar 1 cup coffee	2 drained canned apricot halves ⅓ cup rice with 1 tbsp raisins ½ slice salt-free toast 2 tsp salt-free margarine 1 tbsp jelly ½ cup milk 3½ tsp sugar 1 cup coffee	1 drained canned peach half ½ cup salt-free farina ½ slice salt-free toast 2 tsp salt-free margarine 1 tbsp jelly 3½ tsp sugar ½ cup milk 1 cup coffee
DINNER	1 hard-cooked egg† ¼ cup fried potatoes† ¼ cup drained buttered beets† Drained canned fruit salad (1 slice pineapple, 1 peach half, and 3 tbsp cranberry sauce in center) 1 serving lemon cornstarch pudding with 1 tbsp whipped topping 3½ tsp sugar 1 cup coffee	1 serving "eggs rancheros"† ⅓ cup drained buttered peas† ¼ cup buttered potatoes† 1 serving peach crisp with 1 tbsp whipped topping ½ cup apple juice	1 scrambled egg† ¼ cup fried potatoes† ½ cup drained buttered green beans† 2 drained canned pineapple slices with 2 tbsp raisins 2 spicy cut-out cookies ½ cup grape juice
SUPPER	1 "sunny-side-up" egg† ¼ cup drained buttered tomatoes† ½ cup lettuce with 2 tbsp salt-free mayonnaise ½ slice salt-free bread 2 tsp salt-free margarine 1 tbsp apple jelly 2 drained canned pear halves ½ cup cranberry-apple cocktail	1 fried egg† ⅓ cup drained glazed carrots† ½ cup lettuce with 2 tbsp oil and 2 tbsp vinegar ½ slice salt-free bread 2 tsp. salt-free margarine 1 tbsp jelly 8 drained canned Royal Anne cherries 3½ tsp sugar 1 cup coffee	1 fried egg† ½ cup drained buttered beets† ½ cup shredded lettuce with 1 tbsp oil and 1 tbsp vinegar 1 slice salt-free bread 2 tsp. salt-free margarine 1 tbsp jelly 1 serving peach tart 3½ tsp sugar 1 cup tea
EVENING SNACK	4 drained canned apricot halves 2 lacy sliced cookies	⅓ cup drained canned fruit cocktail 1 slice salt-free toast 2 tsp. salt-free margarine 1 tbsp jelly	⅔ cup canned applesauce 1 slice salt-free bread 2 tsp salt-free margarine

*Reprinted from Mehbod H, Baskin M, and Moss J: Diet in Uremia. AFP 4:75–80, 1971, with permission.
†Prepared without salt

Index